Bedside
Obstetrics and Gynecology
for Postgraduates

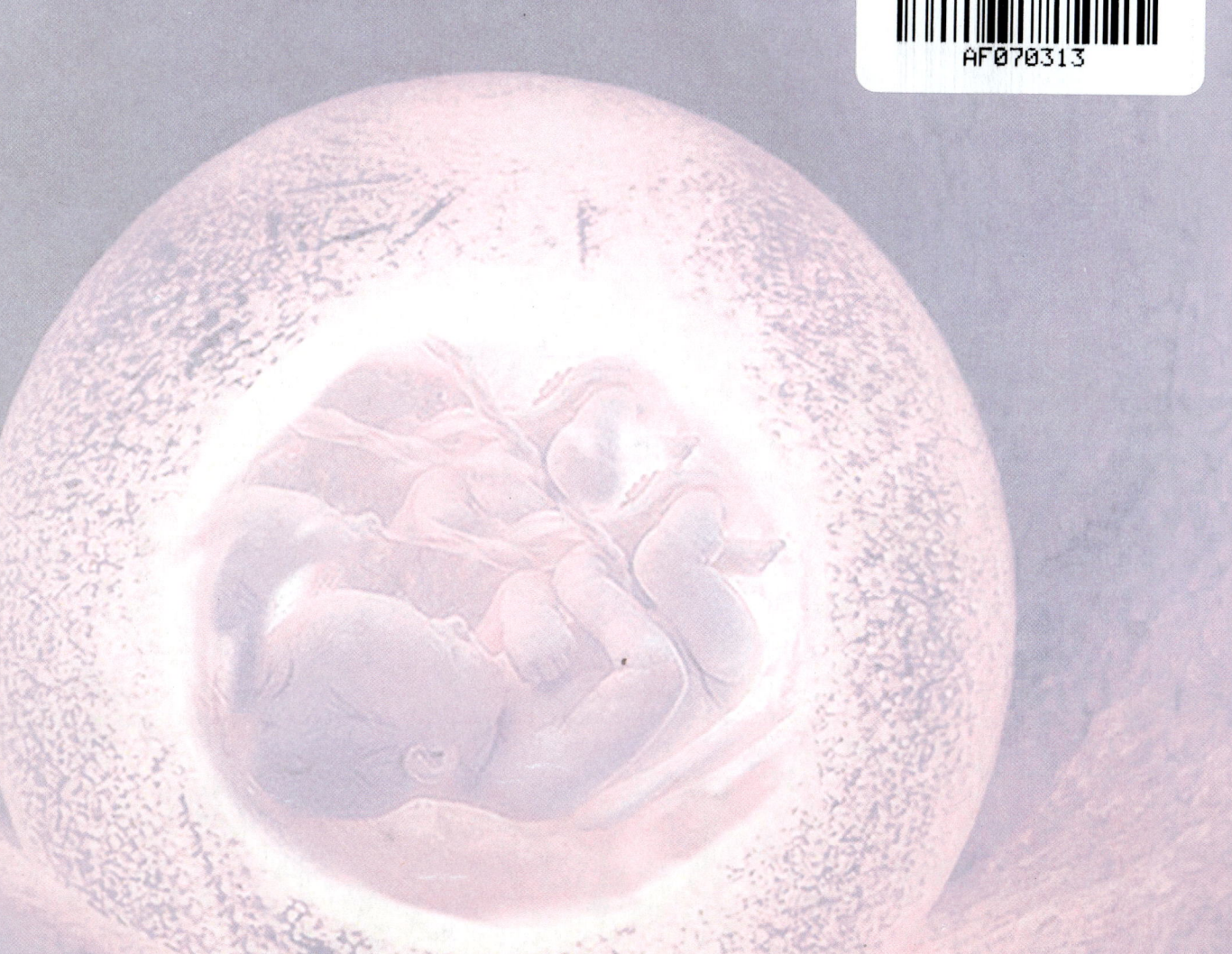

Bedside
Obstetrics and Gynecology
for Postgraduates

THIRD EDITION

Richa Saxena
MBBS MD (Obstetrics and Gynecology)
RCOG Associate
PG Diploma in Clinical Research
Obstetrician Gynecologist—Let's Talk Woman's Health
Mentor—Cracking MRCOG
New Delhi, India

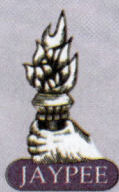

JAYPEE BROTHERS MEDICAL PUBLISHERS
The Health Sciences Publisher
New Delhi | London

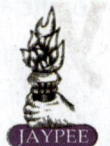 **Jaypee Brothers Medical Publishers (P) Ltd.**

Headquarters
Jaypee Brothers Medical Publishers (P) Ltd
EMCA House, 23/23-B
Ansari Road, Daryaganj
New Delhi 110 002, India
Landline: +91-11-23272143, +91-11-23272703
+91-11-23282021, +91-11-23245672
Email: jaypee@jaypeebrothers.com

Corporate Office
Jaypee Brothers Medical Publishers (P) Ltd
4838/24, Ansari Road, Daryaganj
New Delhi 110 002, India
Phone: +91-11-43574357
Fax: +91-11-43574314
Email: jaypee@jaypeebrothers.com

Overseas Office
JP Medical Ltd.
83, Victoria Street, London
SW1H 0HW (UK)
Phone: +44 20 3170 8910
Fax: +44 (0)20 3008 6180
Email: info@jpmedpub.com

Website: www.jaypeebrothers.com
Website: www.jaypeedigital.com

© 2023, Jaypee Brothers Medical Publishers

The views and opinions expressed in this book are solely those of the original contributor(s)/author(s) and do not necessarily represent those of editor(s) or publisher of the book.

All rights reserved. No part of this publication may be reproduced, stored or transmitted in any form or by any means, electronic, mechanical, photocopying, recording or otherwise, without the prior permission in writing of the publishers.

All brand names and product names used in this book are trade names, service marks, trademarks or registered trademarks of their respective owners. The publisher is not associated with any product or vendor mentioned in this book.

Medical knowledge and practice change constantly. This book is designed to provide accurate, authoritative information about the subject matter in question. However, readers are advised to check the most current information available on procedures included and check information from the manufacturer of each product to be administered, to verify the recommended dose, formula, method and duration of administration, adverse effects and contraindications. It is the responsibility of the practitioner to take all appropriate safety precautions. Neither the publisher nor the author(s)/editor(s) assume any liability for any injury and/or damage to persons or property arising from or related to use of material in this book.

This book is sold on the understanding that the publisher is not engaged in providing professional medical services. If such advice or services are required, the services of a competent medical professional should be sought.

Every effort has been made where necessary to contact holders of copyright to obtain permission to reproduce copyright material. If any have been inadvertently overlooked, the publisher will be pleased to make the necessary arrangements at the first opportunity.

Inquiries for bulk sales may be solicited at: jaypee@jaypeebrothers.com

Bedside Obstetrics and Gynecology for Postgraduates

First Edition: 2010

Second Edition: 2014

Third Edition: **2023**

ISBN: 978-93-5465-984-3

Printed at: Sterling Graphics Pvt. Ltd.

Dedicated to
My Mother, Mrs Bharati Saxena
and all the Mothers
Who have undergone much pain and sufferings for their children.

A mother is the most trusted friend we have, when trials, heavy and sudden, fall upon us;
When adversity takes the place of prosperity;
When friends who rejoice with us in our sunshine, desert us;
When troubles thicken around us, still she will cling to us
and counsel to dissipate the clouds of darkness, causing peace to return to our hearts;
and has proven time and time again that no matter whatever circumstances may come
between mother and her children, their lives are interwoven forever

—Washington Irving

Preface to the Third Edition

Medicine is learned by the bedside and not in the classroom. Let not your conceptions of disease come from words heard in the lecture room or read from the book. See and then reason and compare and control. But see first

–William Osler

The third edition of the book, *Bedside Obstetrics and Gynecology for Postgraduates,* is motivated by the enormous popularity of the past editions and a commitment for maintaining the fundamentals of clinical examination that cannot be overlooked. In the changing world of artificial intelligence and virtual reality, dependency on technology in the diagnostic processes has increased drastically and bedside time with patients has reduced. However, it is pertinent that diagnostic imaging must be complementary and not a replacement for clinical examination. Through this book, I have endeavored to draw attention towards the importance of eliciting the clinical signs and symptoms more than pathology or radiology, especially for the postgraduate students.

Though the text in the third edition has been greatly revamped and updated with recent guidelines in the field of Obstetrics and Gynecology, the concept and focus, however, remains the same. The book, like its earlier editions, highlights the age-old traditional concept of history-taking and clinical examination. Keeping these in mind, all important *Long Cases in Obstetrics and Gynecology* have been described under the following headings: Case study, introduction, history and clinical presentation, general physical examination, specific systemic examination, differential diagnosis, management, investigations, treatment (obstetric/gynecological management), complications, and evidence-based clinical trials. Questions from past 10-year papers have been incorporated in each chapter at topic level for the postgraduate students to prepare and pass the practical examination as well as the university examination with utmost ease. To further emphasise the fact that the book is focused towards the postgraduates, the term "postgraduate" has been inserted in the previous title, "*Bedside Obstetrics and Gynecology*".

While firmly holding on to traditional case-based approach, the third edition equally emphasizes on the evidence-based medicine, providing a wholesome learning to the postgraduates and residents. In line with this, evidence-based clinical trials have been added at the end of each chapter, which can be accessed by scanning a QR code given at the end of each chapter as well as at the end of table of contents on page XII. Each reference is linked to the source article, thereby allowing interested students to access the complete article or its abstract from there in just one click and remain updated with the recent advancements and developments in the field of obstetrics and gynecology. In the third edition, two new chapters "cephalopelvic disproportion", and "adenomyosis", have been added based on the reviews and feedback provided by the students who read this book and teachers/professors who reviewed the script. Keeping up with the updates, as the term, *Dysfunctional Uterine Bleeding* has become obsolete now, the redundant chapter has been removed in this edition. The textual matter of the book has been updated extensively with all new NICE/GTG guidelines including the new WHO portogram (WHO Care Guide, 2020), revised treatment and staging of malignancies including molecular staging of endometrial cancer, new management protocols for Rh negative pregnancy, preeclampsia, gestational diabetes, etc.

This book would serve as a valuable resource for the postgraduate students and residents, containing all the common and important case studies in the field of both Obstetrics and Gynecology, which they might encounter during the practical examinations, university examinations and clinical practice. Though mainly catering to postgraduate students, residents and practitioners, some intellectual undergraduate students who ultimately want to pursue their career in Obstetrics and Gynecology are also likely to find this book very useful.

Writing a book is a herculean task. It can never be completed without divine intervention and approval. Therefore, I have decided to end this preface with a small prayer of thanks to the Almighty, which I was taught in my childhood.

"Father, lead me day by day, ever in thy own sweet way. Teach me to be pure and good and tell me what I ought to do."

–Amen

Simultaneously, I would like to extend my thanks and appreciation to all the related authors and publishers whose references have been used in this book. Book creation is teamwork and I acknowledge the way the entire staff of M/s Jaypee Brothers Medical Publishers (P) Ltd, New Delhi, India, worked hard on this manuscript to give it a final shape. I would especially like to thank Shri Jitendar P Vij (Group Chairman), Mr Ankit Vij (Managing Director), Mr MS Mani (Group president), Ms Chetna Malhotra (Senior Director—Professional Publishing, Marketing and Business Development), Ms Pooja Bhandari (Production Head), Ms Suchita Gera (Development Editor), Mr Ashwani Singh (Manager), Mr Rakesh Kumar (Typesetter), Ms Nirmal (Editorial Coordinator) and Ms Seema Dogra (Cover Designer) for publishing the book.

I would also like to especially thank the content strategists (Dr Mansy Gupta, Ms Isha Sindhwani, Ms Soumya Yadav) for helping me in refining the manuscript.

I strongly believe that writing a book involves a continuous learning process. Though extreme care has been taken to maintain accuracy while writing this book, constructive criticism would be greatly appreciated. Please e-mail me your comments at *richa@drrichasaxena.com*. Also, please feel free to visit my website, *www.drrichasaxena.com* for obtaining information related to various books written by me, projects that I am involved in for promotion of woman's health, and for making use of the free online resources available.

Richa Saxena
richa@drrichasaxena.com
www.drrichasaxena.com

Preface to the First Edition (Extract)

The concept of a bedside book is not new, but is a novel one and unique in itself. It may sound funny, but when I told a nonmedical editor from a reputed publishing house that I was writing a book titled, "Bedside Obstetrics and Gynecology", he laughed asking whether the book is meant to remain at the bedside of the patient or the doctor? Jokes apart, who else other than the medical personnel would know the importance of the education which takes place at the patient's bedside. In today's world of scientific advancement and technology, the clinical art of medicine is sadly dying off ...

The doctors today do not believe in auscultating the patient's chest or merely palpating the patient's abdomen. A stethoscope can diagnose a consolidated lung suggestive of Kochs at a much earlier stage than a chest X-ray or even a bronchoscopic-guided biopsy. Hence, it is important for the medical personnel to become acquainted with the skills of taking history and performing a clinical examination. The purpose of the book is to promote the art of good history taking and clinical examination, and reaching the final diagnosis by obtaining only a few selective investigations or special evaluations. The book highlights the classical and systematic approach towards diagnosis of the disease. Each case study has been carefully designed to simulate the clinical practice scenarios as far as possible in order to evoke the right patient approach and clinical decision making. Unlike the small clinical vignettes described in most other books, detailed explanation of the pathology relevant to the case study in question has been described in all the chapters. One of the key features of this book is its versatility. Not only will the book be useful to the undergraduates who are required to get acquainted with the clinical examination skills but also for the busy postgraduates who are in the rush to go through the clinical scenarios.

Richa Saxena

Contents

PART I: OBSTETRICS

Section 1: Normal and Abnormal Presentations

1. Normal Pregnancy 3
2. Normal Labor in Occipitolateral Position 31
3. Breech Presentation 65
4. Transverse Lie 89
5. Occipitoposterior Position 99
6. Cephalopelvic Disproportion 112

Section 2: Complications of Pregnancy

7. Early Pregnancy Bleeding due to Miscarriage 125
8. Antepartum Hemorrhage 142
9. Multifetal Gestation 166
10. Rh-Negative Pregnancy 187
11. Previous Cesarean Section 204
12. Hydatidiform Mole 227
13. Bad Obstetric History 244
14. Postpartum Hemorrhage 266
15. Intrauterine Growth Restriction 295
16. Preterm Labor 318
17. Postdated Pregnancy and Intrauterine Death 339

Section 3: Medical Disorders Related to Pregnancy

18. Preeclampsia 355
19. Gestational Diabetes 388
20. Anemia in Pregnancy 417
21. Heart Disease During Pregnancy 442

PART II: GYNECOLOGY

Section 4: Normal and Abnormal Menstruation

22. Normal Gynecological Examination 465
23. Abnormal Uterine Bleeding due to Endometrial Cancer 486
24. Heavy Menstrual Bleeding due to Leiomyoma 515
25. Menopause 554

Section 5: Abnormalities of the Vagina and Cervix

26. Vaginal Discharge 573
27. Cervical Intraepithelial Neoplasia (Abnormal Pap Smear) 596
28. Cancer Cervix (Postcoital Bleeding) 619

Section 6: Uterine, Ovarian, and Tubal Pathology

29. Prolapse Uterus 641
30. Pelvic Pain 665
31. Abdominal Lump (Ovarian Cancer) 685
32. Ectopic Pregnancy 713
33. Adenomyosis 739

Section 7: Abnormalities in Conception

34. Infertility 749
35. Amenorrhea 792

Index 809

Online References
(To access the references of all chapters online, kindly scan the QR code)

Introduction

As previously described, this book emphasizes the patient's clinical conditions rather than the disease. For example, a patient may be presenting with jaundice, fever, and malaise, but the actual diagnosis may turn out to be hepatitis. So simply knowing about hepatitis is not enough, one needs to have the ability to diagnose the condition based on the findings of history and clinical examination.

Promoting clinical acumen is the basic purpose of this book. Each chapter has been written keeping in mind the clinical presentation of the patient. Various clinical scenarios have been divided into seven sections in all, out of which the first three deal with obstetrics and last four with gynecology. All the chapters have been divided into various subparts with the help of the symbols as described below:

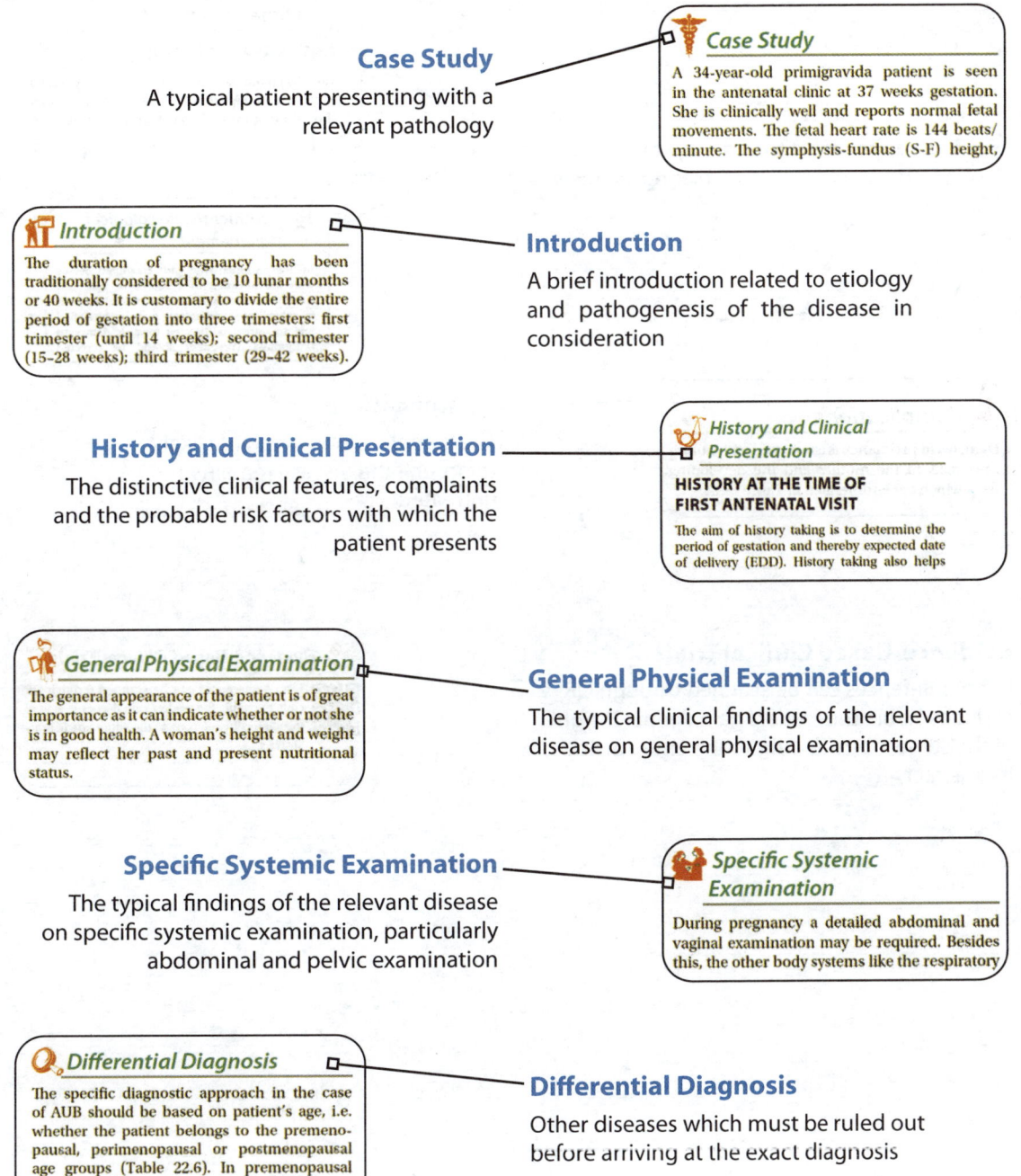

Case Study
A typical patient presenting with a relevant pathology

Introduction
A brief introduction related to etiology and pathogenesis of the disease in consideration

History and Clinical Presentation
The distinctive clinical features, complaints and the probable risk factors with which the patient presents

General Physical Examination
The typical clinical findings of the relevant disease on general physical examination

Specific Systemic Examination
The typical findings of the relevant disease on specific systemic examination, particularly abdominal and pelvic examination

Differential Diagnosis
Other diseases which must be ruled out before arriving at the exact diagnosis

Management
Plan of management of the relevant disease

Investigations
The investigations which may be ordered to confirm the correct diagnosis

Treatment
Most appropriate treatment strategy for the diagnosed disease

Complications
The complications which are likely to occur if the disease remains untreated

Evidence-Based Clinical Trials
List of references can be scanned through QR code to enable the readers gain deeper insight of the subject by referring to the entire article or its abstract

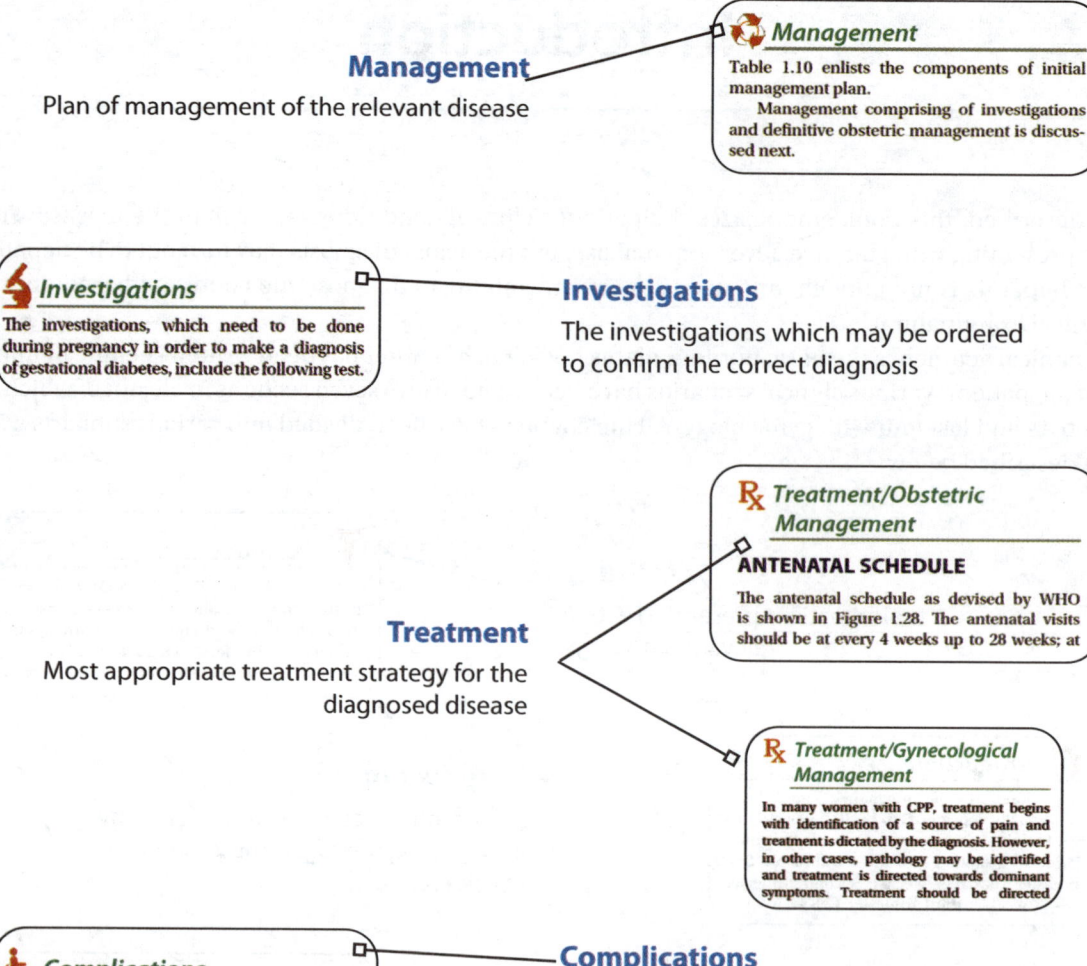

Abbreviations

ACOG:	American College of Obstetricians and Gynecologists	FHR:	Fetal Heart Rate
AFI:	Amniotic Fluid Index	FHS:	Fetal Heart Sound
AFV:	Amniotic Fluid Volume	FIGO:	International Federation of Gynecology and Obstetrics
AIDS:	Acquired Immune Deficiency Syndrome	FISH:	Fluorescent in situ Hybridization
ANC:	Antenatal Care	FMH:	Fetomaternal Hemorrhage
AP:	Anteroposterior	FNAC:	Fine-needle Aspiration Cytology
APH:	Antepartum Hemorrhage	FSH:	Follicle-stimulating Hormone
APLS/APS:	Antiphospholipid Antibody Syndrome/ Antiphospholipid Syndrome	GDG:	Guideline Development Group
		GFR:	Glomerular Filtration Rate
ARDS:	Acute Respiratory Distress Syndrome	GI:	Gastrointestinal
ARM:	Artificial Rupture of Membranes	GnRH:	Gonadotrophin-releasing Hormone
AST:	Aspartate Aminotransferase	GP:	General Practitioner
BCSH:	British Committee for Standards in Hematology	GPE:	General Physical Examinaion
		GTG:	Green-top Guideline
BMI:	Body Mass Index	GUM:	Genitourinary Medicine
BP:	Blood Pressure	Hb:	Hemoglobin
BPM:	Beats Per Minute	HIV:	Human Immunodeficiency Virus
BPP:	Biophysical Profile	HR:	Heart Rate
CBC:	Complete Blood Count	HRT:	Hormone Replacement Therapy
CDC:	Center of Disease Control and Prevention	ICU:	Intensive Care Unit
CI:	Confidence Interval	Ig:	Immunoglobulin
CNS:	Central Nervous System	IM:	Intramuscular
CO:	Carbon Monoxide	IUCD:	Intrauterine Contraceptive Device
CPR:	Cardiopulmonary Resuscitation	IUGR:	Intrauterine Growth Restriction/ Retardation
CRP:	C-reactive protein		
CS:	Cesarean Section	IV:	Intravenous
CST:	Contraction Stress Test	IVF:	In Vitro Fertilization
CT:	Computed Tomography	KFT:	Kidney Function Test
CTG:	Cardiotocography	L:S ratio:	Lecithin:Sphingomyelin ratio
CVS:	Chorionic Villus Sampling	LFT:	Liver Function Test
D&C:	Dilatation and Curettage	LH:	Luteinizing Hormone
DFMC:	Daily Fetal Movement Count	LMP:	Last Menstrual Period
DIC:	Disseminated Intravascular Coagulation	MAS:	Meconium Aspiration Syndrome
DLC:	Differential Leukocyte Count	MCH:	Mean Corpuscular Hemoglobin
DVT:	Deep Vein Thrombosis	MCHC:	Mean Corpuscular Hemoglobin Concentration
ECG:	Electrocardiogram		
ECV:	External Cephalic Version	MCV:	Mean Corpuscular Volume
ELISA:	Enzyme-linked Immunosorbent Assay	MRI:	Magnetic Resonance Imaging
ERCS:	Elective Repeat Cesarean Section	MS:	Multiple Sclerosis
ESR:	Erythrocyte Sedimentation Rate	MTC:	Mother-to-child

NICE:	National Institute for Health and Care Excellence
NICU:	Neonatal Intensive Care Unit
NSAIDs:	Nonsteroidal Anti-inflammatory Drugs
NST:	Nonstress Test
NT:	Nuchal Thickness
OCPs:	Oral Contraceptive Pills
OPD:	Outpatient Department
OR:	Odds Ratio
OT:	Operation Theater
PC:	Platelet Count
PCOS/PCOD:	Polycystic Ovarian Syndrome/Polycystic Ovarian Disease
PCR:	Polymerase Chain Reaction
PE:	Pulmonary Embolism
PID:	Pelvic Inflammatory Disease
PIH:	Pregnancy-induced Hypertension
PO:	Per Orally or Per os
POG:	Period of Gestation
PPH:	Postpartum Hemorrhage
PROM:	Premature Rupture of Membranes
PV:	Per Vaginally
RBC:	Red Blood Cell
RCOG:	Royal College of Obstetricians and Gynecologists
RCT:	Randomized Controlled Trial
RDS:	Respiratory Distress Syndrome
RIA:	Radioimmunoassay
ROM:	Rupture of Membranes
ROS:	Reactive Oxygen Species
RPF:	Renal Plasma Flow
SC:	Subcutaneous
SL:	Sublingual
SOGC:	Society of Obstetricians and Gynecologists of Canada
STD:	Sexually Transmitted Disease
T_3:	Triiodothyronine
T_4:	Thyroxine
TAS:	Transabdominal Scan
TLC:	Total Leukocyte Count
TORCH:	Toxoplasmosis, Other Infections, Rubella, Cytomegalovirus, Herpes Simplex Virus
TSH:	Thyroid-stimulating Hormone
TT:	Thrombin Time
TVS:	Transvaginal Scan or Sonography
TVT:	Tension-free Vaginal Tape
UFH:	Unfractionated Heparin
US:	Ultrasonography
UTI:	Urinary Tract Infection
UV:	Ultraviolet
VBAC:	Vaginal Birth after Cesarean
VDRL:	Venereal Disease Research Laboratory
VTE:	Venous Thromboembolism
WBC:	White Blood Cell
WHO:	World Health Organization

PART I: OBSTETRICS

SECTION 1

Normal and Abnormal Presentations

1. Normal Pregnancy
2. Normal Labor in Occipitolateral Position
3. Breech Presentation
4. Transverse Lie
5. Occipitoposterior Position
6. Cephalopelvic Disproportion

CHAPTER 1

Normal Pregnancy

CASE STUDY

A 34-year-old primigravida patient is seen in the antenatal clinic at 37 weeks' gestation. She is clinically well and reports normal fetal movements. The FHR is 144 beats/min. The symphysis-fundus (S-F) height, which was 35 cm at the time of previous antenatal visit, last week, is presently 34 cm. Also, at the time of the previous visit, the fetal head was freely ballotable above the pelvic brim and presently is just two-fifth above the brim. The patient is reassured that she and her fetus are healthy, and she is asked to attend the antenatal clinic again in a week's time.

INTRODUCTION

The duration of pregnancy has been traditionally considered to be 10 lunar months or 40 weeks. It is customary to divide the entire period of gestation into three trimesters: first trimester (until 14 weeks), second trimester (15–28 weeks), and third trimester (29–42 weeks). During the antenatal period, planned antenatal care is the care given to a pregnant woman in order to ensure good maternal and neonatal outcome.

There is no fixed timing or frequency for antenatal visits. The number of antenatal visits may vary from center to center. Increased number of visits may be required in a patient with a high risk of complications.

HISTORY AND CLINICAL PRESENTATION

HISTORY AT THE TIME OF FIRST ANTENATAL VISIT

The aim of history taking is to determine the period of gestation and thereby the expected date of delivery (EDD). History taking also helps in determining if the pregnancy is associated with any high-risk factors. Taking appropriate history helps the obstetrician determine the further management and mode of delivery. A full history comprising the following needs to be elicited:

- Menstrual history
- Previous obstetric history
- Present obstetric history
- Medical history
- Treatment history
- Surgical history
- Family history
- Social history
- Personal history

Menstrual History

It is important to elicit the proper history regarding the last (normal) menstrual period. It is also important for the obstetrician to find out if the previous cycles were normal and regular or not. It may be difficult to establish the LMP accurately when the woman had been previously experiencing irregular cycles. The obstetrician must also enquire about the length of periods and amount of bleeding. Excessive amount of menstrual blood loss in previous cycles may be associated with anemia.

The last menstrual period can be used for calculating the EDD. To calculate the EDD, 7 days are added to the first day of LMP and then 9 months are added to this date. For example, if the LMP was on 2-2-2009, the EDD will be on 9-11-2009. If the LMP was 27-10-2008, the EDD will be 3-8-2009. This method of estimating EDD is known as Naegele's rule. This rule can also be applied by adding 7 days to the first day of LMP, subtracting 3 months, and then adding 1 year to this. This rule should be used to measure the duration of pregnancy, only if the patient had been having regular menstrual cycles previously.

The history of using steroidal contraception prior to conception is important as in this case EDD may not be accurately determined with the help of Naegele's rule. This is so as ovulation may not immediately resume following withdrawal bleeding; there may be a delay of 2–3 weeks.

Previous Obstetric History

The woman's past obstetric history must be denoted by the acronym GPAL, where G stands for gravida, P for parity, A for number of abortions, and L for number of live births. It is also important to ask the woman how long she has been married.

- *Gravida:* This refers to the number of pregnancies, including the present pregnancy, the woman has ever had. This is irrespective of the fact whether the pregnancies were viable at the time of birth or not.
  - *Nulligravida:* This implies a woman who has never been pregnant.
  - *Primigravida:* This stands for a woman who is pregnant for the first time (gravida 1).
  - *Multigravida:* This stands for a woman who has had at least one previous pregnancy, irrespective of whether it was viable or not (depending on the number of previous pregnancies, she could be gravida 2, 3, or more). For example, a woman has had three previous pregnancies and is now pregnant for the fourth time will be gravida 4.
- *Abortions:* Number of pregnancies, which have terminated before reaching the point of viability (20 weeks). The obstetrician must ask their exact gestational period and also mention whether they were spontaneous or induced abortions; the reason for the induced abortion also needs to be asked.
- *Viability:* This refers to the ability of the fetus to live outside the uterus after birth.
- *Parity:* This refers to the number of previous viable pregnancies (including infants who were either stillborn or born alive). Parity is determined by the number of viable pregnancies and not by the number of fetuses delivered. Thus, parity does not change even if twins or triplets are born instead of a singleton fetus. Previous multiple viable pregnancies are shown as twins +1, triplets +2, etc. For example, if one of the viable pregnancies of this female produced twins, alive or stillborn, she will be gravida 4, para 2+1. If the first viable pregnancy produced twins and the second viable pregnancy produced quadruplet, she will be gravida 4 para 2+1+3.
  - *Nullipara:* A woman who has never carried a previous pregnancy to a point of viability (para 0)
  - *Primipara:* Woman who has had one previous viable pregnancy (para 1). For example, if the woman is gravida 4 and only two of the previous pregnancies of this woman were viable, she would be gravida 4, para 2.
  - *Multipara:* Woman who has had two or more previous viable pregnancies (para 2, 3, or more)
  - *Grand multipara:* Woman who has had five or more previous viable pregnancies (para 5, 6, or more)

A woman is considered as a high-risk mother if she is either a primigravida or nullipara over the age of 30 or if she is a young, teenaged primigravida or if she is a grand multipara.

It is important to take the history of previous pregnancies including history of previous abortions (period of gestation < 20 weeks), precipitate labor, preterm pregnancies (period of gestation < 37 completed weeks), abnormal presentations, preeclampsia or eclampsia, cesarean section, retained placenta, postpartum hemorrhage, stillbirths, history of episiotomies, perineal tears, history of receiving epidural anesthesia during previous pregnancies, etc. History about any episodes of hospitalization during previous pregnancies can be helpful. History of complications during previous pregnancy, such as preeclampsia, placenta previa, abruption placenta, IUGR, polyhydramnios, or oligohydramnios is important because many complications in previous pregnancies tend to recur in subsequent pregnancies. For example, patients with a previous history of perinatal death or spontaneous preterm labor are at a high risk of perinatal death or preterm labor during their future pregnancies, respectively. Patients who develop preeclampsia before 34 weeks' gestation have a greater risk of preeclampsia in further pregnancies. Multiple pregnancy, especially the previous history of nonidentical twins, tends to recur in subsequent pregnancies. It is also important to take the history of previous pregnancy losses. A history of three or more successive first trimester miscarriages suggests a possible genetic abnormality in the father or mother. Previous mid-trimester miscarriages could be associated with cervical incompetence. The patient may often forget to give the history about previous miscarriages and ectopic pregnancies. Therefore, the obstetrician needs to ask specifically about the history of previous miscarriages and ectopic pregnancies. Approximate birth weights of previous children and the approximate period of gestation, especially if the infant was low birth weight or preterm, are useful. Low birth weight at the time of birth is indicative of either IUGR or preterm delivery. On the other hand, large-sized infants point toward the possibility of maternal diabetes.

It is important to know if the woman has had a long labor during her previous pregnancy, as this may indicate cephalopelvic disproportion. History of previous birth in the form of assisted delivery, including forceps delivery, vacuum application, and cesarean section, suggests that there may have been cephalopelvic disproportion. In case of previous cesarean delivery, a detailed history of the previous surgery needs to be taken. The patient should always be asked if she knows the reason for having had a cesarean section. She should be asked to show the hospital notes related to the surgery. This may help provide some information regarding the type of incision made in the uterus, any complications encountered during the surgery, etc. Detailed history of previous live births as well as previous perinatal deaths is important. The following points need to be elicited:

- *Birth weight of each infant born previously:* This is important as previous low-birth-weight infants or spontaneous preterm labors tend to recur during future pregnancies. Also, history of delivering a large-sized baby in the past is suggestive of maternal diabetes mellitus or gestational diabetes, which may recur during subsequent pregnancies.
- *Method of delivery of each previous infant:* The type of previous delivery is also important because a forceps delivery or vacuum extraction may suggest that some degree of cephalopelvic disproportion may have been present. If the patient had a previous cesarean section, the indication for the cesarean section must be determined.
- *History of previous perinatal deaths:* Previous history of having had one or more perinatal deaths in the past places the patient at a high risk of future perinatal deaths. Therefore, every effort must be made to find out the cause of any previous deaths. If no cause can be found, then the risk of a recurrence of perinatal death is even higher.

Present Obstetric History

Regarding the present pregnancy, the following points need to be considered:

- The first day of the LMP must be determined as accurately as possible. The obstetrician must ask the patient how long she had been married or has been in a relationship with the present partner. The obstetrician must also ask the woman if she had previously received any treatment for infertility. The patient must be asked if the present pregnancy is a planned one and since how long she had been planning this pregnancy. Did she ever use any contraceptive agents in the past?
- The obstetrician needs to take the history of any medical or obstetric problems which the patient has had since the start of this pregnancy, e.g., pyrexial illnesses (such as influenza) with or without skin rashes, symptoms suggestive of a urinary tract infection, and history of any vaginal bleeding.
- Enquiry must be also made regarding normal symptoms related to pregnancy, which the patient may be experiencing, e.g., nausea and vomiting, heartburn, and constipation.

Medical History

Patients must be specifically asked about the previous medical history of diabetes, epilepsy, hypertension, renal disease, rheumatic disease, heart valve disease, epilepsy, asthma, tuberculosis, psychiatric illness, or any other significant illness she may have had in the past. She should also be asked if she had any allergies (specifically allergy to penicillin) in the past.

Treatment History

The woman must be asked if she has previous history of receiving immunization against tetanus, or administration of Rhesus (Rh) immunoglobulins during her previous pregnancies. The patient must be asked if she had received any treatment in the past (e.g., hypoglycemic drugs, and antihypertensive drugs). Certain drugs may be teratogenic to the fetus during the first trimester of pregnancy, e.g., retinoids, which are used for acne, and anticoagulant drugs such as warfarin. Also, certain drugs, which the women may be regularly taking prior to pregnancy, are relatively contraindicated during pregnancy, e.g., antihypertensive drugs such as angiotensin-converting enzyme (ACE) inhibitors and β-blockers.

History regarding any previous hospital admission, surgery, blood transfusion, etc. also needs to be taken. It is important to elicit the patient's medical history as some medical conditions may become worse during pregnancy, e.g., a patient with heart valve disease may go into cardiac failure, while a hypertensive patient is at a high risk of developing preeclampsia.

Surgical History

The woman must be enquired if she ever underwent any surgery in the past such as cardiac surgery, e.g., heart valve replacement, and operations on the urogenital tract, e.g., cesarean section, myomectomy, cone biopsy of the cervix, operations for stress incontinence, and vesicovaginal fistula repair.

Family History

Family history of medical conditions such as diabetes, multiple pregnancy, bleeding tendencies, or mental retardation increases the risk for development of these conditions in the patient and her unborn infant. Since some birth defects are inherited, it is important to take the history of any genetic disorder, which may be prevalent in the family.

Social History

It is important to elicit information regarding the patient's social circumstances. The patient should be specifically asked if she has been smoking or consuming alcohol. Smoking and alcohol both may cause IUGR. Additionally, alcohol may also cause congenital malformations. The mother should be asked if she has social or family support to help her bring up the baby, e.g., a working mother may require assistance to help her plan the care of her infant. Social problems such as unemployment, poor housing, and overcrowding increase the risk of the mother developing medical complications such as tuberculosis, malnutrition, and IUGR. Patients living in poor social conditions need special support and help. Sometimes it may become difficult

6 Normal and Abnormal Presentations

TABLE 1.1A: Modified Kuppuswamy's socioeconomic scale (updated January 2018).

Social class	Score	Socioeconomic class
I	26–29	Upper (I)
II	16–25	Upper middle (II)
III	11–15	Lower middle (III)
IV	5–10	Upper lower (IV)
V	Below 5	Lower (V)

Source: Saleem S. Kuppuswamy scale updated for the year 2018. Indian J Res. 2018;7(3)

TABLE 1.1B: Occupation of the head of the family.

Occupation of the head	Score
Legislators, senior officials, or managers	10
Professionals	9
Technicians and associate professionals	8
Clerks	7
Skilled workers and shop and market sales workers	6
Skilled agricultural and fishery workers	5
Crafts and related trade workers	4
Plant and machine operators and assemblers	3
Elementary occupation	2
Unemployed	1

TABLE 1.1C: Education of the head of the family.

Education of the head	Score
Professional or honors	7
Graduate	6
Intermediate or diploma	5
High school certificate	4
Middle school certificate	3
Primary school certificate	2
Illiterate	1

TABLE 1.1D: Total monthly income of the family.

Updated monthly family income in ₹ (2012)	Updated monthly family income in ₹ (2016)	Updated monthly family income in ₹ (2018)	Score
>30,375	≥40,430	>126,360	12
15,188–30,374	20,210–40,429	63,182–126,356	10
11,362–15,187	15,160–20,209	47,266–63,178	6
7,594–11.361	10,110–15,159	31,591–47,262	4
4,556–7,593	6,060–10,109	18,953–38,589	3
1,521–4,555	2,021–6,059	6,327–18,949	2
≤520	≤2,020	≤6,323	1

to ask the patient directly regarding her socioeconomic status. In these cases, taking history regarding the occupation of the husband or partner is likely to give clues regarding the patient's socioeconomic history. Classification of the women based on their socioeconomic status is usually done using Kuppuswamy Prasad's classification system* (revised for 2018), which is based on the total score **(Table 1.1A)**, calculated with the help of parameters such as occupation of the head of the family **(Table 1.1B)**, education of the head of the family **(Table 1.1C)**, and monthly income of the family **(Table 1.1D)**.

Personal History

Personal history includes behavioral factors (smoking or tobacco usage, alcohol usage, utilization of prenatal care services, etc.).

Family Planning

The patient's family planning needs and wishes should be discussed at the first antenatal visit. If she is a multipara having at least two live babies, she should be counseled and encouraged for postpartum sterilization. In case the woman is not willing to undergo permanent sterilization procedure, the patient's wishes should be respected; she can be offered temporary methods of contraception such as oral contraceptive pills and Cu-T.

■ CLINICAL PRESENTATION

> **Q.** Write a long essay on changes occurring in the genital organs during pregnancy.

Clinical presentation during various trimesters of pregnancy is given in the following text.

First Trimester of Pregnancy

- *Cessation of menstruation:* Cessation of menstrual cycles in a woman belonging to the reproductive age group, who had

---

*Kuppuswamy Prasad's classification system is applicable only for the Indian population. Per capita income is calculated by dividing total income of the household by the number of individuals.

previously experienced spontaneous, cyclical, predictable periods, is the first most frequent symptom of pregnancy. Since there may be considerable variation in the length of ovarian and thus menstrual cycle among women, amenorrhea is not a reliable indicator of pregnancy, until 10 days or more after the onset of expected menses.

- *Nausea and vomiting:* Also known as morning sickness, these symptoms appear 1 or 2 weeks after the period is missed and last until 10–12th week. Its severity may vary from mild nausea to persistent vomiting, e.g., hyperemesis gravidarum.
- *Urinary symptoms:* Increased frequency of urination during the early months of pregnancy is due to the relaxant effect of progesterone on the bladder, in combination with the pressure exerted by the gradually enlarged uterus on the bladder.
- *Mastodynia:* Mastodynia or breast discomfort may be present in early pregnancy and ranges in severity from a tingling sensation to frank pain in the breasts.
- *Cervical mucus:* Presence of progesterone during pregnancy helps in lowering the concentration of NaCl in cervical mucus, which prevents the formation of ferning pattern; instead, the cervical mucus shows a characteristic crystallization or beading or an ellipsoid pattern due to the presence of progesterone when the cervical mucus (secreted during pregnancy) is spread over the glass slide and dried.

Second Trimester of Pregnancy

There is disappearance of subjective symptoms of pregnancy such as nausea, vomiting, and frequency of micturition. Other symptoms, which may appear, include the following:
- *Abdominal enlargement:* Progressive enlargement of the lower abdomen occurs due to the growing uterus.
- *Quickening:* Fetal movement (quickening) can usually be seen or heard between 16 and 18 weeks of gestation in a multigravida. A primigravida, on the other hand, is capable of appreciating fetal movements after approximately 2 weeks (i.e., 18–20 weeks).

- *Fetal heart sounds:* This is the most definitive clinical sign of pregnancy and can be detected between 18 and 20 weeks of gestation. The rate usually varies from 120 to 160 beats/min.
- *Palpation of fetal body parts:* The fetal body can usually be palpated by 18–20 weeks of gestation unless the patient is obese; there is abdominal tenderness or an excessive amount of amniotic fluid.
- *External ballottement:* This can be elicited as early as 20th week of gestation because the size of the fetus is relatively smaller in comparison to the amniotic fluid **(Fig. 1.1)**.
- *Internal ballottement:* This can be elicited between 16 and 28 weeks of gestation **(Figs. 1.2A and B)**.
- *Skin changes:* There is an appearance of pigmentation over the forehead and cheeks by 24th week of gestation. There is appearance of linea nigra and striae gravidarum over the abdomen.

Changes in the Third Trimester

- *Abdominal enlargement:* There occurs progressive enlargement of the abdomen, which can result in the development of symptoms of mechanical discomfort such as palpitations and dyspnea. Lightening is another phenomenon, which occurs at approximately 38 weeks of

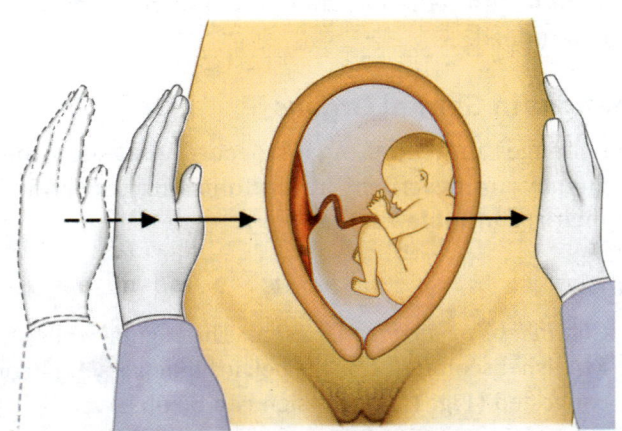

Fig. 1.1: External ballottement.

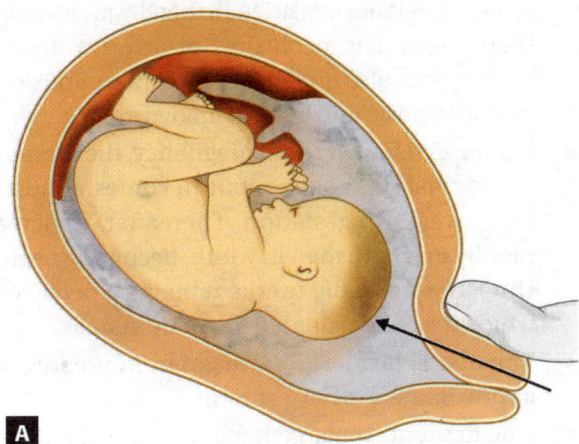
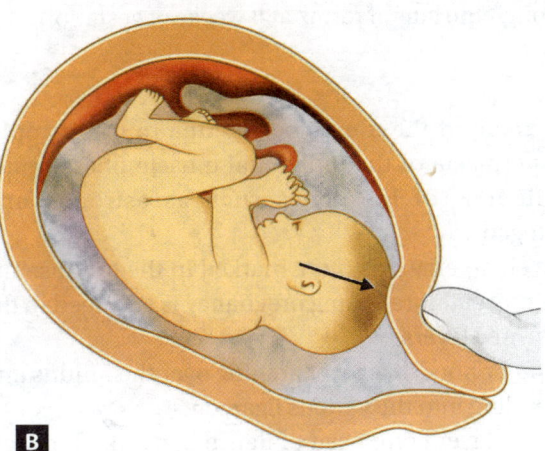

Figs. 1.2A and B: Internal ballottement.

8 Normal and Abnormal Presentations

TABLE 1.2: Changes occurring in genital organs during pregnancy.

Uterus	Cervix	Vagina

• Uterine enlargement
• Becomes palpable per abdominally
• Changes in the uterine tissues:
  – Increased vascularity
  – Increased uteroplacental blood flow
  – Increased hypertrophy
  – Increased weight of the uterus
• *Hegar's sign:* Due to the softening of uterine isthmus
• *Palmer's sign:* Regular rhythmic uterine contractions
• Braxton Hicks contractions
• *Uterine soufflé:* Due to increased blood flow through the umbilical arteries
	• *Goodell's sign:* Softening of the cervix
	• Filling up of the cervical canal with a thick mucus plug
	• Increase in cervical discharge, leukorrhea
	• Characteristic crystallization or beading pattern of cervical discharge when spread on a glass slide
		• *Chadwick's sign:* Increase in vascularity, resulting in bluish discoloration of vaginal walls
		• Vaginal pH rises, and it becomes more susceptible to develop yeast infections

gestation, especially in the primigravida. This results in a slight reduction in fundal height, which provides relief against pressure symptoms.

- *Frequency of micturition:* There is an increased frequency of micturition, which had previously disappeared in the second trimester.
- *Fetal movements become more pronounced:* The fetal movements become more pronounced, and palpation of fetal parts becomes easier.
- Braxton Hicks contractions become more evident.
- Fetal lie, presentation, and period of gestation can be determined.

Changes in Genital Organs

The changes in genital organs occurring at the time of pregnancy are described in the following text and also summarized in **Table 1.2**.

Vagina

- *Chadwick's or Jacquemier's sign:* The vaginal walls show a bluish discoloration as the pelvic blood vessels become congested **(Fig. 1.3)**. This sign can be observed by 8–10 weeks of gestation.
- *Osiander's sign:* There is increased pulsation in the vagina felt through the lateral fornix at 8 weeks of gestation.

Uterus

- Enlargement of the uterus occurs due to hypertrophy and hyperplasia of the individual muscle fibers under the influence of hormones such as estrogen and progestogens.
- Uterine enlargement is more marked in the fundus. The uterine musculature during pregnancy is arranged in the form of three layers:
  1. An outer hood-like layer arching over the fundus and extending into the various ligaments
  2. Middle layer composed of dense network of muscle fibers perforated in all directions by the blood vessels

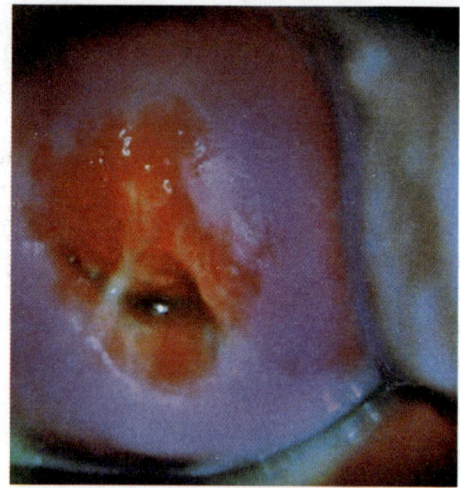

Fig. 1.3: Jacquemier's sign.

  3. An inner layer comprising sphincter-like fibers around the orifices of fallopian tube and internal os of the cervix
- Muscle fibers in the middle layer are arranged in an interlacing, "figure-of-8" manner with blood vessels lying between these fibers **(Fig. 1.4)**.
- As a result, when the uterine musculature contracts following the delivery of the fetus and placenta, the penetrating blood vessels are constricted, thereby preventing excessive blood loss. The occlusion of arteries during uterine contractions also diminishes placental perfusion, resulting in fetal hypoxia and/or fetal bradycardia.
- For the first few weeks of pregnancy, the uterus maintains its original pear shape, but becomes almost spherical by 12 weeks of gestation. Thereafter, it increases more rapidly in length than in width, becoming ovoid in shape. Until 12 weeks, the uterus remains a pelvic organ, after which it can be palpated per abdominally.
- The uterus increases in weight from prepregnant 70 g to approximately 1,100 g at term.
- Due to uterine enlargement, the normal anteverted position gets exaggerated up to 8 weeks. Since the enlarged

uterus lies on the bladder, making it incapable of filling, the frequency of micturition increases. However, after 8 weeks the uterus more or less conforms to the axis of the inlet.
- *Hegar's sign:* At 6–8 weeks of gestation, the cervix is firm in contrast to the soft isthmus. Due to the marked softness of uterine isthmus, cervix and the body of uterus may appear as separate organs. As a result, the isthmus of the uterus can be compressed between the fingers palpating vagina and abdomen, which is known as Hegar's sign **(Fig. 1.5)**.
- *Palmer's sign:* Regular rhythmic uterine contractions, which can be elicited during the bimanual examination, can be felt as early as 4–8 weeks of gestation.
- *Braxton Hicks contractions:* In the early months of pregnancy, uterus undergoes contractions known as Braxton Hicks contractions, which may be irregular, infrequent, and painless without any effect on the cervical dilatation and effacement. Toward the last weeks of pregnancy, these contractions increase in intensity, thereby resulting in pain and discomfort for the patient and may occur after every 10–20 minutes, thereby assuming some form of rhythmicity. Eventually, these contractions merge with the contractions of labor.
- There is hypertrophy of the uterine isthmus to about three times its original size during the first trimester of pregnancy.
- After 12 weeks of pregnancy, the uterine isthmus unfolds downward from above to get incorporated into the uterine cavity and also takes part in the formation of lower uterine segment.
- There is an increase in the uteroplacental blood flow ranging between 450 and 650 mL/min near term. This increase is principally due to vasodilatation.
- *Uterine soufflé:* This is a soft blowing sound synchronous with the maternal pulse or maternal cardiac systole. It is caused by the rush of blood through the arteries of gravid uterus and can be heard upon auscultation of pregnant uterus. On the other hand, fetal soufflé is a sharp whistling sound synchronous with the fetal pulse. It is caused by the rush of blood through the fetal umbilical arteries.

Cervix

- There occur hypertrophy and hyperplasia of the elastic and connective tissue fibers and increase in vascularity within the cervical stroma. This is likely to result in cervical softening (known as Goodell's sign) **(Fig. 1.6)**, which becomes evident by 6 weeks of pregnancy. Increased vascularity is likely to result in bluish discoloration beneath the squamous epithelium of portio vaginalis, resulting in a positive Chadwick's sign.
- With the advancement of pregnancy, there is marked proliferation of endocervical mucosa with downward extension of the squamocolumnar junction. There is copious production of cervical secretions, resulting in the formation of a thick mucus plug which seals the cervical canal. This mucus plug is rich in cytokines and immunoglobulins, and acts as an immunological barrier

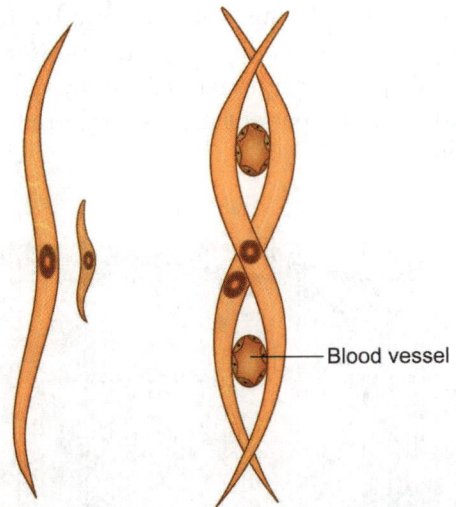

Fig. 1.4: Figure-of-8 arrangement of the uterine muscle fibers.

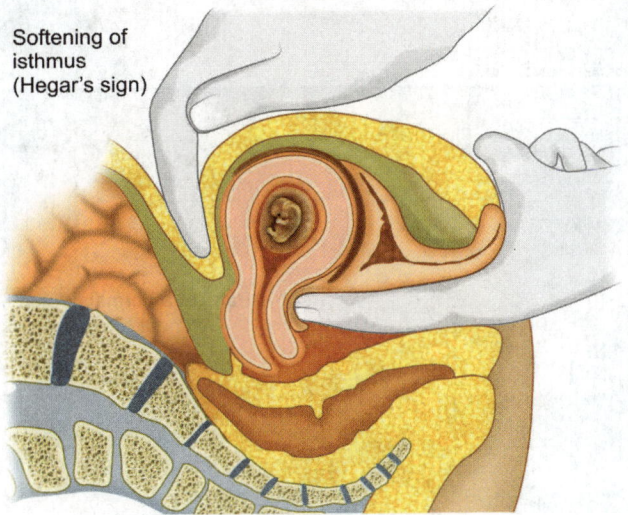

Fig. 1.5: Hegar's sign.

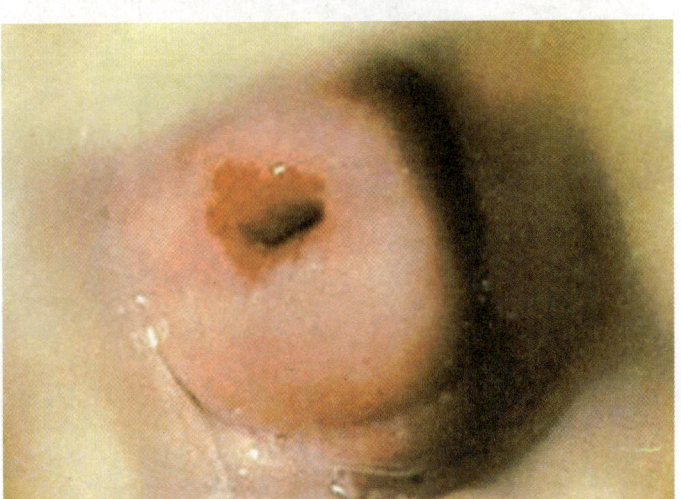

Fig. 1.6: Cervical softening (Goodell's sign).

to protect the uterine contents against infection from the vagina.

- If the history and examination suggest that a patient is pregnant, the diagnosis is easily confirmed by urine pregnancy test. The test becomes positive by the time the first menstrual period is missed. A positive pregnancy test is however produced by both an intrauterine and an extrauterine pregnancy. Extrauterine pregnancy, if undiagnosed, can present as an obstetric emergency. Therefore, it is important to establish whether the pregnancy is intrauterine or not on the clinical examination **(Table 1.3)**. If the clinical examination appears to be suggestive of extrauterine pregnancy, the diagnosis needs to be confirmed by ultrasound examination.

TABLE 1.3: Differentiating between intrauterine and extrauterine pregnancy.

	Intrauterine pregnancy	Extrauterine pregnancy
Size of the uterus	Appropriate for the duration of pregnancy	Uterine size is smaller than the period of gestation
Pain in the abdomen	Absent	Present
Vaginal bleeding	Absent	Present
Vaginal/abdominal tenderness	Absent	Present
Bimanual vaginal examination	No adnexal tenderness or mass	Tender, vague adnexal mass, thickening or fullness is present
Cervical excitation	Absent	Present

GENERAL PHYSICAL EXAMINATION

The general appearance of the patient is of great importance as it can indicate whether or not she is in good health. A woman's height and weight may reflect her past and present nutritional status.

The signs which must be carefully looked for in a pregnant woman include the following:

- Pallor **(Figs. 1.7A to D)**
- Edema **(Figs. 1.8A and B)**
- Jaundice
- Enlarged lymph nodes (neck, axillae, and inguinal areas)
- *The thyroid gland:* The obstetrician must look for an obviously enlarged thyroid gland (goiter). In case there is obvious enlargement of the thyroid gland or it feels nodular, the patient must be referred for further investigations.

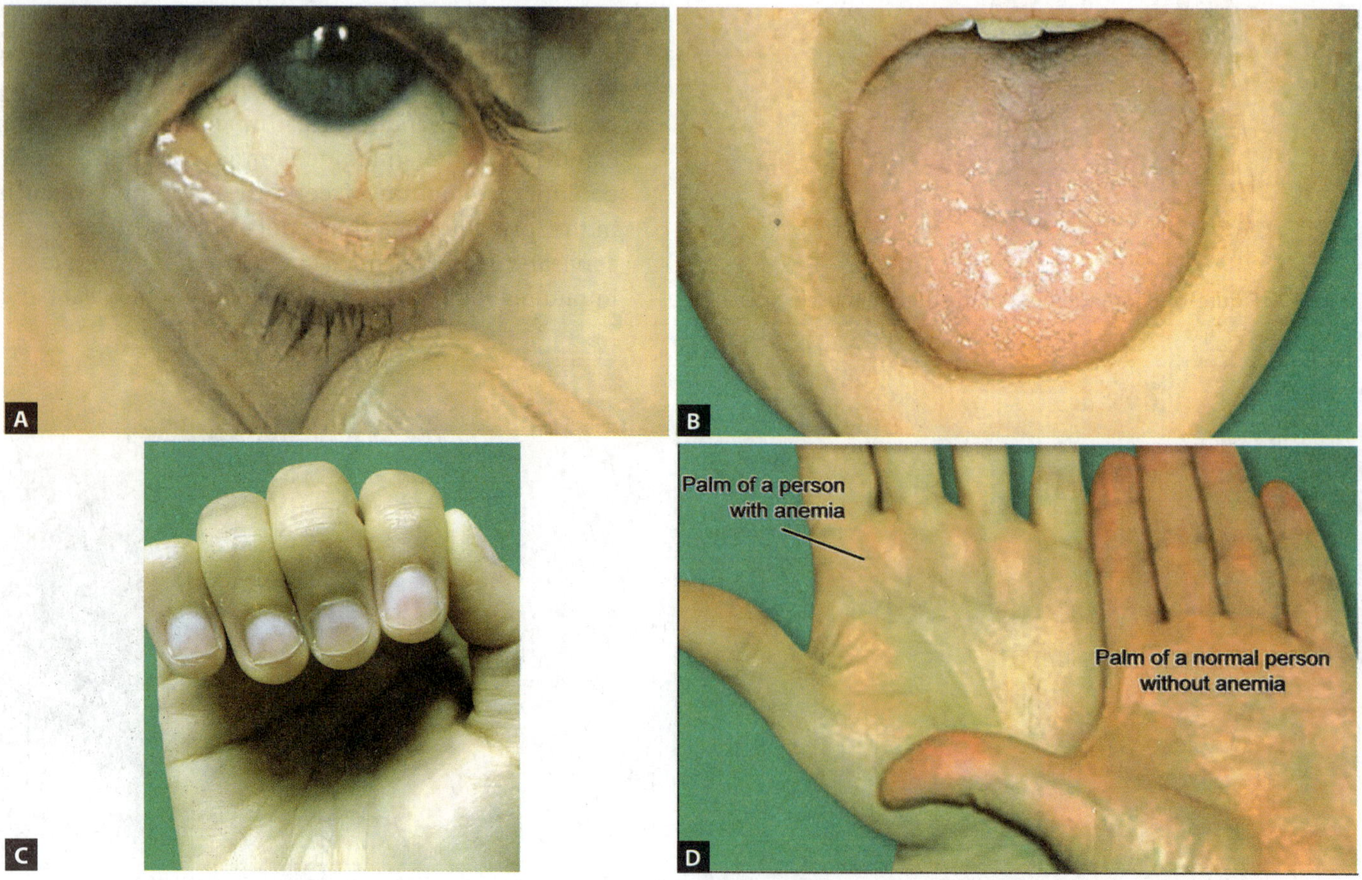

Figs. 1.7A to D: Pallor is observed in (A) Lower palpebral conjunctiva; (B) Tongue; (C) Nail bed; (D) Palm of hands.

Normal Pregnancy

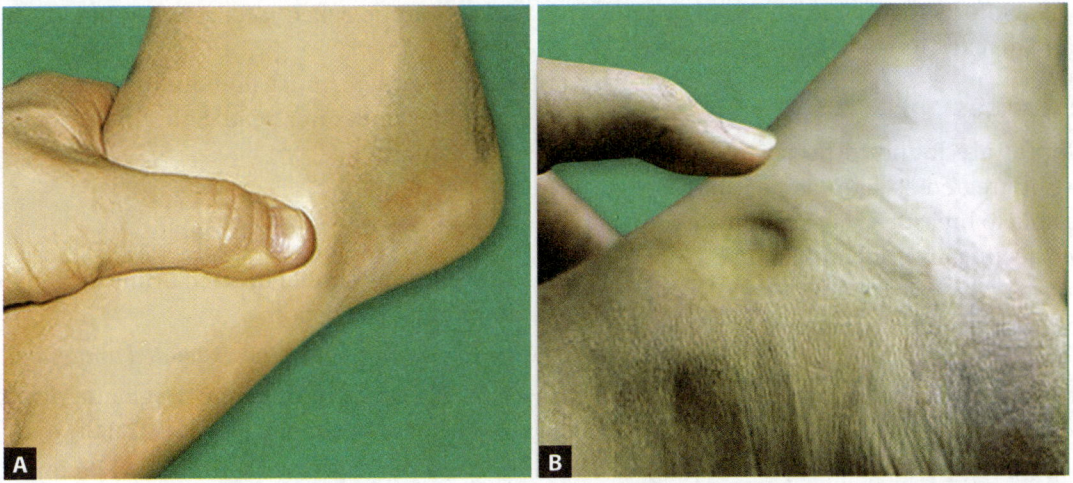

Figs. 1.8A and B: Pedal edema in a pregnant woman. (A) Testing for edema; (B) Presence of pitting edema in the feet.

- *Skin changes:* There may be increased skin pigmentation due to increased production of melanotropin. This may manifest as follows:
  - *Face:* Melasma, a frequently encountered skin change during pregnancy **(Fig. 1.9)**
  - *Breasts:* Darkening of areolas
  - *Abdomen:* Linea nigra

EXAMINATION OF THE BREASTS

Figures 1.10A and B illustrate the changes in breasts occurring during pregnancy. There is pronounced pigmentation of the areola and nipples. There is also the appearance of secondary areola, Montgomery's tubercles, and the presence of increased vascularity. Routine breast examination during antenatal examination is not recommended for the promotion of postnatal breastfeeding. The breasts should be examined with the patient both sitting and lying on her back, with her hands above her head. Changes in the breasts are best evident in the primigravida in comparison to multigravida. The presence of secretions from the breasts of a primigravida who has never lactated is an important sign of pregnancy. Examinations of the breasts involve the following.

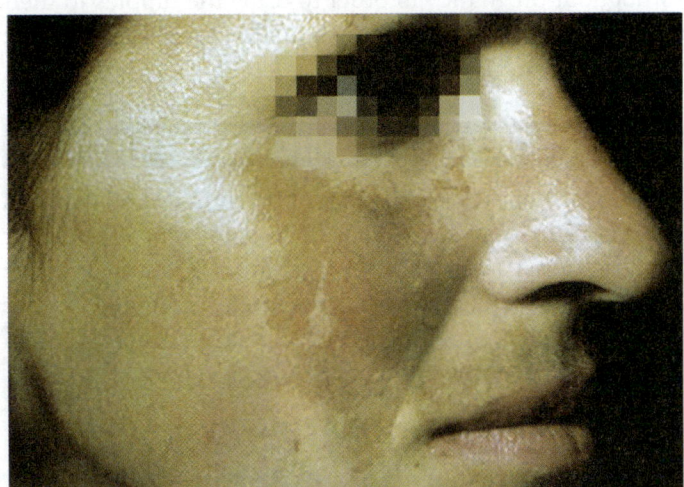

Fig. 1.9: Melasma—skin change during pregnancy.

Inspection

Both the breasts must be inspected for the presence of any obvious gross abnormalities. The obstetrician must particularly look for any distortion of the breasts or nipples. The nipples should be specifically examined with regard to their position and deformity (if any), discharge, inversion, and areola. The presence of any eczema of the areola must also be noted.

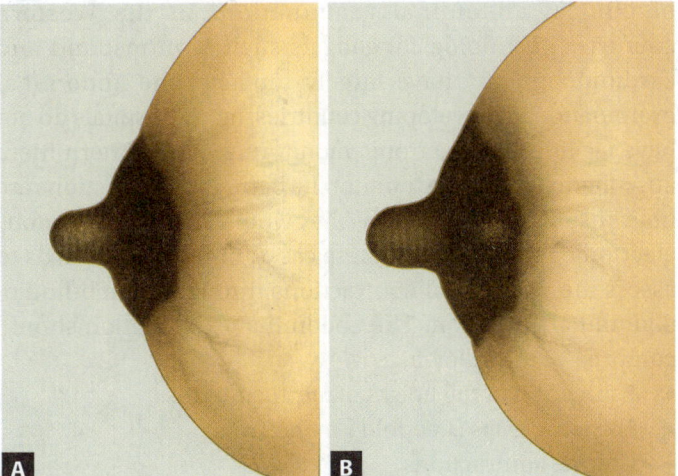

Figs. 1.10A and B: Breast examination of a pregnant woman. (A) Breasts of a nonpregnant woman; (B) Breasts of a pregnant woman.

Palpation

Both the breasts must be palpated with the palm of the hand rather than fingers for the presence of any lumps, masses, etc. In case there is presence of a breast lump or a blood-stained discharge from the nipple, the patient must be sent for a surgical referral and further investigations for diagnosis of a likely malignancy.

Whenever possible, all HIV-negative pregnant women must be advised and encouraged to breastfeed. The clinician must make special efforts to emphasize the importance of breastfeeding and to teach its advantages to women.

Hoffman's Exercises

In case the nipples are found to be inverted or flat, this condition must be treated as soon as possible so that the patient may be able to breastfeed successfully in future. The easiest way of correcting inverted nipples involves the use of Hoffman's exercises, which are performed as described:

- The thumbs are placed on either side of the base of the nipple.
- The thumbs are then moved toward the periphery of the areola. This is done in both vertical and horizontal directions.

This exercise must be repeated several times a day throughout pregnancy in order to bring the nipples in their normal position. The patient should be taught to do these exercises herself.

SPECIFIC SYSTEMIC EXAMINATION

During pregnancy, a detailed abdominal and vaginal examination may be required. Besides this, the other body systems such as the respiratory system and the cardiovascular system must also be briefly examined. In case any pathological sign is observed, a detailed examination of the respective body system must be carried out.

ABDOMINAL EXAMINATION

General Examination of the Abdomen

Even in the present time of technological advancements, the obstetricians must not underestimate the importance of clinical abdominal examination. In the Western countries, technological gadgets such as ultrasound and cardiotocography have largely replaced the abdominal examination. In developing countries, many hospitals do not have facilities for electronic monitoring. When intermittent auscultation is used to monitor the baby, the contractions are not constantly monitored, as they would be with continuous electronic monitoring. In these cases, the clinician needs to assess the abdominal contractions through the method of abdominal palpation. The abdominal examination should comprise of the following:

- Estimation of the height of uterine fundus
- Obstetric grips (Leopold's maneuvers)
- Uterine contractions
- Estimation of fetal descent
- Auscultation of fetal heart

Each of these is described next in detail.

Preparation of the Patient for Examination

- Before starting the abdominal examination, the clinician should ensure that the patient's bladder is empty; she should be asked to empty her bladder in case it is not empty.
- The patient must lie comfortably on her back with a pillow under her head. She should not lie in a left lateral position.

Inspection of the Abdomen

The following should be specifically looked for at the time of abdominal inspection:

- *Shape and size of the distended abdomen:*
  - In case of a singleton pregnancy and longitudinal lie, the shape of the uterus is usually oval **(Fig. 1.11)**.
  - The shape of the uterus will be round with multiple pregnancy or polyhydramnios.
  - The flattening of the lower part of the abdomen suggests a vertex presentation with an occipito-posterior position [right occipitoposterior (ROP) or left occipitoposterior (LOP)].
  - A suprapubic bulge is suggestive of a full bladder.
- *Presence or absence of scars:* In case scar marks as a result of previous surgery are visible **(Fig. 1.12)**, a detailed history must be taken. This should include the reasons of having the surgery and the type of surgery performed [myomectomy or previous lower segment cesarean section (LSCS)]. In case the scar is related to previous LSCS, detailed history as described in Chapter 11 needs to be taken.
- *Presence of striae gravidarum and linea nigra:* In many pregnant women, a black-brownish colored line may sometimes develop in the midline of the abdomen. This is known as linea nigra **(Fig. 1.13)**. In many women, in later months of pregnancy, stretch marks called striae gravidarum **(Fig. 1.14)** may develop over the skin of abdomen, breast, or thighs.

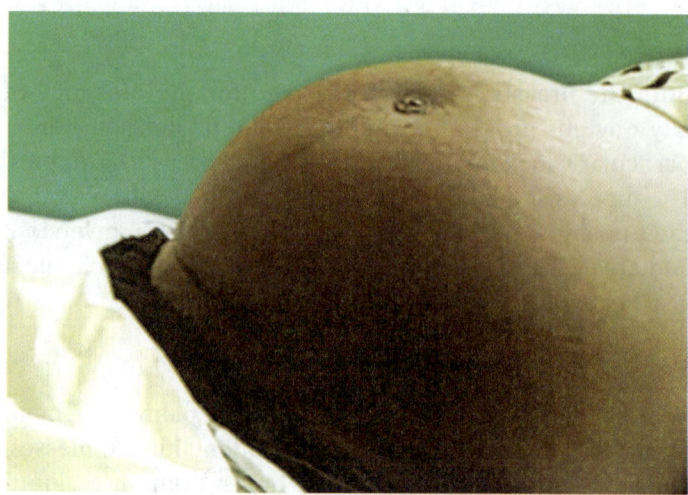

Fig. 1.11: Abdominal distention.

Normal Pregnancy 13

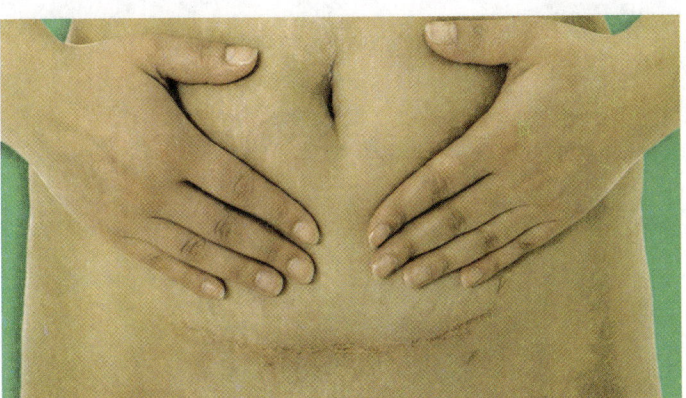

Fig. 1.12: Presence of previous cesarean scar over the abdomen.

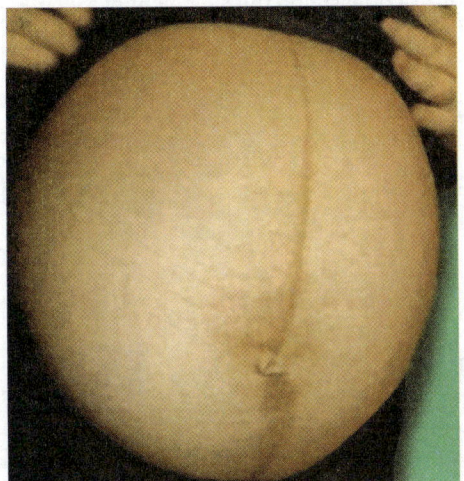

Fig. 1.13: Linea nigra.

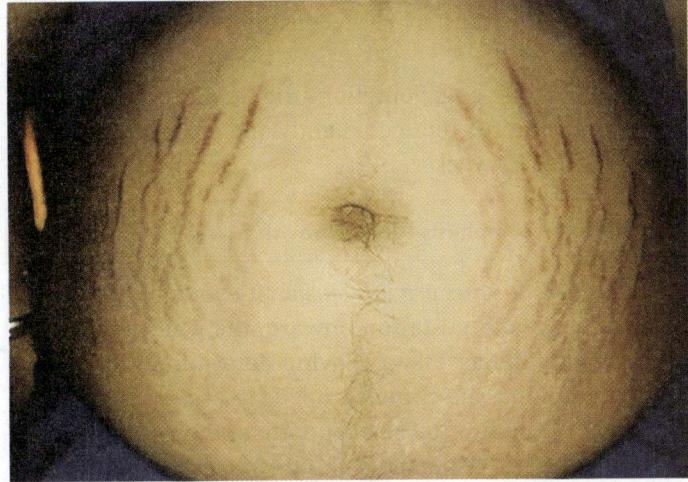

Fig.1.14: Striae gravidarum over the abdomen.

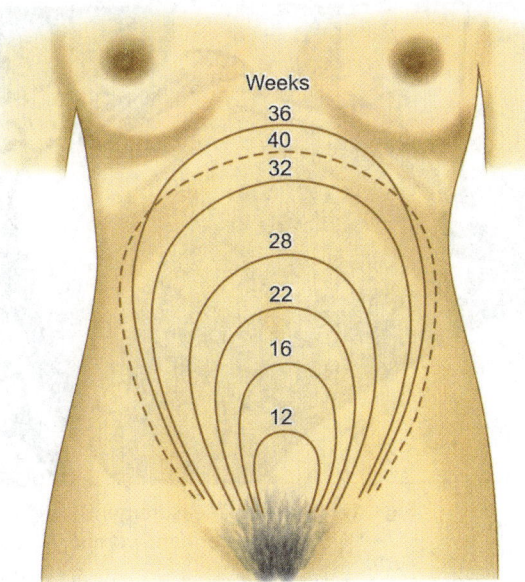

Fig. 1.15: Abdominal measurement of period of gestation.

The presence of an enlarged organ, or a mass, should be appropriately followed-up.

Examination of the Uterus and the Fetus

- The clinician must firstly check whether the uterus is lying in the midline of the abdomen or it is dextrorotated either to the right or to the left. In case the uterus is dextrorotated, it needs to be centralized.
- The wall of the uterus must be palpated for the presence of any irregularities. An irregular uterine wall may be suggestive of the presence of either myomas or a congenital abnormality such as a bicornuate uterus. Uterine myomas may enlarge during pregnancy and become painful.

Determining the Fundal Height

In the first few weeks of pregnancy, there is primarily an increase in the anterior–posterior diameter of the uterus. By 12 weeks, the uterus becomes globular and attains a size of approximately 8 cm. On the bimanual examination, the uterus appears soft, doughy, and elastic. In the initial stages of pregnancy, the cervix may appear firm. However, with increasing period of gestation, the cervix becomes increasingly softer in consistency. From the second trimester onward, the uterine height starts corresponding to the period of gestation. The rough estimation of fundal height with increasing period of gestation is shown in **Figure 1.15**.

Measurement of Symphysis-Fundus Height

The method of measuring the S-F height is shown in **Figures 1.16A and B**. After centralizing the dextrorotated uterus, the upper border of the fundus is located by the ulnar border of left hand, and this point is marked by placing one finger there. The distance between the upper border of the

Abdominal Palpation

Besides the fetal and uterine palpation, other abdominal organs such as the liver, spleen, and kidneys must also be specifically palpated. The presence of any other abdominal mass should also be noted.

14 Normal and Abnormal Presentations

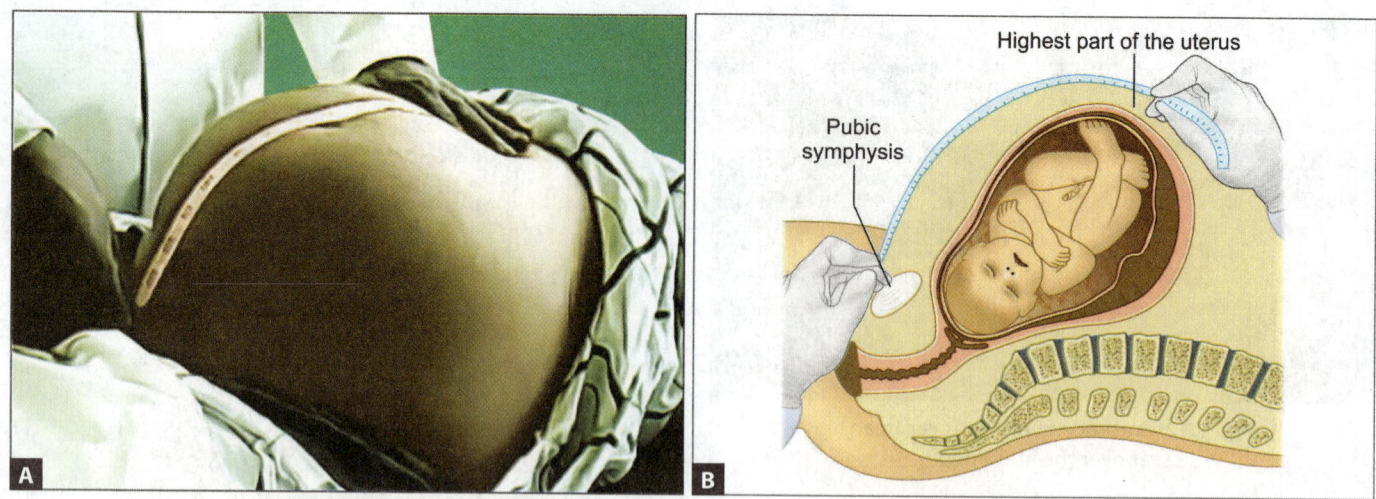

Figs. 1.16A and B: Measurement of symphysis-fundus (S-F) height. (A) Measuring the S-F height of a pregnant woman; (B) Diagrammatic representation of S-F height.

symphysis and the marked point is measured in centimeter with the help of a measuring tape. After 24 weeks, the S-F height, measured in centimeters, corresponds to the period of gestation up to 36 weeks. Though a variation of 2 cm (more or less) is regarded as normal, there are numerous conditions where the height of uterus may not correspond to the period of gestation.

Therefore, estimation of the period of gestation from the fundal height is not a foolproof method as there are certain conditions where height of the uterus can be more than the period of gestation as well as the conditions where height of the uterus is less than the period of gestation.

Determining the Size of the Uterus through Estimation of Fundal Height

- After centralizing the dextrorotated uterus with right hand, the upper border of the uterus is estimated with the ulnar border of left hand. Anatomical landmarks used for determining the size of uterus through estimation of fundal height mainly include the symphysis pubis and the umbilicus:
    - If the fundus is palpable just above the symphysis pubis, the gestational age is probably 12 weeks.
    - If the fundus reaches halfway between the symphysis and the umbilicus, the gestational age is probably 16 weeks.
    - If the fundus is at the same height as the umbilicus, the gestational age is probably 22 weeks (one finger under the umbilicus = 20 weeks and one finger above the umbilicus = 24 weeks).
    - The distance between the xiphisternum and umbilicus is divided into three equal parts. Upper one-third corresponds to 28 weeks, upper two-third corresponds to 32 weeks, whereas the tip of xiphisternum corresponds to 36 weeks. At 40 weeks

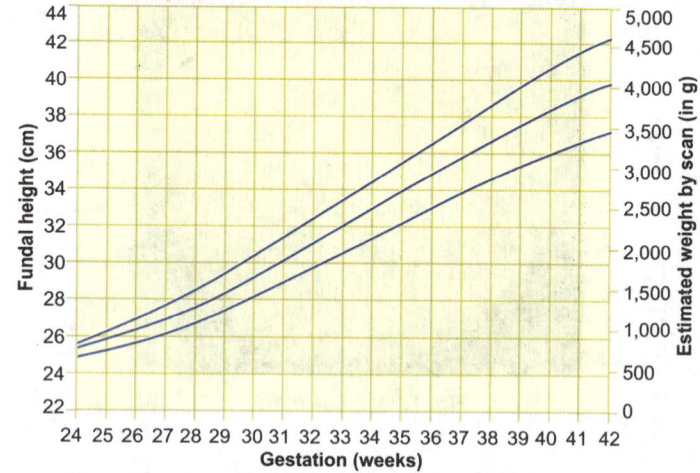

Fig. 1.17: Symphysis-fundus growth curves.

due to the engagement of the fetal head, the height of the uterus reduces slightly and corresponds to the level of 32 weeks.

Q. What is symphysis-fundus growth curve?

- *Symphysis-fundus growth curve:* At every antenatal visit from 28 weeks' gestation onward, the well-being of the fetus must be assessed. Having determined the height of the fundus, the clinician needs to assess whether the height of the fundus corresponds to the patient's dates and to the size of the fetus. From 18 weeks, the S-F height must be plotted on the S-F growth curve to determine the gestational age. This method is, therefore, only used once the fundal height has reached 18 weeks, in other words, when the S-F height has reached 2 finger-widths under the umbilicus.

The S-F growth curve helps in comparing the S-F height with the period of gestation. The growth curve should ideally form part of the antenatal card (**Fig. 1.17**). In this figure, there are three lines of which the middle one represents the 50th centile, the upper one 90th centile, and the lower one 10th centile, respectively. If intrauterine growth is normal, the S-F height will fall between the 10th centile and the 90th centile. In a normal pregnancy, between 18 weeks and 36 weeks of pregnancy, the S-F height normally increases at the rate of about 1 cm a week.

Palpation of the Fetus

The lie and presenting part of the fetus only become important when the gestational age reaches 34 weeks. The following must be determined:

Fetal Lie

Fetal lie refers to the relationship of cephalocaudal axis or long axis (spinal column) of the fetus to the long axis of the centralized uterus or maternal spine. The lie may be longitudinal, transverse, or oblique **(Table 1.4 and Figs 1.18A to C)**.

- *Longitudinal lie:* The fetal lie can be described as longitudinal when the maternal and fetal long axes are parallel to each other.
- *Transverse lie:* The fetal lie can be described as transverse when the maternal and fetal long axes are perpendicular to each other.
- *Oblique lie:* The fetal lie can be described as oblique when the maternal and fetal long axes cross each other obliquely or at an angle of 45°. The oblique lie is usually unstable and becomes longitudinal or transverse during the course of labor.

Fetal Presentation

Fetal presentation can be described as the fetal body part, which occupies the lower pole of the uterus and thereby first enters the pelvic passage. Fetal presentation is determined by fetal lie and may be of three types: cephalic, podalic (breech), or shoulder **(Table 1.5 and Figs. 1.19A to E)**.

Cephalic or the head presentation is the most common and occurs in about 97% of fetuses. Breech and shoulder presentations are less common and may pose difficulty for normal vaginal delivery. Thus, these two presentations are also known as malpresentations. As described previously, in cephalic presentation, the fetal head presents first. Depending on the part of fetal head presenting first, cephalic presentation can be divided as follows:

- *Vertex or occiput presentation:* When the head is completely flexed onto the chest, the smallest diameter of the fetal head (suboccipitobregmatic diameter) presents. In these cases, the occiput is the presenting part. Usually, the occiput presents anteriorly. In some cases, occiput may be present posteriorly **(Figs. 1.20A and B)**. This type of presentation is known as occipitoposterior position. Though most of the cases with occipitoposterior position undergo normal vaginal delivery, labor is usually prolonged in these cases. In some cases with occipitoposterior presentation, cesarean delivery may be required.
- *Face presentation:* When the fetal head is sharply extended, occiput and the back are in contact with one another. In these cases, face is the foremost part of the fetal head inside the birth canal, and it presents first.
- *Brow presentation:* When the fetal head is only partially extended, fetal brows are the foremost part of the fetal

TABLE 1.4: Types of fetal lie.	
Types of fetal lie	**Description**
Longitudinal lie	Spinal columns of mother and fetus are parallel to each other
Transverse lie	Spinal columns of mother and fetus are perpendicular to each other
Oblique lie	Spinal columns of mother and fetus cross each other obliquely at an angle of 45°

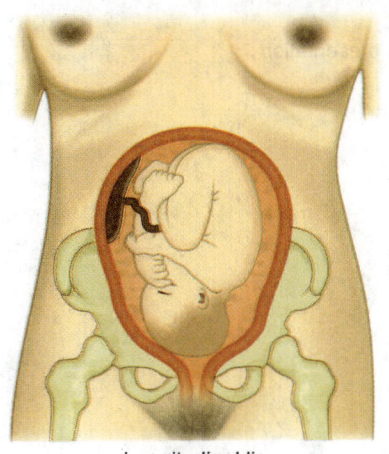
A Longitudinal lie
Vertex presentation

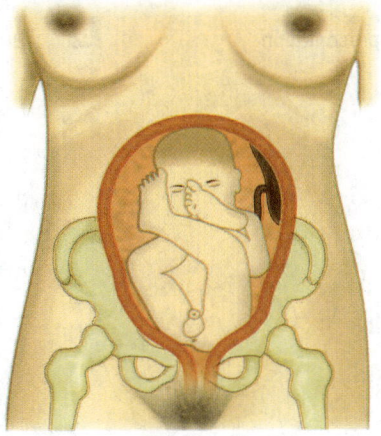
B Longitudinal lie
Breech presentation

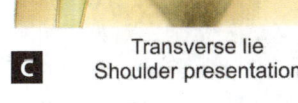
C Transverse lie
Shoulder presentation

Figs. 1.18A to C: Types of fetal lie.

head inside the birth canal, and they present first. Brow presentation is usually transient because with the progress of labor, as further extension of neck takes place, brow presentation almost invariably gets converted into face presentation. If the brow presentation remains persistent, the labor gets arrested and a cesarean section is invariably required.

- *Sinciput presentation:* When the fetal head is only partially flexed, the anterior fontanel or bregma is the foremost inside the birth canal, and it presents. With progress of labor, as the flexion of neck takes place, sinciput presentation almost invariably gets converted into vertex presentation.
  - *Compound presentation:* It is a term used when more than one part of the fetus presents **(Fig. 1.21)**, e.g., the presence of fetal limbs alongside the head in case of a cephalic presentation or one or both arms in case of breech presentation. This can commonly occur in case of preterm infants.

Since fetal presentation can undergo a change in the early weeks of gestation, it should be reassessed by abdominal palpation at 36 weeks or later, when fetal presentation is unlikely to change by itself and it is likely to influence the plans for the birth. In case of suspected fetal malpresentation, an ultrasound examination must be performed to confirm the presentation.

Presenting Part

The presenting part can be defined as the part of fetal presentation which is foremost within the birth canal and is therefore first felt by the obstetrician's examining fingers **(Table 1.6)**.

Fetal Attitude

Fetal attitude refers to the relationship of fetal parts to each other **(Figs. 1.22A to D)**. The most common fetal attitude is that of flexion in which the fetal head is flexed over the fetal neck; fetal arms are flexed unto the chest and fetal legs are flexed over the abdomen.

Denominator

Denominator can be described as an arbitrary fixed bony point on the fetal presenting part **(Table 1.7)**.

Fetal Position

Fetal position can be defined as the relationship of the denominator to the different quadrants of maternal pelvis (anterior, transverse, and posterior). Since the presenting part would be either directed to the left or right side of

TABLE 1.5: Types of fetal presentation.	
Types of fetal presentation	**Presenting part**
Cephalic presentation	Fetal head
Breech presentation	Fetal podalic pole (either buttocks or lower extremities)
Shoulder presentation	Fetal shoulders

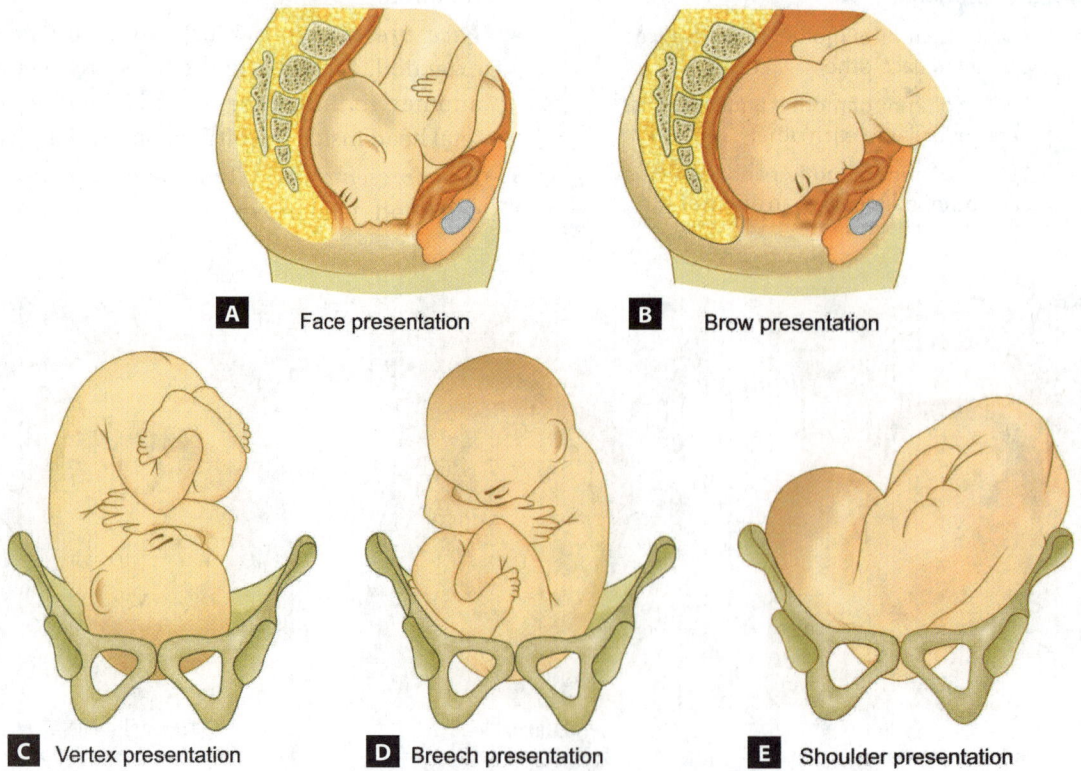

Figs. 1.19A to E: Various types of fetal presentation.

Normal Pregnancy

maternal pelvis, six positions would be possible for each of the fetal presentation **(Table 1.8 and Fig. 1.23)**. For example, with vertex presentation, the six positions that would be possible are left occiput anterior (LOA), right occiput anterior (ROA), left occiput transverse (LOT), right occiput transverse (ROT), left occiput posterior (LOP), and right occiput posterior (ROP). The fetal position gives an idea regarding whether the presenting part is directed toward the front, back, left, or right of the birth passage. Different positions possible with various other presentations are shown in **Figure 1.24**.

Diagnosis of Fetal Presentation and Position

It is most important for the obstetrician to correctly identify the fetal presentation and position. This is usually done by performing Leopold's maneuvers on abdominal examination or via vaginal examination.

Obstetric Grips or Leopold's Maneuvers of Abdominal Palpation

> **Q.** Write a long essay regarding the diagnosis of fetal presentation and positions while performing Leopold's maneuvers.

Obstetric grips which help in determining fetal lie and presentation are also known as Leopold's maneuvers. Leopold's maneuvers basically include four steps and must be performed while the woman is lying comfortably on her back. The examiner faces the patient for the first three maneuvers and faces toward her feet for the fourth. Obstetric grips must be conducted when the uterus is relaxed and not when the woman is experiencing contractions **(Figs. 1.25A and B)**.

Maternal position: The mother should be comfortably lying in supine position and her abdomen is to be bared. She should be asked to semiflex her thighs in order to relax the abdominal muscles.

These maneuvers can be performed throughout the third trimester and between the contractions, when the patient is in labor. These grips help in determining fetal lie

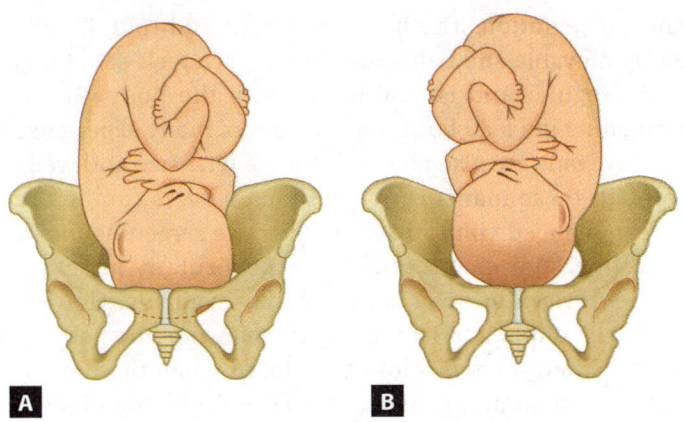

Figs. 1.20A and B: Occipitoposterior position.

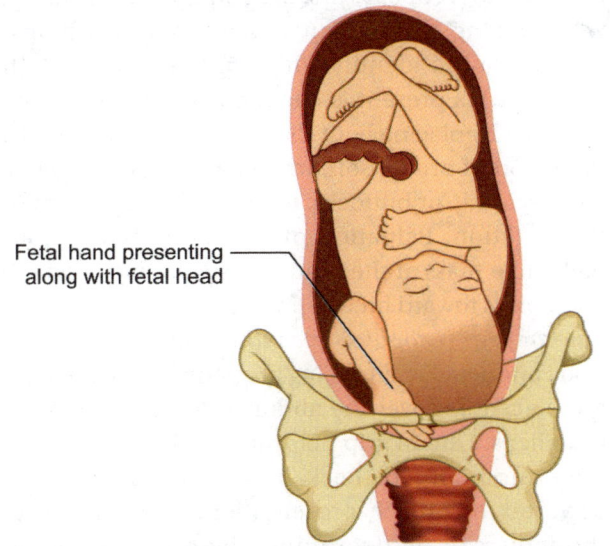

Fig. 1.21: Compound presentation.

TABLE 1.6: Fetal presenting parts.	
Fetal presentation	*Fetal presenting part*
Cephalic	*Vertex:* Completely flexed fetal head *Sinciput:* Deflexed fetal head *Brow:* Partially extended fetal head *Face:* Completely extended fetal head
Breech	Sacrum
Shoulder	Fetal back

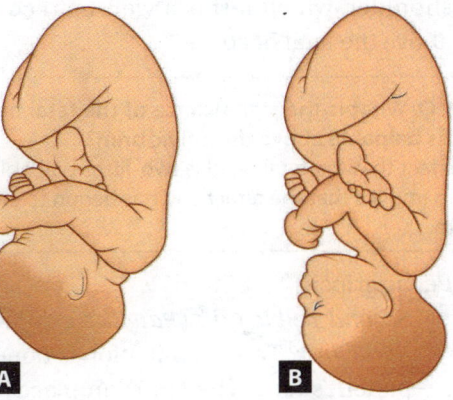
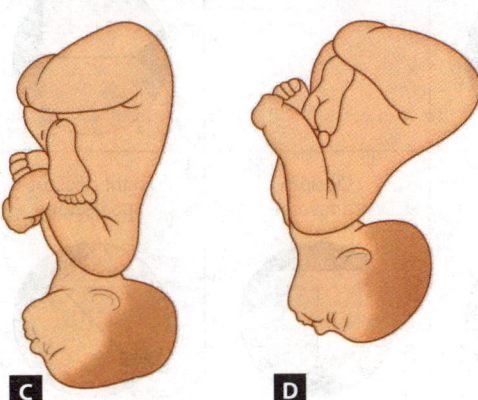

Figs. 1.22A to D: Different types of fetal attitudes. (A) Complete flexion; (B) Moderate flexion; (C) Poor flexion; (D) Hyperextension.

TABLE 1.7: Fetal denominators in relation to fetal presenting parts.

Fetal presenting part	Denominator
Vertex	Occiput
Face	Mentum
Brow	Frontal eminence
Breech	Sacrum
Shoulder	Acromion

TABLE 1.8: Various fetal positions in relation to the fetal denominator.

Fetal denominator	Fetal positions
Occiput	LOA, ROA, LOT, ROT, LOP, ROP
Mentum	LMA, RMA, LMT, RMT, LMP, RMP
Sacrum	LSA, RSA, LST, RST, LSP, RSP
Acromion	Dorsoanterior (R or L), dorsoposterior (R or L), dorsosuperior (R or L), and dorsoinferior (R or L)

(L: left; LMA: left mentum anterior; LMP: left mentum posterior; LMT: left mentum transverse; LOA: left occiput anterior; LOP: left occiput posterior; LOT: left occiput transverse; LSA: left sacrum anterior; LSP: left sacrum posterior; LST: left sacrum transverse; R: right; RMA: right mentum anterior; RMP: right mentum posterior; RMT: right mentum transverse; ROA: right occiput anterior; ROP: right occiput posterior; ROT: right occiput transverse; RSA: right sacrum anterior; RSP: right sacrum posterior; RST: right sacrum transverse)

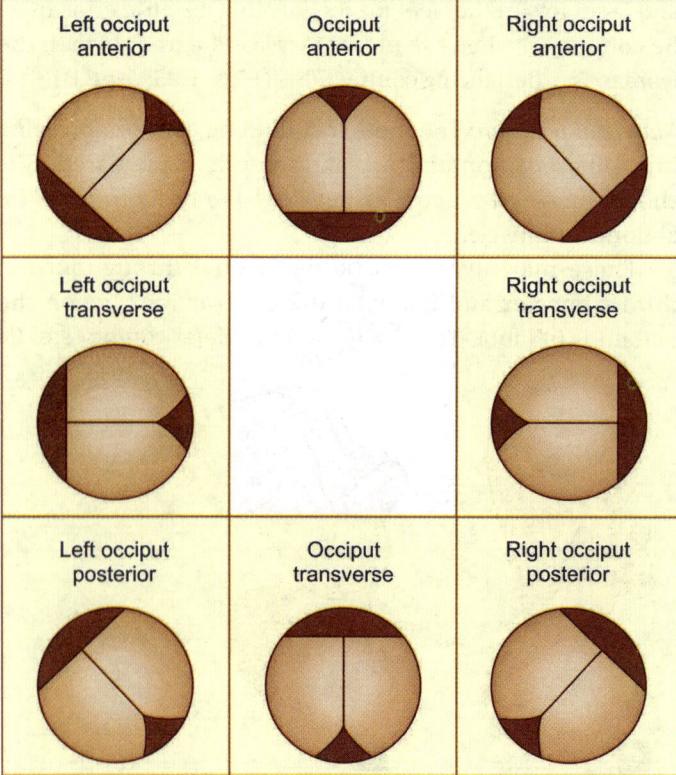

Fig. 1.23: Various positions possible in case of vertex presentation.

and presentation. The head feels hard and round, and is easily movable and ballotable. The breech feels soft, broad, and irregular and is continuous with the body. Besides estimating the fetal lie and presentation, many experienced obstetricians are also able to estimate fetal size and weight through these maneuvers. These maneuvers can be used by experienced clinicians as an effective screening tool for detecting fetal malpresentations, particularly in settings where ultrasound may not be readily available. However, it may be difficult to feel the fetus well when the patient is obese, when there is a lot of liquor, or when the uterus is tight, as in some primigravidas. The following obstetric grips/Leopold's maneuvers are carried out:

- *Fundal grip (Leopold's first maneuver):* This is conducted while facing the patient's face. This grip helps the obstetrician to identify which of the fetal poles (head or breech) is present at the fundus. The fundal area is palpated by placing both the hands over the fundal area. Palpation of broad, soft, irregular mass is suggestive of fetal legs and/or buttocks, thereby pointing toward head presentation. Palpation of a smooth, hard, globular, ballotable mass at the fundus is suggestive of fetal head and points toward breech presentation.
- *Lateral grip (Leopold's second maneuver):* This grip is also conducted while facing the patient's face. The hands are placed flat over the abdomen on either side of the umbilicus. Lateral grip helps the clinician in identifying the position of fetal back, limbs, and shoulder in case of vertex or breech presentation. The orientation of the fetus can be determined by noting whether the back is directed vertically (anteriorly, posteriorly) or transversely. In case of transverse lie, hard, round globular mass suggestive of fetal head can be identified horizontally across the maternal abdomen. The fetal back can be identified as a smooth curved structure with a resistant feel. The position of the fetal back on the left or right side of the uterus would help in determining the position of the presenting part. The fetal limbs would be present on the side opposite to the fetal back and present as small, round, knob-like structures. After identifying the back, the clinician should try to identify the anterior shoulder, which forms a well-marked prominence just above the fetal head.

> **Q. What is the significance of the fetal head, which is two-fifths palpable above the pelvic brim?**
> The fact that the fetal head is two-fifths palpable above the pelvic brim implies that the fetal head has begun to engage in the pelvic brim.

- Pelvic grips:
  - *Second pelvic grip (Pawlik's grip) or third Leopold's maneuver:* This examination is done while facing the patient's face. The clinician places the outstretched thumb and index finger of the right hand, keeping the

Normal Pregnancy

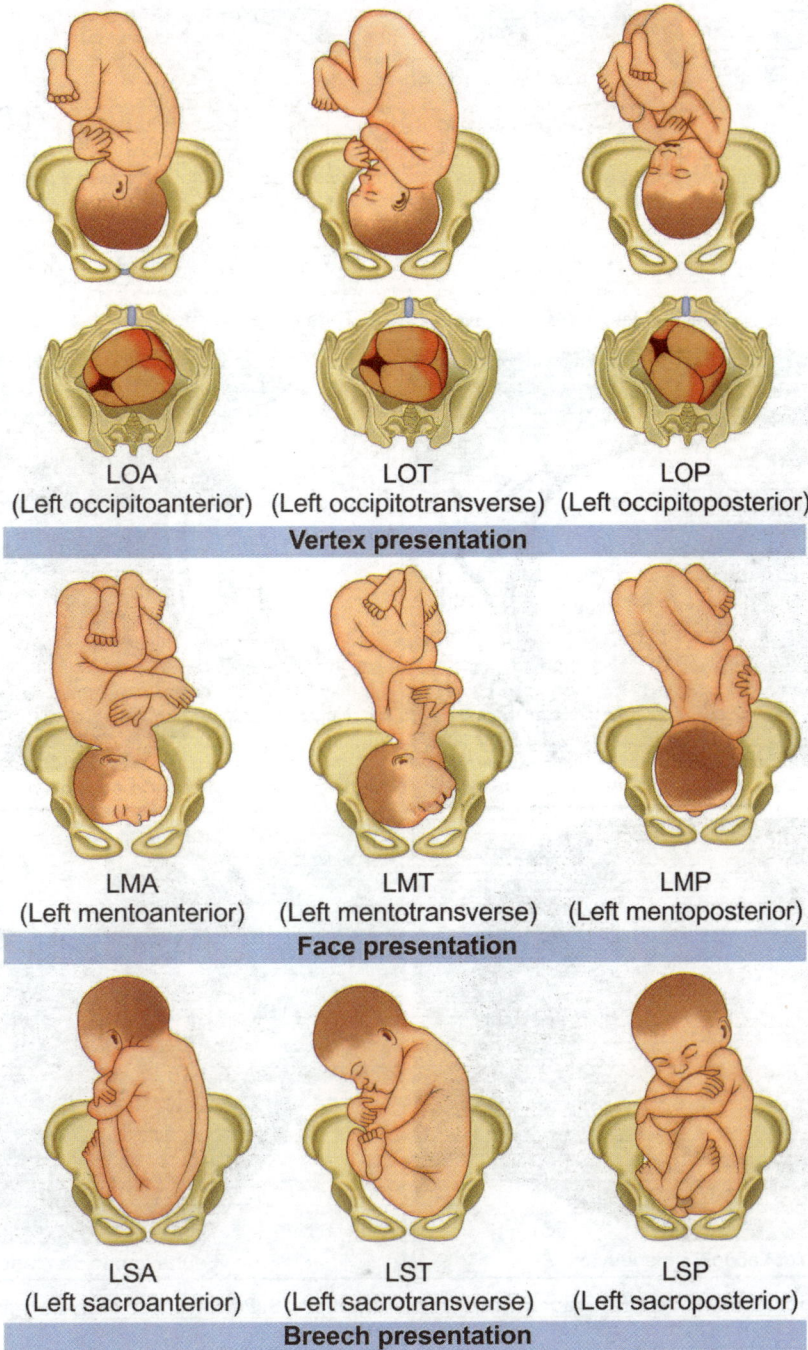

Fig. 1.24: Different positions possible with various presentations.

ulnar border of the palm on the upper border of the patient's pubic symphysis. If a hard globular mass is gripped, it implies vertex presentation. A soft, broad part is suggestive of fetal breech. If the presenting part is not engaged, it would be freely ballotable between the two fingers. If the presenting part is deeply engaged, the findings of this maneuver simply indicate that the lower fetal pole is in the pelvis. Further details would be revealed by the next maneuver. In case of transverse presentation, the pelvic grip is empty. Normally, the size of head in a baby at term would fit in the hand of the examining clinician.

- *First pelvic grip (fourth Leopold's maneuver):* The objective of this step is to determine the amount of head palpable above the pelvic brim in case of a cephalic presentation. First pelvic grip is performed while facing the patient's feet. Tips of three fingers of each hand are placed on the either side of the midline in downward and backward directions in order to deeply palpate the fetal parts present in the lower pole of the uterus. The fingers of both the hands should be placed parallel to the inguinal ligaments, and the thumbs should be pointing toward the umbilicus on both the sides. In case of vertex presentation, a

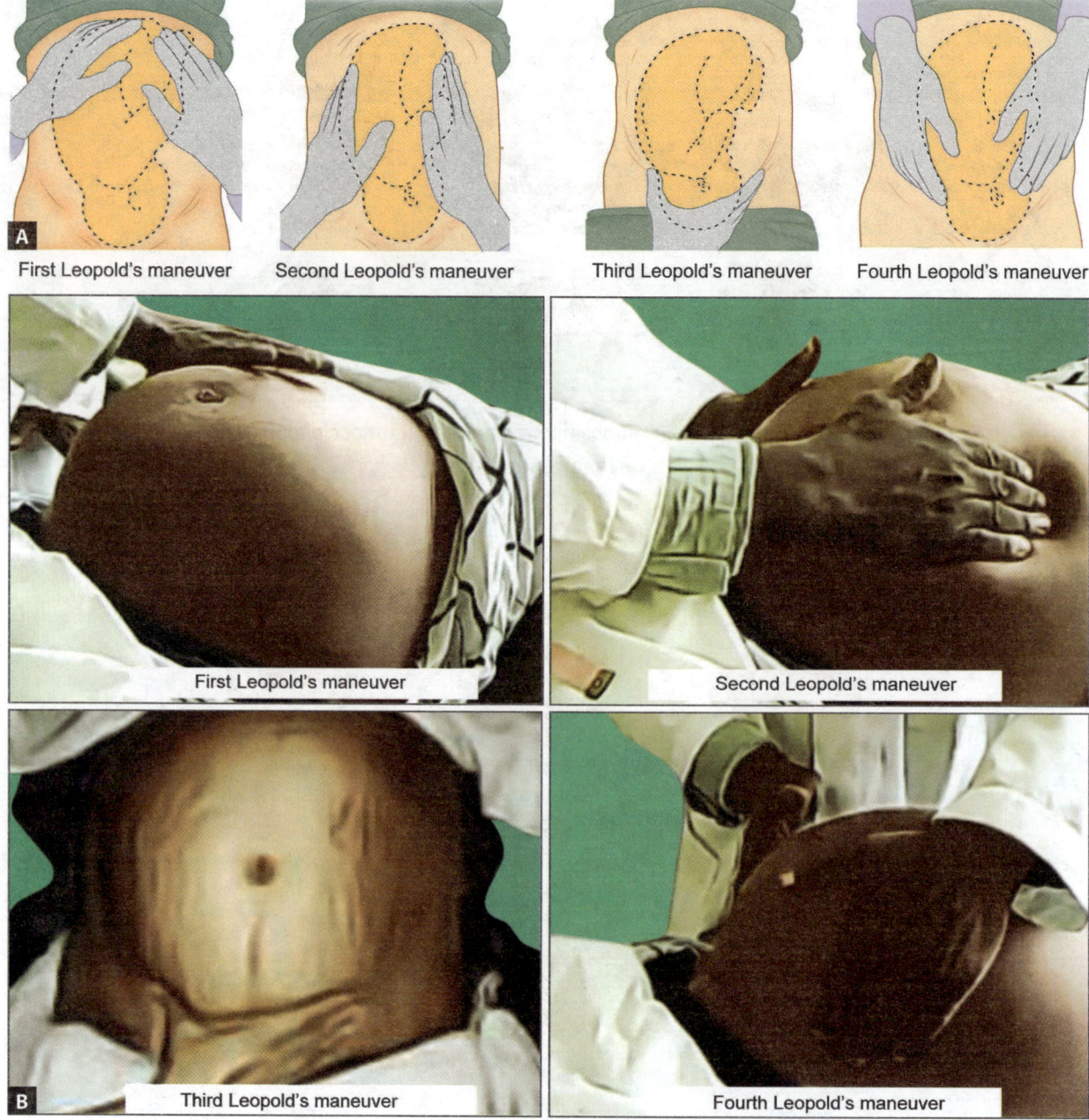

Figs. 1.25A and B: Leopold's maneuvers. (A) Diagrammatic representation; (B) Performance of these maneuvers on the patient.

hard smooth globular mass suggestive of fetal head can be palpated on pelvic grip. In case of breech presentation, broad, soft, irregular mass is palpated.

Auscultation of Fetal Heart

The fetal well-being is usually assessed by listening to the fetal heart. The auscultation of the fetal heart will also give some idea regarding the fetal presentation and position. The region of maternal abdomen where the heart sounds are most clearly heard would vary with the presentation and extent of descent of the presenting part **(Figs. 1.26A and B)**. The fetal heart is most easily heard by listening over the back of the fetus. The FHR can be monitored either through electronic fetal monitoring, using an external fetal monitor, or through intermittent auscultation, using a Doppler instrument or Pinard fetoscope or even an ordinary stethoscope. Normal FHR varies from 100 to 140 beats/min with the average being 120 beats/min.

Auscultation of the FHR is particularly important in cases where the woman is unable to perceive the fetal movements. To make sure that the clinician is not accidentally listening to the mother's heart instead of the fetal heart, the maternal pulse must also be simultaneously palpated. In normal cases, the FHR must be auscultated as described next.

- *During the first stage of labor:* Every 30 minutes, followed by every 15 minutes during the second stage of labor
- In high-risk cases (e.g., preeclampsia), the FHR must be auscultated every 15 minutes during the first stage

Normal Pregnancy

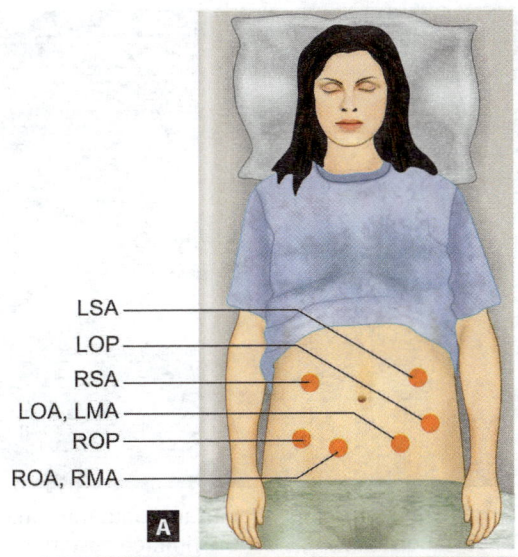

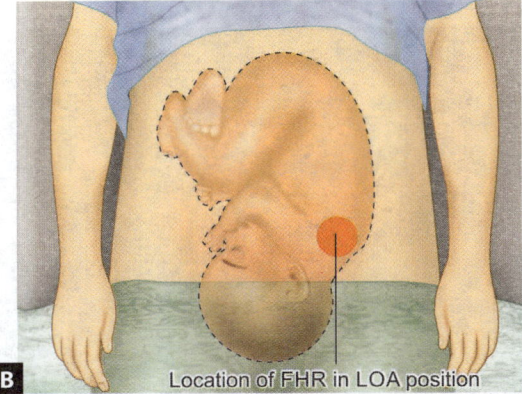

Figs. 1.26A and B: (A) Location of FHR; (B) Location of FHR in LOA position. (LMA: left mentum anterior; LOA: left occiput anterior; LOP: left occiput posterior; LSA: left sacrum anterior; RMA: right mentum anterior; ROA: right occiput anterior; ROP: right occiput posterior; RSA: right sacrum anterior)

TABLE 1.9: Indications for vaginal examination during the antenatal period.

At the time of first ANC visit	Subsequent antenatal visits
• Diagnosis of pregnancy • Assessment of the gestational age • Detection of abnormalities in the genital tract • Investigation of a vaginal discharge • Cervical examination	• Investigation of a threatened abortion • Confirmation of preterm rupture of the membranes with a sterile speculum • Confirmation of the diagnosis of preterm labor • Identification of the fetal presenting part in the pelvis

and every 5 minutes during the second stage of labor. Preferably electronic fetal monitoring must be employed in high-risk cases.

VAGINAL EXAMINATION

Indications for vaginal examination during the antenatal period are listed in **Table 1.9**.

Pelvic examination: Since the routine antenatal pelvic examination does not accurately assess gestational age, nor does it accurately predict preterm birth or cephalopelvic disproportion, it is not recommended in routine clinical practice.

MANAGEMENT

 Q. In the case study described in the beginning of the chapter, there has been a decrease in S-F height by 1 cm over the past week. Should it be a cause of worry? Was the obstetrician correct in assuring the woman that everything was fine?
A slight decrease in S-F height at 37 weeks of gestation is a normal phenomenon, which indicates that the fetal head is descending normally in the pelvis. This also helps in ruling out the cephalopelvic disproportion. The obstetrician was absolutely correct in assuring the women that everything was fine.

Q. What should be the next line of management in the patient described at the beginning of this chapter?
An external cardiotocographic trace should be carried out in this patient. The patient must be reassured that she and her fetus are healthy, and she must be asked to attend the antenatal clinic again in a week's time.

Q. Discuss in detail the various parameters to determine the gestational age. Also discuss the management of a previously booked primigravida at 36 weeks of gestation.

Box 1.1 enlists the components of initial management plan.

Management comprising of investigations and definitive obstetric management is discussed next.

INVESTIGATIONS

Pregnancy can be confirmed with the help of the tests mentioned as follows:

PREGNANCY TEST

Pregnancy test is based on the detection of human chorionic gonadotropin (hCG) in the patient's urine. β-hCG is a glycoprotein hormone produced by the trophoblastic cells and prevents the involution of corpus luteum during early pregnancy. Corpus luteum is the principal site of progesterone production during the first 6 weeks of gestation. In normal pregnancy, β-hCG levels start increasing from the day of implantation and reach their peak by 60–70 days. Thereafter, the levels start decreasing until a nadir is reached by 14–16 weeks of gestation. During early pregnancy, the doubling time of β-hCG is nearly 1.4–2.0 days. The earliest that the β-hCG test can be expected to be positive is 8–10 days following ovulation. The test normally becomes positive by the time a pregnant woman first misses her period. If the test is negative and the woman is not having her period yet, the test should be repeated after 48 hours. The pregnancy test must be performed on a fresh urine specimen (first morning specimen).

The pregnancy test can be considered as negative if only the control band nearest to the upper blue part of the test

BOX 1.1: Components of the initial management plan.
- Review of previous records
- Calculation of expected date of delivery and estimated gestational age from last menstrual period
- Checking various parameters on general physical examination such as weight gain, blood pressure, edema, etc.
- Palpation of the uterus to determine S-F height, uterine size, fetal lie, presentation, position, FHR, etc.
- Developing a plan for delivery
- Scheduling the antenatal visits

strip becomes pink. It can be considered as positive if two pink bands are visible and as uncertain if none of the pink bands are seen. Uncertain test implies that either the test was not performed correctly or the test strip is damaged. In these cases, the test must be repeated with another test strip.

If possible, all pregnant patients should have a midstream urine specimen examined for asymptomatic bacteriuria.

ULTRASOUND EXAMINATION

Ultrasound examination in the first trimester is crucial in establishing intrauterine pregnancy, gestational age, and early pregnancy failure, and to exclude other causes of bleeding such as ectopic and molar pregnancies, missed abortion, and incomplete abortion. A first trimester ultrasound examination helps in accurate estimation of the period of gestation. During normal pregnancy, at the time of transvaginal sonography, the gestational sac appears first by 4.5–5 weeks **(Fig. 1.27)**, yolk sac by 5–5.5 weeks, fetal pole by 5.5–6 weeks, and fetal heartbeat by 6 weeks. All these findings are likely to appear 1 week later on the transabdominal scan. Double-rimmed gestational sac can be considered as a sign of intrauterine pregnancy during early weeks of gestation (4–6 weeks) in cases where the embryo or yolk sac has yet not made its appearance. In cases of normal intrauterine pregnancy, hyperechogenic ring of decidua capsularis is surrounded by another hyperechogenic ring (decidua parietalis). The gestational sac appears double-rimmed because these two layers of decidua are separated by an anechoic space and fluid within the uterine cavity. Ultrasound screening at 11–13 weeks may also be useful for the measurement of nuchal thickness (NT), which may be a useful screening test for Down syndrome (DS) **(Fig. 1.28)**.

A second-trimester ultrasound examination performed between 18 and 22 weeks is helpful in excluding multiple pregnancy, placental localization, determining period of gestation, and screening for gross fetal abnormalities. An ultrasound examination done after the second trimester is too unreliable for estimating the duration of pregnancy. However, it may help in confirming the fetal presentation, placental localization, amount of liquor, etc.

Once the pregnancy has been confirmed, the requirement for antenatal care for every patient needs to be emphasized so that most high-risk cases can be identified early in pregnancy. The advantages of hospital delivery should be stressed upon. Even if the woman is not delivered

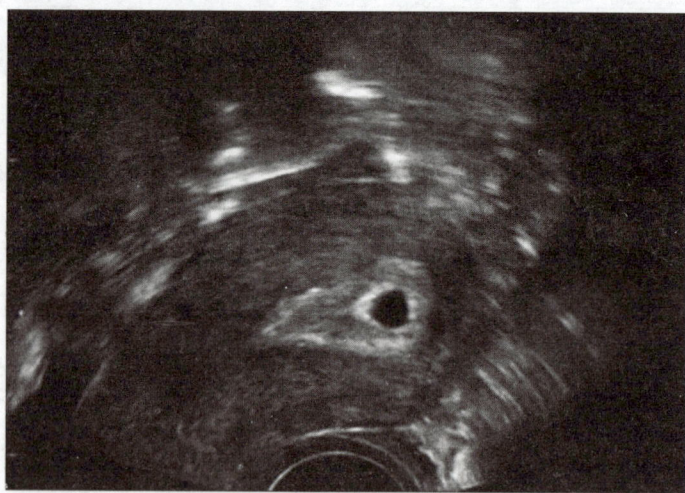

Fig. 1.27: Transvaginal scan demonstrating an intrauterine pregnancy at 5 weeks of gestation showing a double-rimmed gestational sac.

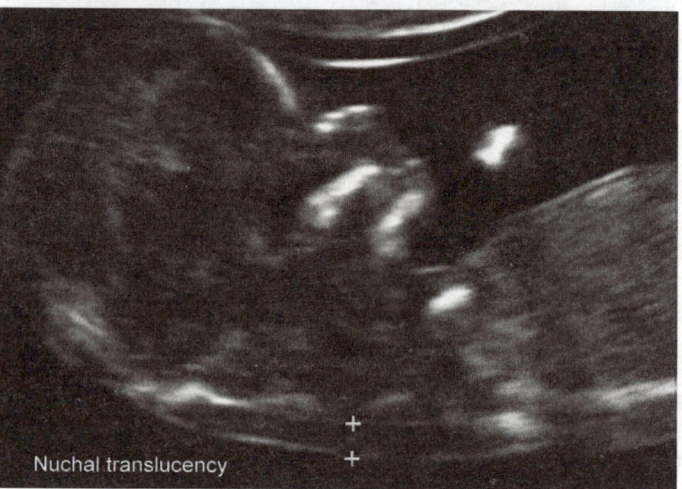

Fig. 1.28: Measurement of nuchal translucency.

in the hospital, she should at least have a trained birth attendant present at the time of birth. The investigations, which need to be done at the time of the first antenatal visit, have been enumerated in **Box 1.2** and those which need to be performed during each subsequent antenatal visit are enlisted in **Box 1.3**.

℞ TREATMENT/OBSTETRIC MANAGEMENT

ANTENATAL SCHEDULE

Q. How is the information recorded on the antenatal card?

Q. Write a long essay discussing the components of antenatal checkup.

Q. Write a short essay on basic components of antenatal checkup.

Q. Briefly describe the aim and objectives of antenatal care.

Q. Write a long essay discussing the aims of antenatal care and its relevance in prevention of various obstetric complications.

Normal Pregnancy

BOX 1.2: Routine investigations to be done during the first antenatal visit.

- Determination of the patient's blood group (ABO and Rh)
- Hemoglobin estimation
- Universal screening for gestational diabetes using a single step DIPSI criteria (for details see Chapter 19)
- Urine test for protein and glucose
- Serological screening test for syphilis (VDRL)
- A rapid HIV screening test after pretest counseling and written consent
- Screening for hepatitis B surface antigen (HbsAg) and hepatitis C virus
- Wet smear of any symptomatic vaginal discharge (i.e., itching, burning, or offensive) must be examined under a microscope
- Screening for asymptomatic bacteriuria
- Screening for Down syndrome, if available
- First trimester ultrasound scan for gestational age assessment
- Ultrasound screening for structural anomalies (20 weeks)

BOX 1.3: Investigations to be performed during each subsequent antenatal visit.

- Packed cell volume, hemoglobin estimation
- Blood pressure, amount of weight gain
- Urine test for proteins and glucose
- Abdominal examination (measurement and plotting of the S-F height from second trimester onward)

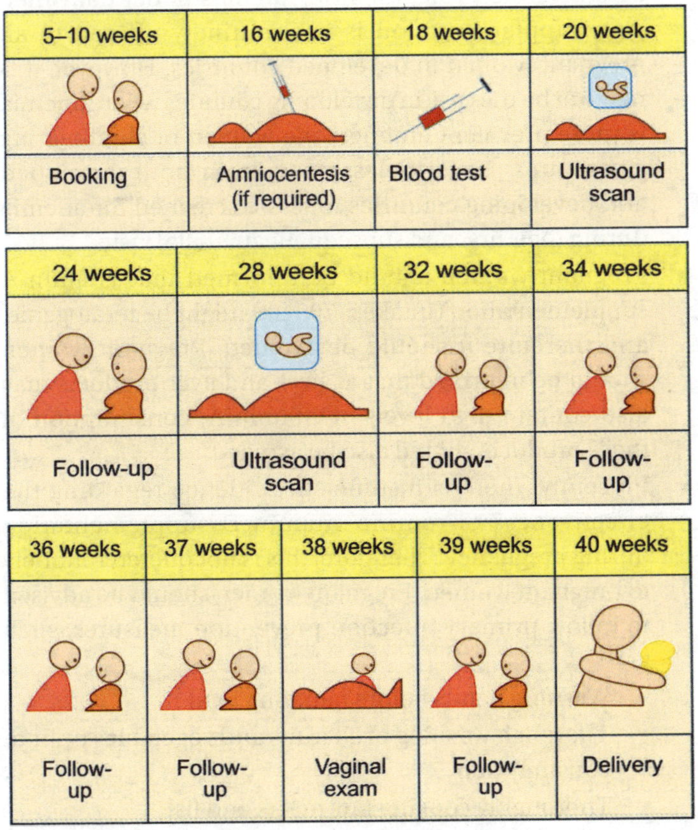

Fig. 1.29: Antenatal schedule.

The antenatal schedule as devised by the WHO is shown in **Figure 1.29**. The antenatal visits should be at every 4 weeks up to 28 weeks, at every 2 weeks up to 36 weeks, and thereafter weekly till the EDD. A minimum of four visits are recommended by the WHO—first at the 16th week, second at 24–28 weeks, third at 32 weeks, and fourth at 36 weeks. The various antenatal visits have now been described in detail.

First Antenatal Visit

The woman must be called for the first antenatal visit preferably before 12 weeks of gestation. However, if this is not possible, the woman can be seen any time. Since detailed history including previous medical and obstetric history needs to be taken, this visit takes about 30–40 minutes. The woman should be given an opportunity to discuss issues and ask questions. The presence of pregnancy needs to be confirmed during this visit. The accurate period of gestation can be established by first trimester ultrasound examination. A complete general physical examination must be performed. Advice regarding diet, exercise, and folic acid intake must be given. She should be offered verbal information supported by written information (leaflets, brochures, etc.) on topics such as diet and lifestyle considerations. She should be advised to stop smoking and consuming alcohol if previously doing so. High-risk women who may require additional care, need to be identified, and pattern of care for the pregnancy needs to be planned. The investigations which need to be performed during the first antenatal visit are listed in **Box 1.2**.

Second Antenatal Visit

Second antenatal visit must be scheduled at about 26 weeks of gestation. This visit is much shorter and lasts for about 20 minutes. A hemoglobin level of <10 g/dL needs to be investigated and oral hematinics (iron supplements) be started. At 18–20 weeks, an ultrasound scan should be performed for the detection of structural anomalies. For a woman whose placenta is found to be extending across the internal cervical os during this time should be offered another scan in third trimester and the results of this scan reviewed at next appointment. Anti-D immunoglobulins must be offered to the Rh-negative women where available and indicated (at 28 weeks of gestation).

Third Antenatal Visit (30–36 weeks)

The obstetrician needs to review, discuss, and document the results of screening tests undertaken during previous visits. Planned pattern of care for the pregnancy needs to be reassessed, and the women who require additional care need to be identified. Investigations mentioned in **Box 1.3** need to be done.

Fourth Antenatal Visit (36–40 weeks)

During this last visit, the position of the baby needs to be checked. In case of suspected malpresentation, ultrasound examination must be performed to confirm the fetal position. For women whose babies are in the breech presentation, external cephalic version can be considered after 37 completed weeks of gestation. Ultrasound scans may be required to confirm the placental position if the placenta had extended over the internal cervical os during the previous ultrasound scans. She should be asked to revisit her obstetrician in case she does not deliver until 41 weeks. Fetal heart rate monitoring needs to be done in these cases. Induction may be considered, if the cervix is inducible and favorable.

ROUTINE ANTENATAL CARE

Throughout the entire antenatal period, healthcare providers/obstetricians should remain alert regarding the development of signs or symptoms of conditions which affect the health of the mother and fetus, such as anemia, preeclampsia, diabetes, malpresentations, and IUGR. If any of the high-risk factors are detected, further management under expert guidance is required.

Antenatal Card

- An antenatal card carrying all the relevant information related to the woman's pregnancy must be designed in such a way so as to facilitate early detection of important and clearly defined conditions related to her pregnancy, which are likely to result in well-defined and beneficial actions with respect to maternal and fetal well-being.
- In the front of the antenatal card, the patient's details including history; any significant findings on general physical, abdominal, and vaginal examination; special investigations; LMP; EDD; and future plan of management need to be mentioned. The back of the antenatal card is used to record the observations made at each antenatal visit throughout the pregnancy.
- *These include the following:* Date of examination, blood pressure, the presence of proteinuria or glycosuria on urine examination with the help of dipstick, fetal movements from 28 weeks onward, fetal presenting part from 34 weeks onward, hemoglobin concentration at 28 and 34 weeks, and the S-F height from 18 weeks onward.

Pregnancy Dating

- The average duration of human pregnancy is 280 days from the first day of the LMP until delivery. EDD is most commonly calculated using Naegele's rule.
- *Naegele's rule:* Using Naegele's rule, the EDD is calculated by adding 9 calendar months and 7 days to the first day of the LMP (28-day cycle). For in vitro fertilization pregnancies, the date of LMP is 14 days prior to the date of embryo transfer.
- *Ultrasonographic dating:* This is the most accurate from 7 to 11 weeks of pregnancy.

Nutrition

> Q. Write a long essay discussing about nutrition in pregnancy and lactation.
>
> Q. Write a short note discussing diet in pregnancy.
>
> Q. Write a long essay discussing folic acid supplementation in pregnancy and its importance.

- Pregnant women require 15% more kilocalories than nonpregnant women, usually 100–300 kcal more per day, depending on the patient's weight and activity.
- Supplementation with iron, folic acid, protein, and calcium is required during pregnancy. The woman should be informed that dietary supplementation with folic acid, before conception and up to 12 weeks' gestation, helps in reducing the risk of having a baby with neural tube defects (anencephaly, spina bifida). The recommended dose is 400 µg/day. Consumption of iron-containing foods should be encouraged. As per WHO, iron supplements containing 120 mg of elemental iron is prescribed daily, starting from second trimester onward. For calcium, the prenatal daily requirement is 1,200 mg. Care should be taken to see that the woman is taking appropriate quantities of proteins, carbohydrates, calcium, iron, and fats in her daily diet. Iron supplementation is not routinely offered to all pregnant women in developed countries. However, this may not be the case in developing counties where anemia is more prevalent amongst the women of childbearing age groups. Nevertheless, women in both developed and developing countries must be screened for anemia during their first and subsequent antenatal visits.
- Pregnant women should be informed that vitamin A supplementation (intake > 700 µg) might be teratogenic, and therefore it should be avoided. Pregnant women should be informed that as liver and liver products may also contain high levels of vitamin A, consumption of these products should also be avoided.
- Presently, there is insufficient evidence regarding the effectiveness of routine vitamin D supplementation during pregnancy. Therefore, this is not offered routinely to pregnant women. Pregnant women should be advised to follow primary infection prevention measures, such as:
  - Washing hands before handling food
  - Thorough washing of all fruits and vegetables prior to consumption
  - Thoroughly cooking raw meats and fish
  - Wearing gloves and thoroughly washing hands after handling soil and farming
  - Avoiding contact with cat/cow feces in litter or soil
  - Avoiding consumption of uncooked meat due to the risk of toxoplasmosis

Normal Pregnancy

Rhesus Blood Grouping and Red Cell Alloantibodies

- Women should be offered testing for blood group and RhD status in early pregnancy.
- Women should be screened for atypical red cell alloantibodies in early pregnancy and again at 28 weeks regardless of their RhD status.
- Routine antenatal anti-D prophylaxis is recommended for all nonsensitized pregnant women who are RhD negative.
- Pregnant women with clinically significant atypical red cell alloantibodies should be offered referral to a specialist center for further advice on subsequent antenatal management.

Weight Gain

The total weight gain recommended during pregnancy based on the prepregnancy body mass index is described in **Table 1.10**. Gestational weight gain amounts to about 28–29 pounds. Distribution of weight gain during pregnancy is described in **Figure 1.30**.

TABLE 1.10: Recommended total weight gain for pregnant women based on their prepregnancy body mass index for singleton gestation.

Weight for height	Body mass index (kg/m²)	Recommended total weight gain (kg)	(lb)
Underweight	<19.8	12.5–18	28–40
Normal weight	19.8–26.0	11.5–16	25–35
Overweight	26.0–29.0	7–11.5	15–25
Obesity	>29	<7	<15
Twin gestation	–	15.5–20.4	35–45

The physiological average weight gain in healthy primigravid women eating without restriction is expected to be about 12.5 kg, of which 1 kg is gained during the first trimester. Approximately 7 lbs. (3.2 kg) is gained at 10–20 weeks and approximately 10 lbs. (4.6 kg) at 20–30 weeks.

Exercise and Employment

In the absence of obstetric or medical complications, most pregnant women are able to work throughout the entire pregnancy. Heavy weightlifting and excessive physical activity should be avoided. Pregnant women should also be informed that beginning or continuing a moderate course of exercise during pregnancy is not associated with adverse outcomes. She should be informed about the potential dangers of certain activities during pregnancy, e.g., contact sports, high-impact sports, and vigorous racquet sports that may involve the risk of abdominal trauma, falls, or excessive joint stress. Scuba diving, which may result in fetal birth defects and fetal decompression disease, must also be avoided during pregnancy.

Prescribed Medicines

The use of prescription medicines during pregnancy should be limited to circumstances where the benefit outweighs the risk. Pregnant women should be informed that only a few over-the-counter (OTC) medicines have been established as being safe during pregnancy. OTC medicines should be therefore used as little as possible during pregnancy. Pregnant women should also be informed that only a few complementary therapies have been established as being safe and effective during pregnancy. Women should not assume that such therapies are safe, and they should be used as little as possible during pregnancy.

Immunizations

> **Q.** Write a long note on immunization in pregnancy.

- All women of childbearing age should be immune to measles, rubella, mumps, tetanus, diphtheria, poliomyelitis, and varicella through natural or vaccine-conferred immunization.
- All pregnant women should be screened for hepatitis B surface antigen. Pregnancy is not a contraindication to the administration of hepatitis B virus vaccine for hepatitis B.
- All vaccines with a live virus, e.g., rubella and yellow fever, should be avoided during pregnancy.
- *Tetanus toxoid:* According to the recent recommendations by the WHO, all pregnant women should be immunized against tetanus and diphtheria. Places where diphtheria-tetanus toxoid (DT) is not available, immunization should be with tetanus toxoid (TT). For unimmunized

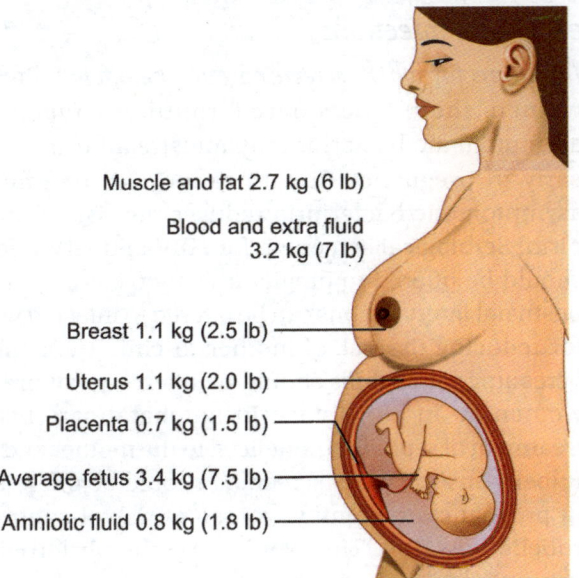

Fig. 1.30: Distribution of weight gain during pregnancy.

- Muscle and fat 2.7 kg (6 lb)
- Blood and extra fluid 3.2 kg (7 lb)
- Breast 1.1 kg (2.5 lb)
- Uterus 1.1 kg (2.0 lb)
- Placenta 0.7 kg (1.5 lb)
- Average fetus 3.4 kg (7.5 lb)
- Amniotic fluid 0.8 kg (1.8 lb)

women, TT or DT must be administered intramuscularly in the dosage of 0.5 mL at 6-weeks interval, with the first dose being administered at 16–24 weeks. For women who have been immunized in the past, a booster dose of 0.5 mL may be administered in the third trimester.
- Varicella zoster immunoglobulin should be administered to any newborn whose mother has developed chickenpox within 5 days before or 2 days after delivery.
- *Coronavirus disease (COVID-19) vaccination:* Considering the recent pandemic of COVID-19, the CDC as well as the RCOG recommends COVID-19 vaccines (first, second, and the booster doses) for pregnant and breastfeeding women. Vaccine is also recommended for infants who are aged 6 months or older and whose mother was vaccinated or suffered from COVID-19 infection prior to or during their pregnancy. While all the available COVID-19 vaccines are considered safe and effective during pregnancy and presently there are no known risks of COVID 19 vaccination during pregnancy, Pfizer or Moderna vaccines should be preferably offered to pregnant women where available. These vaccines should be given preference in pregnant women because presently most of the safety monitoring data during pregnancy available from the studies conducted in the United States and the UK is related to these two vaccines.

Sexual Intercourse

No restriction of sexual activity is necessary for pregnant women. Avoidance of sexual activity must be recommended for women at risk of preterm labor, placenta previa, or women with previous history of pregnancy loss.

Screening during Pregnancy

> Q. Write a short note discussing the screening tests in the first trimester.
> Q. Discuss screening for Down syndrome.
> Q. Write a short note on triple hormone test.

Recommendations for Down Syndrome Screening

According to the current recommendations, a screening test is offered to all women during early pregnancy to evaluate risk of the baby being born with DS. If the woman's screening test shows that she has a high risk of the baby being born with DS, she may be offered a prenatal diagnostic test. The two main prenatal diagnostic tests, which are available, include amniocentesis and chorionic villus sampling.

All pregnant women must preferably be offered first trimester screening by 13^{+6} weeks. However, if first trimester screening could not be performed, provision should be there to perform screening as late as 20^{+0} weeks. Ideally, the combined first trimester screening (NT along with serum markers PAPP-A and hCG) should be offered between 11^{+0} and 13^{+6} weeks of gestation. For women who present for screening in the second trimester, the clinically most effective test (triple test or quadruple test) can be performed between 15^{+0} and 20^{+0} weeks.

Triple test involves with assay of AFP, free β-hCG, and oestriol. Quadruple test includes all the parameters as required for the triple test along with the measurement of serum inhibin levels. In DS, the hCG and inhibin are high, whereas the others are low.

Integrated screening: More complex options for screening of DS have become available in the present times. These mainly include sequential testing and integrated or hybrid testing. In the sequential testing, screening tests are performed at different times during pregnancy and the results are provided to the patient after each test. On the other hand, integrated screening involves performance of screening tests at different times during pregnancy and a single result is provided to the patient only after all tests have been completed.

Fully integrated screening tests (involving the measurement of NT along with the measurement of serum markers in both the trimesters) is likely to be associated with a significantly better performance than either first trimester combined screening or second trimester quadruple screening alone.

A major disadvantage associated with an integrated screening is that it prevents the performance of chorionic villus sampling for early definitive diagnosis because the combined results are available only following the measurement of serum markers in the second trimester.

Noninvasive prenatal testing (NIPT), done by analysing small fragments of fetal DNA in maternal blood, may be sometimes used for determining the risk of fetus being born with DS.

Screening for Infections

- *Infections for which screening must be offered:* Pregnant women should be offered routine screening for asymptomatic bacteriuria by midstream urine culture early in pregnancy. Identification and treatment of asymptomatic bacteriuria reduces the risk of preterm birth. Serological screening for HBV and HIV infection should be offered to pregnant women so that effective postnatal interventions can be offered to infected women for reducing the risk of mother-to-child transmission. Screening for syphilis should be offered to all pregnant women at an early stage in antenatal care because treatment of syphilis is beneficial to the mother and fetus. Rubella-susceptibility screening should be offered early in pregnancy to identify women at risk of contracting rubella infection. This would help the obstetrician in getting the woman vaccinated in the postnatal period for the protection of future pregnancies.

- *Infections for which no screening is required:* No screening is required for infections such as asymptomatic bacterial vaginosis, *Chlamydia trachomatis,* cytomegalovirus, hepatitis C virus, group B *Streptococcus,* and toxoplasmosis because evidence of their clinical effectiveness and cost-effectiveness remains uncertain.

Psychiatric Screening

History of any previous psychiatric illnesses must be taken from the woman. Women having had a past history of serious psychiatric disorder should be referred for a psychiatric assessment during the antenatal period.

Pregnant women should not be offered antenatal education interventions to reduce the development of perinatal or postnatal depression or be offered routine screening with the Edinburgh postnatal depression scale (EPDS) in the antenatal period to predict the development of postnatal depression because these interventions have not been shown to be effective.

Ultrasound Examination

Pregnant women should be offered an early ultrasound scan to determine gestational age, especially if the woman is not sure about her LMP. Pregnant women should be offered an ultrasound scan to screen for structural anomalies, preferably between 18 and 20 weeks' gestation.

Education Regarding Breastfeeding, Birth Spacing, and Contraception

During the antenatal classes, the pregnant women should be taught how to breastfeed their babies and to take care of her own hygiene. The importance of birth spacing should be stressed, and she should be informed about all the methods of contraception that can be safely used during the postpartum period when they are breastfeeding their babies. Various methods of contraception, such as intrauterine contraceptive device, injectable contraceptives, progestogen-only pills, implants, and tubal ligation, must be explained along with their risks, disadvantages, and benefits. Significance of lactational amenorrhea should be stressed for all women, and breastfeeding should be encouraged.

Alcohol and Tobacco Use during Pregnancy

Due to increased fetal risks, it is suggested that women should avoid or limit their alcohol consumption to no more than one standard unit per day when pregnant. One "unit" of alcohol is constituted by the following: a single measure of spirits, one small glass of wine, or a half pint of ordinary strength beer, lager, or cider.

Pregnant women should be informed about the specific risks related to smoking/tobacco use during pregnancy (e.g., risk of having a baby with low birth weight, IUGR, and preterm), and therefore they should be encouraged to quit.

ANTEPARTUM FETAL SURVEILLANCE

> **Q. Write a critical appraisal on the antepartum fetal surveillance tests.**

The management protocol regarding antepartum fetal surveillance in all pregnant women is described in **Flowchart 1.1**.

Methods of Fetal Assessment

> **Q. When are fetal movements first felt?**
>
> **Q. What is the value of assessing fetal movements? Can fetal movements be used to determine the duration of pregnancy accurately?**
>
> Fetal movements are an indicator for fetal well-being. If the patient has reduced perception of the fetal movements, the obstetrician must confirm the fetal well-being using ultrasound examination or electronic fetal monitoring.

Daily Fetal Movement Count

Method: While performing the kick count, the mother must lie on her left side in comfortable location. She is asked to report the time it takes for her to feel 10 movements, no matter how small, and is then instructed to record them in the form of a chart. Whenever she feels a fetal movement, she is instructed to mark each movement on the chart until she has marked 10 movements in all. Then she must note the time. If the women can feel about 10 movements in an hour, it is considered as normal.

Nonstress Test

Nonstress test is a noninvasive test which indicates whether the baby is receiving enough oxygen or not. Reduced oxygen supply to the fetus could be related to placental or umbilical cord problems. NSTs are usually performed after 28 weeks of gestation.

Method of NST: The test involves attaching one belt of an external tocodynamometer to the mother's abdomen to measure the FHR and another belt to measure uterine contractions. Fetal movement, heart rate, and "reactivity" of the fetal heart are measured for 20–30 minutes. The NST is classified as reactive (normal or indicative of fetal well-being) or nonreactive (abnormal or may be indicative of fetal compromise). Kindly refer to Chapter 15 for details.

Biophysical Profile

The biophysical profile has five components altogether, each scored 0 or 2 for a maximum score of 10; these five components are described in detail in Chapter 15. A BPP test score of at least 8 out of 10 is considered reassuring. A score

Normal and Abnormal Presentations

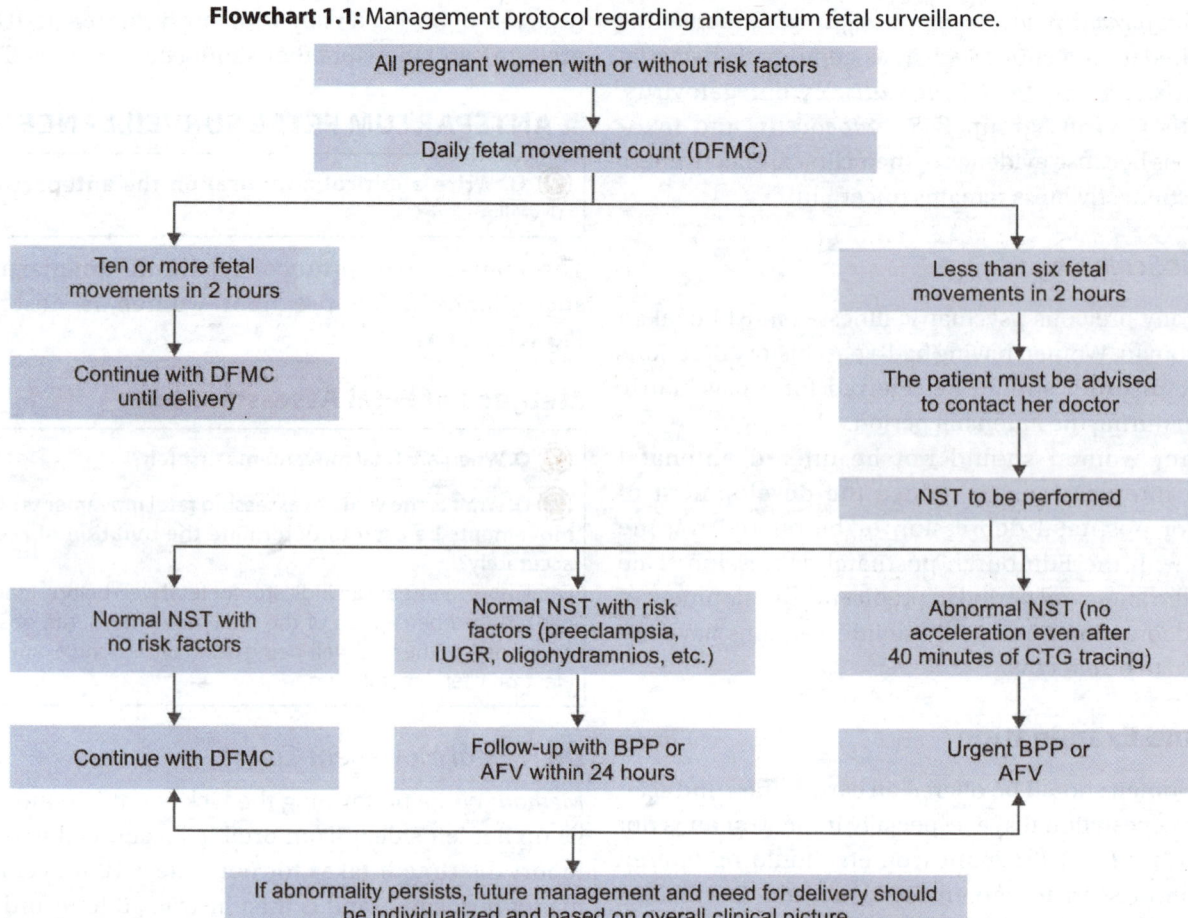

Flowchart 1.1: Management protocol regarding antepartum fetal surveillance.

(AFV: amniotic fluid volume; BPP: biophysical profile; CST: contraction stress test; CTG: cardiotocography; IUGR: intrauterine growth restriction; NST: nonstress test)

of 6 or 7 out of 10 is equivocal, and must be repeated within 24 hours. A score of 4 or less out of 10 is nonreassuring and strongly suggests preparing the patient for delivery.

Doppler Ultrasonography

Doppler ultrasonography is a noninvasive method of assessing fetal vascular impedance **(Fig. 1.31)**. This method helps in assessing fetal–placental unit by detecting the movement of blood flow through the maternal and fetal vessels. Some of the important Doppler indices which help in evaluating the blood flow through uterine and umbilical blood vessels are described in Chapter 15 (IUGR). In normal pregnancy, systolic/diastolic (S/D) ratio and pulsatility index (PI) decrease with an increase in the gestational age. Significant elevations in the S/D ratio have been associated with IUGR, fetal hypoxia or acidosis or both, and higher rates of perinatal morbidity and mortality. Absent and reversed end-diastolic flows are the more extreme examples of abnormal S/D ratio and may prompt delivery in some situations.

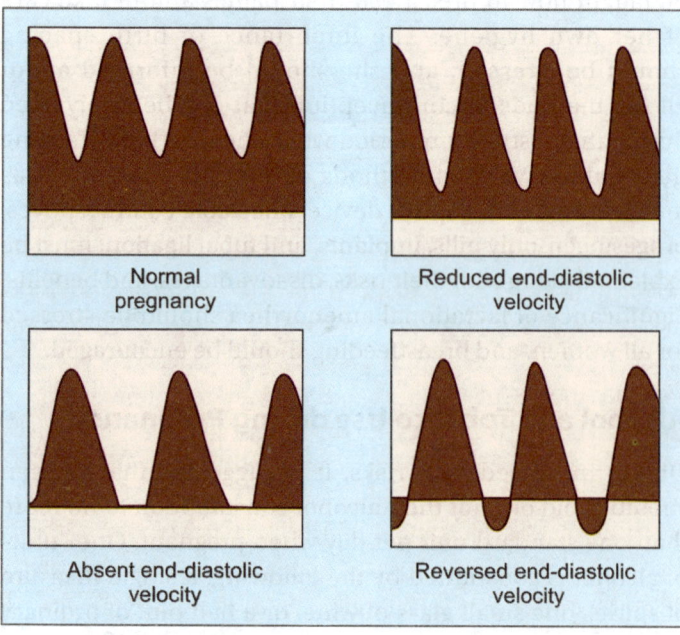

Fig. 1.31: Types of Doppler waveforms.

Assessment of Pulmonary Maturity

Assessment of pulmonary maturity may especially be required in cases where premature fetal delivery is required (e.g., preeclampsia and IUGR). Some such tests of pulmonary maturity are as follows:

- Estimation of the pulmonary surfactant by lecithin/sphingomyelin (L/S) ratio. L/S ratio of >2 is indicative of pulmonary maturity.
- *Clements' shake bubble test*: Increasing dilutions of amniotic fluid are mixed with 96% ethanol and shaken for 15 seconds. Formation of foam or bubbles, which remain stable for about 15 minutes, is a bedside test, which is indicative of pulmonary maturity.
- Presence of phosphatidylglycerol or phosphatidylcholine (>500 ng/mL) in amniotic fluid is indicative of pulmonary maturity.

COMPLICATIONS

> Q. What symptoms or signs, which may indicate the presence of serious complications, must be discussed with patients?

Management of minor pregnancy-related complaints is tabulated in **Table 1.11**.

Pregnant women with the following high-risk conditions may require additional/specialized care in addition to that detailed previously in this chapter. If the patient experiences any of these complaints at any time, she should be asked to immediately contact her obstetrician or visit the hospital:

- Symptoms and signs such as painless vaginal bleeding could be suggestive of placenta previa. On the other hand, symptoms such as vaginal bleeding with persistent, severe abdominal pain could be suggestive of abruptio placenta (see Chapter 8). Severe abruptio placenta may also be associated with reduced fetal movements and/or absent fetal heart sounds.
- Symptoms and signs such as persistent headache, visual disturbances (flashes of light), and sudden severe swelling of the hand, feet, or face may suggest severe preeclampsia (see Chapter 18).
- Symptoms and signs including rupture of the membranes and regular uterine contractions before the EDD suggest preterm labor (see Chapter 16).
- Reduced fetal movements at any time could be indicative of fetal compromise.
- Patient experiences rupture of membranes and finds the liquor to be stained greenish in color. This could be due to meconium-stained liquor, which could be indicative of fetal compromise.

TABLE 1.11: Management of minor pregnancy-related complaints.

Pregnancy-related complication	Management
Nausea and vomiting during pregnancy (morning sickness)	Watchful expectancy, nonpharmacological agents (ginger, P6 acupressure), or safe antiemetics (antihistamines)
Pelvic pain (due to ligamental stretch)	Gentle pelvic exercises/massage therapy
Increased urinary frequency	Urinary tract infection to be ruled out
Ankle swelling (due to inferior vena cava compression)	Woman to be advised to rest in the left lateral position
Varicosities	Compression support stockings
Heartburn	Lifestyle and dietary modifications, antacids
Constipation	Fluids, fiber, fybogel, laxatives such as isabgol (psyllium husk)
Low back pain	Exercising in water, massage therapy, and group or individual back care classes
Dental decay	Dental checkup
Hemorrhoids	Dietary modification, standard hemorrhoid creams
Itching	Ruling out iron deficiency; in case of cholestasis, antihistamines
Stretch marks	Moisturizers, stretch mark-reducing creams
Vaginal discharge	Evaluation and treatment of vaginal infection. A 7-day course of topical clotrimazole may be helpful for candidal infection

COMPLICATED PAST OBSTETRIC HISTORY

- Recurrent pregnancy loss (Chapter 13)
- Preterm birth (Chapter 16)
- Rh-negative isoimmunization (Chapter 10)
- Previous LSCS (Chapter 11)
- Uterine surgery including cesarean section, myomectomy, or cone biopsy
- Puerperal psychosis
- Grand multiparity (more than five pregnancies)
- Previous stillbirth or neonatal death (Chapter 17)
- A baby with a congenital anomaly (structural or chromosomal)

ABNORMAL FETAL PRESENTATIONS

- Breech presentation (Chapter 3)
- Transverse lie (Chapter 4)
- Occipitoposterior position (Chapter 5)

COMPLICATIONS RELATED TO PREGNANCY

- Antepartum hemorrhage (Chapter 8)
- Postpartum hemorrhage (Chapter 14)
- Multifetal gestation (Chapter 9)
- Gestational trophoblastic disease (Chapter 12)
- IUGR (Chapter 15).

PRESENCE OF MEDICAL DISORDERS WITH PREGNANCY

- Preeclampsia (Chapter 18)
- Gestational diabetes (Chapter 19)
- Anemia in pregnancy (Chapter 20)
- Heart disease in pregnancy (Chapter 21)
- Renal disease
- Thyroid dysfunction and other endocrine disorders
- Epilepsy requiring anticonvulsant drugs
- Asthma and other respiratory disorders
- Hematological disorder
- HIV or HBV infection
- Drug abuse such as heroin, cocaine (including crack cocaine), and ecstasy
- Autoimmune disorders
- Psychiatric disorders
- Malignant disease

 EVIDENCE-BASED CLINICAL TRIALS

 List of references can be scanned through QR code to enable the readers gain deeper insight of the subject by referring to the entire article or its abstract.

CHAPTER 2

Normal Labor in Occipitolateral Position

CASE STUDY

A 27-year-old primigravida patient with 38 weeks of gestation presents to the obstetrics and gynecology clinic with complaints of experiencing abdominal cramps since past 2 hours. She is not sure if these are uterine contractions. There is no history of any vaginal bleeding or ROM. She can feel the normal fetal movements. Her antenatal period had been otherwise uneventful, and she had been having regular antenatal checkups.

INTRODUCTION

- Q. Write a long essay on the first stage of labor.
- Q. Write a short essay on the third stage of labor.

Labor comprises a series of events taking place in the genital organs, which help to expel the fetus and other products of conception outside the uterine cavity into the outer world. It can be defined as the onset of painful uterine contractions accompanied by any one of the following: ROM, bloody show, cervical dilatation, and/or effacement. It can be either spontaneous or induced and normally comprises three stages—first stage, second stage, and third stage. Since the most common fetal position is left occipitolateral (transverse) position (**Fig. 2.1**), the mechanism of labor in context to this position comprises the following cardinal movements: engagement, flexion, descent, internal rotation, extension, and external rotation of fetal head. Various stages of labor as described by Friedman (1955) are described in **Table 2.1** and depicted in **Figures 2.2A and B**. Classification of labor depending on the period of gestation has been described in **Table 2.2**.

FIRST STAGE OF LABOR

The first stage of labor begins with the onset of regular uterine contractions and ends with complete dilatation and effacement of cervix. It is divided into two phases.

Latent Phase (Preparatory Phase)

Latent phase begins with the onset of regular contractions, with contractions occurring after every 15–20 minutes, lasting 20–30 seconds. Gradually, the frequency of contractions increases, and they can occur after every 5–7 minutes, lasting for 30–40 seconds. This phase ends when cervix becomes about 3–5 cm dilated. The latent phase lasts for approximately 8–9 hours in the primigravida, and less than 6 hours in multigravida. Prolonged latent phase can be defined as greater than 20 hours in primigravida and greater than 14 hours in the multigravida.

Active Phase

As described by Friedman (1955), active phase begins when the cervix is about 4 cm dilated and ends when it becomes fully dilated. The normal rate of cervical dilatation during this stage is approximately 1–1.5 cm/h. The intensity of contractions increases with the contractions occurring after every 2–3 minutes and lasting for about 40–60 seconds. This stage lasts for an average of 4.6 hours in a primigravida and approximately 2.4 hours in multigravidas.

SECOND STAGE OF LABOR

The second stage of labor begins when the cervical dilatation and effacement are complete and ends with the delivery of

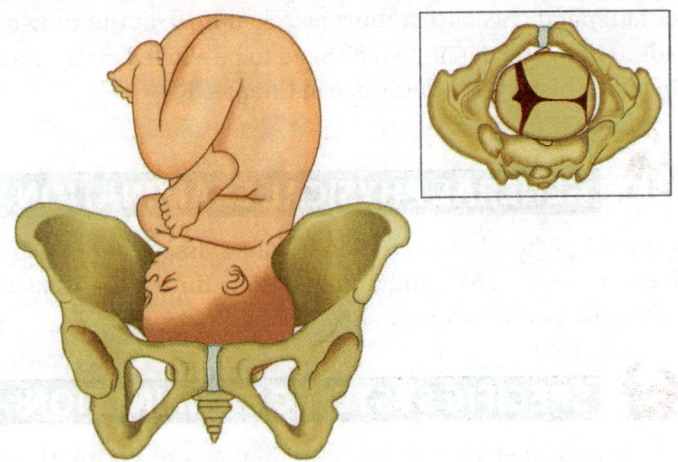

Fig. 2.1: Occipitolateral (transverse) position of the fetal head.

TABLE 2.1: Various stages of labor.

Stages of labor	Description	Characteristics	Duration in primigravida	Duration in multigravida
Stage I	Starts from the onset of true labor pains and ends with complete dilatation of cervix	Can be divided into: • *Latent phase:* Slow and gradual cervical effacement and dilatation (up to 3 cm) • *Active phase:* Active cervical dilatation (3–10 cm) and fetal descent. It comprises: – Acceleration phase – Phase of maximum slope – Deceleration phase	8–20 hours 6–12 hours	6–14 hours 3–6 hours
Stage II	Starts from full dilatation of cervix and ends with expulsion of the fetus from birth canal	–	50–180 minutes	30–50 minutes
Stage III	It begins after expulsion of the fetus and is associated with expulsion of placenta and membranes	–	15 minutes	15 minutes
Stage IV	Stage of observation, which lasts for at least 1 to 2 hours after the expulsion of afterbirths	–	60 minutes	60 minutes

the fetus. Its mean duration is 50 minutes for nullipara and 20 minutes for multipara. During this stage, the woman begins to bear down. The abdominal muscles contract, which helps in the descent of fetal head. When the crowning of fetal head has occurred at vulvar opening, birth of the baby is imminent.

The exact mechanism for the initiation of labor is still unclear. However, the most likely mechanisms are as follows:
- *Mechanical factors:* Uterine distention
- *Endocrine factors:* There is increased cortisol secretion by fetal adrenals and increased production of estrogens and prostaglandins (PGE_2) from the placenta. Together, these cause an increased release of oxytocin from the maternal pituitary and increased synthesis of contraction-associated proteins.

HISTORY AND CLINICAL PRESENTATION

If detailed history had not been taken during the time of antenatal checkup, it must be taken now, at the time of admission. The details, which need to be elicited at the time of taking history, are described in Chapter 1.

GENERAL PHYSICAL EXAMINATION

General physical examination involves assessment of the patient's vital signs, similar to that done during the time of antenatal examination (Chapter 1).

SPECIFIC SYSTEMIC EXAMINATION

Findings of specific systemic examination are summarized in **Table 2.3**.

ABDOMINAL EXAMINATION

The abdominal examination forms an important part of every complete physical examination in labor. It must be done at the time of admission and each time before a vaginal examination is performed. The parameters to be assessed at the time of abdominal examination of a patient who is in labor are similar to those observed at the time of antenatal examination and have been described before. Additionally, descent and engagement of the fetal presenting part, assessment of fetal position, and uterine contractions are especially important when the patient is in labor. The amount of descent and engagement of the presenting part is assessed by feeling how many fifths of the head are palpable above the brim of the pelvis.

Various parameters on abdominal examination, such as estimation of fundal height, detection of fetal lie, presentation, position, conducting the four Leopold's maneuvers, and auscultation of fetal heart rate, have been described in details in Chapter 1. Besides this, other parameters, which need to be assessed at the time of abdominal examination during labor, are given in the following text.

Assessment of Fetal Size

While palpating the fetus, the obstetrician must try to assess the size of the fetus itself. A note should be made regarding the expected fetal weight. This should be later compared with the actual weight of the baby at the time of delivery. Regular use of this practice greatly helps in improving the accuracy of fetal weight estimation. The obstetrician should observe if the uterus appears to be full with the fetus or the fetus feels smaller than what is expected for the particular period of gestation. A fetus, which feels smaller than expected, could be indicative of IUGR or oligohydramnios or wrong dates. A fetus, which feels larger than expected, could

Normal Labor in Occipitolateral Position

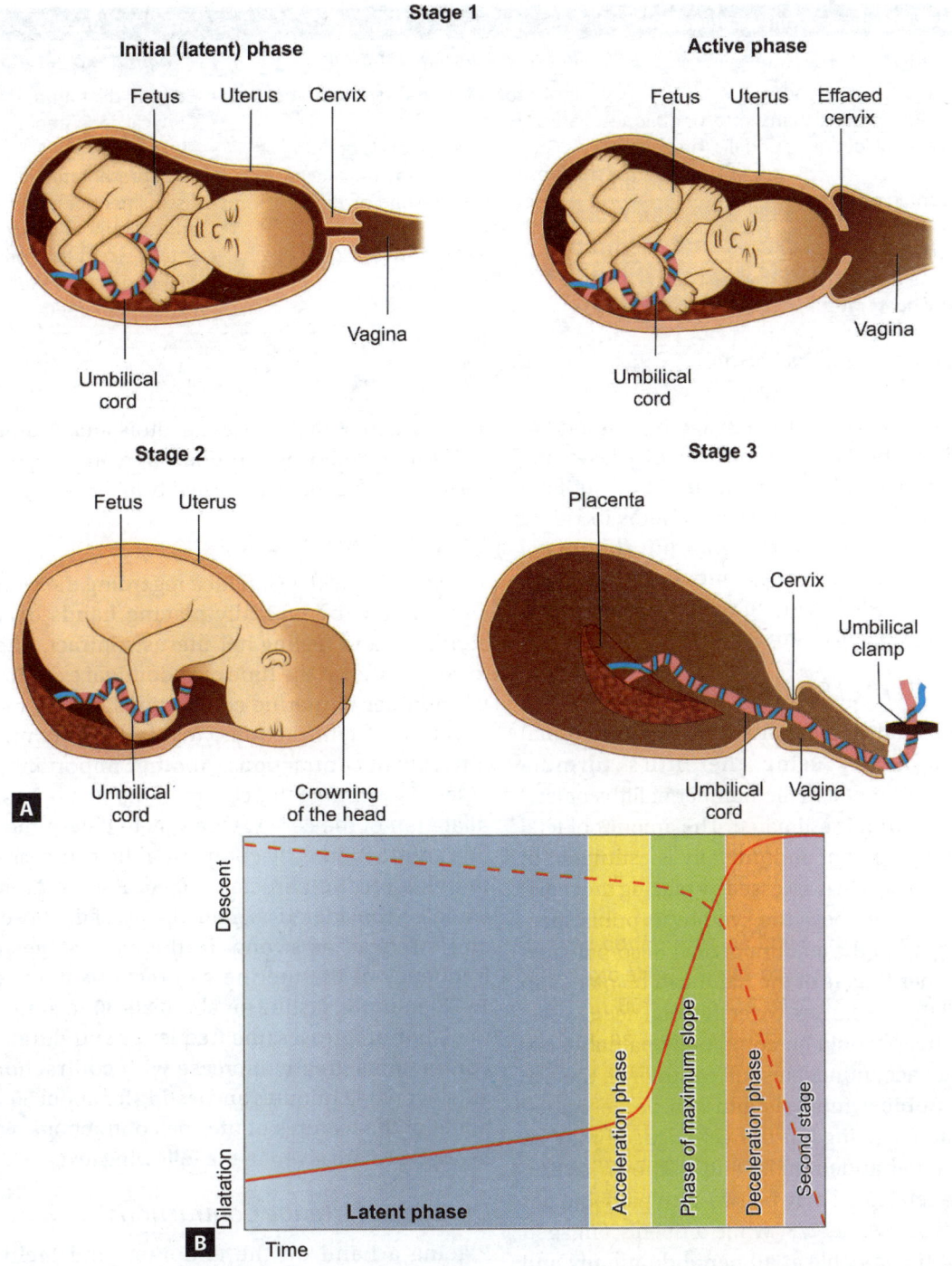

Figs. 2.2A and B: (A) Stages of normal labor; (B) Graphical representation of normal labor as depicted by Friedman (1955).

TABLE 2.2: Classification of labor based on the period of gestation.	
Classification	**Period of gestation**
Preterm labor	Prior to 37 weeks
Term	37–42 weeks
Post-term	After 42 weeks
Postdated	After 40 weeks

be indicative of fetal macrosomia (particularly in association with gestational diabetes), polyhydramnios, or multifetal gestation. In multifetal gestation, though the uterine size is larger than the period of gestation, the size of individual fetuses per se is small.

If the clinician feels that the size of the head appears to be smaller in relation to the period of gestation, he/she must try to assess the size as well as hardness of the fetal head. The fetal head feels harder as the pregnancy gets closer to term. A relatively small fetal head with a hard feel is suggestive of IUGR rather than prematurity.

Engagement

With the progress of second stage of labor, there is progressive downward movement of the fetal presenting

Normal and Abnormal Presentations

TABLE 2.3: Findings of specific systemic examination.

Abdominal examination	Per speculum examination	Per vaginal examination
• Estimation of height of uterine fundus • The fetal lie may be longitudinal, transverse, or oblique • Fetal presentation may be cephalic, podalic (breech), or shoulder • Obstetric grips (Leopold's maneuvers) • Uterine contractions • Estimation of fetal descent • Assessing the engagement of fetal presenting part • Auscultation of fetal heart rate • Assessment of the fetal size • Assessment of the amount of liquor present	Indicators of ruptured membranes are as follows: • Gross vaginal pooling of fluid • Positive results on nitrazine paper test and fern testing of vaginal secretions • Evidence of meconium	• Cervical dilatation • Cervical consistency and effacement • Fetal presentation and position • Assessment of fetal membranes and amount of liquor • Fetal descent (station of fetal head) • Molding of fetal skull • Pelvic assessment

part in relation to the pelvic cavity. Engagement is said to have occurred when the largest diameter of presenting part passes through pelvic inlet. Engagement of the fetal presenting part is of great importance as it helps in ruling out fetopelvic disproportion. It is evident from abdominal and vaginal examinations. Vaginal examination reveals the descent of fetal head in relation to the ischial spines (would be described with the vaginal examination).

Abdominal Assessment of Fetal Descent

The assessment of fetal descent through the abdominal examination is done by using the fifth's formula (**Figs. 2.3A to C**). In this method, the number of fifths of fetal head above the pelvic brim is estimated. The amount of fetal head that can be palpated per abdominally is estimated in terms of finger breadth, which is assessed by placing the radial margin of the index finger above the symphysis pubis successively. Depending upon the amount of fetal head palpated per abdominally, other fingers of the hand can be placed in succession, until all the five fingers cover the fetal head.

A free-floating head would be completely palpable per abdomen. This head accommodates full width of all the five fingers above the pubic symphysis and can be described as 5/5. A head which is fixing but not yet engaged may be three-fifth palpable per abdominally and is known as 3/5. A recently engaged fetal head may be two-fifth palpable per abdominally and is known as 2/5, while a deeply engaged fetal head may not be palpable at all per abdominally and may be described as 0/5.

Assessment of the Amount of Liquor Present

Under normal circumstances, the amount of liquor decreases as the pregnancy approaches term. The amount of liquor can be clinically assessed by feeling the way that the fetus can be balloted while being palpated. Reduced degree of fetal ballottement at the time of abdominal palpation is indicative of reduced amount of amniotic fluid or oligohydramnios. On the other hand, increased degree of fetal ballottement at the time of abdominal palpation is suggestive of increased amount of amniotic fluid or polyhydramnios. Some of the causes for polyhydramnios and oligohydramnios are enumerated in **Table 2.4**. In both the cases an ultrasound examination needs to be performed by a trained person to exclude multiple gestation, congenital abnormality in the fetus, or IUGR.

Uterine Contractions

The clinician will get an idea regarding the woman's uterine contractions by typically placing hands on the patient's abdomen and feeling her uterus contract. The parameters to be assessed at the time of abdominal examination include the number of uterine contractions in a 10-minute period, duration of contractions, regularity of contractions, and intensity of contractions. Another important parameter to assess is whether the contractions result in simultaneous dilatation of the cervix. One way to determine the intensity of a contraction is by comparing the firmness of the uterus to areas on the clinician's face. For example, the cheek could be considered as mild, the tip of the nose as moderate and forehead as strong. In the early stages of labor, the frequency of the uterine contractions may be after every 15–20 minutes, lasting for about 20–30 seconds. However, as the labor progresses, the frequency and duration of uterine contractions greatly increase with contractions occurring after every 1–2 minutes and lasting for about 60–120 seconds. Some of the features of uterine contractions, which need to be assessed are given in the following text.

Duration of Uterine Contractions

Placing a hand on the abdomen and feeling when the uterus becomes hard and when it relaxes help in assessing the length of the uterine contractions. Depending upon the time duration for which the contractions last, they can be classified as strong, moderate, and weak contractions. Grading of the duration of uterine contractions is described in **Table 2.5**.

Strength of Contractions

Measuring the degree of hardness, which the uterus undergoes at the time of contraction, helps in assessing the strength of contractions or their intensity. An experienced obstetrician can estimate the intensity of uterine contractions by palpating the uterine fundus during the contractions.

Normal Labor in Occipitolateral Position

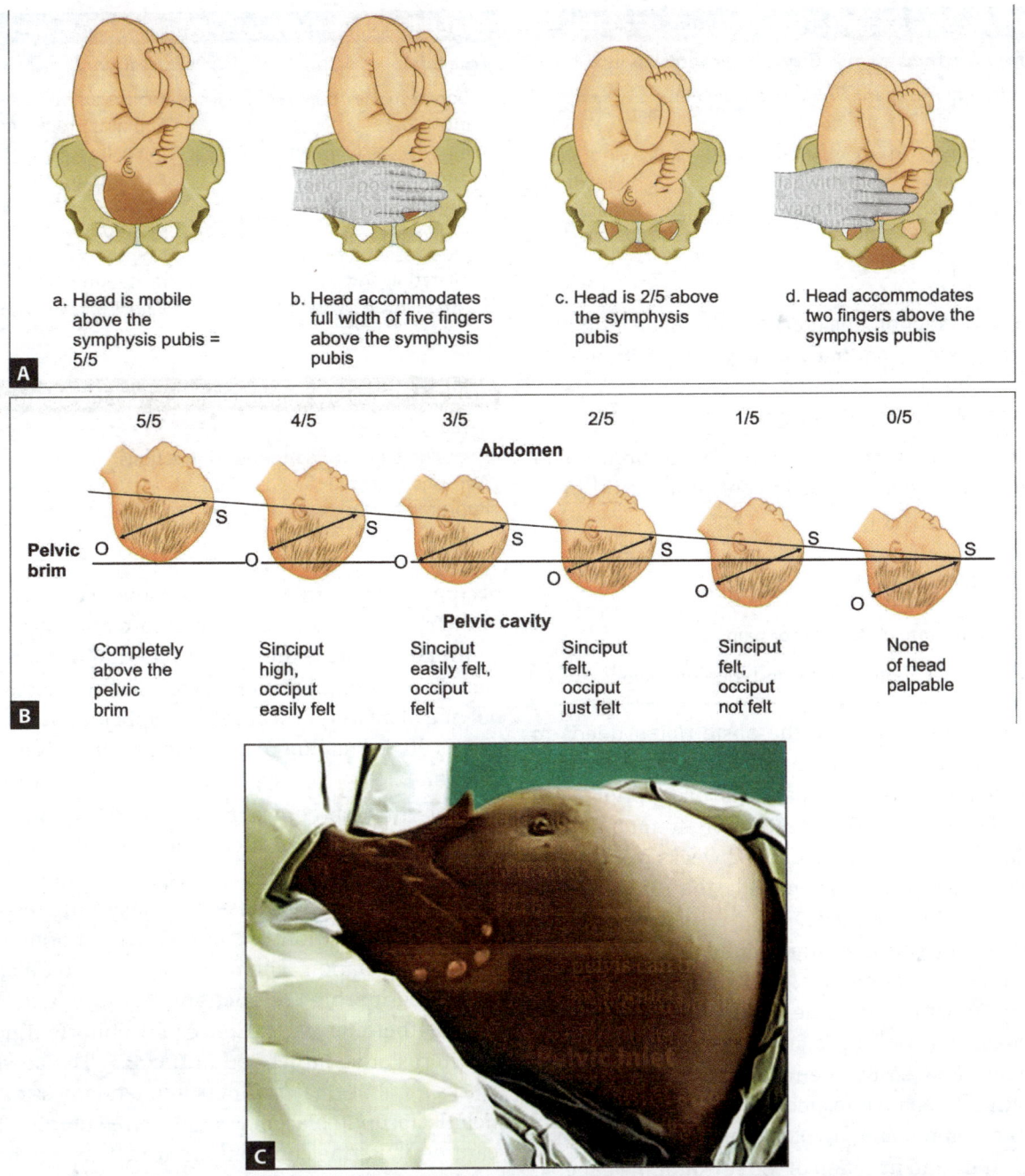

Figs. 2.3A to C: Estimation of the descent of fetal head. (A) Abdominal examination for fetal descent; (B) Stages of fetal descent through the pelvic cavity; (C) Assessment of fetal descent by using the fifth's formula.

TABLE 2.4: Causes for abnormalities in the amount of liquor.	
Causes of polyhydramnios	**Causes of oligohydramnios**
• Multiple gestation • Maternal diabetes • Twin-to-twin transfusion syndrome • Fetal parvovirus B19 infection • Rh blood incompatibilities between the mother and the fetus • Fetal congenital abnormalities (e.g., birth defects) involving the gastrointestinal tract and central nervous system (e.g., esophageal atresia, spina bifida, anencephaly, etc.)	• Intrauterine growth retardation • *Placental dysfunction:* Presence of amnion nodosum (squamous metaplasia of amnion) on the placenta • Premature rupture of the membranes • Birth defects, especially those involving the kidneys and urinary tract, e.g., renal agenesis or obstruction of the urinary tract (posterior urethral valves) • Post-term pregnancy (>40 weeks) • Chronic maternal disorders including gestational diabetes mellitus, preeclampsia, chronic hypertension, systemic lupus erythematosus, etc. • Medications including angiotensin-converting enzyme inhibitors (such as captopril), prostaglandin inhibitors (aspirin, etc.)

Normal and Abnormal Presentations

TABLE 2.5: Grading the duration of contractions.

Duration of contractions	Grading of contractions
Contractions lasting less than 20 seconds	Weak contractions
Contractions lasting for 20–40 seconds	Moderate contractions
Contractions lasting more than 40 seconds	Strong contractions

During a mild contraction, the uterine wall can be indented, whereas during a strong contraction, it cannot be indented.

Frequency of Uterine Contractions

Frequency of uterine contractions measures the number of times the uterine contractions occur in a period of 10 minutes.

True/False Labor Pains

 Q. Write a short note on false labor pains.
 Q. Discuss in brief about the lower uterine segment.

During the first stage of labor, the obstetrician needs to determine whether the woman is having true or false uterine contractions. False labor pains can occur prior to the onset of true labor pains. They occur more frequently in a primigravida where they may occur 1–2 weeks prior to the onset of true labor pains. In multigravida, they may precede the true labor pains by a few days.

The false labor pains are usually dull in nature and are confined to the lower abdominal and groin regions. They have no relation with the uterine contractions and do not cause any effect on cervical dilatation and effacement. This pain is usually relieved by enema and administration of sedatives. False labor pain is related to the formation of lower uterine segment and taking up of cervix, which may cause cervical stretching and irritation of the surrounding ganglia. Difference between true and false labor pain is enumerated in **Table 2.6**.

On the other hand, true labor pains comprise of painful uterine contractions at regular intervals; these contractions tend to increase in intensity and duration with the progression of labor; they are usually experienced at lower back and radiate to abdomen and tend to become more intense with walking, cervical changes, and fetus moving into the lower pelvis. True labor pains are accompanied with the appearance of show (expulsion of cervical mucus plug mixed with blood) and progressive cervical dilatation and effacement. There also may be the formation of bag of membranes. As the lower uterine segment is stretched, membranes get detached from the decidua. With the progressive cervical dilatation, the membranes tend to become unsupported and bulge into the cervical canal. Due to the rise of intra-amniotic pressure at the time of uterine contractions, these membranes tend to become tense and convex, resulting in the formation of bag of membranes. This bulging of membranes usually disappears as the contraction passes off. Formation of bag of membranes is a certain sign of labor.

TABLE 2.6: Differences between true labor and false labor pain.

True labor	False labor
• Contractions occur at regular intervals	• Occurs at irregular intervals
• Interval gradually shortens	• Remains irregular
• Intensity increases	• Intensity remains same over a period of time
• Duration of contraction increases	• Tends to become shorter in duration over time
• Progressive cervical dilatation and effacement	• No progress in cervical dilatation or effacement
• Not relieved by sedation	• Pain is relieved by sedation

BOX 2.1: Causes for abnormal hardness of the uterus.

Some primigravidas
At the time of strong uterine contractions
Abruptio placenta
Rupture of the uterus

True uterine contractions usually follow a rhythmic pattern, with periods of contractions followed by periods of relaxation in between, which would allow the woman to rest. During the phase of relaxation, restoration of placental circulation occurs, which is important for the baby's oxygenation. The uterus appears to be hard during the strong uterine contractions and it may be difficult to palpate the fetal parts. Causes for abnormal hardness of the uterus are enumerated in **Box 2.1**. The most common causes for abnormal hardness and tenderness of the uterus include abruptio placenta or a ruptured uterus. Some of the features of uterine contractions, which need to be assessed, are described in the following text.

VAGINAL EXAMINATION

Vaginal examination must be performed at the time of admission of the pregnant patient in labor. It is carried out at least once every 4 hours during the first stage of labor or if there is ROM or if any intervention is needed. Preparations for delivery are made as the cervical dilatation and effacement approach completion and/or crowning of the fetal presenting part becomes evident at the vaginal introitus.

Prerequisites for a Vaginal Examination

- The patient must be carefully explained about the examination, prior to performing the examination.
- Adequate permission must be taken from the patient.

- There should be a valid reason for performing the examination.
- A vaginal examination must always be preceded by an abdominal examination.

Indications for a Vaginal Examination in Labor

Indications for performing a vaginal examination during the various periods of pregnancy are enumerated in **Box 2.2**.

Contraindications for Vaginal Examination in Pregnancy

Antepartum hemorrhage (see Chapter 8) and preterm ROM without contractions are conditions in which the vaginal examination is contraindicated. In these cases a sterile speculum examination can be done to confirm or exclude ROM.

Preparation for Vaginal Examination

- The patient's bladder must be empty.
- The procedure must be carefully explained to the patient.
- The patient must be placed in either the dorsal or lithotomy position. In clinical practice, dorsal position is most commonly used because it is more comfortable and less embarrassing than the lithotomy position. Also the lithotomy position usually requires equipment such as lithotomy poles and stirrup, which is not the case with dorsal position.
- If the membranes have not ruptured or are not going to be ruptured during the examination, an ordinary surgical glove can be used and there is no need to swab the patient with antiseptic solution. However, if the membranes have ruptured or are going to be ruptured during the examination, vaginal examination in labor should be performed as a sterile procedure. Therefore, in these cases a sterile tray which contains sterile swabs, sterile gloves, sterile instruments (preferably Kocher's forceps) for performing ARM, an antiseptic vaginal solution (betadine), or sterile lubricant (Savlon) is required.
- The clinicians before performing the vaginal examination must either scrub or thoroughly wash their hands and wear sterile gloves. The patient's vulva and perineum must be swabbed with Savlon or Betadine solution. This is done by first swabbing the labia majora and groin on both sides and then swabbing the introitus while keeping the labia majora apart with the thumb and forefinger.
- A vaginal examination must be preceded by the inspection of the external and internal genitalia, for signs of sexually transmitted diseases such as presence of single or multiple ulcers, a purulent discharge, or enlarged inguinal lymph nodes. The vulva must also be carefully inspected for any abnormalities, e.g., scars, warts, varicosities, congenital abnormalities, ulcers, or discharge. Vagina and cervix can be inspected by performing a per speculum examination. The vagina must be assessed for the presence or absence of the following features: vaginal discharge, a full loaded rectum, vaginal stricture or septum, or prolapse of the umbilical cord through the vaginal introitus.
- Presence of a wart-like growth or an ulcer on the cervix may be suggestive of cervical carcinoma. The cervical surface can also be assessed while performing a vaginal examination. A bimanual examination helps in assessing the cervical dilatation and effacement, the size of the uterus, and masses in the adnexa (ovaries and fallopian tubes).

> **BOX 2.2:** Indications for vaginal examination in labor.
> - Assessment of the ripeness of the cervix prior to induction of labor
> - Performance of artificial rupture of the membranes to induce labor
> - Detection of cervical effacement and/or dilatation
> - Identification of the fetal presenting part
> - Performance of pelvic assessment
> - To note progress of labor
> - Following rupture of membranes to rule out cord prolapse
> - Whenever interference is contemplated
> - To confirm the second stage of labor

In the first trimester of pregnancy, a bimanual examination helps in assessment of the uterine size in comparison with the period of amenorrhea. After the first trimester, the uterine size is primarily assessed on abdominal examination. Lastly, the fornices are palpated to exclude any masses, the most common of which is an ovarian cyst or tumor.

Special care must be taken when performing a vaginal examination late in pregnancy, especially in the presence of a high presenting part. The nonengagement of the presenting part could be due to an undiagnosed placenta previa. If this is suspected, the finger must not be inserted into the cervical canal. Instead, the presenting part is gently palpated through all the fornices. If any bogginess is noted between the fingers of the examining hand and the presenting part, the examination must be immediately abandoned and the patient must be referred urgently for an ultrasound examination.

Parameters to be Observed during Vaginal Examination

> **Q.** Discuss in detail changes in the uterine cervix during pregnancy and labor.

The parameters to be observed while performing a vaginal examination are described in **Box 2.3** and include the following:
- Consistency and position of cervix
- Degree of effacement and dilatation of cervix
- To note whether the cervix/vagina is well applied to the presenting part
- Station and position of presenting part

- Whether the membranes are present or absent
- Assessment of pelvis and to rule out cephalopelvic disproportion (CPD)

Cervical Dilatation and Effacement

Cervical dilatation **(Figs. 2.4A to D)** must be assessed in centimeters and is best measured by assessing the degree of separation of the fingers on vaginal examination.

The cervix undergoes progressive shortening or effacement in early labor **(Figs. 2.5A and B)**. The cervical effacement is measured by assessing the length of the endocervical canal.

> **BOX 2.3:** Parameters to be observed while performing a vaginal examination.
> - Consistency of cervix
> - Cervical dilatation
> - Cervical effacement
> - Fetal presentation
> - Position
> - Assessment of fetal membranes
> - Assessment of liquor
> - Fetal descent (station of fetal head)
> - Molding of fetal skull
> - Pelvic assessment

Cervical effacement refers to the distance between the internal os and the external os on digital examination. In an uneffaced cervix, the endocervical canal is approximately 3 cm long. However, when the cervix becomes fully effaced there will be no endocervical canal, only a ring of thin cervix. The cervical effacement is measured as a percentage.

Evaluation of the state of cervix: This is done by calculation of the Bishop's score **(Table 2.7)**. A maximum score of 13 is possible with this scoring system. Labor is most likely to commence spontaneously with a score of 9 or more, whereas lower scores (especially those <5) may require cervical ripening and/or augmentation with oxytocin.

Fetal Presentation

An abdominal examination performed earlier helps in determining the fetal lie and the presenting part. The presenting part of the fetus can be confirmed on vaginal examination. The presenting part could be head, breech, or shoulder. If the head is presenting, the exact fetal presentation, e.g., vertex, brow, or face, needs to be determined.

- *Features of a vertex presentation:* The posterior fontanel is normally felt. It is a small triangular space. In contrast, the anterior fontanel is diamond-shaped. If the head is

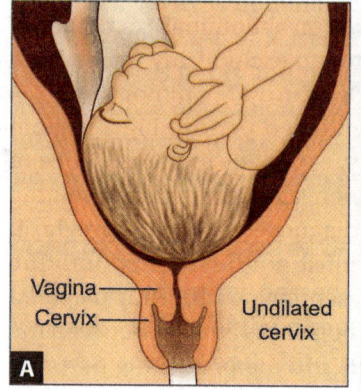 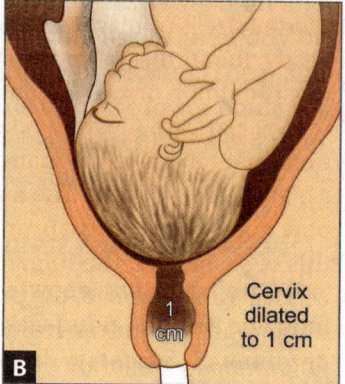 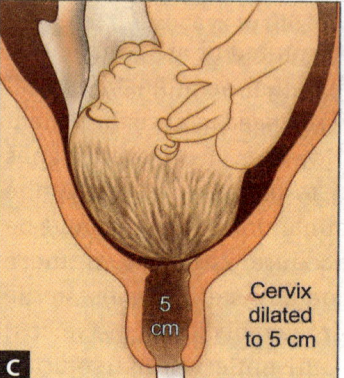 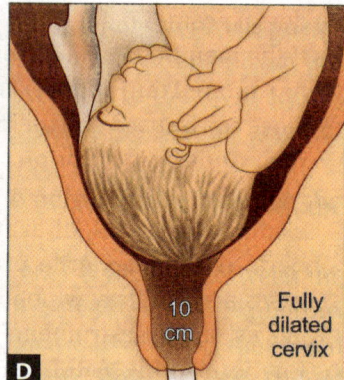

Figs. 2.4A to D: Cervical dilatation.

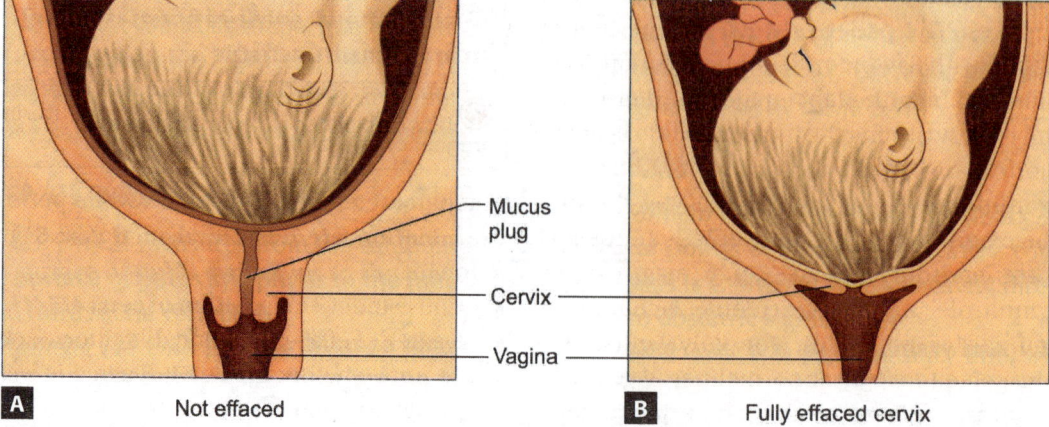

Figs. 2.5A and B: Cervical effacement.

TABLE 2.7: Bishop's score (modified).

Score	Dilation (cm)	Effacement (%)	Station of the presenting part	Cervical consistency	Position of cervix
0	Closed	0–30	–3	Firm	Posterior
1	1–2	40–50	–2	Medium	Mid position
2	3–4	60–70	–1, 0	Soft	Anterior
3	>5	>80	+1, +2	–	–

well flexed, the anterior fontanel will not be felt. If the anterior fontanel can be easily felt, the head is deflexed.

- *Features of a face presentation:* On abdominal examination the presenting part is the head. However, on vaginal examination the following features are observed:
  - Instead of a firm skull, something soft is felt.
  - The gum margins distinguish the mouth from the anus.
  - The cheek bones and the mouth form a triangle.
  - The orbital ridges above the eyes can be felt.
  - The ears may be felt.
- *Features of a brow presentation:* The presenting part is high. The anterior fontanel is felt on one side of the pelvis, the root of the nose on the other side, and the orbital ridges may be felt laterally.
- *Features of a breech presentation:* On abdominal examination the presenting part is the breech (soft and triangular). On vaginal examination, instead of a firm skull, something soft is felt; the anus does not have gum margins; the anus and the ischial tuberosities form a straight line.
- *Features of a shoulder presentation:* On abdominal examination, the lie will be transverse or oblique. Features of a shoulder presentation on vaginal examination will be quite easy if the arm has prolapsed. The shoulder is not always that easy to identify, unless the arm can be felt. The presenting part is usually high. For details related to shoulder presentation, kindly refer to Chapter 4.

Fetal Position

Fetal position refers to relationship of the designated landmark on the fetal presenting part with the left or right side of the maternal pelvis. Fetal position has been described in detail previously in Chapter 1.

Assessment of the Membranes

Drainage of liquor indicates that membranes have ruptured. However, even if the liquor is obviously draining, the obstetrician must always try to feel for the presence of membranes overlying the presenting part. If the presenting part is high, it is usually quite easy to feel intact membranes. However, it may be difficult to feel the membranes, if the presenting part is well applied to the cervix. In this case, one should wait for a contraction when some liquor often comes in front of the presenting part, allowing the membranes to be felt. If the membranes are intact, and the patient is in the active phase of labor, the membranes should be ruptured. However, if the presenting part is high, there is always the danger that the umbilical cord may prolapse, with the ARM. Following precautions should therefore be taken while performing an ARM in a patient with high presenting part:

- Before doing an ARM, the fetal head must be stabilized using the abdominal hand in order to minimize the chances of cord prolapse.
- Fetal heart rate should be heard following the ARM. Decline in fetal heart rate could be indicative of fetal distress resulting from cord prolapse.
- A vaginal examination must be performed following ARM, in order to exclude the possibility of cord presentation.

Membranes are normally not ruptured in HIV-positive patients unless there is poor progress of labor.

Condition of the liquor when the membranes rupture: An important parameter, which must be assessed at the time of assessing the membranes, is the condition of liquor following ROM. Clear-colored liquor following ROM is indicative of a normal healthy fetus. Greenish colored liquor is suggestive of the presence of meconium. The presence of meconium may change the management of the patient as it indicates the presence of fetal distress. In these cases, it may be required to expedite the delivery.

Determining the Descent and Engagement of the Head

The engagement of the fetal head is assessed on abdominal and not on vaginal examination. However, the vaginal examination does help in assessing the descent of fetal presenting part. The level of the fetal presenting part is usually described in relation to the ischial spines, which is halfway between the pelvic inlet and pelvic outlet. When the lowermost portion of the fetal presenting part is at the level of ischial spines, it is designated as "zero" station. The ACOG has devised a classification system that divides the pelvis above and below the spines into fifths. This division represents the distance in centimeters above and below the ischial spine. Thus, as the presenting fetal part descends from the inlet toward the ischial spine; the designation is –5,

–4, –3, –2, –1, and then 0 station. Below the ischial spines, the fetal head passes through +1, +2, +3, +4, and +5 stations till delivery **(Fig. 2.6)**. +5 station represents that the fetal head is visible at the introitus. If the leading part of the fetal head is at the zero station or below, the fetal head is said to be engaged. This implies that the biparietal plane of the fetal head has passed through the pelvic inlet. However, in the presence of excessive molding or caput formation, engagement may not have taken place even if the head appears to be at zero station.

Molding

> Q. With help of a short essay discuss about molding and its clinical significance.

Molding is the overlapping of the fetal skull bones at the regions of sutures, which may occur during labor due to the head being compressed as it passes through the maternal pelvis. Molding results in the compression of the engaging diameter of the fetal head with the corresponding elongation of the diameter at right angles to it **(Fig. 2.7)**. For example, if the fully flexed fetal head engages in the suboccipito-bregmatic diameter, this diameter gets compressed. At the same time, the mentovertical diameter (which is at right angles to the suboccipitobregmatic diameter) gets elongated.

- *Diagnosis of molding:* In a cephalic (head) presentation, molding is diagnosed by feeling the overlapping of the sutures of the skull on vaginal examination and assessing whether or not the overlap can be reduced (corrected) by pressing gently with the examining finger.

  The presence of caput succedaneum (soft-tissue edema of fetal scalp) can also be felt as a soft, boggy swelling, which may make it difficult to identify the presenting part of the fetal head clearly. With severe caput, the sutures may be impossible to feel.

- *Grading the degree of molding* **(Fig. 2.8)**: The occipitoparietal and sagittal sutures are palpated, and the relationship or closeness of the two adjacent bones is assessed. The degree of molding is assessed according to the scale described in **Table 2.8**.

■ PELVIC ASSESSMENT

While assessing the pelvis, it is important to adopt a step-by-step method, i.e., first assessing the size and shape of the pelvic inlet, then the midpelvis, and lastly the pelvic outlet.

Assessment of Pelvic Inlet

For assessment of pelvic inlet, the sacral promontory and the retropubic areas are palpated.

Assessment of Midpelvis

For assessment of the midpelvis, the curve of the sacrum, the sacrospinous ligaments, and the ischial spines are palpated.

Assessment of the Pelvic Outlet

For assessment of the pelvic outlet, the subpubic angle, intertuberous diameter, and mobility of the coccyx are determined.

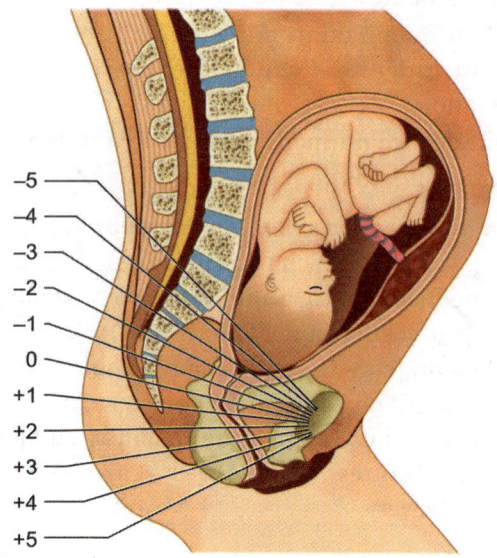

Fig. 2.6: Fetal descent.

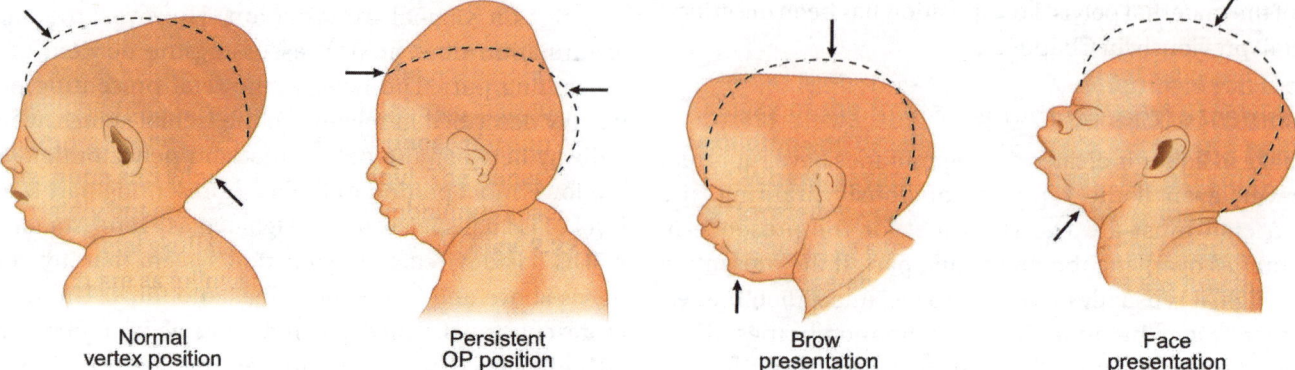

Fig. 2.7: Pattern of molding in different types of cephalic presentations.

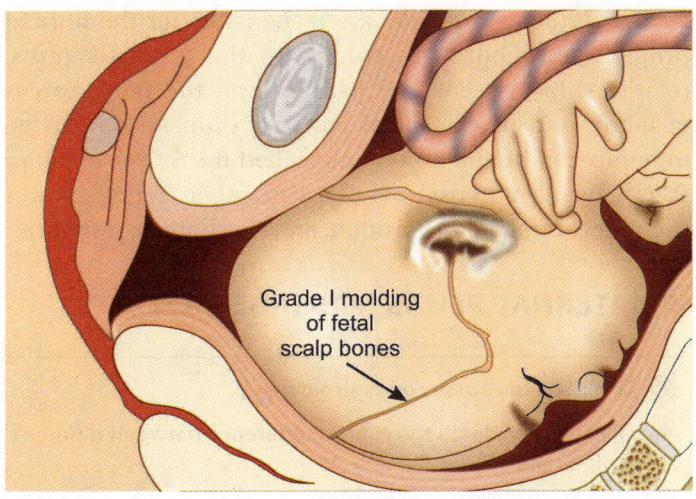

Fig. 2.8: Grade I molding of fetal scalp bones.

TABLE 2.8: Degree of molding of fetal skull.

Degree of molding	Description
0 (normal)	Normal separation of the bones with open sutures
1+ (mild molding)	Bones touching each other
2+ (moderate molding)	Bones overlapping, but can be separated with gentle digital pressure
3+ (severe molding)	Bones overlapping, but cannot be separated with gentle digital pressure

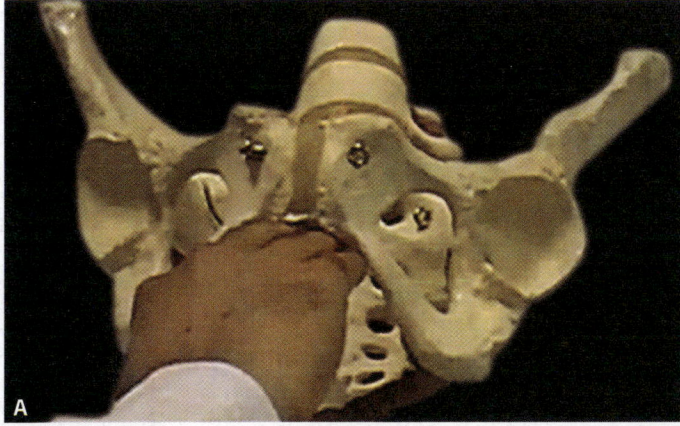

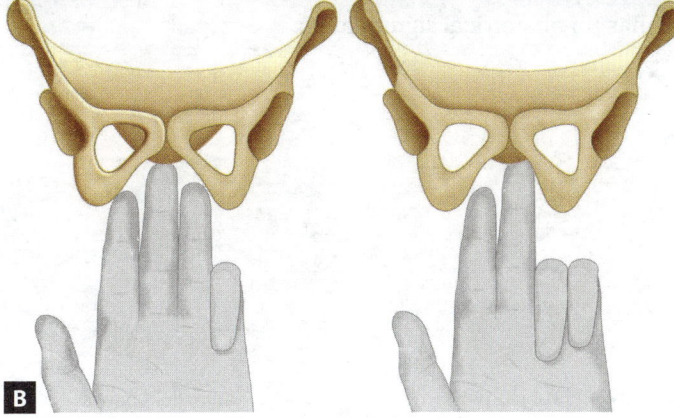

Figs. 2.9A and B: Assessment of subpubic angle.

Normal Labor in Occipitolateral Position

The obstetrician must begin the pelvic assessment by starting with the sacral promontory and then following the curve of the sacrum down the midline. In an adequate pelvis, the promontory cannot be easily palpated, the sacrum is well curved, and the coccyx cannot be felt. In case of an inadequate pelvis, the sacral promontory is easily palpated and prominent, the sacrum is straight, and the coccyx is prominent and/or fixed. After assessing the sacrum, the obstetrician must move his/her fingers lateral to the midsacrum where the sacrospinous ligaments can be felt. If these ligaments are followed laterally, the ischial spines can be palpated. In an adequate pelvis, the sacrospinous ligaments are 3 cm or longer, i.e., at least two of the obstetrician's fingers can be placed over the sacrospinous ligaments. In case of an inadequate pelvis, it may not be possible to place two fingers over the sacrospinous ligaments; the ligaments usually allow less than two fingers. Also, the ischial spines may appear sharp and prominent. Next, the retropubic area is palpated. For this the obstetrician must put two examining fingers with the palm of the hand facing upward, behind the symphysis pubis. The hand is then moved laterally to both sides. In case of an adequate pelvis, the retropubic area is flat. In case of an inadequate pelvis, the retropubic area is angulated. To measure the subpubic angle, the examining fingers are turned so that the palm of the hand faces downward. At the same time, the third finger is also held out at the vaginal introitus, and the angle under the pubis is felt. If three fingers can be placed under the pubis, the subpubic angle is approximately 90°, which can be considered as adequate **(Figs. 2.9A and B)**. If the subpubic angle allows only two fingers, the subpubic angle is about 60°, which is indicative of an inadequate pelvis. Finally, as the obstetrician's hand is withdrawn from the vaginal introitus, the intertuberous diameter is measured with the knuckles of the closed fist of the hand placed between the ischial tuberosities. If the pelvis is adequate, the intertuberous diameter allows four knuckles. In case of an inadequate pelvis, the intertuberous diameter allows less than four knuckles.

MANAGEMENT

Management comprising investigations and definitive obstetric management is discussed next.

INVESTIGATIONS

The investigations which need to be done during the antenatal period have been discussed in Chapter 1. In case these investigations have not been done previously due to some reason or an unbooked patient without the history of previous antenatal visits presents for the first time in labor, these investigations need to be done at the time of admission.

General principles of care to be observed at the time of labor are enlisted in **Box 2.4**.

TREATMENT/OBSTETRIC MANAGEMENT

Q. What should be the next step of management in the case study described in the beginning of the chapter?

The following need to be done in the above-mentioned case study:

- Detailed history must be taken if not had been taken previously in the antenatal period.
- A general physical, vaginal, and abdominal examination must be done. Cervix must be checked for dilatation, effacement, position, and consistency. In this case, the patient was having regular uterine contractions after every 10–15 minutes with each contraction lasting for about a minute. The cervix was dilated by 3–4 cm, was 50–60% effaced, head was at −1 station, and membranes were absent. The baby's head was in occipitoanterior position.
- A management plan for normal vaginal delivery was formulated in this case, following which the patient was admitted to the labor and delivery unit.
- Consent forms must be signed for delivery and potential blood transfusion by the patient and her husband/partner.
- Nonstress test must be performed.
- The patient must be placed on a clear diet and intravenous fluids.
- Intermittent fetal heart monitoring to be done every 30 minutes during the active phase of the first stage, after every contraction during the second stage, and immediately following the spontaneous ROM.
- Patient must be given a choice of whether she wants epidural analgesia or not.

BOX 2.4: General principles of care to be observed at the time of labor.

- Antenatal summary card to be reviewed
- Antenatal visits and investigations to be reviewed
- General physical examination, vital signs, obstetric examination including per speculum examination (especially if leaking is present), and a per vaginal examination needs to be performed

Five important factors are responsible for the normal progress of labor. These include the passage, fetus, relationship between the passage and the fetus, forces of labor, and psychosocial considerations. This can be remembered by the mnemonic called the 5 "Ps" of labor: *P*assageway (maternal pelvis), *P*assenger (fetus), *P*ower (uterine contractions), *P*osition, and *P*sychologic responses.

■ MATERNAL PELVIS (PASSAGEWAY)

Q. Write a long essay on android pelvis.

Q. Discuss in detail the clinical difference between different types of female pelvis.

Q. Discuss maternal pelvis in brief.

The birth passage comprises three parts, namely the pelvic inlet, pelvic cavity, and the pelvic outlet. The bony pelvis can be classified into four types: gynecoid, android, anthropoid, and platypelloid **(Figs. 2.10 and Table 2.9)**. Of these, the gynecoid type of pelvis is the most common, with the diameters favorable for vaginal delivery. The anterior view of maternal gynecoid pelvis is shown in **Figure 2.11**. Gynecoid pelvis is an ideal type of pelvis and is characterized by the presence of the following features:

- The pelvic brim is almost round in shape, but slightly oval transversely.
- Ischial spines are not prominent.
- Subpubic arch is rounded and measures at least 90° in size.
- Obturator foramen is triangular in shape.
- Sacrum is wide with average concavity and inclination.
- Sacrosciatic notch is wide.

The pelvic brim **(Fig. 2.12)** divides the pelvis into false pelvis and true pelvis. The boundaries of the pelvic brim or inlet include the following: sacral promontory, sacral alae, sacroiliac joints, iliopectineal lines, iliopectineal eminence, upper border of superior pubic rami, pubic tubercles, pubic crest, and upper borders of pubic symphysis.

- *False pelvis:* False pelvis lies above the pelvic brim and has no obstetrical significance.

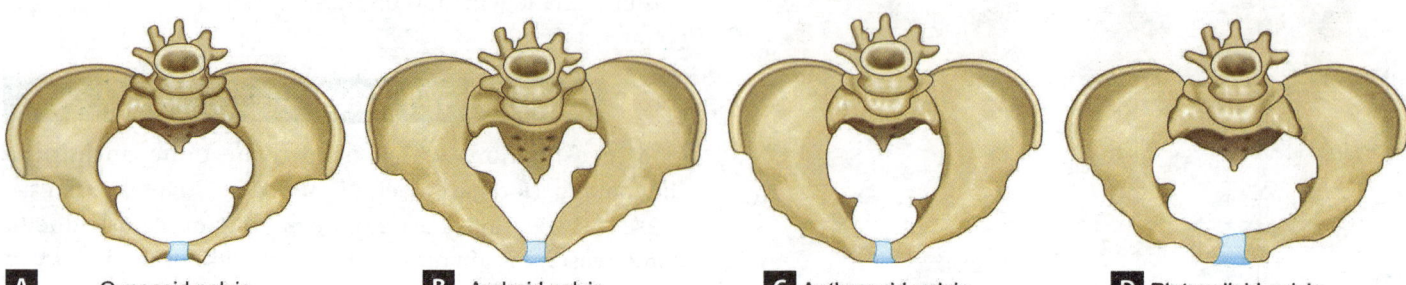

Figs. 2.10A to D: Caldwell and Moloy's classification of pelvis.

TABLE 2.9: Various pelvic dimensions in different types of pelvis.

Part of pelvis	Dimension	Gynecoid	Anthropoid	Android	Platypelloid
Pelvic inlet	Widest diameter of pelvic inlet	12 cm	<12 cm	12 cm	12 cm
	Shape of the pelvic inlet	Oval at the inlet with anterior–posterior diameter being just slightly less than the transverse diameter	Oval, long, and narrow; the anterior–posterior diameter of the inlet exceeds the transverse diameter, giving it an oval shape	Heart-shaped/triangular with the base toward the sacrum. As a result, posterior segment is short, and anterior segment is narrow	Pelvic brim is flat and transverse kidney-shaped. Transverse diameter is much larger than the anterior–posterior diameter
	Anteroposterior diameter of inlet	11 cm	12 cm	11 cm	10 cm
	Forepelvis	Wide	Divergent	Narrow	Straight
Pelvic midcavity	Sidewalls	Straight	Narrow	Convergent (widest posteriorly)	Wide (diverge downward)
	Sacrosciatic notch	Wide and shallow	Wider and more shallow	Narrow and deep	Slightly narrow and small
	Inclination of sacrum	Sacrum is well-curved, and sacral angle exceeds 90%	Sacrum is long and narrow with usual curve; sacral angle is >90°	Sacrum is inclined forward and straight; sacral angle is <90°	The sacrum is prominent and the sacral promontory tends to encroach upon the area of the hind pelvis; sacral angle is >90°
	Ischial spines	Not prominent	Not prominent	Prominent	Not prominent
Pelvic outlet	Subpubic arch	Wide and curved subpubic arch (subpubic angle is not <85°)	Subpubic arch is long and narrow; subpubic angle may be slightly narrowed	Long and straight subpubic arch, narrow subpubic angle	The subpubic arch is generally wide, and the subpubic angle is in the excess of 90°
	Transverse diameter of the outlet	10 cm	10 cm	<10 cm	10 cm

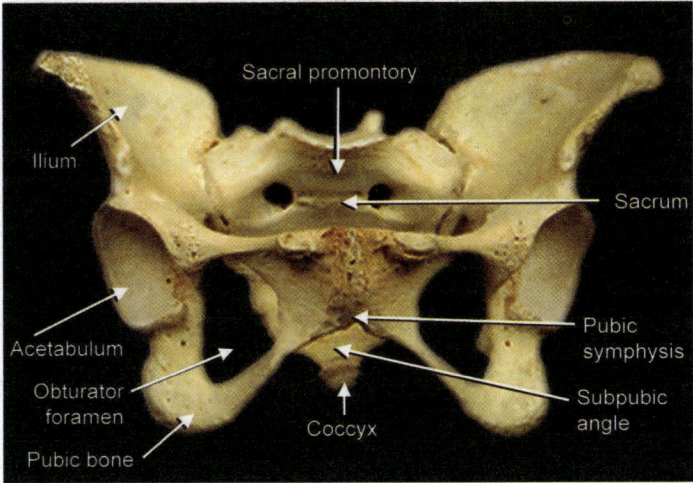

Fig. 2.11: Anterior view of maternal pelvis.

- *True pelvis:* True pelvis lies below the pelvic brim and plays an important role in childbirth and delivery. It forms a bony canal through which the fetus passes at the time of labor. It is formed by the symphysis pubis anteriorly and sacrum and coccyx posteriorly. The true pelvis can be divided into three parts: pelvic inlet, cavity, and outlet.

Pelvic Inlet

Pelvic inlet is round in shape and is narrowest in the anteroposterior dimension and widest in the transverse diameter. The fetal head enters the pelvic inlet with the longest diameter of the fetal head (AP diameter) in the widest part of the pelvic inlet (transverse diameter) **(Figs. 2.13A to C)**.

The plane of the pelvic inlet (also known as superior strait) is not horizontal, but is tilted forward. It makes an angle of 55° with the horizontal. This angle is known as the angle of inclination. Radiographically, this angle can be measured by measuring the angle between the front of the vertebra L5 and plane of inlet and subtracting this from 180°. Increase in the angle of inclination has obstetric significance as this may result in delayed engagement of the fetal head and delay in descent of fetal head. Increase in the angle of inclination also favors occipitoposterior position. On the other hand, the reduction in the angle of inclination may not have any obstetric significance.

44 Normal and Abnormal Presentations

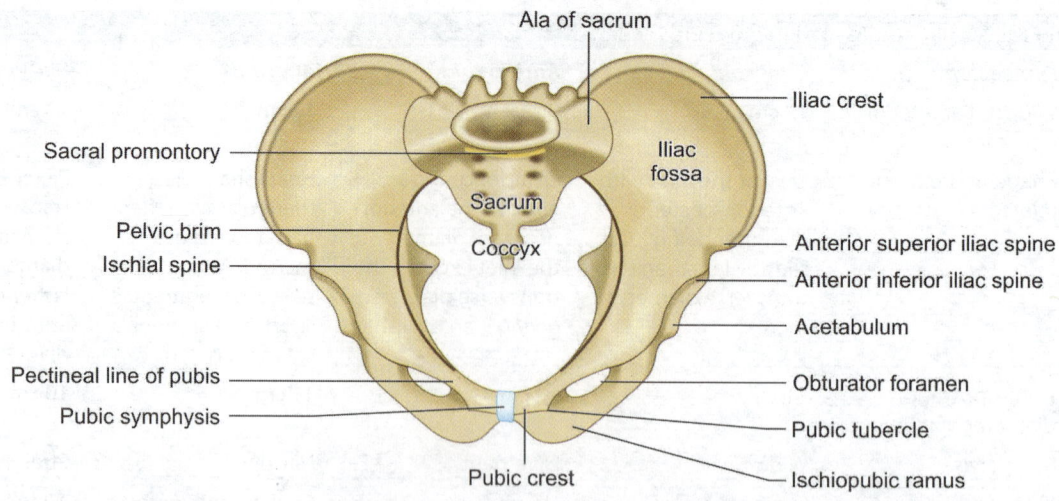

Fig. 2.12: Boundaries of the pelvic brim.

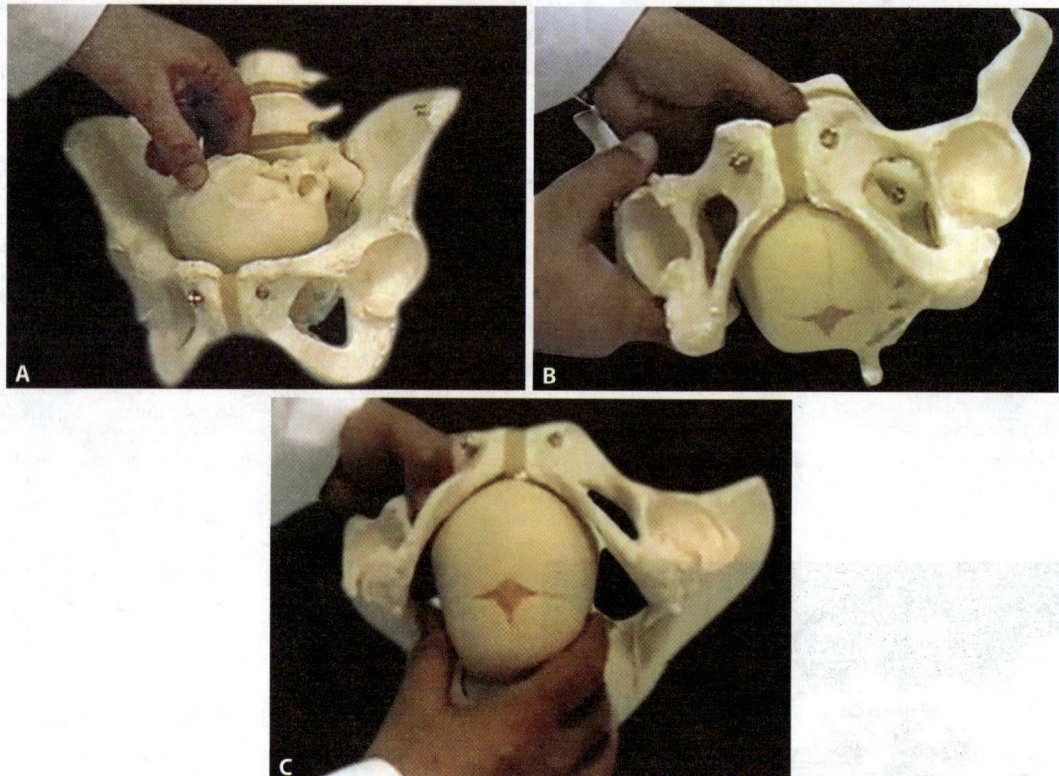

Figs. 2.13A to C: Entry of fetal head into the maternal pelvis. (A) The engaging diameter of fetal head engages in the transverse diameter of the inlet; (B and C) The fetal head undergoes internal rotation by 90° inside the pelvic cavity so that the longest diameter of fetal head engages in AP diameter of the outlet, which is its largest diameter.

The axis of the pelvic inlet is a line drawn perpendicular to the plane of inlet in the midline **(Fig. 2.14)**. It is in downward and backward directions. Upon extension, this line passes through the umbilicus anteriorly and through the coccyx posteriorly. For proper descent and engagement of fetal head, it is important that the uterine axis coincides with the axis of inlet.

Diameters of the Pelvic Inlet AP Diameter

- *AP diameter (true conjugate or anatomical conjugate = 11 cm):* This is measured from the midpoint of sacral promontory to the upper border of pubic symphysis **(Fig. 2.15)**.
- *Obstetric conjugate (10.5 cm):* It is measured from the midpoint of sacral promontory to the most bulging point on the back of symphysis pubic. This is the shortest AP diameter of the pelvic inlet and measures about 10.5 cm.
- *Diagonal conjugate (12.5 cm):* It is measured from the tip of sacral promontory to the lower border of pubic symphysis.

Out of the three AP diameters of pelvic inlet, only diagonal conjugate can be assessed clinically during the late

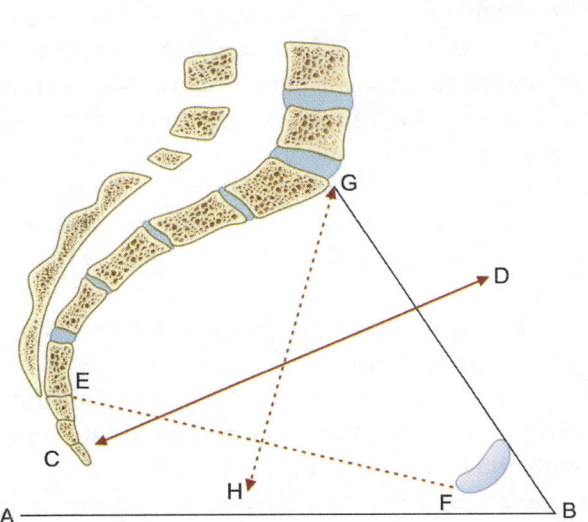

Fig. 2.14: Different planes and axes of the pelvis AB—horizontal line; GB—plane of inlet; FE—plane of obstetric outlet; DC—axis of the inlet; GH—axis of obstetrical outlet.

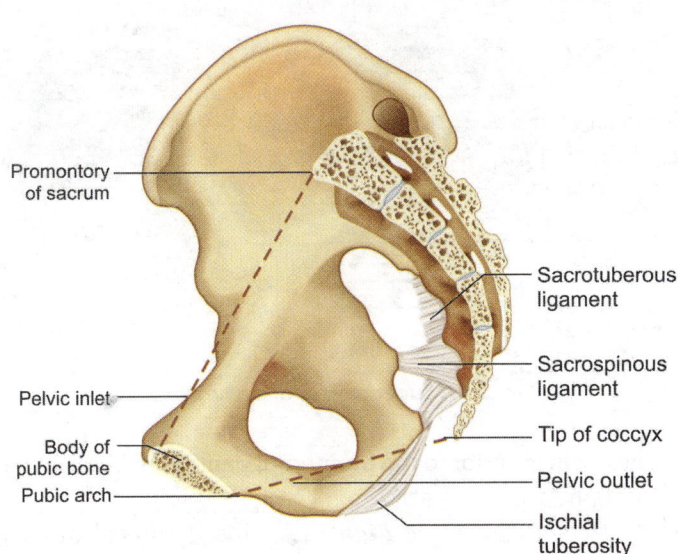

Fig. 2.15: Medial view of maternal pelvis (from left).

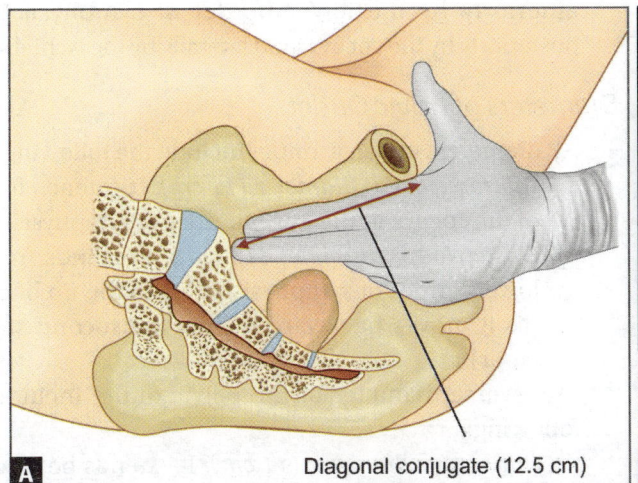
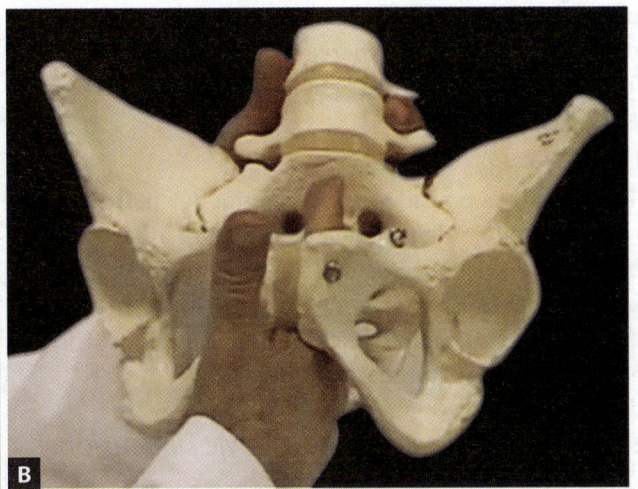

Figs. 2.16A and B: Measurement of diagonal conjugate.

pregnancy or at the time of the labor. Obstetric conjugate can be calculated by subtracting 1.5–2 cm from the diagonal conjugate. Also, the true conjugate can be inferred by subtracting 1.2 cm from the diagonal conjugate.

Measurement of the Diagonal Conjugate

After placing the patient in dorsal position and taking all aseptic precautions, two fingers are introduced into vagina. The clinician tries to feel the anterior sacral curvature with these fingers **(Figs. 2.16A and B)**. In normal cases, it will be difficult to feel the sacral promontory. The clinician may be required to depress the elbow and wrist while mobilizing the fingers upward in order to reach the promontory. The point at which the bone recedes from the finger is sacral promontory. A marking is placed over the gloved index finger by the index finger of the other hand. After removing the fingers from the vagina, the distance between the marking and the tip of the middle finger is measured in order to obtain the measurement of diagonal conjugate. In clinical situations, it may not always be feasible to measure the diagonal conjugate. In these cases, if the middle finger fails to reach the sacral promontory or reaches it with difficulty, the diagonal conjugate can be considered as adequate. Under normal circumstances, an adequate pelvis would be able to allow an average-sized fetal head to pass through.

Transverse Diameter of Pelvic Inlet

- *Anatomical transverse diameter (13 cm)*: It is the distance between the farthest two points on the iliopectineal line **(Fig. 2.17)**. It is the largest diameter of the pelvic inlet and

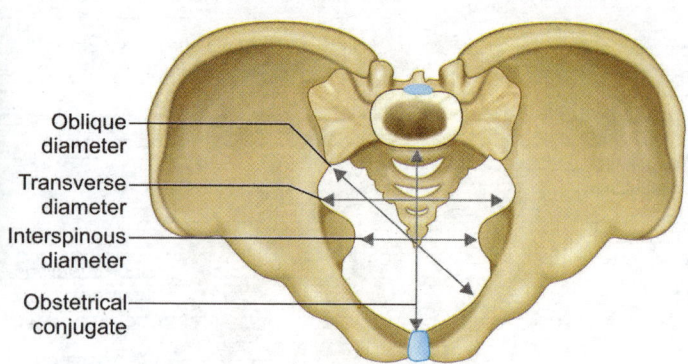

Fig. 2.17: Superior view of pelvic inlet.

lies 4 cm anterior to the promontory and 7 cm behind the symphysis.
- *Obstetric transverse diameter:* This diameter passes through the midpoint of true conjugate and is therefore slightly shorter than the anatomical transverse diameter.

Oblique Diameters of Pelvic Inlet

There are two oblique diameters, right and left (12 cm). The right oblique diameter passes from right sacroiliac joint to the left iliopubic eminence, whereas the left diameter passes from left sacroiliac joint to the right iliopubic eminence.

Pelvic Cavity

The pelvic cavity is bounded above by the pelvic brim and below by the plane of least pelvic dimension, anteriorly by the symphysis pubis and posteriorly by sacrum. The plane of least pelvic dimension extends from the lower border of pubic symphysis to the tip of ischial spines laterally and to the tip of fifth sacral vertebra posteriorly.

Plane of Cavity (Plane of Greatest Pelvic Dimensions)

The plane of cavity passes between the middle of the posterior surface of the symphysis pubis and the junction between second and third sacral vertebrae. Laterally it passes through the center of acetabulum and the upper part of greater sciatic notch. Since this is the roomiest plane of pelvis, it is also known as the plane of greatest pelvic dimensions. This is almost round in shape. Internal rotation of the fetal head occurs when the biparietal diameter of the fetal skull occupies this wide pelvic plane while the occiput is on the pelvic floor, i.e., at the plane of least pelvic dimensions.

Diameters of Pelvic Cavity

- *AP diameter (12 cm):* It measures from the midpoint on the posterior surface of pubis symphysis to the junction of second and third sacral vertebrae.
- *Transverse diameter (12 cm):* It is the distance between two farthest points laterally. Since there are no bony landmarks, the diameter cannot be exactly measured and can be roughly estimated to be about 12 cm.

Pelvic Outlet

- *Anatomical outlet:* It is a lozenge-shaped cavity bounded by anterior border of symphysis pubis, pubic arch, ischial tuberosities, sacrotuberous ligaments, sacrospinous ligaments, and tip of coccyx.
- *Plane of anatomical outlet:* It passes along with the boundaries of the anatomical outlet and consists of two triangular planes with a common base, which is the bituberous diameter.
- *Anterior sagittal plane:* Its apex is at the lower border of the symphysis pubis.
- *Anterior sagittal diameter (6–7 cm):* It extends from the lower border of the pubic symphysis to the center of bituberous diameter.
- *Posterior sagittal plane:* Its apex lies at the tip of the coccyx.
- *Posterior sagittal diameter (7.5–10 cm):* It extends from the tip of the sacrum to the center of bituberous diameter.
- *Obstetric outlet:* It is bounded above by the plane of least pelvic dimensions, below by the anatomical outlet, anteriorly by the lower border of symphysis pubis, posteriorly by the coccyx, and laterally by the ischial spines.

Diameters of Pelvic Outlet

- AP diameters of pelvic outlet include the following:
  - *Anatomical AP diameter (11 cm):* It extends from tip of the coccyx to the lower border of symphysis pubis.
  - *Obstetric AP diameter (13 cm):* It extends from the lower border of symphysis pubis to the tip of coccyx (as it moves backward during the second stage of labor).
- Transverse diameter of the pelvic outlet includes the following:
  - *Bituberous diameter (11 cm):* It extends between the inner aspects of ischial tuberosities. The bituberous diameter is measured with the knuckles of the closed fist of the hand placed between the two ischial tuberosities **(Fig. 2.18)**. If the pelvis is adequate, the intertuberous diameter allows four knuckles.
  - *Bispinous/interspinous diameter (10.5 cm):* It extends between the tips of ischial spines.
  - Measurement of various pelvic diameters is summarized in **Table 2.10**.

Pelvic Axis

- *Anatomical axis:* This is an imaginary line joining the central points of the planes of inlet, cavity, and outlet. This axis is C-shaped with concavity directed forward. It has no obstetric significance.
- *Obstetric axis:* It is an imaginary line, which represents the direction in which the head passes during the labor. It is J-shaped and passes downward and backward along the axis of the inlet till the ischial spines are reached, after

Normal Labor in Occipitolateral Position

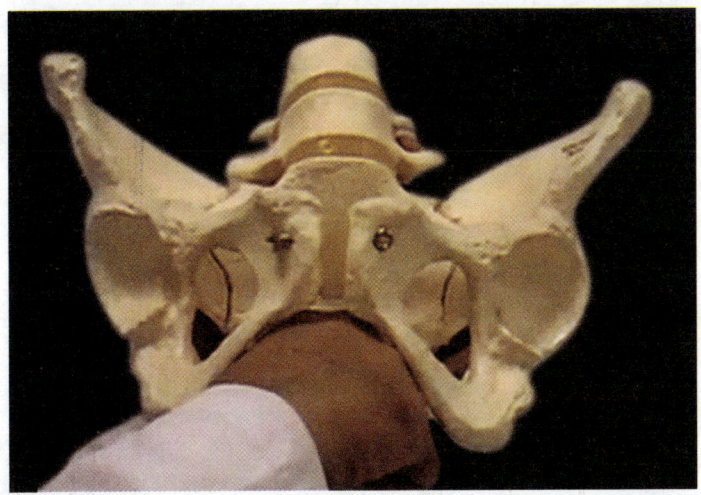

Fig. 2.18: Measurement of transverse diameter of the outlet.

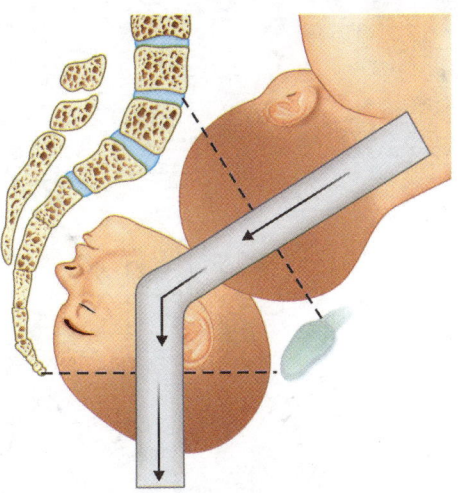

Fig. 2.19: Obstetric axis.

TABLE 2.10: Summary of the measurement of the diameters of the pelvis.

Diameter	Pelvic brim	Pelvic cavity	Pelvic outlet
Anteroposterior	11 cm	12 cm	13 cm
Oblique	12 cm	12 cm	–
Transverse	13 cm	12 cm	11 cm

which it passes downward and forward along the axis of pelvic outlet **(Fig. 2.19)**.

Midpelvis

Midpelvic plane: This plane is bounded anteriorly by the lower margin of symphysis pubis. It extends through the ischial spines to the junction of S4 and S5 or the tip of fifth sacral piece, depending upon the structure of the sacrum. If this plane meets at the tip of the S5 sacral piece, this plane becomes same as that of the plane of least pelvic dimensions; otherwise it forms a wedge posteriorly.

Diameters of Midpelvis

- *AP diameter (11.5 cm):* It is measured from the lower border of the symphysis pubis to the junction of S4 and S5 or the tip of S5, whichever is applicable.
- *Bispinous or transverse diameter (10.5 cm):* It is the distance between two ischial spines. Ischial spines are palpated for the assessment of midpelvis. After assessing the sacrum, the obstetrician must move his/her fingers lateral to the midsacrum where the sacrospinous ligaments can be felt. If these ligaments are followed laterally, the ischial spines can be palpated **(Fig. 2.20)**.
- *Subpubic angle:* It is the angle between two pubic rami. It varies from 85 ± 5°.

Interspinous/Bispinous Diameter

Q. Write a long essay on ischial spine.

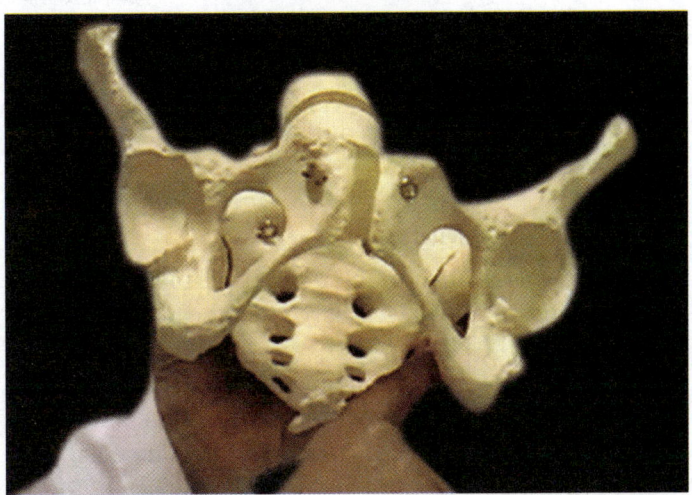

Fig. 2.20: Assessment of ischial spines.

Interspinous diameter is the distance between the two ischial spines and represents the smallest diameter of the maternal pelvis. It corresponds to the transverse diameter of midpelvis and is also known as the plane of least pelvic dimensions. Interspinous diameter is important because of the following reasons:

- Internal rotation occurs at this level.
- The obstetric axis of the pelvis changes its direction; it marks the beginning of the forward curve of pelvic axis.
- Most cases of obstructed labor or deep transverse arrest (DTA) occur at this level.
- Ischial spines correspond to the zero station of fetal presenting part.

The head is considered engaged when the vault is felt at or below this level. It also corresponds to the origin of levator ani muscles, and its ischiococcygeus part is attached to the ischial spines. Ischial spine can be considered as a landmark for giving pudendal block.

Forceps are applied only when the head is at this level or lower. External os of the cervix is located at this level. The ring pessary should be applied above this level for the treatment of prolapse.

48 Normal and Abnormal Presentations

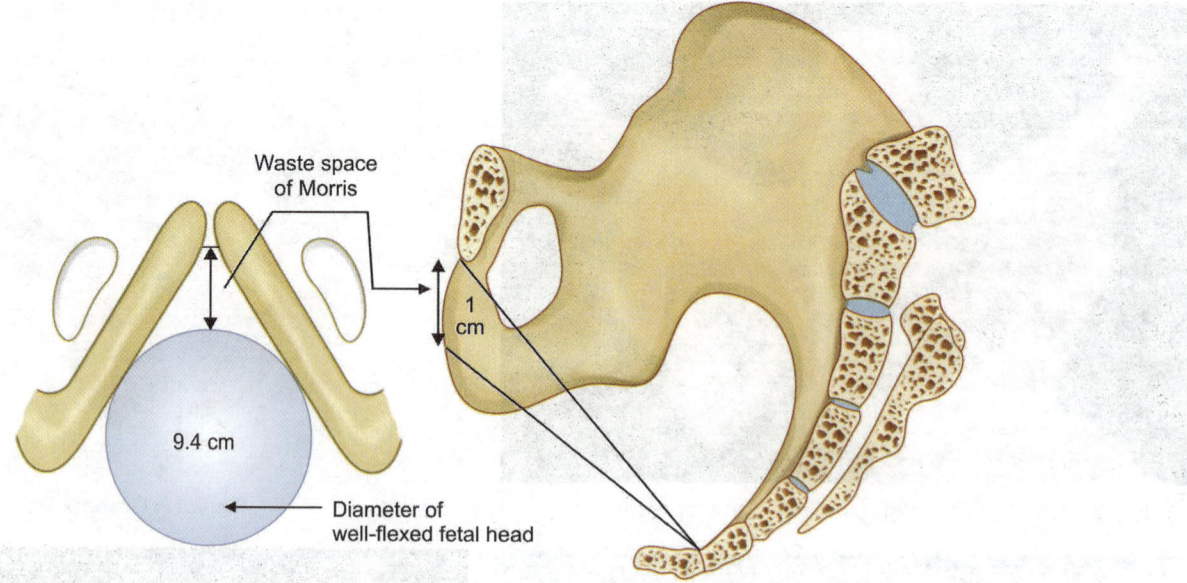

Fig. 2.21: Waste space of Morris.

The plane of obstetric outlet (plane of least pelvic dimensions) is at this level.

Waste Space of Morris

Normally the width of the pubic arch is such that a round disc of 9.4 cm (diameter of a well-flexed head) can pass through the pubic arch at a distance of 1 cm from the midpoint of the inferior border of the symphysis pubis. This distance is known as the "waste space of Morris" **(Fig. 2.21)**. In case of an inadequate pelvis with narrow pubic arch, the fetal head would be pushed backward and the waste space of Morris would increase. As a result, reduced space would be available for fetal head to pass through, due to which the fetal head would be forced to pass through a smaller diameter termed as the "available AP diameter." This is likely to injure the perineum or sometimes cause the arrest of fetal head.

■ PASSENGER: FETUS

 Q. Write a long essay on fetal skull.

Obstetrically, the head of fetus is the most important part, since an essential feature of labor is an adaptation between the fetal head and the maternal bony pelvis. Only a comparatively small part of the head of the fetus at term is represented by the face; the rest is composed of the firm skull, which is made up of two frontal, two parietal, and two temporal bones, along with the upper portion of the occipital bone and wings of the sphenoid. The bones are not united rigidly but are separated by membranous spaces, the sutures. The fetal skull has four main sutures **(Figs. 2.22 and 2.23)**, which are as follows:

1. *Sagittal or longitudinal suture:* This suture lies longitudinally across the vault of the skull in midline. It lies between the two parietal bones.

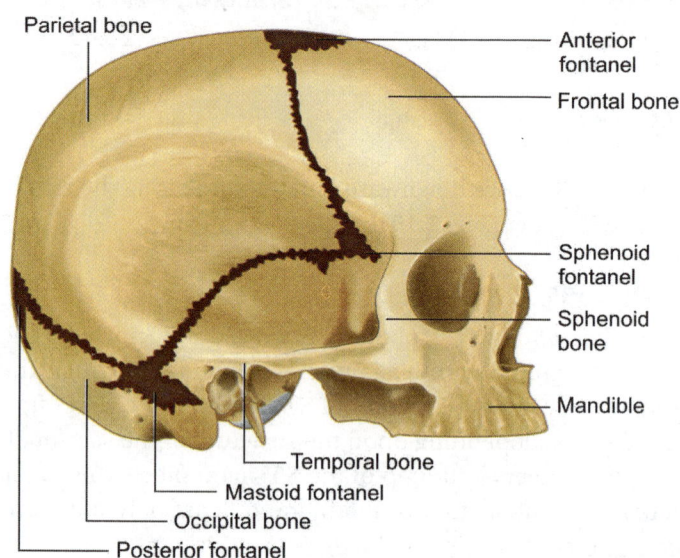

Fig. 2.22: Important sutures and bones of fetal skull.

2. *Coronal sutures:* These sutures are present between the parietal and frontal bones and extend transversely on either side from the anterior fontanel.
3. *Lambdoid suture:* This suture separates the occipital bone from the two parietal bones and extends transversely both on the right and on the left side from the posterior fontanel.
4. *Frontal suture:* This suture is present between the two halves of the frontal bone in the skull of infants and children and usually disappears by the age of 6 years.

Where several sutures meet, an irregular space is formed, which is enclosed by a membrane and designated as a fontanel. The greater or anterior fontanel is a lozenge-shaped space situated at the junction of the sagittal and coronal sutures **(Fig. 2.24)**. The lesser or posterior fontanel is represented by a small triangular area at the intersection of the sagittal and lambdoid

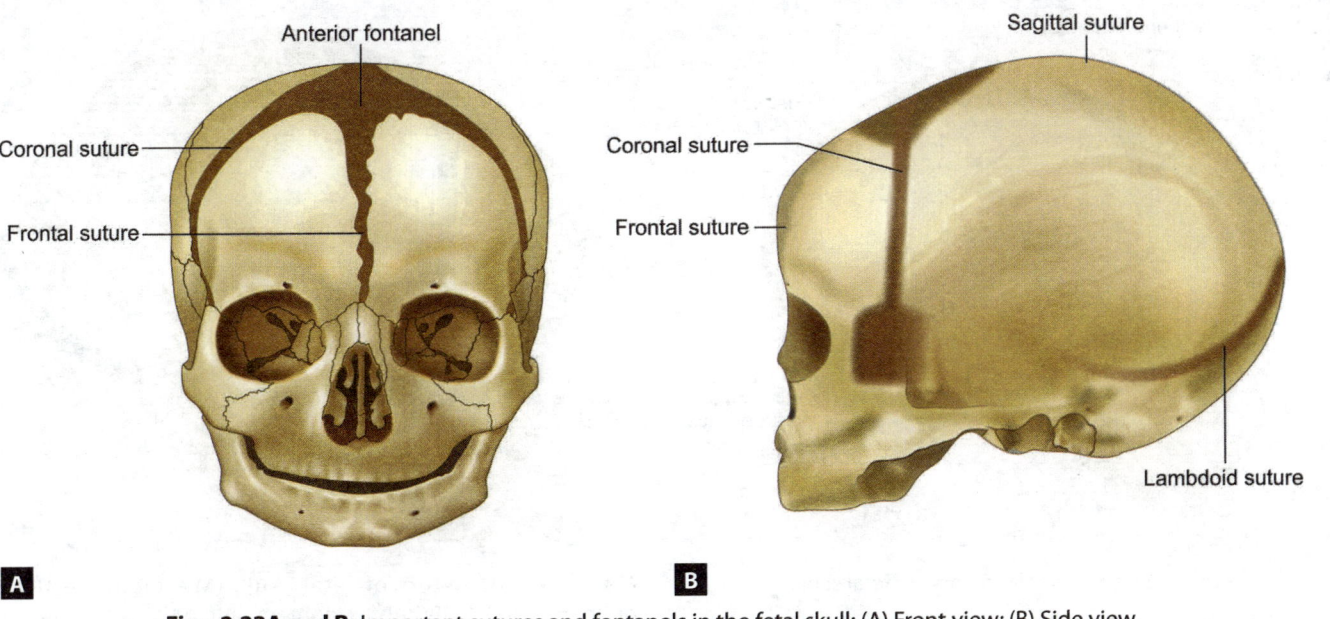

Figs. 2.23A and B: Important sutures and fontanels in the fetal skull: (A) Front view; (B) Side view.

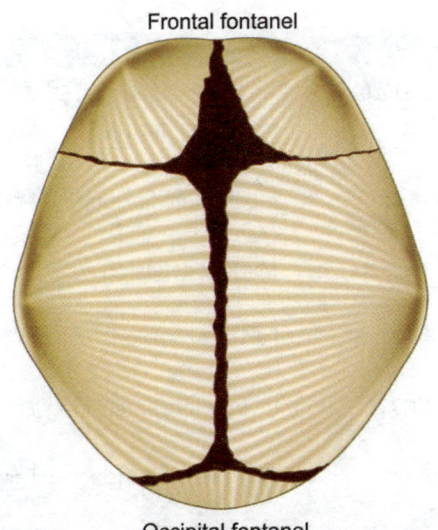

Fig. 2.24: Anterior and posterior fontanels in fetal head.

sutures. Both may be felt readily during labor, and their recognition gives important information concerning the presentation and position of the fetus. The two main fontanels having obstetric significance in the fetal head are anterior fontanel (bregma) and posterior fontanel (lambda). Anterior fontanel is formed by joining of four sutures: frontal suture (anteriorly), sagittal suture (posteriorly), and coronal sutures on the two sides (laterally). The palpation of anterior fontanel on vaginal examination is of great obstetric significance **(Box 2.5)**. On the other hand, posterior fontanel is formed by the joining of three sutures: sagittal suture (anteriorly) and lambdoid sutures on the two sides.

Presenting Parts of Fetal Skull

Presenting parts of the fetal skull include the following **(Fig. 2.25)**:

> **BOX 2.5:** Obstetric significance of the anterior fontanel.
> - Palpation of anterior fontanel indicates degree of flexion of fetal head
> - It facilitates molding of fetal head
> - The membranous nature of anterior fontanel helps in accommodating the rapid growth of brain during neonatal period
> - Floor of the anterior fontanel reflects the intracranial status. The floor may be depressed in case of dehydration and elevated in case of hydrocephalus or other conditions with raised intracranial tension

- *Vertex:* This is a quadrangular area bounded anteriorly by bregma (anterior fontanel) and coronal sutures, posteriorly by lambda (posterior fontanel) and lambdoid sutures, and laterally by arbitrary lines passing through the parietal eminences. When vertex is the presenting part, fetal head lies in flexion.
- *Face:* This is an area bounded by the root of the nose along with the supraorbital ridges and the junction of the chin or floor of mouth with the neck. Fetal head is fully extended during this presentation.
- *Brow:* This is an area of forehead extending from the root of nose and supraorbital ridges to the bregma and coronal sutures. The fetal head lies midway between full flexion and full extension in this presentation.

Some other parts of fetal skull, which are of significance, include the following:
- *Sinciput:* Area in front of the anterior fontanel corresponding to the forehead
- *Occiput:* Area limited to occipital bone
- *Mentum:* Chin of the fetus
- *Parietal eminences:* Prominent eminences on each of the parietal bones
- *Subocciput:* Junction of fetal neck and occiput, sometimes also known as the nape of the neck
- *Submentum:* Junction between the neck and chin

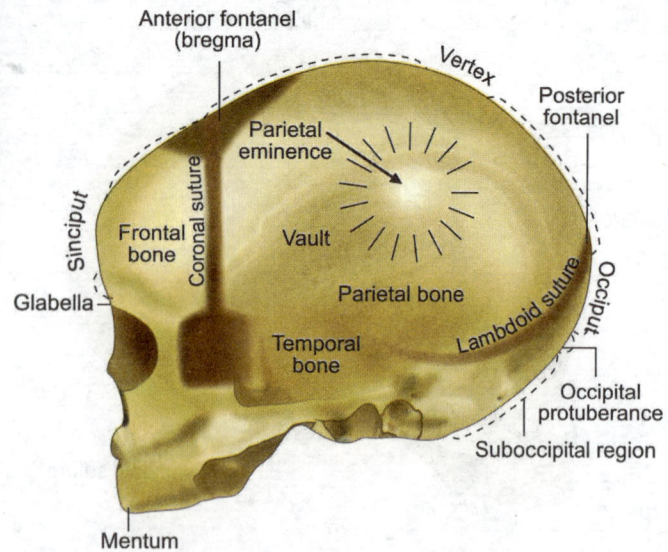

Fig. 2.25: Important landmarks of fetal skull.

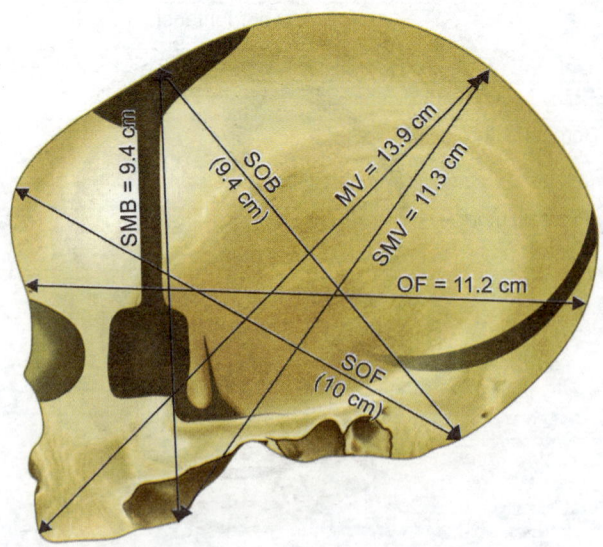

Fig. 2.26: Diameters of fetal skull. (MV: mentovertical; OF: occipitofrontal; SMB: submentobregmatic; SMV: submentovertical; SOB: suboccipitobregmatic; SOF: suboccipitofrontal)

TABLE 2.11: AP diameters of the fetal head, which may engage.

Diameter	Extent	Length	Attitude of head	Presentation
Suboccipitobregmatic	Extends from the nape of the neck to the center of bregma	9.4 cm	Complete flexion	Vertex
Suboccipitofrontal	Extends from the nape of the neck to the anterior end of anterior fontanel or center of sinciput	10 cm	Incomplete flexion	Vertex
Occipitofrontal	Extends from the occipital eminence to the root of nose (glabella)	11.2 cm	Marked deflexion	Vertex
Mentovertical	Extends from midpoint of the chin to the highest point on sagittal suture	13.9 cm	Partial extension	Brow
Submentovertical	Extends from the junction of the floor of the mouth and neck to the highest point on sagittal suture	11.3 cm	Incomplete extension	Face
Submentobregmatic	Extends from the junction of the floor of the mouth and neck to the center of bregma	9.4 cm	Complete extension	Face

Important Diameters of Fetal Skull

AP Diameters

The important AP diameters of the fetal skull are suboccipitobregmatic (9.4 cm), suboccipitofrontal (10 cm), occipitofrontal (11.2 cm), mentovertical (13.9 cm), submentovertical (11.3 cm), and submentobregmatic (9.4 cm). These diameters are described in **Table 2.11** and **Figure 2.26**.

Transverse Diameters

- *Biparietal diameter (9.5 cm):* It extends between the two parietal eminences. This diameter nearly always engages.
- *Supersubparietal diameter (8.5 cm):* It extends from a point placed below one parietal eminence to a point placed above the other parietal eminence of the opposite side.
- *Bitemporal diameter (8 cm):* Distance between the anteroinferior ends of the coronal sutures
- *Bimastoid diameter (7.5 cm):* Distance between the tips of the mastoid process. This diameter is nearly incompressible.

The fetal head is said to be engaged when maximum transverse diameter of fetal head can pass through the pelvic brim. The shape and diameter of the circumference of the fetal skull varies with the degree of flexion and hence the presentation. A normal pelvis would easily be able to permit the engagement of the fetal skull in vertex and face presentations. This is so as in case of vertex and face presentations; the engaging AP diameters of fetal skull are suboccipitobregmatic (9.4 cm) and submentobregmatic (9.4 cm), respectively **(Table 2.12)**. However, the passage of the fetal head in brow presentation would not be able to take place in a normal pelvis as the engaging AP diameter of fetal skull is mentovertical (13.9 cm) in this case. Therefore, arrest of labor occurs when the fetal head is in brow presentation **(Figs. 2.27A to D)**.

MECHANISM OF NORMAL LABOR

Figure 2.28 illustrates the mechanism of normal labor. In normal labor the fetal head enters the pelvic brim most commonly through the available transverse diameter of the pelvic inlet. This is so because the most common fetal position is occipitolateral (transverse position). In some cases, the fetal head may enter through one of the oblique diameters. The fetal head with left occipitoanterior position enters through right oblique diameter, whereas that with right occipitoanterior position enters through left oblique diameter of the pelvic inlet. Left occipitoanterior position is slightly more common than the right occipitoanterior position as the left oblique diameter is encroached by the rectum. The engaging AP diameter of the fetal head is suboccipitobregmatic (9.4 cm) in position of complete flexion. The engaging transverse diameter of the fetal head is biparietal diameter (9.5 cm). As the occipitolateral position of the fetal head is most common, the mechanism of labor in this position would be discussed. The cardinal fetal movements during the occipitolateral position comprise the following: engagement, flexion, descent, internal rotation, crowning, extension, restitution, external rotation of the head, and expulsion of the trunk.

- *Engagement:* In primigravida, the engagement of fetal head usually occurs before the onset of labor, while in multigravida, it may occur only during the first stage of labor, following ROM.

TABLE 2.12: Plane of engagement of fetal head depending upon its attitude.

Attitude of head	Plane of shape	Engagement
Complete flexion	Biparietal-suboccipitobregmatic	Almost round
Deflexion	Biparietal-occipitofrontal	Oval
Incomplete extension	Biparietal-mentovertical	Bigger oval
Complete extension	Biparietal-submentobregmatic	Almost round

- *Asynclitism of the fetal head:* At the time of engagement, the head may have a lateral inclination due to which the sagittal sutures may not strictly correspond with the available transverse diameter of the pelvic inlet. As a result, the head may be either deflected anteriorly toward the pubic symphysis or posteriorly toward the sacral promontory. This lateral deflection of the fetal head in relation to the pelvis is known as asynclitism **(Figs. 2.29A to C)**. When the sagittal sutures lie anteriorly, the posterior parietal bone becomes the leading presenting part, and this is known as posterior asynclitism or posterior parietal presentation or Litzmann obliquity. This is commonly encountered in the primigravida due to the good tone of the abdominal muscles and uterus. If the sagittal sutures lie posteriorly, the anterior parietal bone becomes the leading part, and this is known as anterior parietal presentation or anterior asynclitism or Naegele's obliquity. This is more common amongst the multigravida. While mild degrees of asynclitism are common, severe degrees indicate CPD. In case of posterior parietal presentation, the posterior lateral flexion of the head occurs to glide the anterior parietal bone past the pubic symphysis. In the anterior parietal presentation, lateral flexion of the head occurs in opposite direction. Following this movement, synclitism occurs. In nearly one-fourth of the cases, the head on its own enters the brim in synclitism, i.e., sagittal sutures correspond with the diameter of engagement.

- *Descent:* Descent of the fetal head is a continuous process that occurs throughout the second stage of labor in such a way that toward the end of second stage, crowning of fetal head occurs.

- *Flexion:* In normal cases, increased flexion of fetal chin against chest helps in presenting the smallest fetal diameter. Flexion of the head occurs as it descends and meets the pelvic floor, bringing the chin into contact with the fetal thorax. Adequate flexion of the fetal head produces the smallest diameter of presentation, i.e.,

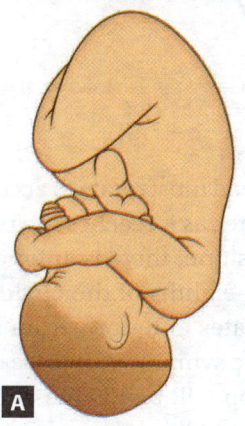 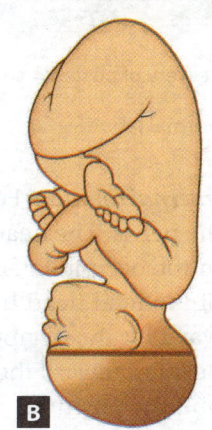 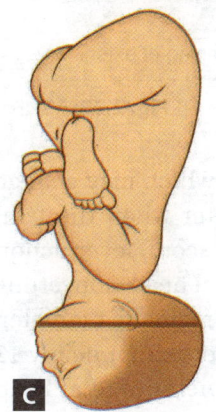 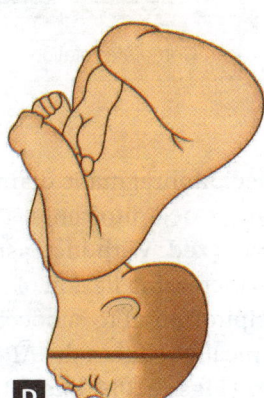

Figs. 2.27A to D: Engaging diameters of fetal head depending on the position of presenting part. (A) Vertex suboccipitobregmatic; (B) Sinciput suboccipitofrontal; (C) Brow mentovertical; (D) Face submentobregmatic.

52 Normal and Abnormal Presentations

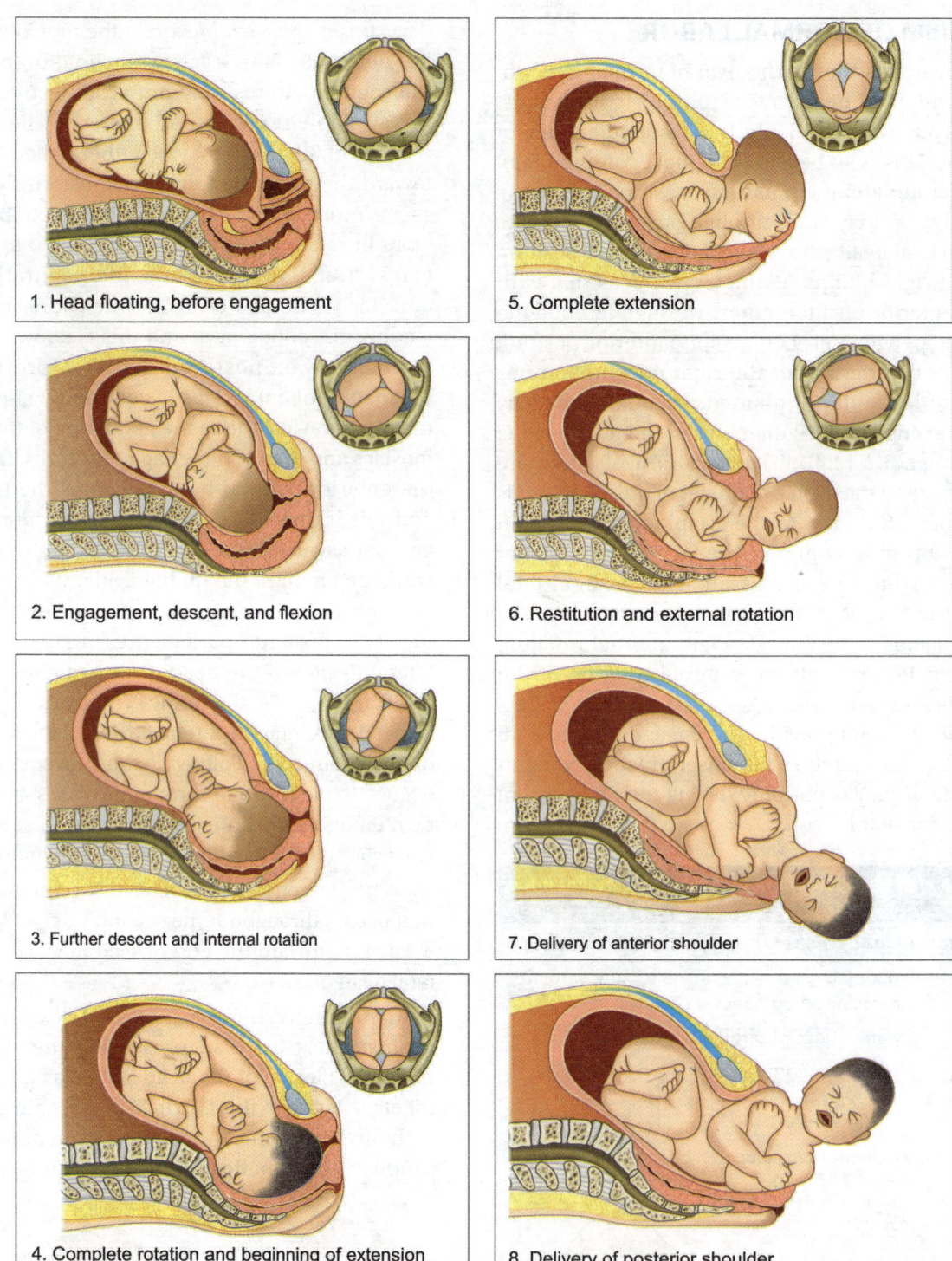

Fig. 2.28: Mechanism of normal labor.

the suboccipitobregmatic diameter, which may change to the larger occipitofrontal diameter when the fetal head is deflexed. With increasing descent, lever action produces increasing flexion of the fetal head, converting from occipitofrontal to suboccipitobregmatic diameter, which typically reduces the AP diameter from nearly 12 to 9.5 cm **(Figs. 2.30A and B)**. Diameter of fetal head entering the pelvis depending upon the degree of flexion is illustrated in **Figures 2.31A to D**.

- *Internal rotation:* Fetal head must rotate to accommodate the pelvis. The head rotates as it reaches the pelvic floor. In the occipitolateral position, there is anterior rotation of the fetal head by two-eighths of the circle in such a way that the occiput rotates anteriorly from the lateral position toward the pubic symphysis. In case of anterior oblique position, rotation will be by one-eighth of the circle placing the occiput behind the pubic symphysis. There always occurs some descent with internal rotation.

Normal Labor in Occipitolateral Position

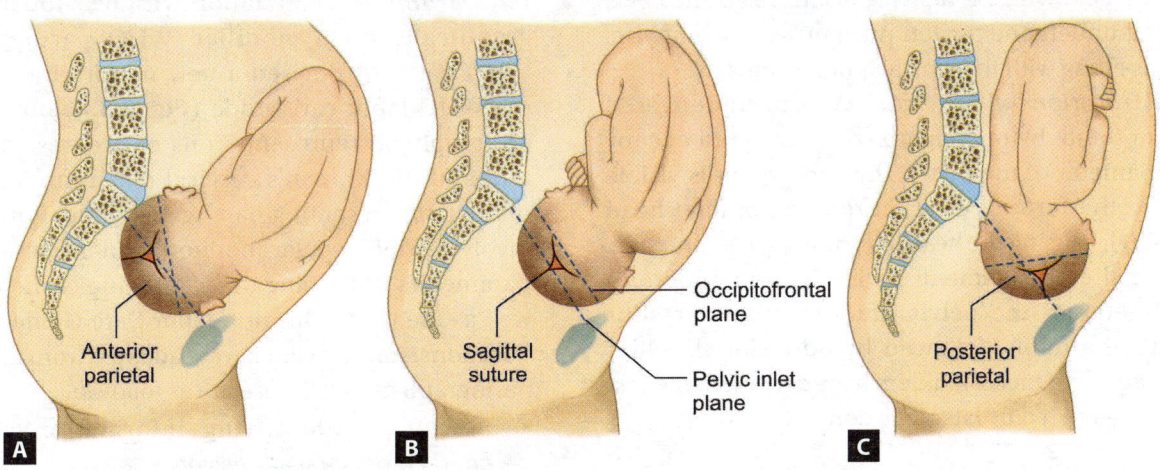

Figs. 2.29A to C: (A) Anterior asynclitism (Naegele's obliquity); (B) Normal synclitism; (C) Posterior asynclitism (Litzmann obliquity) ear presentation.

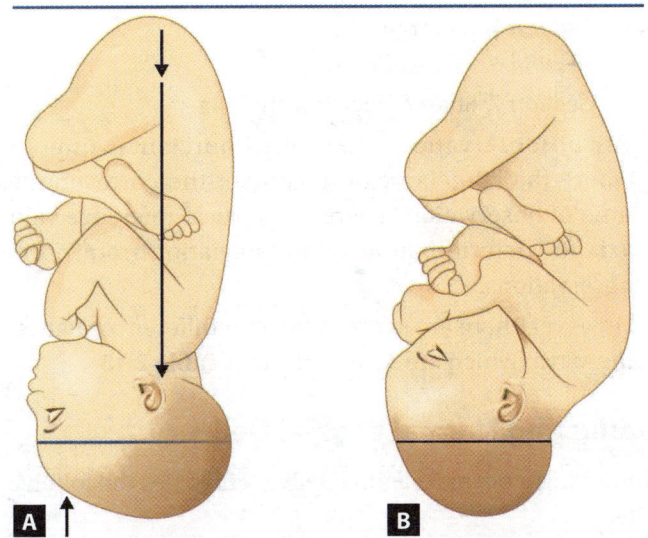

Figs. 2.30A and B: Lever action producing flexion of the head; conversion from occipitofrontal to suboccipitobregmatic diameter, typically reducing the AP diameter from nearly 12 to 9.5 cm.

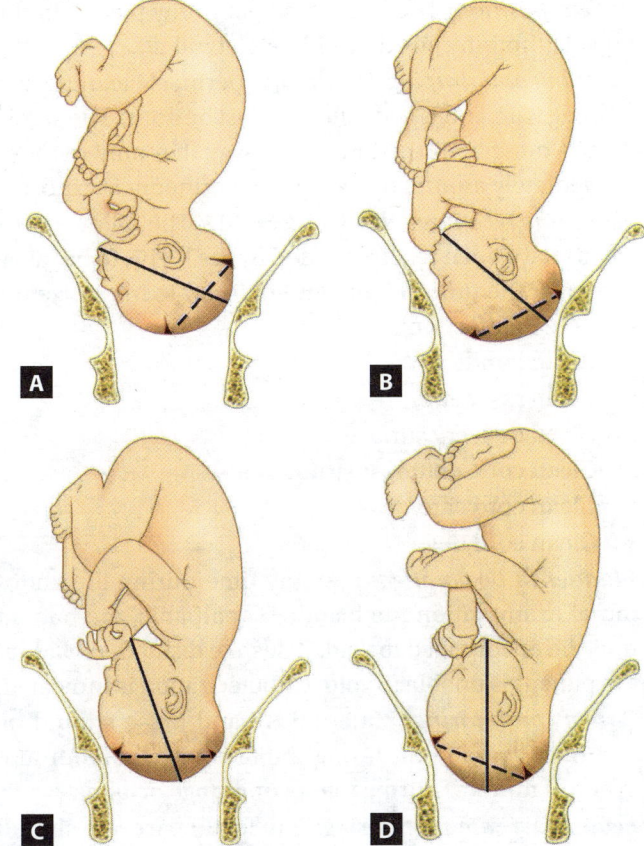

Figs. 2.31A to D: Diameter of fetal head entering the pelvis depending upon the degree of flexion. Four degrees of head flexion are indicated by the solid line (the occipitomental diameter); the broken line connects the center of the anterior fontanel with posterior fontanel. (A) Poor flexion; (B) Moderate flexion; (C) Advanced flexion; (D) Complete flexion.

Torsion of fetal neck is a phenomenon, which will inevitably occur during internal rotation of the fetal head. In case of occipitolateral position, the internal rotation of the fetal head by two-eighths of the circle is likely to cause torsion of fetal neck by two-eighths of the circle. Since the neck would not be able to sustain this much amount of torsion, there would be simultaneous rotation of the fetal shoulders in the same direction by one-eighth of the circle. This would cause the torsion on the fetal neck to get reduced to one-eighth of the circle and would place the shoulders in an oblique diameter, i.e., right oblique with right occipitolateral and left oblique with left occipitolateral.

- *Crowning:* With increasing descent of the fetal head, crowning occurs. During this stage, the biparietal diameter of the fetal head stretches the vaginal introitus. Even as the uterine contractions cease, the head would not recede back during the stage of crowning **(Figs. 2.32A and B)**.
- *Extension:* Fetal head pivots under symphysis pubis and emerges out through extension, followed by occiput, then the face, and finally the chin **(Fig. 2.32C)**.

- *Restitution:* Following the delivery of fetal head, the neck, which had undergone torsion previously, now untwists and aligns along with the long axis of the fetus.
- *External rotation of the head:* As the undelivered shoulders rotate by one-eighth of the circle to occupy the AP diameter of the pelvis, this movement is visible outside in the form of external rotation of fetal head **(Fig. 2.32D)**, causing the head to further turn to one side.

Following the engagement of the fetal shoulders in the AP diameter of the pelvis anterior shoulder slips under symphysis pubis, followed by posterior shoulder **(Figs. 2.32E and F)**. Once shoulders have delivered, the rest of the trunk is delivered by lateral flexion.

NORMAL VAGINAL DELIVERY

Predelivery Preparation

- *Patient position:* The patient is commonly placed in the dorsal lithotomy position with left lateral tilt.
- *Cleaning and draping:* Vulvar and perineal cleaning and draping with antiseptic solution must be done. The sterile drapes must be placed in such a way that only the area immediately around the vulva and perineum is exposed.
- *Six cleans recommended by the WHO:* The following six cleans have been recommended by the WHO, to be taken care of at the time of labor and delivery to minimize the chances of infection:
  - Clean hands
  - Clean perineum
  - Clean delivery surface
  - Clean cord-cutting instruments
  - Clean cord care
  - Clean cord ties
- *Bladder to be emptied:* If at any time during the abdominal examination the bladder is palpable, the patient must be encouraged to void. If despite distended bladder the patient is unable to void, catheterization is indicated.
- *Patient monitoring:* Maternal BP and pulse should be recorded every hour during the first stage of labor and every 10 minutes during the second stage of labor.
- *Fetal heart rate monitoring:* The fetal heart rate should be recorded immediately after a contraction at least every 30 minutes during the active phase of the first stage of labor and at least every 15 minutes (or after every contraction) during the second stage.
- *Induction of labor:* This is required to make the cervix soft and pliable and/or to induce uterine contractions.

> **Q. Discuss the role of partogram in the management of labor.**
>
> **Q. Discuss briefly about partogram and its clinical significance.**

- *Partogram:* Normal labor was previously plotted graphically on a modified WHO partograph. The WHO has now devised a new monitoring tool called the WHO labor care guide **(Fig. 2.33)**. Both the tools are graphical representations of progress of labor in terms of the woman's cervical dilatation and descent of the fetal presenting part against time. Both the tools involve formal regular monitoring of important clinical parameters describing the well-being of the mother as well as the baby. This new labor Care Guide comprises 7 sections, some of which were adapted from the previous partograph design. These are as follows:
  - *Section 1:* Identifying information and labor characteristics at admission
  - *Section 2:* Supportive care
  - *Section 3:* Care of the baby
  - *Section 4:* Care of the woman
  - *Section 5:* Labor progress
  - *Section 6:* Medication
  - *Section 7:* Shared decision-making

For all observations, there is a horizontal time axis where the clinician can document the corresponding time of observation. There is a vertical reference values axis for determination of any deviation from normal observations.

However, there are some important differences between these two which are summarized in **Table 2.13**.

Conducting Normal Vaginal Delivery

Conducting a normal vaginal delivery involves the following steps:

1. *Delivery of fetal head:* With the increasing descent of the head, the perineum bulges and thins out considerably. As the largest diameter of the fetal head distends the vaginal introitus, the crowning is said to occur **(Figs. 2.32A and B)**.
2. As the head distends the perineum and it appears that tears may occur in the area of vaginal introitus, mediolateral surgical incision called episiotomy **(Figs. 2.34A to C)** may be given. Episiotomy is no longer recommended as a routine procedure and is performed only if the obstetrician feels its requirement.
3. As the fetal head progressively distends the vaginal introitus, the obstetrician in order to facilitate the controlled birth of the head must place the fingers of one hand against the baby's head to keep it flexed and apply perineal support with the other hand. Increasing flexion of the fetal head would facilitate the delivery of the smallest diameter of fetal head. This can be achieved with the help of Ritgen maneuver. In this maneuver, one of the obstetrician's gloved hand is used

Normal Labor in Occipitolateral Position

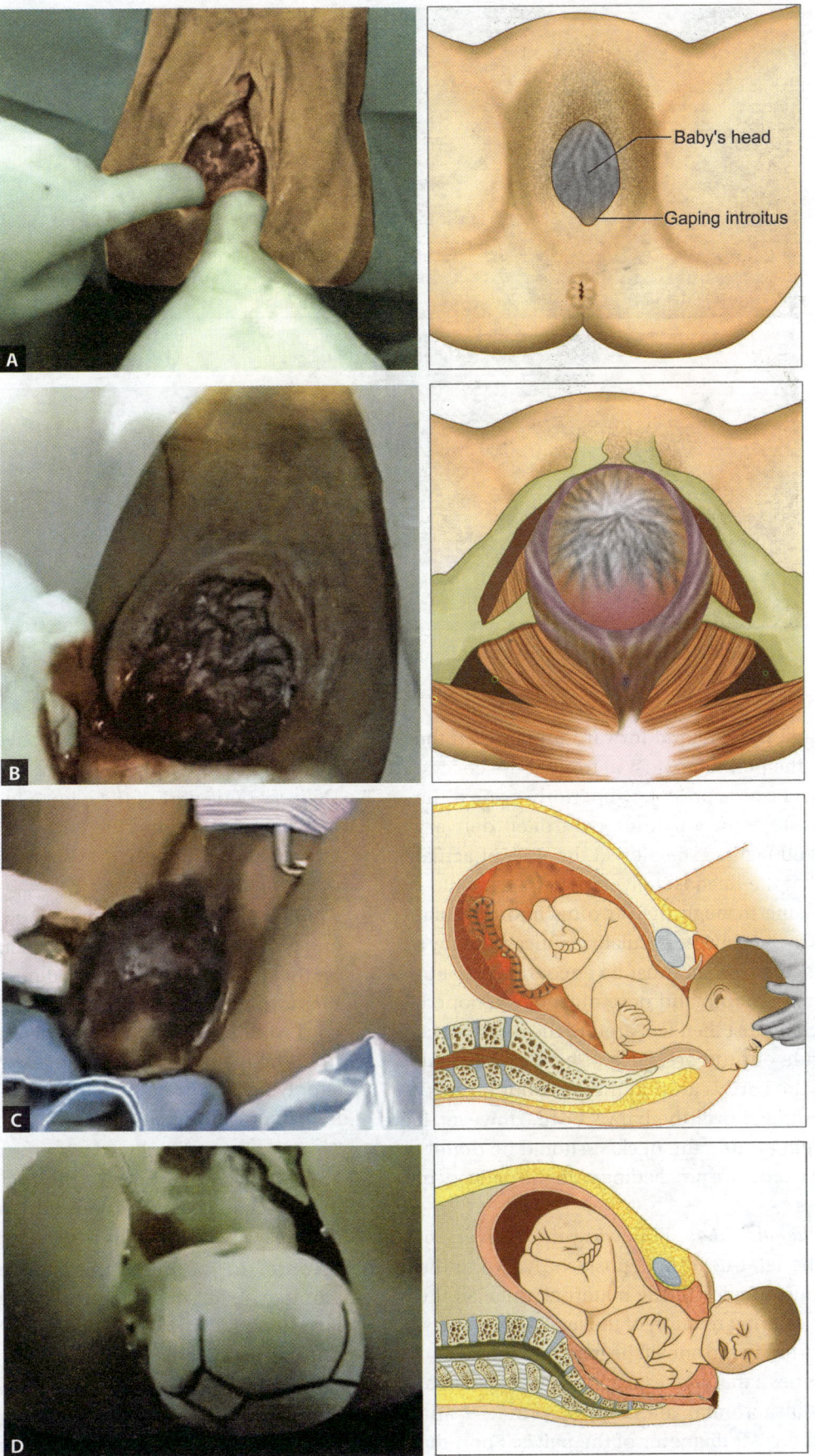

Figs. 2.32A to D: (A) Baby's head visible through the vaginal introitus; (B) Crowning of the fetal head; (C) Delivery of the fetal head; (D) External rotation of head allowing delivery of shoulders.

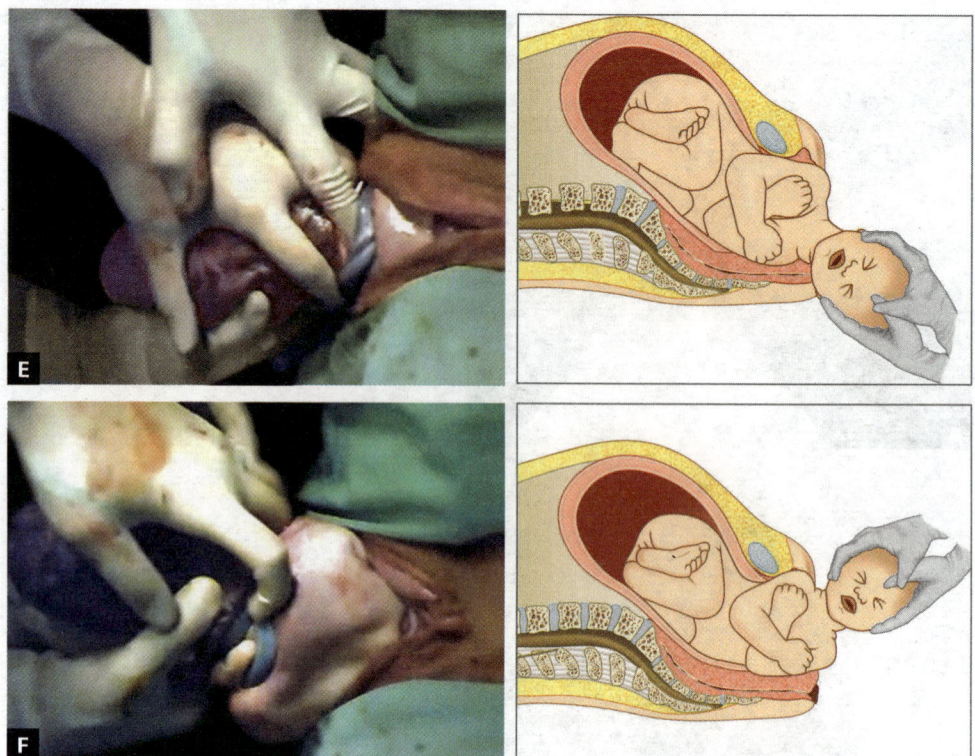

Figs. 2.32E and F: (E) Delivery of anterior shoulder; (F) Delivery of posterior shoulder.

for exerting a downward and forward pressure on the chin through the perineum, just in front of the coccyx. The other hand exerts pressure superiorly against the occiput. This helps in providing controlled delivery of the head and favors extension at the time of actual delivery so that the head is delivered with its smallest diameter passing through the introitus and minimal injury occurs to the pelvic musculature. Once the baby's head delivers, the woman must be encouraged not to push. The baby's mouth and nose must be suctioned. The obstetrician must then feel around the baby's neck in order to rule out the presence of cord around the fetal neck. If the cord is around the neck but is loose, it should be slipped over the baby's head. However, if the cord is tight around the neck, it should be doubly clamped and cut before proceeding with the delivery of fetal shoulders.

4. *Delivery of the shoulders*: Following the delivery of fetal head, the fetal head falls posteriorly, while the face comes in contact with the maternal anus. As the restitution or external rotation of the fetal head occurs, the occiput turns toward one of the maternal thighs and the head assumes a transverse position. This movement implies that bisacromial diameter has rotated and has occupied the AP diameter of the pelvis. Soon the anterior shoulder appears at the vaginal introitus. Following the delivery of the anterior shoulder, the posterior shoulder is born. The obstetrician must move the baby's head posteriorly to deliver the shoulder that is anterior.

5. *Delivery of the rest of the body*: This is followed by the delivery of the rest of the body. The rest of the baby's body must be supported with one hand as it slides out of the vaginal introitus.

6. *Clamping the cord*: The umbilical cord must be clamped and cut if not done earlier. Two clamps must be placed on the umbilical cord and cord must be cut in between them with the help of scissors. Delayed clamping of the cord would help in transferring about 80 mL of blood from the placenta to the neonate, which would help in supplying 50 mg of iron to the fetus. This strategy would help in preventing the development of anemia.

7. The baby must be placed over the mother's abdomen and then handed over to the assisting nurse or the pediatrician. The baby's body must be thoroughly dried, the eyes wiped, and baby's breathing must be assessed.

8. In order to minimize the chances of aspiration of amniotic fluid, soon after the delivery of the thorax, the face must be wiped and the mouth and fetal nostrils must be aspirated.

9. The baby must be covered with a soft, dry cloth and a blanket to ensure that the baby remains warm and no heat loss occurs. Following the delivery of the baby, the placenta needs to be delivered. The obstetrician must look for signs of placental separation following the delivery of the baby.

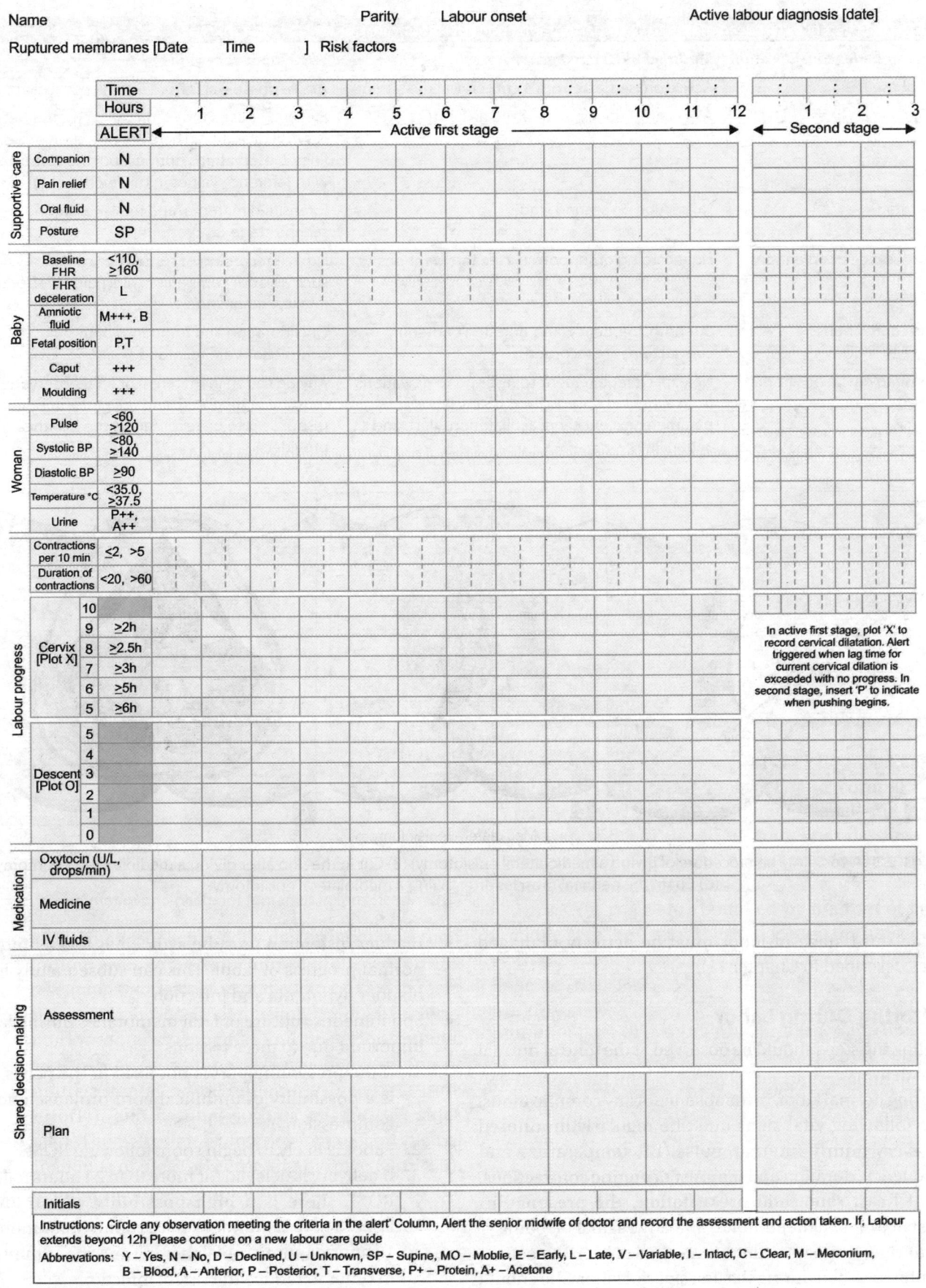

Fig. 2.33: The WHO labor guide.
Source: World health organization. (WHO, 2021). WHO labour care guide: user's manual. [Online]. Available from https://www.who.int/publications/i/item/9789240017566 [Accessed December, 2022].

TABLE 2.13: Differences between modified WHO partograph and WHO labor care guide.

Parameter under consideration	Modified WHO partograph	WHO labor care guide
Active phase	Active phase starts from 4 cm cervical dilatation	Active phase starts from 5 cm cervical dilatation
Alert and action lines	Alert and action lines are fixed at 1 cm/h	Evidence-based time limits at each centimeter cervical dilatation. There are no action or alert lines. Observations during labor are compared with reference values in the "Alert" column
Second stage	No section on second stage	Intensified maternal and fetal monitoring in the second stage
Supportive care interventions	No recording of supportive care interventions	Explicit recording of supportive care interventions such as labor companionship, pain relief, oral fluid intake, and posture
Uterine contractions	Strength, frequency, and duration of uterine contractions are recorded	Only duration and frequency of uterine contractions are recorded
Response to deviations from expected observations	No explicit requirement to respond to deviations from expected observations of any labor parameter except cervical dilatation, alert, and action lines	Any deviation in maternal or fetal observation must be highlighted, and the corresponding response is to be recorded by the healthcare provider

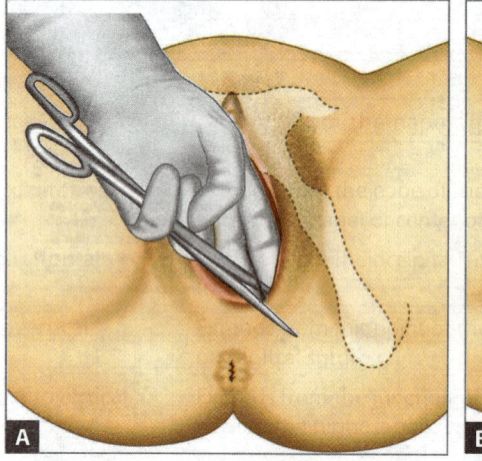
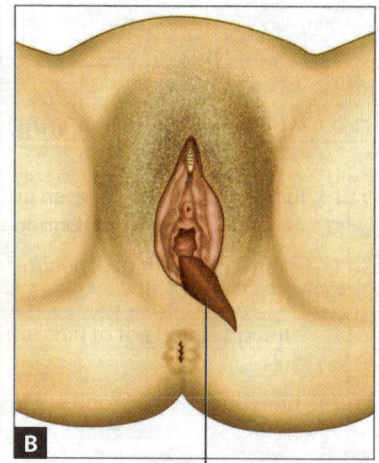
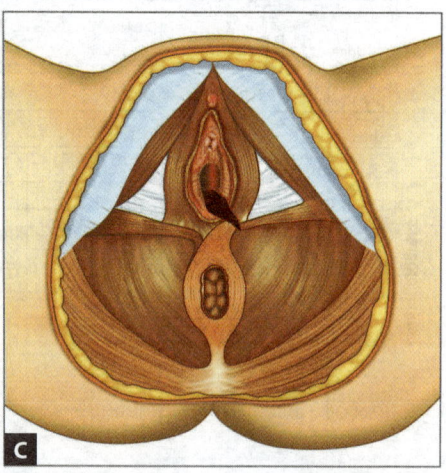

Mediolateral episiotomy

Figs. 2.34A to C: (A) The procedure of giving a mediolateral episiotomy; (B) Cut in the skin after giving a mediolateral episiotomy; (C) Cut in the perineal muscles after giving a mediolateral episiotomy.

10. The third stage of labor must be actively managed (as described in Chapter 14).

Monitoring During Labor

The following steps should be observed at the time of normal vaginal delivery:

- During normal labor, in the absence of any complications, the following vital signs must be regularly monitored at every hourly interval: pulse, BP, temperature and frequency, duration and intensity of uterine contractions, fetal heart rate, fetal presentation, the presence or absence of fetal membranes, and any vaginal bleeding.
- In normal pregnancy, there is no need to keep the patient confined to bed during the first stage of labor. She should be encouraged to move about in the labor room or sit on a birthing ball. She can assume any position in which she is comfortable in the bed.
- Bladder distention must be avoided as it can hinder the normal progress of labor. This can subsequently lead to bladder hypotonia and infection.
- Spontaneous rupture of fetal membranes during labor is important due to three reasons:
  1. If the presenting part is not fixed in the pelvis, there is a possibility of umbilical cord prolapse and cord compression.
  2. Labor is likely to begin soon, following ROM.
  3. If delivery is delayed for more than 24 hours following ROM, there is a high possibility of intrauterine infection. If membranes have ruptured for more than 18 hours, antimicrobial therapy must be administered in order to reduce the risk of infection.
- During the second stage of labor, the woman must be encouraged to push down with each uterine contraction and then relax at the time the contractions stop. During

this period of active bearing down, the fetal heart rate must be auscultated following each uterine contraction. Though FHS may be slow immediately following a contraction, it must normally recover in the time interval before the next contraction begins.

Induction of Labor

 Q. Write a short note on cervical ripening.
 Q. Discuss the methods to prime the cervix at term.

Induction of labor can be defined as commencement of uterine contractions before the spontaneous onset of labor with or without ruptured membranes. It is indicated when the benefits of delivery to the mother or fetus outweigh the benefits of continuing the pregnancy. Induction of labor comprises cervical ripening and labor augmentation. While cervical ripening aims at making the cervix soft and pliable, augmentation refers to stimulation of spontaneous uterine contractions, which may be considered inadequate due to failed cervical dilation or fetal descent. Indications for induction of labor are listed in **Table 2.14**. Various methods for induction of labor are enumerated in **Box 2.6**.

Pharmacological methods for labor induction commonly comprise prostaglandins [dinoprostone (PGE_2) or misoprostol (PGE_1)] and/or oxytocin. Dinoprostone helps in cervical ripening and is available in the form of gel (Prepidil or Cerviprime) or a vaginal insert (Cervidil). Prepidil comprises 0.5 mg of dinoprostone in a 2.5 mL syringe. The gel is injected intracervically every 6 hours for up to three doses in a 24-hour period.

Cervidil, on the other hand, is a vaginal insert containing 10 mg of dinoprostone. The main advantage of Cervidil is that it can be immediately removed in case it causes hyperstimulation. The use of misoprostol for cervical ripening is an off-label use, which is still considered controversial by some clinicians. However, its use is recommended by the ACOG. A dose of 25 μg is placed transvaginally at every 3-hour interval for a maximum of four doses, or it may be prescribed in the oral dosage of 50 μg orally at every 4-hour interval.

Oxytocin is a uterotonic agent, which stimulates uterine contractions and is used for both induction and augmentation of labor. It can be started in low dosage regimens of 0.5–1.5 mU/min or high dosage regimen of 4.5–6.0 mU/min, with incremental increases of 1.0–2.0 mU/min at every 15–40 minutes. If an intrauterine pressure catheter is in place, measurement of intrauterine pressure ranging between 180 and 200 Montevideo units/period is an indicator of adequate oxytocin dosing.

Intracervical application of dinoprostone (PGE_2, 0.5 mg gel) is the gold standard for cervical ripening. 100 μg of oral or 25 μg of vaginal misoprostol has been found to be similar in efficacy to intravenous oxytocin for labor induction.

Epidural Analgesia

Epidural analgesia has presently become a commonly employed technique for providing pain relief during labor. It should be administered only once the diagnosis of labor has been established and the patient requests for pain relief. It should be provided by practitioners only in settings where facilities for resuscitation are immediately available. This technique involves injection of a local anesthetic agent [approximately 10 mL of 0.25% bupivacaine (Marcaine) or 0.25% of ropivacaine, with or without a small dose of a lipid-soluble opioid (e.g., fentanyl or sufentanil)] into the epidural space (between the dura mater and the ligamentum flavum) in the space between vertebrae L3 and L4 (**Fig. 2.35**). An indwelling catheter is usually kept in place for repeat injections or continuous infusion. Epidural analgesia must not be administered in the presence of active maternal hemorrhage, coagulation disorders, maternal septicemia, and/or infection at the insertion site. It is indicated for the following conditions:

- Provision of pain relief during first and second stages of labor
- Facilitation of patient cooperation during labor and delivery
- Provision of anesthesia for episiotomy or forceps delivery or extension for cesarean delivery

During the second stage of labor, it is important to ensure that the segmental extent of epidural analgesia has spread to include the S2–4 nerve roots in order to maintain analgesia in the perineal region.

TABLE 2.14: Indications for induction of labor.

Maternal indications	Fetal indications
• Ruptured membranes with preeclampsia or eclampsia or nonreassuring fetal heart status • Diabetes mellitus • Renal disease • Abruptio placenta • Rh isoimmunization	• Postmaturity • Intrauterine growth restriction • Premature rupture of membranes • Fetus with congenital anomalies • Intrauterine death
Indications specific to pregnancy	
• Oligohydramnios • Polyhydramnios	

BOX 2.6: Methods for induction of labor.

Medical methods:
- Pitocin
- Vaginal prostaglandins [dinoprostone (PGE_2) or misoprostol (PGE_1)]

Surgical methods:
- Low rupture of membrane and stripping of membranes
- Mechanical dilation (through use of dilators, osmotic dilation with laminaria tents, balloon catheters, etc.)

PG: prostaglandin

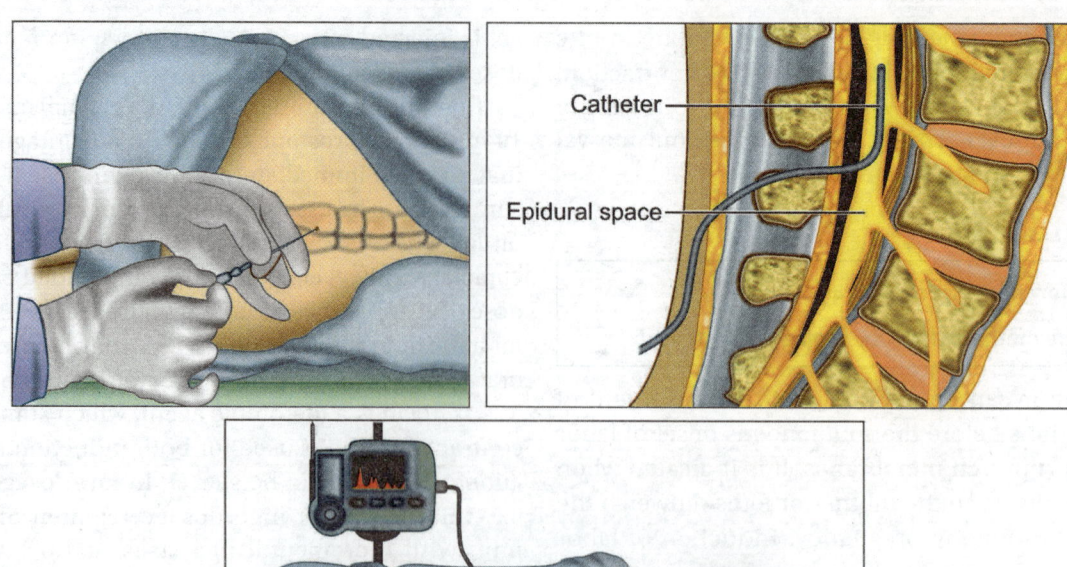
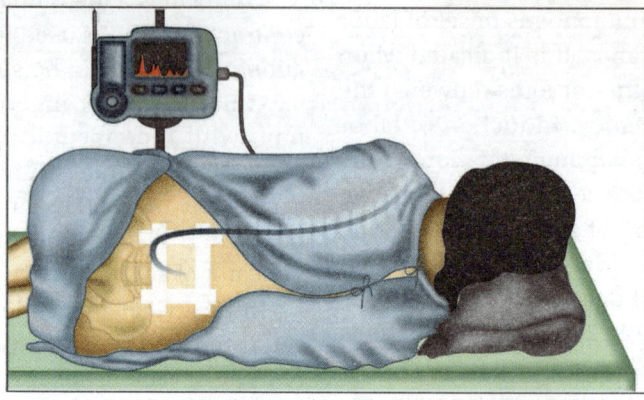

Fig. 2.35: Administration of epidural analgesia.

COMPLICATIONS

DYSTOCIA

Dystocia means difficult labor and can be defined as abnormally slow progress of labor. This could be due to abnormalities in power (abnormal uterine contractions), passage (bony pelvis), or the passenger (fetus). The term dysctocia has now become outdated and replaced by the terminology, "prolonged labor."

PROLONGED LABOR

If a woman's cervix fails to dilate as per the standards of Friedman's curve, she is traditionally assigned to the diagnosis of failure to progress and is usually delivered by cesarean section. 'Failure to progress' is one of the most important causes for unplanned cesarean deliveries in the United States. Though the Friedman's curve was published nearly 60 years ago, it continues to serve as the basis of how most physicians describe normal labor. According to the Friedman's curve, abnormal progress of labor can be defined as the lack of changes or minimal change in cervical dilatation or effacement during a 2-hour period (for each of the phase: latent and active phase) in a woman having regular uterine contractions before the beginning of second stage of labor or as a descent of ≤1 cm/h in nullipara and ≤2 cm/h in multipara during the second stage of labor (from complete cervical dilatation to delivery). Indicators for abnormal labor have been described in **Table 2.15**.

Modern researchers, however, feel that the Friedman's curve can no longer be applied to today's women because there have been many changes in the medical practice since 1955. Women are no longer sedated during labor. However, epidurals are commonly used. Use of epidural analgesia is likely to lengthen both the first and second stages of labor. Also, oxytocin is much more frequently used for both labor induction and augmentation. Women in labor tend to belong to older age groups in comparison to the average age of 20 years included in the Friedman's study.

A study by Zhang et al. (2010) has shown that in the modern times, mothers do not rapidly start dilating at 3 cm as was observed by Dr Friedman in 1955. Instead, most modern women (both nullipara and multipara) begin active labor when they are 6 cm dilated. Before the cervical dilatation of 6 cm was reached, the progress in both nulliparas and multiparas appeared at a similar pace. However, after 6 cm, labor accelerated at a much faster pace in multiparas in comparison to the nulliparas. Majority of women took less than 2 hours to dilate by 1 cm during the active phase of labor. Interestingly, no dilatation occurred in many women for long periods, nevertheless they had a normal vaginal delivery.

The average rate of dilatation for the modern women was 1.2 cm/h during the active stage of labor. These results were different from those described by Friedman, according

TABLE 2.15: Diagnostic criteria for abnormal labor based on Friedman's labor graph.

Indicator	Nullipara	Multipara
Prolonged latent phase	>20 hours	>14 hours
Average second stage	50 minutes	20 minutes
Prolonged second stage without (with) epidural	>2 hours (>3 hours)	>1 hour (>2 hours)
Protraction disorders		
Protracted active phase dilation	<1.2 cm/h	<1.5 cm/h
Protracted descent	≤1 cm/h	≤2 cm/h
Arrest disorders		
Prolonged deceleration	>3 hours	>1 hour
Secondary arrest of dilation*	>2 hours	>2 hours
Arrest of descent*	>1 hour	>1 hour
Failure of descent	No descent in the deceleration phase or the second stage of labor	
Third-stage disorders		
Prolonged third stage	>30 minutes	>30 minutes

*Adequate contractions >200 Montevideo units per 10 minutes for 2 hours

to whom 1.2 cm/h was the lowest acceptable rate of cervical dilation. In other words, what Friedman considered as slow labor is actually the normal rate of dilatation in the present time. Due to this discrepancy in Friedman's data and that in the modern times, many women may be incorrectly diagnosed as having failure to progress, when in fact they may be having normal labor.

The average duration of second stage of labor for nulliparous women was 1.1 hours with an epidural and 0.6 hours without an epidural. On the other hand, the average duration of second stage of labor for multiparous women was less than 0.5 hours with an epidural and about 0.25 hours without an epidural.

In the year 2012, the American College of Obstetricians and Gynecologists (ACOG), the Society for Maternal-Fetal Medicine, and the National Institute for Maternal and Child Health came together in a joint workshop and proposed new definitions for abnormal and arrested labor **(Table 2.16)**.

Etiology

Various causes for abnormal progress of labor include abnormalities in the passage (bony pelvis and the soft tissues within the semirigid structure), passenger (baby), and the power (expulsive uterine contractions). These comprise of the following abnormalities:

- *Abnormalities in expulsive forces:* These include—
  - Hypotonic uterine dysfunction (uterine inertia)
  - Hypertonic uterine dysfunction
  - Poor maternal expulsive efforts (related to maternal fatigue or epidural analgesic use).
- *Fetal abnormalities:* These include—
  - Abnormalities in fetal size (e.g., fetal macrosomia, with fetal weight ≥4,000 g)
  - Abnormalities in fetal presentation (e.g., brow, shoulder, and face)
  - Abnormalities in fetal position (e.g., occiput posterior, etc.): Fetal malpresentations and malpositions may cause larger diameter of the fetal presenting part to present at the pelvic inlet. This may interfere with the rotation of fetal head, thereby impeding progress
  - Abnormalities in fetal attitude (extension, asynclitism, etc.)
  - Fetal congenital abnormalities (anencephaly, fetal ascites, fetal tumors, etc.).
- *Pelvic abnormalities:* These include—
  - Cephalopelvic disproportion (CPD)
  - Cervical dystocia.

Deformities of bony pelvis are rare in developed countries where the nutritional status during childhood is adequate. However, this may not be the situation in developing countries like India. Also, soft tissue abnormalities can also influence the outcome of labor, e.g., abnormalities in the remodelling of cervix and space-occupying lesions in the pelvis such as cervical fibroids, ovarian cysts, etc.

Diagnosis

Clinical Presentation

These include the following:

- Lack of change or minimal change in cervical dilatation or effacement during a 2-hour period (for each of the phase: latent and active phase) in a woman having regular uterine contractions before the beginning of the second stage of labor.
- Descent of ≤1.0 cm/h in nullipara and ≤2.0 cm/h in multipara during the second stage of labor.

Abdominal Examination

- Establishing and documenting an estimated fetal weight
- Monitoring the FHR and uterine contraction patterns.

Vaginal Examination

Vaginal examination should be regularly performed to monitor the progress of cervical dilation and descent of the fetal presenting part as described in the clinical presentation.

Vaginal examination should also involve the following:

- *Clinical pelvimetry:* This is important for assessing the pelvic type (android, gynaecoid, platypelloid, and anthropoid) and the presence of CPD, if any.
- *Evaluation of the position of fetal head:* This should be preferably done early in labor, because as labor

Normal and Abnormal Presentations

TABLE 2.16: New definitions for abnormal and arrested labor.

Condition describing abnormal labor	Old definition (based on the ACOG Practice Bulletin, 2003)	New evidence-based definition (Joint Workshop, 2012)
Labor dystocia	Slow, abnormal progression of labor	This terminology is no longer used
Failure to progress	A vague term implying lack of progressive cervical dilatation, lack of descent of the baby's head or both	The workshop authors recommend that adequate time must be allowed for the normal latent and active phases of the first stage and for the second stage as long as the maternal and fetal conditions remain within normal limits
Active labor	A woman is said to be in active labor after she attains a dilatation of about 3–4 cm. This is the time after which there should be a rapid increase in cervical dilatation	A woman is said to be in active labor after she attains a dilatation of about 6 cm. Multiparous women are likely to progress faster in comparison to the nulliparous women after this point
Arrest of first stage of labor	Labor in the first stage is diagnosed as arrested when the woman in active labor has no change in cervical dilatation even after 2 hours despite of having adequate contractions	• Labor in the first stage is diagnosed as arrested when the woman with cervical dilatation of 6 cm and with ruptured membranes has no cervical changes for 4 hours or more despite of having adequate contractions for 6 hours or more of inadequate contractions • In case the woman's cervix has dilated less than 6 cm, she requires additional time and interventions before arrest of labor can be diagnosed
Arrest of second stage of labor	This can be diagnosed in the presence of following conditions: • >3 hours in a nulliparous woman with an epidural • >2 hours in a nulliparous woman without an epidural • >2 hours in a multiparous woman with an epidural • >1 hour in a multiparous woman without an epidural	This can be diagnosed in the presence of following conditions provided there is no descent or rotation of the baby: • After ≥4 hours in nulliparous women with an epidural • After ≥3 hours in nulliparous women without an epidural • After ≥3 hours in multiparous women with an epidural • After ≥2 hours in multiparous women without an epidural
Failed induction of labor	Progression of labor differs significantly for women with an elective induction of labor in comparison with women who have had a spontaneous onset of labor. At least 12–18 hours of latent labor must be allowed before arriving at the diagnosis of failed induction. This practice may help in reducing the rate of cesarean deliveries	Failure to have regular contractions (every 3 minutes) and failure of the cervix to change after at least 24 hours of oxytocin (and ruptured membranes, if possible). This time should be measured following the completion of cervical ripening

(ACOG: American College of Obstetricians and Gynecologists).

progresses, caput and moulding may interfere with the correct assessment.

Investigations

- *Imaging studies:* X-ray pelvimetry and CT pelvimetry may be helpful for assessment of the maternal bony pelvis. These studies will help to reassure the clinician regarding pelvic adequacy and for ruling out CPD as the probable cause of abnormal labor.
- *Partogram:* The simplest test used for evaluating abnormal progress of labor is to plot the patient's progress (cervical dilation and the decent of fetal presenting part) on a partogram (especially the new WHO care guide).
- *Cardiotocography:* Intermittent auscultation and cardiotocography can be used for monitoring the FHR, especially when the labor is progressing abnormally. The clinician should make sure that the fetal heart tracing remains reassuring throughout the course of labor. Cardiotocography also helps in the evaluation of uterine contractions (especially their strength and frequency).
- *Ultrasound:* Examination by ultrasound helps in confirming an abnormal position, e.g., occiput posterior position as a cause of abnormal progress of labor. This may be sometimes useful when the diagnosis by clinical examination appears questionable.

Management

Patients with prolonged latent phase can be managed in the following ways:

- *Optimisation of maternal wellbeing:* This can be ensured by provision of maternal hydration, pain relief, and provision of one-to-one care or professional maternal companion, if not already provided. The carer need not necessarily be the midwife and should not be the husband or partner. Meta-analysis of randomised controlled trials has shown that the continuous presence of a caregiver or continuous support during labor is likely to improve outcomes for women and infants including increased rate of spontaneous vaginal delivery and reduced likelihood of medication for pain relief, instrumental vaginal delivery, cesarean section, and a 5-minute APGAR score of less than 7. Presently, there is no evidence of any harm caused by continuous support during labor.

- *Amniotomy:* Though amniotomy is traditionally practiced to shorten the duration of labor, meta-analysis has shown that amniotomy is not associated with a statistically significant reduction in the duration of first stage in nulliparous or multiparous women. Amniotomy is therefore not recommended to be used routinely as part of standard labor management and care.
- *Mobilisation during labor:* According to the present recommendations, women in low-risk labor should be informed about the benefits of upright positions, and encouraged and assisted to assume whatever positions they choose.
- *Stimulation with oxytocin:* It is possible to manipulate the component of 'power' or abnormalities in expulsive function to some extent. The frequency, intensity, and duration of uterine contractions can be augmented through the use of oxytocin. However, use of oxytocin may not be practical in all situations. Also, it has the potential for inducing iatrogenic fetal compromise. Women with dysfunctional labor are likely to gain some benefit.

Use of oxytocin is encouraged by National Institute for Health and Care Excellence (NICE) (2014) for nulliparous women and has been shown to shorten the duration of labor. However, it is not likely to bring down the rate of first-stage cesarean sections. Moreover, in case of multiparous women, if there are chances of obstructed labor, forcing uterine contractions with oxytocin can result in uterine rupture. Therefore, NICE has recommended that oxytocin should only be started in multiparous women once the obstetrician has made full assessment. Current guidelines do not recommend the use of syntocinon in the second stage whether or not the regional anesthesia is in place. The only exception to this would be cases where there are poor contractions at the beginning of second stage in nulliparous women with regional anesthesia.

In cases of uterine hypocontractility, oxytocin (30 units diluted in 500 mL of saline) must be started at a rate of 0.5–1.0 mU/min and gradually increased by 1–2 mU/min at every 20–30 minutes, until an adequate pattern of contractions is achieved. Oxytocin should be titrated to provide a contraction frequency of 4–5 per 10 minutes with each contraction lasting for approximately 40 seconds. Oxytocin takes 30–45 minutes to reach the steady state levels following intravenous administration. Increment of oxytocin dosage should not be performed more frequently than half-hourly intervals.

Such regimen has been found to be compatible with normal progress of labor with minimal adverse sequela. Appropriate steps must be taken if signs of maternal or fetal distress appear at any time. Amniotomy can also be tried in cases with reduced uterine activity. If there is no response even after 3 hours of augmentation with oxytocin, cesarean section may be required in most of the cases due to the possibility of an underlying CPD.

Continuous fetal monitoring is required with the use of oxytocin irrespective of the patient's parity. Once oxytocin has been commenced, vaginal examination must be done at every 4-hourly intervals. If there has been less than 2 cm progress, decision should be made regarding the requirement for cesarean section. Presently, there is paucity of evidence demonstrating that the use of oxytocin for augmenting labor is likely to improve either maternal or fetal outcome.

- *Assisted vaginal delivery:* Assisted vaginal delivery in the form of vacuum or forceps application can serve as a good option in cases of delayed second stage.
- *Cesarean section:* This may appear to be treatment of choice when vaginal delivery appears to be unsafe.

Complications

Maternal Complications

There is an increased incidence of the following:

- Traumatic injuries (cervical tears, uterine rupture, etc.)
- Increased incidence of operative deliveries
- Chorioamnionitis
- Postpartum hemorrhage
- Puerperal sepsis, subinvolution.

Fetal Complications

These include:

- Fetal hypoxia, thick meconium-stained liquor
- Intracranial stress or hemorrhage
- Variable or delayed decelerations
- Fetal acidosis
- 5-minute APGAR score of less than 7
- Increased rate of admission to the NICU
- Increased perinatal morbidity and mortality.

Conclusion

The Friedman's criteria for normal labor, which is currently being used by most of the healthcare providers, have now largely become obsolete. The new, evidence-based definitions of normal labor, labor arrest, and failed induction, which have been proposed by ACOG, the Society for Maternal Fetal Medicine, and the National Institute for Maternal and Child Health in a joint workshop (2012), should now be adopted by the obstetricians.

As long as mother and baby are both healthy, and as long as the length of labor does not qualify for being labeled as 'arrested labor,' laboring women should be treated as if they are having normal progression of labor. More time must be allowed to women, who are being medically induced, for completion of the early phase of labor.

Essentially, 6 cm and not 3–4 cm should be considered as the beginning of the active phase. Caregivers should always remember that during the normal latent phase of labor (before the dilatation of 6 cm), sometimes there may be no change in the cervical dilation for several hours.

Immobilization in the first stage has been associated with longer duration of labor and NICE discourages women from staying supine. Not lying down in supine position and not being in lithotomy position has been associated with shorter duration of second stage and lower rates of cesarean section. The present evidence indicates that walking and upright positions in the first stage of labor is likely to reduce the duration of labor, the risk of cesarean birth, and the requirement for epidural analgesia. Moreover, this does not seem to be associated with increased requirement for intervention or cause any adverse effect on maternal and neonatal well-being. Better quality trials are still required in future to confirm the true risks and benefits of upright and mobile positions in comparison with recumbent positions for all women during labor.

Women should be given an adequate time for both the first and second stages of labor. An 'adequate' time in labor is much longer than what has traditionally been allowed by Friedman in the past. Regardless of parity, delivery should be accomplished preferably within 4 hours of full dilatation. The evaluation of the descent of fetal head may be complicated due to development of moulding and caput formation. In nulliparous patients, inadequate uterine activity is a common cause of primary dysfunctional labor, while in multiparous patients, CPD is the common cause.

PRECIPITATE LABOR

Q. Write a short essay on precipitate labor.

Precipitate labor is normally very short, lasting for <2–3 hours. It can be defined as the type of labor where the total duration of first and second stages of labor is <2 hours.

Etiology

Precipitate labor occurs due to causes which result in strong uterine contractions and reduced soft-tissue resistance, e.g., multiparity.

Diagnosis

Pelvic examination: Rate of cervical dilatation is 5 cm or more per hour for nulliparous women.

Management

Obstetric management in these cases with previous history of precipitate labor comprises the following steps:
- Uterine contractions can be suppressed by administration of magnesium sulfate or ether.
- Delivery of fetal head should be controlled.
- Liberal episiotomy should be given to prevent tears.
- Augmentation with oxytocin must be avoided.

Complications

Maternal Complications

Maternal complications include:
- Extensive lacerations of vagina and perineum, and cervical tears
- Postpartum hemorrhage due to uterine atony
- Uterine inversion or uterine rupture
- Infection
- Amniotic fluid embolism

Fetal Complications

Fetal complications include:
- Intracranial hemorrhage
- Erb–Duchenne brachial palsy
- Injury to the fetal head, especially if delivery occurs in the standing position

OBSTRUCTED LABOR

Kindly refer to Chapter 6 for details related to obstructed labor.

EVIDENCE-BASED CLINICAL TRIALS

List of references can be scanned through QR code to enable the readers gain deeper insight of the subject by referring to the entire article or its abstract.

CHAPTER 3

Breech Presentation

CASE STUDY

A 30-year-old primigravida patient with 39 completed weeks of gestation having breech presentation as diagnosed by ultrasound examination had presented for regular antenatal checkup. No other abnormality was detected on the ultrasound.

INTRODUCTION

DEFINITION OF BREECH PRESENTATION

The fetus lies longitudinally with the buttocks and/or feet presenting in the lower pole of the uterus. The incidence of breech presentation may be 20% at 28 weeks of gestation, which reduces to 3–4% at term. Irrespective of the mode of delivery, cesarean or vaginal birth, term babies presenting by breech have a worse outcome than the cephalic ones. The different types of breech presentations are shown in **Figures 3.1A to C** and are described in the following text.

Frank Breech

Frank breech is the most common type of breech presentation (50–70% cases). Buttocks present first with flexed hips and legs extended on the abdomen. This position is also known as the pike position.

Complete Breech

Also known as the cannonball position, this type of presentation is present in 5–10% cases. In this, the buttocks present first with flexed hips and flexed knees. Feet are not below the buttocks.

Footling Breech

One or both feet present as both hips and knees are in extended position. As a result, feet are palpated at a level lower than the buttocks. This type of presentation is present in 10–30% cases.

The denominator of breech presentation is considered to be the sacrum. Depending on the relationship of the sacrum with the sacroiliac joint, the following positions of the breech are possible **(Fig. 3.2)**. These include the left sacroanterior (LSA) position, right sacroanterior (RSA) position, right sacroposterior (RSP) position, and left sacroposterior (LSP) position. LSA position is the most common position. In general, the sacroanterior positions are more common than the sacroposterior positions because in these positions, the concavity of fetal front fits into the convexity of the maternal spine.

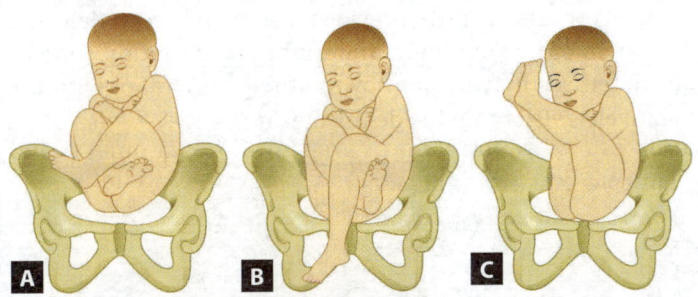

Figs. 3.1A to C: Different types of breech presentation. (A) Complete breech; (B) Footling; (C) Frank breech.

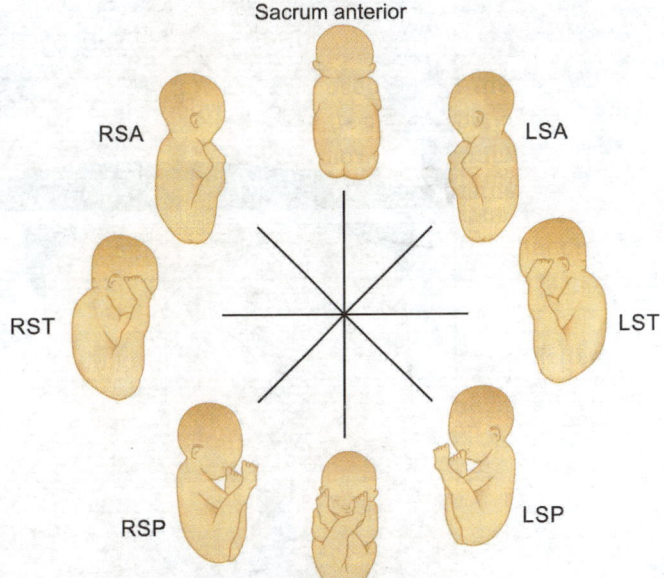

Fig. 3.2: Different positions of the breech. (LSA: left sacroanterior; LSP: left sacroposterior; LST: left sacrum transverse; RSA: right sacroanterior; RSP: right sacroposterior; RST: right sacrum transverse)

HISTORY AND CLINICAL PRESENTATION

RISK FACTORS

Q. Write a short note on the causes of breech presentation.

Normally, the fetus is adapted to the pyriform shape of the uterus, with the larger buttocks in the fundus and smaller head in the lower uterine segment. Any factor which interferes with this adaptation, allows free mobility, and prevents spontaneous version can be considered as a cause for breech presentation.

Maternal Factors

Maternal risk factors for breech presentation include cephalopelvic disproportion, contracted maternal pelvis, liquor abnormalities (polyhydramnios, oligohydramnios), uterine anomalies (bicornuate or septate uterus), space-occupying lesions (e.g., fibroids in the lower uterine segment), placental abnormalities (placenta previa, cornuofundal attachment of placenta), multiparity (especially grand multiparas), cord abnormalities (very long or very short cord), previous history of breech delivery, presence of pelvic tumor, and multifetal gestation (one or more fetuses may present by the breech to adapt with the relatively small room inside the uterine cavity.)

Fetal Factors

Fetal risk factors for breech presentation include prematurity, fetal anomalies (e.g., neurological abnormalities, hydrocephalus, anencephaly, and meningomyelocele), intrauterine fetal death, etc.

GENERAL PHYSICAL EXAMINATION

No specific finding is observed on general physical examination.

SPECIFIC SYSTEMIC EXAMINATION

ABDOMINAL EXAMINATION

Inspection of the Abdomen

A transverse groove corresponding to the fetal neck may be seen above the umbilicus. In a patient with thin built, the fetal head may be seen as a localized bulge in one hypochondrium.

Abdominal Palpation

Fetal lie is longitudinal with fetal head on one side and breech on the other side **(Figs. 3.3A to D)**.

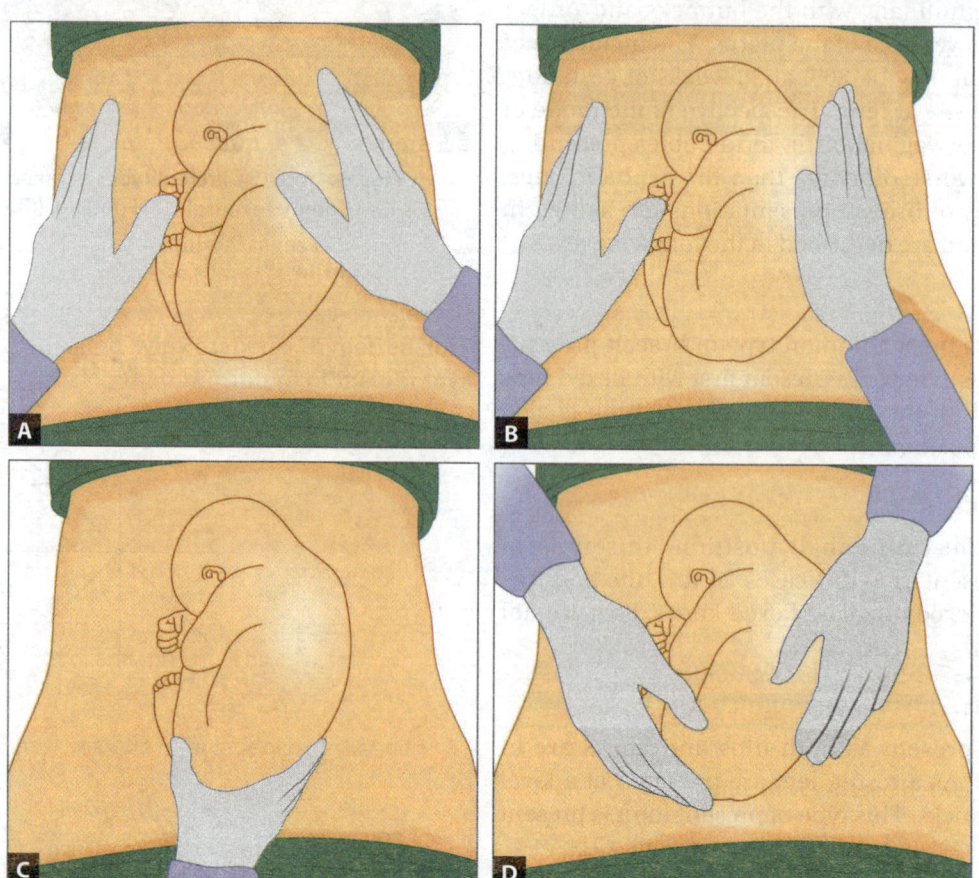

Figs. 3.3A to D: Various Leopold's maneuvers demonstrating abdominal palpation in case of breech presentation. (A) Fundal grip; (B) Lateral grip; (C) Leopold's third maneuver; (D) Leopold's fourth maneuver.

First Leopold Maneuver/Fundal Grip

A smooth, hard, ballotable structure, often tender, is suggestive of fetal head.

Second Leopold Maneuver/Lateral Grip

A firm, smooth board-like fetal back is identified on one side and knob-like structures suggestive of fetal limbs on the other side. A depression corresponding to the fetal neck may also be identified.

Leopold's Third Maneuver

If the engagement has yet not occurred, the breech is movable above the pelvic brim. The breech is felt as a smooth soft mass continuous with the back. Trials to do ballottement of the breech show that the movement is transmitted to the whole trunk.

Leopold's Fourth Maneuver

Head is not felt in pelvis; instead, an irregular, soft, nonballotable structure suggestive of fetal buttocks and/or feet may be felt.

Fetal Heart Auscultation

In case the engagement has not occurred, FHS is just heard above the umbilicus; if the engagement has occurred, the FHS is heard just below the umbilicus.

VAGINAL EXAMINATION

Following features may be observed on vaginal examination:
- Palpation of three bony landmarks of the breech, namely, ischial tuberosities and sacral tip (**Fig. 3.4**)
- Feet may be felt besides the buttocks in cases of complete breech.
- Fresh meconium may be found on the examining fingers; the presence of thick, dark meconium is a normal finding in cases of breech presentation.
- Palpation of the male genitalia

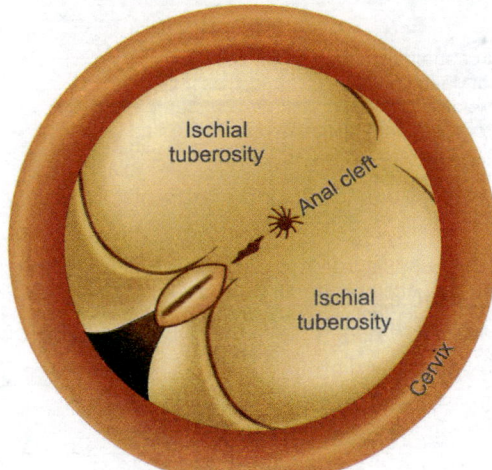

Fig. 3.4: Picture on vaginal examination in case of frank breech.

MANAGEMENT

> Q. Write a long essay critically evaluating the management options in breech presentation.

Management comprising investigations and definitive obstetric management is discussed next.

INVESTIGATIONS

ULTRASOUND EXAMINATION

Ultrasound helps in confirming the type of breech presentation (**Fig. 3.5**). The other things which can be seen on the ultrasound include the following:
- Presence of uterine and/or fetal anomalies
- *Extension of fetal head:* "Stargazing sign" on ultrasound examination can be observed if the degree of extension of fetal head is more than 90°.
- Fetal maturity
- Placental location and grading
- Adequacy of liquor
- Detection of gestational age and fetal weight
- Ruling out multiple gestation (diagnosis of unsuspected twins)
- Exclusion of congenital abnormalities

TREATMENT/OBSTETRIC MANAGEMENT

MANAGEMENT DURING PREGNANCY

> Q. During a routine ANC at 36 weeks, you detect breech presentation in a second gravida. How would you proceed to manage her? Describe with the help of a long essay.

> Q. With the help of a long essay, discuss the management of a primigravida with breech presentation at 37 weeks.

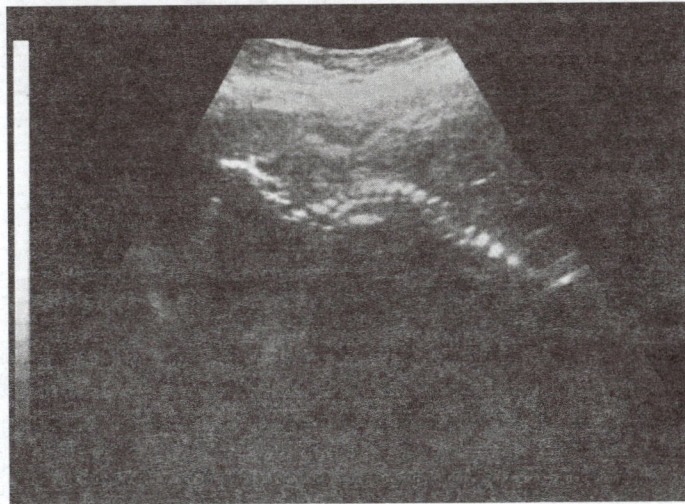

Fig. 3.5: Ultrasound examination showing breech gestation.

68 Normal and Abnormal Presentations

> **Q.** Discuss the management of a primigravida with breech presentation at 38 weeks with the help of a long essay.
>
> **Q.** G2P1L1 with previous normal delivery presents with breech presentation at term. Write a long essay describing the clinical management in this case.
>
> **Q.** Write a short essay on term breech presentation.
>
> **Q.** Describe the management of the case study presented in the beginning of the chapter.
>
> **Q.** Write a short essay on breech delivery in a primary healthcare center (PHC).

The management options for breech presentation include external cephalic version (ECV) during pregnancy or delivery by cesarean section or a breech vaginal delivery at term **(Flowchart 3.1)**. Each of these management options would be described below in detail.

If a patient with breech presentation visits a PHC (primary healthcare center), she should be referred to a community health center (CHC) having facilities for obstetric care and specialist consultations by an obstetrician gynecologist. Facilities for both assisted vaginal breech delivery and cesarean section are available there. Therefore, management options in these patients remain the same as described above.

External Cephalic Version

> **Q.** Write a short essay on ECV: Indications, timing, procedure, and complications.

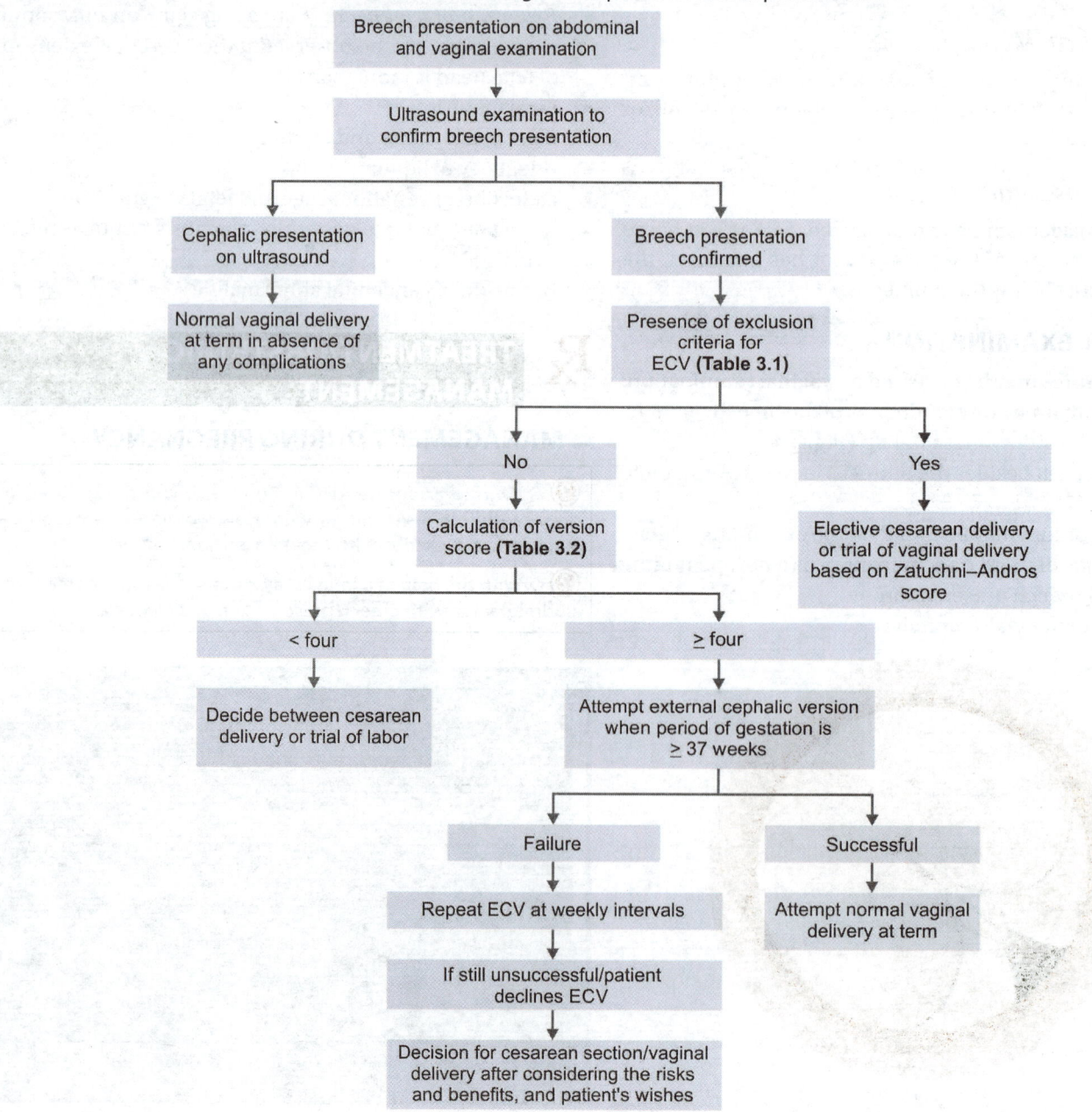

Flowchart 3.1: Management options for breech presentation.

(ECV: external cephalic version)

Definition

External cephalic version is a procedure in which the clinician externally rotates the fetus from a breech presentation into a cephalic presentation. As per the latest RCOG guidelines (2017), women with breech presentation must be offered an ECV if there is an absence of any absolute contraindication for the same. Routine use of external version has been observed to reduce the rate of cesarean delivery by about two-thirds. Therefore, this procedure must become a routine part of obstetric practice. The use of ECV, by reducing the rate of cesarean section, also helps in considerable cost savings. Some clinicians are against the use of ECV due to the assumption that an external version converts only those fetuses to vertex that would have converted spontaneously anyway.

Women need to be counseled that with appropriate precautions, ECV is a safe procedure and is likely to be associated with a very low complication rate. However, they need to be informed that it can be a painful procedure. ECV should only be performed by a trained practitioner or by a trainee working under direct supervision. The use of ECV is associated with minimal risks, including rare complications such as umbilical cord entanglement, abruption placenta, preterm labor, PROM, transient fetal heart changes, and severe maternal discomfort.

Timing for ECV

As per the latest recommendations by the RCOG (2017), ECV should be offered at term from 37^{+0} weeks of gestation. In nulliparous women, it may be offered from 36^{+0} weeks of gestation. The most important reason to wait until the fetus is at term is to avoid iatrogenic prematurity in case emergency delivery is required. This can happen if an attempt at external version results in complications such as active labor, ruptured membranes, and fetal compromise.

Women need to be informed that the success rate of ECV is approximately 50%. They need to be counseled that following an unsuccessful attempt of ECV at 36^{+0} weeks of gestation or later, only a few babies presenting by the breech will spontaneously turn to cephalic presentation. The vice versa is also true, i.e., following a successful attempt at ECV, only a few babies may revert back to breech. A successful ECV is likely to reduce the requirement for a cesarean section for the breech presentation. Women, however, need to be informed that labor after ECV may be associated with a slightly increased rate of cesarean section and instrumental delivery in comparison with spontaneous cephalic presentation. ECV should not be performed in women having contraindications mentioned in **Table 3.1**. However, there is no consensus regarding the eligibility for, or contraindications to, ECV. As per the RCOG guidelines (2017), women should be informed that the risk of scar rupture during ECV after one previous cesarean delivery is no greater than that with an unscarred uterus.

TABLE 3.1: Contraindications for external cephalic version.

Absolute contraindications	Relative contraindications
• Multiple gestations with a breech presenting fetus • Herpes simplex virus infection • Placenta previa • Nonreassuring fetal heart tracing • Premature rupture of membranes • Presence of another obstetric indication for cesarean delivery • Major uterine and/or fetal anomalies • Antepartum hemorrhage within the last 7 days or recurrent antepartum hemorrhage during pregnancy	• Amniotic fluid abnormalities (polyhydramnios or oligohydramnios) • Evidence of uteroplacental insufficiency (small for gestational age fetus with abnormal Doppler parameters, preeclampsia, etc.) • Maternal cardiac disease • Women with a uterine scar

Prerequisites for ECV

Before the performance of ECV, the following prerequisites should be fulfilled:

- The place where ECV is being performed should have all facilities available for fetal monitoring as well as for cesarean section or emergency breech vaginal delivery, in case it is required. There is always a possibility for emergency cesarean section during the procedure in case there is a decline in FHR. Continuous electronic fetal monitoring is required after the procedure.
- Blood grouping and cross-matching should be done in case an emergency cesarean section is required.
- In case the mother is Rh-negative, administration of 50 µg of anti-D immunoglobulin is required after the procedure to prevent the risk of isoimmunization. Anesthetists must be informed well in advance. Maternal intravenous access must be established.
- The woman is not required to be nil by mouth for the procedure.
- An ultrasound examination must be performed to confirm breech, check the rate of fetal growth, amniotic fluid volume, and rule out anomalies associated with breech.
- A nonstress test or a biophysical profile must be performed prior to ECV to confirm fetal well-being.
- Though ECV can be performed by a clinician single-handedly, an assistant is also required.
- Before performing an ECV, a written informed consent must be obtained from the mother.
- Use of tocolysis with betamimetics is likely to improve the success rates of ECV by producing uterine relaxation. A tocolytic agent such as terbutaline in a dosage of 0.25 mg may be administered subcutaneously.

- Routine use of regional analgesia or neuraxial blockade is not recommended but may be considered in cases for a repeat attempt or in cases where the women are unable to tolerate ECV without the use of analgesics. The main disadvantage of these regional analgesic procedures is that the lack of maternal pain could potentially result in excessive force being applied to the fetus without the knowledge of the operator.
- Whether the process has been successful or has failed, a nonstress test and ultrasound examination must be performed after each attempt of ECV and after the end of the procedure to rule out fetal bradycardia and to confirm successful version.
- If ECV is unsuccessful, then the obstetrician can discuss further options with the woman. These include repeat ECV attempt, vaginal breech delivery, or an elective cesarean section.

Procedure

- The patient is placed in a supine or slight Trendelenburg position to facilitate disengagement/mobility of the breech.
- Ultrasonic gel/talcum powder, almond or vegetable oil are applied liberally over the abdomen in order to decrease friction and reduce the chances of an over-vigorous manipulation. External cephalic version can be performed by a clinician experienced in the procedure along with his/her assistant.
- Initially, the degree of engagement of the presenting part should be determined, and gentle disengagement of the presenting part is performed if possible.
- While performing the ECV, the clinician helps in gently manipulating the fetal head toward the pelvis while the breech is brought up cephalad toward the fundus. Two types of manipulation of fetal head can be performed: a forward roll or a backward roll. The clinician must attempt a forward roll first and then a backward roll, if the initial attempt is unsuccessful. Though it does not matter in which direction the fetus is flipped, most physicians tend to start with a forward roll.
- The forward roll (**Figs. 3.6A to D**) is usually helpful if the spine and head are on opposite sides of the maternal midline.
- If the spine and head of the fetus are on the same side of the maternal midline, then the backflip may be attempted (**Figs. 3.7A to C**). If the forward roll is unsuccessful, a second attempt is usually made in the opposite direction. The use of an acoustic stimulator has been described by some researchers to help change the position of the fetal spine from midline to lateral,

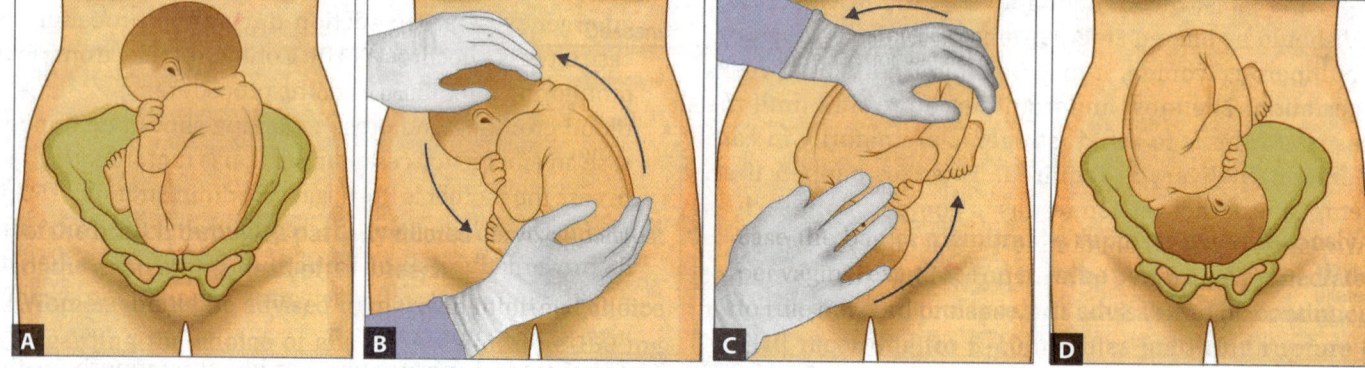

Figs. 3.6A to D: External cephalic version through forward roll. (A) Baby in breech presentation; (B) Forward roll: The breech is disengaged and simultaneously pushed upward; (C) The vertex is gently pushed toward the pelvis; (D) Forward roll is completed.

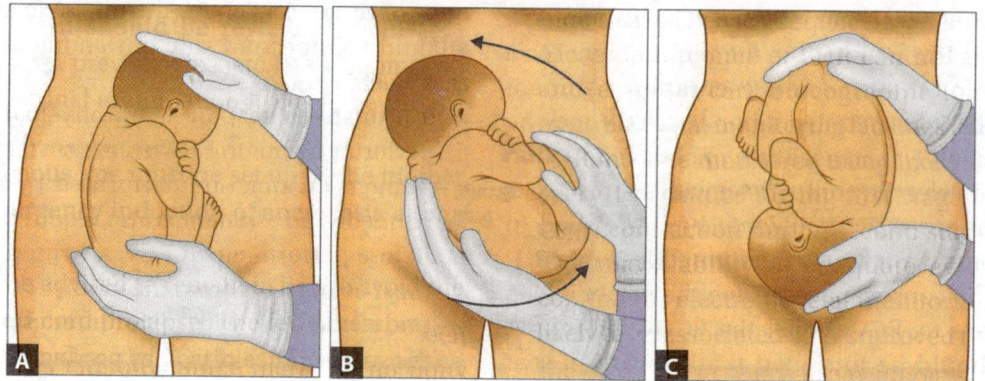

Figs. 3.7A to C: External cephalic version through backflip. (A) Disengaging the breech; (B) Pushing the breech upward and gently guiding the vertex toward the pelvis; (C) Completing the backflip.

thereby improving the chances of success. However, the advantages of the routine use of acoustic stimulation in the clinical practice have not yet been proven.
- While doing the ECV, the fetus should be moved gently rather than using forceful movements.
- If unsuccessful, the version can be reattempted at a later time. The procedure should only be performed in a facility equipped for emergency cesarean section.
- No consensus has been reached regarding how many ECV attempts are appropriate at one particular time. At a particular time setting multiple attempts can be made, making sure that the procedure does not become uncomfortable for the patient. Also, FHR needs to be assessed after each attempt at ECV. Usually, no more than three attempts should be made at a particular sitting.
- If an attempt at ECV proves to be unsuccessful, the practitioner has the option of either sending the patient home and adopting an expectant management policy or proceeding with a cesarean delivery. Expectant management also involves repeat attempts of ECV at weekly intervals. With expectant management, there is also a possibility that the fetus would undergo spontaneous reversion into cephalic position.

Complications of ECV

Though ECV is largely a safe procedure, it can rarely have some complications, including the following:
- Premature onset of labor
- Premature rupture of the membranes
- A small amount of fetomaternal hemorrhage. This is especially dangerous in cases of Rh-negative pregnancies as it can result in the development of Rh isoimmunization. Therefore, in cases of Rh-negative pregnancy, anti-D immunoglobulins must be administered to the mother following the procedure of ECV.
- Fetal distress leading to an emergency cesarean delivery
- *Failure of version:* The baby might turn back to the breech position after the ECV is done. ECV is associated with high rate of spontaneous reversion into breech presentation if performed before 36 weeks of gestation.
- *Risk of cord entanglement:* If fetal bradycardia is detected after a successful version, it is recommended that the infant be returned to its previous breech presentation with the hope of reducing the risk of a tangled cord.
- Transient reduction of the FHR, probably due to vagal response related to head compression with ECV

Indicator of Successful ECV

Some of the indicators of successful ECV include the following:
- *Multiparity:* ECV is more likely to be successful in multiparous women.
- *Nonfrank breech:* ECV is more likely to be successful in nonfrank breech (complete breech) pregnancies in

TABLE 3.2: The external version score.

Parameter	0	1	2
Parity for external cephalic version (ECV)	0	1	≥2
Dilatation	≥3 cm	1–2 cm	0 cm
Estimated fetal weight	<2,500 g	2,500–3,500 g	>3,500 g
Placenta	Anterior	Posterior	Fundal
Station	≥–1	–2	≥–3

comparison to frank breech pregnancies. This is so as the splinting action of the spine in a frank breech gestation is likely to prevent movement of the fetus.
- *Unengaged breech:* Engaged fetus in breech presentation is less likely to undergo version in comparison to the unengaged fetus in breech presentation.
- *Adequate liquor:* Presence of reduced (oligohydramnios) or excessive liquor (polyhydramnios) is likely to interfere with successful version.
- *Fetal acoustic stimulation and transabdominal amnioinfusion of saline:* Their role in improving the success rate of ECV has yet not been proven.

External Version Score

The external version score **(Table 3.2)** helps in predicting the success rate of ECV. Five factors (parity, placental location, dilatation, station, and estimated fetal weight) are used for calculating this score. A higher version score (≥4) is associated with an increased likelihood of successful breech version.

The type of breech (frank, complete, or footling) is not a factor in determining eligibility for ECV. ECV has also been found to be safe in those who have a history of cesarean birth in the past and are the candidates for VBAC. External version has been used successfully in VBAC candidates without any increase in the incidence of adverse effects including uterine rupture.

■ MANAGEMENT DURING LABOR

> Q. With the help of a long essay, discuss breech vaginal delivery and the causes of perinatal morbidity and mortality, which may be present in these cases.

Mode of Delivery

Women who have declined ECV or in whom ECV has been unsuccessful, and eventually present with breech at term, must be given two choices regarding the mode of delivery: breech vaginal delivery (also known as trial of breech) or an elective cesarean section. There has been much controversy for choosing the best option for delivery. Women must be counseled regarding the risks and benefits of each. They need to be informed that planned cesarean section is likely to result in a small reduction in perinatal mortality compared with planned vaginal breech delivery. The reduced risk occurs due to the avoidance of stillbirth after 39 weeks of gestation, the avoidance of intrapartum risks, and the risks associated with the vaginal breech birth. The decision to perform a cesarean section must be taken after balancing the benefits of cesarean section versus the adverse consequences resulting from this. Women also need to be informed that successful vaginal birth is associated with least complications for the mother. On the other hand, planned cesarean section is associated with a higher risk for the mother, with the risk being highest with an emergency cesarean section. An emergency cesarean section may be required in approximately 40% of women planning a vaginal breech birth. Cesarean birth is likely to increase the risk of complications in future pregnancies, such as requirement of cesarean section in future pregnancies, increased risk of complications during repeat cesarean section, and the risk of an abnormally invasive placenta. If a vaginal breech delivery is planned, the healthcare provider must document a detailed informed consent, explaining the higher risks of perinatal or neonatal mortality or short-term serious neonatal morbidity in comparison to a planned cesarean delivery.

Presently, the trend for term breech presentation is elective cesarean section. With an increase in the rates of cesarean sections for breech presentation, vaginal breech deliveries are being performed at a much lower rate. The breech scoring system by Zatuchni and Andros **(Table 3.3)** can be also used for deciding whether to perform a vaginal or an abdominal delivery. If the woman has a score of 3 or less in this scoring system, it means that she should probably be delivered by a cesarean section, which would be associated with a lower degree of fetal morbidity and mortality in comparison to vaginal delivery. Higher scores, although not guarantying a safe vaginal delivery, suggest that a trial of labor (TOL) with close monitoring can be considered. Women should be informed that a planned vaginal breech birth is likely to be associated with a higher risk in the presence of factors mentioned in the **Box 3.1**.

If the woman is diagnosed to be having persistent breech presentation, she should be assessed for risk factors associated with poor outcomes in case of planned vaginal breech birth. In the presence of any risk factor, women should be counseled that planned vaginal birth is likely to be associated with increased perinatal risk. In such cases, delivery by cesarean section is recommended.

Choosing the Route of Delivery for a Woman with Breech Presentation at Term

Vaginal breech deliveries had been routinely used in the past. The question regarding the use of vaginal route or abdominal route for delivery of the fetuses in breech presentation has been associated with much controversy. This controversy was particularly flared up after the declaration of the results of "the term breech trial (TBT)" (2000), a large multicentric randomized controlled trial, designed to determine the safest mode of delivery for a term breech fetus. The results of this trial showed that perinatal mortality and morbidity were significantly lower for women with breech presentation undergoing planned cesarean delivery in comparison to those having planned vaginal delivery. In breech presentation, a sudden delivery of fetal head can cause excessive pressure on the aftercoming head of the breech, resulting in a high risk for tentorial tears and intracranial hemorrhage in comparison to the fetuses in cephalic presentation. After the declaration of these results, it was proposed that all breech presentations should be delivered abdominally to reduce the rates of perinatal morbidity and mortality. As a result, there was an abrupt shift in clinical practice, and term breech cesarean section rates increased around the world. Following the publication of TBT (2000), both the ACOG and the RCOG guidelines recommended that the best method of delivering a term frank or complete breech singleton pregnancy is by planned cesarean section.

However, some authorities still favor vaginal route for breech delivery because numerous weaknesses have also been identified since the publication of TBT despite its various strengths. The recommendations for cesarean delivery were made based on the short-term outcomes.

TABLE 3.3: Zatuchni and Andros score.

Parameter	0 point	1 point	2 points
Parity	Primigravida	Multigravida	–
Gestational age	39 weeks or more	38 weeks	37 weeks
Estimated fetal weight	>8 pounds (3,690 g)	7–8 pounds (3,176–3,690 g)	<7 pounds (<3,176 g)
Previous breech > 2,500 g	None	One	Two or more
Cervical dilatation on admission by vaginal examination	2 cm or less	3 cm	4 cm or more
Station at the time of admission	–3 or higher	–2	–1 or lower

BOX 3.1: Risk factors associated with poor outcomes in case of breech vaginal delivery.

- Poor obstetric history
- Pelvic abnormality
- Previous cesarean section
- Medical maternal conditions, e.g., diabetes and preeclampsia
- Fetal weight estimated to be more than 3,800 g or less than 10th centile
- Presence of hyperextended neck on ultrasound
- Footling presentation
- Antepartum/intrapartum fetal compromise

However, based on the follow-up data from the past 2 years, assessing the long-term outcomes, there appears no evidence to recommend planned cesarean section. It is also recognized that some women will choose to deliver vaginally and not opt for a planned cesarean section. Furthermore, some labor too quickly even when an elective cesarean delivery has been planned. The second study limitation is that larger sample size is required to report accurately on perinatal and maternal mortality rates. Thirdly, there were difficulties in maintaining standardized management protocols across a multitude of sites. Some of these difficulties included variable practitioner experience, requirement of the staff to follow rigid protocols with which they were unfamiliar, unequal access to prenatal diagnosis, electronic FHR monitoring, etc. Fourthly, less than 10% of women in the trial underwent pelvimetry using plain radiography, CT, or MRI scanning. Moreover, in more than 30% cases, attitude of fetal head was determined only using clinical methods and not through ultrasound.

In response to the TBT, Goffinet et al. (2006) published the PREMODA study, a multicenter descriptive study four times larger than the TBT. In this study, data was collected from 8,105 women across 174 centers in France and Belgium. The outcomes of PREMODA study were in stark contrast with those of the TBT. There was no difference in the rates of perinatal mortality or serious neonatal morbidity amongst the groups undergoing TOL or planned cesarean delivery.

As per the Cochrane review (2015), planned cesarean delivery is associated with reduced perinatal or neonatal mortality or serious neonatal morbidity in comparison to the planned vaginal birth. However, this reduction occurs at the expense of somewhat increased maternal morbidity. Moreover, over a 2-year follow-up period, no significant difference in long-term neurodevelopmental delay was observed amongst the two groups.

Years after the analysis of follow-up data from the TBT, both RCOG (2017) and ACOG (2018) recommended that decision regarding the mode of delivery depends upon the patient's preferences, and the experience and judgment of the healthcare provider. Planned vaginal delivery of a singleton breech fetus may be a reasonable option under hospital-specific protocol guidelines. Before deciding the mode of delivery, women should be informed about the benefits and risks, both for the current and future pregnancies, of planned cesarean section versus planned vaginal delivery for breech presentation at term. All women should be given information related to ECV, which must be used as an option unless it is contraindicated, or woman refuses to give her consent.

Though the publication of the TBT has been followed by a large reduction in the incidence of planned vaginal births, vaginal breech births continue to occur mainly due to the reason of maternal choice and to a lesser extent due to factors such as failure to detect breech presentation, presentation of undetected breech in labor, and the limitations of ECV.

Management of Preterm Breech

> **Q.** With the help of a long essay, describe how you shall manage a case of primigravida with breech presentation at 34 weeks.
>
> **Q.** With the help of a short essay, describe the management of a primigravida with breech presentation at 34 weeks' gestation.

There is insufficient evidence to support routine cesarean section for preterm breech deliveries. The mode of delivery for preterm delivery should be individualized for each woman based on the clinical situation (such as stage of labor, type of breech presentation, and fetal well-being), availability of a healthcare provider skilled in conducting vaginal breech delivery, and the wishes of the woman and her partner. The parents should be informed about the perinatal risks associated with breech vaginal delivery.

Women should be informed that planned cesarean section is recommended for preterm breech presentations where the patient needs to be delivered immediately in view of maternal or fetal compromise.

The main problem encountered during preterm breech delivery is entrapment of head due to the delivery of the trunk through an incompletely dilated cervix. It is particularly important for preterm breech vaginal deliveries that the obstetrician confirms the second stage by vaginal examination before the patient starts pushing. If the obstetrician is unable to prevent the patient from pushing before full dilatation occurs, then an epidural should be encouraged. If there occurs head entrapment during a preterm (or term) breech vaginal delivery, lateral incisions to the cervix should be considered. In case of head entrapment at the time of cesarean section, extension of the vertical uterine incision may be used, with or without tocolysis. A senior obstetrician and a senior pediatrician must be present at the delivery of all babies with less than 34 weeks of gestation. Since the same maneuvers which are used for delivery of fetal head during breech delivery are used for delivery of fetal head during the cesarean section for breech presentation, there appears to be an equal chance of fetal head entrapment with both the modes of delivery.

Management of Twin Breech

In case of the first twin presenting as a breech, the mode of delivery should be individualized based on parameters such as cervical dilatation, station of the presenting part, type of breech presentation, fetal well-being, and availability of a healthcare provider skilled in taking breech vaginal delivery. Even though there is an absence of sufficient evidence, a planned cesarean section is recommended in case of a twin pregnancy where the first twin is presenting as a breech. In these cases, cesarean delivery is likely to improve neonatal APGAR score at 5 minutes. A cesarean section for the first twin in breech presentation may also prevent the extremely rare complication of "interlocking" if the second twin is vertex. However, if the woman with the first twin in breech has presented in spontaneous labor, routine emergency cesarean section is not recommended.

In case of breech presentation of the second twin, routine cesarean section is not recommended in either term or preterm deliveries.

Management of the Undiagnosed Breech in Labor

Where a woman presents with an undiagnosed breech in labor, discussion between the woman and the senior obstetrician should take place regarding the mode of delivery. The risks related to both cesarean mode of delivery and vaginal delivery should be explained to help the woman make her choice regarding the delivery option.

Elective Cesarean Delivery

The proponents of "elective cesarean section" support cesarean section because of the concern for birth asphyxia and a possibility of an unexpected arrest of fetal parts at the time of vaginal delivery. Increased risk of medicolegal litigations is another factor associated with the rising incidence of elective breech cesarean deliveries. Thus, the management of term breech fetus has largely shifted from routine vaginal breech delivery to elective cesarean delivery for all. In the developing part of the world, it may sometimes not be possible to resort to cesarean delivery in every case of breech presentation. Under nonideal situations, most obstetricians prefer a cesarean delivery. Some of the absolute indications for cesarean section in cases of breech presentation are enumerated in **Box 3.2**. Most obstetricians also consider a cesarean delivery in cases of primigravidas because in these cases, the maternal passages have not been tested for delivery before. However, presently there are no studies to support this. Cesarean delivery is also considered in pregnancies complicated with diabetes, hypertension, placenta previa, prelabor premature rupture of membranes (≥ 12 hours), post-term pregnancy, IUGR, placental insufficiency, etc.

Trial of Breech (Vaginal Breech Delivery)

> Q. With the help of a long essay, discuss breech vaginal delivery and the causes of perinatal morbidity and mortality, which may be present in these cases.

Vaginal breech delivery may become unavoidable in certain situations, e.g., gravidas presenting in advanced labor with a term breech and imminent delivery or in case of a nonvertex second twin. Certain indications for breech vaginal delivery are described in **Box 3.3**.

The major difference between breech vaginal delivery and normal vaginal delivery in cephalic presentation is based on the fact that in cephalic presentation, the head which is the largest and least compressible structure of the fetus is delivered first, followed by the rest of the body. Once the head has delivered in cases of cephalic presentation, the rest of the body follows without much difficulty. On the other hand in breech presentation, the buttocks which are compressible structures are delivered first, followed by the head. This can result in the entrapment of fetal head. The criteria for defining entrapment of fetal head are described in **Box 3.4**. The maximum danger for entrapment of fetal head is the case of footling presentation. In these cases, the fetal leg and foot can deliver through partially dilated cervix followed by entrapment of fetal head. Also, breech presentation is a slow dilator of cervix. Due to an irregular-fitting presenting

---

BOX 3.2: Indications for cesarean section.

- Cephalopelvic disproportion (any degree)
- Placenta previa
- Estimated fetal weight > 4 kg
- Hyperextension of fetal head (as detected on ultrasound examination)
- Susceptibility to cord prolapse
- Footling breech (danger of entrapment of head in an incompletely dilated cervix)
- Severe IUGR
- Clinician not competent with the technique of breech vaginal delivery
- A viable preterm fetus in active labor
- Early bearing down, which causes the foot to pass through the partially dilated cervix and reach the perineum
- Uterine dysfunction

(IUGR: intrauterine growth restriction)

BOX 3.3: Indications for vaginal breech delivery.

- Frank or complete breech (not footling)
- Estimated fetal weight between 1.5 and 3.5 kg
- Gestational age (36–42 weeks)
- Well-flexed fetal head (no evidence of hyperextension of the fetal head)
- Adequate pelvis (no fetopelvic disproportion)
- Normal progress of labor on partogram
- Uncomplicated pregnancy (no contraindications to vaginal birth, e.g., placenta previa and severe IUGR)
- Multiparas
- No obstetric indication for cesarean section (e.g., cephalopelvic disproportion and placenta previa)
- An experienced obstetrician
- Presence of severe fetal anomaly or fetal death
- Mother's preference for vaginal birth
- Delivery is imminent

(IUGR: intrauterine growth restriction)

BOX 3.4: Criteria for describing the entrapment of fetal head.

- More than 90 seconds have elapsed between delivery of fetal head and the body
- Need for additional or unusual maneuvers to affect the delivery of fetal head
- In case of cesarean section, more than 4 minutes have elapsed from the time of uterine incision to the delivery of fetal head

fetal part, the risk of PROM and cord prolapse is increased. Therefore, with breech vaginal delivery anytime during vaginal delivery, a situation may arise when the clinician might have to resort to cesarean section for fetal or maternal sake. Thus, the vaginal breech birth should take place in a hospital with facilities for emergency cesarean section. Risk factors associated with poor outcomes in case of breech vaginal delivery are described in **Box 3.1**.

If a woman with breech presentation, presents with an unplanned labor, plan for management is based on the following:

- *Stage of labor:* Women near or in an established active second stage of labor should not be routinely offered cesarean delivery.
- Factors associated with poor outcomes in case of vaginal birth
- Availability of appropriate clinical expertise on part of the healthcare provider
- Informed consent by the mother

In cases where adequate time is available and circumstances are appropriate, ultrasound should be used to estimate the position of the fetal neck and legs, and fetal weight should be estimated using ultrasound. Based on the findings of clinical assessment and ultrasound, the woman must be counseled like those with planned breech birth.

It has been argued that the maneuvers used for the delivery of aftercoming head of the breech in case of vaginal delivery, including the maneuvers such as Mauriceau–Smellie–Veit maneuver, Burns–Marshall technique, maneuvers for delivering the shoulders and arms, and Pinard's maneuver, may be associated with an increased risk of perinatal and neonatal injuries.

A possibility of entrapment of head can still occur during cesarean delivery as the uterus contracts after delivery of the body up to the level of shoulders. The chances of head entrapment are higher with preterm breeches, especially when a low transverse uterine incision is used at the time of cesarean section. Due to this, some practitioners have routinely started performing low vertical uterine incisions for preterm breeches prior to 32 weeks' gestation to avoid head entrapment. Low vertical incisions may require extension up to the corpus, thereby mandating the requirement for cesarean delivery in all future deliveries.

Certain precautions which a clinician can take to prevent head entrapment include the following:

- At the time of cesarean delivery, the physician must try to keep the membranes intact as long as possible. He/she should move quickly once the breech has been extracted in order to deliver the aftercoming head before the uterus begins to contract. The clinician should make sure that not more than 4 minutes elapse from the time of uterine incision to the delivery of fetal head.
- The transverse uterine incision can be extended vertically upward (T-shaped incision) or laterally while curving upward (J-shaped incision) if any difficulty occurs with delivery of the fetal head.
- A short-acting dose of nitroglycerin can be used to relax the uterus and cervix in order to facilitate delivery.

Vaginal breech delivery may become unavoidable in certain situations, e.g., gravidas presenting in advanced labor with a term breech and imminent delivery or in case of a nonvertex second twin. Certain indications for breech vaginal delivery are described in **Box 3.3**.

While in cephalic presentation, the head delivers gradually after undergoing molding; in breech presentation, the fetal head delivers suddenly. As a result, sudden excessive pressure on the aftercoming head of the breech is associated with a high risk of tentorial tears and intracranial hemorrhage in comparison to the fetuses in cephalic presentation.

Mechanism of Breech Vaginal Delivery

The breech most commonly presents in LSA position, which causes the bitrochanteric diameter of the buttocks (9.5 cm) to enter through the pelvic inlet in the right oblique diameter of the pelvic brim (**Fig. 3.8A**). Once the bitrochanteric diameter has passed through the oblique diameter of pelvis, engagement is said to occur (**Fig. 3.8B**). With full dilatation of the cervix, the buttocks descend deeply into the pelvis. The descent of remaining fetal parts is however slow. The descent of anterior hip is faster than that of posterior hip.

When the buttocks reach the pelvic floor, the anterior hip, which reaches the pelvic floor first, internally rotates through 45° so that the bitrochanteric diameter lies in the AP diameter of the pelvic outlet.

With continuing fetal descend, the anterior buttock appears at the vulva. With further uterine contractions, the buttocks distend the vaginal outlet. There is delivery of anterior hip followed by that of posterior hip by lateral flexion. The anterior hip slips out under the pubic symphysis, followed by the lower limbs and feet (**Fig. 3.8C**).

Following the delivery of buttocks and legs, sacrum rotates by 45° in the direction opposite to the internal rotation, resulting in the external rotation of the breech. This causes the back to turn anteriorly (**Fig. 3.8D**). With continuing descent, the bisacromial diameter (12 cm) of the shoulders engages in right oblique diameter of the pelvis and descent continues (**Fig. 3.8E**). On touching the pelvic floor, the anterior shoulders undergo internal rotation by 45° so that the bisacromial diameter lies in the AP diameter of the outlet. Simultaneously, the buttocks and sacrum externally rotate anteriorly through 45°.

As the anterior shoulder impinges under the pubic symphysis, the posterior shoulders and arm are born over the perineum, followed by the delivery of anterior shoulder. Following the delivery, anterior shoulders undergo restitution

76 Normal and Abnormal Presentations

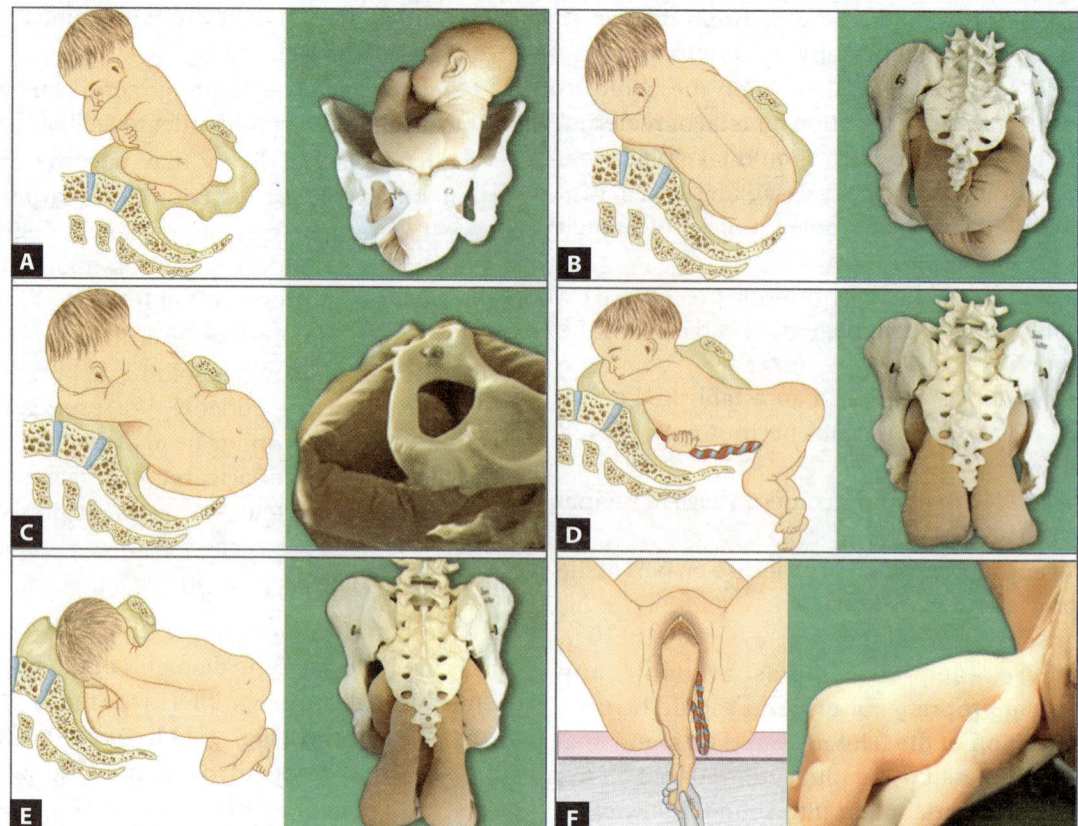

Figs. 3.8A to F: Mechanism of breech vaginal delivery. (A) Descent of buttocks through the pelvic inlet; (B) Engagement of breech; (C) Delivery of hips, lower limbs, and feet; (D) External rotation of breech (back/sacrum turns anteriorly); (E) Engagement of the bisacromial diameter in the right oblique diameter of pelvis followed by the delivery of arms and shoulders; (F) Suboccipitobregmatic diameter of the baby's head engages in left oblique diameter of the pelvis.

through 45° and assume a right oblique position. At the same time the neck undergoes torsion of 45°. As a result, the engaging diameter of the head (suboccipitofrontal diameter, 10.5 cm) or suboccipitobregmatic diameter engages in the left oblique diameter of the pelvis **(Fig. 3.8F)**. Descent into the pelvis occurs with flexion of the fetal head. The flexion of fetal head is often maintained by uterine contractions aided by suprapubic pressure applied by the delivery assistant at the time of delivery. When the head reaches the pelvic floor, it undergoes internal rotation by 45° so that the sagittal sutures lie in the AP diameter of the pelvis, with the occiput present anteriorly and brow in the hollow of the sacrum. As the nape of the neck impinges against the pubic symphysis, the chin, mouth, nose, forehead, bregma, and occiput are born over the perineum by flexion.

Types of Breech Vaginal Delivery

Three types of vaginal breech deliveries are described below:
1. *Spontaneous breech delivery:* No traction or manipulation of the infant by the clinician is done. The fetus delivers spontaneously on its own. This occurs predominantly in very preterm deliveries.
2. *Assisted breech delivery:* This is the most common mode of vaginal breech delivery and is illustrated in **Figures 3.9A to N**. In this method, a "no-touch technique" is adopted in which the infant is allowed to spontaneously deliver up to the umbilicus, and then certain maneuvers are initiated by the obstetrician to aid in the delivery of the remainder of the body, arms, and head.
3. *Total breech extraction:* In this method, the fetal feet are grasped, and the entire fetus is extracted by the clinician. Total breech extraction should be used only for a noncephalic second twin (see Chapter 9); it should not be used for singleton fetuses because the cervix may not be adequately dilated to allow passage of the fetal head.

Intrapartum Care for Patients Undergoing Breech Vaginal Delivery

Intrapartum care for patients undergoing breech vaginal delivery has been described in **Flowchart 3.2**.
- Informed consent must be taken from the patient after explaining that the trial of breech can fail in 20% cases, thereby requiring a cesarean section.
- Breech presentation should be confirmed by an ultrasound examination in the labor ward.
- Plan for vaginal breech delivery must be clearly documented in the mother's notes.

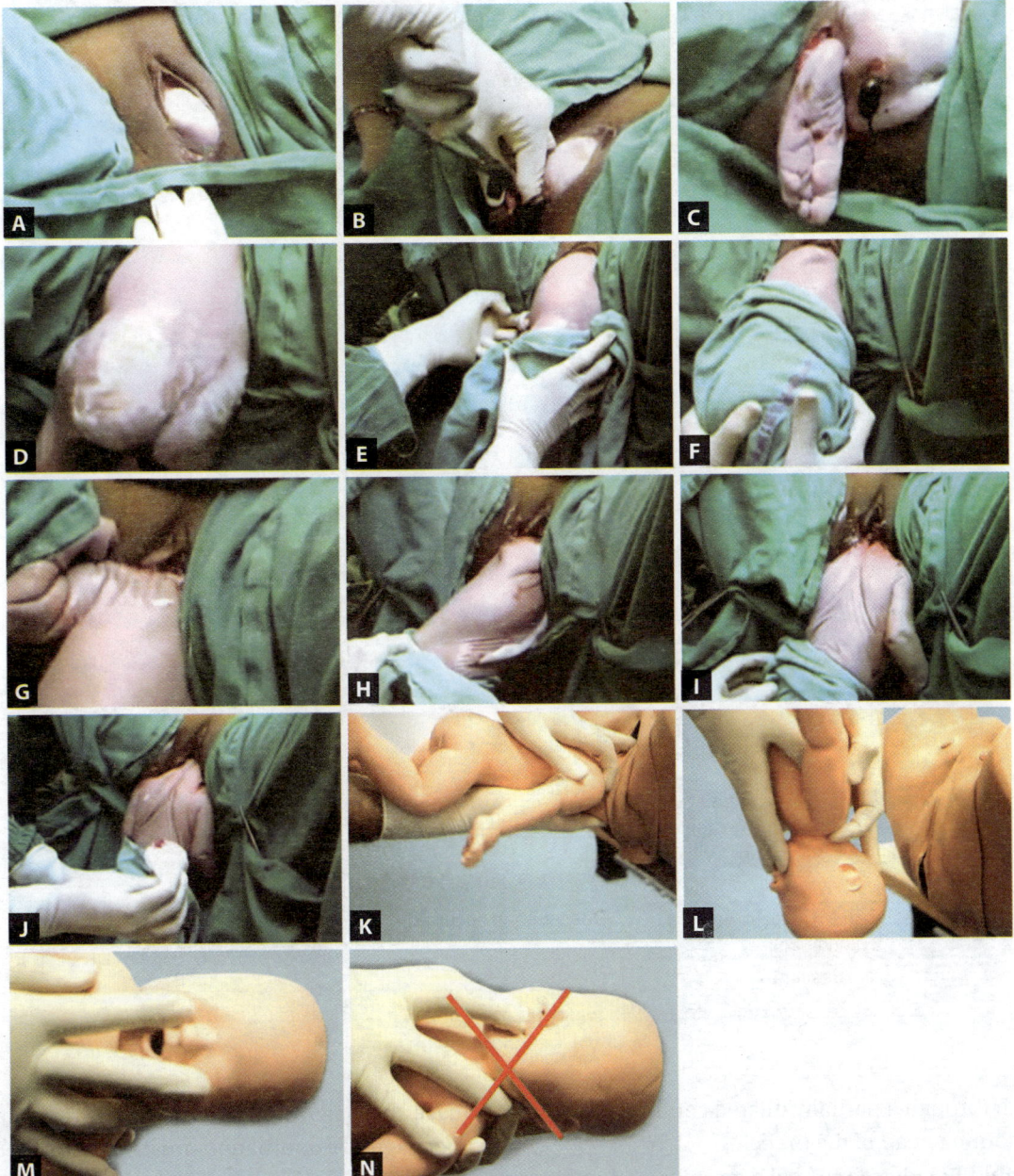

Figs. 3.9A to N: Steps of assisted breech vaginal delivery in case of frank breech. (A) Breech is observed climbing the perineum, i.e., the fetal presenting part does not recede back into the perineum even after the contraction stops; (B) Episiotomy is often performed in cases of assisted vaginal delivery to prevent soft-tissue dystocia; (C) A no-touch policy is adopted while the baby's buttock and external genitalia are observed to be descending; (D) No outward/downward traction is applied until the fetus has delivered up to the level of umbilicus; (E) Towel is wrapped around the fetal hips and the baby's back is turned anteriorly; (F) Slight gentle traction is applied in downward and outward directions in conjunction with uterine contractions until the fetal scapulae are visible; (G) The fetus is rotated by 90° to deliver the anterior shoulder. The baby's arm is swept out of the vagina; (H) The fetus is rotated by 180° to deliver the posterior shoulder; (I) Delivery of the posterior arm and forearm; (J) The baby is allowed to hang by its own weight until the nape of neck is visible; (K and L) Delivery of the head is completed by Mauriceau–Smellie–Veit maneuver; (M) Correct method of application of the obstetrician's fingers over the baby's maxilla and face; (N) Wrong method of application of fingers over the baby's face. The obstetrician's finger must not be inserted in the baby's mouth at the time of Mauriceau–Smellie–Veit maneuver.

- Care should be provided by an experienced obstetrician and midwife. Anesthetist and pediatrician must also be present. A pediatrician is needed because of the higher prevalence of neonatal depression and an increased risk for unrecognized fetal anomalies. An anesthesiologist may be needed if intrapartum complications develop, and the patient requires general anesthesia.

- Early assessment by an anesthetist is recommended. Presently, the effect of epidural analgesia on the success of vaginal breech birth is not clear. However, it is likely to increase the risk of intervention. Lumbar epidural analgesia is likely to provide pain relief and prevent voluntary bearing-down efforts prior to complete dilatation of cervix. This is likely to help prevent slipping

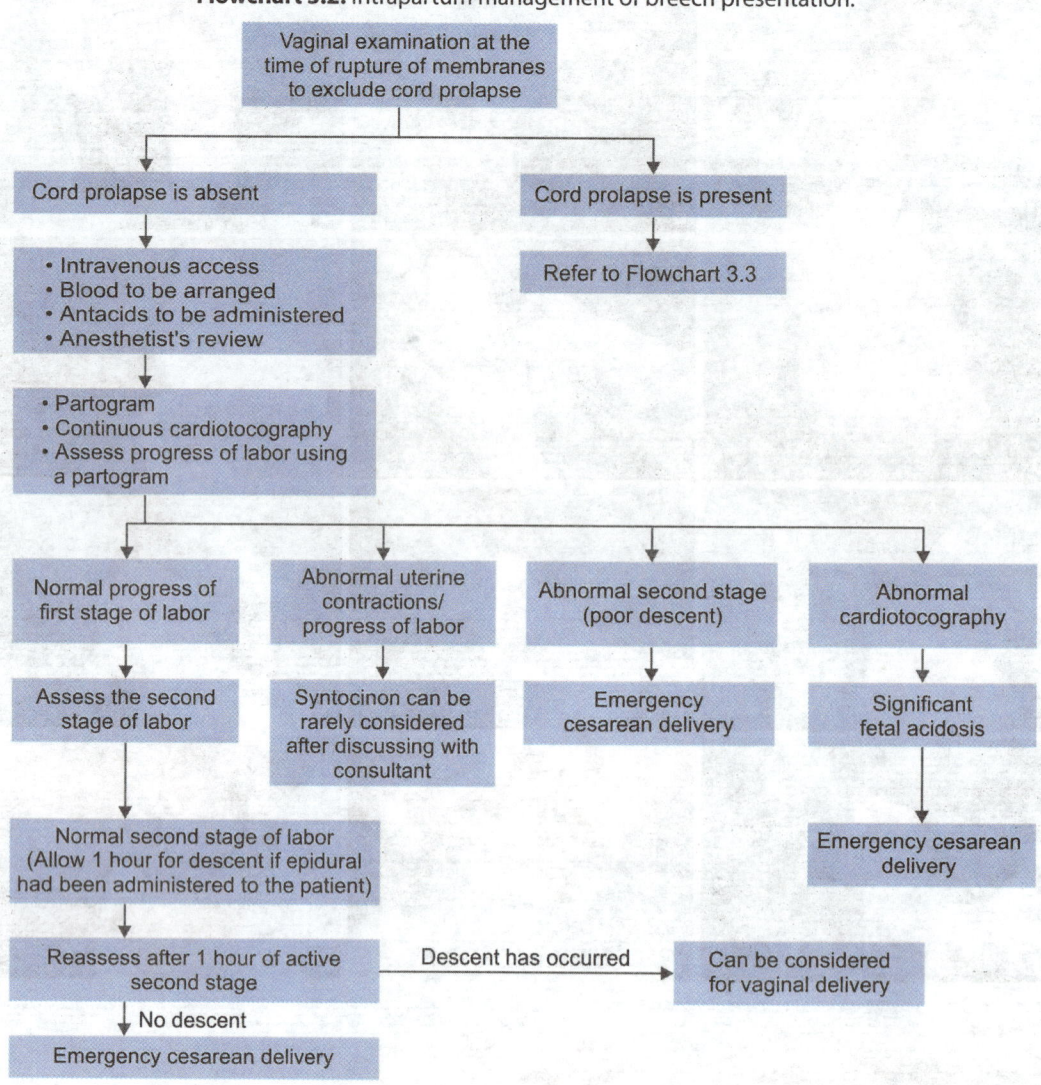

Flowchart 3.2: Intrapartum management of breech presentation.

of the breech through a partially dilated cervix and arrest of the aftercoming head of the breech.

- Women should be advised to make an informed choice regarding the choice of analgesia. Ranitidine 150 mg orally must be administered every 6 hours in case cesarean delivery is required in future.
- At the time of labor, the risk factors for the presence of breech presentation should be reviewed again (the presence of placenta previa, twins, etc.) and a complete abdominal and vaginal examination needs to be carried out.
- Maternal intravenous line must be set up as the mother may require emergency induction of anesthesia at any time.
- Women should be advised to remain in bed to avoid the risk of PROM and cord prolapse. The fetal membranes must be left intact as long as possible; they must not be ruptured artificially, but allowed to rupture on their own in order to prevent the hazard of overt cord prolapse. In case the bag of membranes ruptures spontaneously, a per vaginal examination must be performed immediately to rule out cord prolapse. It is advisable to do continuous FHR recording for 5–10 minutes following rupture of membranes to rule out occult cord prolapse.
- Active management of labor preferably using a partogram needs to be done. A satisfactory progress of labor is indicative of pelvic adequacy.
- Close surveillance of FHR can be done using internal and external cardiotocographic techniques. In case electronic fetal monitoring facilities are not available, the FHR must be monitored using intermittent auscultation every 15 minutes during first stage of labor and after every contraction during second stage of labor. Despite the unavailability of adequate evidence, the use of continuous electronic fetal monitoring in these cases is likely to be associated with improved neonatal outcomes.
- In case of suspected fetal acidosis, fetal blood sampling from the buttocks is not advised due to an insufficient evidence base for this technique.

- Use of oxytocin induction and augmentation for breech presentation is controversial. Many clinicians fear that forceful uterine contractions induced by oxytocin could result in an incompletely dilated cervix and an entrapped head. Induction of labor is usually not recommended. Slow progress of labor with low frequency of contraction in the presence of epidural analgesia may be augmented with oxytocin.
- At the time of delivery, mother should adopt either a semirecumbent or an all-fours position based on her preference and the experience of the attendant. If the mother adopts an all-four position, she should be advised that she may have to adopt the semirecumbent position during delivery, if required.
- Routine episiotomy for every breech vaginal delivery is not required. However, if the clinician feels that the birth passage is too small, he/she must use his/her own discretion in giving an episiotomy. Administration of an episiotomy helps in preventing soft-tissue dystocia.
- In case of breech footling presentation, if the fetal feet prolapse through the vagina, treat expectantly as long as the FHR is stable to allow the cervix to completely dilate around the breech.
- Delivery should be conducted in the operation theater by "assisted breech vaginal delivery" and an anesthetist standby.
- Cesarean section should be considered if there is delay in the descent of the breech in the first or second stage of labor.

Prerequisites for a Vaginal Delivery

Vaginal delivery should be undertaken if the conditions mentioned in **Box 3.5** are fulfilled. Trial of vaginal breech delivery however continues to be offered to women who fulfill the criteria mentioned in **Box 3.5**. These women should be explained about the benefits and risks of both breech vaginal delivery and cesarean section and allowed to choose between the two. The decision for breech vaginal delivery or cesarean section is made based on the type of breech, degree of flexion of fetal head, fetal size, size of maternal pelvis, etc.

Steps for an Assisted Breech Vaginal Delivery

1. Once the buttocks have entered the vagina and the cervix is fully dilated, the woman must be advised to bear down with the contractions.

BOX 3.5: Prerequisites for breech vaginal delivery.

- Facilities for cesarean section are available
- Anesthetist, operation theater staff, and pediatrician have been informed
- Facilities are available for continuous monitoring of FHR and ultrasonography
- Clinician and other healthcare staff, well versed in the technique of vaginal breech delivery and facilities for safe emergency cesarean delivery, are available

(FHR: fetal heart rate)

2. Episiotomy may be performed, if the perineum appears very tight.
3. *Delivery of buttocks and lower back:* A "no-touch policy/hands off the breech policy" must be adopted by the clinician until the buttocks and lower back deliver till the level of umbilicus. At this point, the baby's shoulder blades can be seen.
4. Sometimes the clinician may have to make use of maneuvers such as Pinard's maneuver and groin traction (will be described later), if the legs have not delivered spontaneously.
5. The clinician should be extremely careful and gently hold the baby by wrapping it in a clean cloth in such a way that the baby's trunk is present anteriorly. This will allow the fetal head to enter the pelvis in occipitoanterior position.
6. The baby must be held by the hips and not by the flanks or abdomen as this may cause kidney or liver damage. At no point must the clinician try to pull the baby out, rather the patient must be encouraged to push down.
7. In order to avoid compression on the umbilical cord, it should be moved to one side, preferably in the sacral bay.
8. *Delivery of fetal shoulders and arm:* Appearance of axilla at the vulval outlet indicates that the time has come for the delivery of fetal shoulders. Two methods can be used:
    a. In the first method, once the scapula is visible at the vulval outlet, the trunk is rotated in clockwise direction by 90° in such a way that the anterior shoulder and arm appear at the vulva (**Figs. 3.10A to E**). It can then be easily released and delivered. The body of the fetus is then rotated similarly in the reverse direction (anticlockwise) to deliver the other arm and shoulder.
    b. Second method is employed if the first method is unsuccessful. In the second method, the posterior shoulder is delivered first (described later in the text). Following the delivery of posterior arm, the body of the fetus is depressed to allow the anterior arm to slip out spontaneously. If this does not work, the obstetrician can use two fingers of right hand to sweep the anterior arm down over the thorax.
9. *Nuchal arms:* Sometimes due to inappropriate traction and rotational maneuvers, the shoulder is extended and elbow is flexed. In these cases, the forearm gets trapped behind the occiput. If the obstetrician tries to hook down the trapped arm, there may occur fracture of the humerus. Therefore, in these cases, the following maneuver (**Figs. 3.11A and B**) can be used—the fetus is rotated in the direction in which the baby's hand is pointing. This would cause the occiput to slip past the forearm. Friction of the rotation causes the shoulder to flex and become accessible for delivery.

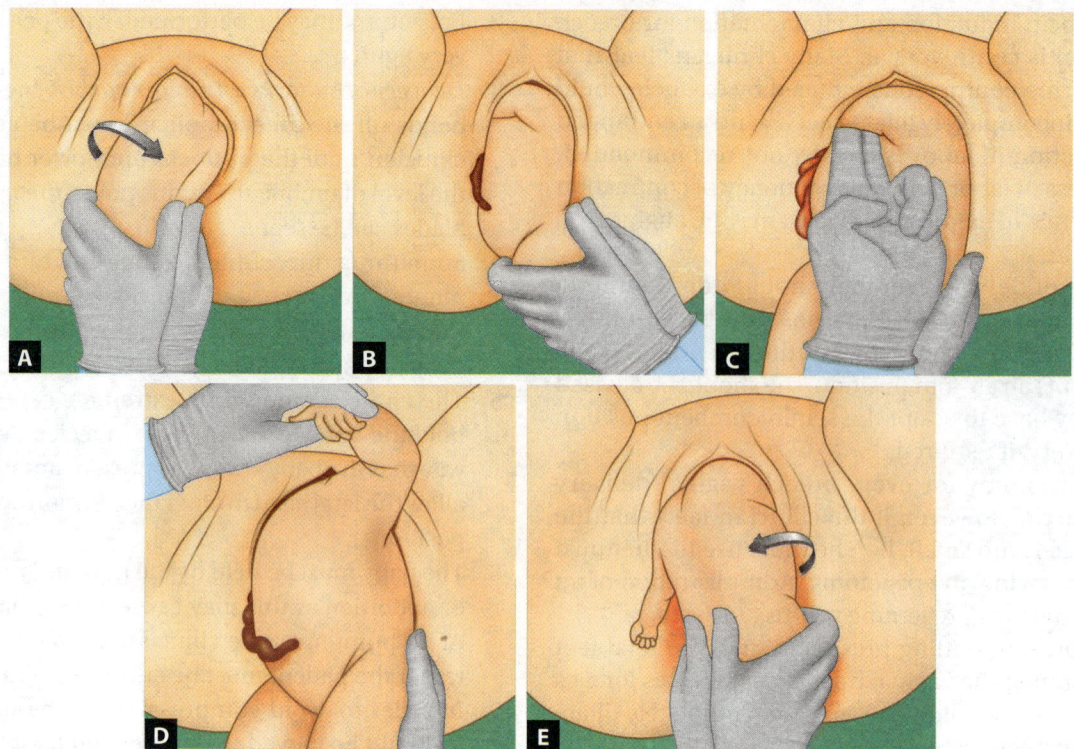

Figs. 3.10A to E: Delivery of fetal shoulders and arms. (A) Rotation of fetal pelvis by 90° in clockwise direction; (B to D) Application of gentle traction to deliver the anterior shoulder, arm, and forearm; (E) Rotation of the fetal pelvis in anticlockwise direction to deliver the posterior arm and forearm.

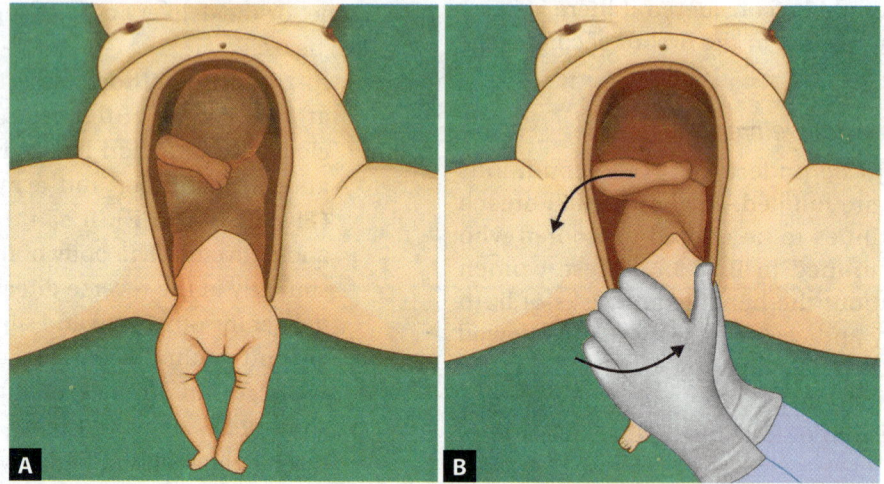

Figs. 3.11A and B: Delivery of nuchal arm. (A) Forearm is trapped behind the occiput; (B) Rotation of fetal body in the direction in which the baby's hand is pointing.

10. The obstetrician must wait to deliver the shoulders until axilla is visible. Attempts must not be made to release the arms immediately after the emergence of costal margins.
11. The clinician must wait for the arms to deliver spontaneously. If arms are felt on chest, the clinician must allow the arms to disengage spontaneously one by one. Assistance should be provided only if necessary. After spontaneous delivery of the first arm, the buttocks must be lifted toward the mother's abdomen to enable the second arm to deliver spontaneously. If the arm does not spontaneously deliver, place one or two fingers in the elbow and bend the arm, bringing the hand down over the baby's face.
12. If the arms still do not deliver, the clinician must reach into the vagina to determine their position. If they are flexed in front of the chest, gentle pressure must be applied to the crook of the elbow to straighten the arm and aid delivery.
13. The same maneuver must be repeated with the other arm.
14. The clinician needs to be aware that there are other maneuvers to deliver the arms and shoulders if needed, including Løvset's maneuver (described later) to deliver

the extended arms, which are stretched above the baby's head.

15. Once the shoulders are delivered, the baby's body with the face down must be supported on the clinician's forearm. The clinician must be careful not to compress the umbilical cord between the infant's body and their arm.

16. One of the following maneuvers, which would be described next, can be then used for delivery of aftercoming head of the fetus.

Maneuvers for Delivery of the Aftercoming Head

Burns–Marshall Technique

Following the delivery of shoulders and both the arms, the baby must be let to hang unsupported from the mother's vulva. This would help in encouraging flexion of fetal head **(Fig. 3.12A)**. The nursing staff must be further advised to apply suprapubic pressure in downward and backward directions, in order to encourage further flexion of the baby's head. As the nape of baby's neck appears, efforts must be made by the clinician to deliver the baby's head by grasping the fetal ankles with the finger of right hand between the two. Then the trunk is swung up, forming a wide arc of the circle, while maintaining continuous traction when doing this **(Fig. 3.12B)**. The left hand is used to provide pelvic support and clear the perineum off successively from the baby's face and brow as the baby's head emerges out.

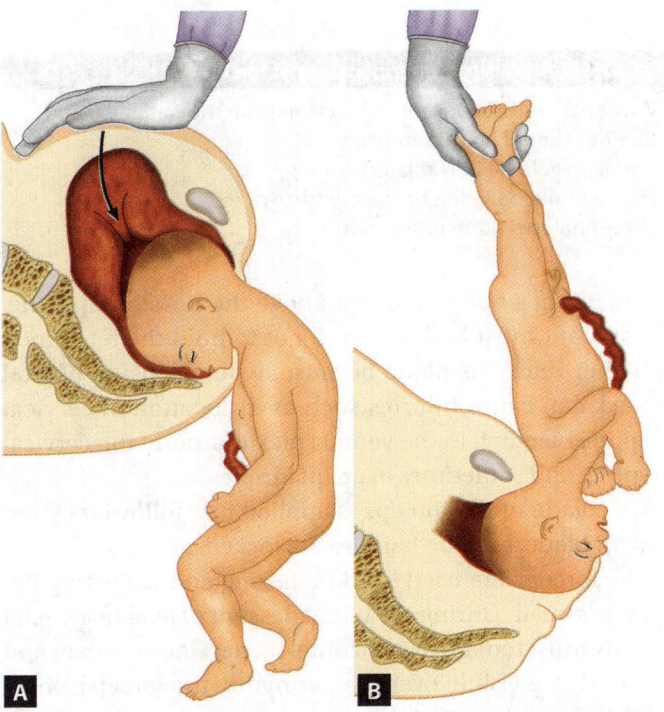

Figs. 3.12A and B: Burns–Marshall technique. (A) Baby is let to hang unsupported from the maternal vulva; (B) As the nape of fetal neck appears, efforts are made to deliver the fetal head by grasping the fetal ankles and swinging the trunk up by forming a wide arc of circle.

Mauriceau–Smellie–Veit Maneuver

The Mauriceau–Smellie–Veit maneuver is another commonly used maneuver for the delivery of aftercoming fetal head and is named after the three clinicians who had described the method of using this grip. This maneuver comprises the following steps:

1. The baby is placed face down with the length of its body over the supinated left forearm and hand of the clinician.
2. The clinician must then place the first (index) and second fingers (middle finger) of this hand on the baby's cheekbones and the thumb over the baby's chin. This helps in facilitating flexion of the fetal head. In the method originally described by Mauriceau, Smellie, and Veit, the index finger of the left hand was placed inside the baby's mouth. This is no longer advocated as placing a finger inside the infant's mouth is supposed to stimulate the vagal reflex. An assistant may provide suprapubic pressure to help the baby's head remain flexed.
3. The right hand of the clinician is used for grasping the baby's shoulders. The little finger and the ring finger of the clinician's right hand is placed over the baby's right shoulder, the index finger over the baby's left shoulder, and the middle finger over the baby's suboccipital region **(Figs. 3.13A to C)**. With the fingers of right hand in this position, the baby's head is flexed toward the chest. At the same time, left hand is used for applying downward pressure on the jaw to bring the baby's head down until the hairline is visible.
4. Thereafter the baby's trunk is carried in upward and forward directions toward the maternal abdomen, till the baby's mouth, nose, brow, and lastly the vertex and occiput have been released.
5. In this maneuver, the clinician uses both the arms simultaneously, in synchronization, to exert gentle downward traction at the same time both on the fetal neck and maxilla.

Delivery of Aftercoming Head Using Forceps

Application of forceps **(Fig. 3.14)** is the technique of choice to ensure safe delivery of baby's head because it provides protection to the fetal head from sudden forces of compression and decompression. Also, the use of forceps helps in better maintenance of flexion of fetal head and helps in transmitting the force to the fetal head rather than the neck. This helps in reducing the risk of fetal injuries. Furthermore, flexion of fetal head helps in reducing the diameter of fetal head, thereby aiding descent. Prerequisites for application of forceps are enumerated in **Box 3.6**. For delivery of fetal head using forceps, the following steps are required **(Figs. 3.15A to G)**:

1. Ordinary forceps or Piper's forceps (specially designed forceps with absent pelvic curve) or divergent Laufe's forceps can be used.

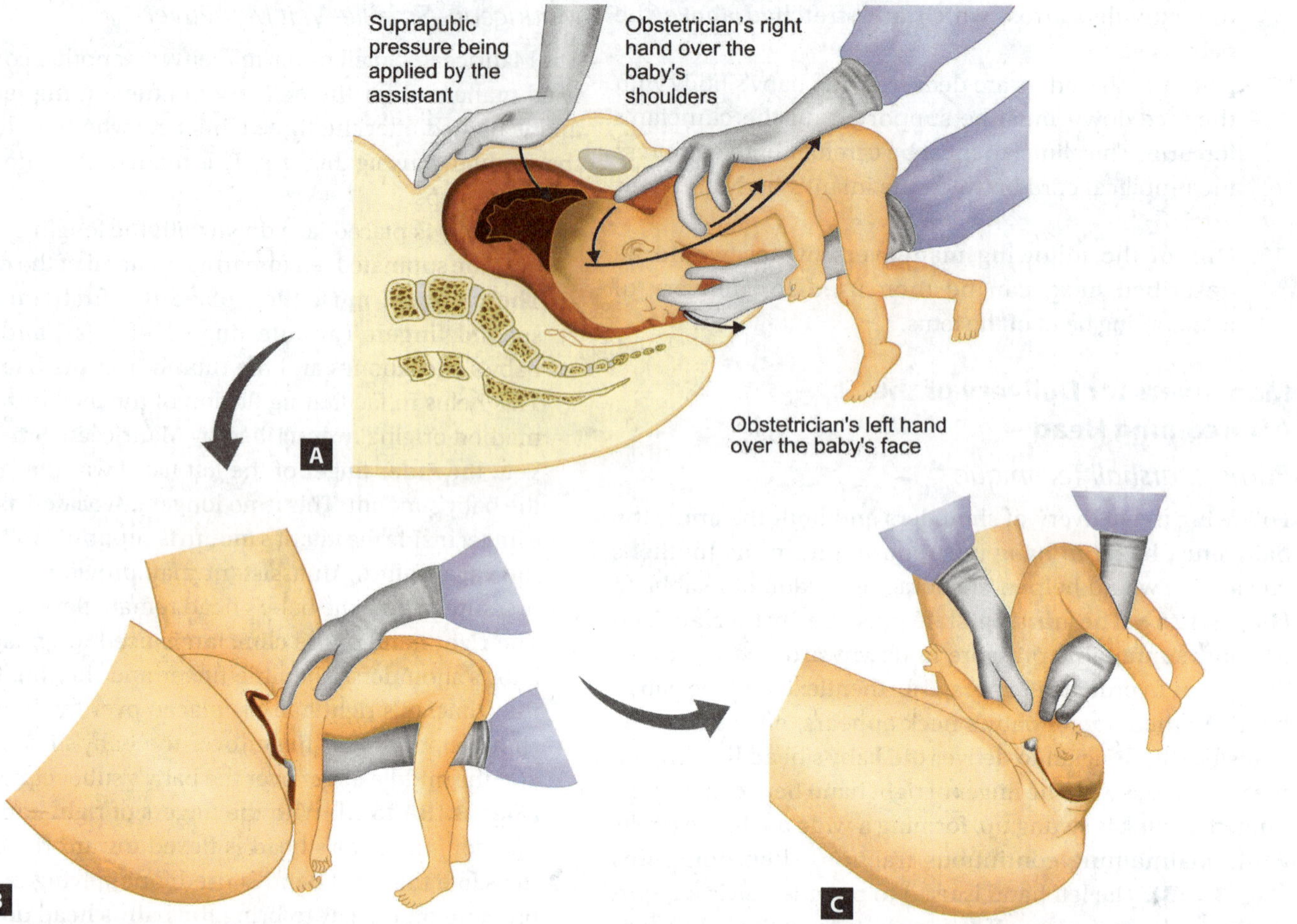

82 Normal and Abnormal Presentations

Figs. 3.13A to C: Mauriceau–Smellie–Veit maneuver. (A) The baby is laid flat over the obstetrician's forearm with the fingers of left hand over the baby's face and right hand over the occiput; (B) The baby's head is gradually flexed; (C) The baby's trunk is carried upward and forward to deliver the fetal head.

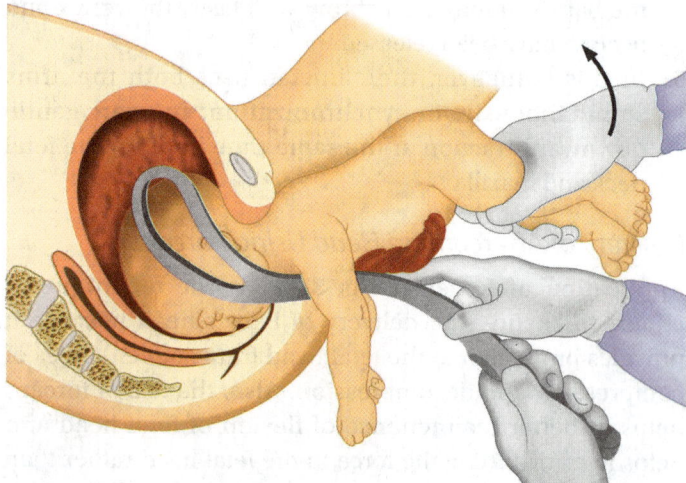

Fig. 3.14: Delivery of aftercoming head of the breech using forceps.

> **BOX 3.6:** Prerequisites for application of forceps.
> - Written or verbal consent to be taken from the patient
> - Bladder should be catheterized
> - Cervix should be fully dilated
> - Head should be in the pelvic cavity
> - No cephalopelvic disproportion

2. While the clinician is applying forceps, the baby's body must be wrapped in a cloth or towel and held on one side by the assistant. Suspension of the baby in a towel prior to application of forceps helps in effectively holding the baby's body and keeping the arms out of the way. At the time of application of forceps, the assistant must hold the infant's body at or just above the horizontal plane. Assistant must be instructed not to hold the fetal body higher than this plane because hyperextension of fetal neck can cause injuries such as dislocation of cervical spine, bleeding in the venous plexus around the cervical spine, and sometimes even quadriplegia.
3. Left blade of the forceps is applied first followed by the right blade, and the handles are locked.
4. The forceps are used for both flexing and delivering the baby's head. During the initial descent of fetal head, fetal body must remain in horizontal plane. Once the chin and mouth are visible over the perineum, the forceps, body, and legs of the fetus are raised to complete delivery.
5. The head must be delivered slowly over 1 minute in order to avoid sudden compression or decompression of fetal head, which may be a cause for intracranial hemorrhage.

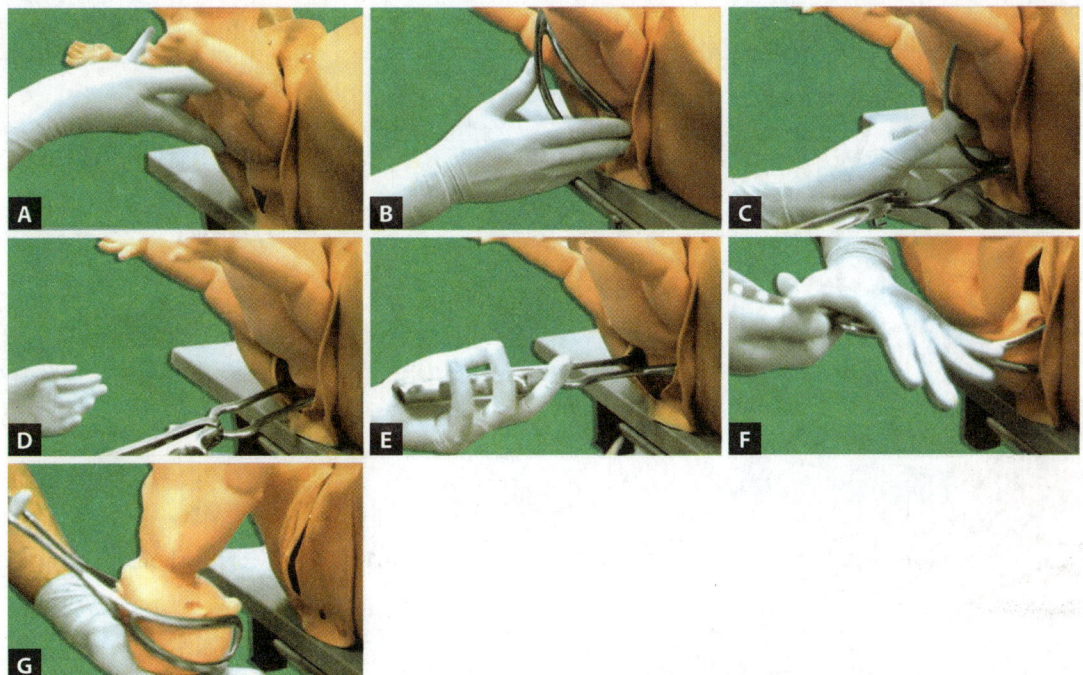

Figs. 3.15A to G: Steps of application of forceps in case of aftercoming head of breech. (A) Before application of forceps, the baby is held by feet on one side by the clinician; (B) Application of the left blade of the forceps; (C) This is followed by the application of the right blade; (D) Locking of the blades of forceps; (E and F) Application of traction over the baby's head; (G) The baby's head is delivered out due to the application of traction.

Delivery of Baby's Shoulders

Reverse Prague's Maneuver

At times, the back of fetus may fail to rotate anteriorly. In these cases, stronger traction on fetal legs or bony pelvis may be applied to turn the back anterior. If the baby's back still remains posterior, head can be extracted using Mauriceau maneuver and delivering the baby with back down. Alternatively, modified Prague's maneuver can be used **(Fig. 3.16)**. In this maneuver, two fingers of obstetrician's one hand grasp the shoulders of back down fetus from below and exert traction in downward and backward directions. Simultaneously, the other hand draws the feet up over the maternal abdomen to flex the infant and aid the delivery of the occiput.

Løvset's Maneuver

If the baby's arms are stretched above the head, the maneuver called Løvset's maneuver is used for delivery of fetal arms. This maneuver is based on the principle that due to the curved shape of the birth canal, when the anterior shoulder is above the pubis symphysis, the posterior shoulder would be below the level of pubic symphysis. The maneuver should be initiated only when the fetal scapula becomes visible underneath the pubic arch and includes the following steps **(Figs. 3.17A to C)**:

1. First, the baby is lifted slightly to cause lateral flexion of the trunk.
2. Then the baby, which is held by pelvifemoral grip, is turned by half a circle, keeping the back uppermost.

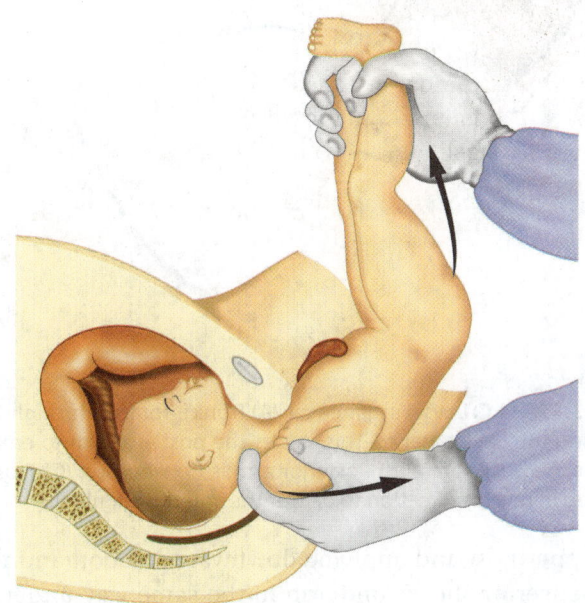

Fig. 3.16: Prague's maneuver.

Simultaneously downward traction is applied so that the arm that was initially posterior and below the level of pubic symphysis now becomes anterior and can be delivered under the pubic arch.

3. Delivery of the arm can be assisted by placing one or two fingers on the upper part of the arm. Then the arm is gradually drawn down over the chest as the elbow is flexed, with the hand sweeping over the face.
4. In order to deliver the second arm, the baby is again turned by 180° in the reverse direction, keeping the back

84 Normal and Abnormal Presentations

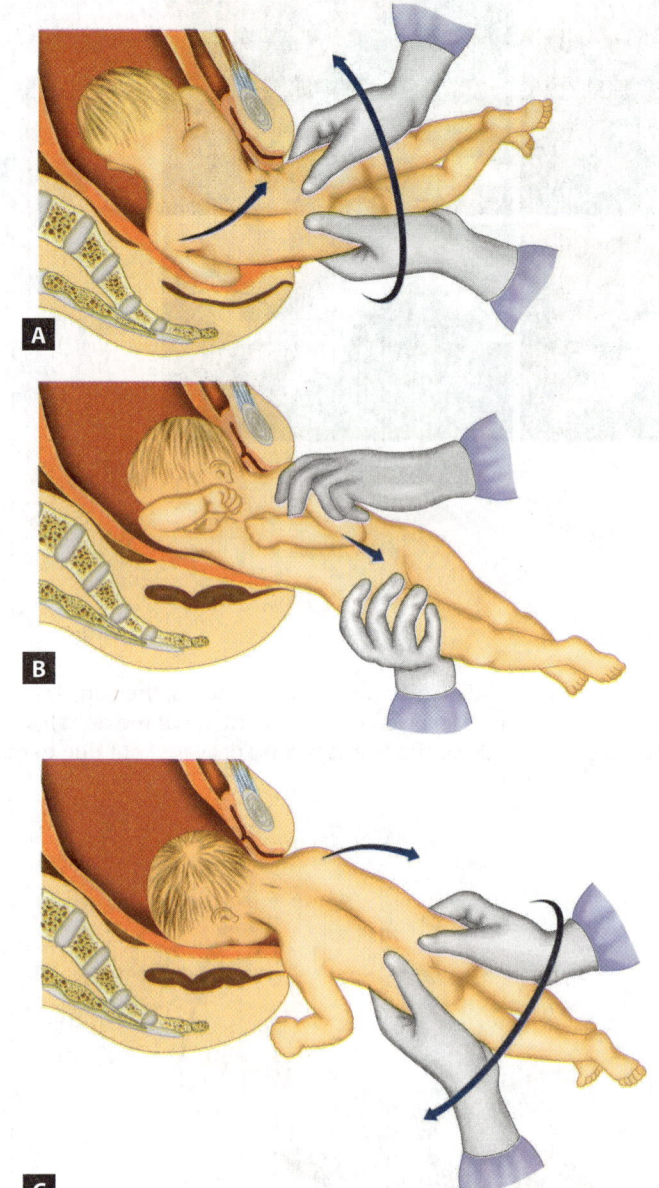

Figs. 3.17A to C: Løvset's maneuver. (A) Trunk is rotated through 180°, keeping the back anterior. This causes the posterior arm to emerge under the pubic arch; (B) Posterior arm is hooked out; (C) Trunk is rotated in reverse direction to deliver the anterior shoulder.

uppermost and applying downward traction and then delivering the second arm in the same way under the pubic arch as the first arm was delivered.

Delivery of the Posterior Shoulder

If the clinician is unable to turn the baby's body to deliver the arm that is anterior first, through Løvset's maneuver, then the clinician can deliver the shoulder that is posterior first **(Fig. 3.18)**. Delivery of the posterior shoulder involves the following steps:

1. The clinician must hold and lift the baby up by the ankles. At the same time, the baby's chest must be moved toward the woman's inner thighs. The clinician must then hook the baby's shoulder with fingers of his/her hand. This

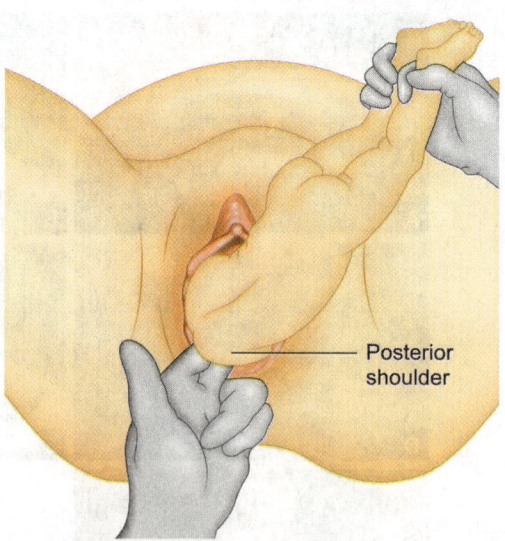

Fig. 3.18: Delivery of the shoulder that is posterior.

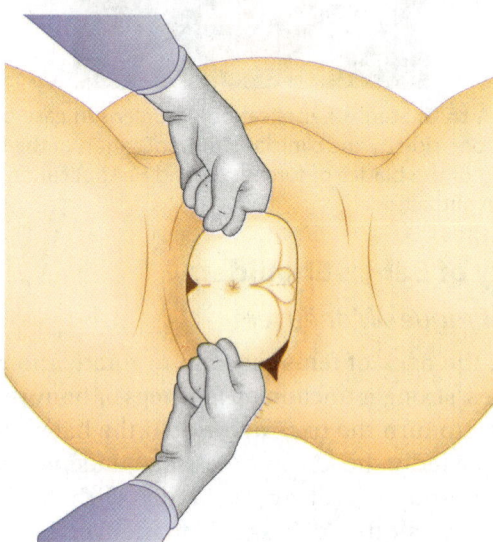

Fig. 3.19: Application of groin traction.

would help in delivering the shoulder that is posterior, followed by the delivery of arm and hand.

2. Then the baby's back should be lowered down, still holding it by ankles. This helps in the delivery of anterior shoulder followed by the arm and hand.

Delivery of Baby's Legs

Groin Traction

If the buttocks and hip do not deliver by themselves, the clinician can make use of simple maneuvers including groin traction or Pinard's maneuver to deliver the legs. Groin traction could be of two types: single or double groin traction. In single groin traction, the index finger of one hand is hooked in the groin fold and traction is exerted toward the fetal trunk rather than toward the fetal femur, in accordance with the uterine contractions. In double groin traction, the index fingers of both the hands are hooked in the groin folds and then traction is applied **(Fig. 3.19)**.

Pinard's Maneuver

In Pinard's maneuver, pressure is exerted against the inner aspect of the knee (popliteal fossa), with help of the middle and index fingers of the clinician **(Fig. 3.20A)**. As the pressure is applied, the knee gets flexed and abducted. This causes the lower leg to move downward, which is then swept medially and gently pulled out of the vagina **(Figs. 3.20B and C)**.

Postdelivery Care

- The baby's mouth and nose must be suctioned.
- The cord must be clamped and cut.
- Active management of the third stage of labor needs to be done.
- The cervix and vagina must be carefully examined for the presence of any tears, and the episiotomy must be repaired.

COMPLICATIONS

Q. Write a short essay on intrapartum complications of breech delivery.

FETAL COMPLICATIONS

Low APGAR Scores

Low APGAR scores, especially at 1 minute, are more common with vaginal breech deliveries and could be related to birth asphyxia. Increased risk of birth asphyxia in cases of breech vaginal delivery could be due to the following causes:
- Cord compression
- Cord prolapse
- Premature attempts by the baby to breathe while the head is still inside the uterine cavity
- Delay in the delivery of the head, often due to head entrapment

Fetal Head Entrapment

Fetal head entrapment may result from an incompletely dilated cervix and head that lacks time to mold to the maternal pelvis. This occurs in 0–8.5% of vaginal breech deliveries. This percentage is higher with preterm fetuses (<32 weeks), when the head is larger in comparison to the rest of the body. In most of the cases, fetal head entrapment is also associated with umbilical cord compression. Therefore, this condition must be dealt with urgently.

Sometimes, with gentle traction on the fetal body, the cervix can be manually slipped over the occiput. If this does not work, Dührssen's incisions, i.e., 1–3 cm deep cervical incisions made through several portions of the cervical canal (to facilitate delivery of the fetal head), may be necessary to relieve cervical entrapment **(Fig. 3.21)**. However, severe hemorrhage and extension can occur into

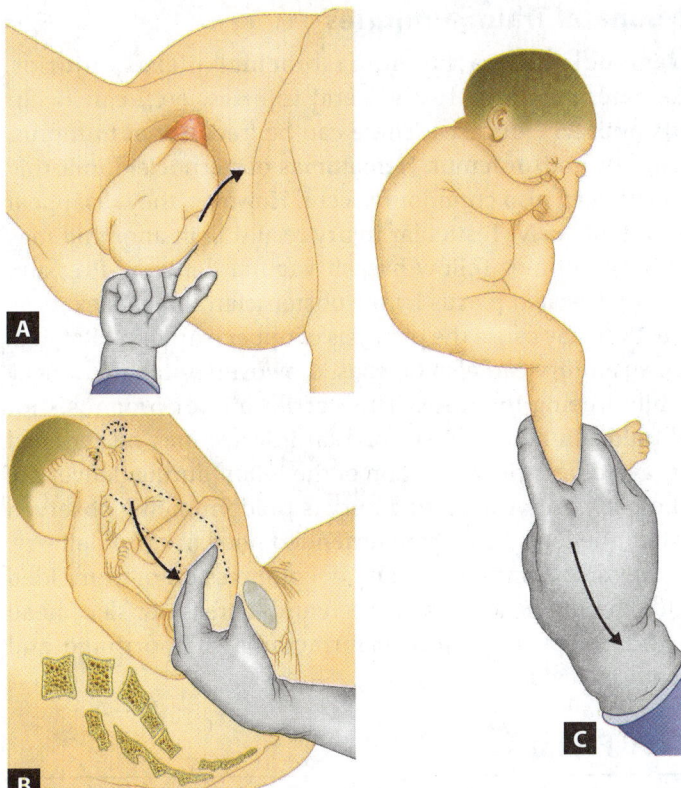

Figs. 3.20A to C: Pinard's maneuver. (A) Pressure is exerted against the popliteal fossa; (B) Due to application of pressure, the fetal knee gets flexed and abducted; (C) As the fetal leg moves downward, it is pulled out by the clinician.

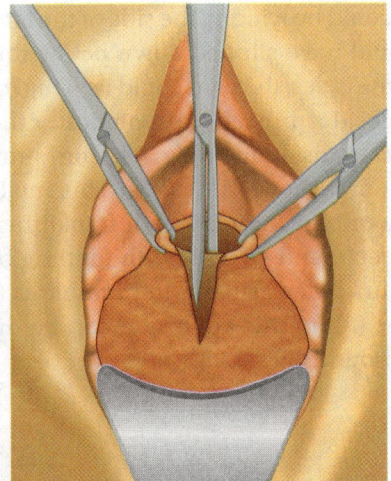

Fig. 3.21: Dührssen's incision.

the lower segment of the uterus. Therefore, the operator must be equipped to deal with this complication. Alternatively, 100 µg of intravenous nitroglycerin can be used to provide cervical relaxation. General anesthesia can also be used in extreme cases.

Preterm Birth

Preterm birth (delivery of baby at <28 weeks) commonly occurs in breech presentation. It can often result in complications related to prematurity.

Neonatal Trauma/Injuries

Neonatal trauma including brachial plexus injuries, hematomas, fractures, visceral injuries, etc., can occur in about 25% of cases. There can be fractures of humerus, clavicle, and/or femur. Hematomas of sternocleidomastoid muscle can also commonly occur. However, they disappear spontaneously. Testicular injury resulting in anorchia may also sometimes follow breech vaginal delivery. Pressure on the brachial plexus by the obstetrician's fingers exerting traction may cause the paralysis of upper extremity. Brachial plexus injury can also be caused by overstretching of neck while freeing the arms. This carries a poor prognosis for shoulder function. Risks of fetal injuries may be reduced by avoiding rapid extraction of the infant during delivery of the body. Cervical spine injury is predominantly observed when the fetus has a hyperextended head prior to delivery. Successive compression and decompression of unmolded aftercoming head of the breech and increased risk of head entrapment can result in intracranial hemorrhage and tentorial tears.

Cord Prolapse

> **Q. Write a short essay on the management of cord prolapse.**

Cord prolapse is a condition associated with abnormal descent of the umbilical cord before the descent of the fetal presenting part **(Fig. 3.22)**.

The cord could be lying by the side of the fetal presenting part, or it could have slipped down below the presenting part. In extreme cases, the cord could be lying totally outside the vagina. Besides breech presentation, other causes of cord prolapse are listed in **Table 3.4**. Cord prolapse occurs in 7.5% of all breeches **(Table 3.5)**. This incidence varies with the type of breech: 0–2% with frank breech, 5% with complete breech, and 10–15% with footling breech. Cord prolapse occurs twice as often in multiparas (6%) than in primigravidas (3%). This condition can be diagnosed on Doppler ultrasound **(Fig. 3.23)**.

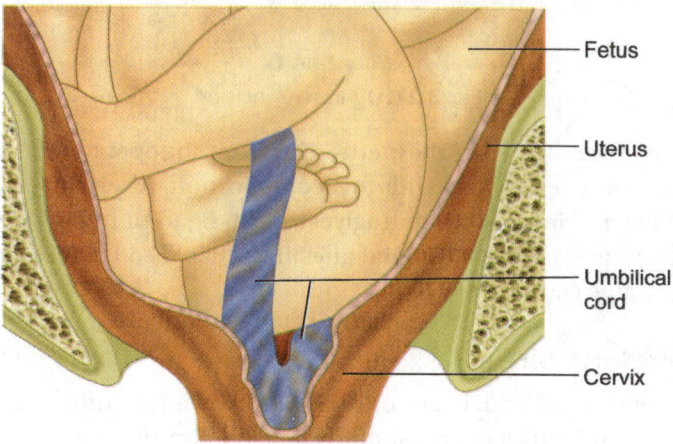

Fig. 3.22: Cord prolapse.

The management for cord prolapse is described in **Flowchart 3.3**. If the cord has already prolapsed at the time of examination, no attempt must be made to replace the cord back. Urgent delivery of the baby (by any route) is required in these circumstances. If urgent vaginal delivery is not possible or is contraindicated, immediate preparations for an emergency cesarean delivery must be made. While preparations for cesarean delivery are being made, attempts must be made to minimize cord compression. This can be achieved in the following ways:

- *Lifting the presenting part off the cord:* This can be either done manually by the clinician **(Fig. 3.24A)** or by filling the bladder with normal saline **(Fig. 3.24B)**. In the manual method, after taking complete aseptic precautions, the clinician's gloved fingers are inserted inside the vagina. Then the clinician applies pressure in an upward direction in order to push the fetus upward and away from the cord. In the other method involving bladder filling, the bladder is filled with approximately 500–750 mL of 0.9% normal saline using a Foley's catheter. Following this, the balloon of Foley's catheter is inflated and the catheter is clamped. The obstetrician must, however, remember to empty the bladder prior to the cesarean delivery.
- *Postural treatment:* Changing the maternal position **(Figs. 3.25A and B)** is also likely to help lift the presenting part off the cord. Some of the commonly adopted maternal positions include exaggerated and elevated Sims position, Trendelenburg position, and knee–chest position. There is no clear-cut evidence regarding the success rates of this method. Moreover, adoption of a specific posture, especially knee–chest position, even

TABLE 3.4: Causes of cord prolapse with breech presentation.

Fetal causes	Maternal causes	Other predisposing factors
• Malpresentations (complete or footling breech, transverse lie, etc.) • Prematurity or low birth weight • Polyhydramnios • Multiple pregnancy • Anencephaly	• Contracted pelvis • Pelvic tumors	• Low-grade placenta previa • Long cord • Sudden rupture of membranes in polyhydramnios

TABLE 3.5: Incidence of cord prolapse with breech presentation.

Type of breech presentation	Incidence of cord prolapse (%)
Frank breech	0–2
Complete breech	5
Footling breech	15

Breech Presentation

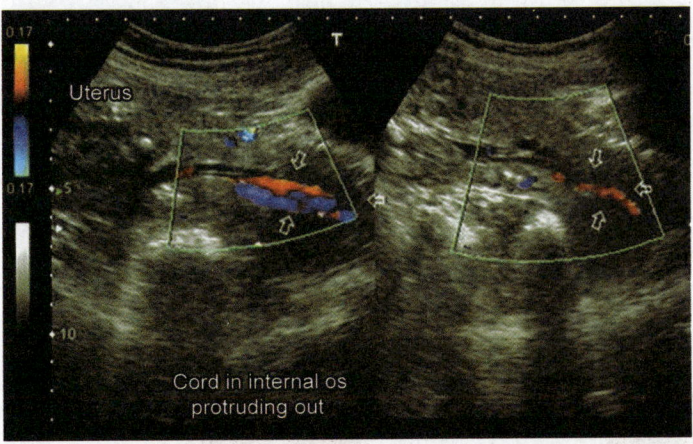

Fig. 3.23: Color Doppler ultrasound showing cord prolapse. Internal os appears dilated with umbilical cord inside the cervix; this finding is diagnostic of cord prolapse.

Flowchart 3.3: Management of cord prolapse.

```
Breech presentation with cord prolapse
         │
    ┌────┴────┐
    │         │
Baby alive:              Baby dead/congenital anomaly:
• Cord is pulsating      • Cord pulsations are absent
• Fetal heart sounds     • Absent fetal heart sounds
  are heard
    │                         │
┌───┴────┐                    │
│        │                    │
Immediate   Immediate      Wait for
vaginal     vaginal        spontaneous
delivery    delivery       delivery
appears     appears
likely      unlikely
│           │
Breech      
extraction  
(delivery of the
aftercoming
head by forceps)
            │
     ┌──────┴──────┐
     │             │
Preliminary      Definitive
management       management
(while making
arrangements
for cesarean
delivery)
                     │
                An emergency cesarean delivery
                • Abdomen to be marked to show
                  that the bladder is full
                • Bladder to be emptied prior to
                  the cesarean section

The presenting part to be lifted
off the cord using bladder filling
or manually (Figs. 3.24A and B)

Administration of intravenous
Ringer's lactate

Oxygen to be given by
face mask

Discontinuation of oxytocin
infusion (if was being
previously administered)

Postural treatment: Exaggerated
and elevated Sims position,
Trendelenburg's position
or knee–chest position
(Figs. 3.25A and B)
```

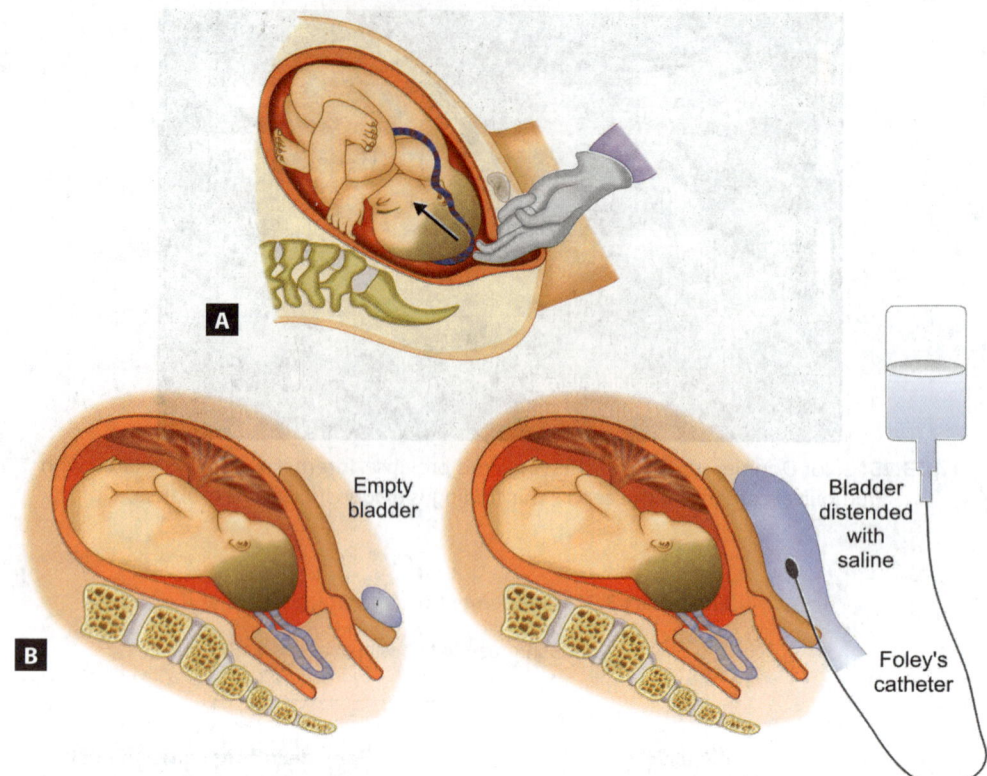

Figs. 3.24A and B: Lifting the presenting part off the cord: (A) A gloved hand in the vagina pushes the fetus upward and off the cord; (B) Bladder filling to lift the presenting part off the cord; bladder can be filled with approximately 500 mL of 0.9% normal saline using a Foley's catheter; the balloon is then inflated and catheter is clamped, and drainage tubing and urine bag are attached.

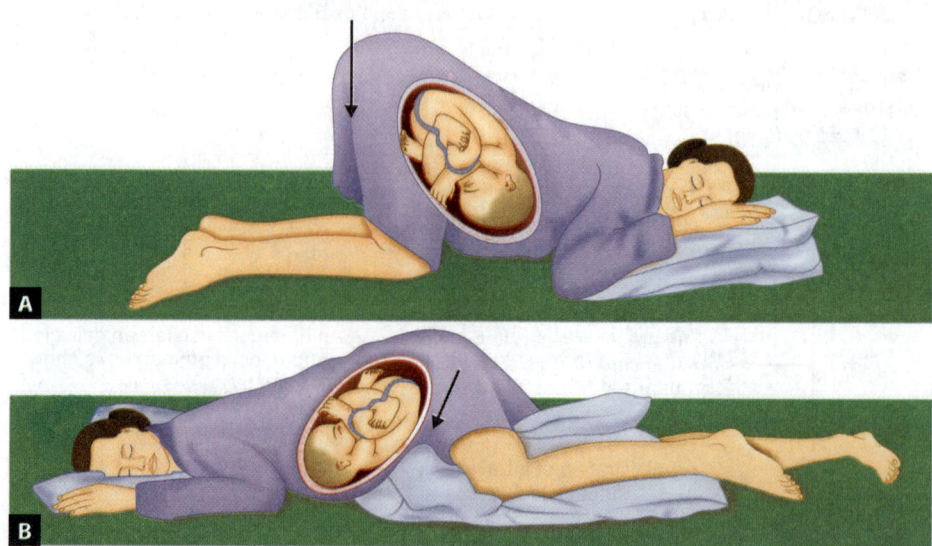

Figs. 3.25A and B: Use of appropriate maternal position to help prevent compression of the cord. (A) Use of knee–chest position to help shift the fetus out of pelvis. The mother's chest should be flat on the bed and her thighs should be at right angles to the bed; (B) Trendelenburg position, along with the elevation of hips with the help of pillows.

for a short duration of time can be cumbersome and uncomfortable for the mother.

MATERNAL COMPLICATIONS

- Increased rate of maternal morbidity and mortality due to an increased incidence of operative/difficult delivery
- Traumatic injuries to the genital tract

EVIDENCE-BASED CLINICAL TRIALS

List of references can be scanned through QR code to enable the readers gain deeper insight of the subject by referring to the entire article or its abstract.

CHAPTER 4

Transverse Lie

CASE STUDY

A 28-year-old primigravida patient with 36 completed weeks of gestation having fetus with shoulder presentation (diagnosed by ultrasound examination at previous antenatal visit) presented for a routine antenatal checkup.

INTRODUCTION

DEFINITION

Transverse lie is an abnormal fetal presentation in which the fetus lies transversely with the shoulders presenting at the lower pole of the uterus. Most fetuses in transverse lie, early in pregnancy, convert to a cephalic (or breech) presentation by term. In this presentation, long axis of the fetus is perpendicular to the maternal spine. As a result, the presenting part becomes the fetal shoulder. The denominator is the fetal back. Depending on whether the position of the fetal back is anterior, posterior, superior, or inferior **(Figs. 4.1A and B)**, the following positions are possible:
- *Dorsoanterior:* This is the most common position where the fetal back is anterior.
- *Dorsoposterior:* Fetal back is posterior.
- *Dorsosuperior or "back-up":* Fetal back is directed superiorly. In this case, the fetal small parts present at the cervix.
- *Dorsoinferior or "back-down":* Fetal back is directed inferiorly. In this case, the fetal shoulder presents at the cervix.

Depending on the position of the fetal head, the fetal position can be described as right or left.

HISTORY AND CLINICAL PRESENTATION

RISK FACTORS

The following maternal and fetal risk factors need to be elicited in the history.

Maternal Factors
- Cephalopelvic disproportion, contracted maternal pelvis
- Liquor abnormalities (polyhydramnios, oligohydramnios)
- Uterine anomalies (bicornuate, septate)
- Space-occupying lesions (e.g., fibroids in the lower uterine segment, presence of pelvic tumor)

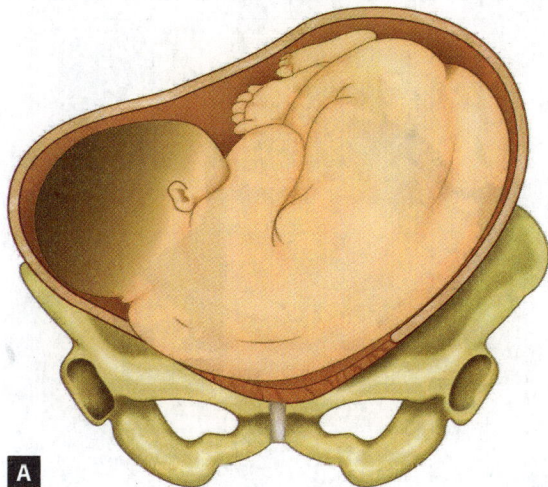
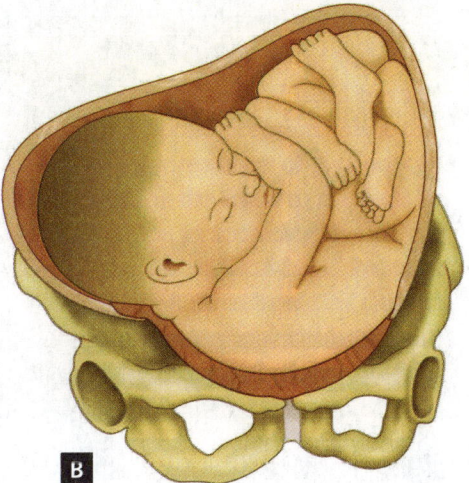

Figs. 4.1A and B: Different positions of transverse lie. (A) Dorsoanterior position; (B) Dorsoposterior position.

- Placental abnormalities (placenta previa, cornuofundal attachment of placenta)
- Multiparity (especially grand multiparas)

Fetal Factors
- Prematurity
- Multifetal gestation
- Hydramnios
- Intrauterine fetal death, fetal anomalies, etc.

GENERAL PHYSICAL EXAMINATION

No specific finding is observed on general physical examination (GPE).

SPECIFIC SYSTEMIC EXAMINATION

ABDOMINAL PALPATION

Transverse lie should be suspected if firm resistance of the fetal head is not detected above the pubis symphysis. The diagnosis of transverse lie is further confirmed when the fetal head is palpated in one or the other of the mother's flanks. If transverse lie is suspected by abdominal palpation, a vaginal examination should be postponed until placenta previa has been excluded. On abdominal palpation, the following findings can be elicited:
- Fetal lie is in the horizontal plane with fetal head on one side of the midline and podalic pole on the other.
- The abdomen often appears barrel-shaped and is asymmetrical.
- Fundal height is less than the period of amenorrhea.

The diagnosis of transverse lie can be made by abdominal palpation utilizing Leopold's maneuvers **(Figs. 4.2A to D)**.

Leopold's First Maneuver/Fundal Grip

No fetal pole (either breech or cephalic) is palpable on the fundal grip. In case of dorsoinferior ("back-down") position, nodulations due to the presence of baby's feet may be palpated on fundal grip. In case of dorsosuperior position, a wide convexity of fetal back may be palpated on fundal grip.

Leopold's Second Maneuver/Lateral Grip

Soft, broad, smooth irregular part suggestive of fetal breech is present on one side of the midline, while a smooth, hard, globular part suggestive of the fetal head is present on the

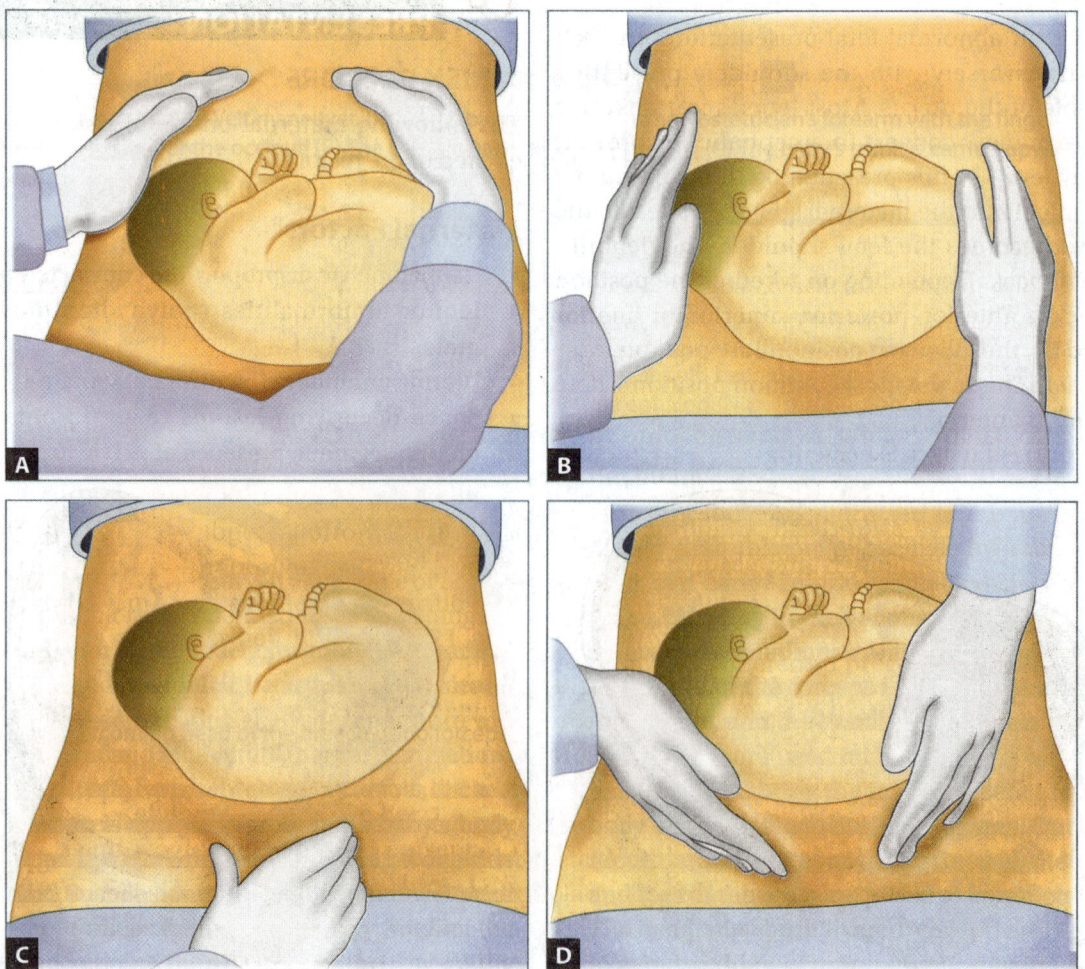

Figs. 4.2A to D: Leopold's maneuvers in case of transverse lie. (A) Fundal grip; (B) Lateral grip; (C) Second pelvic grip; (D) First pelvic grip.

other side of the midline. The fetal head is usually placed at a level lower than the rest of the body and is usually confined to one iliac fossa. In case of dorsoanterior position, back may be felt anteriorly in the midline on the lateral grip. In case of dorsoposterior position, small, irregular, knob-like structures, suggestive of the fetal limbs, are felt anteriorly in the midline while performing lateral grip.

Leopold's Third Maneuver

Pelvic grip appears to be empty during the time of pregnancy. It may be occupied by the shoulder at the time of labor.

Leopold's Fourth Maneuver

No appreciable mass to indicate fetal descent may be identified on Leopold's fourth maneuver.

Fetal Heart Auscultation

Fetal heart rate is easily heard much below the umbilicus in dorsoanterior position. On the other hand, in dorsoposterior position, the fetal heart may be located at a much higher level and is often above the umbilicus.

VAGINAL EXAMINATION

On vaginal examination during the antenatal period, the pelvis appears to be empty. Even if something is felt on vaginal examination, no definite fetal part may be identified **(Fig. 4.3)**.

At the time of labor, on vaginal examination, fetal shoulder including scapula, clavicle, humerus, and grid iron feel of fetal ribs can be palpated **(Figs. 4.4A and B)**. Due to ill-fitting fetal part, an elongated bag of membranes may be felt on vaginal examination. If the membranes have ruptured, the fetal shoulder can be identified by feeling the acromion process, scapula, clavicle, axilla, ribs, and intercostal spaces. Ribs and intercostal spaces upon palpation give a feeling of grid iron. If the arm prolapse has occurred, the fetal arm might be observed lying outside the vagina. If still inside the vagina, a prolapsed arm must be distinguished from a leg. The elbow is sharper than the knee. Moreover, there is no heel, and abduction of the thumb will help in distinguishing hand from foot.

MANAGEMENT

Management comprising investigations and definitive obstetric management is discussed next.

INVESTIGATIONS

ULTRASOUND EXAMINATION

Ultrasound examination is used for confirming the diagnosis of transverse lie and determining the precise fetal position

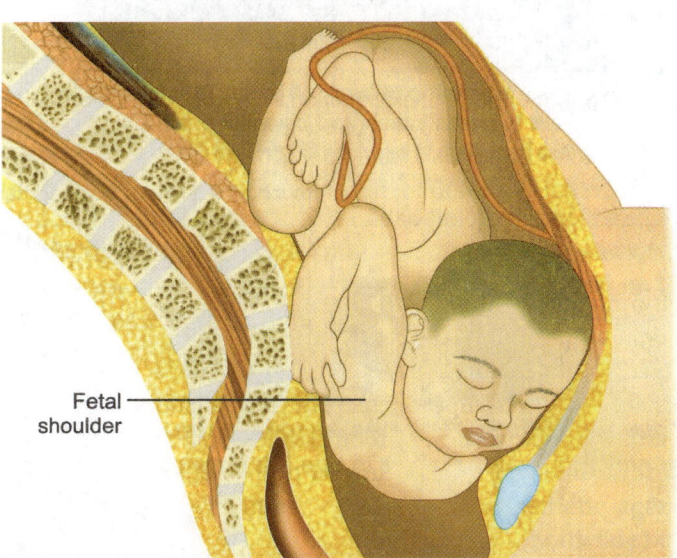

Fig. 4.3: Fetal shoulder presentation.

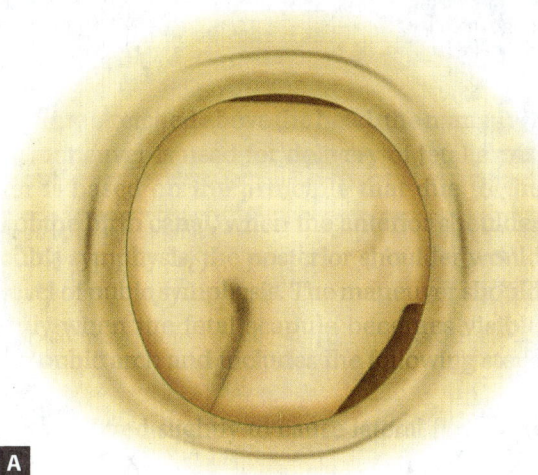

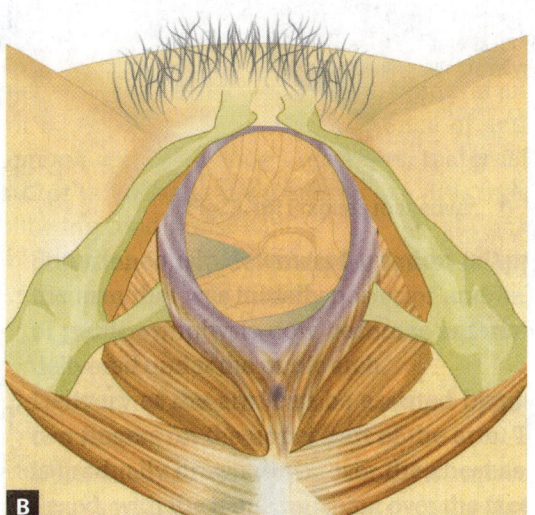

Figs. 4.4A and B: Fetal shoulder as identified on vaginal examination. (A) Vaginal touch picture in case of shoulder presentation; (B) Fetal shoulder as identified on vaginal examination.

(**Fig. 4.5**). Besides confirming the transverse lie, other things which can be observed on the ultrasound include the following:
- Presence of uterine and/or fetal anomalies
- Fetal maturity
- Placental location and grading
- Adequacy of liquor
- Ruling out multiple gestation

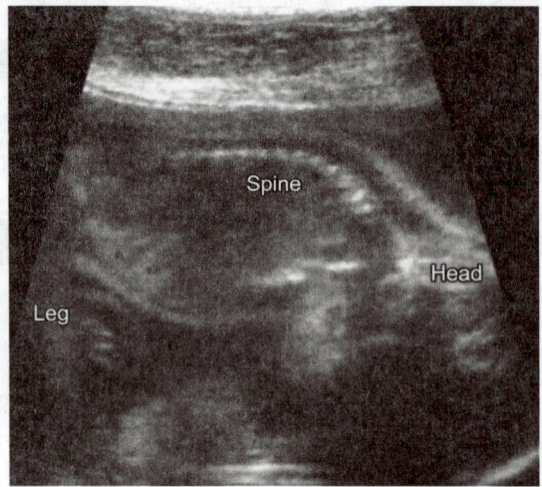

Fig. 4.5: Ultrasound examination at 24 weeks' gestation showing transverse lie.

TREATMENT/OBSTETRIC MANAGEMENT

Q. Describe the management of the case study presented in the beginning of the chapter.

There is no mechanism of labor for a fetus in transverse lie, which remains uncorrected until term. A cesarean section is required to deliver the baby with shoulder presentation.

MANAGEMENT DURING PREGNANCY

- The management options for transverse lie include external cephalic version (ECV) during pregnancy or delivery by cesarean section (elective or an emergency). At some centers, stabilizing induction is used for converting transverse to cephalic presentation at the time of labor. **Flowchart 4.1** illustrates the algorithm for management of fetus in transverse lie.

Flowchart 4.1: Algorithm for management of a fetus in transverse lie.

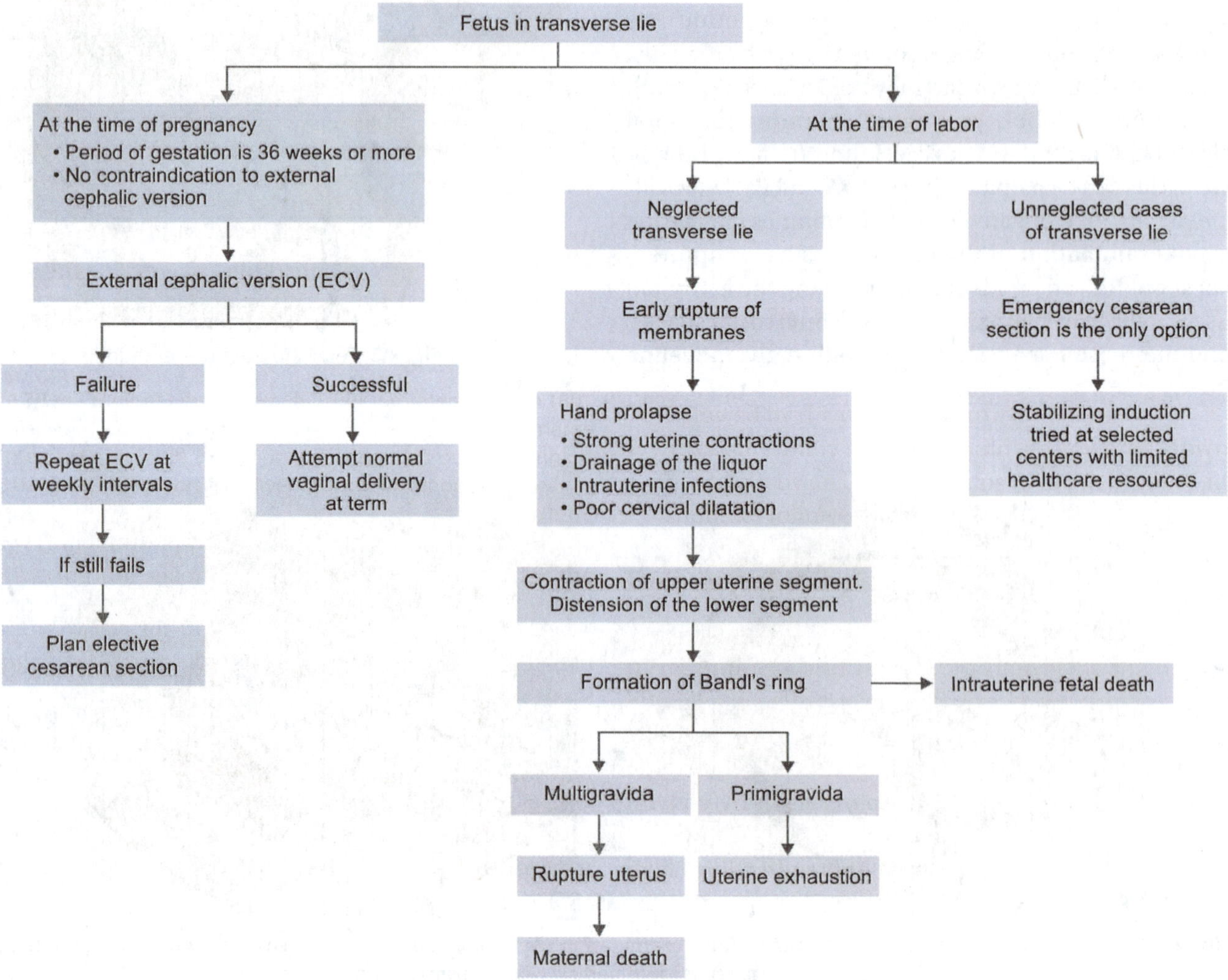

- When transverse lie is diagnosed prior to the onset of labor and there is absence of contraindications to a vaginal delivery, external version to cephalic presentation must be attempted at 38–39 weeks of gestation. Since successful ECV of a transverse lie is frequently followed by spontaneous reversion of the fetus to an unstable lie, successful external version in cases of transverse lie may be followed by artificial rupture of the membranes while the vertex is held in position and the labor is induced.
- If the vertex is high in the pelvis when membranes are to be ruptured, the procedure should be performed in a delivery room and with careful needle punctures to control the flow of amniotic fluid and reduce the risk of cord prolapse.
- If labor has begun or membranes have ruptured and the fetus is viable, a cesarean delivery must be performed. However, if labor has begun, but membranes are still intact, external version to either a cephalic or breech presentation may be considered.
- If external version is unsuccessful, the only option for delivering a viable fetus in transverse lie is performing a cesarean delivery. The only cases where vaginal delivery can be considered in patients with transverse lie in modern obstetrics are as follows:
  - *Labor occurs with a previable fetus or dead fetus very early in gestation, and placenta previa has been ruled out:* In these cases of transverse lie, vaginal delivery can be attempted because the small, collapsed fetal body can often pass through the birth canal.
  - *Delivery of second twin in transverse lie where the first twin has been delivered vaginally:* The second twin can be delivered vaginally with internal podalic version and total breech extraction.

Each of the management options for transverse lie is described next in detail.

External Cephalic Version

 Q. Write a short note on external cephalic version.

Definition

External cephalic version is a procedure in which the clinician externally rotates the fetus from a transverse lie into a cephalic presentation. The use of ECV helps in producing considerable cost savings in the management of the fetus in transverse lie by reducing the rate of cesarean section.

Prerequisites for ECV

Before the performance of ECV, the following prerequisites should be fulfilled:
- The place where ECV is being performed should have all facilities available for cesarean section. There is always a possibility for emergency cesarean section during the procedure, in case there is a decline in fetal heart rate.
- Blood grouping and cross-matching should be done in case an emergency cesarean section is required. In case the mother is Rh-negative, administration of anti-D immunoglobulin is required after the procedure in order to prevent the risk of isoimmunization.
- The patient should have nothing by mouth for at least 8 hours prior to the procedure.
- An ultrasound examination must be performed to confirm the shoulder presentation, check the rate of fetal growth, amniotic fluid volume, and rule out the presence of any associated anomalies.
- A nonstress test or a biophysical profile must be performed prior to ECV to confirm fetal well-being.
- Though ECV can be performed by a clinician single-handedly, an assistant is usually required.
- Before performing an ECV, a written informed consent must be obtained from the mother.
- A tocolytic agent such as terbutaline in a dosage of 0.25 mg may be administered subcutaneously. By producing uterine relaxation, administration of this drug is supposed to help increase the success rate of procedure. The use of oral, parenteral, or general anesthesia should be avoided due to an increased risk of complications.
- Whether the process has been successful or has failed, a nonstress test and an ultrasound examination must be performed after each attempt of ECV and after the end of the procedure in order to rule out fetal bradycardia and confirm successful version. Some contraindications for the procedure are described in **Table 4.1**.

Procedure

- The patient is placed in a supine or slight Trendelenburg position. Ultrasonic gel is applied liberally over the abdomen in order to decrease friction and to reduce

TABLE 4.1: Contraindications for external cephalic version.

Absolute contraindications	Relative contraindications
• Multiple gestation with a fetus presenting as a transverse lie • Herpes simplex virus infection • Placenta previa • Nonreassuring fetal heart rate tracing • Premature rupture of membranes • Significant third-trimester bleeding (placenta previa, etc.)	• Uterine malformation • Evidence of uteroplacental insufficiency (IUGR, preeclampsia, etc.) • Fetal anomaly • Maternal cardiac disease

the chances of an overvigorous manipulation. External version can be performed by a clinician who is experienced in the procedure along with his/her assistant.

- Initially, the clinician grasps the fetus from its two poles.
- While performing the ECV, the clinician helps in gently manipulating the fetal head towards the pelvis while the podalic pole is brought up cephalad towards the fundus **(Figs. 4.6A to D)**.
- While doing the ECV, the fetus should be moved gently rather than using forceful movements.
- If unsuccessful, the version can be reattempted at a later time. The procedure should only be performed in a facility equipped for emergency cesarean section.
- No consensus has been reached regarding how many ECV attempts are appropriate at one particular time. At a particular time setting, multiple attempts can be made ensuring that the procedure does not become uncomfortable for the patient. Also, fetal heart rate needs to be assessed after each attempt at ECV.
- If an attempt at ECV proves to be unsuccessful, the practitioner has the option of either sending the patient home after fixing the date for elective cesarean delivery or proceeding with a cesarean delivery.

Complications of ECV

Though ECV is largely a safe procedure, it can be associated with complications, some of which are mentioned in **Box 4.1**.

Internal Podalic Version

> **Q. Is there any scope for internal version for management of transverse lie in modern obstetrics?**
>
> **Q. A 27-year-old primigravida with preterm gestation (28 weeks) presented with an intrauterine death with transverse lie having uterine contractions. What would be further management in this case?**

Internal podalic version involves manipulating the fetus with the help of the operator's one hand introduced inside

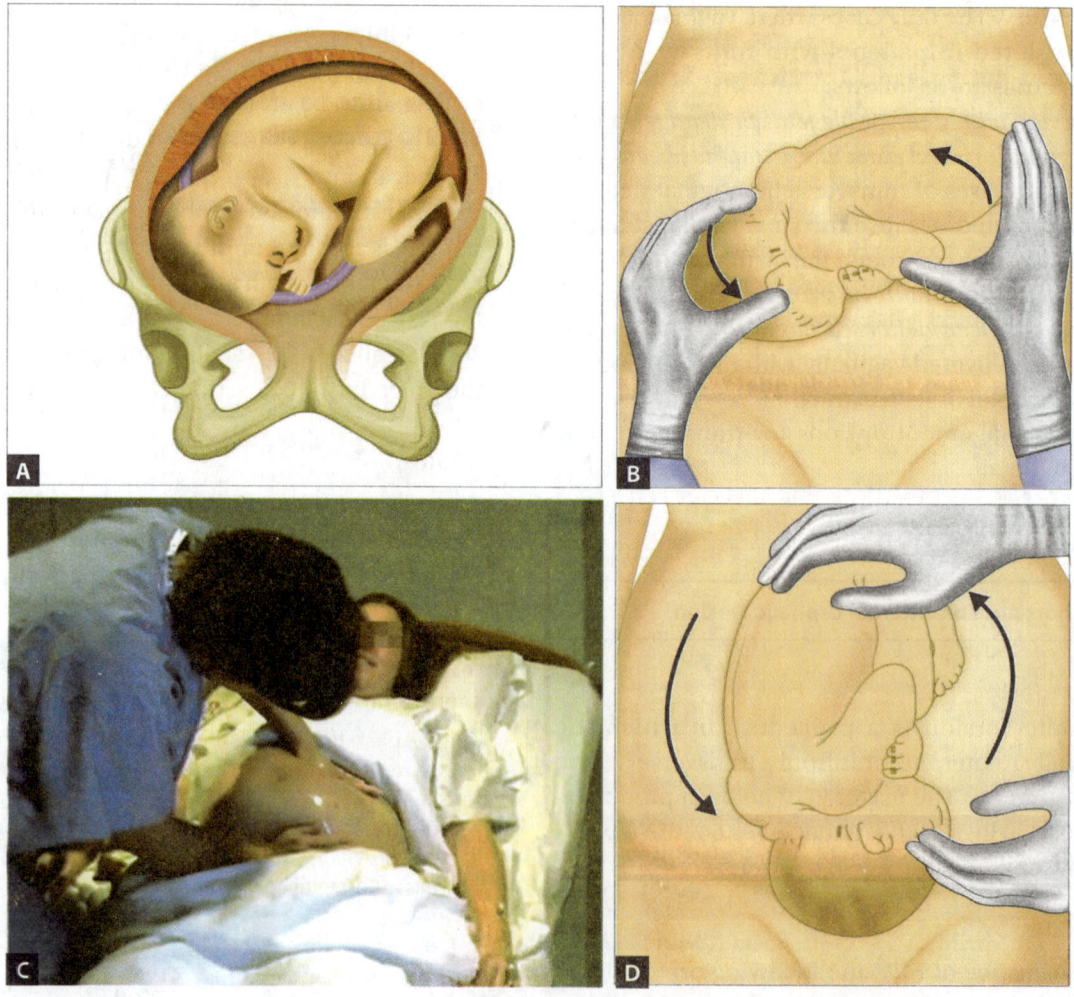

Figs. 4.6A to D: Procedure for ECV in case of transverse lie. (A) A fetus originally in RDA; (B) The procedure of ECV; (C) Photograph showing an obstetrician perform ECV on a woman; (D) The presence of fetus in longitudinal lie after version. (ECV: external cephalic version; RDA: right dorsoanterior position)

BOX 4.1: Complications of external cephalic version.
- Premature onset of labor, premature rupture of the membranes
- Fetomaternal hemorrhage (danger of development of Rh isoimmunization in Rh-negative pregnancies)
- Fetal distress (e.g., cord entanglement resulting in fetal bradycardia)
- Transient reduction of the fetal heart rate
- *Failure of version*: Spontaneous reversion into transverse presentation

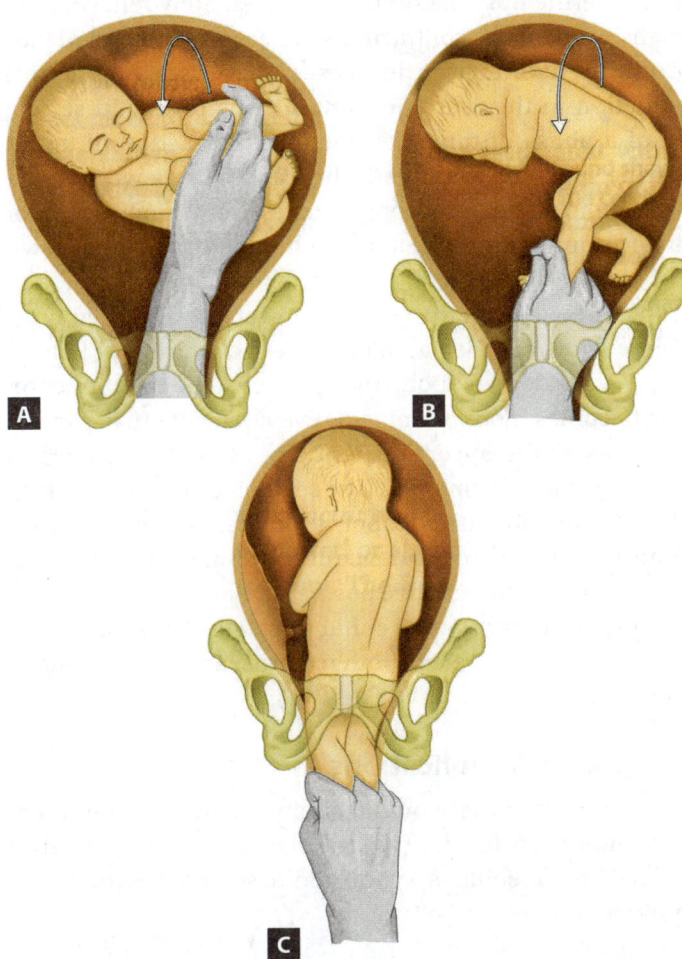

Figs. 4.7A to C: Technique of internal podalic version.

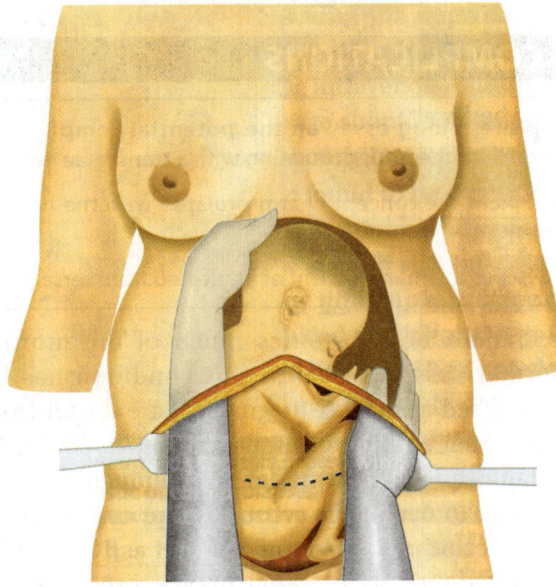

Fig. 4.8: Intra-abdominal version of the fetus (in transverse lie) to longitudinal lie by the assistant at the time of cesarean section. The fetus is later extracted as breech by the surgeon through the transverse lower uterine incision (dotted line).

the uterus to help bring down the podalic pole of the fetus into the lower pole of the uterus **(Figs. 4.7A to C)**. This is completed with the breech extraction of the baby.

Indication: In modern obstetrics the only indication for internal version is fetus in transverse lie in case of second baby in twin gestation.
- Besides this indication, this technique is rarely employed in obstetric practice.
- This technique must never be employed in case of obstructed labor.

MANAGEMENT DURING LABOR

There is hardly any scope for ECV in labor as fetal manipulation at this time is likely to rupture the membranes and cause drainage of amniotic fluid, increasing the further risk for development of complications. Therefore, if the maternal and fetal conditions are stable, the best option would be to perform a cesarean section. However, at some healthcare centers with limited resources, clinicians opt for a stabilizing induction in which ECV is used for converting transverse lie into a cephalic presentation and ensuring that the fetus remains in that position by starting an oxytocin drip immediately following the procedure of version. The labor is closely monitored and an ARM is done when the head is engaged. Labor follows in normal fashion and is usually followed by a normal vaginal delivery in cephalic presentation.

Cesarean Delivery

In case of dorsosuperior position, the fetus may be delivered as a footling breech through a low transverse incision in a well-developed lower uterine segment. However, it may be difficult to deliver a fetus through a low transverse incision in case of dorsoinferior position, due to potential technical difficulties associated with extraction of the fetus. In these cases the obstetrician may find it difficult to grasp the fetal feet and effect a footling breech extraction. A vertical incision in the lower uterine segment may be employed in these cases. Alternatively, if the fetal membranes are intact at the time of cesarean delivery, intra-abdominal version of the fetus can convert the transverse lie to a cephalic or breech presentation, allowing delivery through a low-segment transverse incision **(Fig. 4.8)**. A vertical incision, even in the lower uterine segment is less desirable as it increases the risk of uterine rupture in a subsequent pregnancy.

96 Normal and Abnormal Presentations

> **COMPLICATIONS**
>
> **Q.** Write a long essay on the potential complications associated with the fetus presenting with a transverse lie.
>
> **Q.** Explain the concept of arm prolapse with the help of a short essay.
>
> **Q.** Discuss the management of neglected transverse lie.

Though in modern obstetrics much of the morbidity and mortality associated with this condition has been considerably reduced, these pregnancies are at an increased risk of maternal and perinatal morbidities in comparison to pregnancies in which the fetus is cephalic or breech presentation. In developed countries, the most important causes of morbidity in cases of transverse lie are related to conditions such as placenta previa, prolapse of the umbilical cord, fetal trauma, and prematurity. In developing countries, increased morbidity and mortality are related to complications of neglected transverse lie such as arm prolapse, obstructed labor, and ruptured uterus.

■ MATERNAL COMPLICATIONS

Arm Prolapse
Due to the ill-fitting fetal part, the sudden rupture of membranes can result in the escape of a large amount of liquor and the prolapse of fetal arm **(Figs. 4.9A and B)**. Prolapse of fetal arm is often accompanied by a loop of cord. The consequences of a neglected arm prolapse are shown in **Flowchart 4.2**.

Obstructed Labor
If the transverse lie with or without a prolapsed arm is left neglected, a series of complications including obstructed labor can occur **(Flowchart 4.2)**. In primigravidas, as a result of obstructed labor, features of maternal exhaustion and sepsis are apparent. However, the uterus becomes inert. On the other hand, in multigravidae, the uterus responds vigorously in the face of obstruction. In order to push out the fetus, the upper uterine segment thickens whereas the lower uterine segment distends. A retraction ring forms at the junction of upper and lower uterine segments **(Fig. 4.10)**. If the uterine obstruction is not immediately relieved, the intensity of uterine contractions increases. As the frequency of uterine contraction increases, there is a progressive reduction in the relaxation phase. This results in setting up of a phase of tonic contractions. Retraction of upper uterine segment continues. This causes the lower uterine segment to elongate, become progressively thinner in order to accommodate the fetus which is being pushed down from the upper segment, resulting in formation of a circular groove between the upper and lower uterine segments. This is known as the pathological retraction ring or Bandl's ring. As the degree of obstruction increases, the retraction ring becomes more prominent. Eventually, there is rupture of uterus as the lower segment gives way due to marked thinning of the uterine wall. The sequence of changes taking place during obstructed labor is illustrated in **Figure 4.11**. There is an increased incidence of dehydration, ketoacidosis, septicemia, rupture uterus, postpartum hemorrhage, shock, peritonitis, injury to the genital tract, etc. All these factors result in increased rate of both maternal and fetal morbidity and mortality.

Long-term Complications
Long-term maternal complications include development of genitourinary fistulas **(Fig. 4.12)**, secondary amenorrhea (related to Sheehan's syndrome associated with PPH), hysterectomy, etc.

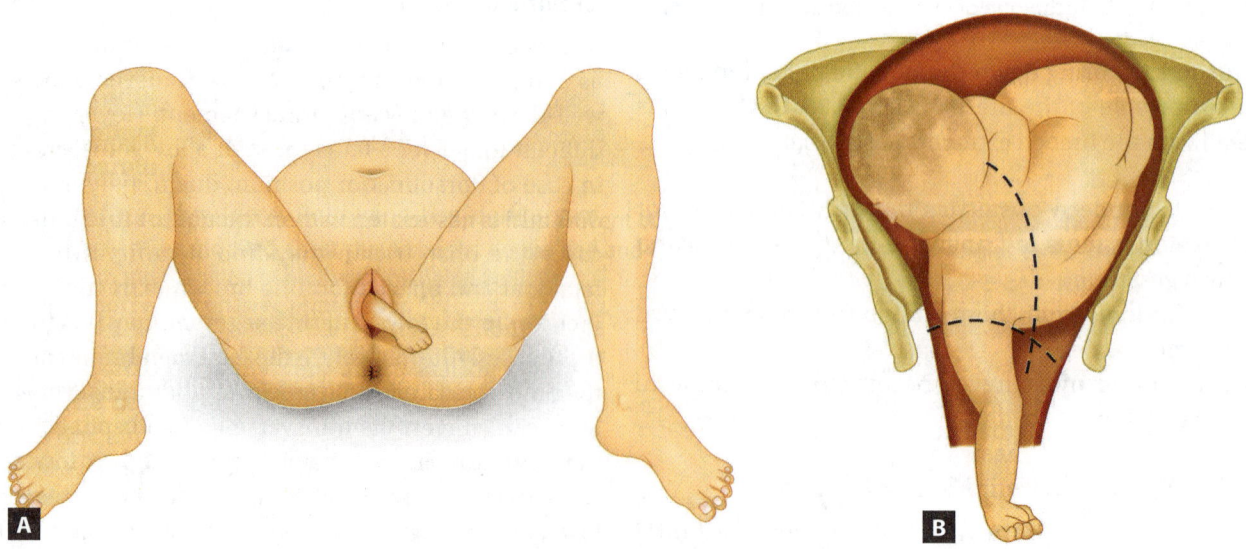

Figs. 4.9A and B: Arm prolapse.

Flowchart 4.2: Consequences of a neglected arm prolapse.

```
Transverse lie
      ↓
 Arm prolapse
      ↓
   ┌──┴──────────────────────┐
Neglected           Managed with an
                    emergency cesarean section
   │
┌──┴──────────────┐
Primigravida    Multigravida
   ↓                ↓
Uterus becomes    Upper uterine segment thickens
inert              ↓
   ↓              Lower uterine segment thins out,
Uterus does not   stretches and elongates
rupture but other  ↓
complications such Formation of pathological retraction ring
as maternal       or Bandl's ring
exhaustion,        ↓
ketoacidosis,     Uterine rupture
sepsis occur       ↓
   ↓              Maternal complications such as shock,
Increased         sepsis and peritonitis
maternal           ↓
morbidity         Increased maternal mortality
```

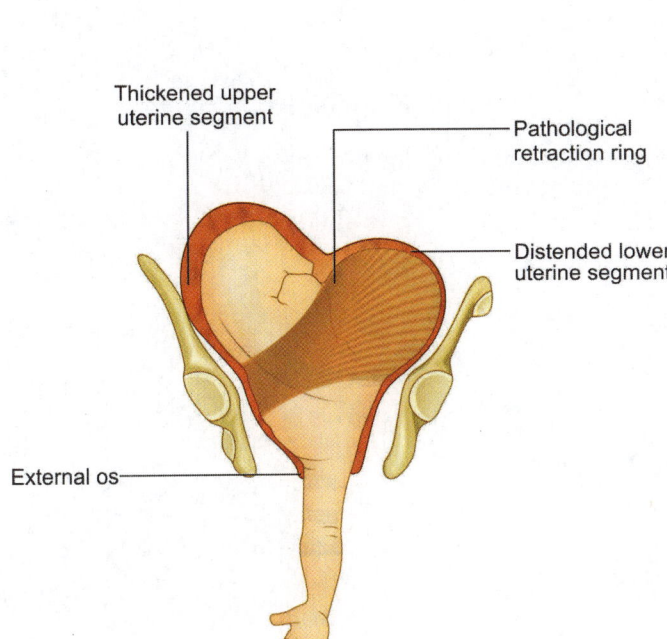

Fig. 4.10: Formation of retraction ring.

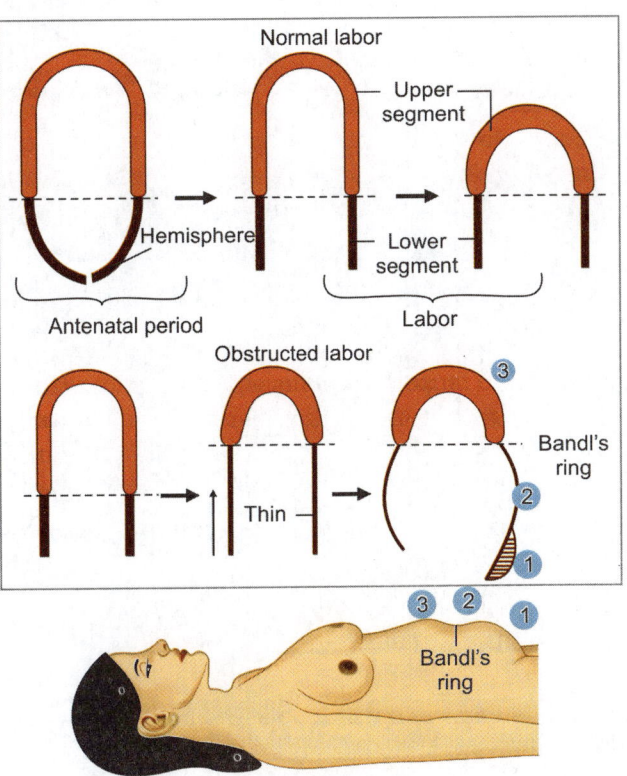

Fig. 4.11: Obstructed labor. [① Edematous bladder; ② Overstretched lower segment (impending rupture); ③ Thickened upper segment]

98 Normal and Abnormal Presentations

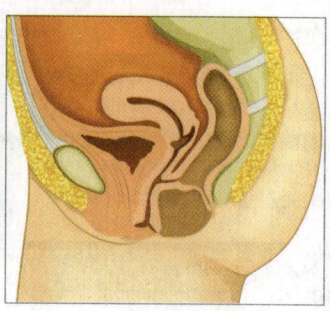
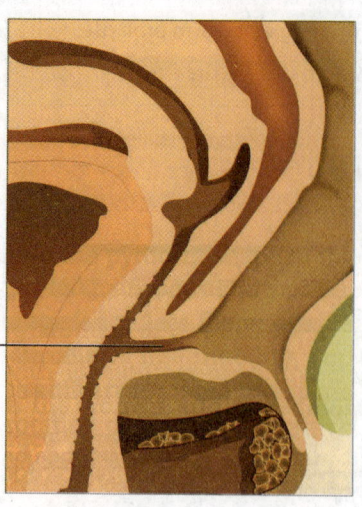

Fistula between rectum and vagina (rectovaginal)

Fig. 4.12: Genitourinary fistula.

FETAL COMPLICATIONS

Fetal Asphyxia

Tonic uterine contractions can interfere with uteroplacental circulation, resulting in fetal distress. Other fetal complications may include preterm birth, premature rupture of membranes, intrauterine fetal death, and increased fetal mortality.

EVIDENCE-BASED CLINICAL TRIALS

List of references can be scanned through QR code to enable the readers gain deeper insight of the subject by referring to the entire article or its abstract.

CHAPTER 5

Occipitoposterior Position

CASE STUDY

A 26-years-old primigravida patient presented at 37 weeks of gestation with the complaints of abdominal pain intermittently since past few hours. She has been complaining of severe back pain since morning. She also gave a history of rupturing the membranes half an hour back, following which she was rushed to the hospital. On GPE, the patient's vitals were stable. On abdominal examination, fundal height corresponded to 38 weeks of gestation. The fetal head was palpated on pelvic grip and it was not engaged. On vaginal examination, cervix was 4 cm dilated, 70–80% effaced, and the head was palpated at –1 station. The fetal occiput could be palpated and was present posteriorly.

INTRODUCTION

This is a type of abnormal position of the vertex where the occiput is placed over the left sacroiliac joint [left occipitoposterior (LOP) or 4th position of vertex] or right sacroiliac joint [right occipitoposterior (ROP) or third position of vertex] **(Figs. 5.1A and B)** or directly over the sacrum (direct OP position). ROP is more common than the LOP position as dextrorotation of the uterus favors ROP, if the back is on right side. Also, the left oblique diameter is slightly reduced in size due to the presence of sigmoid colon due to which the right oblique diameter is slightly longer than the left oblique diameter. OP position can be considered as an abnormal position of the vertex rather than an abnormal presentation. It can be of two types:

1. *Primary:* Occurrence of the OP position before the onset of labor and during the antenatal period.
2. *Secondary:* Occurrence of the OP position during the labor.

Cesarean section is not indicated per se in the cases of OP position. Most of the fetuses in OP position before labor rotate back into occipitoanterior (OA) position in the intrapartum period. Persistence of the OP position is important because it can be associated with labor abnormalities and numerous maternal and neonatal complications (e.g., birth trauma, neonatal acidosis, etc.).

The likely outcomes in case of OP position are summarized in **Flowchart 5.1**.

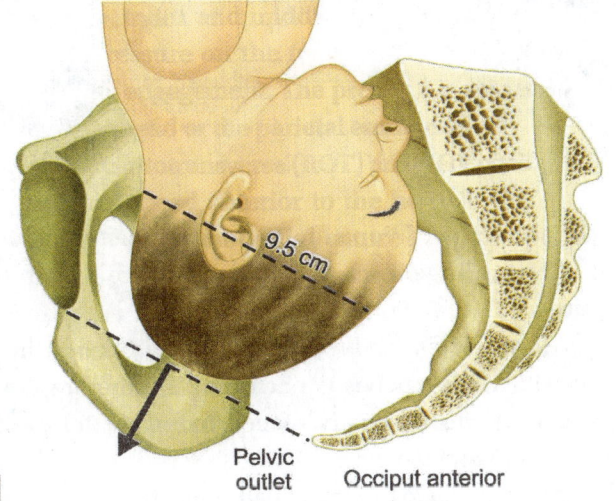 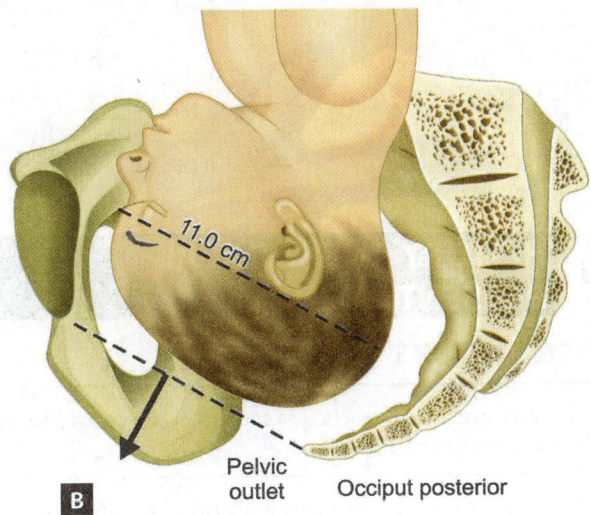

Figs 5.1A and B: (A) Left occipitoanterior position and; (B) Left occipitoposterior position.

Flowchart 5.1: Occipitoposterior position and its likely outcomes.

Occipitoposterior position
Lie: longitudinal; presentation: vertex; denominator: occiput
Presenting part: Anterior (left) parietal bone (in ROP)
Diameter of engagement: Right oblique diameter in ROP and left oblique diameter in LOP
Engaging diameter: The engaging transverse diameter is biparietal diameter (9.5 cm) and that of anterior posterior diameter is either occipitofrontal diameter (11.5 cm) or suboccipitofrontal (10 cm)

- Favorable conditions:
  - Pelvis is adequate
  - Good uterine contractions
    - Increasing flexion with engagement of fetal head
    - Rotation of fetal head by three-eighths of circle
    - Expectant management
    - Spontaneous vaginal delivery
      - Pelvis is adequate
        - The following options can be used:
          - Ventouse
          - Manual rotation and forceps application
          - Forceps (Keilland's) rotation and extraction (only in expert hands)
      - Pelvis is inadequate
        - Cesarean section

- Unfavorable conditions:
  - Plevis is inadequate
  - Uterine inertia
    - Engagement of head is delayed, deflexion persists
      - Short anterior rotation → Deep transverse arrest
      - Short posterior rotation → Persistent occipitoposterior position
        - Spacious gynecoid pelvis → Face-to-pubis delivery
        - Arrest in descent
          - Following options can be used:
            - Ventouse/forceps delivery
            - Manual rotation and forceps applications
          - Station of fetal head above the ischial spines → Cesarean delivery
          - Station of fetal head below the ischial spines → Ventouse or forceps with deep episiotomy
      - Nonrotation → Oblique posterior arrest
        - Further progress of labor is unlikely
          - Pelvis is adequate
          - Pelvis is not adequate → Cesarean delivery

(LOP: left occipitoposterior; ROP: right occipitoposterior)

HISTORY AND CLINICAL PRESENTATION

RISK FACTORS

Q. Enumerate the risk factors for development of occipitoposterior position.

It is now believed that the OP position is actually often the result of malrotation from an OA position. Most of the cases of OP position are idiopathic. Various risk factors associated with the pathogenesis of OP position are illustrated in **Figures 5.2A to D**. Some of these include:

- *Presence of an anthropoid or android pelvis:* In these cases, the forepelvis is narrow and therefore the wide occiput can be easily placed in the wider posterior segment of the pelvis.
- Marked deflexion of fetal head
- High pelvic inclination

Occipitoposterior Position

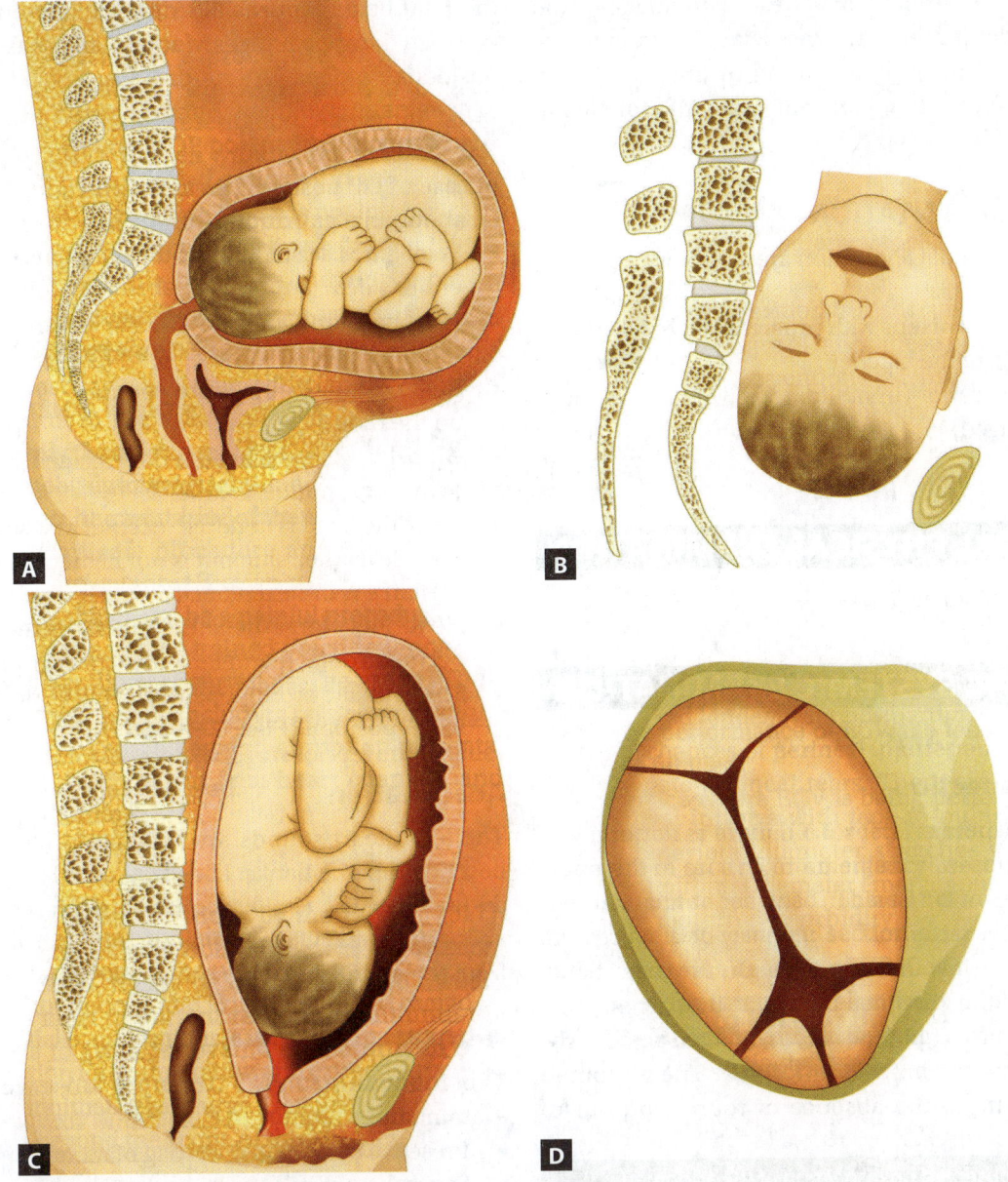

Figs. 5.2A to D: Causes of occipitoposterior position. (A) Pendulous abdomen found in multipara; (B) Flat sacrum with deflexed head leads to further deflexion and occipitoposterior position; (C) Placenta placed on the anterior abdominal wall; and (D) Android pelvis.

- Attachment of placenta on the anterior uterine wall
- Brachycephaly of fetal head
- *Abnormal uterine contractions:* If the uterine contractions are not strong enough to cause descent and flexion of the fetal head, the head may remain deflexed and present as OP position.
- Nulliparity
- Maternal age > 35 years
- Obesity
- African–American race
- Previous OP delivery
- Decreased pelvic outlet capacity
- *Maternal kyphosis:* The convexity of fetal back fits with the concavity of maternal spine (created due to maternal lumbar kyphosis)
- Gestational age ≥41 weeks
- Birth weight ≥ 4,000 g
- Prolonged first and/or second stage of labor
- *Epidural analgesia in causation of OP position:* Whether epidural analgesia has a causative role in OP position at delivery remains a matter of controversy. Many studies have demonstrated that the women with OP position had epidural anesthesia in place. It is still not very clear whether the epidural anesthesia is a cause or effect of OP position. It is possible that under the effect of the epidural anesthesia, the relaxation of pelvic musculature either promotes fetal rotation of OA position to OP or inhibits rotation from OP to OA position. Alternatively, OP position is associated with more painful and prolonged labors, thereby increasing the requirement of epidural

anesthesia for pain control. These data suggest that pelvic musculature relaxation associated with epidural analgesia leads to malpositioning of the fetal head, and this is an important mechanism for OP position at delivery.

CLINICAL PRESENTATION

Symptoms suggestive of OP position are as follows:
- Early ROM
- Backache which worsens with progress of labor
- Frequent filling of the bladder
- Prolongation of labor (in nulliparous women, the labor may be prolonged)

GENERAL PHYSICAL EXAMINATION

No specific finding is observed on GPE.

SPECIFIC SYSTEMIC EXAMINATION

ABDOMINAL EXAMINATION

Abdominal Inspection

On abdominal inspection **(Box 5.1)**, there is flattening of the abdominal contour from the umbilicus up to the pubic symphysis in cases of OP position. The abdominal contour may appear concave (scaphoid). There may be a depression at or immediately below the umbilicus. On the other hand, there is fullness of the abdomen below the umbilicus in OA position. In OP position, the fetal back is directed posteriorly, whereas the limbs are directed anteriorly. The abdomen looks flattened due to the absence of round contour of the fetal back. **Figures 5.3A and B** show the comparison between the appearances of abdomen in cases of OP and OA positions.

Abdominal Palpation

In case of OP position, the following findings are observed on abdominal palpation **(Box 5.2)**:
- Fetal limbs are palpated more easily near the midline on either side.
- Fetal back and anterior shoulders are far away from the midline.
- ROP position being more common, the fetal back is felt on the right side.
- On pelvic grip, the head is not engaged. Head is often felt high and is nonballotable.
- Since the head is deflexed, occiput and sinciput are at the same level (i.e., sinciput is not higher than the occiput as seen in a well-flexed head).
- Head feels large because it is deflexed and the large occipitofrontal diameter (11.5 cm) is gripped.
- The cephalic prominence is not felt as prominently as felt in OA position **(Figs. 5.4A and B)**.

Auscultation

The fetal heart sounds are difficult to locate and may be best heard in the flanks. Localization of fetal heart sounds is difficult because fetal limbs are between the fetal chest and abdominal wall. On auscultation, FHS is usually heard away from the middle line below the umbilicus.

VAGINAL EXAMINATION

The following findings may be observed on vaginal examination:
- Presence of an elongated bag of membranes
- Sagittal sutures occupy any of the oblique diameters of the pelvis.
- Posterior fontanel and lambdoid suture are felt near the sacroiliac joint.

BOX 5.1: Findings observed on inspection of the abdomen.
- Flat abdomen below the umbilicus
- Subumbilical transverse groove
- Scaphoid abdominal contour below the umbilicus

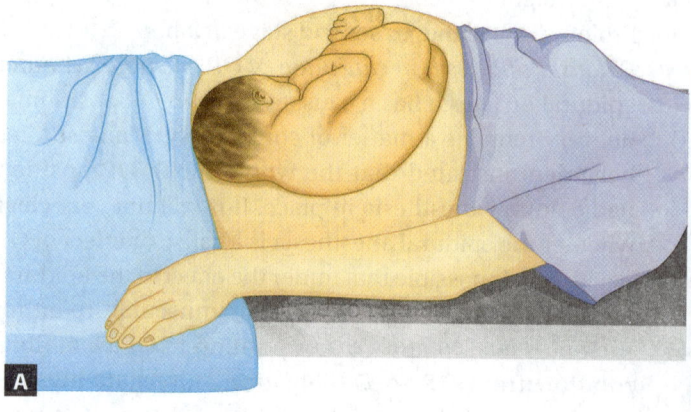
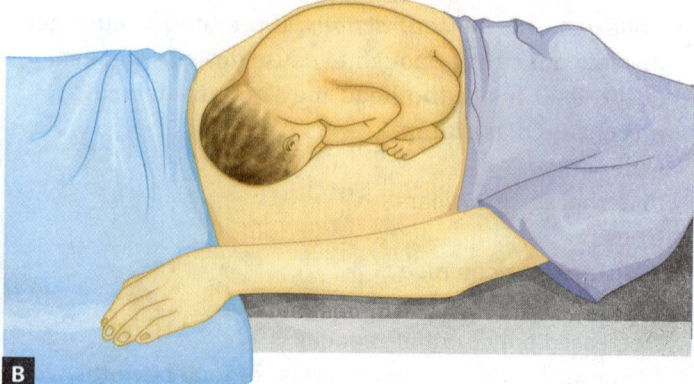

Figs. 5.3A and B: Comparison between occiput anterior and occiput posterior position on abdominal examination. (A) Occiput posterior position; (B) Occiput anterior position.

Occipitoposterior Position

> **BOX 5.2:** Findings observed on palpation of abdomen in case of occipitoposterior position.
> - *Fundal grip:* Soft, bulky, irregular, and nonballotable mass suggestive of breech
> - *Lateral grip:* Fetal back is away from the middle line and may be felt with difficulty in one of the flanks. Fetal limbs are near the midline
> - *First pelvic grip:* The head is usually not engaged
> - *Second pelvic grip:* Head is usually deflexed

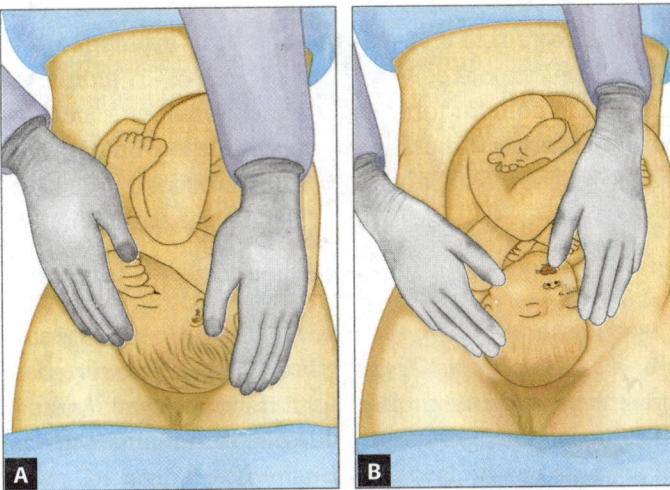

Figs. 5.4A and B: Palpation of the fetal head (third pelvic grip). (A) Occipitoanterior position; (B) Occipitoposterior position.

- Anterior fontanel can be felt more easily due to the deflexed head and at times it may be at a lower level than the posterior one. Anterior fontanel would be felt anteriorly, while the posterior fontanel would be posterior and hence difficult to feel, especially if the head is deflexed.
- Sagittal sutures would be in one of the oblique diameters of maternal pelvis (e.g., right oblique diameter in case of ROP position).
- Cervix may not be well applied to the presenting part.
- With the progress of labor, posterior fontanel is felt laterally and then anteriorly.

In addition to the above, vaginal examination also shows the following:
- Degree of deflexion of fetal head
- Degree of molding of fetal head (presence of caput succedaneum)
- Degree of cervical dilatation and effacement
- Rupture of membranes and cord prolapse
- Direction of the occiput
- Exclusion of contracted pelvis

In late labor, diagnosis may be difficult due to considerable molding and formation of caput succedaneum over the presenting part which obliterates the sutures and the fontanels. In these cases, the occiput can be identified by the direction of the unfolded pinna, which points toward the occiput. If the pinna of the ear is observed to be pointing toward the mother's sacrum, it indicates an OP position.

MANAGEMENT

Management comprising of investigations and definitive obstetric management is discussed next.

INVESTIGATIONS

Diagnosis of OP position is generally made by digital examination, but in case of uncertainty in diagnosis, ultrasound examination is both useful and accurate.

ULTRASONOGRAPHY

Ultrasound examination can be useful in the following:
- Confirmation of the diagnosis
- Other parameters such as fetal weight, fetal well-being, placental localization, and amniotic fluid volume can be determined.

TREATMENT/OBSTETRIC MANAGEMENT

> **Q.** Describe the management of the case study presented in the beginning of the chapter.
>
> **Q.** With the help of a short note, discuss the likely outcomes in case of occipitoposterior position.

In the OP position, a certain degree of deflexion of fetal head is present due to the opposition of the convexities of maternal and fetal spine. Due to the deflexion of fetal head, occipitofrontal diameter (11.5 cm) or suboccipitofrontal diameter (10 cm) enters the pelvis, resulting in delayed engagement. The likely consequences related to OP position are shown in **Figure 5.5** and are based on the rule that part of the fetus which meets the pelvic floor first shall rotate anteriorly. Long anterior rotation of fetal head by three-eighths of the circle occurs in 90% of cases and is the most favorable outcome.

FAVORABLE OUTCOME

In majority of cases, good uterine contractions result in the flexion of fetal head. Descent occurs and the occiput undergoes long anterior-rotation by three-eighths of the circle to lie behind the pubic symphysis, resulting in an OA position. Various factors which can affect (either favor or interfere) with long anterior rotation of fetal head are enlisted in **Table 5.1**.

UNFAVORABLE OUTCOME

In a small number of cases, the outcome may be unfavorable, resulting in short anterior rotation, nonrotation, or short posterior rotation.

104 Normal and Abnormal Presentations

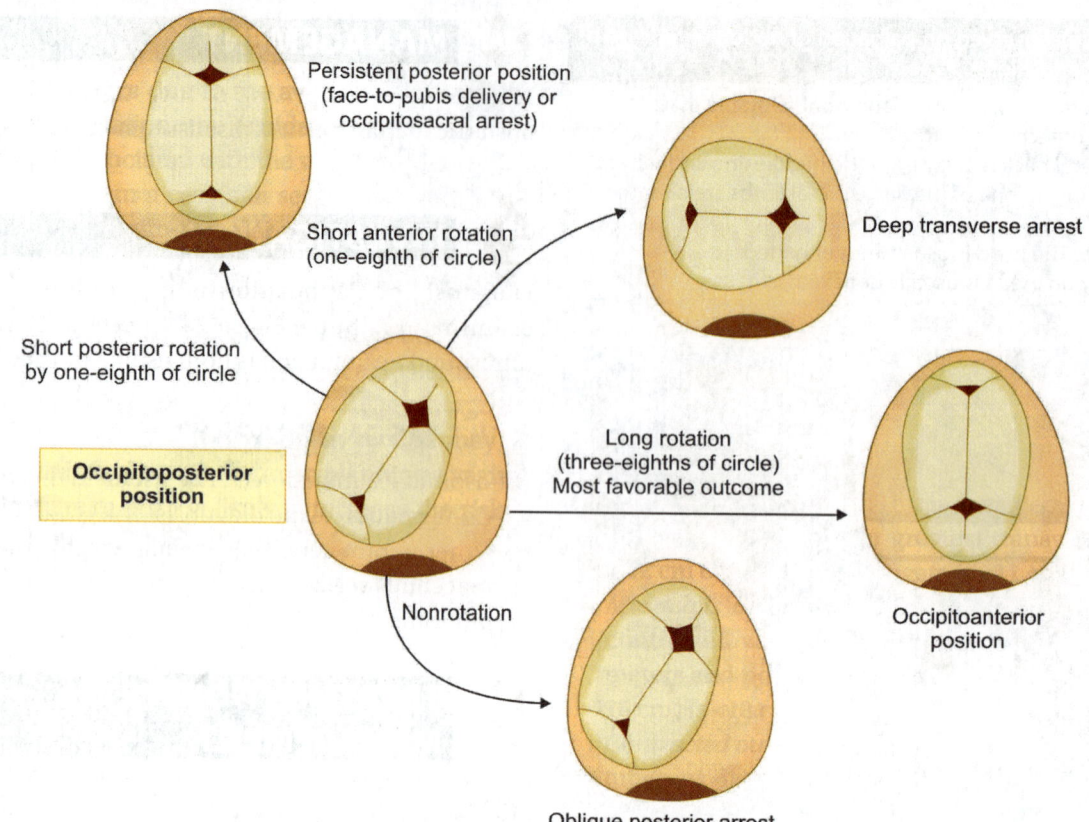

Fig. 5.5: Consequences related to occipitoposterior position.

TABLE 5.1: Factors affecting long anterior rotation.	
Factors favoring long anterior rotation	**Factors interfering with long anterior rotation**
• Strong uterine contractions • Correction of deflexion • Adequate pelvis • Strong pelvic floor • Intact membranes • Epidural anesthesia	• Uterine inertia • Persistent deflexion • Contracted pelvis • Lax or rigid pelvic floor • ROM

(ROM: rupture of membranes)

Short Anterior Rotation

In case of short anterior rotation, the occiput rotates through one-eighth of the circle anteriorly so that the sagittal sutures lie in the bispinous diameter. This position is known as the "deep transverse arrest".

Deep Transverse Arrest

 Q. Write a short note on deep transverse arrest.

In these cases, the occipitofrontal diameter is caught at the narrow bispinous diameter of the outlet. This occurs in about 1% cases. The head is placed deep inside the pelvic cavity, sagittal suture is placed in the transverse bispinous diameter and there is no progress in the descent of fetal head even after half an hour to 1 hour of full cervical dilatation. Some likely causes of deep transverse arrest are enumerated in **Box 5.3**.

> **BOX 5.3:** Causes of deep transverse arrest.
> • Faulty pelvic architecture (prominent ischial spines, flat sacrum, convergent side walls, narrow pubic arch, etc.)
> • Deflexed fetal head
> • Weak uterine contractions
> • Laxity of pelvic floor muscles

Nonrotation of the Occiput

In case of nonrotation of the occiput, sagittal sutures lie in the oblique diameter. Further progress of labor is unlikely and this is known as oblique posterior arrest.

Short Posterior Rotation

Short posterior rotation occurs when the sinciput reaches the pelvic floor first and rotates forward. On the other hand, the occiput fails to rotate. In this case, posterior rotation of the sinciput occurs by one-eighth of the circle, placing the occiput in the sacral hollow. At the same time, sinciput rotates forward to lie under the pubic symphysis. This position is known as persistent occipitoposterior position (POP) **(Figs. 5.6A and B)**. Under favorable conditions with an average-sized baby, spacious pelvis and good uterine contractions, spontaneous face-to-pubis delivery can occur. As a result, the baby is born facing the pubic bone (face-to-pubis delivery). This can occur in 6% cases. Due to deflexed head, the occipitofrontal diameter (11.5 cm) enters the pelvis leading to delayed engagement. Face-to-pubis or direct OP spontaneous delivery or by the aid of forceps usually occurs.

If conditions are not favorable, delivery may not occur, resulting in an occipitosacral arrest. Even if normal vaginal delivery occurs in case of POP position, the labor is generally prolonged.

Persistent Occipitoposterior Position

Course of labor in case of POP is described in **Box 5.4**. In most of the cases, an expectant management is all that is required to achieve spontaneous normal vaginal delivery.

Vaginal examination: The following findings may be observed on vaginal examination:

- In case of POP, on vaginal examination, the anterior fontanel is felt behind the pubic symphysis. However, this may be sometimes masked due to the presence of a large caput succedaneum.

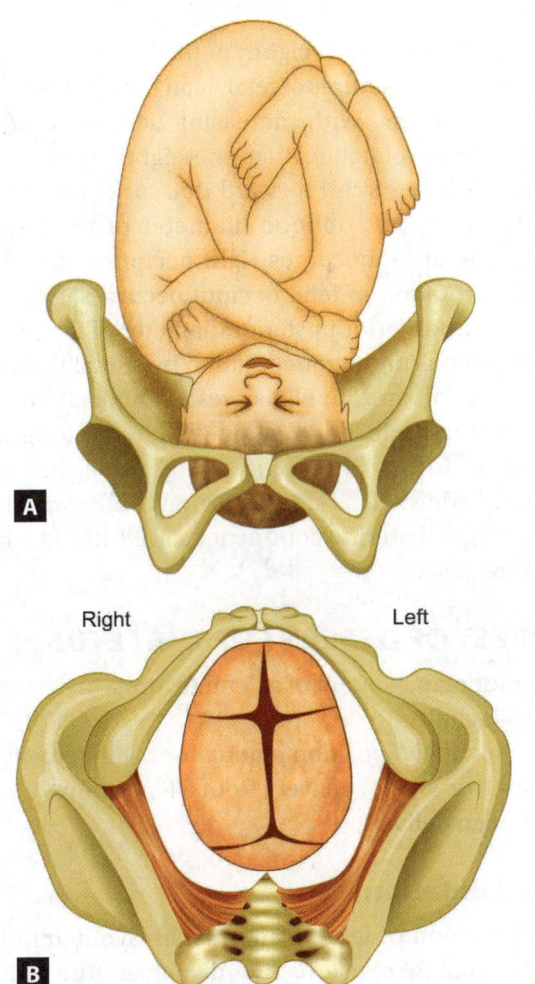

Figs. 5.6A and B: Persistent occipitoposterior position.

BOX 5.4: Course of labor in case of occipitoposterior position.
• Delayed engagement as there is a degree of deflexion • Prolonged labor • Uterine inertia • Premature ROM

- Characteristic molding is present with caput succedaneum on the anterior part of the parietal bone.
- The long occipitofrontal diameter causes considerable anal dilatation and vaginal gaping, while the fetal head is barely visible. The broad biparietal diameter distends the perineum and may cause excessive bulging.

Delivery of the baby: At the time of delivery of fetal head, the following must be done:

- The sinciput emerges from under the pubic symphysis as far as the root of the nose. The assistant must try to promote flexion of fetal head and restrain the head from escaping further than the glabella. This would allow the occiput to sweep the perineum and be born.
- The assistant must extend the head by grasping it and bringing the face down under the pubic symphysis.

EXPECTANT MANAGEMENT

With expectant management, >50% multiparous women and >25% nulliparous women with OP fetuses are likely to achieve spontaneous vaginal delivery. Prerequisites for expectant management of OP position are as follows:

- Presence of a reassuring fetal heart rate
- Average-sized baby and spacious pelvis
- Continued progress in the second stage
- Multiparous women with persistent OP fetuses

Intrapartum Management

Intrapartum management in the cases of OP position comprises of following steps.

First Stage of Labor

Occipitoposterior position may be commonly associated with conditions such as contracted pelvis, cord presentation, or cord prolapse. Therefore, pelvis must be assessed for adequacy and cord presentation or prolapse must be ruled out at the time of vaginal examination. Since cases of OP position are more liable to poor and abnormal progress of labor, PROM and abnormal and/or incoordinate uterine action, the following steps must be taken:

- Intravenous infusion of ringer lactate must be started in anticipation of prolonged labor.
- Due to high chances of PROM, the steps mentioned in **Box 5.5** must be advised to avoid early ROM.
- There may be marked backache. Therefore, analgesic drugs in form of pethidine or epidural analgesics may be administered.

BOX 5.5: Steps to be taken to avoid early ROM.
• Bed rest • Maternal straining to be avoided even there is premature urge to bear down • High enema must be avoided • Vaginal examination must be minimized

BOX 5.6: Contraindication of oxytocin infusion.

- Pelvic disproportion
- Incoordinate uterine action
- Previous uterine scar (previous cesarean delivery, hysterectomy, myomectomy, metroplasty, etc.)
- Grand multipara
- Fetal distress

- Since uterine inertia and prolonged labor are expected, oxytocin infusion must be started unless there is some contraindication present **(Box 5.6)**.
- Watchful expectancy must be observed for around 1 hour hoping for long anterior rotation of the occiput, which will result in normal delivery in 90% of the cases.

Second Stage of Labor and Delivery of the Baby

- During the second stage of labor, mother and fetus must be carefully assessed.
- Oxytocin can be used to combat inertia unless there is some contraindication to the use of oxytocin **(Box 5.6)**.
- Liberal episiotomy should be given to prevent perineal tears.
- Since in the majority of cases, long anterior rotation of head occurs, delivery, occurs spontaneously or with low forceps or ventouse.
- In cases of occipitotransverse or oblique OP positions, ventouse application can be done. In cases of POP, under favorable conditions with an average-sized baby, spacious pelvis and good uterine contractions, spontaneous face-to-pubis delivery, or vaginal delivery with the aid of forceps/ventouse can occur.
- Manual rotation of fetal head or rotation using Kielland's forceps, both of which were previously performed are no longer done nowadays.
- Nowadays, cesarean section is the most commonly used mode of delivery in cases of POP (occipitosacral arrest) or deep transverse arrest.

Molding of fetal head following POP: In cases of fetal head in POP, characteristic molding of head is observed with the caput succedaneum present on the anterior part of the parietal bone. On vaginal examination, anterior fontanel is felt behind the pubic symphysis and a large caput succedaneum may be seen masking this **(Fig. 5.7)**. If the pinna of the ear is observed to be pointing toward the mother's sacrum, it indicates an OP position.

Mechanism of Vaginal Delivery in Case of Occipitoposterior Position

Figures 5.8A to D demonstrate the mechanism of normal vaginal delivery in cases of ROP position. Descent of the head occurs with increased flexion. As the fetal head enters the maternal pelvis, sagittal sutures are in right oblique diameter of the pelvis. With the increasing descent, occiput and shoulders rotate by one-eighth of the circle forward due to which the sagittal sutures of fetal head occupy the transverse diameter of pelvis. With increasing descent, occiput and shoulders have rotated further one-eighth of circle (total of two-eighths of a circle) forward due to which the sagittal sutures occupy left oblique diameter of the pelvis. The position therefore becomes right occipitoanterior (ROA). As further rotation of fetal occiput occurs, sagittal sutures now lie in the anterior posterior diameter of the pelvis. This way occiput has undergone rotation by a total three-eighths of the circle forward. In 90% cases of OP position, delivery occurs normally through vaginal route as long anterior rotation occurs by three-eighths of circle, bringing the occiput anteriorly. This kind of favorable outcome occurs in cases with good uterine contractions, well-flexed fetal head, and roomy pelvis.

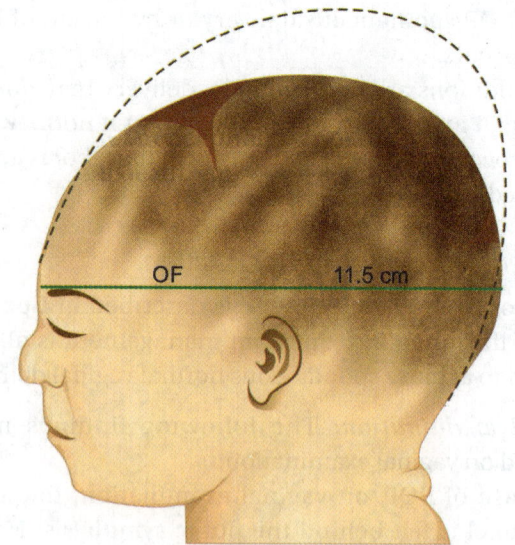

Fig. 5.7: Molding of fetal head following persistent occipitoposterior position. (OF: occipitofrontal)

ARREST OF DESCENT OF THE FETUS

Options for management of a definite arrest of descent of the OP fetus include:

- Rotation to OA position manually or with forceps
- Operative vaginal delivery from OP position
- Cesarean delivery

Manual Rotation

Manual rotation of fetal head must be avoided in the first stage of labor because it may disengage the fetal head, which could lead to prolapse of the umbilical cord or small parts. Rotation is more likely to be successful in the second stage of labor when the cervix has fully dilated. The optimum time for rotation during the second stage has yet not been decided. However, performing prophylactic manual rotation prior to the arrest of descent is likely to be more successful than the procedure performed after arrest of descent.

Occipitoposterior Position

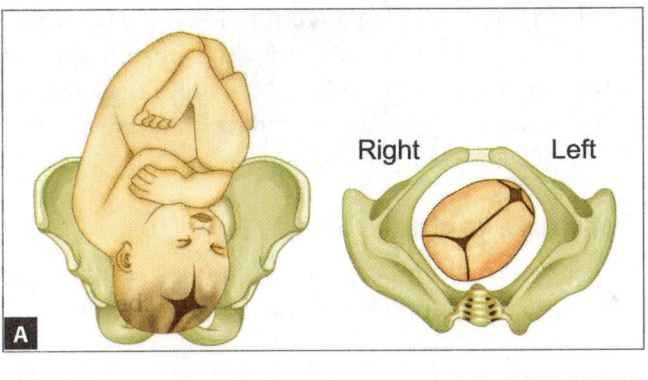
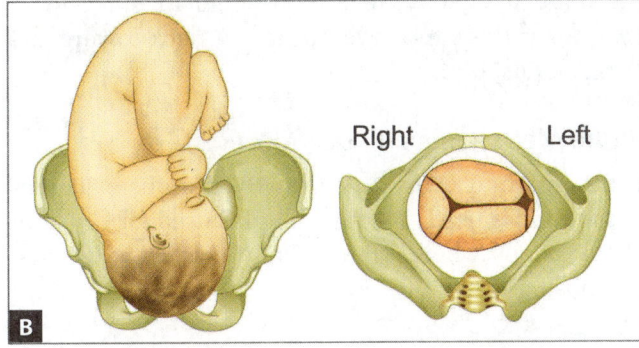
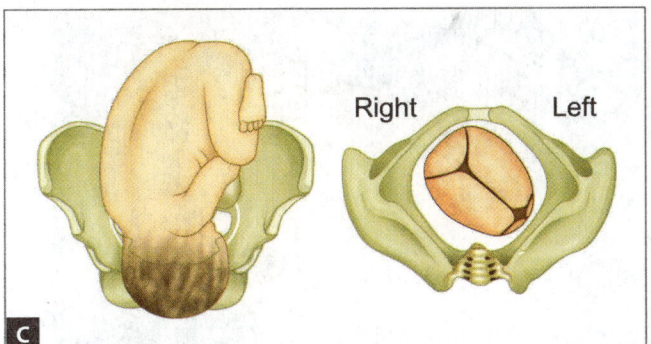
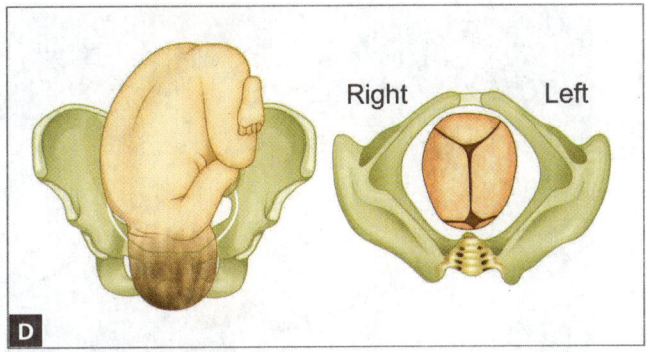

Figs. 5.8A to D: Mechanism of vaginal delivery in case of occipitoposterior position.

Prerequisites

- The maternal bladder must be emptied prior to the procedure.
- The procedure is usually performed under general anesthesia.
- The patient must be placed in lithotomy position.
- Complete surgical asepsis must be maintained.
- Vaginal examination must be performed prior to the procedure to identify the direction of occiput.

Procedure of Three-finger Rotation

- In the procedure of three-finger rotation of fetal head **(Figs. 5.9A and B)**, the obstetrician uses tips of his/her thumb, index and middle fingers of the right hand to apply pressure on the fetal head at the level of the diameter of engagement. The pressure is applied on the side of fetal head or the parietal eminence.
- In right occipitotransverse (ROT) and ROP positions, the fingers are placed anterior to the head in the anterior segment of the lambdoidal suture near the posterior fontanel. Pressure is applied by the ulnar border of hand to perform digital rotation.
- In left occipitotransverse (LOT) and LOP positions, the fingers are placed posterior to the head and the pressure is applied by the radial border of the hand.
- After flexing and slightly dislodging the vertex, the obstetrician then rotates the fetal head to the OA position by rotating his/her hand and forearm.

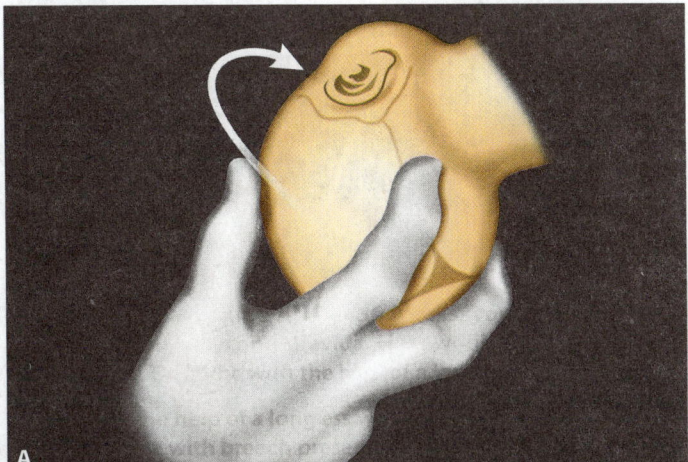
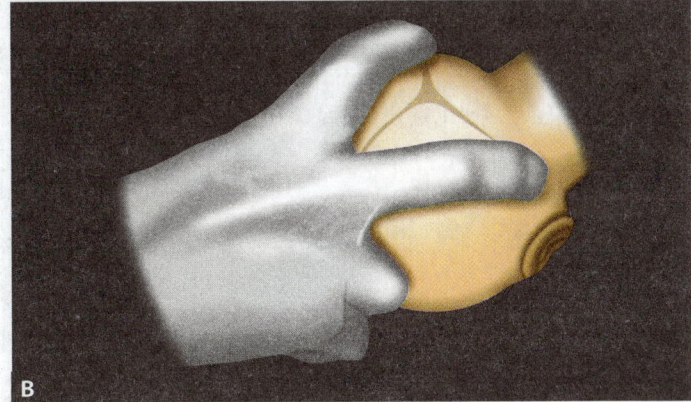

Figs. 5.9A and B: Procedure of three-finger rotation of fetal head. The tips of the index and middle fingers are placed in the anterior segment of the lambdoidal suture near the posterior fontanels. The fingers are used for rotating the fetal head to the occipitoanterior position via rotation of the operator's hand and forearm.

- The fetal head may need to be held in place for a few contractions to prevent rotation back toward the posterior position.

Full-hand Method (Five-finger Rotation)

- In this method **(Figs. 5.10A to F)**, the obstetrician's whole hand is used. The right hand is used for LOP and LOT positions, whereas the left hand is used for ROP and ROT positions.

- The maneuvers of manual rotation must be performed only by skilled and experienced obstetricians, fully conversant in this technique. Nowadays, these maneuvers are rarely used in clinical practice and have been largely replaced by cesarean section.

Operative Vaginal Delivery

Forceps or vacuum can be sometimes used to deliver the fetus from the direct OP position without using the

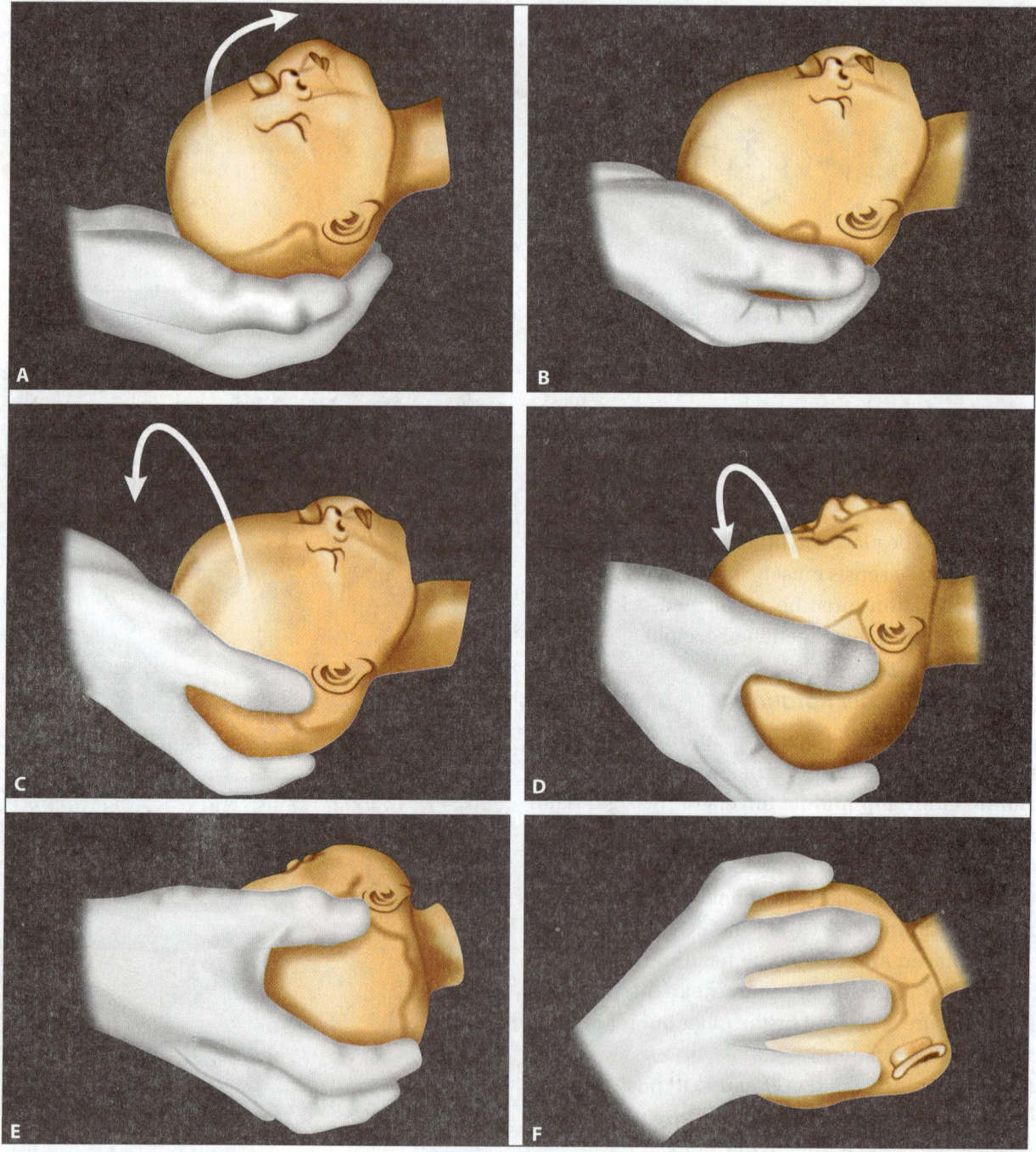

Figs. 5.10A to F: The procedure of five-finger rotation of fetal head. (A) The operator places four fingers behind the posterior parietal bone with the palm up and the thumb over the anterior parietal bone. The head is grasped with the tips of the fingers and thumb; (B to F) During a contraction, the patient is encouraged to push and the operator attempts to flex and rotate the fetal head to the OA position. (OA: occipitoanterior)

procedure of manual rotation. This is probably preferable in those women where the pelvis is too narrow to permit anterior rotation (women with an anthropoid pelvis with a narrow transverse diameter and women with an android pelvis having a narrow arch). OP position is associated with a significantly higher rate of failed operative vaginal delivery in comparison to the OA position. There is no demonstrated advantage of forceps over vacuum delivery for OP fetuses. The choice is usually made based on individual patient factors and clinical situation. Operative vaginal delivery should not be attempted above +2 stations.

Forceps Extraction Following Manual Rotation

Once the fetal head has been manually rotated into OA position, and the obstetrician's right hand is placed on the left side of the pelvis, the left blade of the forceps is applied, followed by the right blade.

In case the obstetrician's left hand is placed on right side of pelvis, right blade of the forceps is applied followed by the left blade which is introduced from underneath the right blade. While introducing the blades, the head is fixed by application of suprapubic pressure by the assistant. Following application, the two blades are locked and traction applied to extract out the fetal head.

Rotation with Forceps

Forceps Rotation

The performance of rotation using forceps (e.g., Kielland's forceps) should be reserved for use by those obstetricians who are highly experienced and skilled in this art due to the high risk of potential complications. Kielland's forceps are used for single application for both rotation and extraction because this forceps has minimal pelvic curve. Detailed description of this procedure is beyond the scope of this chapter.

Scanzoni's Double Application

First the forceps are applied to rotate the occiput anteriorly. Then the forceps are removed and reapplied so that the pelvic curve of the forceps is directed anteriorly. The head is then extracted out. This method is not used in modern obstetrics as it is hazardous to both mother and fetus.

Cesarean Section

The indications for cesarean delivery in case of OP position are listed in **Box 5.7**. Nowadays, cesarean delivery is preferred over manual rotation or application of forceps.

> **BOX 5.7:** Indications for cesarean delivery.
> - Failure of manual rotation or rotation using forceps
> - Contracted pelvis
> - Placenta previa
> - Prolapsed pulsating cord
> - Elderly primigravida

COMPLICATIONS

Various complications associated with OP position are enlisted in **Table 5.2**.

■ MATERNAL

The maternal complications associated with OP position are as follows:
- Since the OP position is associated with prolonged first and second stages of labor, these patients are more likely to undergo interventions, such as ARM, augmentation with oxytocin, operative delivery (vaginal and abdominal), and delivery-related complications such as anal sphincter injury. Prolonged duration of both first and second stages of labor (due to labor dystocia; delayed engagement of the fetal head and abnormal uterine contractions with slow dilatation of cervix) may occur.
- Early ROM
- Extreme degree of molding of fetal skull can result in tentorial tears.
- Increased tendency for postpartum hemorrhage
- High chances of perineal injuries and trauma including complete perineal tears. There are higher chances of perineal injuries with face-to-pubis delivery because the biparietal diameter stretches the perineum and occipitofrontal diameter emerges out of the introitus.
- High maternal morbidity due to increased rate of operative delivery.

Conversion to Face or Brow Presentation

In case the head is deflexed at the onset of labor, it may occasionally extend, especially in case of multiparas. If the

TABLE 5.2: Complications associated with occipitoposterior position.

Maternal	Fetal
• Prolonged labor and/or maternal distress	• Fetal asphyxia
• Infection (intrauterine infection, infections of urinary tract, general infections, and puerperal infections)	• Fetal intracranial injuries (e.g., tears of tentorium cerebelli, cerebral edema, hemorrhage, etc.)
• Injuries to the birth canal	• Excessive molding of fetal head resulting in cerebral edema and hemorrhage
• Atonic and traumatic postpartum hemorrhage	• Cord prolapse
• Obstructed labor	• Fetal and neonatal infections
• Lacerations and damage to soft tissues, extension of episiotomies, bruising, tears of vagina, hematoma formation, etc.	• Potential fetal injuries due to instrumental delivery
• Puerperal sepsis due to prolonged ROM	

extension occurs completely, a face presentation may result. In case of incomplete extension of the face, head is arrested at the brim resulting in brow presentation.

Face Presentation

Face presentation is an abnormal fetal position characterized by an extreme extension of the fetal head so that the fetal face rather than the fetal head becomes the presenting part and the fetal occiput comes in direct contact with the back **(Fig. 5.11)**. Ultrasonography must be performed in order to assess fetal size and to rule out the presence of any bony congenital malformations.

Different Positions in Case of Face Presentation

Denominator in the cases of face presentation is mentum or chin. Four positions are possible depending on the position of the chin with left or right sacroiliac joints **(Figs. 5.12A and B)**:

- Right mentoposterior position (deflexed left OA)
- Left mentoposterior position (deflexed ROA)
- Left mentoanterior position (deflexed ROP)
- Right mentoanterior position (deflexed LOP).

Most common type of face presentation is left mentoanterior position.

Abdominal Examination

In case of mentoanterior positions, the fetal limbs can be palpated anteriorly. Fetal chest is also present anteriorly against the uterine wall. The FHS is thus clearly audible. On abdominal palpation, the groove between the head and neck is not prominent and cephalic prominence lies on the same side as the fetal back. On pelvic grip, the head is not engaged. In case of mentoposterior positions, the back is better palpated toward the front.

Vaginal Examination

The following structures can be felt—alveolar margins of the mouth, nose, malar eminences, supraorbital ridges, and the mentum **(Fig. 5.13)**. Also, there is absence of meconium staining on examining fingers, which helps differentiate mouth from anus.

Management

Delivery occurs spontaneously in most of cases of face presentation. In presence of normal cervical dilatation and descent, there is no need for the obstetrician to intervene. Labor will be longer, but if the pelvis is adequate and the head rotates to a mentoanterior position, a vaginal delivery can

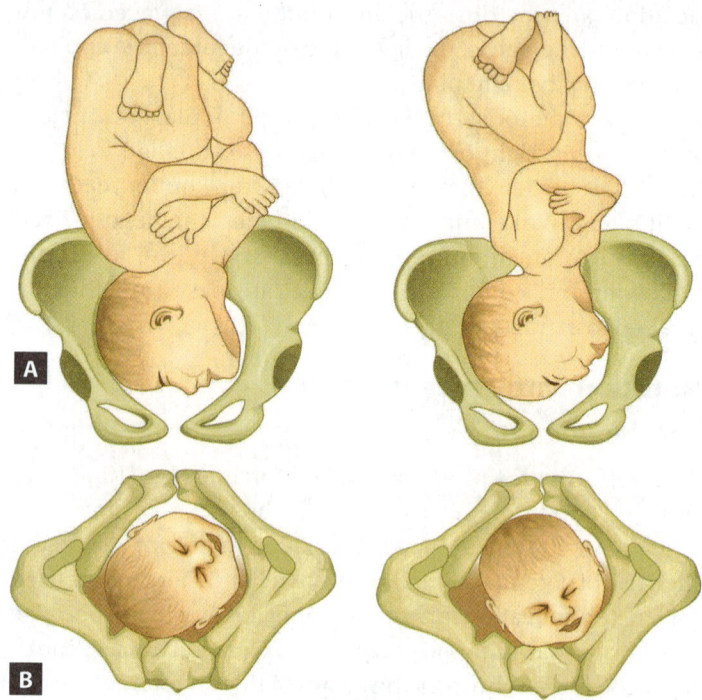

Figs. 5.12A and B: Different positions in case of face presentation. (A) Left mentoanterior position; (B) Left mentoposterior position.

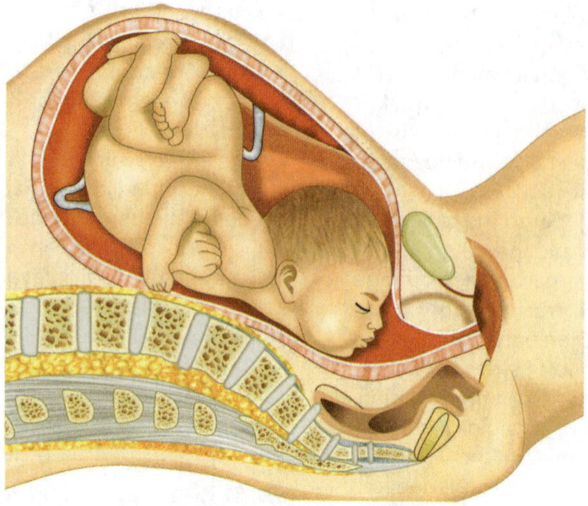

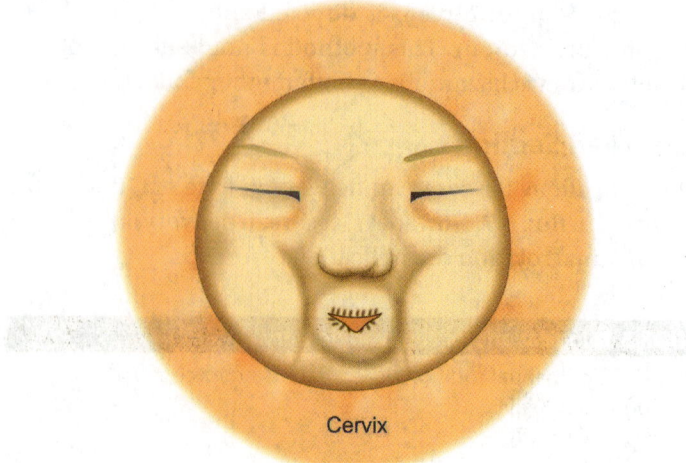

Fig. 5.11: Face presentation.

Fig. 5.13: Vaginal touch picture in case of face presentation.

be expected. The mechanism of delivery and corresponding body movements in case of anterior face presentations are similar to that of the corresponding OA position. The only difference being that delivery of head occurs by flexion rather than extension. The engaging diameter is submentobregmatic in case of a fully extended head.

If the head rotates backward to a mentoposterior position, a cesarean section may be required. In case of posterior face presentations, the mechanism of delivery is same as that of OP position except that the anterior rotation of the mentum occurs in only 20–30% of the cases. In the remaining 70–80% cases, there may be incomplete anterior rotation, no rotation, or short posterior rotation of mentum. There is no possibility of spontaneous vaginal delivery in case of persistent mentoposterior positions. Cesarean section may be required in these cases.

Brow Presentation

This is a type of cephalic presentation where the fetal head is incompletely flexed as shown in the **Figure 5.14**. The head is short of complete extension, which could have resulted in a face presentation. As a result, presenting part becomes the brow. On vaginal examination, the occiput and sinciput are palpated at the same level.

Since the engaging diameter of the head is mentovertical (14 cm), there would be no mechanism of labor with an average-sized baby and a normal pelvis. Vaginal delivery may be the possible option only in cases where there is spontaneous conversion to face or vertex presentation. Therefore, after ruling out the cephalopelvic disproportion and fetal congenital anomalies, the obstetrician must await for spontaneous vaginal delivery. In cases where this does not occur, cesarean section is the best method for delivery.

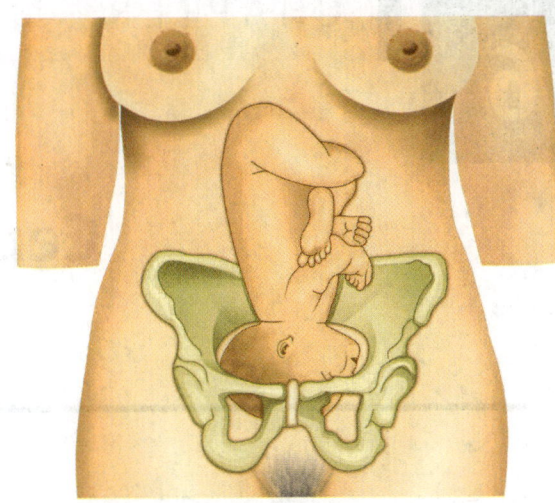

Fig. 5.14: Brow presentation.

FETAL

Neonatal complications associated with delivery in the OP position include a higher risk of 5 minutes Apgar score <7, umbilical artery acidemia, meconium-stained amniotic fluid, birth trauma, and neonatal intensive care admission. There is increased perinatal morbidity and mortality due to asphyxia or trauma.

EVIDENCE-BASED CLINICAL TRIALS

List of references can be scanned through QR code to enable the readers gain deeper insight of the subject by referring to the entire article or its abstract.

CHAPTER 6

Cephalopelvic Disproportion

CASE STUDY

A 34-year-old, short-statured primigravida patient is seen in the antenatal clinic at 38 weeks' gestation for a routine antenatal check-up. She is clinically well and reports normal fetal movements. The fetal heart rate is 144 beats/minute. On examination, she is found to have a singleton fetus with cephalic presentation in a right occipitoanterior (ROA) position. The fetal head appears deflexed, and is four-fifths palpable per abdomen.

INTRODUCTION

Q. Write a short essay on obstructed labor.

Cephalopelvic disproportion (CPD) occurs when there is mismatch between the size of the fetal head and size of the maternal pelvis. It could be due to an average-sized baby with a small pelvis or due to a big baby with normal-sized pelvis (e.g., hydrocephalus, macrosomia, etc.) or a combination of both. Any of these situations may result in failure to progress in labor or abnormally slow progress of labor or dystocia. If undiagnosed and untreated, obstructed labor can jeopardize the lives of both mother and fetus and is associated with significant maternal and perinatal mortality and morbidity. In these cases, it becomes challenging and sometimes even impossible for the baby to be delivered vaginally.

CPD occurs rarely. According to the American College of Nurse-Midwives (ACNM), CPD occurs in 1 out of 250 pregnancies. Having CPD in one pregnancy does not imply that the woman would be at risk of this problem in future deliveries.

On the other hand, contracted pelvis may result in CPD even with an average-sized baby. In cases of contracted pelvis, one of the essential diameters of the pelvis may be reduced by 1 cm or more in one or more planes. Obstetrically, contracted pelvis may be defined as an alteration of sufficient degree in the size or shape of pelvis so as to alter the normal mechanism of labor in case of an average-sized baby. The various types of pelvic contractions are as follows:

- *Pelvic inlet contraction:* This is considered when obstetric conjugate is < 10 cm or greatest transverse diameter is < 12 cm or diagonal conjugate is <11 cm.
- *Midpelvis contraction:* Midpelvis is considered to be contracted when the sum of inter ischial spinous diameters and posterior diameter of midpelvis (10.0 + 5.0 = 15 cm) is <13 cm.
- *Contracted outlet:* This is suspected when the interischial tuberous diameter is 8 cm or less. A contracted outlet is likely to be associated with midpelvic contraction.

ETIOLOGY

Q. Write a short essay on the causes and management of obstructed labor.

Likely causes of CPD could be due to the defects in pelvis or abnormalities with the baby **(Table 6.1)**.

TABLE 6.1: Likely causes of cephalopelvic disproportion.

Defects in the pelvis	Abnormalities with the baby
• A history of pelvic surgery or injury • Small pelvis • Abnormally shaped pelvis (android or platypelloid) • Development defects in the pelvis [Naegele's pelvis (obliquely contracted pelvis characterized by the arrested development of one lateral half of the sacrum), Robert's pelvis (narrowed transversely due to the almost complete absence of the alae of the sacrum) **(Figs. 6.1A and B)** etc.] • *Osteomalacic pelvis* **(Fig. 6.2)**: Occurs due to the softening of pelvic bones, the sacral promontory is pushed downward and forward. Also, the lateral pelvic walls are pushed inward causing the anterior wall to form a beak. Sacrum is markedly softened, while the coccyx is pushed forward	• Large-sized baby having weight ≥ 4 kg (hereditary factors, gestational diabetes, postmaturity, etc.) • Abnormal presentation (transverse lie, brow presentation, and compound presentation) • Congenital malformations of the fetus (hydrocephalus) • Abnormal fetal positions (occipitoposterior position, etc.) • Conjoint twins

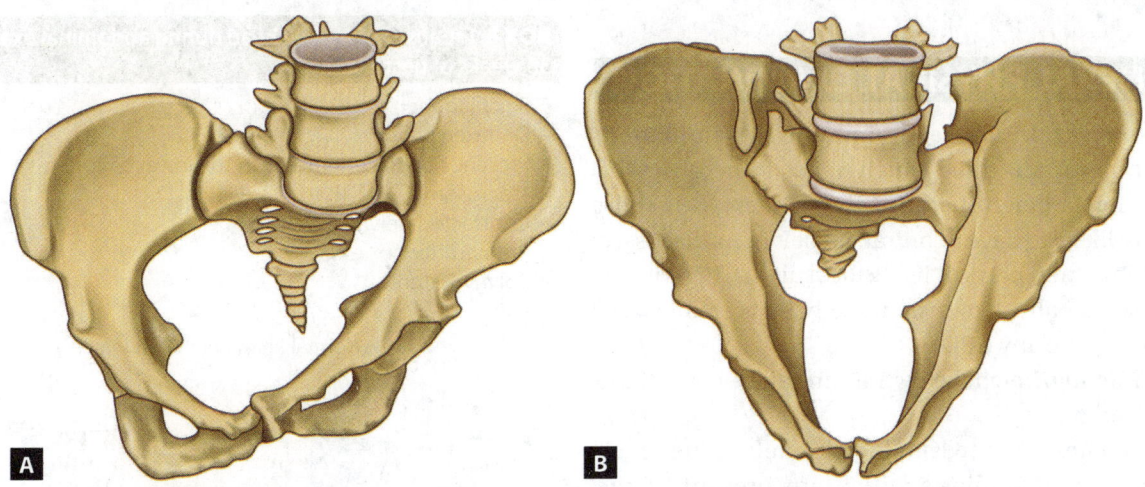

Figs. 6.1A and B: Development defects in pelvis: (A) Naegele's pelvis—Absence of one ala of sacrum; (B) Robert's pelvis—Absence of entire ala of sacrum.

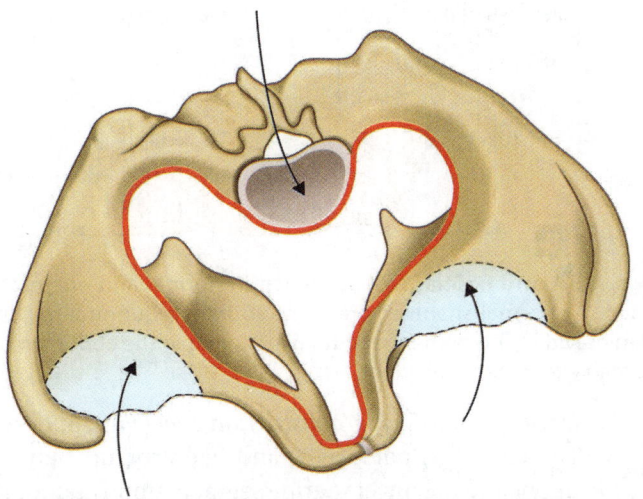

Fig. 6.2: Osteomalacic pelvis.

HISTORY AND CLINICAL PRESENTATION

There may not be any specific complaints related to CPD. The woman may be admitted at term with uterine contractions or in labor.

MENSTRUAL HISTORY

Kindly refer to Chapter 1 for elicitation of such history.

MARITAL HISTORY

Kindly refer to Chapter 1 for elicitation of such history.

PAST OBSTETRIC HISTORY

The clinician needs to ask the history of previous deliveries, if any:
- In case of past history of vaginal delivery, the following history needs to be taken:
  - History of prolonged labor
  - History of instrumental delivery (forceps or vacuum)
  - History of difficult labor (history of tears, lacerations, PPH, fistulas, etc.)
- In case of past history of cesarean delivery, the following history needs to be taken:
  - Emergency or elective
  - Indication of cesarean delivery—was cesarean section done due to prolonged labor as a result of CPD or due to a history of malpresentation.
- *Weight of the baby born:* If the woman had an uncomplicated previous normal vaginal delivery without any complication and delivered an average-sized baby, cephalopelvic disproportion is unlikely.

MEDICAL HISTORY

In consideration of CPD, the history of the following pathologies needs to be elicited:
- Rickets/osteomalacia
- Tuberculosis of hip/pelvic joints/spine
- Poliomyelitis of the lower limb

Elicitation of this history assumes importance because these pathologies are likely to be associated with bony deformities and malformations.

SURGICAL HISTORY

The clinician needs to ask the following from the patient:
- Past history of fracture in the spine/pelvis which may affect the pelvic configuration.
- Fracture of the lower limb resulting in shortening of lower limbs/contracted pelvis.

FAMILY HISTORY

Kindly refer to Chapter 1 for elicitation of such history.

PERSONAL HISTORY

Kindly refer to Chapter 1 for elicitation of such history.

GENERAL PHYSICAL EXAMINATION

- *Patient's height:* In the general physical examination, the most important thing which needs to be observed is the patient's height because the women with short stature are likely to have a contracted pelvis. As discussed before, contracted pelvis is likely to result in CPD with an average-sized baby. However, if the baby is small sized, there may not be any CPD.
- In Indian setting, height below 145 cm can be considered as short stature.
- *Spine:* The clinician needs to look for deformities such as kyphosis and scoliosis which are present at the thoracolumbar level. Other deformities in the spine could include spondylolisthesis, coccygeal deformity, etc.
- *Pelvic bones/hip bones:* Deformities of pelvic bones or hip joints may be associated with CPD.
- *Ribs:* To look for rachitic rosary or beading of the ribs which refer to the permanent knobs of bone at the osteochondral junction in patients with rickets.
- *Lower limbs:* Shortening of the lower limbs could be due to fracture/poliomyelitis, etc. One needs to remember that the cases of rickets and polio are not commonly seen nowadays.
- *Dystocia dystrophy syndrome:* This syndrome refers to short stocky individuals having male pattern of hair distribution and an android pelvis and is commonly encountered amongst the elderly primigravida. Such women are more exposed to occipitoposterior position and bony dystocia.
- *Gait:* Look for limping/exaggerated or waddling gait of the patient. These could be related to neurological or musculoskeletal disorders.

SPECIFIC SYSTEMIC EXAMINATION

ABDOMINAL EXAMINATION

Inspection

As the patient walks in the clinic/hospital, her pendulous abdomen which is hanging loosely may be observed. Pendulous abdomen may be indicative of inlet contraction.

Palpation

- *Mobility of fetal head:* In cases of primigravida with vertex presentation, the head is likely to have engaged by 38 weeks. In case the fetal head is still mobile at 38 weeks of gestation, CPD could be a likely cause. On the other hand, in cases of multigravida, engagement of fetal head usually occurs during labor.
- Other likely causes of mobile head are listed in **Box 6.1**.

BOX 6.1: Causes of mobile head during abdominal examination at 38 weeks of gestation.

- Full bladder
- Deflexed head
- Presence of placenta/mass in the lower segment
- Macrosomia
- Contracted pelvis
- Prematurity
- Polyhydramnios

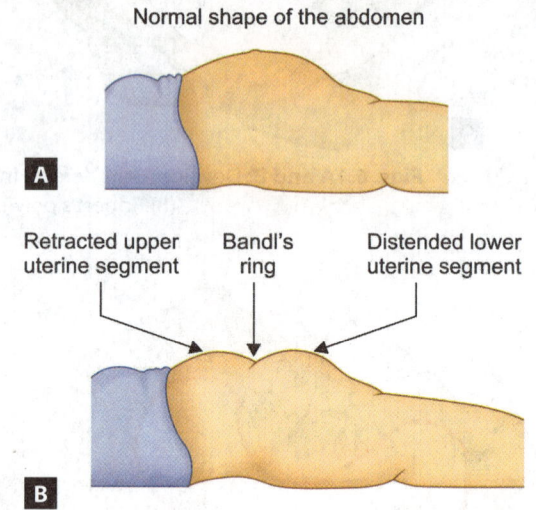

Figs. 6.3A and B: Shape of abdomen in normal and obstructed labor. (A) Normal shape of pregnant abdomen during labor, in a primigravida lying on her back; (B) Bandl's ring in the abdomen of a woman with obstructed labor.

- *Presence of Bandl's ring/constriction ring* (**Figs. 6.3A and B**): This can be palpated as a band-like structure between the upper and the lower uterine segment upon abdominal palpation. The lower segment may appear thin and stretched out. This is a sign of obstructed labor and in case the obstructed labor is allowed to progress, the Bandl's ring can be seen ascending upward toward the umbilicus.
- *Malpresentations:* Fetal malpresentations are more common with CPD.

Methods for Assessment of Fetopelvic Disproportion

The following methods can be used for the assessment of fetopelvic disproportion:

- *Abdominal method:* Abdominal method can be used as a screening method because it does not involve insertion of fingers into the vagina. However, it may be difficult to perform in obese patients, in cases of deflexed or high-floating head or in cases of thick abdominal wall.

In this method, the patient is asked to empty her bladder and then placed in dorsal position with thighs slightly flexed and abducted. The index and the middle fingers of the right hand are placed above the pubic symphysis over the abdomen in such a way that the inner surface of the middle finger is in line with the anterior surface of pubic symphysis (**Fig. 6.4A**). The fetal head is grasped by the obstetrician's left hand and pushed down towards the pelvis. Fingers

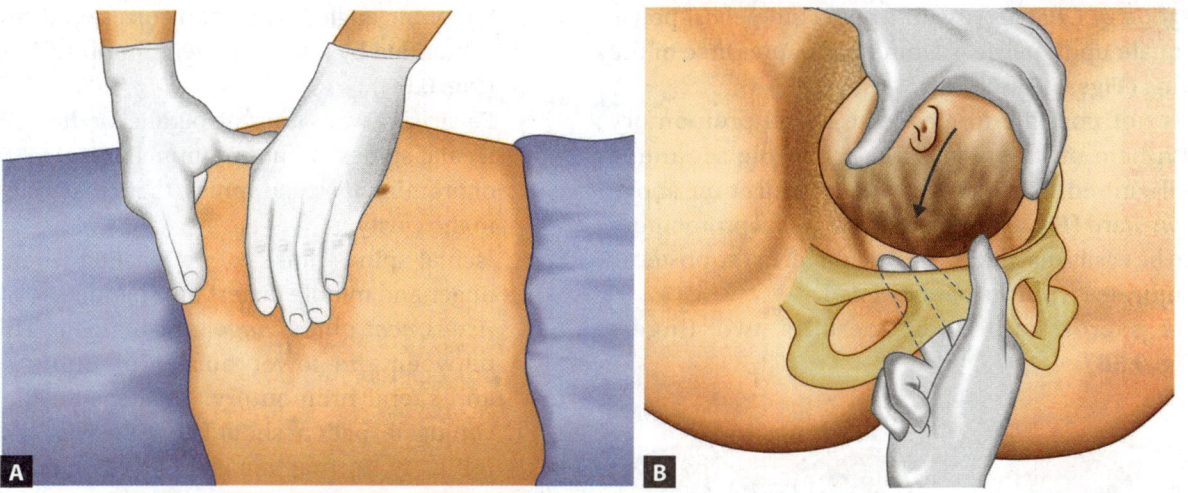

Figs. 6.4A and B: (A) Abdominal method; (B) Abdominal vaginal (Müller–Munro Kerr) method.

of the right hand placed on the pubic symphysis help in interpretation of CPD in the following ways:
- *No CPD:* If the head can be pushed into the pelvis.
- *Mild CPD:* Head can be only slightly pushed into the pelvis and is flushed with symphysis pubis.
- *Major CPD:* Head cannot be pushed into the pelvis and there is over-riding of head over the pubic symphysis.

- *Abdominal vaginal (Müller-Munro Kerr) method:* This is a bimanual method **(Fig. 6.4B)** for assessing the pelvis and comprises the following steps:

The patient is asked to empty her bladder and then placed in dorsal position with thighs slightly flexed and abducted. After observing all aseptic precautions, the obstetrician introduces index finger and middle finger of the right hand inside the vagina with tips of the fingers placed at the level of ischial spines and thumb above the symphysis pubis. The fetal head is then grasped by the left hand and pushed in a downward and backward direction (along the curve of Carus) into the pelvis.

The conclusions which can be reached depending upon the findings on the abdominovaginal examination are:
- *No disproportion:* Fetal head can be pushed down up to the level of ischial spines without any overlapping of the parietal bones.
- *Slight or moderate disproportion:* The head can be pushed down a little but not up to the level of ischial spines and there is only a slight overlapping of the parietal bones. However, it still remains flushed with the thumb.
- *Severe disproportion:* The fetal head cannot be pushed down and instead the parietal bone overhangs the symphysis pubis.

PER VAGINAL EXAMINATION

The following need to be assessed on per vaginal examination:

- Bishop's score
- Station of fetal head
- Excessive amount of caput and molding of fetal head
- Position of fetal head (anterior, posterior, and transverse)
- Nonprogression of the fetal presenting part despite of good uterine contractions.

PELVIC EXAMINATION

Pelvic examination or clinical pelvimetry involves manual assessment of the various pelvic diameters. In case of primigravida, this may be done at 38 weeks of gestation. However, it may be difficult to assess CPD at this time because the cervix may be uneffaced at this time. Therefore, CPD is best assessed at the time of labor.

Prerequisites for Pelvic Examination

- *Excellent dates:* Before assessing the pelvis, the clinician should ensure that the patient's dates are excellent. The patient's date of LMP is considered excellent if she had experienced three regular menstrual cycles previously; there is no history of intake of OCPs and dates by her LMP corresponds with her first trimester scan.
- Patient's bladder must be empty.
- Patient must lie in dorsal position.
- Pelvic examination must be done after observing all aseptic precautions.
- Middle and index fingers of right hand are introduced into the vagina.

Indications of Pelvic Examination

- Assessment of Bishop's score
- Evaluation of the type of pelvis [gynecoid (50%), anthropoid (25%), android (20%), or platypelloid pelvis (5%)]. Caldwell and Moloy's classification of pelvis according to its shape is described in Chapter 2.

- *Evaluation of CPD:* In case of a gynecoid pelvis, pelvis is adequate upon pelvic examination in presence of the following **(Figs. 6.5 and 6.6)**:
  - It is not possible to reach the sacral promontory with help of the middle finger and the sacrum is well-curved from side to side as well from above downward **(Fig. 6.5A)**. In case the sacral promontory can be easily reached, the AP diameter or the obstetric conjugate is likely to be shortened.
  - The sacrosciatic notch permits two fingers **(Fig. 6.5B)**.
  - Subpubic angle is wide and corresponds to the angle subtended by fully abducted thumb and index finger **(Fig. 6.5C)**.
  - Pelvic side walls must be parallel or divergent.
  - Ischial spines are not prominent **(Fig. 6.5D)**. In case of prominent ischial spines, there may be contraction in the cavity.
  - Ischial spines must not be reached when the index finger and middle fingers are spanned.
  - *Assessment of the diagonal conjugate:* This extends between the lower border of pubic symphysis and sacral promontory. To measure the diagonal conjugate, patient should be at the edge of examining table. It normal measures 12.5 cm. For details regarding measurement of the diagonal conjugate, kindly refer to Chapter 2. Obstetric conjugate can be estimated by subtracting 1.5–2 cm from the diagonal conjugate. Obstetric conjugate of length 10.5 cm is considered as normal.
  - Intertuberous diameter must permit four knuckles.

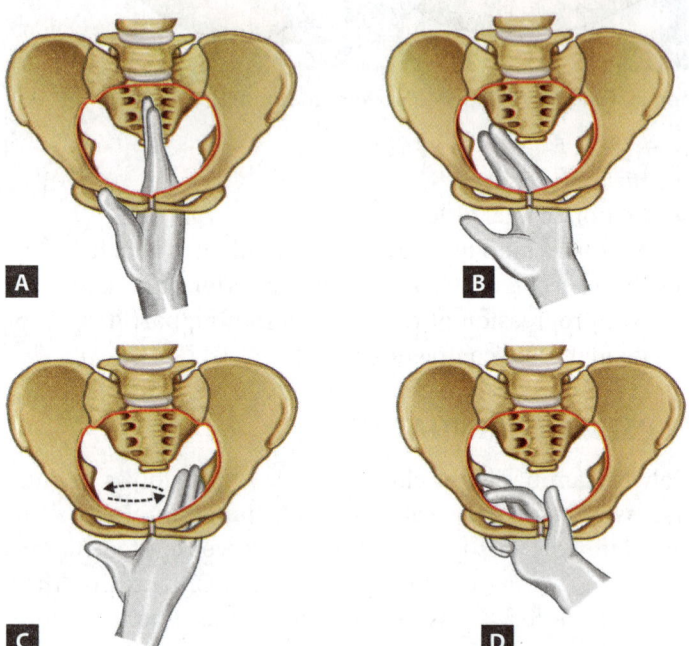

Figs. 6.5A to D: Pelvic assessment: (A) Assessment of sacral promontory; (B) Assessment of right ischial spine; (C) Assessment of left ischial spine; and (D) Evaluation of the sacrosciatic notch.

MANAGEMENT

> **Q.** A 28-year-old primigravida with term gestation has been referred as a case of obstructed labor. Write a long essay discussing the causes, prevention, and management of obstructed labor.
>
> **Q.** Write a long essay on prevention and management of the cases of obstructed labor.
>
> **Q.** Discuss the management of case study described in the beginning of the chapter.

Management comprising of diagnosis (investigations) and definitive obstetric management would be discussed next.

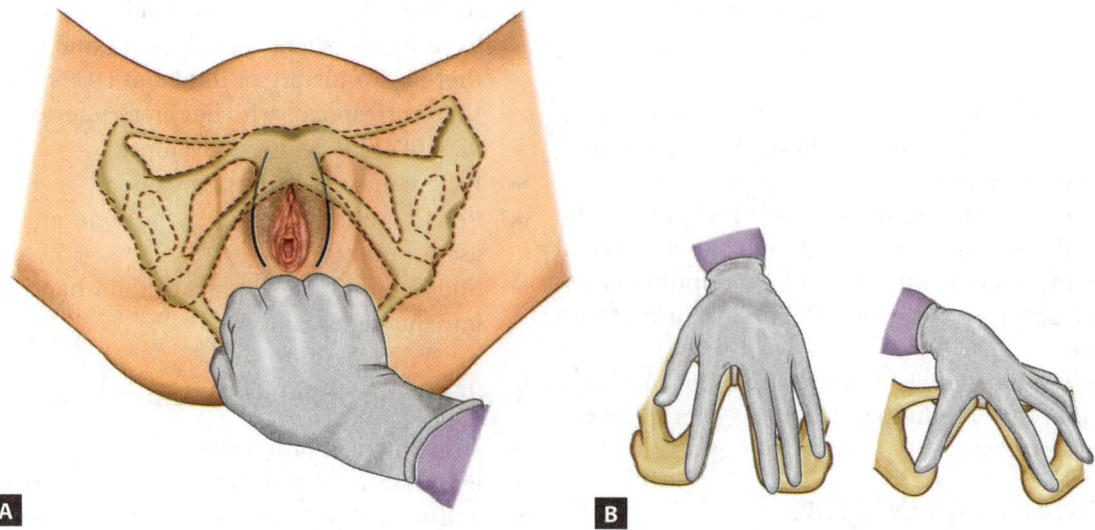

Figs. 6.6A and B: Pelvic outlet evaluation: (A) Evaluation of intertuberous diameter (transverse diameter of outlet); (B) Evaluation of the subpubic angle.

Cephalopelvic Disproportion

INVESTIGATIONS

The methods for diagnosing CPD are as follows:

■ CLINICAL ASSESSMENT

Cephalopelvic disproportion is usually diagnosed clinically during labor when the baby is not progressing naturally through the birth process. The obstetrician must suspect CPD in case of signs mentioned in **Box 6.2**.

■ RADIOLOGIC PELVIMETRY

Radiologic pelvimetry is a type of imaging technology that helps in measuring the dimensions of the mother's pelvis, for predicting or confirming CPD. In this technique, various imaging modalities like ultrasound, MRI, CT, or X-rays can be used for estimating the dimensions of pelvis as well as the size and position of the baby's head. However, the available evidence has demonstrated a poor correlation between the use of imaging technologies and labor outcomes. This could be due to the fact that the bones in the fetal skull are capable of undergoing slight change in shape by a process known as molding in order to negotiate through the birth canal. Moreover, the imaging technologies do not provide an accurate estimate of the baby's size. They only provide an estimate of the baby's size, not the exact measurements. As a result, the imaging technologies are not commonly used in clinical practice. Brief description of these modalities is as follows:

- *Clinical pelvimetry:* This method is used for assessing various diameters of pelvis using the fingers at the time of vaginal examination and/or with a pelvimeter.
- *Pelvimetry by MRI:* This is used for assessment of the dimensions of pelvis, determining the baby's position, and examining the maternal as well as fetal soft tissues.
- *Ultrasound pelvimetry:* A routine ultrasound examination can be used for measuring the negotiating diameter of the baby's head (biparietal diameter) as well as the baby's weight. There measurements can be compared with the readings against standardized growth charts to determine the relative risk of CPD at the time of delivery. The most reliable ultrasound measurement (using transperineal ultrasound) for assessing the progression of fetal head in labor is the angle of progression **(Fig. 6.7)**. The angle of progression is the angle extending between a straight line drawn along the longitudinal axis of the pubic bone and a line drawn from the inferior edge of the pubic bone to the leading edge of the fetal cranium.
- *X-ray or CT pelvimetry:* This is a radiographic examination for determining the dimensions of the maternal pelvis and the biparietal diameter of the fetal head. The benefits of X-ray/CT pelvimetry need to be weighed against the risk of radiation exposure to the mother and the fetus.

TREATMENT/OBSTETRIC MANAGEMENT

The goal of management is to have a safe delivery, without any complications for the mother as well as the baby. In case of major CPD, where the vaginal delivery appears unlikely, the obstetrician has no choice, but to proceed with a cesarean delivery. In case of mild degree CPD, where the obstetricians feel that it may be possible for the patient to deliver vaginally, they may go ahead with the trial of labor. The goal of treatment is to have a safe delivery, so that the clinician can decide how to treat the condition based on the progress of labor.

■ TRIAL OF LABOR

In cases of mild CPD, the clinician may opt for trial of labor and let the labor and delivery progress vaginally. Trial of labor must be undertaken in tertiary care settings having a double setup, with facilities available for an emergency cesarean delivery in case it is required. If the woman's labor continues to progress well, the obstetrician must keep assisting with the process of vaginal delivery. However, if at any point the obstetrician observes signs of obstruction, an urgent decision for emergency cesarean delivery must be taken. When risk factors for CPD are present, it is essential for the obstetrician to carefully monitor the mother and baby very closely and be vigilant in anticipation for an emergency cesarean delivery. Indications and contraindications for trial of labor are listed in **Table 6.2**.

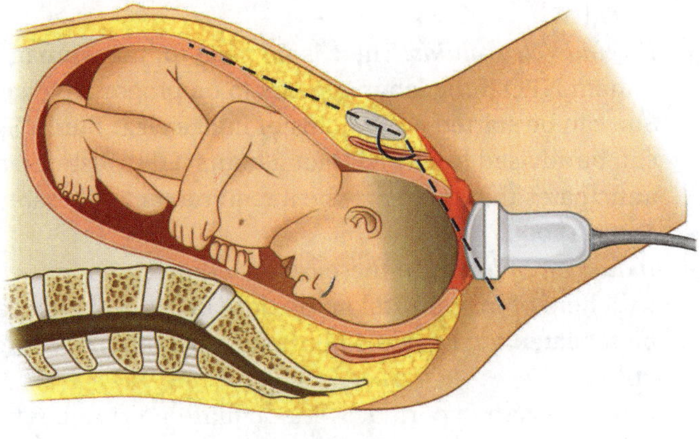

BOX 6.2: Signs suggestive of cephalopelvic disproportion.
- The labor is prolonged or lasting longer than expected
- Uterine contractions are not strong enough to keep the labor moving forward
- Cervical dilatation and effacement is occurring slowly or not at all
- The fetal head is not engaging
- The fetal head is not progressing down through the pelvic stations despite of adequate uterine contractions
- Signs of fetal distress (due to oxygen deprivation because of prolonged and arrested labor)

Fig. 6.7: Transperineal ultrasound to measure the angle of progression.

TABLE 6.2: Indications and contraindications for trial of labor.

Indications	Contraindications
• Mild-to-moderate degree of cephalopelvic disproportion • Average-sized baby • Absence of any obstetric complications	• Elderly primigravida • Major degree CPD (obstetric conjugate <9 cm) • Presence of obstetric or medical complications • Fetal macrosomia • Outlet contraction

(CPD: cephalopelvic disproportion)

BOX 6.3: Unfavorable signs of trial of labor.

- Ineffective uterine contractions
- Head remaining high despite full cervical dilatation and efficient uterine contractions
- Loosely hanging cervix, not well applied to fetal head
- Rupture of membranes prior to full cervical dilatation
- Maternal or fetal distress
- No progress of cervical dilatation or failure of fetal descent

Trial of labor may have a favorable outcome in cases of mild CPD due to the following reasons:

- Good uterine contractions and maternal effort may help to facilitate fetal descent by encouraging flexion of fetal head. Flexion of fetal head may convert occipitofrontal diameter to occipitobregmatic thereby reducing the fetal diameter of engagement by a few mm.
- Molding of fetal head may further help in reducing the fetal diameter of engagement by a few mm. Up to 4 mm of molding is considered acceptable, whereas that >4 mm is likely to be associated with increased chances of hypoxic-ischemic encephalopathy.
- Pelvis gives way during labor thereby helping in increasing the pelvic diameter by a few mm.

These above factors help in accommodating the fetal head, enabling it to pass through the maternal pelvis, thereby allowing normal vaginal delivery in cases of mild CPD.

First Stage of Labor

While assisting with the process of vaginal delivery, the obstetrician must perform the following steps:

- *Patient counseling:* Prior to undertaking trial of labor, the woman and her partner needs to be counseled that at any time there is possibility for failure of trial of labor and requirement of an emergency cesarean delivery.
- *Double set-up:* Trial of labor must be preferably performed in a double set-up with facilities for emergency cesarean delivery in case it is required.
- Blood grouping and cross-matching must be done in advance.
- *IV fluids/clear fluids:* There is no need for the woman to remain NPO if the labor appears to be progressing well. She can be started on IV fluids or intake clear fluids. She can be advised to stay NPO for 2 hours if the obstetrician anticipates that there may be a requirement of cesarean section soon.
- *Induction of labor:* In these cases, labor can be induced with help of misoprostol in the dose of 25 µg, which can be repeated after every 4 hours for a maximum of three doses.
- If the woman experiences inadequate uterine contractions even after administration of misoprostol, syntocinon must be started. Oxytocin infusion pump can be used to deliver oxytocin in the dose of 1 mIU/mL (5 U/500 mL of normal saline). For this, the pump must be set at the rate of 6 mL/h. In case of inadequate uterine contractions, the infusion rate can be doubled after 20–30 minutes.
- Close monitoring of the uterine contractions and abdominal examination for assessing the extent of fetal head palpable per abdomen. The woman must be experiencing 4–5 contractions in 10 minutes, with each contraction lasting for 30–40 seconds. If the fetal head is not at all palpable per abdomen, the head is likely to be deeply engaged.
- The labor must be preferably monitored using the new WHO partograph or care chart (kindly refer to Chapter 2 for details).
- Close monitoring of the fetal movements and the fetal heart rate.
- Confirmation of the baby's position with a vaginal examination. Assessing the progress of labor by evaluating cervical dilation and effacement.
- Other tests such as X-ray, ultrasound, or MRI pelvimetry can be used for assessment of the baby's head and maternal pelvis.
- While progressing with trial of labor the mother can be advised to adopt the position suitable for her, for example sitting, squatting, lying on left lateral position, or using a birthing ball.

Second Stage of Labor

Prolonged second stage of labor is defined as the second stage of labor lasting ≥ 3 hours (without an epidural) or lasting for ≥ 4 hours (in presence of an epidural) in case of a primigravida.

If labor continues, and the fetal head has reached +1 station, outlet forceps or vacuum can be applied to deliver the deliver the fetal head. However, if the woman experiences unfavorable signs such as ineffective contractions, slow dilation and effacement, no descent, or fetal distress **(Box 6.3)**, the obstetrician may have to immediately end the trial, and take up the woman for an emergency cesarean delivery.

Failure of Progress of Labor

As per the new guidelines by WHO, active phase of labor begins at 5–6 cm (in comparison to the previously used cut-off of 3–4 cm). Failure of progress of labor is defined if even after 4 hours of good uterine contractions and absent membranes in the active phase of labor (cervical dilatation of ≥ 6 cm), there is no descent of fetal head. In case of inadequate uterine contractions and syntocinon supplementation, a time limit of 6 hours rather than 4 hours is used. Other definitions of protracted labor, failure of descent, etc., have now been given up.

CESAREAN SECTION

As previously described, if the trial of labor is not progressing well, the woman may require a cesarean delivery. Other indications for an elective cesarean delivery in these cases are listed in **Box 6.4**. As per the WHO, accepted rate of cesarean delivery is 15%. The obstetricians need to adopt the policy of safe prevention of primary cesarean delivery.

Second Stage Cesarean Section

In cases of failed trial of labor, it is likely that a cesarean delivery may be required when the labor has progressed to the second stage. Since in these cases, the head may have descended and may be deep impacted in the pelvis, problems may be encountered while delivering the fetal head. Some of the maneuvers which can be employed for delivering the fetal head in this case include the following.

Pull Method (Reverse Breech Extraction)

In this method, the operator's right hand is inserted inside the uterine cavity toward the fundus. The fetal feet are grasped, which are then subsequently pulled to deliver the baby using footling breech extraction **(Fig. 6.8)**. When grasping and pulling the feet, the obstetrician must take care to only apply force of traction parallel to the axis of fetal legs to avoid fracturing the tibia and/or fibula. As per SOGC guidelines (2021), the pull technique is likely to be associated with fewer complications in comparison to the abdominovaginal method which involves pushing upward from below. However, both the approaches are considered acceptable.

Push Method or the Abdominovaginal Delivery

In this method, an assistant places his/her gloved hand in a cup-shaped manner inside the vagina and helps gently disengage and push the impacted fetal head up toward the uterine cavity. The fetal head is then subsequently extracted by the operating surgeon via cesarean delivery **(Fig 6.9)**. The assistant uses his/her three or four fingers, which are separated and spread over a large area of fetal skull. This helps in avoiding exertion of excessive focal pressure, which can even be traumatic to the baby. The operating obstetrician also assists from above by providing steady upward traction on the fetal shoulders and by trying to flex the fetal head or preventing further deflexion of fetal head. The mother's legs are abducted into the "Whitmore" or "frog" position to help provide the assistant an easy access into the vagina. To facilitate this, stirrups can also be used for placing the patient in dorsal lithotomy position for delivery.

Once the deeply impacted fetal head has been dislodged, rest of the delivery can be completed in a usual manner. However, this method may be associated with an increased

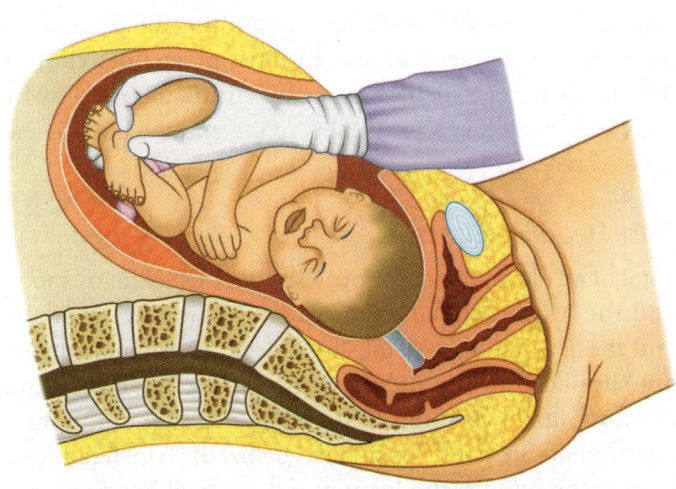

Fig. 6.8: Pull method (reverse breech extraction).

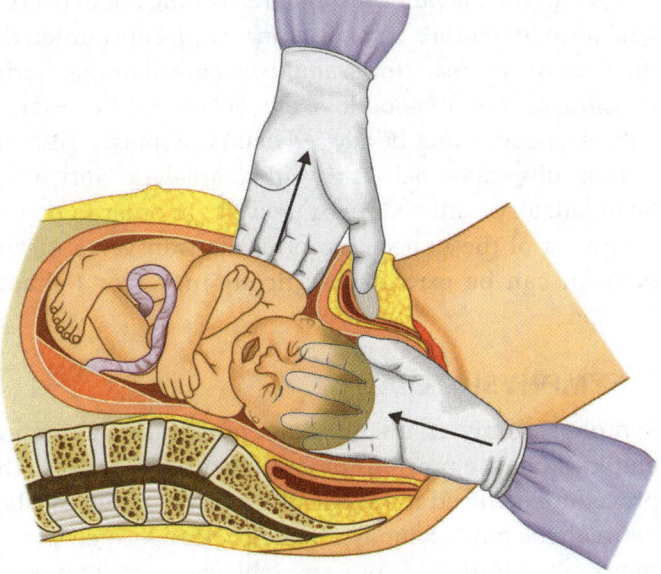

Fig. 6.9: Push method or the abdominovaginal delivery.

> **BOX 6.4:** Indications for an elective cesarean delivery.
> - Previous history of cesarean delivery
> - Previous history of difficult labor or cesarean delivery due to cephalopelvic disproportion
> - Elderly primigravida
> - Occipitoposterior position
> - Post-term baby
> - Fetal macrosomia
> - Medical complications such as preeclampsia
> - Obstetric complications such as placenta previa

risk of extension of the uterine incision. Moreover, it has also been found to be associated with serious fetal morbidity, including skull fracture. Therefore extreme care must be observed by the assistant to avoid excessive pressure on the fetal skull when pushing up from below. Also, this method may be associated with an increased risk of postpartum endometritis probably due to the contamination of the operative field by vaginal flora. To avoid this, abdomen, vagina, and perineum must be prepared using strict aseptic technique. Prophylactic antibiotics must also be administered to the mother to reduce the risk of infection.

Patwardhan's Method

This is the maneuver commonly employed in our set-up for delivering the baby with deeply impacted fetal head. This method involves delivery of anterior shoulder along with the anterior arm by hooking a finger in the elbow. With the application of gentle traction on this shoulder, the posterior shoulder is then delivered. Once both the shoulders have been delivered, the obstetrician must place both thumbs parallel to spine to deliver the baby's trunk followed by the baby's buttocks and legs. Finally, in the end the baby's head is delivered.

Fetal Head Elevators

Fetal head elevators (e.g., Coyne spoon, the Sellheim spoon, and the Murless head extractor) are nowadays available and these function as fetal shoe horns. These instruments are slipped into the uterus, between the fetal head and the anterior lower uterine segment. Subsequently, these instruments are gently positioned below the fetal head. With help of the handle, the instrument and fetal head are then carefully raised out of the pelvis. Following this, the delivery is completed in the usual manner.

Due to the difficulty encountered during the delivery of fetal head, numerous complications may be encountered at the time of cesarean, for example extension of the uterine incision, excessive blood loss, etc. Following the cesarean delivery, patient must be advised that VBAC must be differed during subsequent deliveries and cesarean delivery would be mandatory during her next delivery. In order to prevent extension of the uterine incision, the transverse uterine incision can be extended vertically into T or J-shaped incision.

SYMPHYSIOTOMY

Symphysiotomy is an obsolete procedure commonly employed in the previous times in African countries. This procedure involved the surgical division of pubic cartilage between the pubic symphysis to help widen the pelvis at the time of childbirth. This procedure helped in facilitating the delivery of baby's head in cases of mild CPD.

TABLE 6.3: Complications encountered in cases of CPD.

Maternal	Fetal
• Preterm rupture of membranes • Cord prolapse • Prolonged labor • Increased chances of operative delivery • PPH (atonic and traumatic) • Obstructed labor (associated with complications such as dehydration, ketoacidosis, sepsis, rupture uterus, vesicovaginal fistula, etc.) • Shoulder dystocia • Difficult/prolonged labor • Injuries to the perineum and birth canal • Dystocia • Uterine rupture • Pitocin overdose	• Asphyxia • Hypoxia • Intrapartum death • Tentorial tears • Multiple fractures • Cephalohematoma • Hypoxic ischemic encephalopathy • Extreme molding of the head • Prolapse of the umbilical cord • Fetal distress • Umbilical cord compression

(PPH; postpartum hemorrhage)

COMPLICATIONS

Maternal and fetal complications encountered in cases of CPD are listed in **Table 6.3** and are described next in the text.

■ INCREASED RISK OF CESAREAN DELIVERY

Most women with CPD are likely to have a successful pregnancy outcome after a cesarean delivery. Presently, there is no evidence to suggest that CPD may affect a baby after its birth. However, the woman is likely to be at an increased risk of complications due to cesarean section per se. Kindly refer to Chapter 11 for details.

■ SHOULDER DYSTOCIA

The risk of shoulder dystocia is increased when woman with a mild CPD has a vaginal delivery. In cases of shoulder dystocia, the baby is at risk of developing injuries such as Erb's Palsy or Klumpke's palsy. Kindly refer to Chapter 19 for details related to shoulder dystocia and its management.

■ POSTPARTUM HEMORRHAGE

It is an increased risk of postpartum bleeding. Kindly refer to Chapter 14 for details.

■ OBSTRUCTED LABOR

This can be defined as a condition in which the progressive descent of the presenting part through the maternal genital tract is arrested despite of strong uterine contractions. In primigravidas as a result of obstructed labor, features of maternal exhaustion and sepsis are apparent. However, the uterus becomes inert. On the other hand, in multigravidae, the uterus responds vigorously in face of obstruction, which may eventually lead to the rupture of uterus. Tonic contractions in the face of uterine obstruction result in formation of a circular groove between the upper and lower uterine segment, known as the pathological retraction ring or Bandl's ring. Mechanism of formation of Bandl's ring is shown in the **Figure 6.10**. Eventually, there is rupture of uterus as the lower segment gives way due to marked thinning of the uterine wall. Obstructed labor must be urgently handled like an obstetric emergency. Conscious efforts must be made to exclude rupture of the uterus in every case of obstructed labor.

Etiology

The most common cause of obstructed labor is mechanical obstruction, which results due to a mismatch between the size of fetal presenting part and the maternal pelvis. This could occur due to defects with the passage (bony pelvis) or the passenger (fetus) and are enumerated in **Table 6.4**.

Diagnosis

General Physical Examination

Upon general physical examination, the patient may be in severe pain and features of exhaustion and ketoacidosis may be present.

Abdominal Examination

Upper uterine segment may be hard and tender and a pathological retraction ring (Bandl's ring) is present which may be placed obliquely between the umbilicus and the pubic symphysis and rises in the course of time. Fetal parts may not be well-defined; FHS is usually absent.

Assessment of fetopelvic disproportion: Methods for assessment of CPD (abdominal method and Muller–Munro Kerr method) have been described previously in the text

Vaginal examination: In cases of obstructed labor, vagina may appear to be hot and dry. Cervix may be fully dilated and offensive discharge may be present. Cervix may be hanging loose and not applied firmly against the presenting part. Membranes may be absent. There may be extensive molding of fetal head and caput formation.

Management

- Most important step in the prevention of obstructed labor is early recognition of prolonged labor or abnormal progress of labor by plotting the progress of labor on a partograph.
- Oxytocin must not be used for stimulating uterine contractions in cases of suspected obstruction.
- Taking steps for relieving the obstruction as soon as possible.
- Checking against dehydration and ketoacidosis.
- Controlling sepsis.
- Correction of fluid and electrolyte balance
- *Antibiotics:* Usually, a combination of third-generation cephalosporin (e.g., ceftriaxone) and metronidazole is administered.
- A timely cesarean section gives the best results.

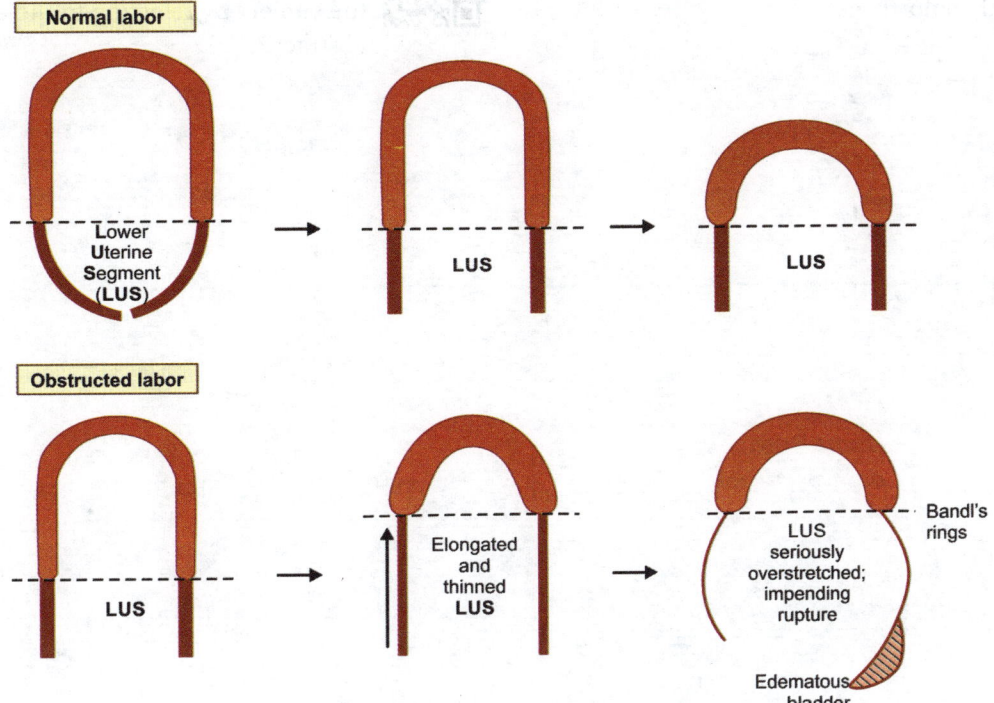

Fig 6.10: Mechanism of development of Bandl's ring.

TABLE 6.4: Etiology of obstructed labor.

Defects with the passage	Defects with the passenger
• Cephalopelvic disproportion • Cervical dystocia due to operative scarring of cervix, cervical or broad ligament fibroids, impacted ovarian tumors, etc.	• Transverse lie • Brow presentation • Congenital malformations of the fetus (hydrocephalus, cystic hygroma of the fetal neck) • Compound presentation • Occipitoposterior position • Conjoint twins

Complications

Complications related to obstructed labor are as follows:
- *Maternal*
  - Pressure necrosis of the bladder base and urethra resulting in the development of genitourinary fistulae, particularly vesicovaginal fistula (more common in the primigravida)
  - Maternal exhaustion, dehydration and/or metabolic acidosis
  - Rupture of the uterus (more common in the multigravida)
  - Postpartum hemorrhage and shock
  - Sepsis
  - High maternal mortality and morbidity
  - Secondary amenorrhea following hysterectomy due to rupture
  - Sheehan's syndrome due to massive postpartum hemorrhage
- *Fetal*
  - Asphyxia
  - Acidosis
  - Intracranial hemorrhage
  - Infection

■ PITOCIN OVERDOSE

One of the major problems with CPD is that physicians may react by administering Pitocin in an effort to speed up delivery. Too much of this drug may cause excessive and traumatic contractions, which can harm the baby.

■ PROLONGED LABOR

Many physicians allow labor to progress for far too long. Labor is a trying time for the baby, and if it is prolonged, oxygen-deprivation injuries may occur. These injuries can lead to hypoxic-ischemic encephalopathy, cerebral palsy, and developmental delays. Furthermore, the trauma from continued labor may result in serious intracranial hemorrhages.

■ UMBILICAL CORD COMPRESSION

When there is decreased space in the uterus, either because of a large baby or a small maternal pelvis, oxygen deprivation may occur due to a trapped umbilical cord.

■ BIRTH INJURIES TO THE BABY

If a cesarean section is not performed on time, the baby may suffer from oxygen deprivation resulting in the development of birth injuries, including cerebral palsy.

EVIDENCE-BASED CLINICAL TRIALS

List of references can be scanned through QR code to enable the readers gain deeper insight of the subject by referring to the entire article or its abstract.

SECTION 2

Complications of Pregnancy

7. Early Pregnancy Bleeding due to Miscarriage
8. Antepartum Hemorrhage
9. Multifetal Gestation
10. Rh-Negative Pregnancy
11. Previous Cesarean Section
12. Hydatidiform Mole
13. Bad Obstetric History
14. Postpartum Hemorrhage
15. Intrauterine Growth Restriction
16. Preterm Labor
17. Postdated Pregnancy and Intrauterine Death

CHAPTER 7

Early Pregnancy Bleeding due to Miscarriage

CASE STUDY

A 22-year-old G2P1A0L1 patient with LMP 9 weeks ago presented to the emergency room with slight spotting and mild pain per abdomen. An ultrasound examination during the last antenatal visit had revealed a gestational sac consistent with 7 weeks of gestation having cardiac activity. The vaginal examination done in the emergency room showed an open cervical os and active vaginal bleeding was present. Products of conception (POC) could be observed to be protruding out from the cervical os. The ultrasound examination revealed an intrauterine gestational sac, but there was no fetal cardiac activity.

INTRODUCTION

Q. Discuss in detail about early pregnancy loss.

According to WHO and Centers for Disease Control and Prevention (CDC), spontaneous abortion (preferably termed as miscarriage) can be defined as the termination of pregnancy prior to 20 weeks of gestation or birth of a fetus weighing <500 g in case the period of gestation is not known. Abortion/miscarriage occurs in about 10–20% of all pregnancies. Birth defects occur in about 3% of all pregnancies, some of which result in spontaneous miscarriage early in pregnancy. On the other hand, presence of chromosomal disorders, such as trisomy 21, 13, 18, monosomy XO, etc., may result in viable pregnancies and are associated with advanced maternal age. Approximately, 75% of miscarriages occur before 16 weeks of gestation and of these nearly three-fourths occur within the first 2 months of pregnancy.

TYPES OF MISCARRIAGE

Various types of spontaneous miscarriages are described in **Table 7.1** and **Figure 7.1**.

Threatened Abortion

Threatened abortion is a type of abortion where the process of abortion has begun, but has yet not progressed to a stage from where the recovery would be impossible (**Fig. 7.2**). In case of threatened abortion, despite of occurrence of bleeding before 20 weeks of gestation, the cervical os is closed. The fetal heart rate is usually present and there may be normal intrauterine growth. The bleeding may sometimes stop on its own and pregnancy may continue normally. If the pregnancy continues, there may be increased chances of preterm labor, intrauterine growth restriction, placenta previa, etc.

Sonography can help differentiate between a viable or nonviable intrauterine pregnancy. Therapy should be directed toward treatment of the underlying cause. Treatment is mostly empirical. Bed rest along with sedation and painkillers is commonly prescribed.

Inevitable Abortion

Inevitable abortion is a type of abortion where the process of abortion has progressed to such an extent that the continuation of pregnancy is not possible (**Fig. 7.3**). It is often associated with pain in abdomen and bleeding. The cervical os is open in these cases. This type of miscarriage may progress into either complete or incomplete miscarriage.

Incomplete Abortion

When the process of inevitable abortion has progressed to such an extent that part of fetal products has been expelled out and part of it is still within the uterine cavity, it is known as incomplete abortion (**Fig. 7.4**). This type of abortion is associated with pain and bleeding. Cervical os is open and some of the fetal tissues may have been passed out.

Missed Abortion

Missed abortion is a condition in which the fetus becomes dead and is retained inside the uterine cavity (**Fig. 7.5**). Beyond 12 weeks of gestation, the liquor amnii gets absorbed and the placenta becomes papery, pale, and adherent. The patient is likely to present with features of threatened miscarriage. There may be presence of brownish vaginal discharge and subsidence of pregnancy symptoms

TABLE 7.1: Various types of miscarriage.

Subcategory	Definition	Clinical characteristics	Ultrasound criteria	Management
Threatened abortion	Bleeding before 20 weeks' gestation with closed cervix; pregnancy viable at time of presentation and may or may not result in a miscarriage	Internal cervical os is closed	Findings appropriate according to the gestational age; subchorionic hemorrhage may be present	Mostly empirical treatment
Inevitable miscarriage	Miscarriage is imminent or is in the process of happening	• Leaking amniotic fluid • Cervical dilatation • Heavy bleeding • Severe pain • Miscarriage is unavoidable • Risk of incomplete abortion or sepsis	Products of conception are visible; fetal cardiac activity may or may not be present	Uterine evacuation
Incomplete abortion	A miscarriage where some parts of the fetus or placenta are unable to be naturally expelled by the mother	• Open internal cervical os • Bleeding • Ultrasound or pelvic examination shows products of conception • Complications such as hemorrhage and sepsis	Heterogeneous and/or echogenic material (suggestive of products of conception) along the endometrial stripe in endometrial cavity or in the cervical canal	Uterine evacuation
Complete abortion	All products of conception have been passed out through the cervical canal	Closed internal cervical os	Empty uterine cavity; endometrial lining may be normal/thickened	No medical or surgical interventions are required because the uterine cavity is already empty
Missed abortion/ embryonic or fetal demise	A confirmed, nonviable pregnancy on ultrasound with no bleeding	• The fetus dies but the woman's cervical os stays closed • There is no bleeding • The fetus continues to stay inside the uterus • May be associated with coagulation defects	Embryonic pole ≥ 5 mm without fetal cardiac activity, or embryonic pole < 5 mm and no interval growth over 1 week	Expectant, medical or surgical management
Anembryonic pregnancy/ empty sac or blighted ovum	Pregnancy in which a gestational sac develops without development of any embryonic structures	• A fertilized egg implants into the uterine wall, but fetal development never begins • There is a gestational sac with or without a yolk sac, but there is an absence of fetal growth	Gestational sac > 13 mm without yolk sac or > 18 mm without embryonic pole, or empty sac beyond 38 days of gestation and no interval growth over 1 week	Expectant, medical or surgical management

such as retrogression of breast changes, cessation of uterine growth, etc. The fetal heart sounds may not be heard and the immunological tests for pregnancy may become negative. The uterus may be small for dates and ultrasound may reveal an empty gestational sac.

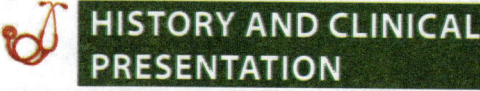

HISTORY AND CLINICAL PRESENTATION

Various causes of miscarriage (**Flowchart. 7.1**) are as follows:

GENETIC CAUSES

Genetic causes commonly include changes in the number of chromosomes, e.g., trisomy, polyploidy, etc., or structural abnormalities of chromosomes, e.g., translocations, deletions, etc. While nearly 33% of pregnancies that abort are anembryonic, 50% cases of spontaneous abortion occur due to chromosomal abnormalities (**Table 7.2**).

ENDOCRINOLOGICAL CAUSES

These include causes such as luteal phase defects, thyroid disorders including both hypothyroidism and hyperthyroidism, diabetes mellitus, etc.

INFECTIONS

Infections include viral causes such as rubella, cytomegalovirus, HIV, etc.; parasitic causes such as Toxoplasma, malaria, etc.; and bacterial causes such as Ureaplasma, Chlamydia, Brucella, etc.

Early Pregnancy Bleeding due to Miscarriage

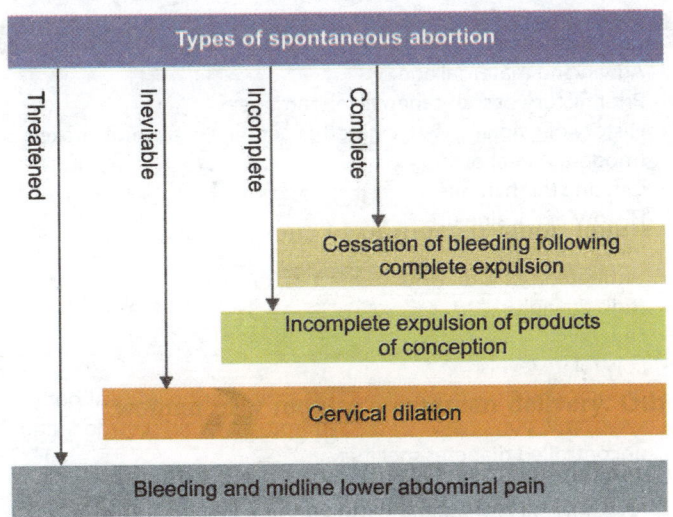

Fig. 7.1: Various types of spontaneous miscarriage.

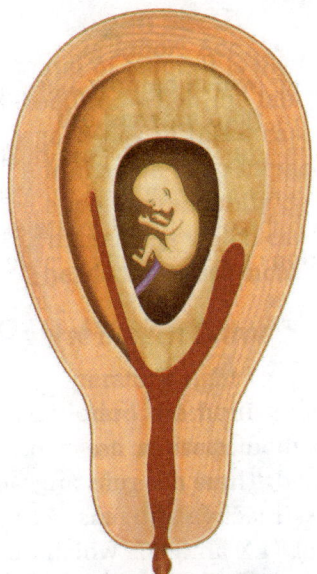

Fig. 7.2: Threatened abortion.

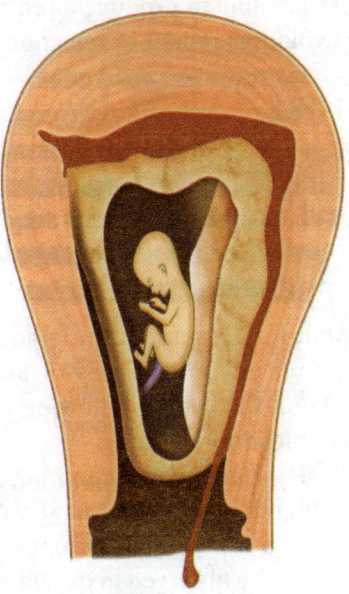

Fig. 7.3: Inevitable abortion.

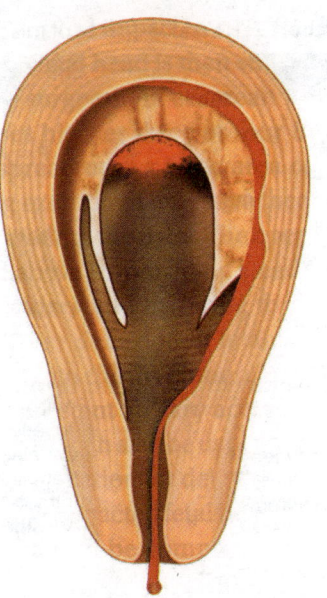

Fig. 7.4: Incomplete abortion.

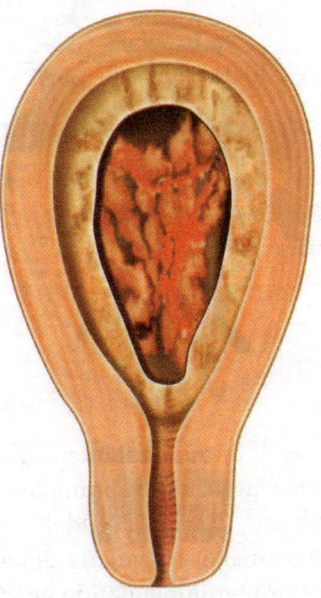

Fig. 7.5: Missed abortion.

IMMUNOLOGICAL CAUSES

Immunological causes include autoimmune diseases, alloimmune diseases, thrombophilias, etc.

ANATOMICAL CAUSES

Anatomical causes can include reproductive tract abnormalities such as congenital uterine anomalies (bicornuate uterus, septate uterus, etc.), leiomyomas, shortened cervical canal (resulting in cervical incompetence), and uterine adhesions.

Various anatomic abnormalities of the uterus are associated with 10–15% cases of recurrent second-trimester miscarriages. Müllerian abnormalities, such as septate uterus and bicornuate uterus, are commonly associated with recurrent miscarriage due to poor blood supply to the

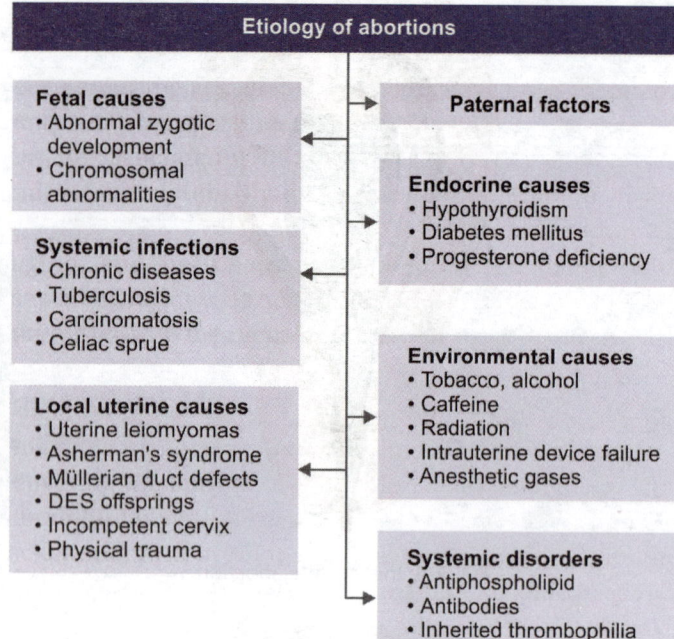

Flowchart 7.1: Various causes of miscarriage.

(DES: diethylstilbestrol)

BOX 7.1: Risk factors for spontaneous miscarriage.

- Advancing maternal age
- Prior history of spontaneous miscarriage
- History of smoking (>10 cigarettes per day) or alcohol intake (moderate intake)
- Caffeine (high intake)
- History of cocaine use
- Maternal weight (BMI < 18.5 or > 25)
- Untreated celiac disease
- High gravidity
- Fever
- Low folate levels
- Chronic maternal diseases such as antiphospholipid antibody syndrome, polycystic ovarian syndrome, thyroid disorders, and uncontrolled diabetes mellitus
- Use of medications such as itraconazole, methotrexate, nonsteroidal anti-inflammatory drugs, paroxetine, and retinoids
- Exposure to toxins and occupational exposure (e.g., ionizing radiation, pesticides, etc.)

TABLE 7.2: Various chromosomal abnormalities which can result in spontaneous miscarriage.

Type of chromosomal abnormality	Incidence (%)
Autosomal trisomies	52
Monosomy X	19
Polyploidies	22
Others	7

conceptus as a result of the implantation of the gestational sac over a relatively avascular septum. Müllerian anomaly, such as bicornuate uterus, could be responsible for producing an abnormal or irregularly shaped uterus, which could result in improper implantation and/or growth of the embryo, thereby resulting in recurrent miscarriages. Uterus didelphys is commonly associated with preterm labor but can also sometimes cause recurrent miscarriage.

Asherman's syndrome, characterized by presence of intrauterine adhesions and synechiae within the uterine cavity, is another cause of recurrent miscarriage. Diagnosis of Asherman's syndrome can be reached by doing tests like hysteroscopy, transvaginal ultrasound examination, hysterosalpingography, etc. Hysterosalpingogram revealing irregular filling defects in the endometrium is suggestive of endometrial adhesions. Hysteroscopic resection of the adhesions can be performed.

ANTIPHOSPHOLIPID ANTIBODY SYNDROME

Antiphospholipid antibody syndrome is an autoimmune condition that has emerged as the most important treatable cause of recurrent miscarriage, early-onset preeclampsia, preterm labor, low birth weight babies, and intrauterine growth restriction. This disease causes miscarriage by forming antibodies against the body's own tissues and placenta, resulting in thrombosis of vessels, placental infraction, fetal hypoxia, and ultimately fetal death. For detailed description of APAS, kindly refer to Chapter 13.

ABSENCE OF BLOCKING ANTIBODIES AS A CAUSE OF MISCARRIAGE

Allotypic antigens in the trophoblast may elicit the production of antibodies, which are cytotoxic to peripheral leukocytes in blood. These antigens are called trophoblast-lymphocyte cross-reactive antigens (TLX). If the embryo contains paternal TLX antigens which do not exist in the mother, it may mount a protective reaction, resulting in abortion. If the mother produces antipaternal blocking antibodies, these are able to produce a protective response, which helps in avoiding pregnancy rejection.

RISK FACTORS

Various risk factors which could be associated with an increased risk of miscarriage and must be elicited while taking history are enlisted in **Box 7.1**.

CLINICAL PRESENTATION

Clinical presentation of a patient undergoing miscarriage is usually after first missed menses or after a period of amenorrhea and may involve the following symptoms:

- First trimester bleeding/spotting
- There may be associated pain/cramping per abdomen.

Pregnancy testing should be done in all women belonging to reproductive age group with abnormal vaginal bleeding. The β-hCG levels may be observed to be falling or abnormally rising. Besides having vaginal bleeding and abdominal pain, patients with early pregnancy loss can have varied clinical presentation including:

- Absent fetal heart tones on Doppler ultrasound
- Size-dates discrepancy on bimanual examination
- Routine ultrasonography indicating a nonviable pregnancy

GENERAL PHYSICAL EXAMINATION

There are no specific signs on general physical examination suggestive of spontaneous pregnancy loss. Clinical signs suggestive of anemia may be present if there has been excessive bleeding (refer to Chapter 20). Changes in vital signs with increasing amount of blood loss and hemodynamic instability have been described in detail in Chapter 14.

SPECIFIC SYSTEMIC EXAMINATION

ABDOMINAL EXAMINATION

Abdominal Palpation

- If an intrauterine pregnancy is >12 weeks of gestation, it may be palpable per abdomen.
- There may be extrauterine tenderness (suggestive of ectopic pregnancy).

VAGINAL EXAMINATION

- Products of conception can be visualized in the cervical os or vaginal vault upon per speculum examination. This is diagnostic of miscarriage (incomplete or inevitable). Any visible lesion on the cervix which may be responsible for producing bleeding (e.g., cervical erosions, polyps, malignancy, etc.) may also be visualized on per speculum examination.
- The cervix and uterus may appear to be soft upon vaginal examination.
- In cases of incomplete or inevitable miscarriage, the internal cervical os would felt to be open on per vaginal examination.
- In cases with early pregnancy bleeding where the internal cervical os is not open or POC cannot be visualized to be protruding from the cervical os, it is essential to rule out the diagnosis of ectopic pregnancy using TVS and determination of serial β-hCG levels, or both.
- A bimanual examination often helps in detecting size-dates discrepancy.

Differential Diagnosis

Bleeding in pregnancy could be commonly due to pregnancy-related causes or rarely due to nonpregnancy-related causes **(Table 7.3)**.

TABLE 7.3: Various causes of bleeding during the early pregnancy.

Pregnancy-related causes	Causes unrelated to pregnancy
• Miscarriage (spontaneous or induced) • Ectopic pregnancy (refer to Chapter 32) • Hydatidiform mole (refer to Chapter 12) • Implantation bleeding • Pregnancy of unknown location	• Vascular erosions • Cervical polyps • Ruptured varicose veins • Malignancy

Pregnancy of Unknown Location

Q. Write a long essay discussing the diagnostic dilemmas associated with pregnancy of unknown location.

This can be defined as a pregnancy where the pregnancy test is positive, yet ultrasound is unable to visualize the pregnancy. Even with the use of TVS, it may not be possible to confirm whether the pregnancy is intrauterine or extrauterine in 8–31% of cases during the first antenatal visit. The threshold hCG levels whereby an intrauterine pregnancy would not be expected to be seen with ultrasound is 1,500–2,000 mIU/mL or IU/L (approximately 1,500 mIU/mL for TVS and 2,000 mIU/mL for TAS). Based on the findings on ultrasound and β-hCG levels, women are likely to experience either of the following five outcomes:

1. *Defined ectopic pregnancy:* Presence of extrauterine gestational sac with a yolk sac and/or embryo with or without cardiac activity
2. *Probable ectopic pregnancy:* Presence of heterogeneous adnexal mass or gestational sac-like structure
3. *Pregnancy of unknown location:* Absence of images pointing toward intrauterine or extrauterine pregnancy
4. *Probable intrauterine pregnancy:* Presence of intrauterine echogenic gestational sac
5. *Defined intrauterine pregnancy:* Presence intrauterine gestational sac with yolk vesicle and/or embryo with or without cardiac activity

MANAGEMENT

Q. What is the probable diagnosis and management in the case study described in the beginning of the chapter?

Q. Write a long essay discussing the implications of first-trimester bleeding and what are the investigations and results which can be correlated with an ultimate outcome?

Management comprising of investigations and definitive obstetric management is discussed next. The diagnosis of miscarriage is made by a combination of patient's history, physical/vaginal examination and clinical investigations. **Flowchart 7.2** illustrates the management protocol for early pregnancy bleeding, whereas **Flowchart 7.3** shows

130 Complications of Pregnancy

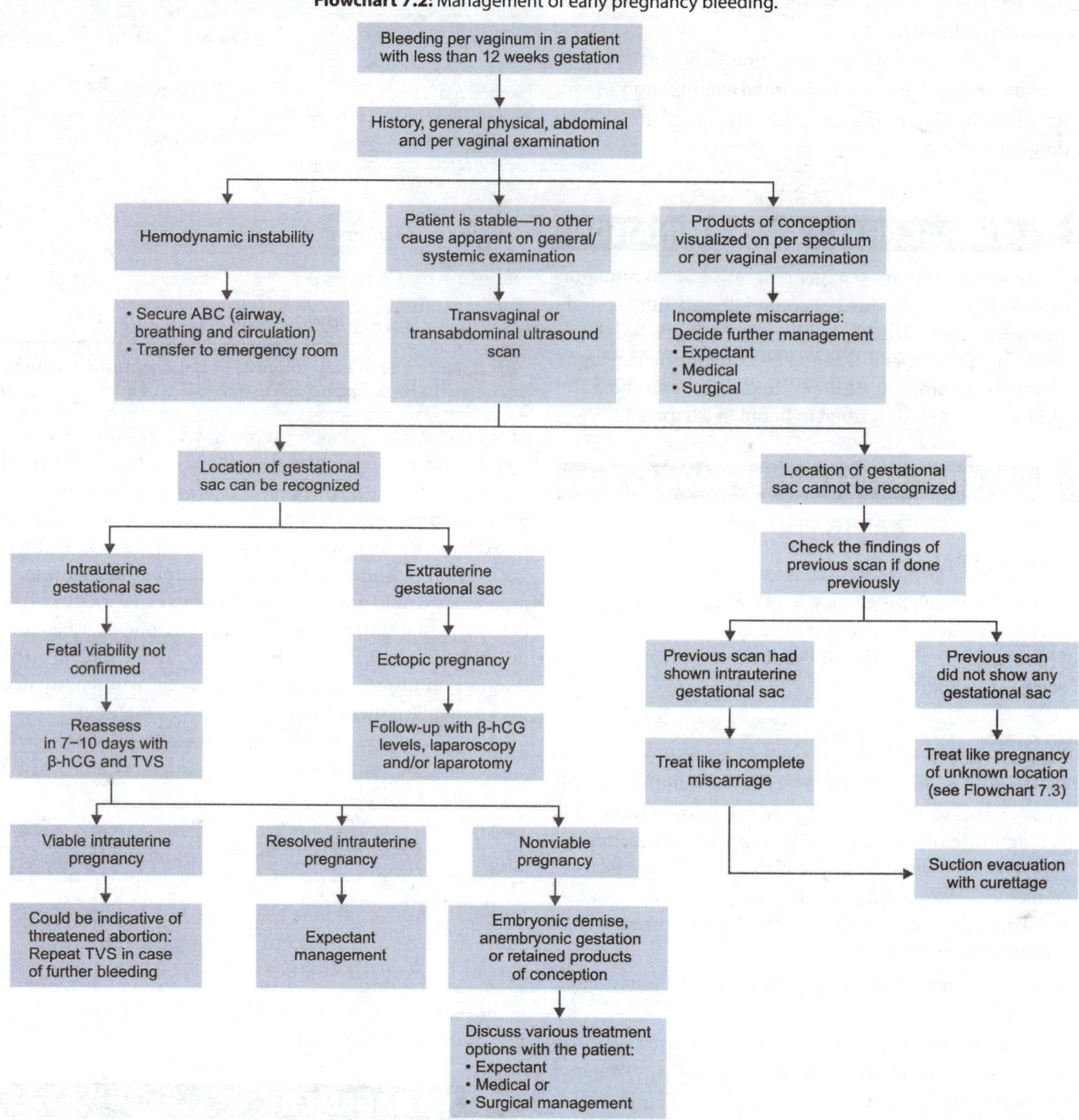

Flowchart 7.2: Management of early pregnancy bleeding.

(hCG: human chorionic gonadotropin; TVS: transvaginal sonography)

management of pregnancy at unknown location. Various medical and surgical techniques used for completion of miscarriage are tabulated in **Table 7.4**.

INVESTIGATIONS

DIAGNOSIS OF MISCARRIAGE USING ULTRASOUND

Ultrasound examination forms an important investigation for arriving at a definitive diagnosis. Both TAS and TVS are complementary to one another in arriving at a diagnosis and the appropriate modality should be used depending upon the clinical situation. TVS has been shown to have a positive predictive value of 98% in confirming the diagnosis of complete miscarriage.

In a normal TVS, the yolk sac is normally visible by 5–5.5 weeks, fetal pole is visible by 5.5–6 weeks, and fetal heart beat by 6 weeks. Gestational sac is the first to appear at 4.5–5 weeks. All these findings are likely to appear 1 week later on the transabdominal scan. Normally, when a gestational sac is observed on TVS, levels of β-hCG in

Flowchart 7.3: Management of pregnancy at unknown location.

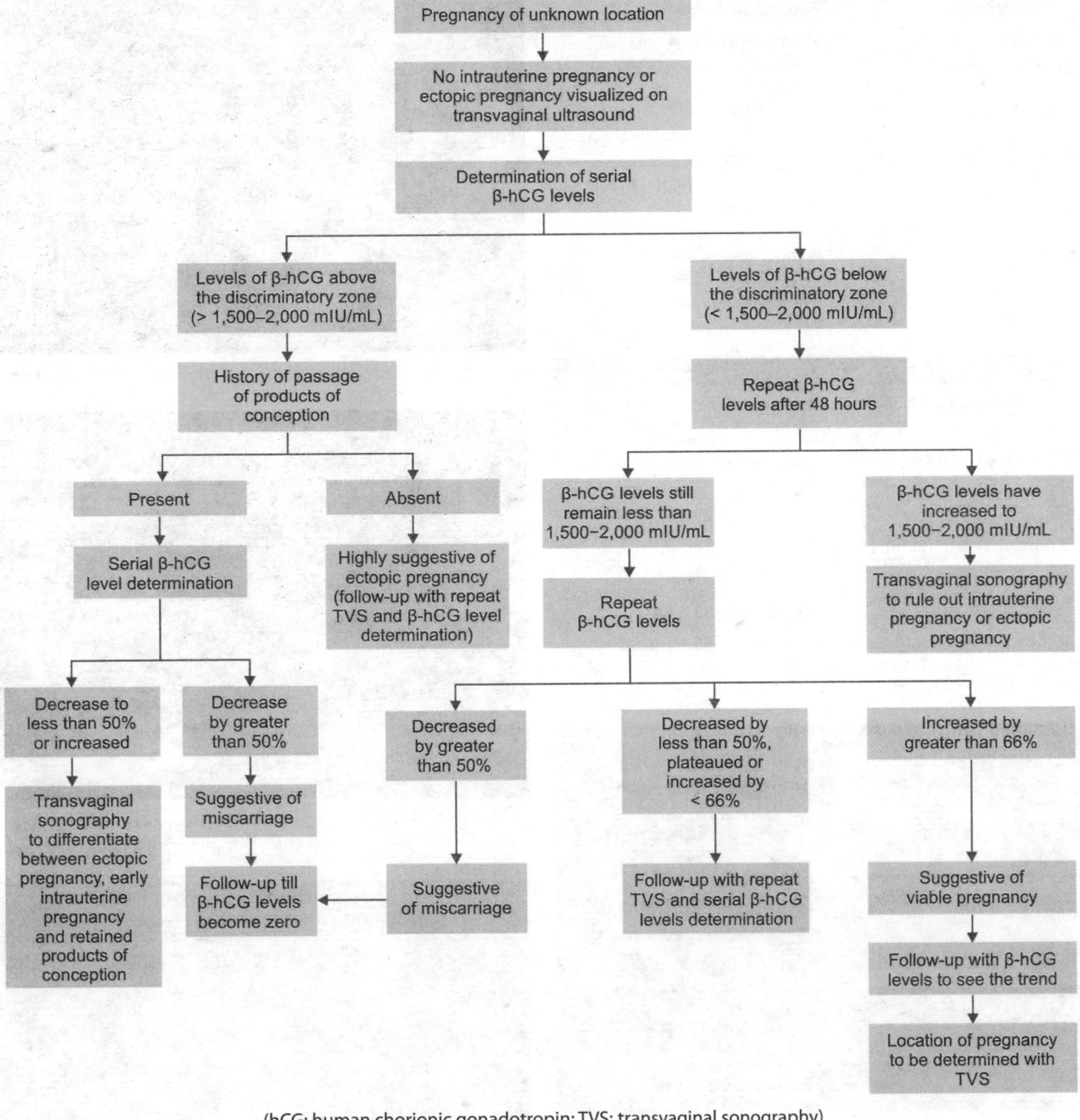

(hCG: human chorionic gonadotropin; TVS: transvaginal sonography)

the serum can vary between 1,500 IU/L and 2,000 IU/L. Features suggestive of nonviable pregnancy on ultrasound examination are described in **Table 7.5**.

Other ultrasound features suggestive of nonviability on ultrasound examination are as follows:
- No embryonic growth on serial ultrasound scans
- Collapsed or distorted gestational sac
- *Abnormalities of the yolk sac or its complete absence:* Absence of yolk sac or presence of an abnormal yolk sac is associated with a positive predictive value of 95%.
- Absence of or an abnormality in fetal heart rate pattern
- Presence of subchorionic hematoma

Figure 7.6 demonstrates the ultrasound findings in case of inevitable abortion. There is a loss of definition of gestational sac, resulting in a smaller diameter of gestational sac. There are no central echoes in the gestational sac which are normally indicative of a healthy pregnancy. Fetal cardiac activity is normally absent. **Figure 7.7** demonstrates the ultrasound findings in case of missed abortion. There was absence of the growth of the fetal pole over 5 days of

TABLE 7.4: Techniques for completion of abortion.

Surgical techniques	Medical techniques

• Cervical dilatation followed by uterine evacuation
• Curettage
• Vacuum aspiration (suction curettage)
• Dilatation and evacuation (D and E)
• Menstrual aspiration
• Laparotomy: Hysterotomy
• Hysterectomy
	• Intravenous oxytocin
	• Intra-amniotic hyperosmotic fluid saline or urea
	• Prostaglandins
	  – Intra-amniotic injection
	  – Vaginal insertion
	  – Parenteral injection
	  – Oral ingestion
	• Antiprogesterones—RU 486, mifepristone, etc.
	• Methotrexate—intramuscular and oral

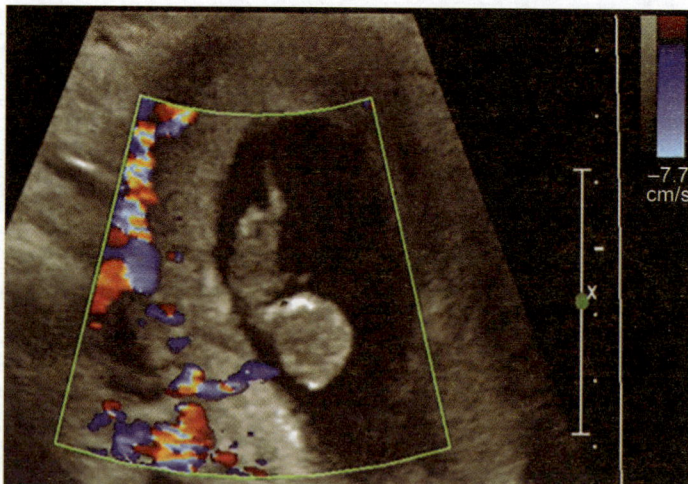

Fig. 7.7: Transvaginal ultrasound showing missed abortion.

TABLE 7.5: Predictors of nonviability on ultrasound examination.

Ultrasound feature which is present	Ultrasound feature which is absent
Gestational sac of 8 mm	No yolk sac
Gestational sac of 16 mm	No demonstrable embryo
Gestational sac diameter > 25 mm (TAS) or > 18 mm (TVS)	Absent fetal poles
Embryo with CRL of > 5 mm	No cardiac activity
7th week of gestation	Heart rate < 85 bpm

(bpm: beats per minute; CRL: crown rump length; TAS, transabdominal sonography; TVS, transvaginal sonography)

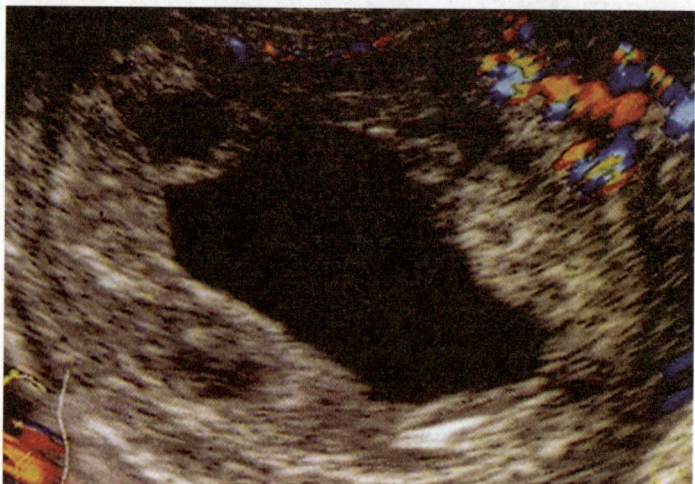

Fig. 7.8: Anembryonic pregnancy as observed on color Doppler ultrasound.

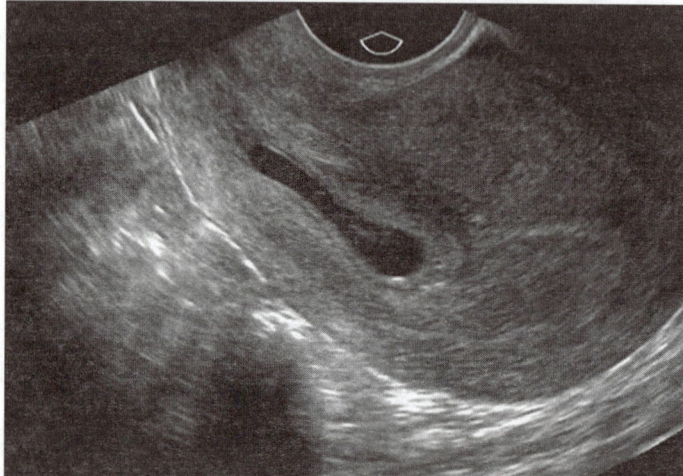

Fig. 7.6: Transvaginal ultrasound in case of inevitable abortion.

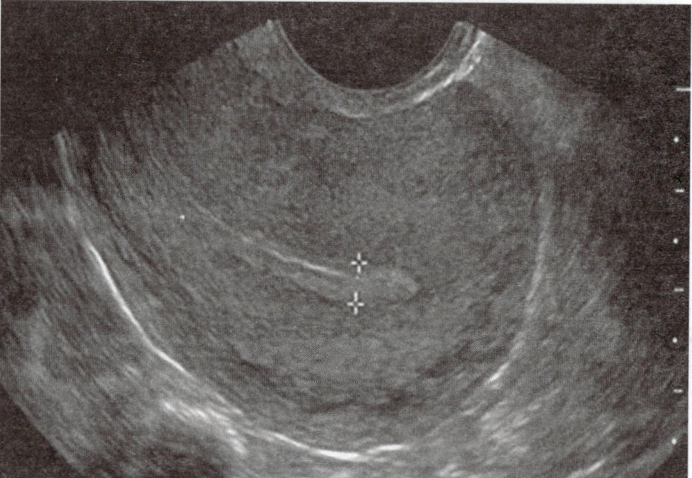

Fig. 7.9: Transvaginal ultrasound image in case of a complete abortion, where the gestational sac and POC have been completely expelled out.

observation period. The fetal heart rate was also absent. **Figure 7.8** shows an anembryonic pregnancy where there is large gestational sac having a size 3 × 2 cm. The gestational sac was empty without having presence of yolk sac or fetal pole. The pregnancy may be deemed abnormal if no yolk sac appears at the gestational sac size of 10 mm or no fetal pole is seen at the gestational sac size of 18 mm. If the gestational sac has an irregular or scalloped appearance that is also abnormal. **Figure 7.9** shows an ultrasound image in case of a complete abortion, where the gestational sac and POC have been completely expelled out. As a result, the triple-line uterine endometrium with an empty uterine cavity can be seen on TVS.

ROLE OF SERIAL hCG ASSESSMENT IN PREDICTING PREGNANCY OUTCOME

Serial serum hCG assay is particularly useful in the diagnosis of cases of asymptomatic ectopic pregnancy. Modern monoclonal antibody-based kits can detect hCG at concentrations of 25 IU/L, a level reached 9 days postconception (day 23 of a 28-day cycle). Normally, a gestational sac would be visualized on transvaginal ultrasonography at β-hCG levels of 1,500–2,000 mIU/mL. This β-hCG level is known as the discriminatory zone and in a normal intrauterine gestation it is usually attained by 5 weeks of gestation. This may, however, vary depending on the quality of the machine and the sonographer's skill. Discriminatory zones for serum hCG should be used to help exclude the diagnosis of possible ectopic pregnancy. At β-hCG levels above 1,500–2,000 IU/L, an ectopic pregnancy will usually be visualized with TVS. However, at the levels of β-hCG below the discriminatory zone, pregnancy of unknown location and miscarriage are both possible outcomes. Although a doubling of hCG titer is often expected to occur in cases of viable pregnancy within 48 hours, this can vary depending on the period of gestation. If the quantitative β-hCG level is > 1,500–2,000 mIU/mL discriminatory zone, the pregnancy is likely to be viable. In these cases, an urgent transvaginal ultrasound examination must be arranged to rule out an ectopic pregnancy and assess viability. If β-hCG levels are below the discriminatory zone, these levels must be followed at every 48 hours intervals until the discriminatory threshold is reached or until the diagnosis is clear from the trend of the β-hCG levels. Declining β-hCG levels are indicative of nonviable pregnancy or a miscarriage.

ROLE OF SERUM PROGESTERONE ASSAY IN PREDICTING PREGNANCY OUTCOME

Measurement of serum progesterone level can be a useful adjunct in cases where ultrasound suggests pregnancy of unknown location. In these cases, TVS, measurement of serial serum hCG levels, and progesterone levels may all be required in order to establish a definite diagnosis. When ultrasound findings suggest pregnancy of unknown location, serum progesterone levels below 25 nmol/L are usually associated with pregnancies subsequently confirmed to be nonviable. However, viable pregnancies have been reported with initial serum progesterone levels <15.9 nmol/L. In most cases, serum progesterone levels above 25 nmol/L are "likely to indicate" and above 60 nmol/L are "strongly associated with" pregnancies subsequently shown to be normal. Therefore, active intervention, and uterine evacuation should not be undertaken based on low initial progesterone levels. Presently, it is not possible to define a specific discriminatory value for a single serum progesterone result that may allow absolute clinical confirmation of viability or nonviability. Therefore at present, pregnancy of unknown location is largely managed by TVS and serial β-hCG level determination.

TREATMENT/OBSTETRIC MANAGEMENT

Treatment is usually directed toward the management of underlying cause. Beyond addressing modifiable risk factors and treating underlying maternal chronic conditions, no interventions have been shown to prevent miscarriage.

Tissue retained inside the uterine cavity as a result of miscarriage is associated with an increased risk of infection and hemorrhage and would not be passed spontaneously. The options for treatment include: expectant management, medical management, and surgical uterine evacuation. A woman should be given the choice of various treatment options and should be counseled to use the treatment option which she considers as the best.

In cases with positive β-hCG results and absence of intrauterine gestational sac, ectopic pregnancy and pregnancy of unknown location must be ruled out **(Flowchart 7.3)**. The patient must be carefully observed for ectopic pregnancy if no POC's are documented upon suction evacuation.

Cochrane reviews have shown that miscarriage is not prevented by strategies such as bed rest, vitamin supplementation, progestogen, or hCG.

Emotional support: The woman undergoing miscarriage must be counseled that it has not occurred due to her fault. It was probably just bad luck, unless some obvious or recurrent cause can be detected, which warrants evaluation or intervention. She should be assured that there is nothing she has done that caused her pregnancy to fail. She must be encouraged to face her family and friends without any guilt. She must be encouraged to allow herself a normal grieving process by taking out time off from work and other commitments. The father/partner must also be involved. The patient may require additional appointments to monitor the grief process and look for signs of depression.

THREATENED ABORTION

Administration of progestogens and hCG may prove to be useful in some cases. Anti-Rh immunoglobulins must be administered to Rh-negative nonsensitized women with symptoms of threatened abortion, at or after 12 weeks of gestation. However, no treatment is available, which can stop the process of abortion.

INEVITABLE ABORTION

In case of excessive bleeding, IV drip should be started with 5% dextrose in water or 5% dextrose in saline. Blood should be arranged and cross-matched, following which it may be transfused. In these cases, an IV injection of oxytocin 5–10 units or ergometrine 0.5 mg could be given. Arrangements should be made to evacuate the uterus as soon as possible. Suction evacuation can be used in case the period of gestation is <12 weeks. If the period of gestation is >12 weeks, the process of abortion can be accelerated using oxytocin infusion.

INCOMPLETE ABORTION

Treatment in cases of incomplete abortion is same as that discussed in cases of inevitable abortion. In case the size of uterus is > 12 weeks, using a single dose of 600 µg misoprostol per orally (PO) or 400 µg sublingually (SL) can facilitate the process of abortion to completion.

MISSED ABORTION

> Q. Write a short essay on missed abortion.

Before 12 weeks of pregnancy, the treatment comprises suction evacuation. Oxytocin can be used for inducing uterine contractions after 12 weeks of gestation. Misoprostol (single oral dose of 600 µg) can be used for inducing uterine contractions both before and after 12 weeks of gestation. Passage of tissues should occur within a few days of receiving medical therapy. If it is not successful, surgical approach can be used to empty the uterine cavity.

TREATMENT OF THE UNDERLYING CAUSE

When a specific cause of spontaneous miscarriage has been identified, treatment of that particular cause must be initiated.

- *Antiphospholipid antibody syndrome:* Patients with recurrent pregnancy loss must be administered a prophylactic dose of subcutaneous heparin (preferably low-molecular-weight heparin) and low-dose aspirin. In patients for whom the treatment with aspirin and heparin is not successful, use of IV immunoglobulins can be used. For details related to treatment of APAS, kindly refer to Chapter 13.
- *Absence of blocking antibodies as a cause of miscarriage:* Immunotherapy with paternal pool leukocytes can be considered as an optimal solution for this problem. However, this therapy is presently in purely experimental stage and can be considered dangerous before further research is conducted.
- *Asherman's syndrome:* The most accurate method for diagnosis of Asherman's syndrome is direct visualization via hysteroscopic resection. These adhesions can also be removed on hysteroscopy. In order to prevent reformation of adhesions following surgery, prescription of estrogen supplementation or placement of a splint, balloon, or copper device may prove useful.
- *Uterine malformations:* Surgical correction of the underlying uterine defect can be undertaken.

BOX 7.2: Prerequisites before using expectant management.
- Less than 13 weeks gestation
- Stable vital signs
- No evidence of infection or hemorrhage
- Patient desires the use of expectant management

TABLE 7.6: Success rate with expectant management in case of various types of miscarriage.

Type of miscarriage	Success rate with expectant management (%)
Incomplete/inevitable abortion	91
Missed abortion	76
Anembryonic pregnancies	66

EXPECTANT MANAGEMENT

Expectant management involves a "wait and watch" policy to ensure that the process of miscarriage gets completed naturally without requiring any intervention. Various prerequisites before using expectant management have been described in **Box 7.2**.

Patient counseling is particularly important for those women with an intact sac who wish to follow an expectant approach. They should be aware that complete resolution may take several weeks and that overall efficacy rates are low. If the patient so desires, she can quit expectant management at any stage and opt for a medical or surgical evacuation at a later date. In women undergoing expectant management, a follow-up visit may be required to assess if the process of expulsion is complete. Success can be defined as absence of gestational sac (or its remnants) and presence of an endometrial thickness ≤15 mm on TVS, 3 days–6 weeks after diagnosis; absence of any vaginal bleeding; and 80% drop in the β-hCG levels 1 week following the passage of tissues. Since vaginal bleeding and positive urine pregnancy test can continue for 2–4 weeks, these cannot be considered as good measures of success.

Most expulsions occur in the first 2 weeks after diagnosis. Prolonged follow-up may be needed. It is acceptable and safe to wait up to 4 weeks postdiagnosis. It is associated with an overall success rate of 81%. Success rates can vary depending on the type of miscarriage. Expectant management is highly effective in cases of incomplete miscarriage **(Table 7.6)**.

MEDICAL MANAGEMENT

> 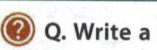 Q. Write a long essay discussing the medical methods of abortion.

Medical management can be offered as an effective alternative in the management of confirmed first-trimester miscarriage and is associated with several advantages **(Box 7.3)**. To avoid unnecessary anxiety, women should be informed that bleeding may continue for up to 3 weeks after medical uterine evacuation. Medical evacuation is an alternative technique that complements, but does not replace, surgical evacuation. Various medical methods (**Box 7.4**) have been described using prostaglandin analogs (gemeprost or misoprostol) with or without antiprogesterone priming (mifepristone). Presently, there is no medical regimen for management of early pregnancy loss that is FDA approved. Misoprostol is a cheap, highly effective prostaglandin analog that is active PO, SL, and per vaginally (PV). In case of missed miscarriages (closed cervix and intact sac), effective regimens involve use of a higher dose of prostaglandin for a longer duration of time or, alternatively, following priming with antiprogesterone. Prerequisites for medical management of spontaneous miscarriage are listed in **Box 7.5**.

For treatment of incomplete abortion <13 weeks of gestation, misoprostol 600 μg orally or 400 μg SL is recommended by WHO (2018). At a period of gestation ≥ 13 weeks, repeated doses of misoprostol in the dosage 400 μg can be administered SL, vaginally or buccally every 3 hours.

For medical management of induced abortion < 12 weeks gestation, WHO (2018) recommends the use of 200 mg mifepristone followed 1-2 days later by 800 μg of misoprostol administered vaginally, SL, or buccally. The minimum recommended interval between the use mifepristone and misoprostol is 24 hours. Mifepristone is progestin antagonist that binds to progestin receptor. It may be used with misoprostol to "destabilize" the implantation site. For misoprostol only regimens, WHO recommends the use of 800 μg of misoprostol administered vaginally, SL, or buccally. Combination regimen is the most recommended because it is likely to be more effective.

For medical management of induced abortions ≥ 12 weeks of gestation, WHO recommends the use of 200 mg mifepristone, followed 1-2 hours later with repeat doses of 400 μg of misoprostol administered vaginally, SL, or buccally every 3 hours. Maximum recommended interval between the use of mifepristone and misoprostol is 24 hours.

For misoprostol only regimens, WHO recommends the use of 400 μg of misoprostol administered vaginally, SL, or buccally every 3 hours.

Despite the use of medical therapy, surgical management may still be used in the following conditions:
- Gestational sac continues to be present (as observed on ultrasound examination)
- Clinical symptoms such as bleeding
- Patient's preference
- It is not possible to wait for 3 weeks or more and immediate results are required.

Besides mifepristone, other drug combinations which can be used are methotrexate and misoprostol. Methotrexate is a folic acid antagonist, which is cytotoxic to the trophoblast. It was initially used for medical management of ectopic pregnancy. It has also been used in combination with misoprostol to treat elective abortion medically. This combination has been found to be associated with success rates up to 98%. Misoprostol is administered 7 days after methotrexate injection.

SURGICAL UTERINE EVACUATION

> Q. Write short essay discussing surgical methods of first trimester medical termination of pregnancy (MTP).
>
> Q. Write a short note on termination of pregnancy prior to 6 weeks.
>
> Q. With help of a long essay discuss different methods of MTP used in first trimester abortion and its complications
>
> Q. Discuss briefly about first trimester MTP.

Surgical uterine evacuation has been the standard treatment offered to women who miscarry. Surgical option should be used in presence of indications mentioned in **Box 7.6**. Surgical management options help in providing immediate therapy and are associated with high success rates varying between 93% and 100%.

Suction and evacuation or vacuum aspiration is a surgical procedure involving cervical dilatation, followed by the use of vacuum or suction to evacuate gestational sac and the products of conception from the uterine cavity. This method is often also used for first trimester MTP. Prostaglandins are commonly administered prior to surgical evacuation.

BOX 7.3: Advantages of using misoprostol.
- May help in avoiding surgery
- Cost effective
- Few side effects (especially with vaginal)
- Stable at room temperature
- Readily available

BOX 7.4: Various options used for medical management of spontaneous abortion.
- Misoprostol
- Mifepristone plus misoprostol
- Methotrexate plus misoprostol

BOX 7.5: Prerequisites for medical management of spontaneous miscarriage.
- Less than 13 weeks gestation
- Stable vital signs
- No evidence of infection
- No history of any allergies to medications used

BOX 7.6: Indications for surgical management.
- Patient is unstable
- Significant medical morbidity
- Excessive and persistent bleeding
- Patient desires immediate therapy
- Presence of retained infected tissue
- Suspected gestational trophoblastic disease

Their use is associated with several advantages such as significant reductions in dilatation force, hemorrhage, and uterine/cervical trauma. Screening for infection, including *Chlamydia trachomatis*, should be considered in women undergoing surgical uterine evacuation, especially in presence of signs and symptoms suggestive of infection. Vaginal swabs can be considered to diagnose bacterial vaginosis, if clinically indicated. Women with *C. trachomatis*, *Neisseria gonorrhoeae*, or bacterial vaginosis in the lower genital tract at the time of induced pregnancy termination are at an increased risk of developing pelvic inflammatory disease at a later stage. Such women must be administered antibiotics for treatment of infection. However, presently there is insufficient evidence to recommend routine antibiotic prophylaxis prior to surgical uterine evacuation. Antibiotic prophylaxis should therefore be administered based on individual clinical indications.

Preoperative Preparation

- *Patient counseling:* Adequate counseling of the woman and her partner is essential, in order to enable her to make a free and fully informed decision. An informed consent from the woman must be taken prior to the procedure. It is the duty of the surgeon to ensure that the woman remains calm and relaxed during the procedure and should adopt a sympathetic attitude toward her.
- *Ultrasound examination:* Ultrasound examination is essential to confirm the diagnosis of the type of miscarriage.
- *History:* A complete medical history must be taken, in order to rule out the presence of the medical diseases, such as asthma, diabetes, and the history of the drug allergy.
- *Investigations:* Simple investigations, such as hemoglobin estimation, urine analysis, and blood grouping (ABO, Rh), need to be routinely done prior to the procedure. In case, the procedure would be carried out under general anesthesia (GA), investigations, such as blood sugar levels, kidney function tests, electrocardiography, and X-ray, may be required.
- *Anesthesia:* The procedure is usually carried out under local anesthesia, using a paracervical block with 20 mL of 0.5% lignocaine. Short GA may be used in the patients, who are very apprehensive. Many patients are likely to experience some discomfort during abortion, although the amount of pain usually varies from mild to moderate. In order to reduce the pain during and after the procedure, nonsteroidal anti-inflammatory drugs, such as naproxen 550 mg, may be commonly prescribed before the procedure. Vasoconstrictive agents, such as vasopressin (2 units) may be added to the local anesthetic agent, which would help in reducing the amount of bleeding in second trimester procedures. Atropine (0.5 mg) can also be mixed with the local anesthetic agent to reduce vagal effects and prevent syncope and nausea.
- *Prophylactic antibiotics:* In cases, where the possibility of intrauterine infection is suspected (e.g., history of prolonged bleeding per vaginum, patient at risk of bacterial endocarditis, etc.), antibiotics can be administered prior to the procedure. Antibiotics are routinely prescribed following the procedure in our set-up. It has also been observed that the routine use of prophylactic antibiotics can help in preventing nearly 50% cases of postabortion endometritis.
- *Bladder catheterization:* Bladder must be emptied prior to the procedure.
- *Cleaning and draping:* Shaving the perineum is not required, but the perineal hair must be trimmed. After taking all aseptic precautions, the area of perineum, mons, and lower part of the abdomen must be cleaned and draped, using povidone-iodine or chlorhexidine solution.
- The surgeon must use the "no-touch" technique, in which he/she must use sterile instruments and sterile gloves and take care never to touch that part of the instrument that would enter the uterus.

Procedure of Vacuum Aspiration

The equipments used for vacuum aspiration are shown in **Figures 7.10A and B**. The procedure of vacuum aspiration comprises the following steps **(Figs. 7.11A to D)**:

- The cervix is exposed after retracting the posterior vaginal wall using Sims vaginal speculum.
- The anterior lip of the cervix is held, using a Vulsellum or tenaculum. Once the cervix has been properly visualized, paracervical block is given.
- The cervix is then serially dilated, using a series of metallic or plastic dilators. Though a variety of dilators are available, Hegar's dilators are most commonly used. While dilating the cervix, the dilators must be held in a pen holding fashion and an undue force must not be applied over the cervix. The dilatation is initially started using smaller dilators and then generally large dilators are used, one after the other. The dilators must be inserted slowly and gently. This practice is both safe and less painful. If resistance is experienced, the operator should return to the previous dilator, reinsert it, and allow it to remain in place for a minute or so before attempting to insert the next large dilator. The rule normally followed is that "the size of the suction cannula to be used for the procedure must be equivalent to the size of the uterus." The dilation of the cervix must be approximately 0.5–1 mm more than the size of suction cannula to be used. Safe dilation depends on the operator's proper determination of the direction of the endocervical canal at the time of bimanual examination. Failure to appreciate that the uterus is retroverted may result in an anterior perforation.

Early Pregnancy Bleeding due to Miscarriage

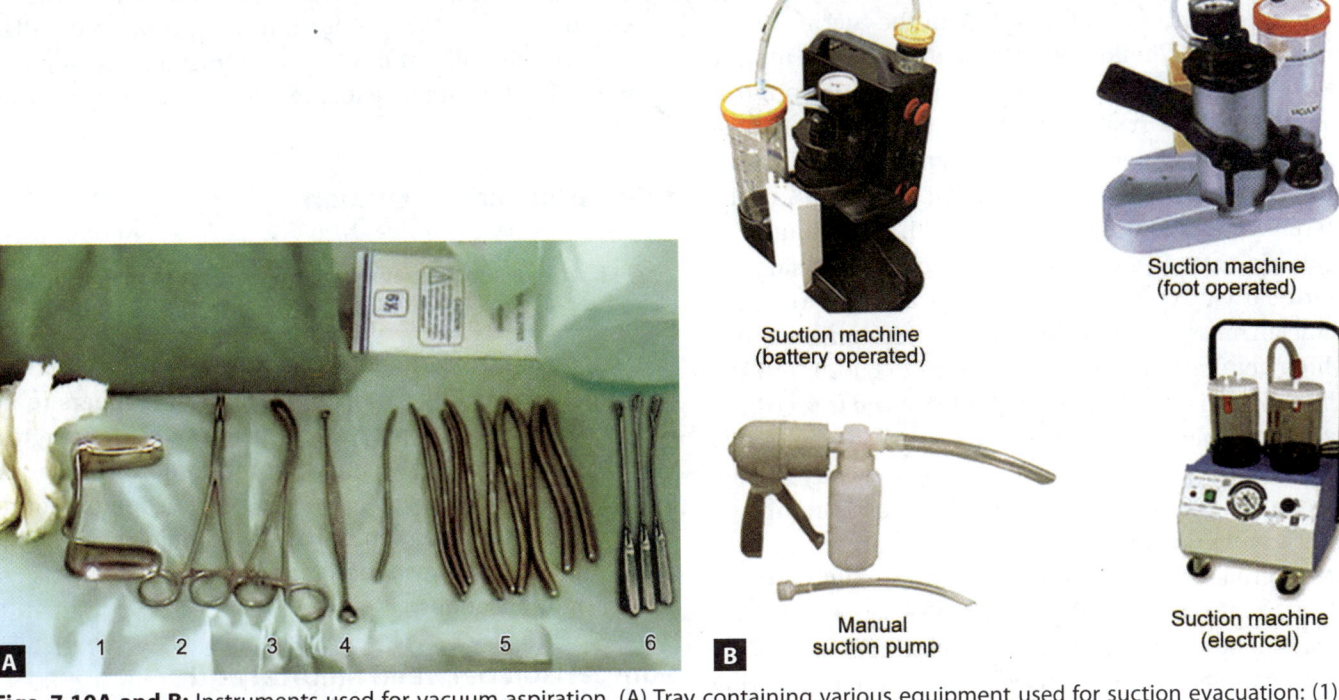

Figs. 7.10A and B: Instruments used for vacuum aspiration. (A) Tray containing various equipment used for suction evacuation: (1) Sim's speculum; (2) Sponge holder; (3) Vulsellum; (4) Anterior vaginal wall retractor; (5) Hegar's dilators of increasing sizes; (6) Uterine curettes of varying sizes; (B) Suction units of various types.

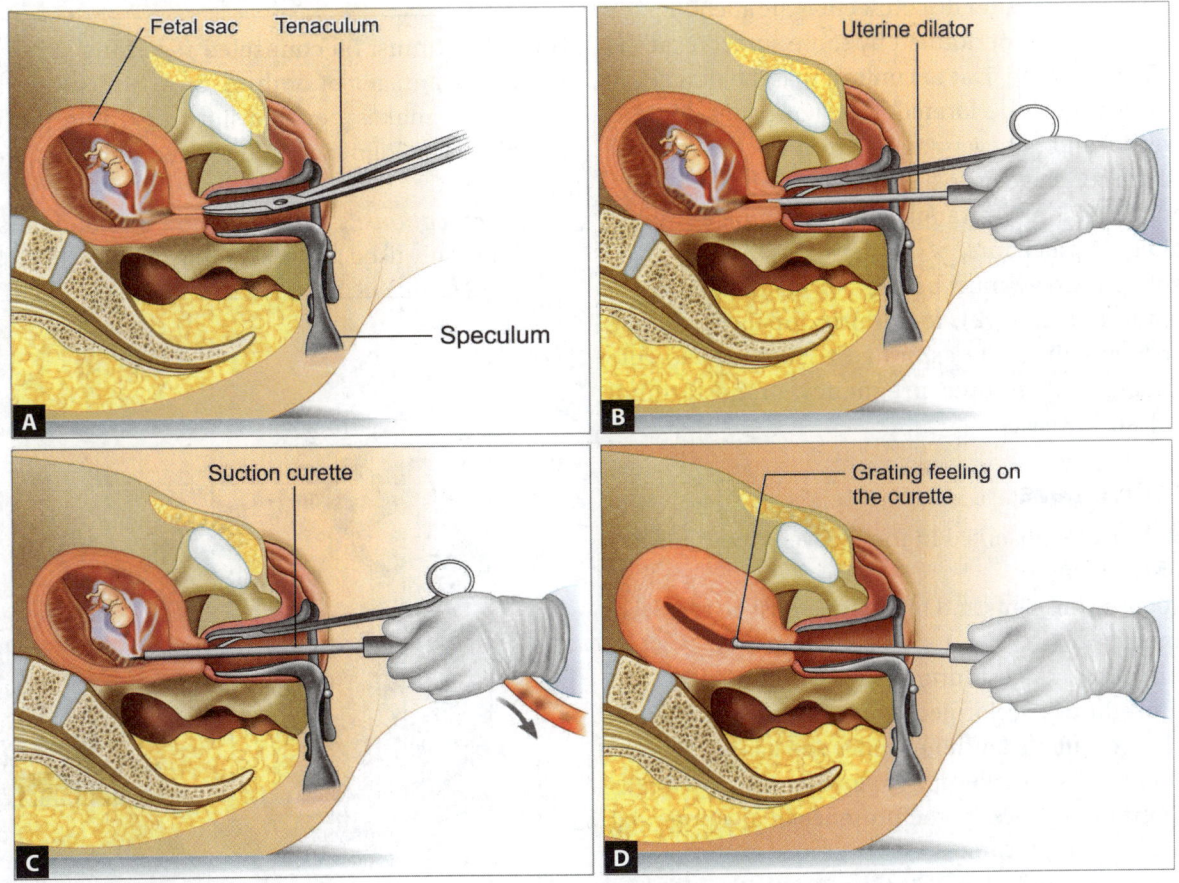

Figs. 7.11A to D: Steps of the procedure of vacuum aspiration. (A) Retracting the posterior wall of the uterus with Sim's speculum and grasping the anterior lip with tenaculum; (B) Dilating the external cervical os with Hegar's dilator; (C) Insertion of Karman's cannula for producing suction; and (D) The evacuation of the uterine contents is almost complete resulting in a grating feeling.

- Some clinicians prefer to use a uterine sound for determining the depth of the uterine cavity. We normally do not perform routine sounding of the uterine cavity in our set-up. Whether or not, the depth of the uterine cavity needs to be measured with a uterine sound is controversial. Most surgeons do not use a sound for fear of perforation. Moreover, uterine sounding provides little information, which could be useful. Up to 25% of the uterine perforations are associated with use of sound.
- A plastic Karman's cannula is then inserted inside the uterine cavity. Once the cannula has been inserted, the clinician must connect the cannula to a suction machine, which generates pressure equivalent to 60–70 mm Hg. The cannula is rotated at an angle of 360° and moved back by 1–2 cm, back and forth, till the entire uterine cavity has been evacuated. The cannula can be gently rotated several times. When one round of suction is complete, the cannula tip is pulled back to the region just above the internal os, but not out of it. Care should be taken not to rotate the cannula inside the cervix. Evacuation is said to be complete, when no more contents are seen coming out of the uterine cavity; instead of the uterine contents, air bubbles start appearing in the cannula and/or the uterine cavity appears to be firm and gritty. Once the surgeon is sure that the procedure is complete, the cannula is removed after disconnecting the suction.
- A sharp curettage is performed by some surgeons at the end of the procedure, just to confirm that the procedure has been completely performed. This step is considered as controversial and not every-one performs it, because the use of sharp curettage may slightly increase the blood loss.
- Methergine 0.25 mg intramuscularly may be administered after the procedure.
- The aspirated tissue must be sent for histopathological examination **(Fig. 7.12)**, to confirm for the presence of chorionic villi in the aspirated tissues and to rule out presence of ectopic pregnancy or gestational trophoblastic disease.

Postoperative Care

The patient must be observed in the recovery room for 2–3 hours before discharge.
- The patient's vital signs and blood loss must be regularly monitored.
- In case of pain, analgesic drugs may be prescribed.
- If the procedure is performed under GA, the patient can be discharged after a few hours, once she has stabilized.
- The patients are scheduled for a follow-up visit, 1–2 weeks after abortion to check for the presence of any potential MTP-related complications.
- *Anti-D immunoglobulins:* Nonsensitized Rh-negative women should receive anti-D immunoglobulin in the following situations—ectopic pregnancy and any miscarriage or termination of pregnancy, regardless of gestational age of the fetus or the method of uterine evacuation. For successful immunoprophylaxis, RhD immunoglobulin should be administered as soon as possible after the sensitizing event, but always within 72 hours.

Dilatation and Evacuation

> Q. Write a short essay discussing the methods of second trimester MTP.

When the period of gestation is >14 weeks, surgical abortion by D&E, preceded by cervical preparation, appears to be the most appropriate procedure. In these cases, surgical abortion is performed using a combination of vacuum aspiration and specialized forceps for evacuation of uterine contents. RCOG recommends that D&E should be preferably performed under ultrasound guidance to reduce the risk of surgical complications.

Comparison between Medical and Surgical Management

> Q. How should the patient be counseled before making a choice between medical and surgical abortion?

The patient must be counseled regarding various benefits and disadvantages of both medical and surgical methods before she makes her decision regarding the treatment modality. The following things need to be explained to the patient:
- *Complications:* Though suction evacuation is the most commonly used method for termination of first trimester

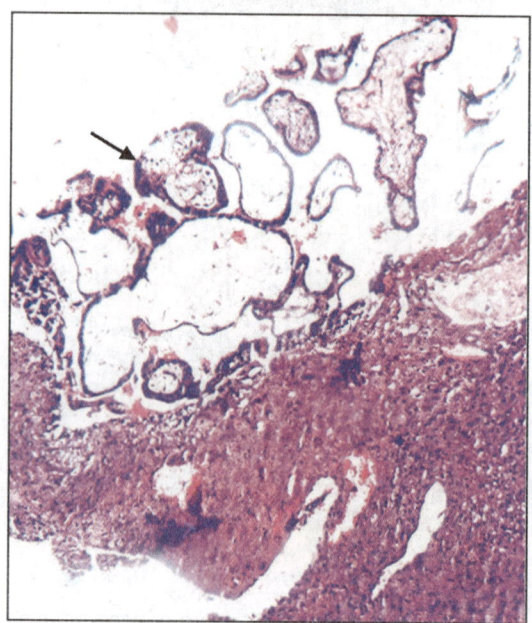

Fig. 7.12: The histopathological appearance of the evacuated products.

pregnancies, being an invasive surgical technique, it may be associated with various complications such as risks of infection, perforation of uterus, incomplete abortion, and postprocedure uterine synechiae formation (Asherman's syndrome). Though the complication rate is higher with surgical method than that of medical method, serious complications usually do not occur in experienced hands.

Medical method, though associated with minor complications is associated with several other disadvantages. It may take several days, is not completely predictable, and may be associated with heavy bleeding and severe cramping, which may last for a longer period and has a higher failure rate in comparison with the surgical method.

- *Period of gestation:* While medical abortion should be only used in cases the pregnancy is ≤7 weeks, vacuum aspiration can be performed, all through the 12 weeks in the first trimester. The chances of failed surgical abortion increase with pregnancy of <6 weeks. While medical abortion can be used only in early pregnancy, vacuum aspiration can be used until late first trimester.
- *Time required:* Medical method has been found to be a safe and noninvasive process but takes longer time for complete termination. The process is more natural and may appear like a miscarriage. With medical method, there is no requirement of anesthesia, vacuum aspiration machine, and other instruments. Medical method usually requires many visits to the healthcare provider. A follow-up visit is essential and is usually fixed at 2 weeks from the time of first appointment. The procedure of surgical abortion, on the other hand, usually requires a single visit to the clinic and takes about 15–20 minutes. Follow-up visit is fixed and must take place at 3–4 weeks following the procedure. However, if the medical method fails, surgical method is required.
- *Duration of bleeding following the procedure:* Medical method may be associated with heavy bleeding and passage of clots for 3–4 days. The bleeding may last for 2 weeks or longer. Vacuum aspiration, on the other hand, is associated with light to moderate bleeding, which may continue for a few days following the procedure.
- *Success rate:* Medical method is successful in 97% cases. It may not be successful, in cases where period of gestation is >7 weeks. If medical method fails, vacuum aspiration becomes essential. On the other hand, vacuum aspiration is more successful, the success rate being almost 99%.

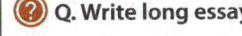
COMPLICATIONS

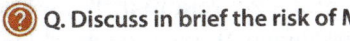 Q. Write long essay on complications and sequelae of MTP.

Q. Discuss in brief the risk of MTP at 18 weeks.

COMPLICATIONS ASSOCIATED WITH THE MISCARRIAGE PROCESS

Septic Abortion/Miscarriage with Sepsis

In these cases, incomplete abortion is associated with ascending infection of the endometrium, parametrium, adnexa uteri, or peritoneum. Ultrasound findings are consistent with those of incomplete abortion. Infection may also be associated with criminal abortion. Various organisms which may be involved include anaerobic bacteria, coliforms, *Haemophilus influenzae, Campylobacter jejuni*, group A streptococcus, etc. Infection, if not timely treated, may be associated with complications such as severe hemorrhage, bacterial shock, acute renal failure, uterine infection, parametritis, peritonitis, endocarditis, septicemia, disseminated intravascular coagulation, infertility, etc. Treatment involves supportive care; use of antimicrobials and evacuation.

COMPLICATIONS ASSOCIATED WITH SURGICAL EVACUATION

Surgical evacuation could be associated with complications mentioned in **Box 7.7**. The risk of these complications is likely to be higher with an increased period of gestation.

Though small amount of cramping, pain, and bleeding can commonly occur for 2–3 days after the procedure, severe degrees of persistent pain, or amount of bleeding more than that associated with normal menstruation, especially in association with fever or fainting could be indicative of the underlying complications. Some of these are discussed here.

Uterine Perforation

The most dreaded complication of the procedure is uterine perforation because the procedure of suction evacuation is essentially a blind one. The risk of uterine perforation becomes greater with the increasing gestational age of the fetus. Most uterine perforations are thought to occur during the process of uterine sounding or cervical dilation because the most common site of perforation is the junction of the cervix and the lower uterine segment. While the midline perforations in this region are usually benign, lateral perforations at this location may be particularly hazardous for the patient because they may extend to the branches of the uterine artery resulting in profuse hemorrhage. A uterine

BOX 7.7: Complications associated with surgical evacuation.
- Uterine perforation
- Infection
- Incomplete evacuation
- Bleeding during and following the abortion
- Failure of the procedure
- Hypotension
- Asherman's syndrome
- Cervical lacerations/cervical incompetence

perforation must be suspected, when no tissue is obtained; when the instruments appear to be inserted deeper than the depth expected, on the basis of the gestational age; when hemorrhage occurs; or when obvious maternal tissues, such as omentum, are obtained.

Sometimes when MTP is being performed during the procedure of laparoscopic sterilization, the perforation may be visualized laparoscopically. Treatment of perforation depends on the expected location, the woman's vital signs and condition and whether the abortion is complete or not. In case of a suspected perforation, the patient must be observed for a few hours for the signs of hypovolemia and shock. Intramuscular oxytocics (methergine) and antibiotics must be administered. If the patient's vitals are stable; the uterine perforation is midline; repeated pelvic examinations are negative; repeat hematocrit results are stable; the uterus is already empty and/or the amount of bleeding is minimal or none, then there is no need for patient hospitalization. The patient may be discharged home in the company of a responsible adult and instructed to visit the hospital immediately, in case she experiences excessive pain or bleeding or some other complication at any time. She must be scheduled for a repeat general physical and pelvic examination, the next day. In case the patient continues to experience bleeding, pain, or her vitals continue to remain unstable, she should be admitted to a hospital for observation and a possible laparoscopic examination. If the abortion is not complete at the time perforation is suspected, it should be completed with the aid of ultrasound or laparoscopy. Laparotomy may be required, in cases where intraperitoneal bleeding or bowel injury is suspected.

Infection

This can be easily avoided by the administration of broad-spectrum antibiotics. In case the infection is as a result of incomplete evacuation, the surgeon first needs to completely evacuate the uterine cavity. Following this, the antibiotics must be given. In the cases of serious infection, IV antibiotics can be given. Laparotomy may be required in cases of peritonitis. If upon examination, the uterus appears to be tender and slightly enlarged, infection is a possibility. Infection in association with the retained POC is likely to result in the development of postabortion endometritis, among women undergoing first trimester surgical abortion. Typically, the woman returns 3 or 4 days, after the procedure with increased cramping and bleeding, sometimes accompanied by fever or nausea. The microorganism commonly involved in such cases is beta (β)-hemolytic streptococci. Endometritis should be treated immediately to avoid progression of infection. In most early cases, hospitalization is not required, and the outpatient treatment proves to be sufficient. Ampicillin usually works against microorganisms such as hemolytic streptococci. In case of infection with organisms, such as *Chlamydia* or bacterial vaginosis or other anaerobic organisms, combination of oral metronidazole and ofloxacin is commonly prescribed.

Incomplete Evacuation

The most common presentation in cases of incomplete evacuation is prolonged bleeding. In these cases, the uterine contents have to be reevacuated, under antibiotic coverage. Typical history suggestive of an incomplete evacuation is a woman returning several days after the procedure with the history of increased bleeding and cramping. On examination, she may have an enlarged uterus or tissue visible in the cervical os. Ultrasound examination is usually performed, but may not be always helpful because blood and debris are commonly present inside the uterus and the amount of retained tissue may be small.

Treatment of incomplete abortion may be pharmacologic. Uterotonic drugs, such as methylergonovine (methergine) may help contract the uterus and expel the residual tissue. This method is appropriate when the amount of retained tissue is small and there are no signs of infection. If this method is chosen, the woman should be called for a follow-up visit within a few days, to make sure that her symptoms have resolved.

If the amount of retained tissue inside the uterine cavity is large or if the woman cannot return for follow-up, then repeat suction should be done. Repeat suction is usually easy because the cervix is dilated and a cannula smaller than that used for the original procedure is adequate.

Bleeding During and Following the Abortion

Most women have minimal bleeding during first trimester abortion. However at times, there may be severe bleeding during and after the procedure. Uterine atony is the most likely cause of heavy and prolonged bleeding in these cases. IV ergometrine (0.2 mg) or oxytocin (10–20 units) may be used to contract the uterus. Alternatively misoprostol, in the dosage of 400 μg may be prescribed either through oral or rectal route. Doses of misoprostol as high as 1000 μg have been used per rectally in cases of atonic uterus. Prostaglandin F2α (carboprost) can be prescribed intramuscularly or into the uterus. In the absence of an obvious cervical or uterine injury, the surgeon should complete the abortion, evacuating the uterus rapidly, but gently. If the bleeding still continues to occur, the uterus is massaged between the two hands, e.g. bimanual compression.

The aspirated tissue is examined to assess gestational age and to confirm that all fetal parts have been removed. If the bleeding still does not stop, the cervix should be explored for the presence of a likely laceration or for bleeding from the tenaculum site. Next, the uterus is gently explored with a sharp curette, preferably under ultrasound guidance, checking for uterine shape and size, retained tissue and uterine wall irregularities or defects. Repeat suction may remove clots and retained tissue and allow the uterus to contract. If bleeding persists even after the uterus has been emptied, the next maneuver is uterine tamponade. For details regarding control of bleeding from an atonic uterus, kindly refer to Chapter 14.

Failure of the Procedure

The procedure, if not performed properly, may result in the continuation of the pregnancy. This may result in cases of very small sized uterus, where the suction cannula fails to suck out the POC. This may also occur in cases associated with a uterine anomaly (e.g., uterus didelphys or bicornuate uterus) or cases of ectopic pregnancy.

Hypotension

This could be related to excessive blood loss or due to a vasovagal response to pain. Management in these cases comprises administration of IV fluids, oxygen, whole blood transfusion, and corticosteroids.

Minor Complications

Minor complications like postoperative nausea and vomiting can be managed with antiemetics such as metoclopramide or ondansetron.

Asherman's Syndrome

This is a delayed complication, which can occur as a result of vigorous curettage. This complication is usually managed by hysteroscopic resection of intrauterine adhesions, followed by insertion of an intrauterine contraceptive device or a Foley's catheter, in order to keep the uterine wall apart.

Cervical Lacerations/Cervical Incompetence

Rarely, vigorous dilatation may result in the development of cervical lacerations and/or cervical incompetence in the subsequent pregnancies. This complication can be avoided by taking a good history and correct estimation of gestational age during the bimanual examination. Overzealous cervical dilation must be avoided. Dilatation is carried out using the smallest-sized dilator. The Hegar's dilators are commonly used. These dilators must be held in a pen holding fashion and must be gently inserted into the cervical canal. Undue force must not be used, while inserting the cannula. The dilatation must be started using the smallest-sized dilator. Gradually, larger-sized dilators must be used. The cervix must be dilated about 0.5–1.0 mm more than the size of the suction cannula to be used. Cervical priming using prostaglandins, prior to the procedure, facilitates the process of dilatation without the use of undue force.

EVIDENCE-BASED CLINICAL TRIALS

List of references can be scanned through QR code to enable the readers gain deeper insight of the subject by referring to the entire article or its abstract.

CHAPTER 8

Antepartum Hemorrhage

ANTEPARTUM HEMORRHAGE

> Q. With help of a long question, discuss the differential diagnosis and management of a multigravida patient presenting with APH at 36 weeks of gestation.
>
> Q. How will you evaluate a case of APH? Discuss in detail the management of a case presenting with accidental hemorrhage.

Hemorrhage has been identified as one of the most important causes of maternal death worldwide. Maternal bleeding in the antepartum period, before the birth of the child, can be considered as one of the most disastrous obstetric emergency which is encountered in clinical practice. This condition can cause a pregnant patient to become exsanguinated and bleed to death within a matter of minutes, thereby resulting in the death of her baby as well. Therefore, all clinicians need to be well versed with the causes and the management of bleeding taking place during the antenatal period, which is also known as APH. APH can be defined as hemorrhage from the genital tract occurring after the 28th week of pregnancy, but before the delivery of baby. It does not include the bleeding which occurs after the delivery of the baby; this bleeding which occurs in the postpartum period after the birth of the baby is known as postpartum hemorrhage (PPH). The 28 weeks interval is arbitrarily taken as a limit while defining APH because the fetus is supposed to have attained viability by that time.

The various causes of APH are illustrated in **Flowchart 8.1**. The antepartum bleeding could be due to placental or extraplacental causes. Besides this, some cases of APH could be due to unexplained causes and are also termed as indeterminate APH: The placental causes of bleeding are termed as true APH and can be due to placenta previa or placental abruption. Extraplacental cause of bleeding is also termed as false APH and includes bleeding related to the presence of cervical polyps, carcinoma cervix, cervical varicosities, etc. Placental causes of bleeding are the most common cause of APH, accounting for nearly 70–75% cases; whereas the extraplacental causes account for 5% cases and unexplained causes for the remaining 20–25%.

PART 1: PLACENTA PREVIA

CASE STUDY

A 32-year-old G2P1L1 lady with 33 weeks of gestation, presented with painless bleeding per vaginum since last 2 hours. This was the first time during the pregnancy that she has experienced this bleeding. According to her, the bleeding was severe, and she gave a history of soaking nearly 5–6 pads in last 2 hours. Her pulse rate is 90 beats/minute and her BP is 110/70 mm Hg.

> Q. What is the likely diagnosis in the above case? Why does this patient need to be assessed urgently?
>
> Q. What is the first step in the management of a patient with APH?

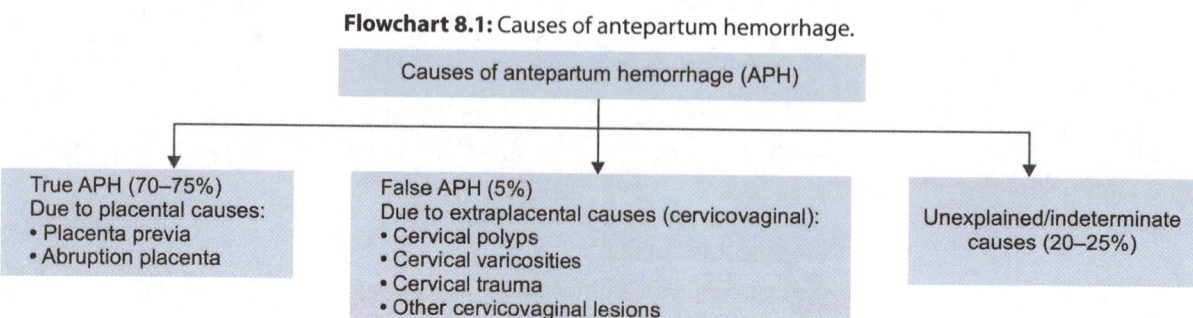

Flowchart 8.1: Causes of antepartum hemorrhage.

Antepartum Hemorrhage

INTRODUCTION

Q. Discuss in detail the management of a G2P1 previous LSCS patient with 34 weeks of gestation presenting with bleeding per vaginum.

Q. A 34-year-old G4P3A0L3 patient presents with painless bleeding per vaginum at 32 weeks of gestation. Discuss the management in such a patient.

Q. Discuss the management of first episode of painless bleeding at 32 weeks of gestation.

Placenta previa is one of the important placental causes of APH and can be defined as abnormal implantation of the placenta in the lower uterine segment **(Fig. 8.1A)**. Depending on the location of placenta in the relation of cervical os, there can be four degrees of placenta previa, which are described in the **Figure 8.1B**. The cause of bleeding is related to mechanical separation of the placenta from the site of implantation.

This usually occurs at the time of formation of the lower uterine segment, during third trimester, or during effacement and dilatation of the cervix at the time of labor. As the lower uterine segment progressively enlarges in the later months of pregnancy, the placenta gets sheared off from the walls of the uterine segment. This causes opening up of uteroplacental sinuses which can initiate an episode of bleeding.

Since the growth of the lower uterine segment is a physiological process, the episode of bleeding becomes inevitable in cases of placenta previa. The episode of bleeding is also triggered off, if placenta is separated from the lower uterine segment due to traumatic acts like vaginal examination, sexual intercourse, etc.

DEGREES OF PLACENTA PREVIA

There are four specific types of placenta previa.

Type 4 Placenta Previa

This is also known as total or central placenta previa **(Fig. 8.2)**. A complete placenta previa can be defined as a condition in which the placenta completely covers the internal os as observed on TVS.

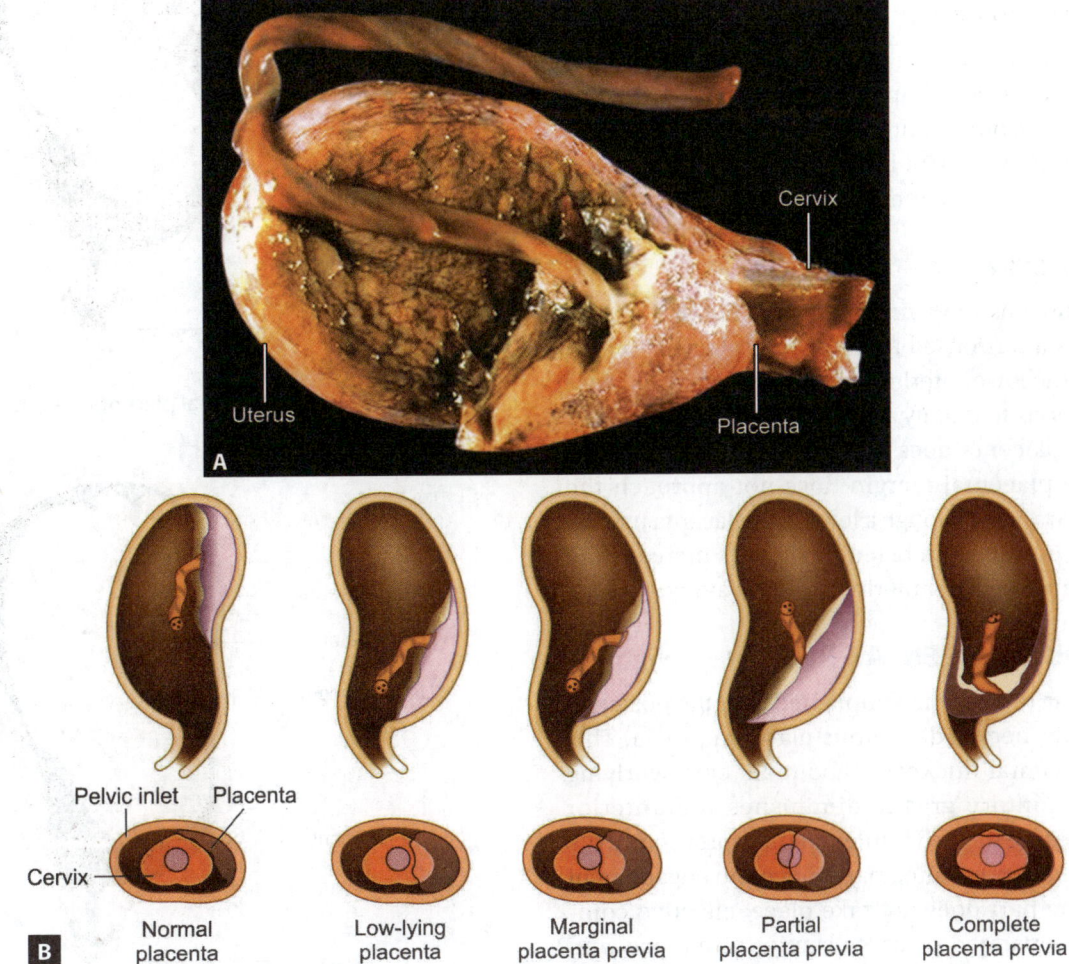

Figs 8.1A and B: Placenta previa. (A) Photograph showing placenta covering the cervical os; (B) Relationship of various degrees of placenta previa with the cervix.

144 Complications of Pregnancy

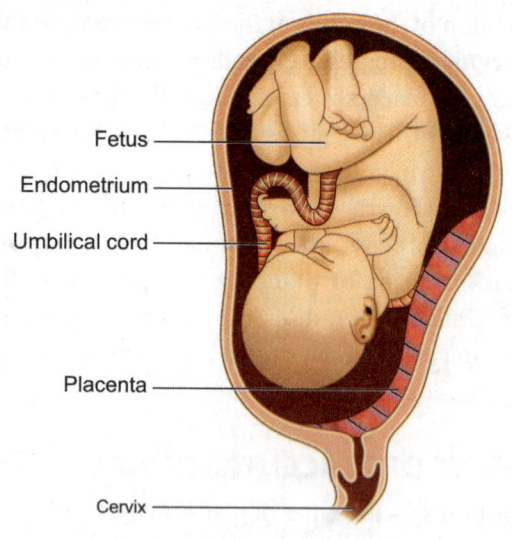

Fig. 8.2: Total placenta previa.

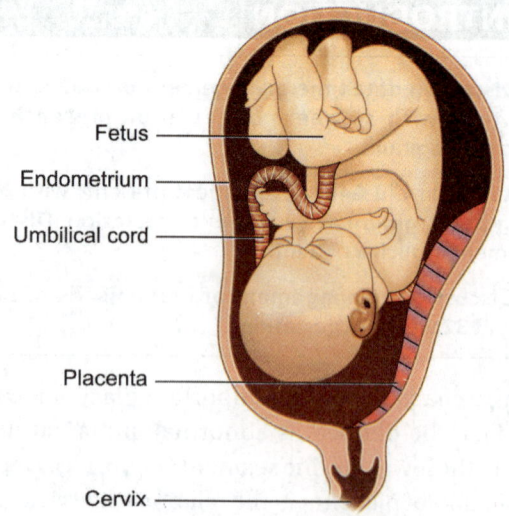

Fig. 8.3: Partial placenta previa.

Type 3 Placenta Previa

This is also known as partial placenta previa (**Fig. 8.3**). In partial placenta previa, the placenta partly covers the cervical os.

Type 2 Placenta Previa

This is also known as marginal placenta previa (**Fig. 8.4**). In marginal placenta previa, the placenta does not in any way cover the cervical os, but it approaches the edge of the cervix. Marginal placenta previa can be defined as one where the placental edge lies ≤2.5 cm from the internal cervical os.

Type 1 Placenta Previa

This is also known as low-lying placenta (**Fig. 8.5**). Low-lying placenta is a term used to describe a placenta which is implanted in the lower uterine segment but is not as close enough to the cervix to qualify as marginal placenta previa.

Though the placenta does lie in close proximity to the internal os, the placental margin does not approach the cervical edge in any way. Though a low-lying placenta usually does not cause intrapartum bleeding, it does increase the risk of PPH because of lower uterine segment atony.

■ DANGEROUS PLACENTA PREVIA

Marginal placenta previa when implanted over the posterior uterine wall is termed as dangerous placenta previa. This is so, as the placental thickness (about 2.5 cm) overlying the sacral promontory greatly diminishes the anterior posterior diameter of the pelvic inlet, thereby preventing the engagement of fetal presenting part. Since the engagement of the presenting part does not take place, effective compression of the separated placenta cannot take place, and the vaginal bleeding continues to occur. In fact, if the vaginal bleeding is allowed to occur, fetal distress may develop soon.

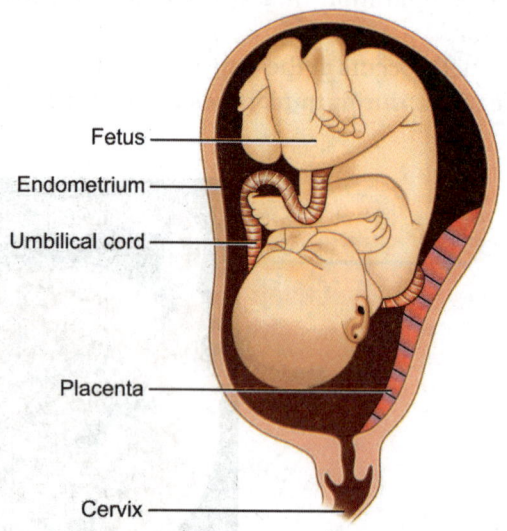

Fig. 8.4: Marginal placenta previa.

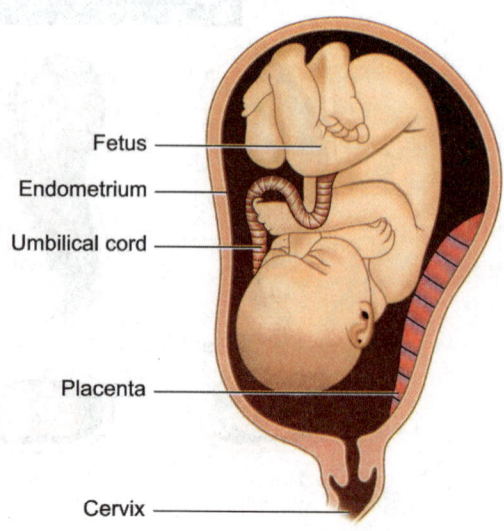

Fig. 8.5: Low-lying placenta previa.

HISTORY AND CLINICAL PRESENTATION

CLINICAL FEATURES

It is important to elicit the characteristics of bleeding in order to arrive at a diagnosis. As previously described, true APH occurs due to two causes—placenta previa and placental abruption. History is one of the most important parameters for differentiating between these two most important causes for bleeding, late in pregnancy. While placenta previa will be discussed in this part, placental abruption would be discussed in part 2 of this chapter.

- *Timing for occurrence of bleeding:* Such patients present with bleeding after 28 weeks of gestation, which is suggestive of APH. The earlier in pregnancy, the bleeding occurs, more likely it is to be due to severe degree of placenta previa.
- *Type of bleeding:* Placenta previa is typically associated with sudden, painless, apparently causeless, recurrent, and profuse bleeding, which is bright red in color.
- *Amount of bleeding:* The amount of bleeding in cases of placenta previa may range from light to heavy. It may stop, but it nearly always recurs days or weeks later. Some women who have placenta previa may also experience uterine contractions with bleeding, especially if they are in labor. The patient may also give a history of experiencing small "warning hemorrhages" before the actual episode of bleeding. The occurrence of these warning hemorrhages must be viewed with greatest suspicion and caution. Also, appropriate steps must be taken to exclude placenta previa. These small episodes of hemorrhage which occur prior to the episode of the major hemorrhage occur at about 34 weeks of gestation or earlier when the lower uterine segment begins to form.

It is also important to take the history regarding the amount of blood loss. Most of the times, it is difficult to rely upon the patient's own estimation regarding the amount of bleeding. An important parameter to help decide the severity of hemorrhage is to ask the patient regarding the number of pads she had to use during the episode of bleeding. A history of passage of clots is also indicative of severe hemorrhage. Presence of blood at the sides of patient's legs, at the time of examination often extending up to the heels is also indicative of severe hemorrhage.

RISK FACTORS

Some risk factors which are associated with an increased incidence of placenta previa and need to be elicited in the history include the following:

- Multiparity
- *Previous history of cesarean delivery:* History of a single previous cesarean section may increase the incidence of placenta previa in a subsequent pregnancy to as much as 5%. The risk further increases as the number of previous cesarean deliveries increase. Previous history of suction curettage is also associated with an increased risk. It is important to elicit the history of previous uterine surgery, as presence of a uterine scar along with placenta previa may be often associated with placenta accreta, increta, or percreta. Women requesting elective cesarean delivery for nonmedical indications should be counseled by informing them about the risk of placenta accreta spectrum and its consequences for subsequent pregnancies.
- *Advanced maternal age:* The risk of placenta previa also increases with advancing maternal age, with the risk increasing by 2% after 35 years of age and by 5% after the age of 40 years.
- History of placenta previa in the previous pregnancy
- History of smoking
- *History of multiple gestations:* Multifetal gestation is usually associated with a large placenta which commonly encroaches upon the lower uterine segment.
- Fetal malpresentation
- Fetal congenital anomaly
- Previous history of assisted reproductive technology

GENERAL PHYSICAL EXAMINATION

- The patient's physical condition is proportional to the amount of blood loss.
- *Anemia or shock:* Repeated bleeding can result in anemia, whereas heavy bleeding may cause shock.
- Profuse hemorrhage can result in hypotension and/or tachycardia.

SPECIFIC SYSTEMIC EXAMINATION

ABDOMINAL EXAMINATION

- Uterus is soft, relaxed, and nontender.
- Uterine contractions may be palpated.
- Size of the uterus is proportional to the period of gestation.
- The fetal presenting part may be high and cannot be pressed into the pelvic inlet due to the presence of placenta.
- Abnormal fetal presentation (e.g., breech presentation, transverse lie, etc.)
- Fetal heart rate is usually within normal limits. Fetal heart tones may be rarely absent in cases of APH due to placenta previa as a result of maternal shock. Slowing of fetal heart rate can sometimes occur in cases of dangerous placenta previa (described previously).

Stallworthy's Sign

In cases of placenta previa, when the head is pushed into the pelvis, there is slowing of fetal heart rate. This usually occurs due to compression of placenta and cord, especially in cases where marginal degree of placenta previa is located posteriorly (dangerous placenta previa).

VAGINAL EXAMINATION

Vaginal examination must never be performed in suspected cases of placenta previa. Instead, an initial inspection must only be performed. On inspection, the following points must be noted:
- To see if bleeding is occurring or not.
- In case the bleeding is occurring, to note the amount and color of the bleeding.

A per speculum inspection using a Cusco's speculum can be performed once the patient has become stable. Performance of per speculum examination helps in ruling out the local causes (e.g., cervical erosions, polyps, etc.) of bleeding per vaginum.

Nowadays, the diagnosis of placenta previa can be confirmed on ultrasound examination. Thus, there is no need to perform a vaginal examination in suspected cases of placenta previa. In case, facilities for ultrasound examination are not available and a vaginal examination is required, it must be performed in the operating room under double set-up conditions (i.e., arrangements for an emergency cesarean delivery are in place). An emergency cesarean section may be required in case the vaginal examination provokes an episode of bleeding. The vaginal examination must be performed just prior to the delivery and the following steps must be taken:
- The obstetrician must scrub up and put on double pair of gloves. If on vaginal examination placenta is felt, the first pair of gloves would be discarded so that the obstetrician can immediately proceed for an emergency cesarean section.
- The OT nurse must be scrubbed up with her trolley ready.
- The patient must be preferably under GA or epidural anesthesia. In case, an emergency cesarean section is required, the anesthetist must be ready to extend the anesthesia.
- An IV drip should be started.
- Arrangements for blood transfusion must be in place at time of examination.
- A careful digital examination is done by the clinician.
  - Firstly, the index finger must be gently introduced inside the vagina. The vaginal fornices must be palpated for presence of any bogginess between the fetal presenting part and the finger.
  - If the fetal presenting part can be palpated through the fornix, the finger can be introduced with some confidence into the cervical canal and a careful examination is done through the cervix.
  - If the placental edge is felt at any point, the examination must be stopped, and the finger must be withdrawn. In these cases, an emergency cesarean section needs to be performed. If no placental edge is palpable, the entire lower segment can be gradually explored.
    In these cases, the membranes can be ruptured with the aim of allowing a vaginal delivery.

RECTAL EXAMINATION

A rectal examination is more dangerous than a vaginal examination and must never be performed in cases of suspected placenta previa. On vaginal examination, it may be sometimes possible to feel the placenta, before it is seriously disturbed.

However, on rectal examination, the gloved finger is covered by rectal wall, vaginal wall, and the intervening fascia before it can feel the placenta. Thus, on rectal examination, it virtually appears to be impossible to detect the placenta before it has separated and has provoked serious bleeding.

DIFFERENTIAL DIAGNOSIS

Various causes for antepartum vaginal bleeding are listed in **Flowchart 8.1**. In the above-mentioned case described in the beginning of the chapter, where the patient presents with the history of bleeding after 28 weeks of gestation, the most important task of the obstetrician is to determine whether the bleeding is due to placental abruption or placenta previa. Another important but rare cause of hemorrhage, where bleeding is of fetal origin rather than from the mother is vasa previa.

VASA PREVIA

 Q. Write a short note on vasa previa.

Vasa previa is an uncommon obstetric complication which may be associated with a high risk of fetal demise, if it is not recognized before rupture of membranes. In vasa previa, umbilical vessels traverse the membranes in the lower uterine segment in front of the fetal presenting part **(Fig. 8.6)**. Neither the umbilical cord nor the placenta supports the vessels. Due to the absence of Wharton's jelly, the vessels may be easily lacerated at the time the membranes rupture.

Also during uterine contractions, fetal vessels can get compressed resulting in fetal hypoxia and death. Some risk factors for vasa previa include bilobed and succenturiate placentas, low-lying placentas, multiple pregnancies, marginal insertion of the cord, velamentous insertion of the cord, etc. Vasa previa is an important cause for fetal mortality. The most important step for reducing blood loss from vasa previa is its prenatal diagnosis. Diagnosis of vasa previa can be made by ultrasound examination, particularly Doppler ultrasound **(Figs. 8.7A and B)**. Presently, there is no definite recommendation regarding the optimal time of delivery in these women. The patient is usually hospitalized at 30–32 weeks and is posted for an elective cesarean delivery at 35–36 weeks' gestation without confirmation of lung maturity by amniocentesis. This strategy helps in reducing the risk related to rupture of membranes before the onset of labor, which may occur in nearly 10% cases and is associated with a high mortality rate.

Patients with vasa previa present with painless vaginal bleeding at the time of spontaneous rupture of membranes or amniotomy. Since the bleeding occurs from fetal vessels, fetal shock, or demise can occur rapidly. When the membranes rupture, a small amount of continuous bright red bleeding occurs. The blood is from the fetal circulation and therefore, the fetus can bleed to death. If the cervix is almost fully dilated, the fetus can be delivered vaginally. If cervix is not completely dilated, an emergency cesarean section must be done to save the fetus. The presence of fetal blood can be confirmed by performing the Apt test. In this test, one drop of blood is added to nine drops of 1% sodium hydroxide in a glass test tube. The color of the test tube must be checked after 1 minute. If the blood is of fetal origin, the mixture remains pink. However, if the blood is of maternal origin, the mixture turns brown in color.

ANTEPARTUM HEMORRHAGE DUE TO PLACENTAL ABRUPTION

This is explained in detail in part 2 of this chapter.

EXTRAPLACENTAL CAUSES OF ANTEPARTUM HEMORRHAGE

Extraplacental causes of hemorrhage, including the presence of cervical polyps, erosion, varicosities, or carcinoma are usually rare and can be ruled out on the per speculum examination.

MANAGEMENT

Management comprising of investigations and definitive obstetric management is discussed below.

INVESTIGATIONS

ABO/RHESUS COMPATIBILITY

At least 4 units of blood need to be cross-matched and arranged. At any time, if severe hemorrhage occurs, the patient may require a blood transfusion.

IMAGING STUDIES

The main way of confirming the diagnosis of placenta previa is by imaging studies, especially ultrasonography. Placenta previa is diagnosed through ultrasound, either during a

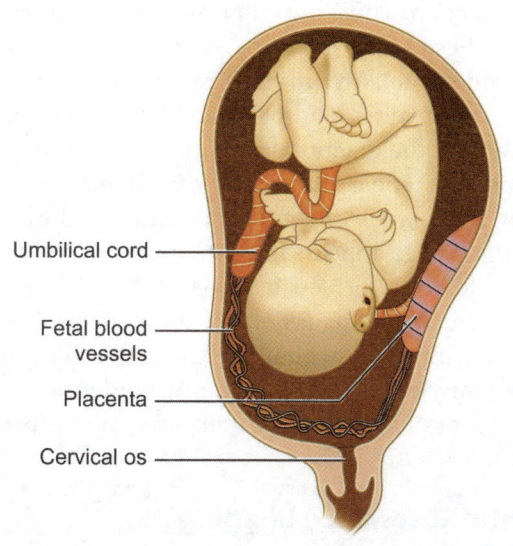

Fig. 8.6: Vasa previa.

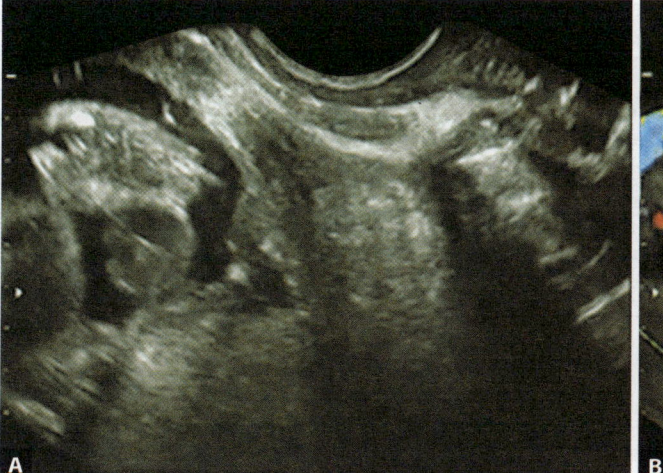
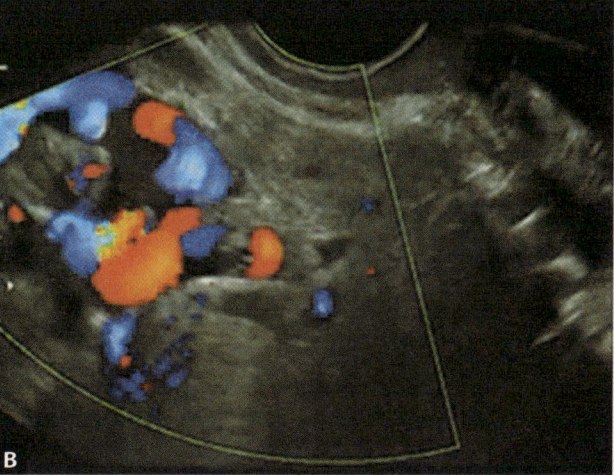

Figs. 8.7A and B: Diagnosis of vasa previa. (A) Transvaginal ultrasound; (B) Doppler ultrasound showing presence of fetal blood vessels in front of the fetal presenting part.

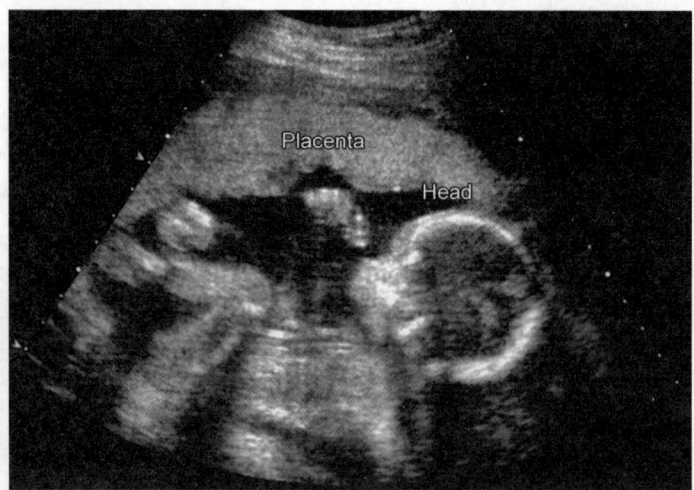

Fig. 8.8: Placental localization on transabdominal imaging.

routine prenatal appointment or following an episode of vaginal bleeding. Ultrasound examination can be of two types—transabdominal and transvaginal ultrasound.

Transabdominal Ultrasonography

Transabdominal sonography (TAS) helps in determining the placental position **(Fig. 8.8)**, fetal maturity, fetal well-being, fetal presentation, and presence of congenital anomalies. TAS is a simple, precise, and safe method of visualizing the placenta, having an accuracy rate of 93–98%

Some of the disadvantages of transabdominal ultrasound include poor visualization of the posterior placenta and influence of many factors on the accuracy of ultrasound examination. Some of the factors which can interfere with the visualization of the lower segment include patient obesity, underfilled or overfilled bladder, and skills of the operator.

Transvaginal Ultrasonography

According to the RCOG (2018), a transvaginal ultrasonography (TVS), if available, must be used to confirm the placental location at any time in pregnancy when the placenta is thought to be low-lying. TVS is considered to be significantly more accurate than TAS. Also, both the approaches, transperineal and transvaginal are considered to be largely safe.

On TVS examination, the actual distance from the placental edge to the margin of internal cervical os must be determined in millimeters. A placental edge exactly reaching the internal os is described as 0 mm.

As per the RCOG guidelines (2018), the terminology, "placenta previa" should be used only in cases where the placenta is present directly over the internal os. The term "low-lying placenta" should be used for pregnancies at >16 weeks of gestation when the placental edge is <20 mm from the internal os as visualized on TAS or TVS. If the diagnosis of placenta previa or low-lying placenta is made at the time of routine fetal anomaly scan, a follow-up ultrasound examination, preferably using a TVS is recommended at 32 weeks of gestation. This would help in establishing the diagnosis of persistent low-lying placenta and/or placenta previa. In these cases, who remain asymptomatic, an additional TVS is recommended at 36 weeks of gestation to help decide regarding the mode of delivery. In asymptomatic women with placenta previa, measurement of cervical length may also help in deciding the management plan. If cervical length on TVS before 34 weeks of gestation is short, this is likely to increase the risk of preterm emergency delivery as well as the risk of massive hemorrhage at the time of cesarean delivery.

The process of placental migration with increasing period of gestation does not occur due to placental movement, rather due to the growth of placenta towards the fundal regions getting a better blood supply in comparison to the lower uterine segment. This process is known as trophotropism. Placental migration, however, is unlikely if the placenta is posterior or if there has been a previous cesarean section. Thus, the clinician needs to remain more vigilant in these cases.

The individuals in whom a major placenta previa is suspected at the time of initial scan at 20–24 weeks, further clarification of the diagnosis is required earlier in gestation and therefore a repeat ultrasound scan should be conducted at around 28–32 weeks. If significant change in the position of the placental edge appears to be occurring over time, a final study should be performed at 36 weeks. The clinician should therefore avoid making a definitive diagnosis of placenta previa in asymptomatic patients before the third trimester, because many cases of placenta previa identified early in pregnancy would resolve on their own as the pregnancy advances.

Magnetic Resonance Imaging

Magnetic resonance imaging has been reported as a safe technique in the diagnosis of placenta previa when the images obtained by ultrasound (both TAS and TVS) have been unsatisfactory. MRI has the advantage of being possible without a full bladder and is not dependent on operator skills. It is also particularly useful in imaging posterior placentas. Since MRI is able to give information regarding myometrial invasion, it has been suggested as a safe and alternate method for determining the presence of placenta accreta. However, future large scale trials for determining the efficacy and safety of the use of MRI during pregnancy need to be performed in future.

Doppler Ultrasound

Antenatal imaging by color flow Doppler ultrasonography is especially useful in women with placenta previa who are at an increased risk of placenta accreta. Women with placenta previa having a previous history of uterine scar are at an increased risk of having a morbidly adherent placenta, especially when there has been a short cesarean to conception interval. Doppler ultrasound examination should be preferably done in such individuals.

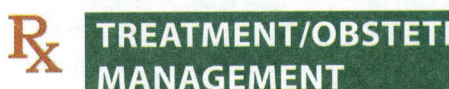
TREATMENT/OBSTETRIC MANAGEMENT

■ PREVENTION

Antenatal Period

There is no treatment available to change the position of the placenta. However, steps can be taken to reduce the development of hemorrhage and other related complications. Important measures, which can be taken in the antenatal period to reduce the complications resulting due to placenta previa include the following:

- *Early hospital admission of woman at risk:* The women at high risk of developing APH should be admitted to the hospital early in the third trimester. These particularly include those patients who have had previous histories of APH; those with high parity; those over the age of 35 years, etc.
- *Prevention of anemia:* It is an obvious fact that greater the degree of anemia, the lower would be the woman's ability to withstand hemorrhage. Therefore, prevention and treatment of anemia in the antenatal period helps in reducing the complications related to APH.
- *Prevention of placental abruption:* Preventive steps like early detection of preeclampsia; avoidance of trauma and avoidance of sudden uterine decompression, all of which can be associated with an increased risk of placental abruption, help in reducing the development of APH in relation to placental abruption.

Intrapartum Period

As previously described, cervical digital and rectal digital examination must never be performed in suspected cases of placenta previa, unless the woman is in the OT, with all the preparations in place for an emergency cesarean delivery. Even the gentlest of cervical examination can sometimes precipitate torrential vaginal bleeding, thereby necessitating an emergency cesarean delivery.

Also, once placenta previa is diagnosed, additional ultrasound examinations must be performed as the placental migration may often take place during the third trimester.

■ DEFINITIVE MANAGEMENT/TREATMENT

In order to decide the final treatment plan for patients with placenta previa, each of the factors described in **Box 8.1** need to be taken into consideration.

Evaluation of the amount of bleeding is an important step in the management of patients with placenta previa. There are no medicines to stop the bleeding but in many cases it stops on its own. Depending on the amount of bleeding present at the time of examination, the management options in a patient with placenta previa are shown in **Flowchart 8.2**.

> **BOX 8.1:** Factors to be considered before deciding the final treatment plan for patients with placenta previa.
> - Amount of vaginal bleeding
> - Whether bleeding has stopped or is continuing
> - Gestational age
> - Fetal condition
> - Maternal health and her preferences
> - Position of the placenta and baby
> - Clinical background
> - Findings on ultrasound (including the distance between the placental edge and the fetal head position relative to the leading edge of the placenta)

Management of Patients with Severe Bleeding

Patients with severe bleeding need to be carefully monitored in the hospital. These women must be transferred to tertiary care units as soon as possible. In cases of severe bleeding, the most important step in management is to stabilize the patient, arrange and cross-match at least four units of blood, and start blood transfusion if required. All efforts must be made to shift her to the OT as soon as possible for an emergency cesarean delivery. The following steps need to be taken:

- Rapid infusion through insertion of one or two large bore IV cannula and IV fluids like ringer lactate must be immediately started. Fluid warming devices should be immediately available.
- Monitoring of pulse, BP and amount of vaginal bleeding to be done at every half hour intervals.
- Input-output charting at hourly intervals
- If the bleeding is severe, a blood transfusion may be required in order to replace the lost blood.
- Once the patient has stabilized, the blood sample should be taken and sent for CBC, blood grouping, and cross-matching. At least four units of blood need to be arranged.
- Sedative analgesics like pethidine can be administered.
- Electronic fetal monitoring needs to be initiated.
- Rhesus (Rh) immunoglobulins must be administered, when appropriate, to Rh-negative, nonimmunized women.
- The definitive cause of the bleeding needs to be addressed after the maternal and fetal conditions have stabilized. If the definitive diagnosis of placenta previa is made and the period of gestation is ≥36 weeks of gestation, delivery is appropriate. In case, the bleeding is excessive or continuous or the fetal heart tracing is nonreassuring, the patient needs to be delivered irrespective of the period of gestation.
- Severe bleeding is usually due to a major degree of placenta previa. The definitive treatment in these cases would be delivery by cesarean section.

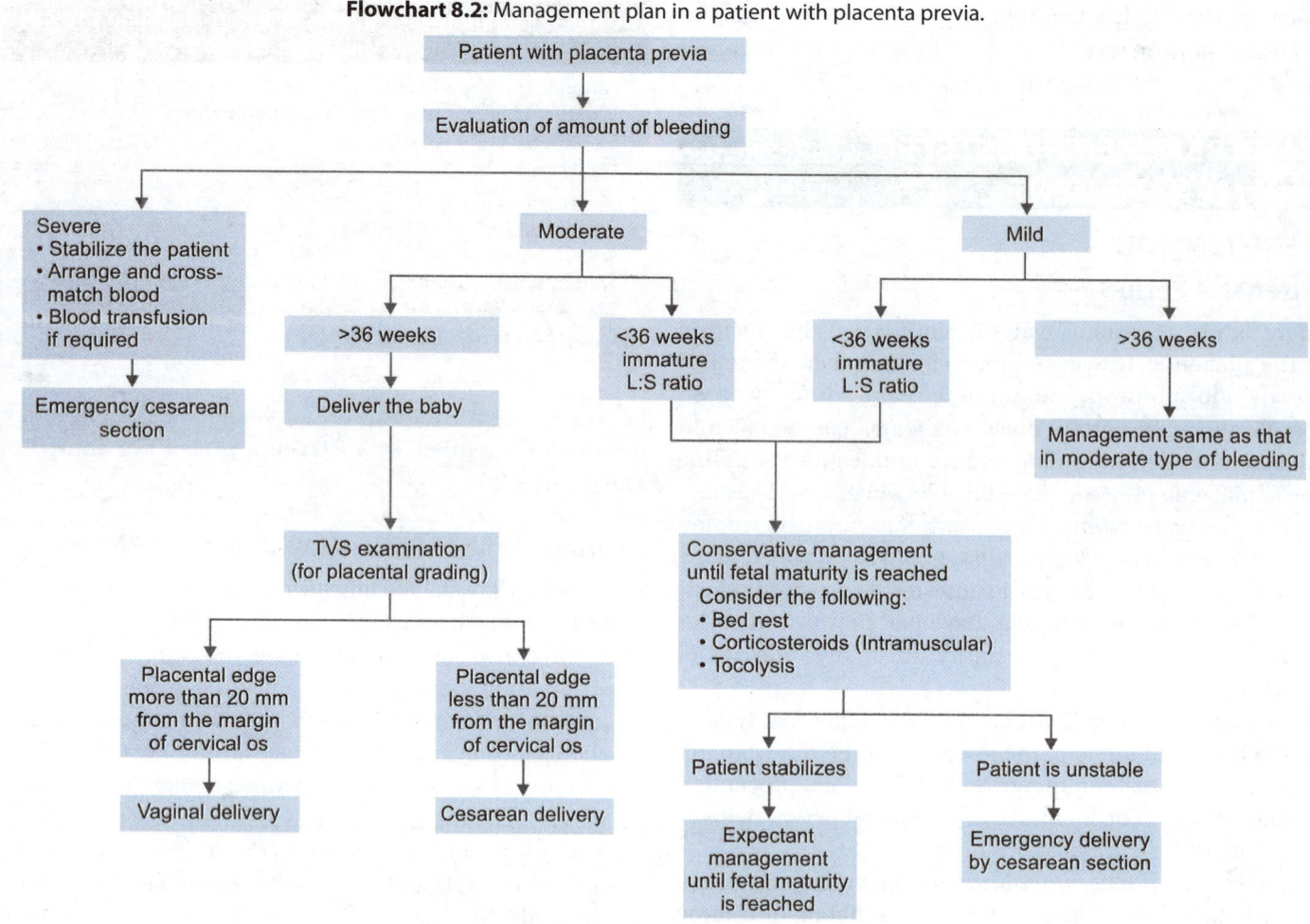

Flowchart 8.2: Management plan in a patient with placenta previa.

(L:S: lecithin:sphingomyelin; TVS: transvaginal sonography)

Management of Patients with Moderate Bleeding

- The initial five steps as mentioned in patients with severe bleeding must be applied at the same time using clinical discretion.
- The timing for delivery in these patients must be based upon the period of gestation as discussed here:

Period of Gestation ≥ 36 Weeks

If the period of gestation is 36 weeks or more, the women must be delivered by performing a cesarean section.

Period of Gestation is Between 32 and 36 Weeks

If the period of gestation is between 32 and 36 weeks, assessment of fetal lung maturity needs to be done using the lecithin-sphingomyelin (L:S) ratio.

The L:S ratio of ≥2 indicates fetal lung maturity, implying that the fetus can be delivered in these cases.

If L:S ratio is <2, the fetal lungs have yet not attained maturity. Intramuscular corticosteroid injection must be given to the mother. Until the complete dose of corticosteroids has been administered, the delivery should be preferably delayed.

During this waiting period, the patient must be kept under intensive monitoring. Though the role of tocolysis remains controversial, tocolytic agents such as β-mimetics and magnesium sulfate can be used to prevent uterine activity. If the patient remains stable for next 24–48 hours, she becomes a candidate for expectant management. If the patient does not remain stable for the next 24–48 hours, she must be delivered by a cesarean section.

Management of Patients with Mild Bleeding

Similar to the patients with moderate bleeding, in the patients with mild bleeding the management is based on period of gestation and fetal pulmonary maturity. Delivery of women presenting with uncomplicated placenta previa should be preferably considered between 36^{+0} and 37^{+0} weeks of gestation. If the period of gestation is <36 weeks or the fetal lungs are immature (i.e., L:S ratio is < 2), the woman becomes a candidate for expectant management. If the fetus has attained maturity, the women can be delivered. The mode of delivery depends upon the grade of placenta previa.

Expectant Management

The expectant management was introduced by Macafee and Johnson and is often also known as Macafee and Johnson's regime. The aim of expectant management is to delay pregnancy until the time fetal maturity is reached.

Prerequisites for Expectant Management

The prerequisites for expectant management are as follows:
- Stable maternal health (Hb > 10%)
- Period of gestation is <37 completed weeks.
- Fetal well-being is assured on ultrasound examination.
- No active bleeding is present.
- Facilities for emergency cesarean section are there, in case it is required.

Steps to be Taken

The expectant management includes the following steps:
- If there is little or minimal bleeding, the woman is advised to limit her physical activity and take bed rest. Bed rest helps in reducing pressure on the cervix, which may help in stopping preterm contractions or vaginal bleeding. Bed rest also helps in increasing blood flow to the placenta, thereby stimulating fetal growth.
- The women must be asked to avoid sexual intercourse, which can trigger vaginal bleeding by initiating contractions or causing direct trauma.
- The woman is also advised not to engage in any type of physical exercise as far as possible.
- The woman should be prescribed iron tablets throughout pregnancy in order to keep the blood hemoglobin levels within the normal range.
- A single course of antenatal corticosteroid therapy can be administered prior to 30^{+0} weeks of gestation or between 34^{+0} and 35^{+6} weeks of gestation
- Tocolysis may be considered for 48 hours to facilitate administration of antenatal corticosteroids. However, tocolysis should not be used for prolonging gestation especially if delivery is indicated based on maternal or fetal concerns.
- Placenta previa is likely to result in fetomaternal hemorrhage. Therefore, all Rh-negative women with placenta previa who bleed must be offered anti-D immunoglobulin injections to prevent the risk of Rh isoimmunization.
- Thromboprophylaxis may be offered to women, based on the risk factor assessment, to reduce the risk of thromboembolism.
- The use of prophylactic technique like cervical cerclage to help reduce the bleeding and prolong the duration of pregnancy is not backed up by sufficient evidence to recommend their routine use.

Hospitalization versus Outpatient Management in Placenta Previa

Once the patient presents to the hospital with an episode of bleeding, she should be observed in the hospital until she is free of bleeding for at least 48 hours. Following the initial period of observation, the expectant management plan can be carried out at home or in the hospital. The indications for hospitalization are described in **Box 8.2**. The major concern in caring for an asymptomatic woman with placenta previa major is that she might suddenly start bleeding heavily at any time, requiring urgent delivery. For this reason, hospitalization is recommended by RCOG during the latter part of the third trimester (commencing from 32–34 weeks) in women with major degrees of placenta previa, who previously had been stable.

Hospitalization is also advised as soon as she experiences heavy bleeding, including spotting, contractions, or vague suprapubic period-like pain, irrespective of the degree of placenta or the period of gestation. For heavy bleeding, bed rest in the hospital may be required, irrespective of the period of gestation. If the patient experiences reduced fetal movements, she must be admitted in the hospital for fetal monitoring and assessment.

If bleeding stops and the fetus has not attained maturity, hospital discharge and outpatient management may be allowed. Some criteria for outpatient management of women with placenta previa are described in **Box 8.3**. It should be made clear to all women, who are being managed

> **BOX 8.2:** Indications for hospitalization in women with placenta previa.
> - Hospitalization at 32–34 weeks is required for women with major degrees of placenta previa, who had been previously stable
> - Severe bleeding irrespective of the period of gestation
> - Patient perceives reduced fetal movements

> **BOX 8.3:** Criteria for outpatient management of women with placenta previa.
> - Woman is in stable condition (Hb > 10 g and hematocrit > 33%)
> - Patient has been observed in the hospital setting for a period of 48–72 hours during which the maternal and fetal conditions were stable.
> - Nonstress test was reactive at the time of discharge
> - No active bleeding
> - Patient willing to take bed rest at home
> - Fetus has not attained maturity
> - Close proximity with the hospital and facilities for transportation to the hospital available, 24 hours all 7 days of the week
> - Constant presence of a companion
> - Telephone communication with the hospital
> - Patient is willing to come for weekly check-ups until the time of delivery
> - Patient has shown acceptance for receiving donor blood or blood products

at home that they must attend hospital immediately if they experience any bleeding, contractions, or pain. They must be advised to report to the hospital even if they experience vague suprapubic aches, similar to that experienced at the time of periods. The women who are being managed at home should have support of a partner or a carer who would bring her to the hospital in case of emergency. The woman's residence must not be too far away from the hospital and she should have facilities of communicating with the hospital through a telephone.

Mode of Delivery

Cesarean delivery is necessary for most cases of placenta previa, especially the major degree placenta previa including type II (posterior), type III, and type IV. Severe blood loss may require a blood transfusion. Prior to delivery, the obstetrician needs to have detailed antenatal discussions with the woman and her partner, regarding the need for cesarean delivery, possibility of hemorrhage, possible blood transfusion, and requirement for major surgical interventions, such as hysterectomy.

Regional anesthesia may be employed for cesarean section in the presence of placenta previa. Delivery of the women with placenta previa must be conducted by the most experienced obstetrician and anesthetist on duty; preferably a consultant obstetrician and anesthetist should be present within the delivery suite. In case of an emergency, the senior obstetrician and senior anesthetist should be alerted immediately and attend urgently. A junior doctor under training should not be left unsupervised while caring for the women with placenta previa.

Indications for Emergency Delivery

Indications for immediate delivery by an emergency cesarean section irrespective of the period of gestation or degree of placenta previa are listed in **Box 8.4**. Some of the steps that can be taken at the time of cesarean section to reduce the chances of bleeding are described in **Box 8.5**. Detailed description of all these techniques has been done in Chapter 13. If all conservative measures mentioned in **Box 8.5** fail and the patient continues to bleed, the obstetrician may have no other alternative left, but to resort to cesarean hysterectomy in order to save the mother's life.

- Cesarean delivery must be undertaken by a senior team of obstetricians because there is a risk of substantial intraoperative hemorrhage.
- Regional anesthesia is usually used in these cases because it is considered safe and is likely to be associated with lower risks of hemorrhage in comparison to general anesthesia. The woman needs to be counseled that it may be necessary to convert to general anesthesia if required and she may be asked to give consent.

BOX 8.4: Indications for an emergency cesarean section.
- Bleeding is heavy
- Bleeding is uncontrolled
- Major degree placenta previa (type II posterior, type III, and type IV)
- Fetal distress
- Obstetric factors like cephalopelvic disproportion, fetal malpresentation, etc.

BOX 8.5: Steps to be taken to control bleeding at the time of cesarean section.
- Use of uterotonic agents to reduce the blood loss
- CHO sutures
- B-lynch sutures
- Bilateral uterine artery or internal iliac artery ligation
- Intrauterine packing
- Hydrostatic balloon catheterization
- Aortic compression
- Pelvic artery embolization

- Preoperative and/or intraoperative ultrasonography can be considered to accurately determine placental location and the optimal place for giving the uterine incision. In most cases, a lower uterine segment incision is appropriate. If the fetus is in transverse lie or is premature, a vertical skin and/or uterine incision can sometimes be given. If the placenta is present anteriorly or it is transected at the time of uterine incision, the surgeon may be required to immediately clamp the umbilical cord to prevent excessive blood loss caused by interruption of the placenta at the time of entry.
- The surgeon must also be prepared to deal with PPH, which may occur due to atony at the placental implantation site. If pharmacological measures are unable to control the hemorrhage at the time of surgery, the obstetrician must initiate intrauterine tamponade and/or surgical hemostatic techniques sooner rather than later. Interventional radiological techniques should also be urgently employed where required. The obstetrician may have to resort to hysterectomy in cases where conservative medical and surgical interventions prove ineffective.

COMPLICATIONS

MATERNAL

Bleeding

One of the biggest concerns with placenta previa is the risk of severe vaginal bleeding (hemorrhage) during labor, delivery, or the first few hours after delivery. The bleeding can be heavy enough to cause maternal shock or even death, necessitating the requirement for a hysterectomy. Therefore, delivery should be arranged in a maternity unit having access to the on-site blood transfusion services and critical care.

Such cases are also at an increased risk of PPH because the placenta is implanted in the lower uterine segment which, normally does not have the same ability as the upper segment to contract and retract after delivery. Due to this, the chances of bleeding following the delivery of the baby are increased. Therefore, measures must be taken in advance to prevent the occurrence of PPH.

Placenta Accreta, Increta, and Percreta

> Q. Briefly discuss about adherent placenta.
>
> Q. Write a long essay on placenta accreta.
>
> Q. Write a short note discussing the management options for placenta accreta.

Pathological adherence of the placenta is termed as invasive or adherent placenta. In this condition, the trophoblastic invasion occurs beyond the normal boundary established by the Nitabuch's fibrinoid layer. While the term "accreta" refers to abnormal attachment of the placenta to the uterine surface, the terms "increta" and "percreta" refer to much deeper invasion of the placental villi into the uterine musculature **(Figs. 8.9 and 8.10)**. Abnormally adherent placenta can result in severe bleeding and, may often require cesarean hysterectomy **(Fig. 8.11)**. In placenta increta, the invasion by the placental villi is limited to approximately half the myometrial thickness. On the other hand, in cases of placenta percreta, there is through and through invasion of the uterine wall. The diagnosis of placental invasion can be made by ultrasound examination, both transabdominal and Doppler ultrasound **(Figs. 8.12 and 8.13)**. MRI also serves as a useful investigation **(Figs. 8.14 and 8.15)**. It proves useful in cases of posterior placenta and in the assessment of myometrial, parametrial, and bladder involvement. It is important to diagnose this condition prior to delivery because of the risk of massive intraoperative hemorrhage. In fact, placenta accreta has been reported as an important cause of emergency peripartum hysterectomy.

History of placenta accreta in a previous pregnancy, previous history of a lower-segment cesarean section or any other uterine surgery, including repeated endometrial curettage are typically associated with an increased risk for placenta previa in the future pregnancies. The risk increases with an increase in the number of previous cesarean deliveries. Though the exact mechanism behind the association of placenta previa with previous scar is poorly

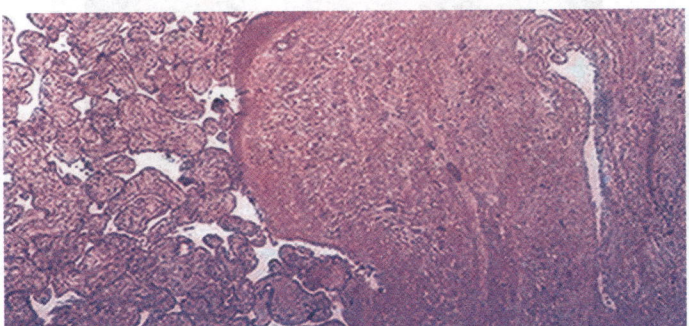

Fig. 8.10: Histological specimen showing placenta increta.

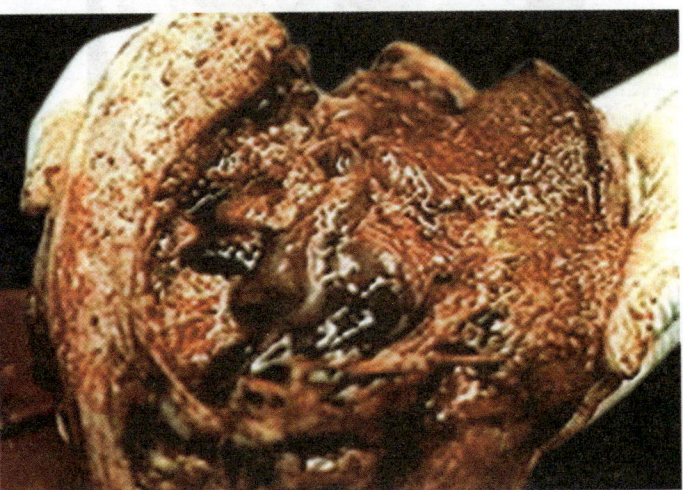

Fig. 8.11: Hysterectomy specimen showing placental invasion of myometrium.

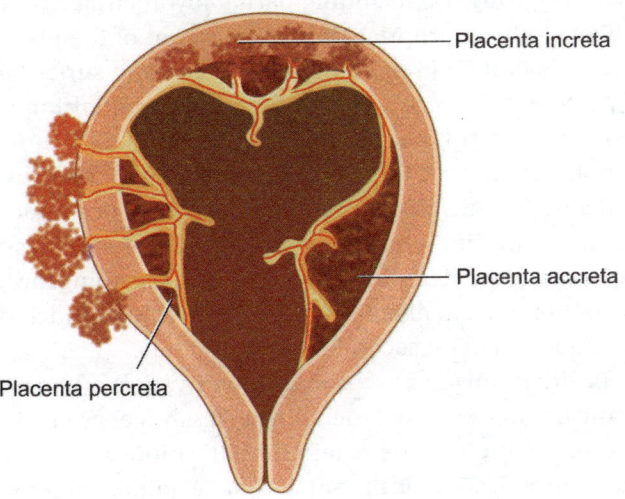

Fig. 8.9: Abnormally adherent placenta.

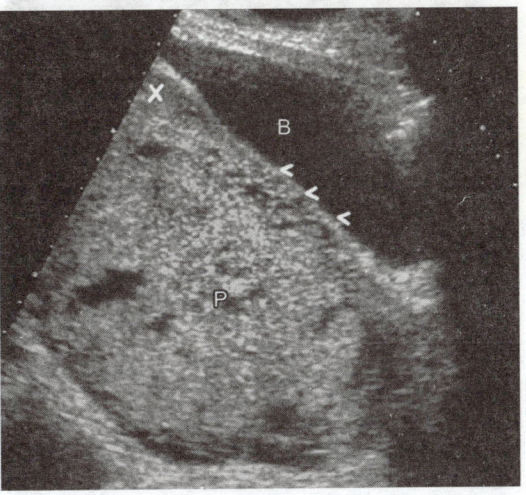

Fig. 8.12: Abdominal sonography at 27 weeks' gestation showing a morbidly adhering placenta. (B: bladder; P: placenta)

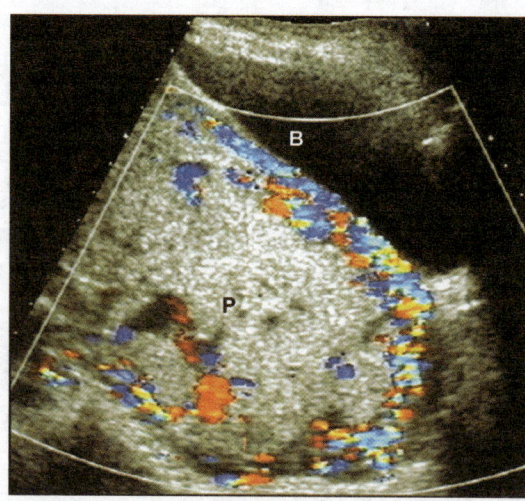

Fig. 8.13: Color Doppler scanning at 27 weeks' gestation in a case of placenta percreta demonstrating prominent placental vessels extending across the myometrium into the bladder wall. (B: bladder; P: placenta)

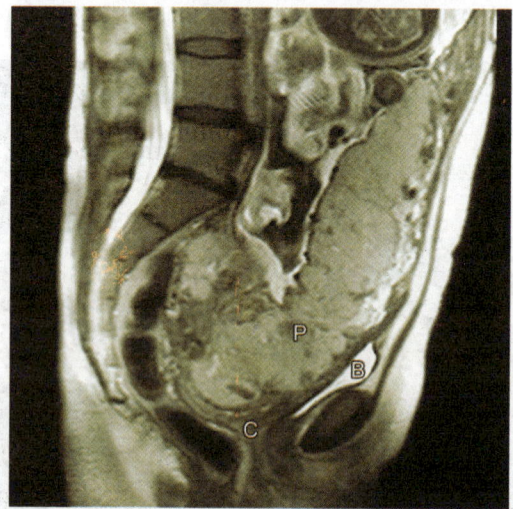

Fig. 8.14: Magnetic resonance imaging of the patient with placenta percreta at 27 weeks of gestation. (B: bladder; C: cervix; P: placenta)

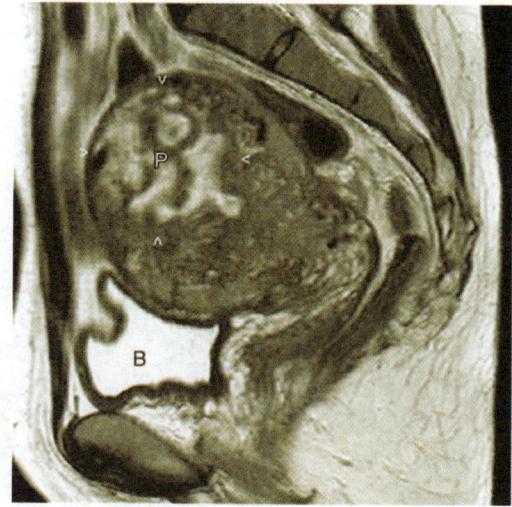

Fig. 8.15: Magnetic resonance imaging of placenta increta at 10 days postpartum. (B: bladder; P: placenta)

understood, it may be due to reduced differential growth of the lower segment resulting in reduced upward shift in placental position with increasing gestation. Presence of placenta previa in association with the previous history of lower uterine scar is typically associated with adherent placentas.

Diagnosis

Diagnosis of placenta accreta spectrum in the antenatal period is important for planning its management. This is likely to reduce maternal morbidity and mortality.

Ultrasound imaging using color Doppler is a highly accurate investigation for establishing the diagnosis of placenta accreta spectrum. However, it should be performed by a skilled operator having the required experience in diagnosing placenta accreta spectrum. If an obstetrician detects any features suggestive of placenta accreta spectrum on ultrasound examination, the woman must be referred to a specialist unit having imaging expertise. Both MRI and ultrasound imaging are likely to have a similar diagnostic ability in detecting placenta accreta spectrum when performed by experts. MRI may be used to complement ultrasound imaging for assessing the depth of myometrial invasion and lateral extension of placental tissue into the myometrium, especially in cases with posterior placentation and/or in women where ultrasound is suggestive of parametrial invasion.

Management

The most commonly used therapeutic option for management of cases with placenta accreta comprises conservative/expectant management, which involves leaving the placenta in situ with preservation of the uterus. Such cases must be regularly reviewed using clinical and ultrasound examination. These women should also have an easy access to emergency care in case they experience complications, such as bleeding or infection. Uterus preserving surgery, including partial myometrial resection is likely to be appropriate when the extent of the placenta accreta is limited in relation to the depth and surface area of placental invasion. Also, the entire placental implantation area must be accessible and visible (i.e., it must be completely anterior, fundal, or posterior) and there must be no deep pelvic invasion. There is limited evidence regarding the use of uterine preserving surgery in cases of placenta percreta and women should be counseled regarding the high risk of peripartum and secondary complications, including the requirement for secondary hysterectomy.

Besides conservative management varied other therapeutic options are used including cell salvage, prophylactic or therapeutic uterine artery embolization, and internal iliac artery ligation at the same time as initial surgery and intramuscular methotrexate injections following delivery of the baby. Use of methotrexate adjuvant therapy for expectant management is presently not indicated because it is associated with unproven benefit and significant adverse effects.

Hysterectomy may sometimes be required in cases with conservative management as a result of delayed hemorrhage. Moreover, sometimes cesarean section hysterectomy with the placenta left in situ is preferable to attempting to separate it from the uterine wall.

When placenta accreta is anticipated, consultant anesthetic and consultant obstetrician need to discuss the plan of delivery. In the absence of risk factors for preterm delivery, delivery should be preferably planned at 35^{+0}–36^{+6} weeks of gestation to achieve the best balance between fetal maturity and the risk of unscheduled delivery.

The consent for cesarean hysterectomy must be taken well in advance. She should be also informed about the specific risks of placenta accreta spectrum including the risks of complications such as massive obstetric hemorrhage, risk of damage to the lower urinary tract, requirement for blood transfusion, etc. Delivery should involve specialized multidisciplinary personnel and should occur in settings having facilities for high-volume blood transfusion, and both adult and neonatal intensive care units.

Anemia and Infection

Excessive blood loss can result in anemia and increased susceptibility to infections.

FETAL

Placenta previa can be commonly associated with neonatal complications such as fetal growth impairment, neurodevelopmental delay, sudden infant death syndrome (SIDS), and iatrogenic prematurity.

Premature Birth

Severe bleeding may force the obstetrician to proceed with an emergency preterm cesarean delivery.

Fetal Death or Fetal Distress

Though chances of fetal distress and fetal death are much less in cases with placenta previa in comparison to that in cases with placental abruption, severe maternal bleeding in cases with placenta previa is sometimes also responsible for producing fetal distress.

PART 2: PLACENTAL ABRUPTION

CASE STUDY

A G4P3L2 patient, who is 32 weeks pregnant, presents with a history of severe vaginal bleeding and abdominal pain. The blood contains dark-colored clots. Since the hemorrhage, the patient has also been complaining of reduced fetal movements. The patient's BP is 80/60 mm Hg and the pulse rate is 120 beats per minute.

INTRODUCTION

DEFINITION

Placental abruption can be defined as abnormal, pathological separation of the normally situated placenta from its uterine attachment **(Figs. 8.16A and B)**. As a result, bleeding occurs from the opened sinuses present in the uterine myometrium. "Abruptio placentae" is a Latin word meaning, "rending asunder of placenta", which denotes a sudden accident. Thus, placental abruption is also known as accidental hemorrhage. Pathophysiology of bleeding related to placental abruption is shown in

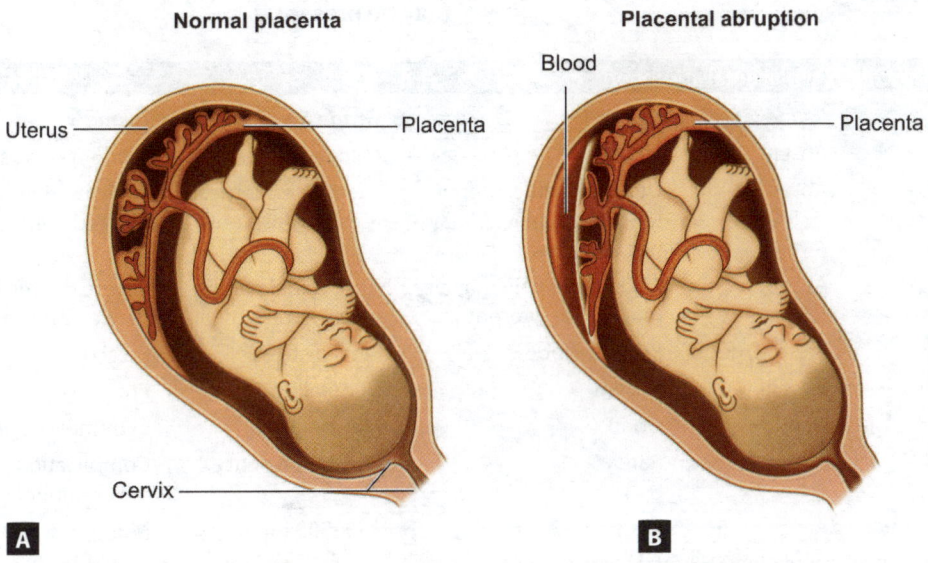

Figs. 8.16A and B: Placental abruption and its comparison with normal placenta.

the **Flowchart 8.3**. Separation of the normally situated placenta results in hemorrhage into the decidua basalis. A retroplacental clot develops between the placenta and the decidua basalis, which interferes with the supply of oxygen to the fetus. As a result, fetal distress can develop.

CLINICAL CLASSIFICATION OF PLACENTAL ABRUPTION

Clinical classification of placental abruption based on degree of disease severity is shown in **Table 8.1**.

Depending on the severity of clinical features, the placental abruption could be of the following types:

Grade 0

No obvious clinical features are present. Diagnosis is made after the inspection of placenta following the delivery of the baby. Sometimes placental abruption is not diagnosed until after delivery, when an area of clotted blood may be found behind the placenta.

Grade 1 (Mild)

There may be slight external bleeding. Uterus may be irritable; uterine tenderness and abdominal pain may or may not be present. FHS is good and shock is absent (no signs of low BP in the mother). The perinatal outcome is usually favorable and volume of retroplacental clot is usually <200 mL.

Grade 2 (Moderate)

In this type of placental abruption, the external bleeding is mild-to-moderate in amount. The uterus is tender and the abdominal pain is often present. Maternal shock is absent; the patient may have tachycardia but does not have signs of hypovolemia. FHS may be present or absent and often there are signs of fetal distress. The perinatal outcome may or may not be favorable and fetal death often occurs. The volume of retroplacental clot may vary from 150–500 mL.

Grade 3 (Severe)

This type of placental abruption is associated with moderate to severe amount of revealed bleeding or concealed (hidden) bleeding. In this condition, more than half of the placenta separates and the volume of retroplacental clot is often > 500 mL. Retroplacental clot volume >2.5 L is usually sufficient to cause fetal death. Tonic uterine contractions (called tetany), abdominal pain, and marked uterine tenderness may be present. The abdominal pain is very severe. On examination, the uterus is tender and rigid; it may be impossible to feel the fetus. Maternal shock is pronounced and the BP may become extremely low. Fetal death commonly occurs. Complications related to severe disease like coagulation failure or anuria may be present.

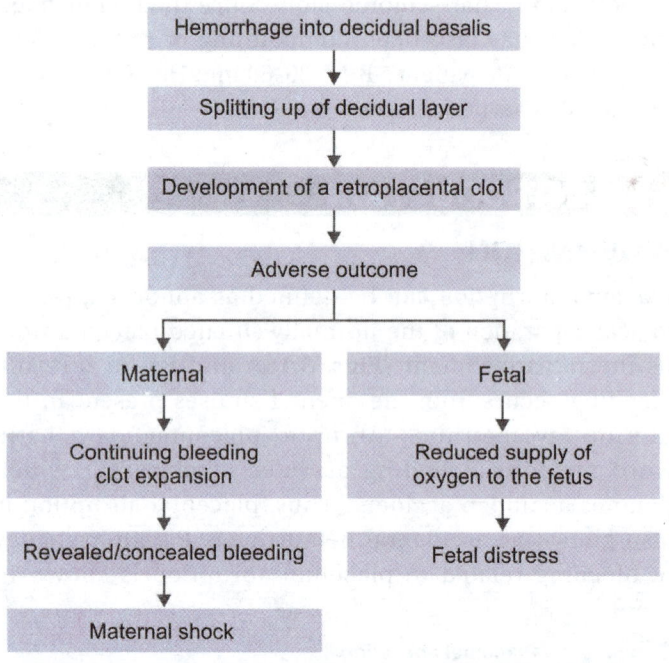

Flowchart 8.3: Pathophysiology of placental abruption.

TABLE 8.1: Clinical classification of placental abruption.				
Parameter	*Grade 0*	*Grade 1*	*Grade 2*	*Grade 3*
External bleeding	Absent	Slight	Mild to moderate	Moderate to severe
Uterine tenderness	Absent	Uterus irritable, uterine tenderness may or may not be present	Uterine tenderness is usually present	Tonic uterine contractions and marked uterine tenderness
Abdominal pain	Absent	Abdominal pain may or may not be present	Abdominal pain is usually present	Severe degree of abdominal pain may be present
FHS	Present, good	Present, good	Fetal distress	Fetal death
Maternal shock	Absent	Absent	Generally absent	Present
Perinatal outcome	Good	Good	May be poor	Extremely poor
Complications	Absent	Rare	May be present	Complications like DIC and oliguria are commonly present
Volume of retroplacental clot	–	Less than 200 mL	150–500 mL	More than 500 mL

(DIC: disseminated intravascular coagulation; FHS: fetal heart sound)

Antepartum Hemorrhage

TYPES OF PLACENTAL ABRUPTION

Based on the type of clinical presentation, there can be three types of placental abruption:

1. *Concealed type* (**Fig. 8.17**): In this type of placental abruption, no actual bleeding is visible. The blood collects between the fetal membranes and decidua in form of the retroplacental clot. Though this type of placental abruption is usually rarer than the revealed type, it carries a higher risk of maternal and fetal hazards because of the possibility of consumptive coagulopathy, which can result in the development of disseminated intravascular coagulation (DIC).
2. *Revealed type* (**Fig. 8.18**): In this type of placental abruption, following placental separation, the blood does not collect between the fetal membranes and decidua but moves out of the cervical canal and is visible externally. This type of placental abruption is more common than the concealed variety.
3. *Mixed type:* This is the most common type of placental abruption and is associated with both revealed and concealed hemorrhage.

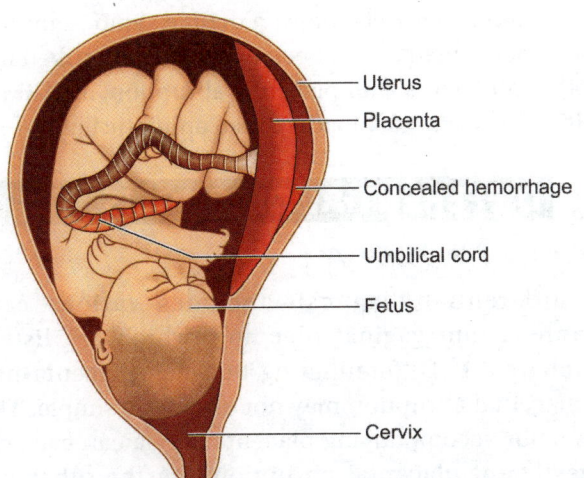

Fig. 8.17: Concealed type of placental abruption.

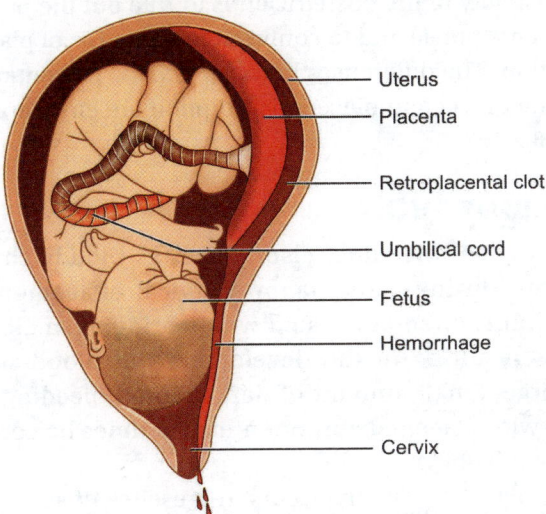

Fig. 8.18: Revealed type of placental abruption.

HISTORY AND CLINICAL PRESENTATION

CLINICAL PRESENTATION

The clinical features depend upon the degree of placental separation and the speed at which the separation occurs and whether it remains concealed or revealed. The clinical evidence of abruption may sometimes appear 24 hours or more after trauma. Therefore, asymptomatic women giving history of trauma or road traffic accident must be observed at least for 6 hours prior to discharge, while those who give a history of bleeding or uterine contractions must be observed for at least 24 hours.

Signs and symptoms of placental abruption are described next.

Vaginal Bleeding

The most common symptom of placental abruption is dark red vaginal bleeding with pain, usually occurring after 28 weeks of gestation. It can also occur during labor. The amount of vaginal bleeding can vary greatly. Bleeding in placental abruption is mainly of maternal origin. The amount of bleeding may not be proportional to the amount of placental separation as in many cases the bleeding may be concealed.

Abdominal Pain

Abdominal and back pain often begins suddenly. Uterine tenderness may be present. There may be tonic uterine contractions in which there are rapid uterine contractions, coming one after another, without any intervening period of relaxation.

Some women may experience slightly different symptoms including, fainting and collapse, nausea, thirst, reduced fetal movements, etc.

If the placenta is present posteriorly, the women may experience severe backache. This pain may further worsen on abdominal palpation because palpation further pushes the fetus against the placenta.

Signs of Hemodynamic Compromise

Hemodynamic compromise may be present in cases of severe placental abruption especially in cases of concealed hemorrhage. Anemia and oliguria may also be sometimes present.

RISK FACTORS

The specific cause of placental abruption is often unknown. Some of the commonly associated risk factors which need to be elicited at the time of history include the following:

- *Trauma or injury to the abdomen:* Injury resulting due to a motor vehicle accident or fall is a common cause for placental abruption. Rarely, placental abruption may be caused by an unusually short umbilical cord or sudden

uterine decompression (as in cases of polyhydramnios) which may cause sudden placental detachment.
- *Increased age and parity:* Increased maternal age (>40 years) and parity (>4) are commonly associated with an increased risk of placental abruption.
- *Previous history of placental abruption:* If the woman has a history of experiencing placental abruption in past, she is at a high risk of experiencing the same condition during her present pregnancy as well. As the number of previously affected pregnancies increase, the risk further increases, with the risk of recurrence increasing to 25% with previous two affected pregnancies.
- *High BP associated with preeclampsia and chronic hypertension:* High BP increases the risk of placental abruption. The Magpie trial has demonstrated that use of magnesium sulfate in women with severe preeclampsia is associated with reduced incidence of placental abruption.
- *Blood clotting disorders:* Blood clotting disorders, e.g., thrombophilias (both inherited and acquired) may also act as risk factors.
- *Multifetal gestation:* Carrying multiple fetuses including twins, triplets, etc., increases the woman's risk of developing placental abruption.
- *Hydramnios:* The women with polyhydramnios are associated with an increased risk of placental abruption.
- *Substance abuse especially cocaine abuse:* Placental abruption is more common in women who smoke, drink alcohol, or abuse drugs like cocaine or methamphetamine during pregnancy.
- *Preterm rupture of membranes:* Sudden preterm rupture of membranes is likely to cause placental separation resulting in placental abruption.
- *Presence of uterine leiomyomas:* Presence of uterine leiomyomas especially at the site of placental implantation is supposed to be associated with an increased incidence of placental abruption.

GENERAL PHYSICAL EXAMINATION

- Most important sign of placental abruption is vaginal bleeding and abdominal and back pain.
- The patient may be in shock (tachycardia and low BP).
- There may be signs and symptoms suggestive of preeclampsia (increased BP, proteinuria, etc.)
- Often the patient's clinical condition is disproportionate to the amount of blood loss, especially in cases of concealed hemorrhage.

SPECIFIC SYSTEMIC EXAMINATION

ABDOMINAL EXAMINATION

- *Uterine hypertonicity and uterine contractions:* Uterine hypertonicity and frequent uterine contractions are commonly present. It may be difficult to feel the fetal parts due to presence of uterine hypertonicity. Uterine rigidity may become apparent on abdominal palpation. The uterus may either be tense and tender upon palpation or it may feel doughy or woody hard due to persistent hypertonus.
- *Severe back ache:* If abruption occurs in a posteriorly located placenta, there may be severe back pain.
- *Absent or slow FHS:* Severe degree of placental abruption may be associated with fetal bradycardia and other fetal heart rate abnormalities. In extreme cases, fetal demise may even be detected at the time of examination. Fetal bradycardia and intrauterine death are relatively less common in cases of placenta previa.

VAGINAL EXAMINATION

Though presence of placental abruption is not a contraindication for vaginal examination, vaginal examination should ideally not be performed in patients with history of APH due to the risk of placenta previa. If the cause of APH turns out to be placenta previa rather than placental abruption, performance of a vaginal examination can provoke an episode of torrential bleeding. In case, vaginal examination needs to be done, a double setup examination must be performed as has been previously described in this chapter. In patients with placental abruption, an ARM may result in the release of blood-stained amniotic fluid.

DIFFERENTIAL DIAGNOSIS

PLACENTA PREVIA

The differential diagnosis includes various causes for antepartum vaginal bleeding, which are listed in **Flowchart 8.1**. Differentiating between placenta previa and placental abruption may not always be simple. This is so as labor accompanying placenta previa can cause pain suggestive of placental abruption. On the other hand, placental abruption may mimic normal labor. Thus, the main responsibility of the obstetrician is to rule out the presence of placenta previa and to confirm the diagnosis of placental abruption. The differences between clinical presentation of placenta previa and placental abruption are enumerated in **Table 8.2**.

BLOODY SHOW

Slight vaginal bleeding, also known as bloody show, is common during active labor. Cervical effacement and dilatation is often associated with tearing of small blood vessels resulting in the development of blood-stained discharge. Small amount of dark-colored bleeding associated with placental abruption may at times be confused with bloody show.

Bloody show usually occurs in presence of active labor and is not associated with uterine tenderness and rigidity.

Antepartum Hemorrhage

TABLE 8.2: Difference between placenta previa and placental abruption.

Parameter	Placenta previa	Placental abruption
Characteristics of bleeding		
Nature of bleeding	Painless, causeless, and recurrent episodes of bleeding	Bleeding is associated with abdominal pain and is usually related to some cause such as trauma or preeclampsia
Color of blood	Blood is bright red in color	Blood is dark colored
Amount of blood loss	Profuse, may be preceded by small amounts of warning hemorrhages	Blood loss may vary from slight in amount to large. In cases of concealed hemorrhages, the blood loss may be disproportionately low in relation to the woman's general physical condition (pallor, shock, etc.)
Abdominal examination		
Fundal height	Fundal height is proportionate to the period of gestation	Uterus may be disproportionately enlarged in cases of concealed hemorrhage
Feel of the uterus	Uterus is soft and relaxed	Uterus is usually tense, tender and rigid
Fetal presentation	Fetal malpresentation is commonly present	Fetal malpresentation is not related to the etiology of placental abruption
Engagement of fetal presenting part	The fetal presenting part remains high up; the engagement of the presenting part does not take place	The fetal presenting part commonly gets engaged
Fetal heart sound	FHS is usually present and is within the normal limits	Fetal bradycardia related to fetal distress may commonly be present
Investigations		
Ultrasound examination	Placenta is present in the lower uterine segment	Normal placental location
Coagulation profile	Usually not affected	May be altered in severe cases of placental abruption associated with DIC

(DIC: disseminated intravascular coagulation; FHS: fetal heart sound)

BOX 8.6: Differential diagnosis for abdominal pain in later half of pregnancy.

- Preterm labor/premature contractions
- Imminent eclampsia right upper quadrant tenderness/epigastric pain
- Chorioamnionitis
- Urinary tract infection
- Red degeneration of fibroids
- Other surgical/medical illness

Also, show has a mucoid character in which the mucus is mixed with blood.

Other differential diagnoses for abdominal pain in later half of pregnancy have been tabulated in **Box 8.6**.

MANAGEMENT

Management comprising of investigations and definitive obstetric management is discussed below.

INVESTIGATIONS

The diagnosis of placental abruption is usually made on history and clinical examination. Ultrasound examination must be performed in order to confirm the diagnosis.

ULTRASOUND EXAMINATION

Ultrasonography examination helps in showing the following details:

- Ultrasound examination may help in showing the location of the placenta and thus would help in establishing or ruling out the diagnosis of placenta previa because many a times it may become clinically impossible to differentiate between placenta previa and placental abruption.
  Therefore, the main use of ultrasound examination is to rule out placenta previa as a cause of hemorrhage.
- Ultrasound examination also helps in visualization of retroplacental clot, which may appear as a sonolucent area **(Fig. 8.19)**, thereby confirming the diagnosis of placental abruption. Blood or collection of blood and clots may be identified on ultrasound examination. There may be presence of "Jello sign". This implies that there may be jiggling of the intrauterine clots when bounced by the transducer.
- Ultrasound also helps in checking the fetal viability and presentation.
- Ultrasound examination is especially important in cases of placental abruption as it may become extremely difficult to palpate the fetal parts due to uterine hypertonicity. Also, it is important to record the fetal

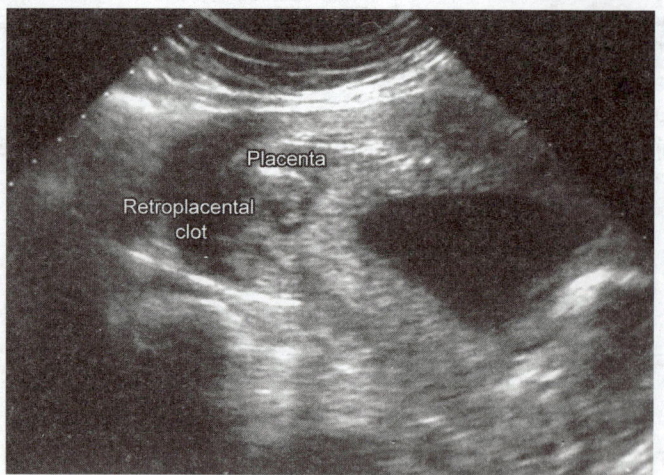

Fig. 8.19: Ultrasound examination in case of placental abruption showing presence of a retroplacental clot.

heart rate as the fetus is quite likely to be at jeopardy in the severe cases of placental abruption.
- In case no blood is retained inside the uterine cavity, there may be no specific sonographic findings. Negative findings with ultrasound examination, therefore, do not exclude placental abruption. There may be no retroplacental collection in revealed type of placental abruption.

CARDIOTOCOGRAPHIC EXAMINATION

Cardiotocography forms an integral component of evaluation of such cases. A variety of abnormalities may be observed on cardiotocographic examination such as variable and late decelerations, poor variability, prolonged bradycardia, sinusoidal pattern, etc. These findings may be indicative of fetal asphyxia.

 ## TREATMENT/OBSTETRIC MANAGEMENT

> **Q.** What should be the initial steps for management in the case study mentioned in the beginning of this topic?
>
> **Q.** How will you diagnose a case of concealed accidental hemorrhage? What are the complications associated with it and how would you about with the management of such a case. Discuss in detail.
>
> **Q.** What are the various causes of APH? Discuss the management of abruptio placentae at 36 weeks of gestation.
>
> **Q.** A 28-year-old primi patient with the history of fall a day back presents with a pregnancy of 8 months duration. She is experiencing pain in the abdomen, vaginal bleeding and absent fetal movements. On examination, FHS is absent. Discuss the diagnosis and management of such a case.
>
> **Q.** A 32-year-old primigravida patient at term presented to the A&E after having a fall on her abdomen. On ultrasound examination, a retroplacental clot was observed and placenta was located posteriorly in the upper uterine segment. Cardiotocography trace showed nonreassuring fetal heart trace. What would be the next step in management in this case?

PREVENTION

Once placental detachment has occurred, there is no treatment to replace the placenta back to its original position. However, some of the following steps can be taken to help reduce its occurrence:
- Early detection and treatment of preeclampsia
- Avoidance of smoking, drinking alcohol, or using illicit drugs during pregnancy
- Avoidance of trauma
- Avoidance of sudden uterine decompression.

The obstetrician needs to remain more vigilant during the antenatal period in the cases associated with high-risk factors for development of placental abruption.

DEFINITIVE TREATMENT

The treatment plan for the patient with placental abruption is shown in **Flowchart 8.4**.

The management plan depends on grade of placental abruption (extent and severity of the disease process) and fetal maturity. Other factors which need to be considered before deciding the specific treatment for placental abruption include maternal condition, amount of maternal bleeding, and fetal condition.

MILD PLACENTAL ABRUPTION

In cases with mild abruption, where fetal maturity has yet not been attained, expectant management can be undertaken until the fetus attains maturity. If at any time severe bleeding occurs; fetal distress appears or maternal condition worsens, an emergency cesarean delivery may be required.

MODERATE PLACENTAL ABRUPTION

A moderate case of placental abruption requires hospitalization and constant fetal monitoring. The expectant management can be continued if the mother remains stable.

In case the maternal condition deteriorates or fetal distress develops, an emergency cesarean delivery may be required. If the uterus remains soft, the pregnancy must be terminated by induction of labor by ARM and oxytocin infusion. Amniotomy helps in the escape of fluid, which might help in reducing the amount of bleeding from the implantation site. It also helps in reducing the entry of thromboplastin into the maternal circulation, thereby preventing the development of DIC. If during labor, the FHR becomes nonreassuring or if the uterus becomes hypertonic, an emergency cesarean section is usually required.

SEVERE PLACENTAL ABRUPTION

If the women presents with severe placental abruption, the following steps need to be urgently undertaken:
- The patient requires an urgent admission to the hospital

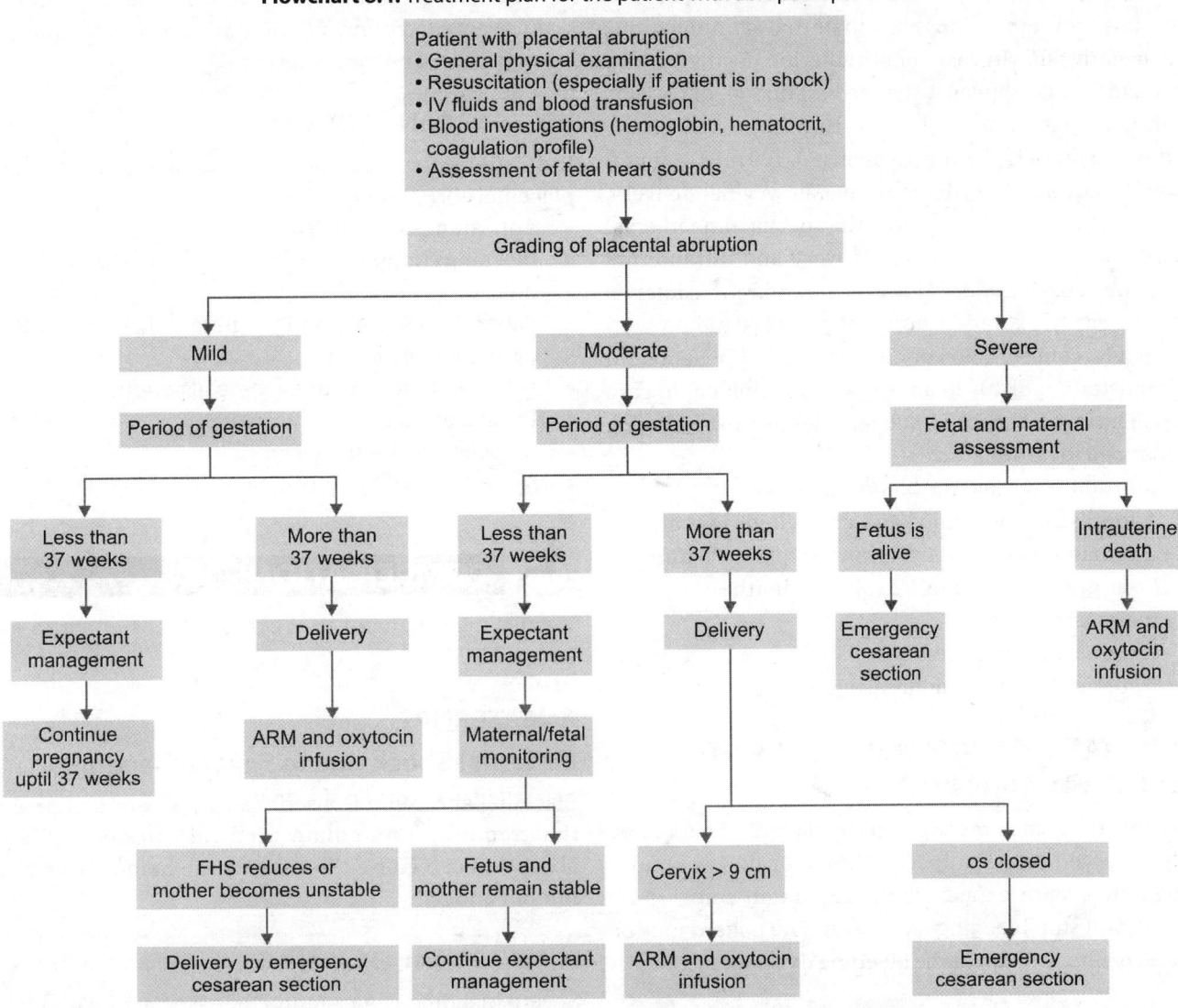

Flowchart 8.4: Treatment plan for the patient with abruption placenta.

(ARM: artificial rupture of membranes; FHS: fetal heart sound; IV: intravenous)

- Insertion of a central venous pressure line, IV line, and a urinary catheter
- Blood needs to be sent for ABO and Rh typing, cross-matching, and CBC. At least four units of blood need to be arranged.
- Blood transfusion must be started if signs of shock are present. Once the patient has stabilized the following investigations need to be sent—clotting time, fibrinogen levels, prothrombin time, activated partial thromboplastin time (APTT) and platelet count.
- Analgesia can be administered.
- Intravenous fluids and blood should be administered in such a way as to a maintain hematocrit at 30% and a urine output of at least 30 mL/hr.
- Inspection of vaginal pads and monitoring of vitals (pulse, BP, etc.) at every 15–30 minutes intervals depending upon the severity of bleeding.
- Blood coagulation profile (fibrinogen, fibrin degradation products (FDP), APTT, prothrombin time, platelet count, etc.) needs to be done at every 2 hours intervals.
- The placental position must be localized using an ultrasound scan. After the patient has stabilized, the cervix must be inspected with the help of a speculum in order to rule out the local causes of bleeding.
- The FHS must be monitored continuously with external cardiotocography.
- Intramuscular corticosteroids need to be administered to the mother in case of fetal prematurity.
- As the chances of the baby being distressed at birth are high, pediatrician and neonatologist need to be informed for resuscitation of the baby, immediately after the delivery.
- Definitive treatment in these cases is the delivery of the baby. In case of severe abruption, delivery should be performed by the fastest possible route. Cesarean delivery needs to be performed for most cases with severe placental abruption.

If the baby is alive, a cesarean section is often the best mode of delivery especially when the cervical os is closed. In conditions where the baby has already died in the womb, urgent delivery is still warranted keeping in view the development of possible maternal complications particularly DIC. In cases of intrauterine death, delivery by vaginal route appears to be the best option. In patients with fetal death and unripe cervix, misoprostol 400 µg intravaginally or high dose oxytocin (50–100 mIU/minute) may be required in order to accelerate vaginal delivery. In the past, it was believed that the specific time interval between obtaining a vaginal delivery and intrauterine death must be 4–6 hours. However, nowadays this interval can be easily extended up to 24 hours. Patients with fibrinogen concentration of <100 mg/dL may benefit from administration of 10–20 units of cryoprecipitate. In case of patients with abruption and fetal demise, the following steps need to be undertaken:

- Infusion of packed red blood cells
- Administration of blood and crystalloids to maintain a hematocrit of 30% and a urine output of 30 mL/h
- Sonography to confirm fetal death and fetal malpresentation
- Obtaining a DIC profile
- Heparin is not to be administered.

EXPECTANT MANAGEMENT FOR MILD PLACENTAL ABRUPTION

A mild abruption may resolve and the patient can often be closely observed on an outpatient basis for the remainder of pregnancy. With expectant management, some small abruption will stop bleeding on its own. The patient may be discharged after 4–5 days if the bleeding does not recur.

Prerequisites for Expectant Management

Before the expectant management can be undertaken, the following conditions need to be fulfilled:

- Fetal maturity is not achieved (fetus < 36 weeks of gestation).
- Bleeding has stopped and there is no active bleeding.
- The fetus is not in distress.
- The mother's vital signs are stable.
- Patient is not in labor.

Steps of Expectant Management

The following steps need to be undertaken:

- Admission to the hospital
- Bed rest must be advised.
- The women must be advised to avoid sexual intercourse.
- Blood investigations need to be done: Blood grouping and cross-matching, hematocrit, and coagulation studies.
- Placenta to be localized by an ultrasound scan
- Once the active bleeding has stopped, cervix needs to be inspected with a speculum.
- The fetal monitoring should be done using daily fetal movement count, ultrasound measurements of fetal growth and nonstress test.

CESAREAN SECTION

Indications for emergency cesarean section in cases of placental abruption are as follows:

- Appearance of fetal distress
- Bleeding continues to occur despite of ARM and oxytocin infusion
- Labor does not seem to progress well, despite ARM and oxytocin infusion.
- Deterioration of maternal or fetal condition
- Presence of fetal malpresentation
- Associated obstetric factors
- Appearance of a complication (DIC, oliguria, etc.).

COMPLICATIONS

Various maternal and fetal complications of abruption are enlisted in **Box 8.7**.

MATERNAL

Maternal Shock due to Severe Bleeding

Placental abruption is a serious complication of pregnancy that requires immediate medical attention. Placental abruption can cause life-threatening hemorrhage for both mother and baby.

MATERNAL DEATH

Severe bleeding, shock, and DIC associated with placental abruption can result in maternal death.

RENAL FAILURE

The likely causes for renal failure in patients with placental abruption are as follows:

- Severe shock resulting from grade 3 placental abruption
- Disseminated intravascular coagulation can also be responsible for development of renal failure.

BOX 8.7: Complications of abruption.

Fetal:
- Prematurity
- Fetal distress
- Fetal death/stillbirths

Maternal:
- Anemia/shock/oliguria (rarely acute renal failure)
- Consumptive coagulopathy
- Couvelaire uterus
- Maternal death
- Postpartum uterine atony and postpartum hemorrhage
- Disseminated intravascular coagulopathy

Antepartum Hemorrhage

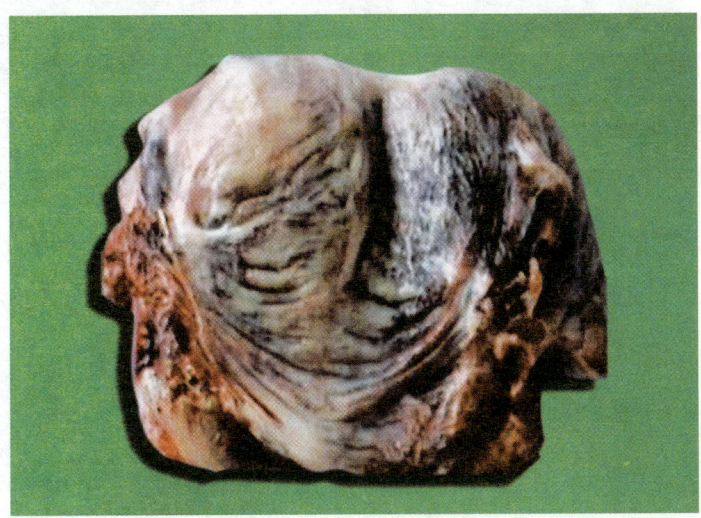

Fig. 8.20: Couvelaire uterus.

- Acute tubular necrosis
- Massive hemorrhage resulting in impaired renal perfusion.
- Frequent coexistence of preeclampsia which is an important cause of renal vasospasm.

COUVELAIRE UTERUS OR UTEROPLACENTAL APOPLEXY

Q. Write a short note on couvelaire uterus.

This condition has been found to be associated with severe forms of concealed placental abruption and is characterized by massive intravasation of blood into the uterine musculature up to the level of serosa (Fig. 8.20). The blood gets infiltrated between the bundles of muscle fibers. As a result, the uterus becomes port wine in color. This is likely to interfere with uterine contractions and may predispose to the development of severe PPH. However, couvelaire uterus per se is not an indication for cesarean hysterectomy.

In couvelaire uterus, there can be effusions of blood beneath the tubal serosa, connective tissues of broad ligaments, substance of the ovaries as well as free blood in the peritoneal cavity. These myometrial hemorrhages may interfere with uterine contractions to produce PPH.

RISK OF RECURRENCE OF ABRUPTION IN FUTURE PREGNANCIES

Recurrence risk of placental abruption varies from 8% to 15%.

POSTPARTUM UTERINE ATONY AND POSTPARTUM HEMORRHAGE

If the woman has suffered a placental abruption, there might be presence of intramuscular hemorrhages within the uterine musculature, which may prevent effective uterine contractions thereby resulting in development of PPH. Due to onset of DIC in cases with severe placental abruption, there might be failure of coagulation due to which the blood may fail to clot. This may be another cause for PPH. Management of PPH has been discussed in detail in Chapter 14.

DISSEMINATED INTRAVASCULAR COAGULATION

Q. With help of a short note, discuss the pathophysiology of DIC in cases of abruptio placentae.

Disseminated intravascular coagulation is a syndrome associated with both thrombosis and hemorrhage. The pathophysiology of DIC is shown in **Flowchart 8.5**. In DIC, initially there is activation of the coagulation pathways, both intrinsic and extrinsic (**Flowchart 8.6**), due to thromboplastin released from the decidual fragments and placental separation. As the process of coagulation continues, it results in consumption of various clotting factors and widespread deposition of fibrin. This can result

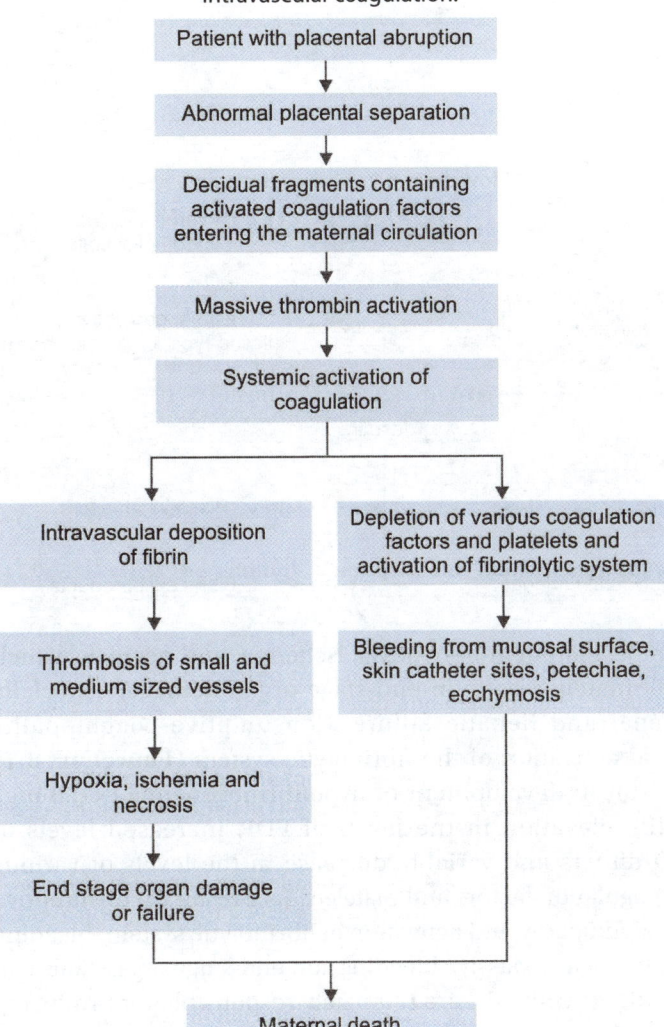

Flowchart 8.5: Pathophysiology of disseminated intravascular coagulation.

Flowchart 8.6: Coagulation pathways.

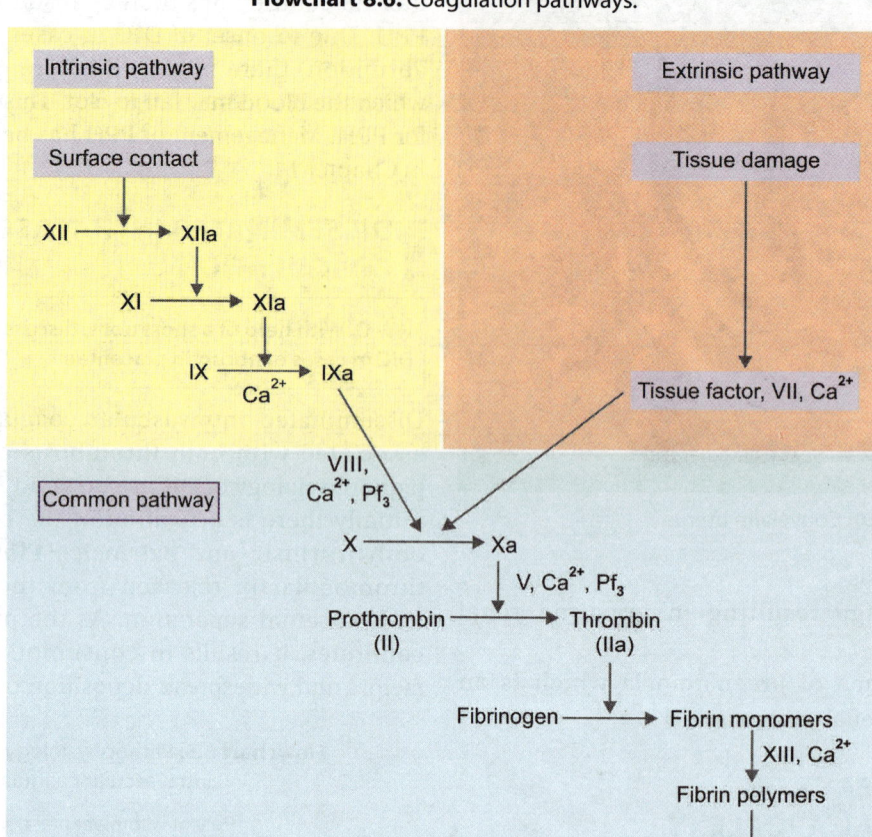

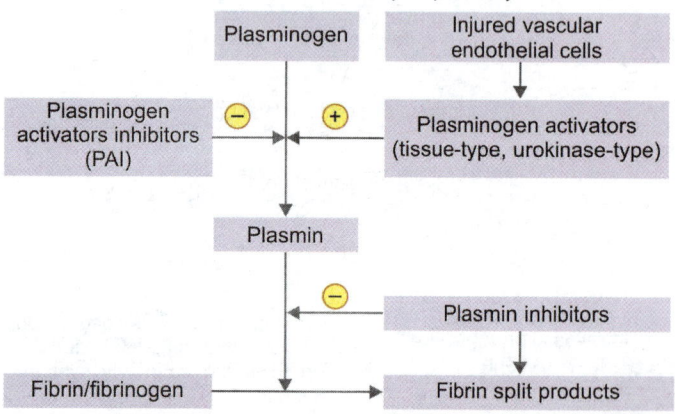

Flowchart 8.7: Fibrinolytic pathway.

> **BOX 8.8:** Various causes for disseminated intravascular coagulation.
>
> - Obstetrical causes (placental abruption, septic abortion, amniotic fluid embolism, and intrauterine death)
> - Infection (bacterial, viral, parasitic, rickettsial, and mycotic)
> - Malignancy (metastatic tumors including those in colon, lungs, breast, prostate, etc.)
> - Transfusion reactions (ABO incompatibility)
> - Vascular disorders (giant hemangiomas, aneurysm, prosthetic grafts, etc.)
> - Massive tissue injury (trauma/burns, etc.)
> - Miscellaneous (snake bites, iron toxicity, pancreatitis, etc.)

in development of hypoxia, ischemia, and necrosis, which ultimately results in end-stage organ damage, especially renal and hepatic failure. Consumptive coagulopathy and activation of the fibrinolytic system **(Flowchart 8.7)** result in development of hypofibrinogenemia (<150 mg/dL), elevation in the levels of FDP, increased levels of D-dimers and variable decrease in the levels of various coagulation factors and platelets. As a result of consumptive coagulopathy and activation of fibrinolytic system, bleeding takes place. Massive bleeding and end-stage organ failure in patients with DIC are ultimately responsible for producing death.

Causes of Disseminated Intravascular Coagulation

Besides placental abruption, there are many causes which may be responsible for producing DIC. Some of these causes for DIC are listed in **Box 8.8**.

Clinical Presentation

Most common sign of DIC is bleeding. It can be manifested in form of ecchymosis, petechiae, and purpura. There can be oozing or frank bleeding from multiple sites. Extremities may become cool and mottled. Pleural and pericardial involvement may be responsible for causing dyspnea

Antepartum Hemorrhage

TABLE 8.3: Abnormal results of coagulation profile in cases of disseminated intravascular coagulation.

Test	Normal	DIC
Fibrinogen	150–600 mg/dL	Reduced (<150 mg/dL)
Prothrombin time	11–16 seconds	Prolonged
APTT	22–37 seconds	Prolonged
TT	15–25 seconds	Prolonged
Platelet count	1.2–1.5 lakh/mm^3	Reduced
D-dimer	< 0.5 mg/L	Increased (>0.5 mg/L)
FDP	< 10 µg/dL	Increased (>10 µg/dL)

(APTT: activated partial thromboplastin time; DIC: disseminated intravascular coagulation; FDP: fibrin degradation products; TT: thrombin time)

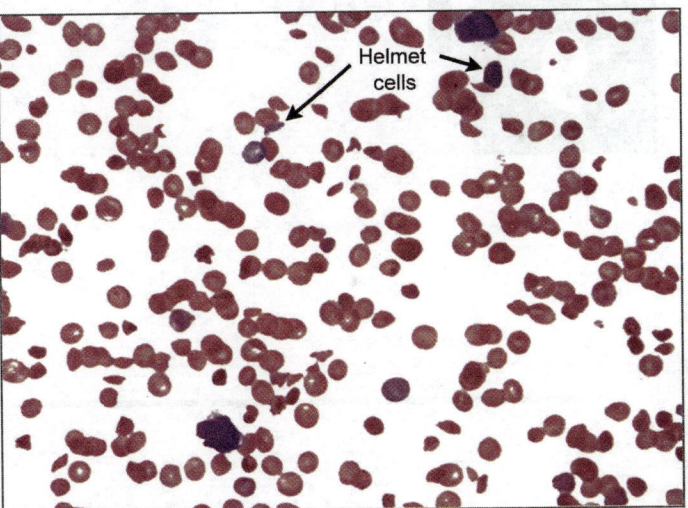

Fig. 8.21: Peripheral smear in patient with disseminated intravascular coagulation, suggestive of hemolytic anemia. The black arrows point towards the helmet cells.

and chest pain respectively. Hematuria is commonly present. Bleeding and renal failure are the most important manifestations in cases with DIC.

Diagnosis

In the cases of DIC, coagulation profile is mainly affected. Abnormal results of various tests in coagulation profile in patients with DIC are shown in **Table 8.3**. Fibrinogen levels are reduced; prothrombin time, APTT, and thrombin time are prolonged; platelet levels are reduced and levels of D-dimer and FDP are increased.

- *Prothrombin time:* It is the time taken by the blood to clot after addition of tissue thromboplastin. It indicates the amount of prothrombin present in the blood.
- *Activated partial thromboplastin time:* Time taken for the blood to clot after addition of phospholipids and calcium
- *Thrombin time:* Time taken for blood to clot after adding thrombin to it.

The findings on peripheral smear **(Fig. 8.21)** in patients with DIC are suggestive of microangiopathic hemolytic anemia. The peripheral smear shows presence of multiple helmet cells, fragmented red blood cells, microspherocytes and schistocytes, and paucity of platelet cells.

Treatment of Disseminated Intravascular Coagulation

Treatment of DIC mainly involves the treatment of the underlying cause. Platelets can be transfused in patients at high risk of bleeding, e.g., those who need to undergo surgery. Replacement therapy with fresh frozen plasma (FFP) may also be administered. FFP is usually administered to maintain fibrinogen levels above 150 mg/dL. FFP usually contains the clotting factors V, VIII, XIII, and antithrombin III. Usual dose of FFP is 10–15 mg/kg body weight. Indications for administration of FFP include prolongation of prothrombin time and fibrinogen levels < 50 mg/dL. Transfusion of platelets, fibrinogen concentrates, and cryoprecipitate is also sometimes given. Cryoprecipitate is composed of fibrinogen and factor VIII. The use of heparin in cases of DIC is largely controversial and is supposed to worsen the bleeding.

FETAL COMPLICATIONS

Fetal Distress

Placental abruption can deprive the baby of oxygen and nutrients and cause heavy bleeding in the mother. If left untreated, placental abruption puts both mother and baby in jeopardy. Decreased oxygen to the brain leads to later development of neurological or behavioral problems. In severe cases, stillbirth is possible.

Premature Delivery

Peak incidence of abruption occurs between 24 and 26 weeks of gestation and is associated with nearly 10% cases of preterm birth. The preterm babies have been found to be at an increased risk of perinatal asphyxia, intraventricular hemorrhage, periventricular leukomalacia, and cerebral palsy.

Stillbirth and Fetal Death

Placental abruption is an important cause of fetal distress, asphyxia, and ultimately intrauterine death. Premature delivery in cases with placental abruption is an important cause of fetal morbidity.

EVIDENCE-BASED CLINICAL TRIALS

List of references can be scanned through QR code to enable the readers gain deeper insight of the subject by referring to the entire article or its abstract.

CHAPTER 9

Multifetal Gestation

CASE STUDY

A 24-year-old G2P1L1 with 36 completed weeks of gestation and previous history of normal vaginal delivery at term presented for an ANC check-up. There is no history of taking any fertility treatment. She gives history of being diagnosed with twin gestation on an ultrasound examination done at 8 weeks.

INTRODUCTION

Development of two or more embryos simultaneously in a pregnant uterus is termed as multifetal gestation (**Figs. 9.1A and B**). Development of two fetuses simultaneously is known as twin gestation; development of three fetuses simultaneously as triplets; four fetuses as quadruplets; five fetuses as quintuplets and so on.

The incidence of twin gestation is about 1 per 80 live births. The incidence varies among different countries and ethnic groups, with the incidence being highest in African countries, lowest in Japan and intermediate amongst Caucasians.

According to the Hellen's rule, the frequency of twins is 1 in 80; frequency of triplets 1 in 80²; frequency of quadruplets 1 in 80³, and so on. The exact cause of multifetal gestation is not known.

TYPES OF TWIN GESTATION

> **Q. Write a short note discussing the etiology of twin gestation.**
>
> **Q. Write a short note on mechanism of twinning.**
>
> **Q. With help of a long essay discuss chorionicity in twins.**

Multifetal twin gestation can be of two types—monozygotic twins and dizygotic twins. The differences between these two are described in **Table 9.1**.

Dizygotic Twins

When two or more ova are fertilized by sperms, the result is development of dizygotic twins or nonidentical twins

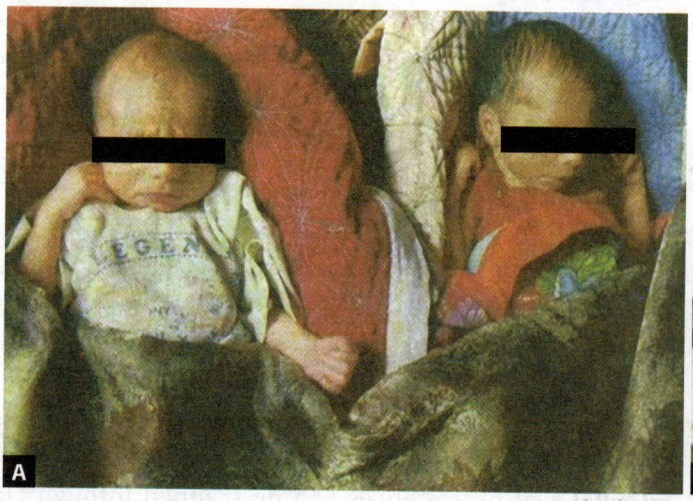
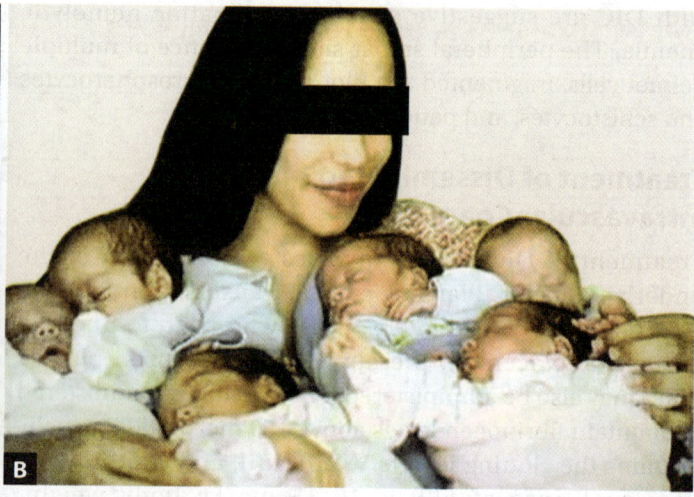

Figs. 9.1A and B: (A) Photograph showing two newly born twin babies; (B) The highest number of babies born to a mother at one time nonuplets—a set of nine children born to Nadya Suleman (California, United States) in 2009. She gave birth to two healthy boys and six girls. All these babies were conceived by in vitro fertilization and survived infancy (The above picture only shows six babies, remaining were in the neonatal intensive care unit).
(*Source:* Mail Today, March 2013)

TABLE: 9.1: Difference between monozygotic and dizygotic twins.		
Parameter	Monozygotic twins (identical twins)	Dizygotic twins (nonidentical or fraternal twins)
Etiology	Division of a fertilized ovum into two	Fertilization of two or more ova by sperms
Sex	Same	Can be different
Placenta	Single	Each fetus has a separate placenta
Communication between fetal vessels	Present	Absent
Genetic features (DNA fingerprinting)	Same	Different
Blood group	Same	Different
Skin grafting	Acceptance by the other twin	Rejection by the twin
Intervening membrane between the two fetuses	*Composed of three layers:* A fused chorion in the middle surrounded by amnion on two sides	*Composed of four layers:* Two chorions in the middle surrounded by amnion on two sides
Fetal growth and congenital malformations	More common	Less common
Incidence	Comprises of one-third of total cases of twins	Comprises of two-thirds of total cases of twins
Frequency	The frequency of monozygotic twin births is relatively constant worldwide and is approximately one set per 250 live births	Variable
Influence of various factors	Though the occurrence of monozygotic twins is largely independent of factors such as race, heredity, age, and parity, there is now increasing evidence that assisted reproductive technology increases the incidence of zygotic splitting	The incidence of dizygotic twinning is greatly influenced by factors such as race, heredity, maternal age, parity, nutrition and, fertility treatment

or fraternal twins (**Figs. 9.2 and 9.3**). As a result of being fertilized by two separate sperms, the two embryos can be of different sexes. Furthermore, in dizygotic twins the two embryos have separate placentae and there is no communication between the fetal vessels of the two embryos.

Monozygotic Twins

Monozygotic twins are formed due to the division of a single fertilized egg (**Figs. 9.3 and 9.4**). In monozygotic multiple pregnancies, different types can result depending on the timing of the division of the ovum (**Fig. 9.5**).

Different Types of Monozygotic Twins

Diamniotic dichorionic monozygotic twin pregnancy (**Fig. 9.6A**): The embryo splits at or before 3 days of gestation. This results in development of two chorions and two amnions. There is development of two distinct placentae or a single-fused placenta. This type of monozygotic twin accounts for nearly 8% of all twin gestations.

Diamniotic monochorionic monozygotic twin pregnancy (**Fig. 9.6B**): The cleavage division is delayed until the formation of inner cell mass and the embryo splits between 4 and 7 days of gestation. This results in development of a single chorion and two amnions. Nearly, 20% of all twins are of this type.

Monoamniotic monochorionic monozygotic twin pregnancy (**Fig. 9.6C**): The embryo splits between 8 and 12 days of

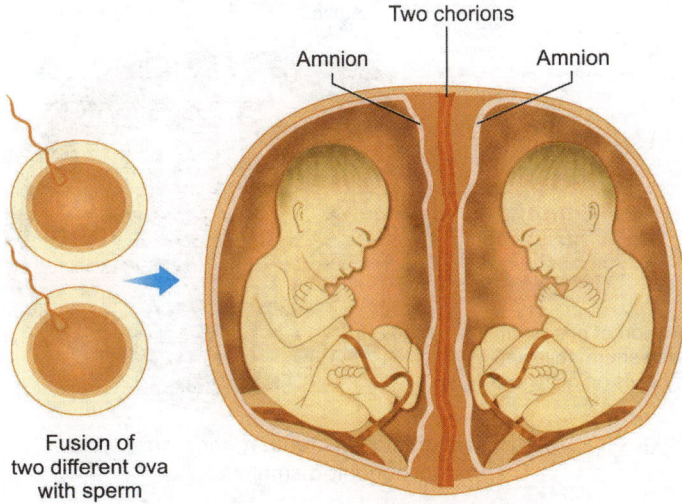

Fig. 9.2: Formation of dizygotic twins.

gestation. This results in development of one chorion and one amnion. Such types of monozygotic twins are rare, accounting for <1% of all twin gestations.

Conjoined or Siamese monozygotic twin pregnancy: The embryo splits at or after 13 days of gestation, resulting in development of conjoined twins, which share a particular body part with each other. Development of such type of monozygotic twins is extremely rare. Joining of the twins can begin at either pole and may be dorsal, ventral, and lateral. Of the various types of conjoined twins, parapagus twins (laterally joined) are the most common type.

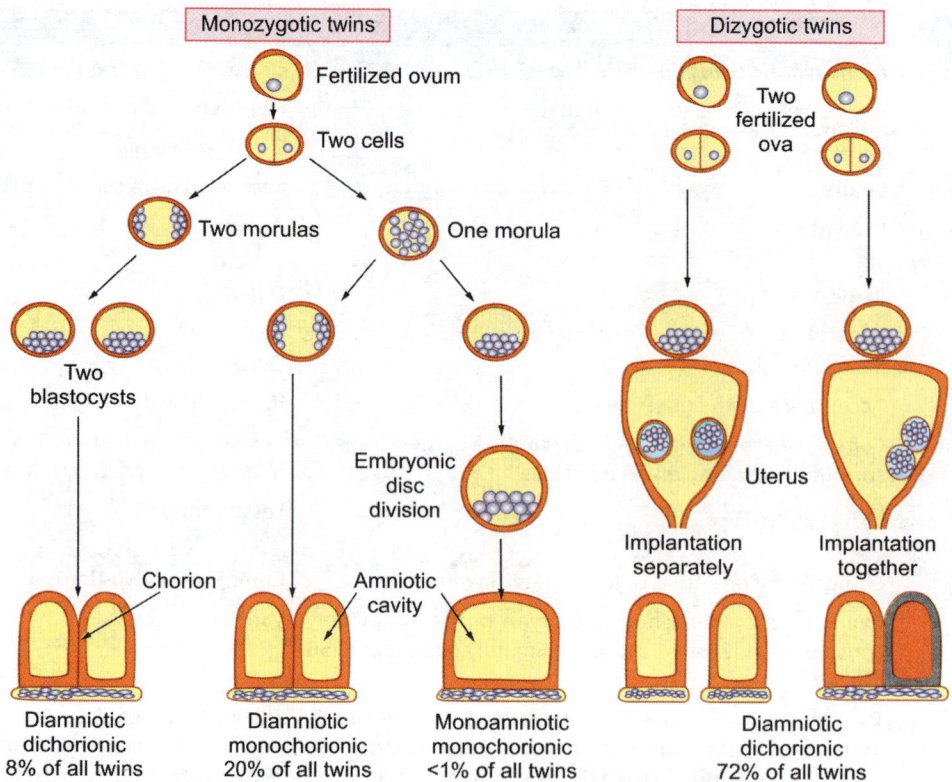

Fig. 9.3: Difference between the monozygotic and dizygotic twins.

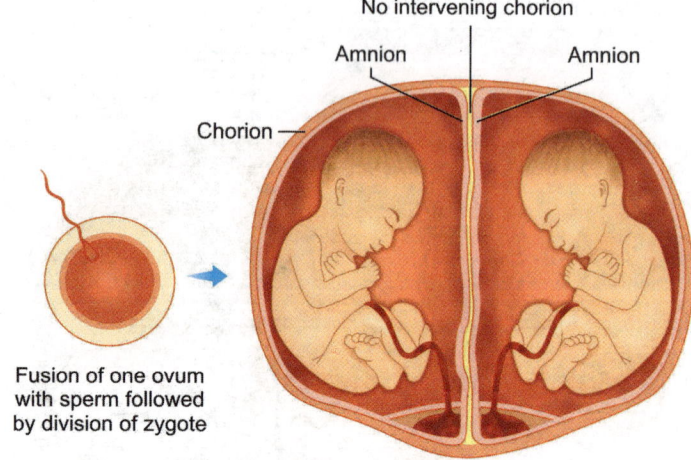

Fig. 9.4: Formation of monozygotic twins (monochorionic diamniotic).

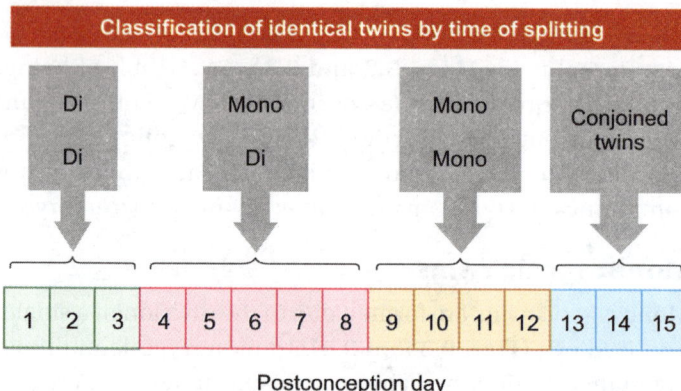

Fig. 9.5: Formation of different types of monozygotic twins. (Di Di: diamniotic dichorionic; Mono Di: monochorionic diamniotic; Mono Mono: monoamniotic monochorionic)

Different types of conjoined twins, which can result, are shown in **Figures 9.7A to C** and are listed in **Table 9.2**. The conjoined twins are diagnosed by ultrasonographic features **(Figs. 9.8A and B)**, some of which are as follows:
- Both the twins appear to be facing one another, with their heads being at the same plane and level.
- The thoracic cages of both the twins appear to be unusually close to one another. Repeat ultrasound examination done at an interval of few days or even few weeks is unable to show any change in the relative positions of the fetuses.
- The fetal heads may appear to be unusually hyperextended. If the pregnancy is allowed to continue, delivery by cesarean section is the only option followed by surgical separation of the babies after birth. Surgical separation of conjoined twins may be successful if the essential organs are not shared. Consultation with a plastic surgeon is often required prior to surgery.

HISTORY AND CLINICAL PRESENTATION

RISK FACTORS

The risk factors which are most likely to result in twin pregnancies and need to be elicited while taking the history include the following:

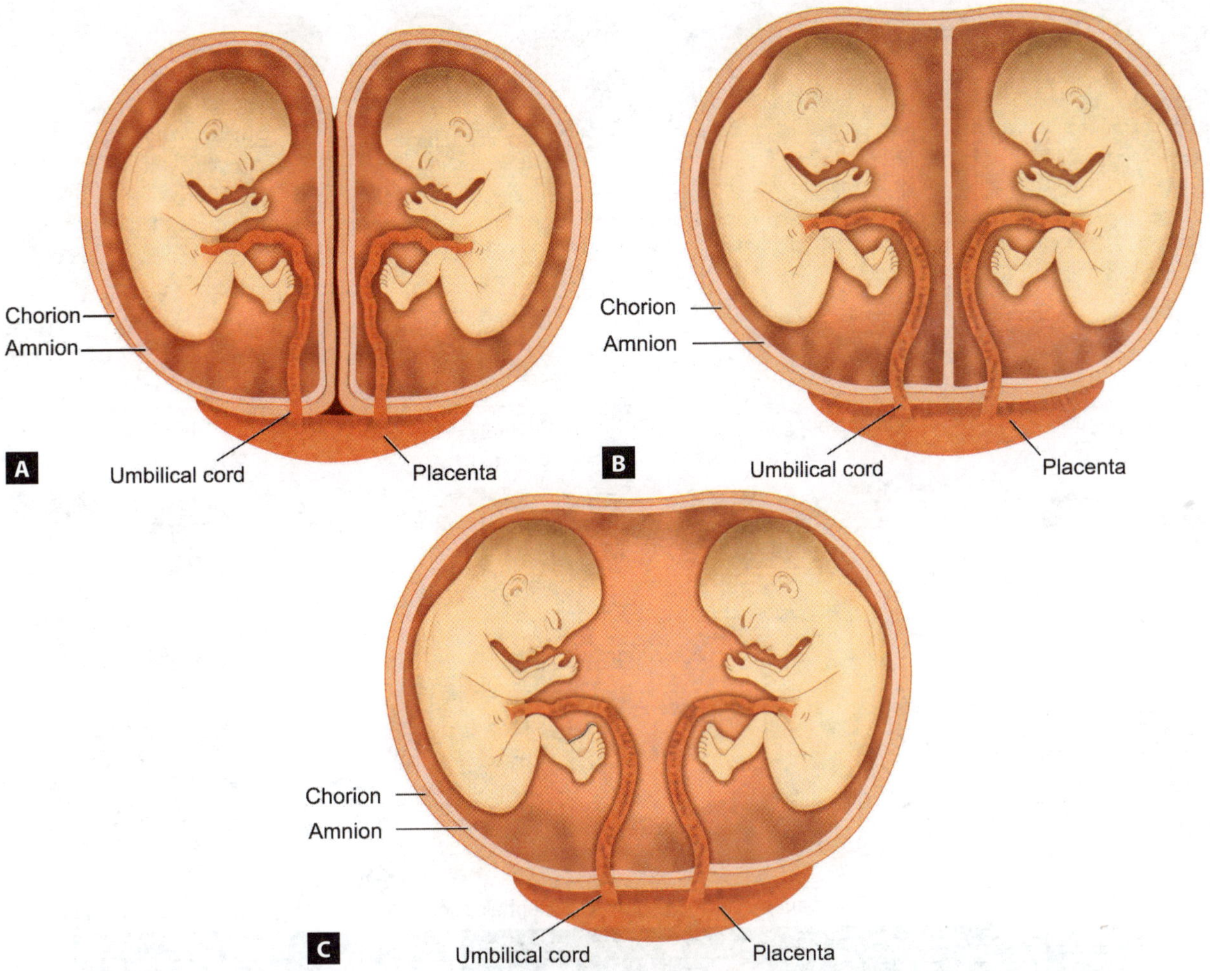

Figs 9.6A to C: (A) Diamniotic dichorionic monozygotic twin pregnancy; (B) Diamniotic monochorionic monozygotic twin pregnancy; (C) Monoamniotic monochorionic monozygotic twin pregnancy.

- Increased maternal age and parity
- Previous history of twin gestation
- Family history of twin gestation (especially on maternal side)
- Conception following a long period of infertility
- Pregnancy attained through use of assisted reproductive technology (ART) (IVF or use of clomiphene citrate)
- Racial origin (twin gestation is more common amongst the women of West African ancestry, less common in those of Japanese ancestry)
- History of using progestational agents or combined oral contraceptives. These are the drugs which are prone to reduce the tubal mobility.

CLINICAL PRESENTATION

The woman may experience exaggeration of symptoms of early pregnancy, including symptoms such as nausea, piles, varicosities, heartburn, shortness of breath, backache, ankle swelling, piles, and varicose veins, due to higher levels of circulating hormones. Pregnancy complications such as preterm labor, preeclampsia, placenta previa, polyhydramnios, and anemia are also more common in twin pregnancies. Nearly, all multiple pregnancies are now diagnosed in the first trimester by ultrasound. However, some twins die and are absorbed in the first half of pregnancy resulting in "the disappearing twin" syndrome. With increasing period of gestation, the woman may experience increased frequency of heartburn; indigestion and urinary frequency as the enlarging uterus presses on other organs. Back pain is common because of the extra load of the enlarging uterus in combination with the relaxation of muscles and ligaments produced by the pregnancy hormones. The women with multifetal gestation may experience early onset of preeclampsia. Hypertensive disorders due to pregnancy are also more likely to develop with multiple fetuses.

GENERAL PHYSICAL EXAMINATION

The signs of anemia may be exaggerated in a woman with multifetal gestation and she may exhibit pallor of extreme degrees. There may be early onset of preeclampsia in these women. As a result, they may show high blood pressure and proteinuria before 20 weeks of gestation.

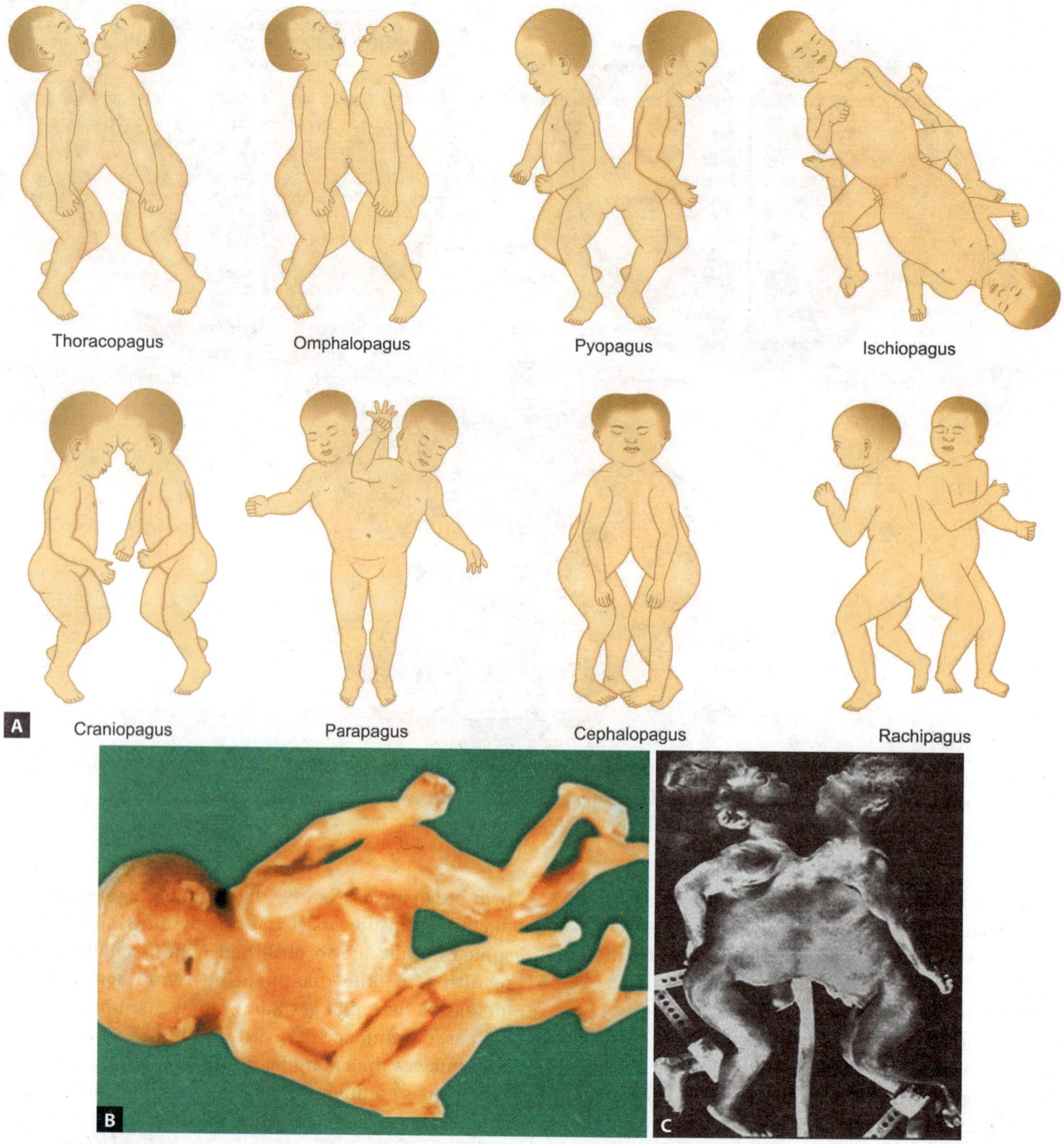

170 Complications of Pregnancy

Figs. 9.7A to C: Conjoined twins. (A) Different types of conjoined twins; (B) Autopsy specimen of craniopagus twins; (C) Autopsy specimen of thoracopagus twins.

TABLE 9.2: Different types of Siamese twins.

Type of Siamese twin	Description
Thoracopagus	Joined at the chest
Omphalopagus	Joined at the anterior abdominal wall
Craniopagus	Joined at the head
Pyopagus	Joined at the buttocks
Ischiopagus	Joined at the ischium

SPECIFIC SYSTEMIC EXAMINATION

ABDOMINAL EXAMINATION

Inspection

Abdominal overdistention (barrel-shaped abdomen) may be present.

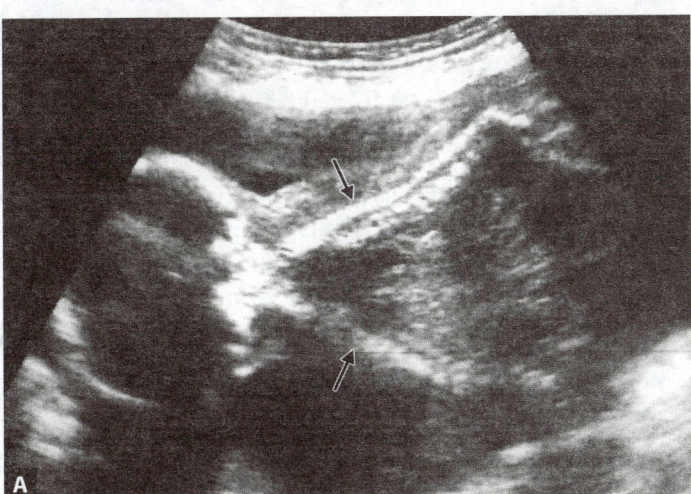
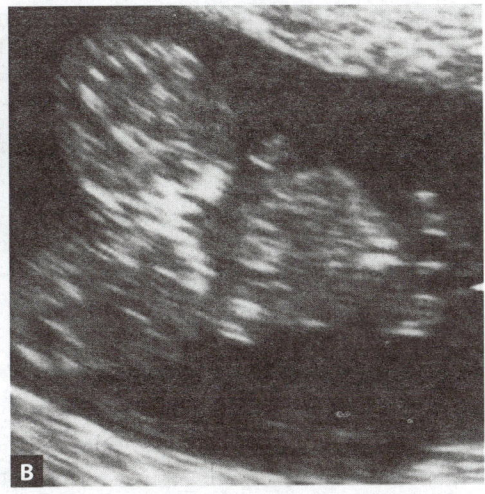

Figs. 9.8A and B: Ultrasound appearance of conjoined twins. (A) Conjoined twins fused in the regions of skull and anterior chest wall; (B) Conjoined twins fused in the region of thorax and abdomen.

Palpation

- The uterus may be palpable abdominally earlier than 12 weeks of gestation.
- In the second half of pregnancy, the women may present with a uterine size more than the period of gestation and/or higher than expected weight gain in comparison to singleton pregnancies. Height of the uterus is greater than period of amenorrhea (fundal height is typically 5 cm greater than the period of amenorrhea in the second trimester).
- Abdominal girth at the level of umbilicus is greater than the normal abdominal girth at term.
- Palpation of multiple fetal parts (e.g., palpation of two fetal heads)
- Presence of hydramnios

Auscultation

Two fetal heart sounds (FHS) can be auscultated, located at two separate spots separated by a silent area in between.

VAGINAL EXAMINATION

Vaginal examination may help in identifying the presenting parts of one or more fetuses.

Designation of twins in utero: In case of twin gestation, the twin which presents first (whose presenting part is palpated first on vaginal examination), is designated as twin A. On the other hand, the twin which presents next (whose presenting part can be palpated on vaginal examination, following the delivery of first twin) is designated as twin B. Following the delivery of twin A and before the delivery of twin B, an abdominal and vaginal examination should be performed to confirm the lie, presentation, and FHS of the second baby. External version at the time of abdominal examination or internal podalic version at the time of vaginal examination can be attempted, in case the lie of twin B is transverse. Vaginal examination also helps in diagnosing cord prolapse,

BOX 9.1: Differential diagnosis of multifetal gestation.

- Hydramnios
- Wrong dates
- Hydatidiform mole
- Uterine fibroids
- Adnexal masses
- Fetal macrosomia
- Elevation of the uterus by a distended bladder

if present. Following the vaginal delivery of first twin, vaginal examination helps in determining the position of second twin.

DIFFERENTIAL DIAGNOSIS

Other causes for fundal height being more than period of amenorrhea are listed in **Box 9.1**.

Ultrasound examination can help in ruling out various other conditions which cause the fundal height to be more than the period of gestation and also help in confirming the diagnosis of multifetal gestation.

MANAGEMENT

Q. Discuss the etiology, diagnosis, and management of a case of twin pregnancy presenting at term.

Q. A G2P1A0L1 with 33 weeks of gestation with twin pregnancy has presented to you. You notice that there is IUD of one fetus. Discuss the counseling and management in such a case.

Q. What would be the further course of management in the case study mentioned in the beginning of the chapter?

Q. Following the delivery of first twin an ultrasound examination was performed. A fetus with breech presentation, having an EFW of 2.4 kg was diagnosed on ultrasound examination. What should be the next step of management?

Q. With help of a long essay write about the diagnosis and management of monochorionic twins.

172 Complications of Pregnancy

Management comprising of investigations and definitive obstetric management is discussed below.

INVESTIGATIONS

ROUTINE ANC INVESTIGATIONS

See Chapter 1

ULTRASOUND EXAMINATION

- *Multiple fetuses:* There may be presence of two or more fetuses or gestational sacs **(Figs. 9.9 to 9.15)**. Two fetal heads or two abdomens should be seen in the same plane, to avoid scanning the same fetus twice and interpreting it as twins. Fetuses with opposite gender are usually dizygotic and therefore dichorionic.

- *Multiple placentas:* There may be two placentas lying close to one another or presence of a single large placenta with a thick dividing membrane. This dividing layer could be composed of maximum up to four membranes (two layers of chorion fused in the middle, surrounded by amnion). In case of dichorionic pregnancies, the dividing membrane is usually 2 mm or more in thickness. On the other hand, in case of monochorionic pregnancies, the dividing membrane is composed of only two layers and may be so thin (<2 mm) that it may not be visualized until the second trimester.

In a woman presenting with a twin or triplet pregnancy after 14^{+0} weeks, ultrasound must be used for determining the chorionicity and amnionicity using the parameters such as number of placental masses, presence of amniotic membrane(s) and membrane thickness, the lambda or T-sign, and discordant fetal sex.

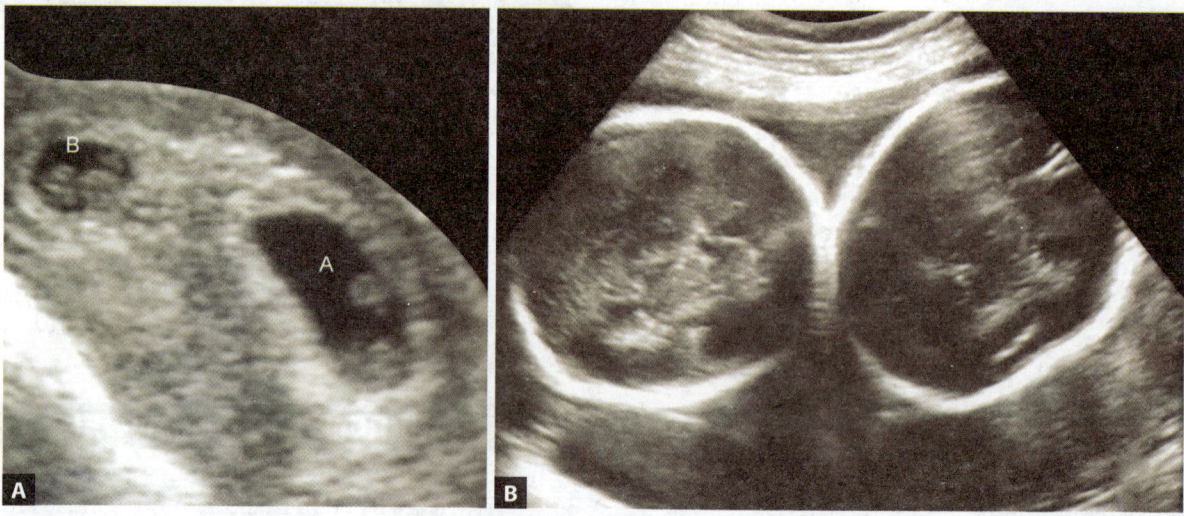

Figs. 9.9A and B: (A) Presence of two gestational sacs on ultrasound, with sac A = 7.6 weeks and sac B = 8.7 weeks; (B) Ultrasound of the same patient at 30 weeks of gestation, showing two fetal heads.

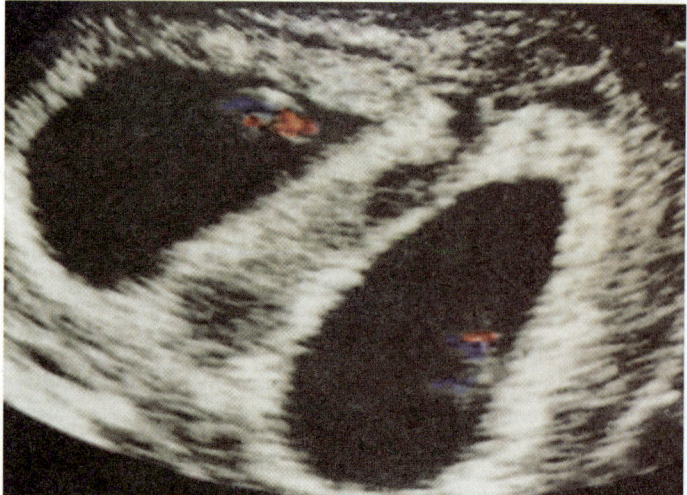

Fig. 9.10: Diamniotic dichorionic twins at 7 weeks of gestation. There are two separate chorionic sacs surrounding each of the two amniotic sacs, with each sac containing an embryo. The intervening membrane between the twins is composed of four layers: two layers of chorion in the middle surrounded by a layer of amnion on either side.

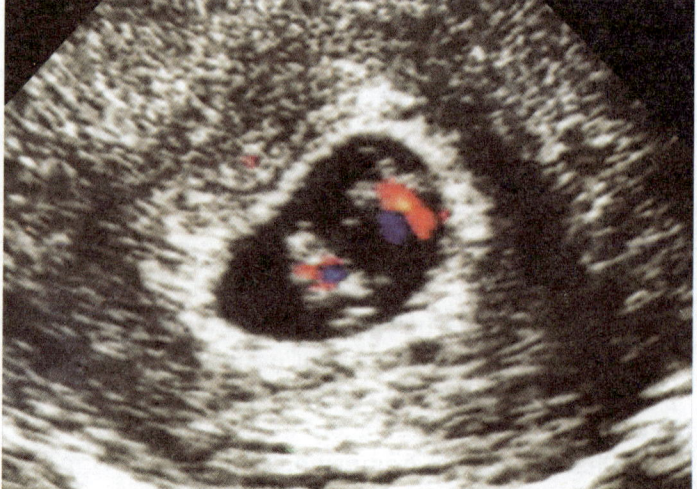

Fig. 9.11: Monoamniotic monochorionic twins at 7 weeks of gestation. In this case, the two embryos are surrounded by a single amnion and a single chorion. Therefore, there is no intervening membrane between the two fetuses.

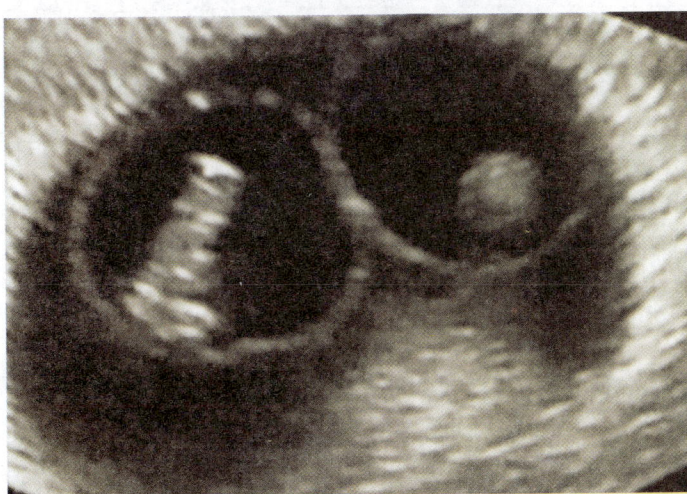

Fig. 9.12: Monochorionic diamniotic twins. In this case, each embryo is surrounded by a separate amniotic sac. There is common chorionic sac which surrounds the two amniotic sacs. Therefore, the intervening membrane between the two twins comprises of two layers of amnion.

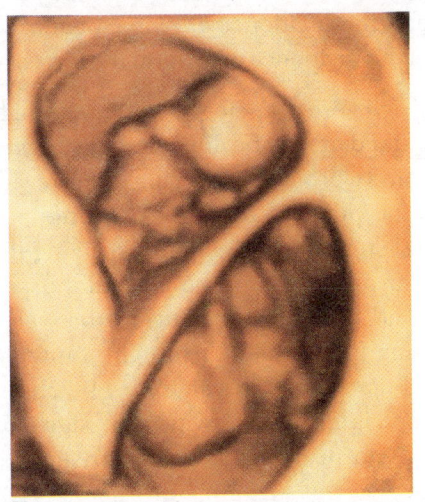

Fig. 9.13: Three-dimensional view of diamniotic dichorionic twins at 10 weeks of gestation. The intervening membrane between the two twins in this case is composed of four layers: two intervening layers of chorion surrounded by a layer of amnion on either side.

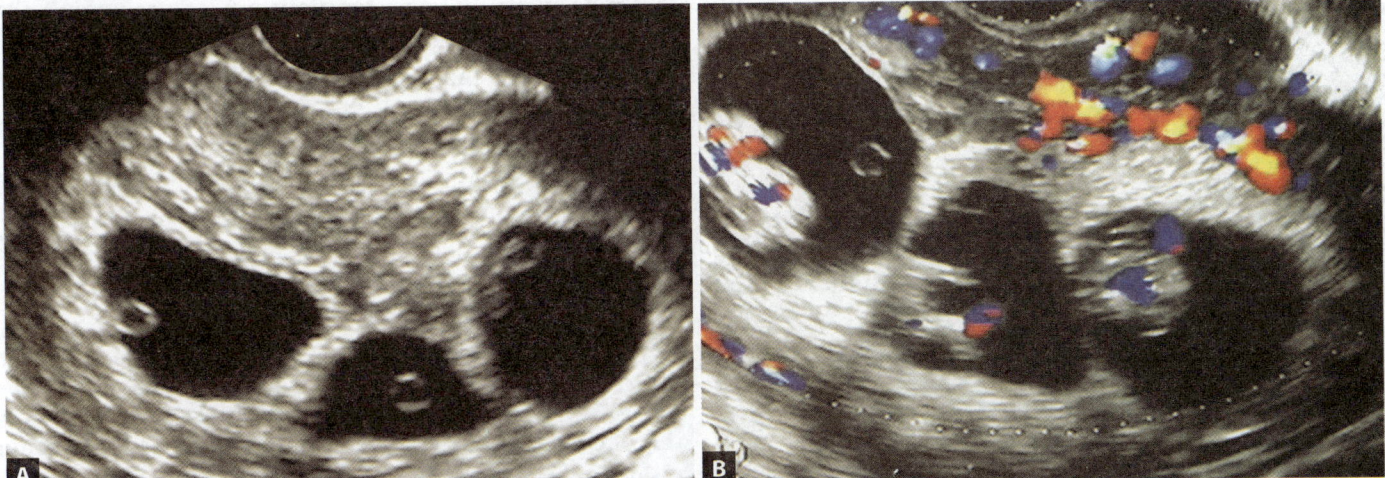

Figs. 9.14A and B: Triplets at 7 weeks of gestation. (A) Transvaginal ultrasound showing three separate gestational sacs; (B) Color Doppler ultrasound in the same patient shows presence of a single placenta.

If it is not possible to determine chorionicity or amnionicity by ultrasound at the time of detecting the twin or triplet pregnancy, woman must be referred to seek a second opinion from a senior sonographer or to a competent healthcare professional. If the chorionicity remains undetermined even after the referral the pregnancy must be managed as a monochorionic pregnancy unless proven otherwise. In case of poor transabdominal scan views, transvaginal ultrasound can be used. However, it is not advisable to use 3-dimensional ultrasound scans for determining chorionicity and amnionicity.

- *Vanishing twins:* One of the twins diagnosed during an ultrasound examination performed in the first trimester may be lost or "vanishes" before the second trimester in up to 20–60% cases of spontaneous twin gestations.

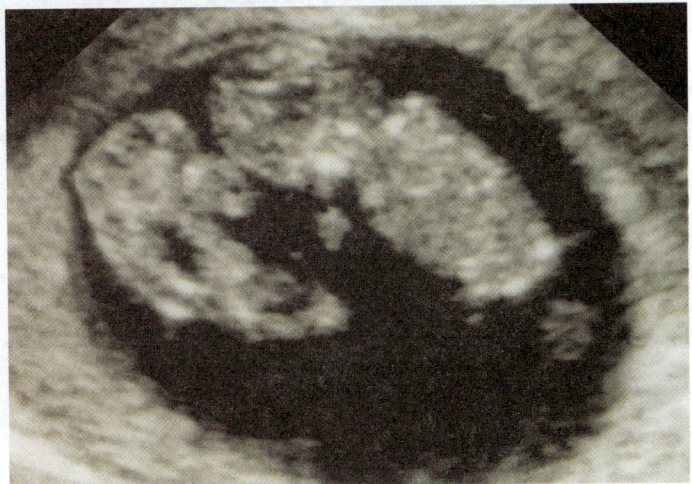

Fig. 9.15: Monochorionic monoamniotic twins. There is absence of any intervening membrane between the two twins, in this case.

Therefore, the incidence of twins diagnosed at birth is less than the incidence of twins at the time of conception.

Twin peak sign: Pregnancies in which a single placental mass is identified, it may be difficult to distinguish one large placenta from two placentas, lying side by side or fused. Examining the point of origin of dividing membrane on the placental surface may help in clarifying the situation. If a triangular projection of the placental tissue is seen to extend beyond the chorionic surface between the layers of the dividing membrane, this might imply the presence of two-fused placentas. This sign may be observed on the ultrasound and is termed as "twin-peak" sign or lambda sign **(Fig. 9.16)**. Twin-peak sign is characteristic of dichorionic pregnancies.

On the other hand, in monochorionic pregnancies, there occurs a right-angled relationship between the membranes and placental tissue and there is no apparent extension of placental tissue between the dividing membranes. This is known as the "T sign" **(Figs. 9.17A and B)**.

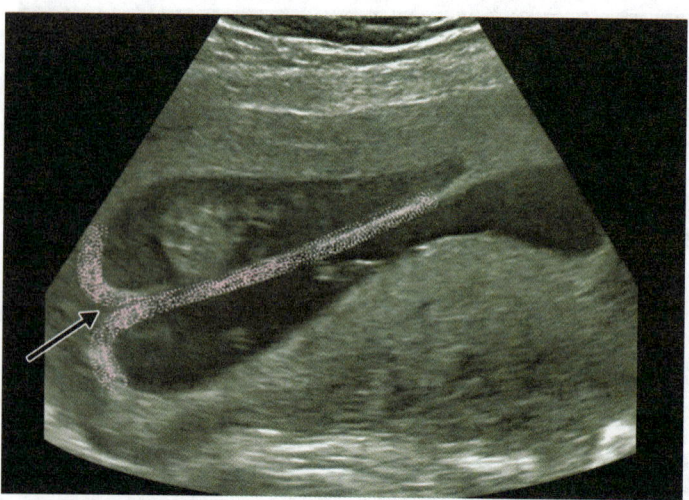

Fig. 9.16: Diamniotic dichorionic pregnancy. Arrow shows the presence of the lambda sign.

TREATMENT/OBSTETRIC MANAGEMENT

Q. Critically evaluate the management options in case of multiple pregnancy.

Q. How will you manage the delivery of second twin?

Q. What is the mode of management of triplets or higher-order gestation?

Q. With help of a short note discuss antepartum management of multiple pregnancy.

Q. Using a short essay discuss the delivery of twins in the second stage.

Q. Write a short essay on internal podalic version in twins.

PREVENTION

Primary Prevention

Methods of primary prevention aim at preventing the occurrence of twin pregnancies in the first place. These include, limiting the number of embryos transferred in IVF and close counseling/monitoring of women using ovulation induction therapies. Since 2001, the Human Fertilisation and Embryology Authority (UK) has recommended that the maximum number of embryos to be transferred per cycle of IVF must be limited to two. Recently, the emphasis is on transferring a single good-quality embryo at the time of IVF.

Secondary Prevention

The methods of secondary prevention aim at reducing the occurrence of twin gestation and other higher order pregnancies, once the formation of multiple gestational sacs has already occurred. This method mainly involves the procedure of multifetal pregnancy reduction (MFPR). This

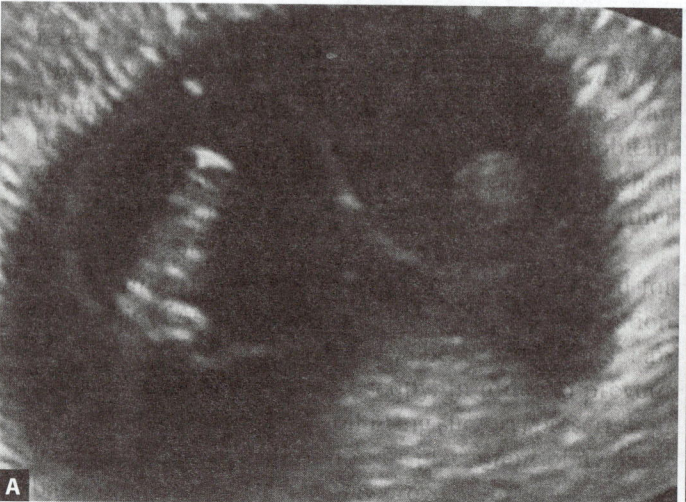 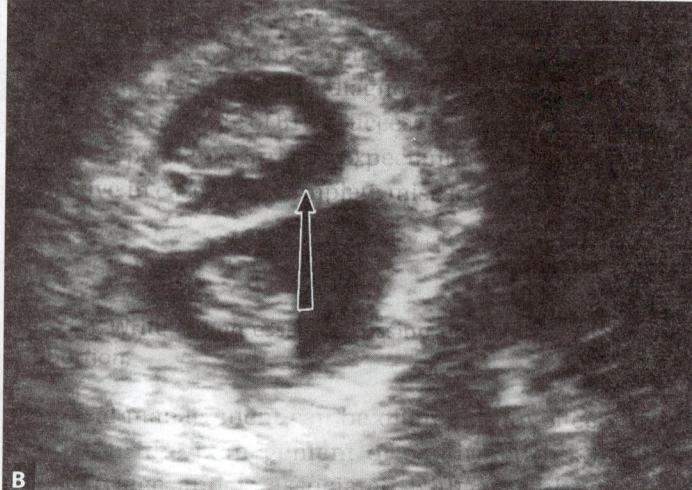

Figs. 9.17A and B: Early monochorionic diamniotic pregnancy. (A) The intertwin membrane is very thin and there is no "twin peak" sign; (B) Presence of T-sign is indicative of monochorionic pregnancy (arrow).

option, however, may not be acceptable to all individuals with a past history of infertility. MFPR is performed early in pregnancy, usually between 9 and 12 weeks. In this procedure, potassium chloride is injected into the selected fetuses under either a transabdominal or transvaginal ultrasound guidance. MFPR may be associated with many risks, including the miscarriage of remaining fetuses, emotional consequences for the parents, and rarely infection.

MANAGEMENT IN THE ANTENATAL PERIOD

Steps for Prevention of Preterm Labor

Women with multifetal gestation are at an increased risk for preterm delivery. Practices such as testing of fetal fibronectin levels or home uterine activity monitoring should not be used for predicting the risk of spontaneous preterm birth in these cases. There is little evidence regarding the usefulness of following strategies to avoid the risk of preterm labor: bed rest, administration of tocolytic agents, prophylactic cervical cerclage, weekly injections of 17-β hydroxyprogesterone caproate, etc.

According to the NICE (2022), guidelines for the use of corticosteroids for attaining pulmonary maturity in cases of multifetal gestation are same as that used for singleton gestation.

Increased Daily Requirement for Dietary Calories, Proteins, and Mineral Supplements

There is an increase in requirement for total dietary calories and proteins. There is an additional calorie requirement to the extent of 300 kcal/day above that required for a normal singleton gestation or 600 kcal more in comparison with the nonpregnant state. There is a requirement for increased iron and folic acid supplements in order to meet the demands of twin pregnancy. Iron requirement must be increased to the extent of 60–100 mg/day and folic acid to 1 mg/day. Calcium also needs to be prescribed above the requirements for a normal singleton gestation.

Increased Frequency of Antenatal Visits

Women with an uncomplicated dichorionic diamniotic twin pregnancy must be offered at least 8 antenatal appointments with a healthcare professional, of which at least 2 should be with the specialist obstetrician. Women with an uncomplicated monochorionic diamniotic twin pregnancy must be offered at least 11 antenatal appointments with a healthcare professional of which at least 2 should be with the specialist obstetrician.

Women with a triplet pregnancy must be offered anywhere between 9 and 11 antenatal appointments depending upon the amnionicity and chorionicity.

Attention should be focused on evaluation of blood pressure, proteinuria, uterine fundus height and fetal movements. The patient should be advised to maintain a daily fetal movement count chart (DFMC chart). The fetal growth should be monitored using an ultrasound examination every 3–4 weeks. Vaginal and bladder infections should be recognized and treated promptly to prevent the risk of preterm labor. The patient should be advised to stop doing extraneous activities and rest in the lateral decubitus position for a minimum of 2 hours each morning and afternoon.

Increased Fetal Surveillance

Since presence of multifetal gestation can produce numerous complications for the fetuses, which can result in significant neonatal morbidity and mortality, stringent fetal surveillance becomes mandatory. Failure of one or both fetuses to thrive must be identified. Fetal monitoring can be done with the help of following tests:

- *Assessment of amniotic fluid volume or index (AFI):* Associated oligohydramnios may be indicative of uteroplacental pathology and should be immediately followed-up by further tests for evaluation of fetal well-being. An AFI of < 8 cm (below the 5th percentile) or > 24 cm (above the 95th percentile) between the gestational ages of 28–40 weeks must be considered as abnormal.
- *Nonstress test or biophysical profile:* The nonstress test or biophysical profile is commonly used in the management of twins or higher-order multiple gestation.
- *Doppler evaluation of vascular resistance:* Increased resistance with diminished diastolic flow velocity on Doppler evaluation is often accompanied with intrauterine fetal growth restriction.

Monitoring for Complications of Monochorionic Multifetal Gestation

Women with monochorionic multifetal gestation must be offered simultaneous monitoring for complications such as feto-fetal transfusion syndrome, fetal growth restriction, and advanced-stage twin anemia polycythemia sequence (TAPS) during each ultrasound assessment. This would ensure effective monitoring for all complications of monochorionicity.

Screening for Chromosomal Disorders

Women with triplet pregnancy must be counseled regarding the greater likelihood for occurrence of chromosomal disorders such as Down's syndrome, Edwards' syndrome, and Patau's syndrome. They are also likely to be associated with increased false positive rates of screening tests, thereby resulting in an increased requirement for invasive testing and thereby increased occurrence of complications associated with this. These women should also be counseled regarding occurrence of physical and psychological risks in relation to selective fetal reduction if required.

Parameters such as nuchal translucency on ultrasound and maternal age should be used to screen for Down's Syndrome. Second trimester serum screening for Down's syndrome in triplet pregnancies should be preferably avoided.

Screening for structural abnormalities (especially cardiac abnormalities) must be offered in multifetal gestation, similar to routine ANC in a singleton pregnancy.

MANAGEMENT IN THE INTRAPARTUM PERIOD

Management in the intrapartum period is demonstrated in **Flowcharts 9.1A and B**. The following precautions need to be observed in the intrapartum period:
- Blood needs to be arranged and kept cross-matched.
- Pediatrician/anesthesiologist needs to be informed.
- An obstetrician skilled in intrauterine identification of fetal parts and in intrauterine manipulation of a fetus should be present.
- Patient should be advised to stay in bed as far as possible in order to prevent premature rupture of membranes.
- Labor should be monitored with help of a partogram and the heart rate of both the fetuses must be monitored preferably using a cardiotocogram. If the membranes have ruptured, the first twin can be monitored with help of internal cardiotocography, whereas the second twin can be monitored with help of external cardiotocography **(Fig. 9.18)**.
- Prophylactic administration of corticosteroids for attaining pulmonary maturity in cases of anticipated preterm deliveries.

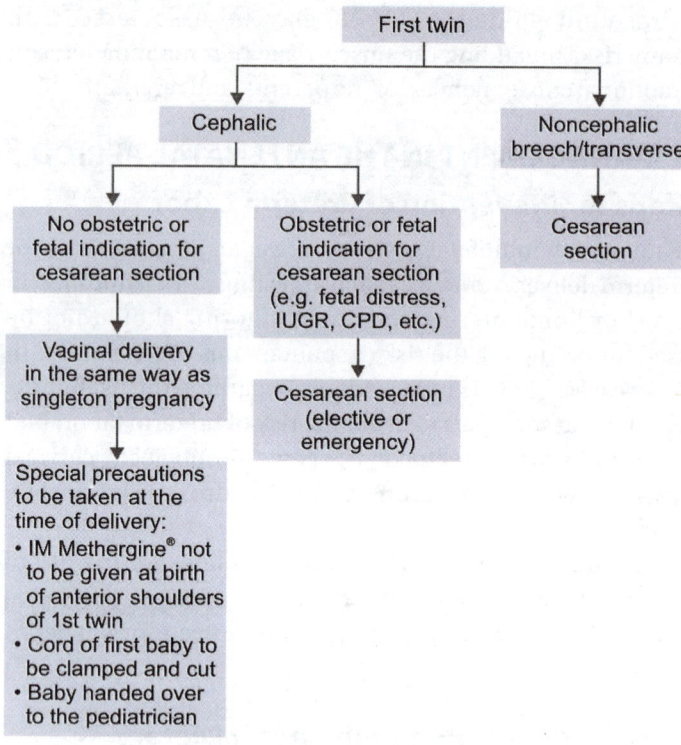

Flowchart 9.1A: Intrapartum management of first twin.

(CPD: cephalopelvic disproportion; IUGR: intrauterine growth retardation)

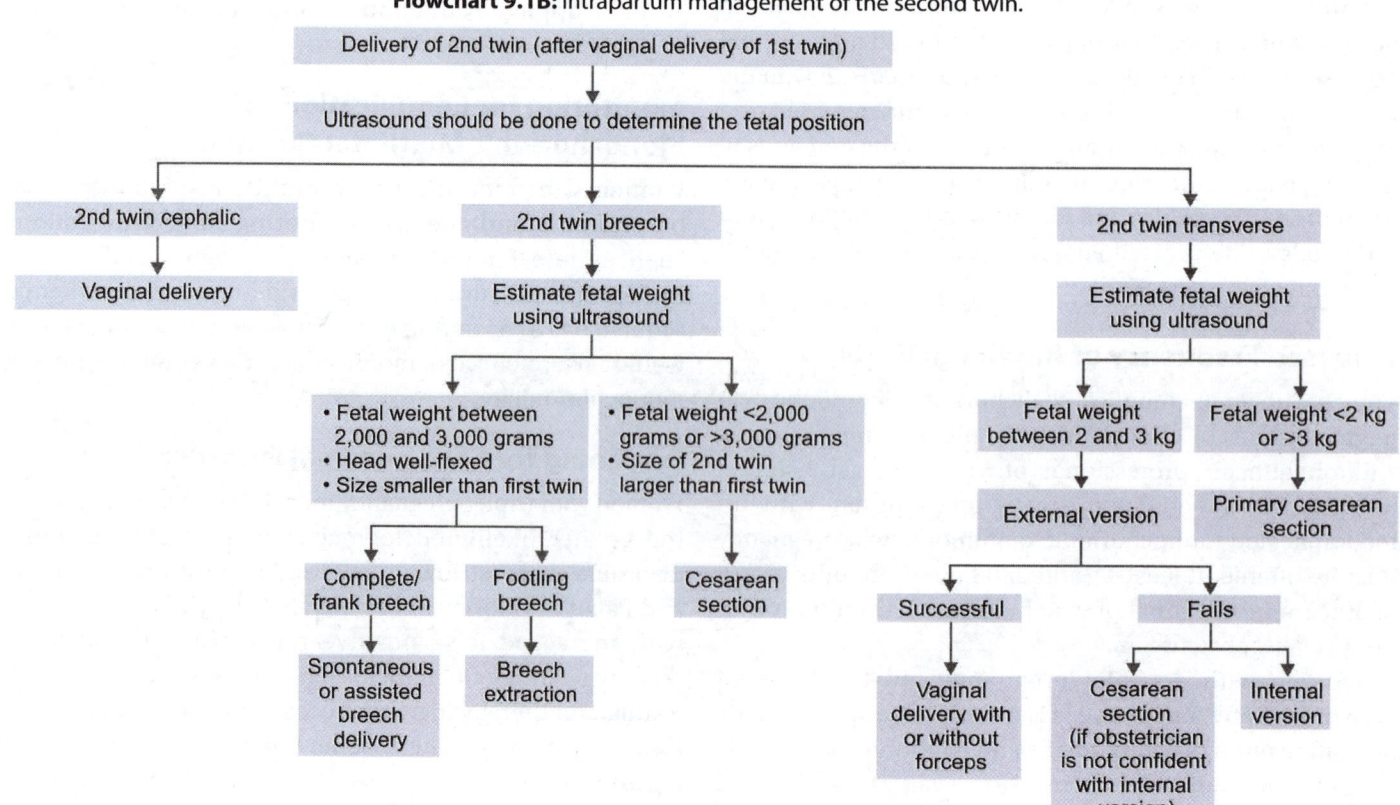

Flowchart 9.1B: Intrapartum management of the second twin.

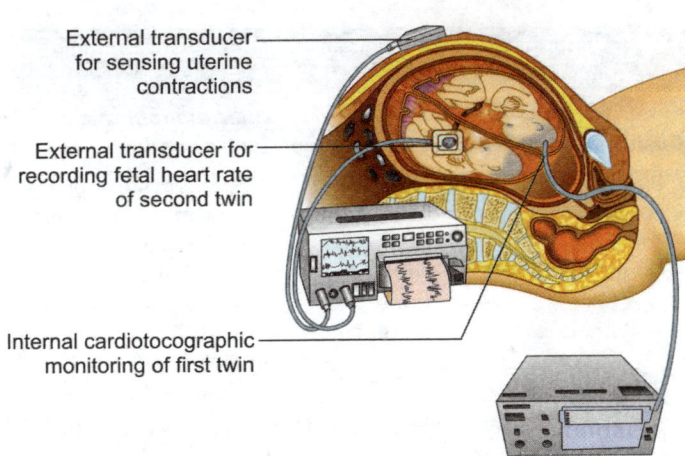

Fig. 9.18: Internal electronic monitoring of the first twin and external electronic monitoring of the second twin.

- Intravenous access in the mother must be established. In the absence of hemorrhage or metabolic disturbances during labor, lactated Ringer or an aqueous dextrose solution may be infused at a rate of 60–120 mL/h.
- Fetal trauma at the time of labor and delivery should be avoided.
- Expert neonatal care must be available.
- Epidural analgesia for relief from pain is preferred as it can be rapidly extended in caudal direction in case a procedure like internal podalic version or cesarean section is required.
- Vaginal examination must be performed soon after the rupture of membranes to exclude cord prolapse and to confirm the presentation of first twin.
- The labor ward where the deliveries of the babies have to take place should be equipped with fetal monitoring equipment. An ultrasonography machine should be readily available to help evaluate the position and status of the remaining fetus(es) after delivery of the first one.
- An experienced anesthesiologist should be immediately available in case some intrauterine manipulation or cesarean delivery is required.
- Two health care professionals (one obstetrician and one pediatrician) should be available for each anticipated fetus. At least one of these persons should be well-versed in neonatal resuscitation.

■ MANAGEMENT AT THE TIME OF DELIVERY

> **Q. What should be the anticipated time of delivery in the case study mentioned in the beginning of the chapter?**

Time of Delivery

Timings for offering planned birth based on the type of twin gestation are tabulated in **Table 9.3**.

An individualized assessment to determine the timing of planned birth must be done in women with any of the following:
- A complicated twin or triplet pregnancy

TABLE 9.3: Timings for offering planned birth based on the type of twin gestation.

Type of twin gestation	Timing for offering planned birth
Uncomplicated dichorionic diamniotic twin pregnancy	37 weeks
Uncomplicated monochorionic diamniotic twin pregnancy	36 weeks
Uncomplicated monochorionic monoamniotic twin pregnancy	32^{+0} and 33^{+6} weeks
Uncomplicated trichorionic triamniotic or dichorionic triamniotic triplet pregnancy	35 weeks

TABLE 9.4: Mode of delivery in case of twin gestation.

Type of twins	Mode of delivery
Both cephalic	Vaginal delivery
First twin cephalic, second twin noncephalic	The obstetrician needs to decide between vaginal delivery and cesarean delivery
First twin noncephalic, second twin cephalic	Cesarean section
Both twins noncephalic	Cesarean section

- A monochorionic triamniotic triplet pregnancy
- A triplet pregnancy that involves a shared amnion.

Mode of Delivery of Twins

Mode of delivery in case of twin gestation is summarized in **Table 9.4**. If both the twins are in cephalic presentation, delivery can usually be accomplished spontaneously or with help of forceps. The optimal route for delivery in case of first twin cephalic, second twin noncephalic presently remains controversial. When the EFW is > 1,500 g, vaginal delivery of a nonvertex second twin is reasonable. If the EFW is < 1,500 g, the vaginal delivery can still be tried based on clinical circumstances. According to the recommendations by the NICE guidelines (2019) cesarean delivery should be the method of choice when the first twin is in nanocephalic presentation. In case of first baby is in breech presentation, problems with vaginal delivery are most likely to occur in circumstances enumerated in **Box 9.2**. If one of these problems occurs or is anticipated to occur, cesarean delivery appears to be the most feasible option, except in cases where the fetus is dead or is not expected to live.

Indications for Vaginal Birth in Twin Gestation

Women with an uncomplicated dichorionic/monochorionic diamniotic twin pregnancy may be offered a vaginal mode of delivery in presence of the following:
- The pregnancy remains uncomplicated and has progressed beyond 32 weeks.

> **BOX 9.2:** Circumstances when the vaginal delivery in case of breech presentation are likely to result in several complications.
>
> - Fetus is unusually large and the aftercoming head of the breech is larger than the capacity of the birth canal
> - Fetus is sufficiently small so that the extremities and trunk are delivered through a cervix inadequately effaced and dilated to allow an easy delivery of the head
> - Prolapse of the umbilical cord

- There are no obstetric contraindications to labor.
- First baby is in a cephalic presentation.
- There is no significant size discordance between the twins.

Indications for Cesarean Section in Twin Gestation

Cesarean section is not required in routine clinical practice for every case of twin gestation. However, in case of presence of an obstetric or fetal indication as shown in **Table 9.5**, a cesarean delivery may be required.

There are some indications specific to twin gestation for cesarean section, which are as follows: monochorionic twins with twin-to-twin transfusion syndrome (TTTS); conjoined twins; locking of twins, etc. The locking of twins usually takes place when the first fetus presents as breech, whereas the second twin presents as cephalic presentation. The aftercoming head of the fetus in breech presentation locks between the neck and chin of the second fetus. Cesarean section is usually recommended in case the potential for locking is identified. Cesarean delivery must also be offered to the women with twin gestation in following circumstances **(Table 9.5)**.

- *Dichorionic/monochorionic diamniotic twin gestation:* Cesarean delivery in required in following circumstances:
  - First twin is not cephalic at the time of planned birth.
  - Women in established preterm labor between and to 32 weeks, the first twin is not cephalic.
- *Monochorionic monoamniotic twin gestation:* Cesarean delivery in required in following circumstances:
  - At the time of planned birth (between 32^{+0} and 33^{+6} weeks) or
  - Presence of any complication in her pregnancy requiring earlier delivery or
  - She is in established preterm labor, and there is a reasonable chance of survival of the babies as per their gestational age and the first twin is not in advanced labor so that the vaginal delivery appears imminent.
- *Triplet Pregnancy:* Cesarean delivery in required in following circumstances:
  - Planned birth at 35 weeks of gestation
  - Presence of any complication in her pregnancy requiring earlier delivery or
  - She is in established preterm labor, and there is a reasonable chance of survival of the babies based on their gestational age.

TABLE 9.5: Indication for cesarean section in cases of multiple gestation.

Obstetric indication	Fetal indication	Indication specific to twin gestation
• Placenta previa • Previous cesarean section • Contracted pelvis	• Twin with IUGR • First fetus with Noncephalic presentation	• First twin noncephalic, second twin cephalic • Both twins noncephalic • Monochorionic twins with TTTS • Locking of twins • Conjoined twins

(IUGR: intrauterine growth restriction; TTTS: twin-to-twin transfusion syndrome)

Most clinicians believe that pregnancies complicated by three or more fetuses are best delivered by cesarean section. Other clinicians believe that vaginal delivery may be safe under certain circumstances (e.g., all fetuses are in cephalic presentation). Vaginal delivery nowadays is usually reserved for those cases where fetal survival is not expected because of marked immaturity of fetuses or in cases where cesarean delivery is likely to result in maternal complications.

Precautions to be taken at the Time of Cesarean Delivery

> Q. What are precautions, which should be taken at the time of cesarean section in case of twins?

Precautions to be taken at the time of cesarean delivery in case of multifetal gestation are as follows:
- It is important to place patients in a left lateral tilt so as to deflect the uterine weight off the aorta to avoid hypotension.
- A transverse incision over the skin and uterus must be given liberally. The uterine incision should be large enough to allow atraumatic delivery of all the fetuses.
- It is important to ensure that the uterus remains well contracted during completion of the cesarean delivery and thereafter.
- The surgeon must remain vigilant regarding the remarkable blood loss, which may be concealed within the uterus and vagina during the time taken to close the incision. Appropriate precautions must be taken to prevent the occurrence of PPH.

Vaginal Delivery of the First Baby

- Delivery of the first baby in cephalic presentation should be conducted according to guidelines for normal pregnancy.
- Ergometrine is not to be given at the birth of first baby.
- Cord of the first baby should be clamped and cut to prevent exsanguination of the second twin in case communicating blood vessels between the two twins exist.

Delivery of Second Baby

The various types of twin presentations, which are possible, are shown in **Table 9.6**. The most common presentations at admission for delivery are cephalic-cephalic, cephalic-breech, and cephalic-transverse. After the delivery of the first baby, the following steps must be taken:

- An abdominal and vaginal examination should be performed to confirm the lie, presentation and FHS of the second baby. External version can be attempted at the time of abdominal examination, in case the lie is transverse.
- Vaginal examination also helps in diagnosing cord prolapse if present.
- If following the delivery of second twin, contractions do not resume within approximately 10 minutes, dilute oxytocin may be used to stimulate contractions.
- Monitoring of fetal heart rate of second twin and observation of mother for presence of vaginal bleeding must be performed.
- Vigilant monitoring in case of nonreassuring fetal heart rate or active vaginal bleeding is required. Hemorrhage may be indicative of placental abruption.

Timing the Delivery of Second Twin

According to the ACOG (1998), the interval between the deliveries of twins is not critical in determining the outcome of twins delivered. The obstetrician must still try to expedite the delivery of second twin as far as possible. However, an urgent delivery of the fetus is not required unless the conditions mentioned in **Box 9.3** are present.

Mode of Delivery of Second Twin

Depending on the presentation of second twin, various options can be adopted as shown in **Flowchart 9.1B**.

TABLE 9.6: Various types of twin presentations.

Types of twin presentation	Frequency
Both vertex	42%
1st vertex, 2nd breech	21%
1st breech, 2nd vertex	6%
1st and 2nd both breech	5%
1st vertex, 2nd transverse	18%
1st breech, 2nd transverse	4%
Both transverse	4%

BOX 9.3: Indications for urgent delivery of second twin.
- Severe bleeding per vaginum
- Cord prolapse of second baby
- Fetal distress of second baby
- Inadvertent use of intravenous ergometrine with the delivery of anterior shoulder of the first baby
- Delivery of the first baby under general anesthesia

Lie is Longitudinal

- *Cephalic:* Low rupture of membranes is done after fixing the presenting part on the pelvic brim. If the patient is not having good contractions, labor can be induced with help of syntocinon. If the head has reached pelvic brim, i.e., the head has engaged and is not progressing beyond this point, outlet forceps or vacuum can be applied.
- *Breech:* In case of breech presentation, delivery is completed by breech extraction (see Chapter 3).

Lie is Transverse

If the lie is transverse, external version must be attempted in order to correct the fetal lie. If the external version fails, internal version under general anesthesia can be attempted. The only indication for internal version in modern obstetrics is the transverse lie of second twin.

Technique for Internal Podalic Version

This technique has been described in Chapter 4. Following the delivery of the baby, routine exploration of the cervicovaginal canal must be done to exclude out any injuries.

Delivery of the Placenta

Following the delivery of the babies, placenta is delivered:
- Placental tissue must be examined carefully in order to determine the zygosity of the twins. If the dividing membrane between the two placentas is composed of two layers of chorion in between, surrounded by amnion on two sides, the zygosity is most likely dizygotic; even though monozygosity is possible.
- Cord blood is to be collected after delivery of both the twins.
- Determination of the blood group of the twins also helps in confirming the zygosity.

Management of Third Stage of Labor

There is an eminent risk for PPH due to uterine atony. Some of steps which can be taken to prevent PPH include the following:
- The options for managing the third stage of labor as well as the potential requirement for blood transfusion, including the need for intravenous access must be discussed with a woman having twin or triplet pregnancy well in advance, preferably by 28 weeks of pregnancy
- Intravenous methergine (0.2 mg) must not be administered with the delivery of anterior shoulder of first twin as this can result in the trapping of second twin inside the uterine cavity.
- However, intravenous methergine must be definitely administered with the delivery of anterior shoulder of the second twin. Oxytocin drip can be continued for about 1 hour following delivery.
- Delivery of placenta must be by controlled cord traction.

COMPLICATIONS

- Q. Discuss the complications of multiple pregnancy.
- Q. What is the cause for increased risk of PPH in twin gestation?
- Q. Why are women with multifetal gestation at an increased risk of development of gestational diabetes?
- Q. Write a long essay on the complications of multiple gestation.
- Q. With help of a long essay, discuss the diagnosis, treatment and outcome of TTTS.
- Q. Write a long note on acardiac twins.
- Q. Write a short essay on discordant twins.

MATERNAL COMPLICATIONS

During Antenatal Period

Multifetal gestation is associated with an increased frequency of pregnancy-related complications in the antenatal period such as:

- *Hypertensive disorders of pregnancy*: Since women with multifetal gestation are at a higher risk for development of hypertension, blood pressure must be measured, and urine tested for proteinuria to screen for hypertensive disorders at the time of each antenatal appointment. Women who are at high risk due to the presence of any of the following: hypertensive disease during a previous pregnancy, chronic kidney disease, autoimmune disease such as systemic lupus erythematosus or antiphospholipid syndrome, type 1 or type 2 diabetes, chronic hypertension, etc., must be advised to take low-dose aspirin in the dose of 75–150 mg daily from 12 weeks until the birth of the babies.
- Spontaneous abortion
- *Anemia:* Due to increased iron requirement by two fetuses, early appearance of anemia is a common complication. This problem can be avoided by increasing the dose of daily iron supplementation.
- *Fatty liver of pregnancy:* It is rare complication that occurs more often in multifetal than in singleton pregnancies.
- *Gestational diabetes:* Increased frequency of gestational diabetes in women with multifetal pregnancy is probably due to the large placental mass-producing large amount of human placental lactogen, a hormone, which is a competitive inhibitor of insulin action.
- Hyperemesis gravidarum
- Polyhydramnios
- Preeclampsia
- Antepartum hemorrhage
- Preterm labor
- Varicosities, dependent edema

During Labor

Multifetal gestation is also associated with a higher rate of complications during labor, such as:

- Fetal malpresentation
- Vasa previa
- Cord prolapse
- Premature separation of placenta, resulting in abruption placenta
- Cord entanglement
- *Postpartum hemorrhage:* Severe postpartum bleeding following the delivery of twin is usually the consequence of uterine atony due to large uterine size. Chances of perineal injury resulting from trauma are small due to small size of the babies. However, there is an increased use of instrumental delivery, which may be the cause of perineal injury and accompanying PPH.
- Dysfunctional uterine contractions
- Increased operative interference

Puerperium

Multifetal gestation can also result in a high rate of complications during the puerperium including complications like:

- Subinvolution
- Infection
- Failure of lactation

FETAL COMPLICATIONS

Fetal Complications due to Twin Gestation

- Miscarriage
- *Prematurity:* Premature labor (onset before 37 completed weeks of gestation) is the main risk of twin pregnancy, probably resulting from overstretching of the uterine cavity. The mean period of gestation for twins has been estimated as 37 weeks and for triplets as 31 weeks. The duration of gestation decreases as the number of fetuses increases.
- The most frequent neonatal complications of preterm birth are hypothermia, respiratory difficulties, persistent ductus arteriosus, intracranial bleeding, hypoglycemia, necrotizing enterocolitis, infections and retinopathy of prematurity, low birth weight babies, etc.
- *Congenital anomalies:* A 2–4 fold increase in the risk of congenital abnormalities has been found to be associated with multiple pregnancies (**Box 9.4**), especially the monozygotic twin pregnancies.
- Intrauterine death
- Intrauterine growth restriction often resulting in low birth weight babies
- Low birth weight babies due to IUGR and preterm delivery.

> **BOX 9.4:** Congenital malformations associated with multifetal gestation.
>
> *Defects resulting from twinning itself*
> - Conjoined twinning
> - Acardiac anomaly
> - Sirenomelia (involving fusion of the lower limbs)
> - Neural tube defects
> - Holoprosencephaly
>
> *Defects resulting from vascular interchange between monochorionic twins*
> - Twin-to-twin transfusion syndrome
> - Acardiac twin or twin reversed arterial perfusion syndrome
> - Twin embolization syndrome
> - Vascular connections resulting in dramatic blood pressure fluctuations may cause defects such as microcephaly, hydranencephaly, intestinal atresia, aplasia cutis, or limb amputation.
>
> *Defects that occur as the result of crowding*
> - Talipes equinovarus (clubfoot)
> - Congenital hip dislocation

FETAL COMPLICATIONS SPECIFIC TO TWIN GESTATION

Discordant Growth

Discordancy refers to the difference in growth rates between the two twins. Grade I discordant growth indicates a difference of 15–20%, whereas grade II discordant growth indicates a difference of >25%. As a result of discordant growth, there can be discrepancy in the weight of the two twins and a discrepancy of 20% or more is usually considered to be significant. The smaller twin is at high risk for perinatal complications. Discordancy is evaluated by using the larger twin as the index and can be calculated using the following formula:

Birth weight discordancy =
$$\frac{\text{Weight of the larger twin} - \text{Weight of the smaller twin}}{\text{Weight of the larger twin}} \times 100$$

- The causes of discordant growth may include factors such as unequal placental mass, genetic syndromes (neural tube defects, cardiac abnormalities, chromosomal defects, etc.) and TTTS. While discordant growth due to unequal placental mass or genetic syndromes can occur in both monochorionic and dichorionic twins that due to TTTS is largely limited to monochorionic twins.
- The earlier in pregnancy, the discordancy develops, more serious is the sequelae. Also, as the weight difference within a twin pair increases, perinatal mortality increases proportionately.
- Several ultrasound criteria have been used to diagnose discordant twin growth before birth. Recently, the criteria used most frequently for diagnosis is a difference of 15–25% in EFW.
- Diagnostic monitoring for fetal weight discordance must be offered to women with a monochorionic twin or triplet pregnancy. This can be done using 2 or more biometric parameters along with the assessment of amniotic fluid levels at the time of ultrasound scan from 16 weeks of gestation onward.
- For assessment of amniotic fluid levels, deepest vertical pocket (DVP) must be measured on either side of the amniotic membrane.
- Diagnostic monitoring can be initially done at biweekly intervals and can be later increased to weekly intervals. This must also include umbilical artery Doppler assessment for each baby, if the weight discordance is 20% or more and/or the EFW of any of the babies is below the 10th centile for gestational age.
- In case of fetal weight discordance of 25% or more and if the EFW of any of the babies is below the 10th centile for gestational age, the woman must be referred to a tertiary level fetal medicine center because these are clinically important indicators for selective fetal growth restriction.
- Urgent delivery is usually not required for size discordancy per se.

Abnormalities Specific to Monozygotic Twins

Spectrum of abnormalities associated with monozygotic, specifically monoamniotic twin include the following:
- Abnormal vascular communication between twins, resulting in TTTS
- Conjoined twins
- Acardiac twins or twin reversed arterial perfusion (TRAP) syndrome
- *External parasitic twin:* In this abnormality, the defective fetus or merely a part of it is attached externally to a relatively normal twin.
- *Fetus-in-fetu:* In this abnormality, one fetus may be enfolded inside the other twin. Normal development of this twin is arrested early in first trimester.

Monoamniotic twins form nearly 1% of all twin gestations. Monoamniotic twins are associated with a high rate of complications such as cord entanglement, TTTS, preterm births, and congenital malformations. Rarely, diamniotic twins can get converted into monoamniotic twins due to the rupture of the intervening membrane.

Twin-to-Twin Transfusion

This is a rare complication that can occur in monozygotic monochorionic diamniotic twins, which cause the blood to pass from one twin to the other (**Figs. 9.19A and B**). This usually occurs due to the presence of placental vascular communication. The placental vascular anastomoses responsible for the development of TTTS could be from artery-to-artery (A-A); artery-to-vein (A-V); or from vein-to-vein (V-V) (**Fig. 9.20**). As a result of the vascular communication, one of the twins, which donates blood (donor twin) becomes thin and undernourished, while the other twin who receives blood (recipient twin) grows at

182 Complications of Pregnancy

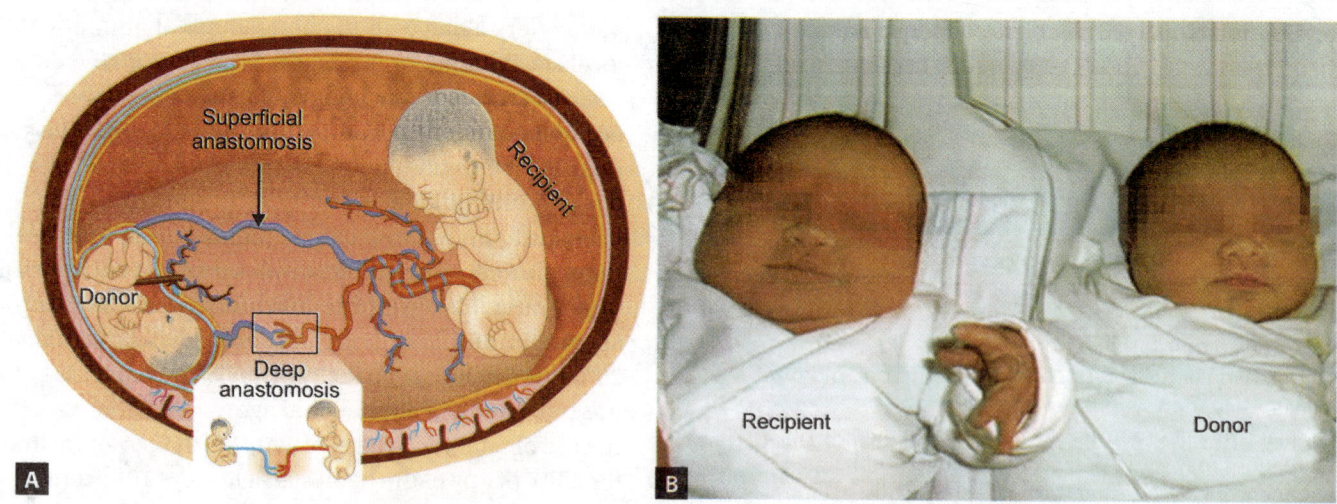

Figs. 9.19A and B: Twin-to-twin transfusion syndrome. (A) Diagrammatic representation; (B) The donor and recipient immediately following the delivery.

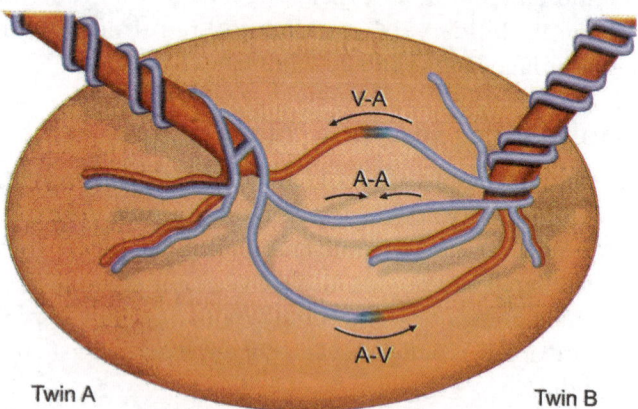

Fig. 9.20: Diagrammatic representation of placenta showing arteriovenous anastomosis.

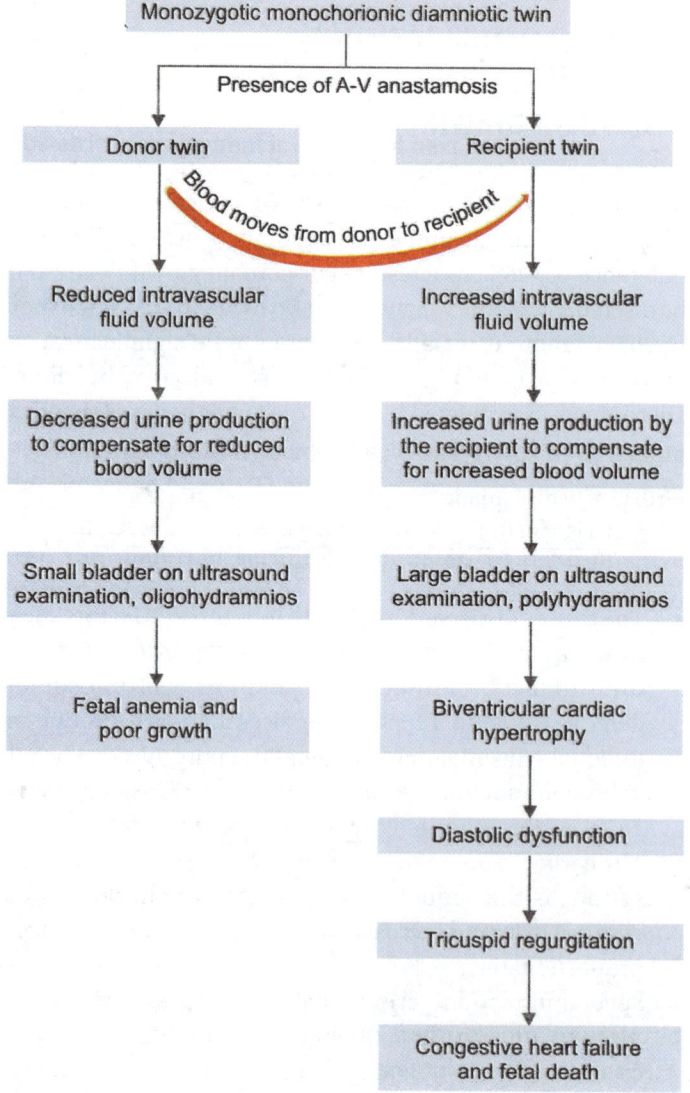

Flowchart 9.2: Pathogenesis of twin-to-twin transfusion syndrome.

the expense of donor twin. The donor twin in TTTS usually shows poor growth, oliguria, anemia and hyperproteinemia, low or absent liquor, resulting in development of oligohydramnios, etc. **(Flowchart 9.2)**.

With the severe disease, the donor may not produce any urine, resulting in oligohydramnios and nonvisualization of urinary bladder on ultrasound examination. In these cases, the twin may become wrapped by its amniotic membrane, resulting in the formation of a "stuck" twin **(Fig. 9.21)**. On the other hand, the recipient twin shows polyuria, polyhydramnios, and an enlarged urinary bladder. In the long run, this twin frequently develops polycythemia, biventricular cardiac hypertrophy, and diastolic dysfunction with tricuspid regurgitation. The death of this twin eventually occurs due to congestive heart failure.

Ultrasound Findings

The fundamental diagnostic criterion in TTTS is the finding of oligohydramnios in one twin and polyhydramnios in the other twin belonging to monochorionic twin gestation. The criterion for the diagnosis of oligohydramnios is no fluid or a pocket of fluid < 2 cm in its largest diameter. The criterion for the diagnosis of polyhydramnios is a pocket of fluid 8 cm or more in its largest diameter. Almost 80–90% of cases of

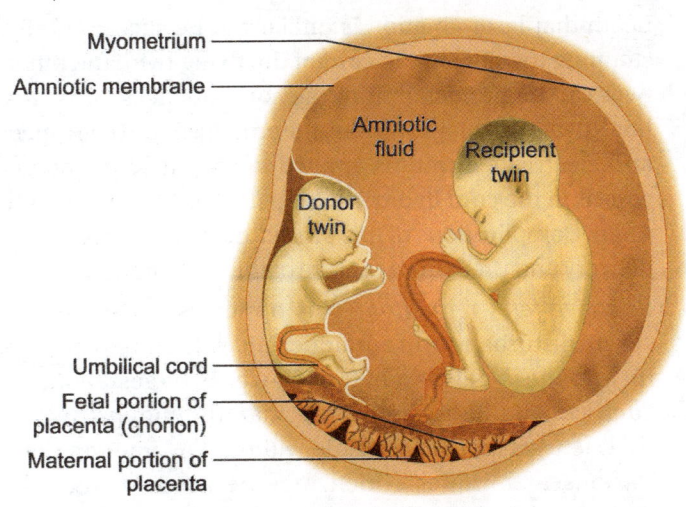

Fig. 9.21: Stuck twin syndrome.

> **BOX 9.5:** Sonographic criteria for the diagnosis of twin-to-twin transfusion syndrome.
>
> - Monochorionic twins
> - Twins having same gender
> - Presence of hydramnios (defined as the largest vertical pocket > 8 cm) in one twin and oligohydramnios (defined as the largest vertical pocket is < 2 cm) in the other twin
> - Discrepancy in the size of umbilical cord between the two twins
> - Cardiac dysfunction in the recipient twin along with the presence of hydramnios
> - Abnormal findings on the Doppler velocimetry of umbilical vessels or ductus venosus
> - Significant discordance of growth amongst the twins

TTTS if left untreated, prior to 24 weeks of gestation are associated with the loss of one or both twins. In case death of one of the twins occurs, the blood vessel connections in the placenta can place the surviving twin at risk for long-term brain damage. Sonographic criteria for the diagnosis of TTTS as proposed by Harkness and Crombleholme (2005) are described in **Box 9.5**.

Quintero Stages of TTTS

- *Stage I:* A small amount of amniotic fluid (oligohydramnios) is found around the donor twin and a large amount of amniotic fluid (polyhydramnios) is found around the recipient twin. However, some urine is still visible sonographically within the donor twin's bladder.
- *Stage II:* In addition to the presence of above findings, there is absence of urine in the bladder of donor twin on ultrasound examination. In these cases, laser photocoagulation may be helpful.
- *Stage III:* In addition to the characteristics of stages I and II, Doppler studies are critically abnormal. Critically abnormal Doppler studies are defined as absent/reverse end-diastolic velocity in the umbilical artery, reverse flow in the ductus venosus, or pulsatile flow in the umbilical vein, ductus venosus, or umbilical artery. Laser photocoagulation is recommended in this situation.
- *Stage IV:* In addition to all of the above findings, the recipient twin shows evidence of heart failure, ascites, or fetal hydrops. Laser photocoagulation may be attempted, but the chance of survival in this stage is much lower.
- *Stage V:* In addition to all of the above findings, one of the twins has died. Usually, the donor twin is the first to die, but death can occur first in either of the twins.

Treatment Options

- Monitoring for feto-fetal transfusion syndrome must be done by visualizing the amniotic membrane within the measurement image using ultrasound. The DVP of amniotic fluid on either side of the amniotic membrane must be measured.
- The woman must be referred to a tertiary level fetal medicine center if the diagnosis of TTTS is made based on difference in DVP of two amniotic sacs, i.e., the amniotic sac of 1 baby has a DVP depth of <2 cm and the amniotic sac of another baby has a DVP depth of over 8 cm before 20^{+0} weeks of pregnancy or over 10 cm from 20^{+0} weeks onward.
- Diagnostic monitoring for feto-fetal transfusion syndrome must be done on a weekly basis for women in their second and third trimesters if there are concerns about differences between the babies' amniotic fluid level (a difference in DVP depth of 4 cm or more). In these cases, Doppler assessment of the umbilical artery flow for each baby must also be included in the scan.
- Monochorionic multifetal pregnancies which are complicated by feto-fetal transfusion syndrome (treated with fetoscopic laser therapy), or selective fetal growth restriction, must be offered weekly ultrasound monitoring from 16 weeks of pregnancy using middle cerebral artery peak systolic velocity (MCA-PSV) to detect more advanced stage of twin anemia polycythemia sequence (TAPS).
- The various therapies that are presently available, either involve balancing the fluid volumes between the two sacs or interrupting the communication of blood vessels between the twins. The treatment options that are currently available are described below in details.
- *Reduction amniocentesis:* Serial amniocentesis involves the removal of the excessive amount of amniotic fluid from the sac of the recipient twin through the process of amniocentesis. This technique may be useful for milder cases of TTTS that occur later in pregnancy. The procedure is generally not thought to be effective for more advanced stages of TTTS (stages III and IV). As a general rule no > 5 L of amniotic fluid is removed at any one time. The procedure is usually by completed within 30 minutes or less. However, the procedure may only temporarily restore the balance in the amniotic fluid in both twins' sacs as the fluid levels may

return back within a few days. Thus, the procedure might require to be repeated after every few days. The procedure of repeated amniocenteses for the treatment of TTTS can result in numerous complications such as premature labor, premature rupture of the membranes, and rarely infection or an abruption. Pregnancies managed with serial reduction amniocentesis on an average deliver by 29–30 weeks of gestation.

- *Septostomy (microseptostomy):* Septostomy involves the creation of a hole in the membrane between the fetal sacs using a needle. This causes the movement of the fluid from the amniotic sac of the donor into the sac with absent or low fluid (recipient's sac). Though the risk for complications such as infection, premature labor, and premature rupture of the membranes are rare, septostomy does carry the additional potential risk for the hole between the two sacs to become too large. Sometimes, it can cause the entire separating membrane to get disrupted, allowing the babies to share the same amniotic space. In the worst case, this could result in entanglement of the umbilical cords of the two twins, resulting in the death of one or both the fetuses. However, the advantage of septostomy over amnioreduction is that the patients undergoing septostomy typically require fewer procedures in comparison to those treated with amnioreduction.
- *Selective laser ablation of the placental anastomotic vessels:* In more advanced stages of TTTS (stage II and higher), ablation of the communicating vessels on the placental surface using laser beams under ultrasound guidance can act as a curative procedure. A fetoscope is introduced in the amniotic cavity after administration of adequate anesthesia to the patient in order to directly visualize the blood vessels on the surface of the placenta. Vessels that are found to communicate between the twins are then ablated using laser light energy. Being a more invasive procedure in comparison to amnioreduction or septostomy, laser ablation is associated with a higher risk of complications such as premature contractions, premature rupture of the membranes (15–20% of cases), placental separation (2%), and infection. In order to prevent these complications, tocolytics to prevent uterine contractions and antibiotics to prevent infection may be given both before and after the procedure. In addition, laser therapy may be associated with unique risks since the laser energy may cause certain areas of the placenta or blood vessels on the surface of the placenta to bleed. Therefore, after laser therapy, close ongoing maternal and fetal surveillance is necessary.
- *Selective cord coagulation:* In this procedure, under ultrasound guidance, one of the twins is purposefully sacrificed in order to save the life of other twin. This procedure is used when laser ablation of the connecting vessels is not possible or if one of the twins is so close to death that laser ablation is unlikely to be successful. By stopping the flow in the cord of the dying twin, the other twin can be protected from the consequences of its sibling's death. In this procedure, the umbilical cord is grasped and electrical current is applied to coagulate the blood vessels in the cord in order to stop the blood flow through them. Complications of this procedure include premature delivery and premature rupture of the membranes.
- *Selective fetal reduction:* This option is considered if severe disturbances in amniotic fluid volume and growth disturbances develop before 20 weeks of gestation. In such cases, due to shared circulation amongst twins, both fetuses typically will die without any intervention. Various techniques which may be used for feticide include injection of an occlusive substance into the selected twin's umbilical vein or radiofrequency ablation, fetoscopic ligation, laser coagulation of one umbilical cord. Despite these procedures, other fetus remains at appreciable risk.

Neurological Damage

Abnormal vascular communication between twins could be responsible for causing neurological complications such as cerebral palsy, microcephaly, porencephaly, and multicystic encephalomalacia. This is usually caused by ischemia. In the donor, ischemia can result from hypotension or anemia, while in the recipient this can develop from blood pressure instability and episodes of severe hypotension.

Acardiac Twin or Twin Reversed Arterial Perfusion Syndrome (TRAP)

This is an unusual form of TTTS, occurring in about 1 in 15,000 pregnancies. In these monochorionic twins, one twin develops normally while the other twin fails to develop a heart as well as other body structures. This abnormal twin, called an acardiac fetus, shows characteristic features, in which the cardiac structures are absent or nonfunctioning and the head, upper body and upper extremities are poorly developed.

The lower body and lower extremities are, however, more or less normal. The acardiac twin acts as a recipient and depends on the normal donor (pump) twin for obtaining its blood supply via transplacental anastomoses and retrograde perfusion of the acardiac umbilical cord. Perfusion of the malformed (acardiac) fetus occurs via A-A and V-V anastomoses between the fetuses. The perfusion pressure of the donor twin overpowers that in the recipient twin, who thus receives reverse blood flow from its twin sibling. Deoxygenated umbilical arterial blood from the donor, thus, flows into the umbilical artery of the recipient, with its direction reversed. In these pregnancies, the umbilical cord from the acardiac twin branches directly from the umbilical cord of the normal twin. This blood flow is reversed from the normal direction leading to the name for this condition—TRAP syndrome **(Figs. 9.22A to C)**. As a result, there is better perfusion of the lower part of the deformed body. On the other hand, the upper part of the body, showing lack of head, heart, and upper extremities remains poorly perfused. Normal twin (donor) eventually develops high-output failure because it is responsible for maintaining the circulation of both the twins. Thus, the circulatory load of the donor twin may become extremely large resulting in heart failure.

Das (1902) established four categories of acardiac twins based on their physical appearance **(Table 9.7)**. There is controversy surrounding the use of these traditional four categories because some cases are so complex that they may not fit into one of Das' four categories.

Doppler verification of reversed flow in the umbilical cord of the acardiac fetus helps confirms the diagnosis. In some cases, the blood flow from the pump twin to the acardiac twin stops on its own and the acardiac twin stops growing. In other cases, the flow continues and the acardiac twin continues to increase in size. This eventually leads to heart failure and polyhydramnios in the pump twin. Without treatment, >50% of cases of TRAP will result in the death of the pump twin. Radiofrequency ablation of a major blood vessel in the acardiac fetus often serves as the therapeutic strategy of choice. This procedure helps in stopping the blood flow and as a result the pump twin (normal twin) has to no longer send the blood to the acardiac twin.

Conjoined Twins

Conjoined twins are the least common form of monozygotic twinning, which is always associated with monochorionic monoamniotic twins. Detailed description of conjoined twins has been done earlier in the text.

Death of One Fetus

In case of death of one of the fetuses, prognosis for the surviving twin depends on the gestational age at the time of the demise, the chorionicity, and the length of time between the demise and delivery of the surviving twin. Early demise of one of the fetuses, such as in case of "vanishing twin" does not appear to increase the risk of death in the surviving fetus after the first trimester. However, the death of

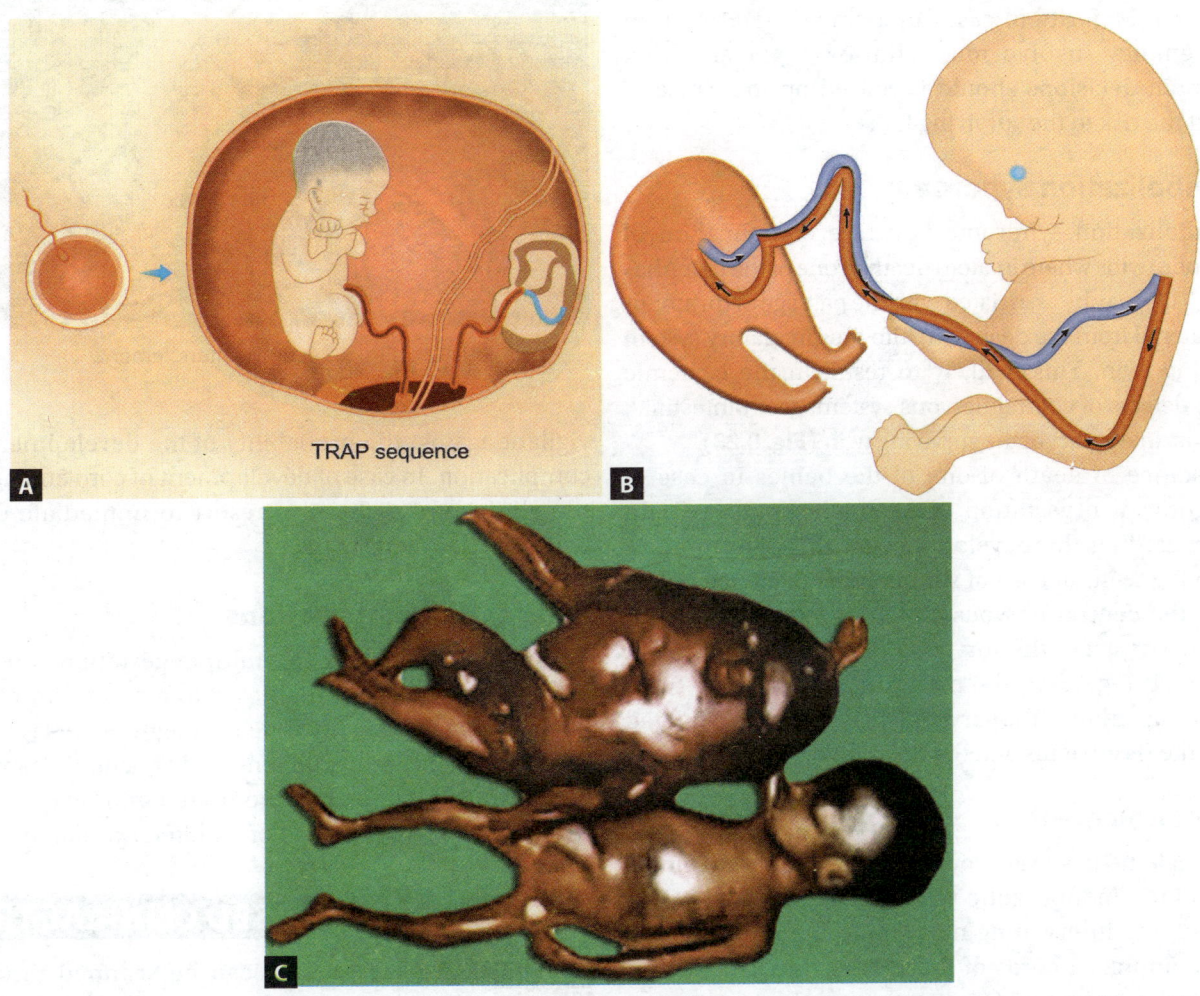

Figs. 9.22A to C: Twin reversed arterial perfusion (TRAP). (A) Diagram showing the TRAP syndrome; (B) Perfusion of the acardiac twin in a retrograde manner with poorly oxygenated blood which should have been delivered to the placenta; (C) Computerized generation of image showing a normal twin and an acardiac twin with poorly developed cephalic end.

TABLE 9.7: Different types of acardiac twins based on Das classification.	
Type of acardiac twin	Characteristics
Acardius acephalus	The most common type of acardiac twin where there is failure or disrupted growth of the head. They may have an underdeveloped skull base. They have legs, but do not have arms
Acardius myelacephalus/ acardius anceps	The most developed form of acardiac twin, it has partially developed head with brain tissues and facial structures and identifiable limbs. This type of acardiac twin is associated with a high risk for complications in the normal twin
Acardius amorphous	Failure of any recognizable structure or human organs. This fetus appears as a disorganized mass of tissues containing skin, bone, cartilage, muscle, fat, blood vessels, etc.
Acardius acormus	The rarest type of acardiac twin, which presents as an isolated head with no body development

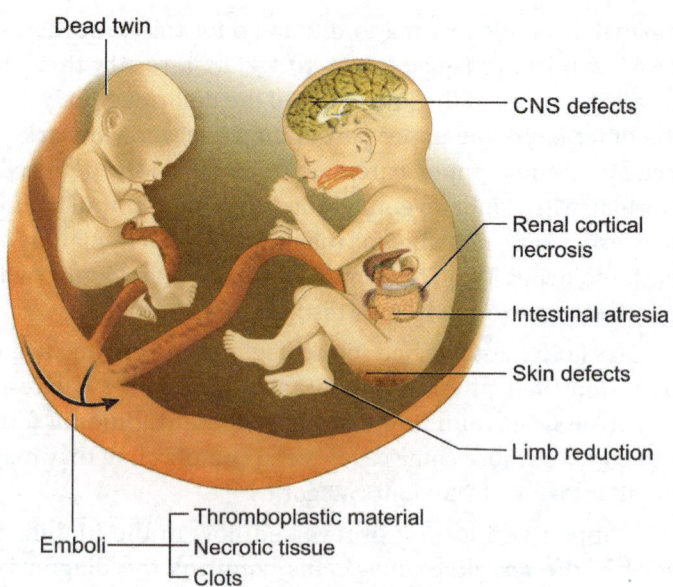

Fig. 9.23: Twin embolization syndrome.

one of multiple fetuses later in gestation could theoretically trigger coagulation defects in the mother resulting in the development of twin embolization syndrome, (explained next in text). Majority of cases of a single fetal death in twin pregnancy involve monochorionic placentation. Management decisions should be based on the cause of death and the risk to the surviving fetus.

Twin Embolization Syndrome

Twin embolization syndrome is a rare complication of monozygotic twins where in utero death of one of the twins has occurred. This may be associated with the passage of thromboplastic material from the dead twin into the circulatory system of surviving twin. This is likely to result in the ischemic structural defects of central nervous system, gastrointestinal, and genitourinary tract of the surviving twin **(Fig. 9.23)**.

In instance of death of one of the babies in case of monozygotic twin gestation, the clinician must remain vigilant regarding the development of this syndrome in the surviving twin. In case of sonographic evidence of any defect in the central nervous system, gastrointestinal or genitourinary tract of the surviving twin, the parents must be counseled regarding the prognosis of surviving twin. Medical termination of the surviving twin can be considered based on the risk to fetus and the decision of parents.

Cord Entanglement

Cord entanglement is a rare complication of monochorionic monoamniotic monozygotic twin pregnancy. Due to the absence of any intervening membrane between the two twins, the umbilical cords of these twins are likely to get entangled with each other **(Fig. 9.24)**.

Doppler ultrasound may help in confirming the diagnosis of cord entanglement. The clinician must remain

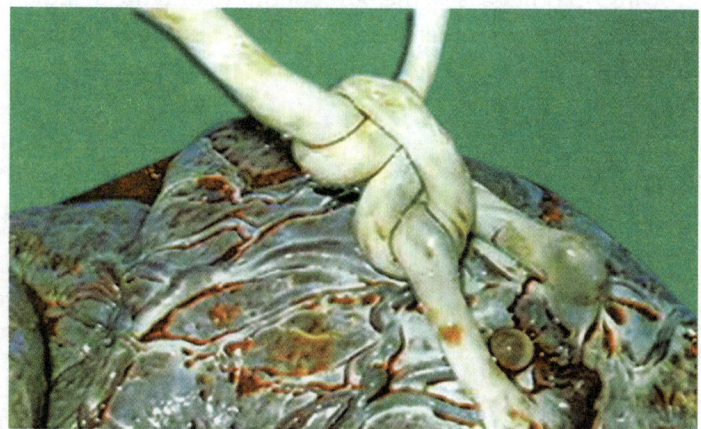

Fig. 9.24: Cord entanglement.

vigilant against the probability of the development of this complication. In case of development of cord entanglement, the clinician may have to resort to immediate cesarean delivery, to save the twins.

Long-term Complications

Complications related to multiple gestations do not end with the birth of the babies. Long-term complications like language and speech delay, cognitive delay or motor problems, behavioral problems, and difficulty in parent-child interactions all appear to be more commonly associated with babies born as a result of multifetal gestation.

EVIDENCE-BASED CLINICAL TRIALS

 List of references can be scanned through QR code to enable the readers gain deeper insight of the subject by referring to the entire article or its abstract.

CHAPTER 10

Rh-Negative Pregnancy

CASE STUDY

A 34-year-old patient (Rh negative, G3P2A0L1) with history of previous pregnancy being affected by anemia presents for antenatal checkup. She gives history of receiving some kind of injection related to Rh-negative blood (probably Rh immunoglobulins) in the previous pregnancy.

INTRODUCTION

Blood groups were discovered by Landsteiner. Two major classification systems are used for grouping blood. They are based on the presence of different antigens in the blood cells. These systems are the "ABO system" and the "Rhesus (Rh) system."

ABO CLASSIFICATION

According to the ABO system, the blood groups can be classified as blood groups A, B, AB, and O **(Table 10.1)**.

Blood Group A

People with blood group A contain antigen A in their blood cells and antibody anti-B in their plasma. They can receive and give blood to people with blood group A only (provided they are compatible for Rh factor).

Blood Group B

People with blood group B contain antigen B in their blood cells and antibody anti-A in their plasma. They can receive and give blood to people with blood group B only (provided they are compatible for Rh factor).

Blood Group AB

People with blood group AB contain both antigens A and B in their blood cells and none of the antibodies in their plasma. They are known as "universal recipients" as they can receive blood from any person belonging to any of the ABO groups (with matching Rh status). This is so as their blood does not contain any antibodies, so there cannot be any reaction with any of the antigens present in the donor's blood.

Blood Group O

People with blood group O contain none of the antigens (A or B) in their blood cells but contain both the antibodies (anti-A and anti-B) in their plasma. They are known as "universal donors" as they can donate their blood to a person belonging to any of the ABO groups (with matching Rh status). Thus, people with O blood type can donate blood to people with blood groups A, B, AB, or O (however, compatibility with other antigens like Rh needs to be matched). This is so as their blood does not contain any antigens, hence there is no reaction with any antibodies present in the recipient's blood.

RHESUS CLASSIFICATION

> **Q. Can Rh-positive ABO compatible blood be transfused to an Rh-negative individual?**

After the ABO blood group system, the next most important blood group system is the Rh blood group system.

TABLE 10.1: ABO system and blood groups.

Blood group	RBC antigen	Plasma antibody	RBC choice	Plasma choice
A	A	Anti-B	A, O	A, AB
B	B	Anti-A	B, O	B, AB
AB	A, B	None	A, B, AB, O	AB
O	None	Anti-A, anti-B	O	O, A, B, AB

Complications of Pregnancy

TABLE 10.2: Rh system and blood grouping.

Rh group	Rh antigen	Rh antibody	RBC choice	Plasma choice
Rh positive	D positive	None	Positive or negative	Either
Rh negative	D negative	Anti-D	Negative	Either

Though the Rh system contains five main antigens (C, c, D, E, and e), antigen D is considered to be the most immunogenic. There is no specific antiserum for "D" antigen. The letter "D" indicates the absence of a discernible allelic product. According to the Rh classification, the blood groups can be basically classified as Rh positive and Rh negative **(Table 10.2)**.

The major Rh system antigen is the D antigen and it is found in 85% of the population. Anti-D antibodies are IgG antibodies that bind to the surface of the red cells, resulting in deformation of cells. These deformed red cells are then sequestered in the spleen, resulting in delayed extravascular hemolysis. It is now known that the Rh system is very complex, and there are other antigens besides D antigen. Some important Rh antigens include C, D, and E. Since there are two possible alleles for each antigen—c or C, d or D, and e or E, one haplotype consisting of c/C, d/D, and e/E is inherited from each parent. The resulting Rh type of the individual depends on their inherited genotype. The haplotypes are given a code based on the Fisher system in **Table 10.3**. If an individual's Rh genotype contains at least one of the C, D, E antigens, they are Rh positive. Only individuals with the genotype cde/cde (rr) are Rh negative. For blood transfusion purposes, donors possessing C or E, even in Rh genotypes r'r (Cde/cde) and r"r (cdE/cde), are classified as Rh positive. Thus, based on Rh classification system, two main types of blood groups are possible: Rh positive and Rh negative. The prevalence of Rh-negative pregnancies in India varies between 5% and 10%. However, the risk of alloimmunization in the population is only 16%. The rest 84% population may be protected from alloimmunization due to the following:

- 30% of the population may be nonresponders.
- Size of the FMH may be small.
- There may be ABO incompatibility.
- Husband may be heterozygous for Rh antigen due to which the baby may be Rh negative.

Rh Positive

Rh-positive people contain Rh antigen in their blood cells. RBCs of such individuals are agglutinated by antiserum against D antigen.

Rh Negative

Rh-negative people do not contain Rh antigens in their blood cells. RBCs of such individuals are not agglutinated by the antiserum. Individuals with Rh-negative blood normally

TABLE 10.3: Haplotypes for three rhesus antigens.

Haplotype	Fisher system	Rh status
CDe	R1	Rh positive
cDE	R2	Rh positive
CDE	Rz	Rh positive
cDe	R0	Rh positive
Cde	r'	Rh positive
cdE	r"	Rh positive
CdE	Ry	Rh positive
cde	r	Rh negative

do not have antibodies against Rh antigens. However, these people may develop "anti-Rh" antibodies if they receive exposure to Rh antigens (e.g., transfusion of Rh-positive blood in a person with Rh-negative status). Thus, people with Rh-positive blood can safely receive blood from people with Rh-negative blood. However, people with Rh-negative blood must not receive blood from Rh-positive people as they will develop anti-Rh antibodies on receiving Rh-positive blood. If these people receive Rh-positive blood the second time, there will be a reaction between the Rh antigens of the donor and the anti-Rh antibodies already present in the recipient.

The above-mentioned scenario can also occur in Rh-negative women if they bear an Rh-positive child. Therefore, transfusion of Rh-positive, ABO compatible blood products should always be avoided in Rh-negative women of childbearing age to prevent the formation of anti-D antibodies prior to pregnancy. However, inevitable Rh incompatibility occurs when Rh-negative mother carries an Rh-positive child.

Rh INCOMPATIBILITY DISEASE

Due to difference in blood groups between the mother and fetus, two types of incompatibility diseases can occur: Rh incompatibility disease **(Flowchart 10.1)** and ABO incompatibility disease. Both diseases have similar symptoms, but Rh disease is much more severe, because anti-Rh antibodies cross over the placenta more readily than anti-A or anti-B antibodies. Rh incompatibility may develop when a woman with Rh-negative blood marries a man with Rh-positive blood and conceives a fetus with Rh-positive blood group (who has inherited the Rh factor gene from the father). Rh-positive fetal RBCs from the fetus leak across the placenta and enter the woman's circulation. Throughout the pregnancy, small amounts of fetal blood can enter the maternal circulation (fetomaternal hemorrhage or FMH),

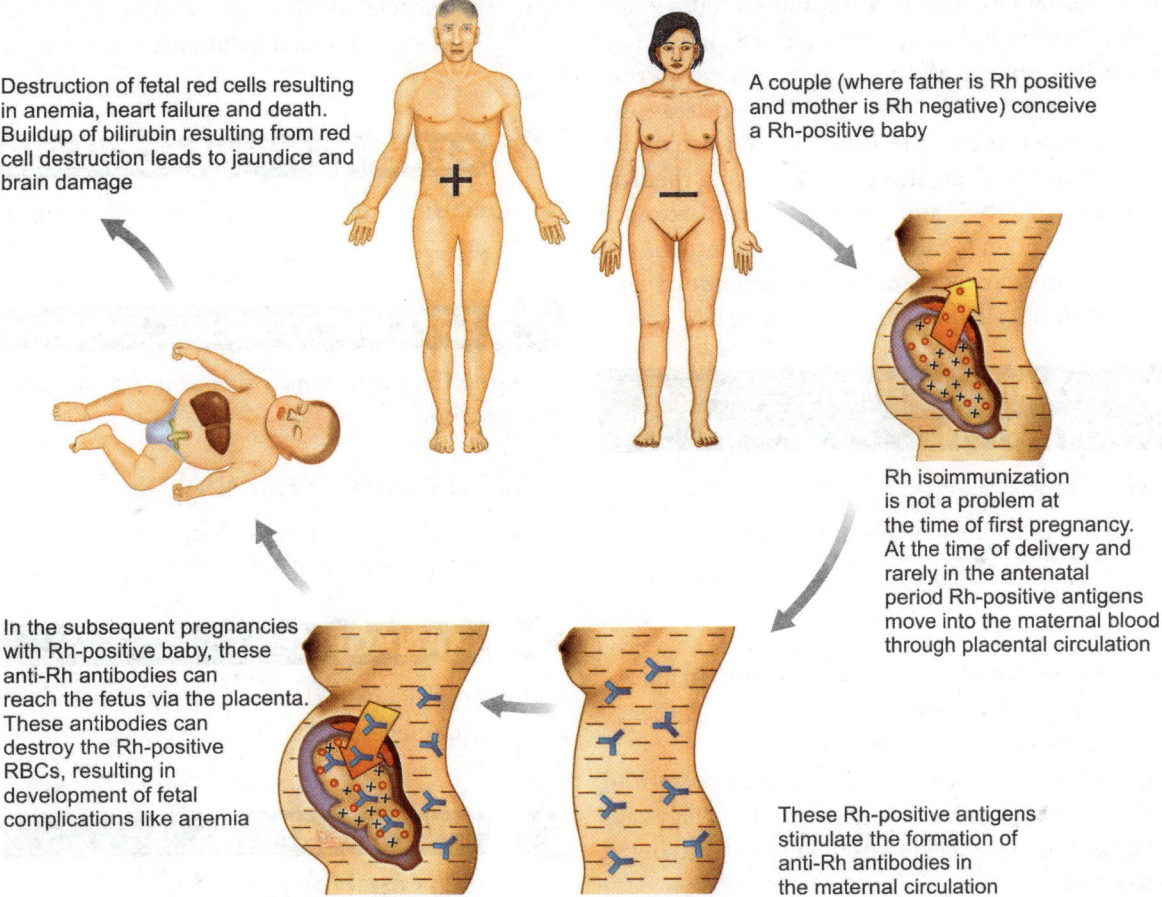

Flowchart 10.1: Pathogenesis of Rh isoimmunization.

with the greatest transfer occurring at the time of delivery or during the third trimester. This transfer stimulates maternal antibody production against the Rh factor, which is called isoimmunization. The process of sensitization has no adverse health effects for the mother. During the time of first Rh-positive pregnancy, the production of maternal anti-Rh antibodies is relatively slow and usually does not affect that pregnancy. Rh incompatibility is not a factor in a first pregnancy, because few fetal blood cells reach the mother's bloodstream until delivery. The antibodies that form after delivery cannot affect the first child. However, if the mother is exposed to the Rh D antigens during subsequent pregnancies, the immune response is quicker and much greater. The anti-D antibodies produced by the mother can cross the placenta and bind to Rh D antigen on the surface of fetal RBCs, causing lysis of the fetal RBCs and resulting in development of hemolytic anemia. Severe anemia can lead to fetal heart failure, fluid retention and hydrops, and intrauterine death. Depending on the degree of erythrocyte destruction, various types of fetal hemolytic diseases can result. An umbrella term for these hemolytic disorders is known as "erythroblastosis fetalis." Clinical manifestations of erythroblastosis fetalis include hydrops fetalis, icterus gravis neonatorum, and congenital anemia of the newborn. Hemolysis often results in hyperbilirubinemia. Low levels

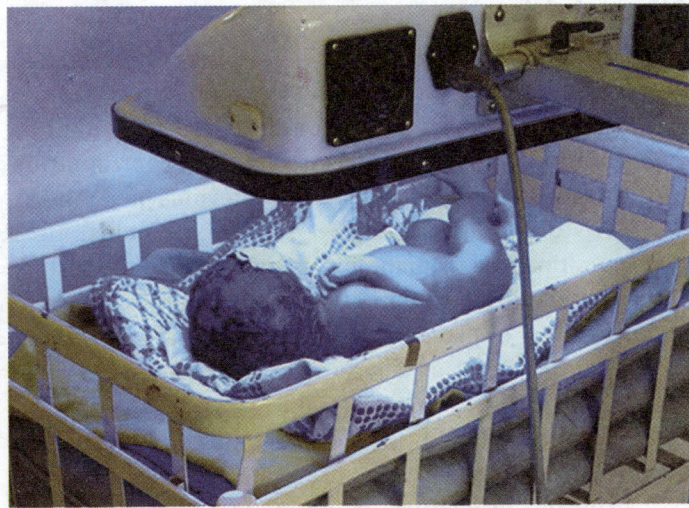

Fig. 10.1: A newborn baby with mild degree of postnatal jaundice being treated with phototherapy.

of jaundice are not harmful but, if left untreated, higher levels may develop resulting in damage to the specific areas of the neonatal brain, causing permanent brain damage (kernicterus). This can lead to a range of neurodevelopmental problems such as cerebral palsy, deafness, and motor and speech delays. Postnatal jaundice can be treated with phototherapy **(Fig. 10.1)** and exchange transfusion.

Isoimmunization depends on the volume of fetal blood entering the maternal circulation and usually occurs when at least 0.1 mL of fetal blood enters the maternal circulation. Chances of Rh isoimmunization in the antenatal period due to FMH are about 1–5%, whereas those during the end of third trimester and at the time of labor are about 10–15%. Isoimmunization can also occur following medical interventions such as CVS, amniocentesis, and external cephalic version, and other medical events such as pregnancy terminations, late miscarriages, antepartum hemorrhage, and abdominal trauma, all of which can cause FMH.

HISTORY AND CLINICAL PRESENTATION

RISK FACTORS

The following risk factors must be elicited on history.

Maternal History

- Rh-negative (dd) blood type
- Younger (<16 years) or older (>35 years) maternal age
- Rh-negative women partnered with Rh-positive father
- History of previous blood transfusion
- History of consanguineous marriage: It is important to elicit this history because consanguineous marriages are associated with increased chances of her husband being Rh negative too.

Obstetric History

- *History of previous pregnancies:* It is important to elicit detailed obstetric history from the patient:
  - History of jaundice, anemia, congenital malformations, hydrops fetalis, stillbirths or intrauterine deaths, neonatal deaths, etc. in previous pregnancies
  - History of FMH in the past pregnancies: In a multiparous woman, this includes taking the history of potential sensitizing events such as manual removal of placenta, retained placenta, antepartum hemorrhage, and cesarean delivery in her past pregnancies.
  - History of having received injection of anti-Rh immunoglobulins in previous pregnancies as a routine procedure or following some sensitizing event such as miscarriage, and invasive procedures such as amniocentesis and CVS
- *History of present pregnancy:* It is important to ask about the following:
  - History of FMH in the present pregnancy: In the first trimester, this could be due to events such as trauma, blood pressure variability (BPV), miscarriage, chorionic villus sampling, ectopic pregnancy, and fetal reduction. In the second trimester, history of amniocentesis could be associated with FMH.

External cephalic version in the third trimester could be associated with a likely FMH.
- Decrease in fetal movements

GENERAL PHYSICAL EXAMINATION

No specific finding is observed on general physical examination.

SPECIFIC SYSTEMIC EXAMINATION

No specific finding is observed on specific systemic examination.

ABDOMINAL EXAMINATION

Normal abdominal and vaginal examinations should be carried out as described in Chapter 1.

MANAGEMENT

Management comprising investigations and definitive obstetric management is discussed next.

INVESTIGATIONS

BLOOD GROUPING

Routine antenatal investigations including ABO and Rh typing must be performed in all women at the time of their first antenatal visit.

Maternal antibody screening, which helps in detecting the presence of anti-D antibodies, must be performed in all pregnant women who turn up to be Rh negative. In this test, the maternal serum is incubated with Rh-positive erythrocytes and Coombs serum (antiglobulin antibodies). The red cells will agglutinate if Rh antibodies are present in the maternal plasma.

TESTS FOR ESTIMATING THE VOLUME OF FETOMATERNAL HEMORRHAGE

Kleihauer–Betke Test

It is important to estimate the volume of FMH to calculate the appropriate dose of anti-D immune globulins to be administered to nonimmunized RhD-negative mothers. Kleihauer–Betke test is the most commonly used quantitative test performed in Rh-negative mothers for measuring the amount of fetal hemoglobin transferred from a fetus to mother's bloodstream as a result of FMH. This test is performed within 2 hours of delivery and helps identify RhD-negative women with a large FMH **(Box 10.1)** who may require additional anti-D Ig. It is based on the principle that fetal hemoglobin is resistant to acid. In this

BOX 10.1: Clinical circumstances that are more likely to be associated with a large fetomaternal bleed.
- Traumatic deliveries including cesarean section
- Manual removal of the placenta
- Stillbirths and fetal deaths
- Abdominal trauma during the third trimester
- Twin pregnancies (at delivery)
- Unexplained hydrops fetalis

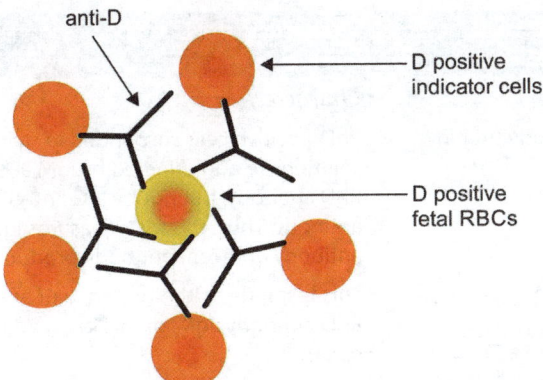

Fig. 10.3: Rosette test.

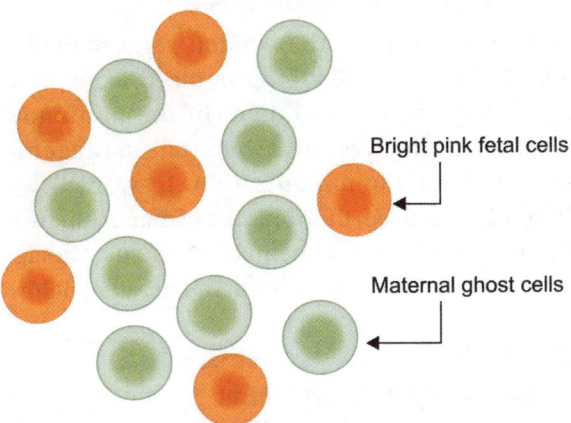

Fig. 10.2: Kleihauer–Betke test.

Rosette Test

Rosette test is a qualitative test for identifying whether fetal RhD positive cells are present in the circulation of Rh-negative mother. Routine 300 µg or 1,500 IU of anti-D is able to neutralize 15 mL fetal RBCs or 30 mL whole blood. In 0.2–0.3% pregnancies, the volume of FMH may exceed 30 mL. A single dose of 300 µg of anti-D may not be sufficient in these situations. Therefore, as recommended by the ACOG (2018), screening of all Rh-negative women must be done using a Rosette test. Only for samples where Rosette test is positive, Kleihauer–Betke test is ordered.

In this test, a sample of maternal blood is mixed with anti-D antibodies. These antibodies will coat any D-positive fetal cells present in the sample. Addition of indicator red cells bearing D antigen will result in the formation of rosettes around the fetal cells because the indicator cells would attach to them through antibodies **(Fig. 10.3)**. Therefore, the presence of rosettes indicates the presence of fetal D-positive cells in the sample.

test, maternal blood smear is exposed to an acidic solution (citric acid phosphate buffer). The acid is able to elute adult hemoglobin, but not fetal hemoglobin, from the RBCs. As a result, on subsequent staining, the fetal cells (containing fetal hemoglobin) appear rose pink in color, while adult RBCs appear as "ghosts" **(Fig. 10.2)**. The fetal cells are counted and expressed as the percentage of adult cells. The fetal blood volume is calculated using the following formula:

$$FBV = \frac{MBV \times \text{maternal hematocrit} \times \text{percentage of fetal cells in Kleihauer–Betke test}}{\text{Newborn hematocrit}}$$

where, FBV = fetal blood volume; MBV = maternal blood volume.

For a normal normotensive pregnant woman at term, the mean MBV is estimated to be about 5,000 mL.

On an average, for the purpose of rough estimation, the presence of 80 fetal RBCs in 50 low power fields is suggestive of 4 mL of FMH.

While this test is routinely performed within 2 hours of delivery in the UK, in some European countries a standard postnatal dose of 1,000–1,500 IU anti D-Ig is used with no requirement for a routine Kleihauer test.

Flow Cytometry

Flow cytometry can be considered as an alternative technique for quantifying the size of FMH. This method uses monoclonal antibodies to hemoglobin F or D antigen. Following the addition of monoclonal antibodies, the degree of fluorescence is measured.

MEASUREMENTS OF ANTIBODIES IN MATERNAL SERUM

Various methods for detecting anti-D antibodies in maternal serum are described in **Table 10.4**. The risk of alloimmunization is dependent on the volume of fetal red cells **(Table 10.5)**.

ULTRASONOGRAPHY

Ultrasound examination can be used for the following:
- To establish the correct gestational age
- To guide invasive procedures (amniocentesis, fetal blood sampling, etc.)
- To Monitor fetal growth and wellbeing

Ultrasonographic parameters for determining fetal anemia are mentioned in **Box 10.2**.

Doppler velocimetry of the fetal middle cerebral artery (MCA): Anemic fetus preserves oxygen delivery to the brain by

Complications of Pregnancy

TABLE 10.4: Methods for detecting anti-D antibodies in maternal serum.

Test	Characteristics
Antibody titer in saline	RhD-positive cells suspended in saline solution are agglutinated by IgM anti-RhD antibody, but not by IgG anti-RhD antibody. Thus, this test measures IgM antibody or recent antibody production
Antibody titer in albumin	This test reflects the presence of any anti-RhD antibody, IgM, or IgG in the maternal serum
Indirect antiglobulin (Coombs) test: Measuring the presence of antibodies, which are present unbound in the maternal serum **(Fig. 10.4A)**	• In this test, RhD-positive RBCs are incubated with maternal serum. Any anti-RhD antibody present in the serum will adhere to the RBCs • The RBCs are then washed and suspended in serum containing anti-human globulin (antiglobulin serum) • Red cells coated with maternal anti-RhD will be agglutinated by the antihuman globulin (positive indirect antiglobulin test)
Direct antiglobulin (Coombs) test: Detecting the antibodies that are bound to the surface of RBCs **(Fig. 10.4B)**	• This is done after birth to detect the presence of maternal antibody on the neonatal RBCs • The infant's RBCs are placed in antiglobulin serum. If the cells are agglutinated, this indicates the presence of maternal antibody

TABLE 10.5: Risk of alloimmunization based on the volume of fetal red cells transferred.

Volume of fetal red cells transferred (mL)	Risk of alloimmunization (%)
0.1	3
0.25–1	25
>5	65

BOX 10.2: Ultrasonographic parameters for determining fetal anemia.

- Umbilical vein diameter
- Hepatic size
- Splenic size
- Polyhydramnios
- Fetal hydrops (e.g., presence of ascites, pleural effusions, and skin edema)

increasing the cerebral blood flow. Besides predicting fetal anemia, Doppler velocimetry also helps in predicting the timing of a second intrauterine fetal transfusion.

INVASIVE TECHNIQUES

Invasive procedures such as fetal blood sampling are often required, especially when there is a suspicion of fetal anemia. Previously used invasive techniques such as amniocentesis and fetal blood sampling have now been largely replaced with noninvasive techniques such as middle cerebral artery peak systolic velocity (MCA PSV).

℞ TREATMENT/OBSTETRIC MANAGEMENT

ANTENATAL MANAGEMENT

In the antenatal period, the women can be divided into two groups: Rh-negative nonimmunized women and the Rh-negative immunized women. In the nonimmunized women, the objective of antenatal management is prevention of Rh alloimmunization. In women who are already alloimmunized, the objective of management is early detection and treatment of anemia in the fetus. Management of both these cases would be discussed in detail below.

MANAGEMENT OF Rh-NEGATIVE NONIMMUNIZED WOMEN

> Q. With help of a long essay discuss the management of a 32 years old G2P1L1 Rh-negative nonimmunized woman.
>
> Q. Write a short essay discussing the management of Rh-negative nonimmunized woman.

Rh-negative nonimmunized women do not show any antibodies in their blood at the time of the initial prenatal evaluation. In these patients, the first step in the management should be the determination of the blood group of the baby's father. If the father's blood group is Rh negative, there is no possibility that the baby would be Rh positive. Such pregnancies should be managed like normal ones, and no further testing of Rh antibodies is required **(Flowchart 10.2)**.

If the father is Rh positive, there is 50–100% chance that the baby born would be Rh positive, with the chance being 100% if the father is homozygous and 50% if the father is heterozygous.

In such cases, it is important to detect the development of antibodies in the mother during the antenatal period and administer routine antenatal anti-D prophylaxis (RAADP) if the antibody screen turns out negative. The maternal antibody screen in order to detect the presence of antibodies needs to be carried out at the first booking visit (first trimester). In case the antibody screen is negative at this time, a repeat antibody test is done at 28 weeks' gestation. Various tests for detecting the presence of these antibodies have already been described in **Table 10.4**.

In case, the antibody screen still turns out negative, the woman must be further managed as nonsensitized pregnancy. Negative antibody titer on indirect antiglobulin test (previously known as the indirect Coombs test) can help identify the fetus that is not at risk. As per the NICE guidelines

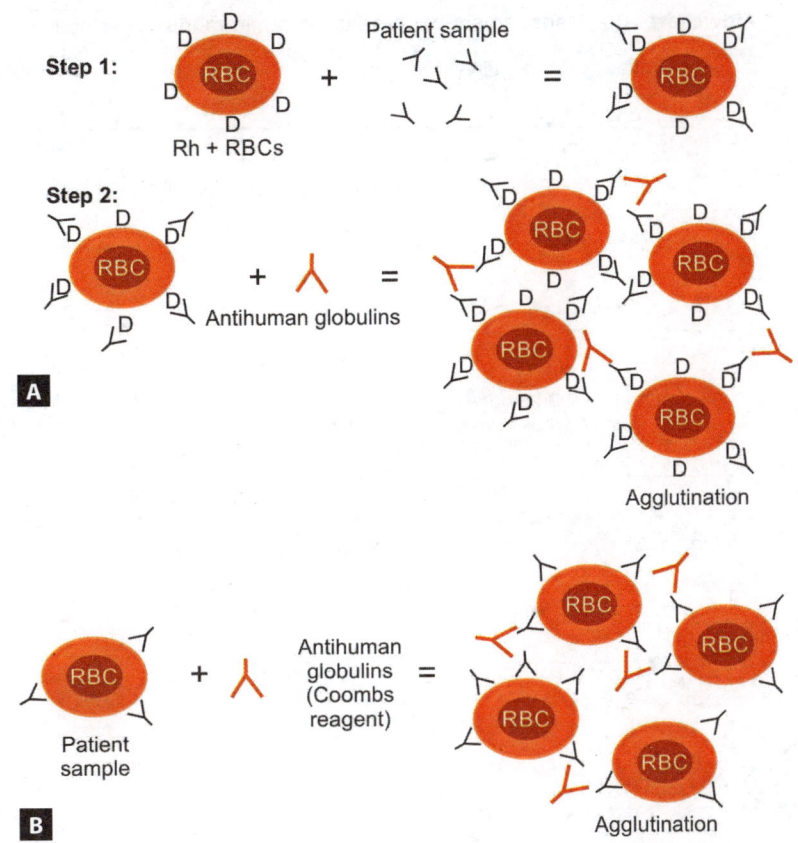

Figs. 10.4A and B: Antiglobulin test. (A) Indirect antiglobulin test; (B) Direct antiglobulin test.

(2002, 2008) all nonsensitized RhD-negative women must be offered RAADP in the third trimester because of the occurrence of small amounts of FMH during this time even in the absence of any sensitizing event. RAADP helps in reducing the incidence of Rh alloimmunization in previously nonsensitized RhD-negative women who deliver an RhD-positive baby.

In case the antibody screen turns out to be positive, the woman must be further managed as Rh-sensitized pregnancy. RAADP is not required in Rh-sensitized women.

The regimens for providing RAADP as recommended by NICE (2008), UK are:
- Two doses of 500 IU antiD Ig at 28 and 34 weeks of gestation
- A single dose of 1,500 IU at 28 weeks or between 28 and 30 weeks of gestation

Presently, there is no evidence to prove if one regimen is more effective than the other. The NICE (2008) recommends that the preparation associated with the lowest cost must be used.

In an Indian setup, 300 µg (where 10 µg is 50 IU) or 1,500 IU of anti-D is administered at 28 weeks of gestation.

Besides the RAADP, anti-D Ig must be additionally administered as soon as possible (preferably within 72 hours) to the nonsensitized Rh-negative women in situations in which FMH is likely, in order to reduce the risk of their sensitization by neutralizing the fetal antigens.

However, if the deadline of 72 hours has not been met for some reason, anti-D Ig must be administered up to 10 days after the sensitizing event because it is still likely to provide some protection. Some of these sensitizing events include miscarriage, version, invasive procedures, abdominal trauma, etc. **(Table 10.6)**. These potentially sensitizing events could be associated with an introduction of a substantial quantity of fetal RhD antigens into the maternal circulation.

In the presence of a sensitizing event, minimum recommended dose of anti-D Ig at less than 20 weeks of gestation ($12–19^{+6}$ weeks) is 250 IU and at more than 20 weeks of gestation is 500 IU. For pregnancies prior to 12 weeks of gestation, anti-D prophylaxis may not be required for all the events. However, it is required following events such as ectopic pregnancy, molar pregnancy, medical termination of pregnancy, and uterine bleeding (which is heavy, repeated, or associated with abdominal pain). In these cases, minimum dose of anti-D Ig required is 250 IU. Also, in case of a sensitizing event prior to 20 weeks, test for FMH is not required. However, for potentially sensitizing events after 20 weeks of gestation, a test for FMH is required.

An intramuscular dose of 500 IU of anti-D Ig will help neutralize an FMH of up to 4 mL. For each mL of FMH in the excess of 4 mL, a further 125 IU of anti-D IgG (if administered intramuscularly) or 100 IU of anti-D IgG (if administered intravascularly) for each mL of fetal RBCs detected is necessary. For successful immunoprophylaxis,

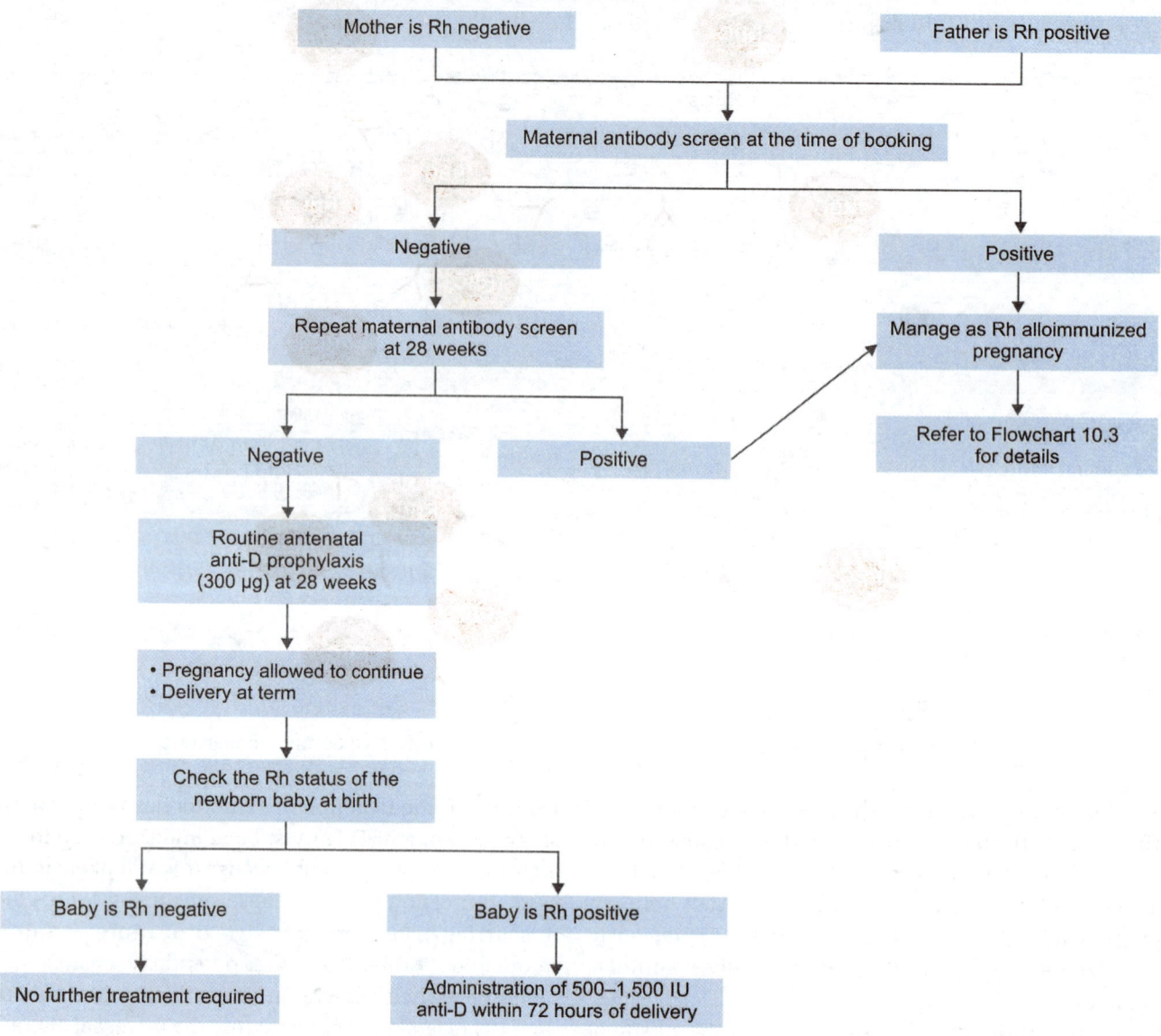

Flowchart 10.2: Management of Rh-negative nonimmunized women.

anti-D Ig should be administered as soon as possible after the potentially sensitizing event but always within 72 hours. If it is not given before 72 hours, every effort should still be made to administer the anti-D Ig as soon as possible. Even a dose given within 10 days may be able to provide some protection.

Administration of these anti-Rh antibodies helps in blocking the recognition of fetal Rh-positive cells by the mother's body by neutralization of maternal antibodies before they can destroy the fetal Rh-positive cells (**Fig. 10.5**). Ideally, anti-D Ig should be administered into the deltoid muscle. In women with bleeding disorders, anti-D Ig can be administered via the subcutaneous or intravenous route.

The woman's eligibility for second dose of anti-D Ig needs to be determined at the time of delivery of the baby (**Box 10.3**). Once the anti-D Ig has been administered to the mother, the anti-D antibodies in her blood would be detected on antibody screening. However, the antibody titer would not be >4 at term in these cases. If the antibody titer is >4, it probably is due to alloimmunization rather than due to administration of the anti-D Ig.

Following the baby's birth, the blood should be drawn from the umbilical cord for carrying out the various tests including ABO and Rh typing. In case the cord blood is found to be Rh positive, all D-negative previously nonsensitized women must be offered at least 500 IU of anti-D within 72 hours of delivery.

Maternal samples must be tested for FMH, and additional dose may be required as guided by FMH. Since the maximum chances of FMH occur at the time of delivery, administration of anti-D Ig to eligible mothers postdelivery helps in reducing the incidence of alloimmunization to about 1–2%. With an additional antenatal anti-D prophylaxis, this risk is further reduced to 0.1%. In the absence of any kind of prophylactic anti-D administration, the risk of alloimmunization can be as high as 16%.

TABLE 10.6: Events requiring the administration of anti-D immunoglobulins.		
Antepartum period	**Intrapartum period**	**Postpartum period**
Spontaneous miscarriage All nonsensitized RhD-negative women who have a spontaneous complete or incomplete miscarriage at or after 12^{+0} weeks of gestation (anti-D Ig is not required for spontaneous miscarriage before 12^{+0} weeks of gestation, provided there is no instrumentation of the uterus because there is evidence which suggests that significant FMH occurs only after curettage to remove products of conception but does not occur after complete spontaneous miscarriages occurring before 12^{+0} weeks of gestation)	• Instrumental delivery • Cesarean delivery • Stillbirths • Multiple pregnancies • Hydrops fetalis • Placental abruption • Manual removal of placenta	Blood transfusion
Medical/surgical evacuation of uterus • Nonsensitized RhD-negative women undergoing surgical evacuation of the uterus, regardless of the period of gestation • All nonsensitized RhD-negative women undergoing medical evacuation of the uterus, regardless of gestation		
Threatened miscarriage All nonsensitized RhD-negative women with a threatened miscarriage after 12^{+0} weeks of gestation. In women in whom bleeding continues intermittently after 12^{+0} weeks of gestation, anti-D Ig should be given at 6-weekly intervals		
Ectopic pregnancy All nonsensitized RhD-negative women who have an ectopic pregnancy, regardless of the modality of management		
Therapeutic termination of pregnancy All nonsensitized RhD-negative women having a therapeutic termination of pregnancy, whether by surgical or medical methods, regardless of gestational age		
Other sensitizing events • Invasive prenatal diagnosis (amniocentesis, CVS, cordocentesis, intrauterine transfusion, etc.) • Other intrauterine procedures (e.g., insertion of shunts, embryo reduction, and laser) • Antepartum hemorrhage • External cephalic version of the fetus • Any abdominal trauma (direct/indirect, sharp/blunt, open/closed) • Fetal death		

(FMH: fetomaternal hemorrhage)

Q. Can indirect Coombs test (ICT) or indirect antiglobulin test (IAT) be positive in a nulliparous woman in her first pregnancy?

It is unlikely for the nulliparous women to be sensitized in her first pregnancy. Few mechanisms are likely to be responsible for this and include the following:

- Occurrence of undetected leakage of fetal RBCs into the maternal circulation during pregnancy
- *Grandmother theory:* Rh-negative woman may have been sensitized from birth by receiving Rh-positive cells from her mother at the time of her own delivery, resulting in an antibody response. This is known as the grandmother theory because the fetus in the current pregnancy is at risk due to the presence of maternal antibodies, which were initially triggered by the Rh-positive erythrocytes of his/her grandmother.
- History of having received transfusion of Rh-positive blood in the past
- History of premarital abortions/delivery of a Rh-positive baby (which the woman may be hiding)

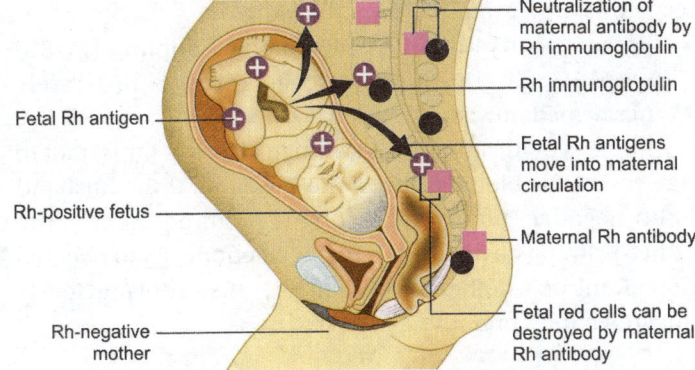

Fig. 10.5: Mechanism of action of anti-D immunoglobulins.

BOX 10.3: Criteria for administration of second dose of anti-D immunoglobulins to Rh-negative nonimmunized women.

- The baby born is Rh positive
- Direct antiglobulin (Coombs) test) on the umbilical cord blood is negative
- The cross-match between the anti-D Ig and mother's red cells is compatible

Rh-NEGATIVE IMMUNIZED WOMEN

> **Q.** With the help of a long essay, discuss the management plan in the case study described in the beginning of the chapter.
>
> **Q.** Discuss the management plan in case of Rh-negative sensitized pregnancy.

Upon confirmation of maternal Rh alloimmunization, identification of fetuses at risk is the main priority. This involves taking a good obstetric history and regular monitoring of maternal antibody titer level. A woman who previously had an affected pregnancy is likely to experience a recurrence in her present pregnancy, if not treated. Therefore, monitoring for fetal anemia in these cases must commence at least 10 weeks earlier than the time of her previously affected pregnancy. Fetal anemia can be diagnosed through the following ways (**Flowchart 10.3**):

- Measurement of the peak systolic velocity (PSV) of the fetal middle cerebral artery (MCA): This is done by Doppler ultrasound. With the advancements in fetomaternal medicine, there is a shift toward the use of noninvasive methods for assessment of fetal anemia. The use of fetal MCA PSV for the diagnosis of moderate-to-severe anemia has therefore emerged as an important noninvasive method for the identification of fetal anemia and helps in avoiding invasive procedures in nearly 70% cases. The risk of fetal anemia is high in fetuses with PSV of 1.5 times the median or higher. Fetuses with values below 1.5 are unlikely to have any anemia or may have only mild anemia.
- *Amniocentesis and amniotic fluid analysis:* This involves determination of bilirubin concentration in the amniotic fluid. Being an invasive test, it is rarely performed nowadays.
- Ultrasound examination of the fetus
- Percutaneous umbilical cord blood sampling (PUBS) (cordocentesis): This is also an invasive test rarely performed nowadays.

In cases of Rh-immunized woman also, it is important to determine the blood group of the husband. If the husband is Rh negative, no further testing is required. In case the father is Rh positive, further management needs to decided depending on whether the woman has a history of previously affected babies or not.

First Affected Pregnancy (No Previous History of Affected Pregnancies)

The risk of fetal anemia is proportional to maternal anti-Rh antibodies titer in the first affected pregnancy and is likely to be associated with minimal fetal or neonatal disease. This relationship is, however, lost in the subsequent pregnancies, and they are likely to be associated with worsening disease.

In case of first affected pregnancy, the maternal antibody titers must be repeated every 2-weekly until term. If the antibody titer remains under the critical level (usually 32) up to 36 weeks of gestation, the woman may be continued until the term. The pregnancy should not be allowed to get postdated, and she should be induced between 38 and 40 weeks of gestation. If there is a sudden rise in the antibody titer at any time, any evidence of fetal anemia must be checked with the help of an ultrasound examination. Serial Doppler of MCA PSV must be performed at every 1–2 weeks' intervals and continued until 35 weeks, following which the delivery can be planned.

Women with a History of Previously Affected Pregnancy

Such pregnancies should be especially referred to the centers having facilities of fetal medicine specialists. It is important in these cases to determine the blood group of the father. If the father is Rh negative, nothing needs to be done. In case the father is Rh positive, determination of the zygosity of paternal phenotype helps in assessing whether the fetus has 100% likelihood of being Rh positive (in case of homozygous paternal phenotype) or 50% likelihood of being Rh positive (in case of heterozygous paternal phenotype). Techniques such as multiplex quantitative PCR can help determine paternal zygosity. In case of heterozygous paternal phenotype, cell-free fetal DNA (cffDNA) or amniocentesis at 15 weeks of gestation can be used for determining the fetal Rh status. PCR analysis of cell-free DNA from maternal plasma or serum is likely to be associated with an accuracy of 99–100%.

In these cases, anti-D titers are unable to predict the development of fetal anemia. Therefore, other tests are required to predict the development of fetal anemia, some of which are as follows:

- *Ultrasound:* Ultrasound examination in the first trimester helps in an accurate estimation of the gestational age. The ultrasound may reveal the evidence of hydrops fetalis and fetal anemia. There could be a presence of polyhydramnios and increased placental thickness (>4 cm). The fetus may show pericardial effusion, ascites or pleural effusion, and/or echogenic bowel. There could be splenomegaly and hepatomegaly along with the dilatation of cardiac chambers. Some tests for estimation of fetal hemoglobin include immunofluorescent flow cytometry or DNA analysis using PCR.
- *Tests for fetal surveillance:* The earliest warning of fetal anemia may be experienced by the mother in the form of reduced fetal body movements. External CTG may show evidence of sinusoidal fetal heart rate patterns (**Fig. 10.6**), and fetal biophysical profile may be affected.
- *MCA PSV on Doppler ultrasound:* This is a noninvasive method for detection of fetal anemia. There is a strong correlation between the high PSV in the MCA and the low levels of fetal hemoglobin.

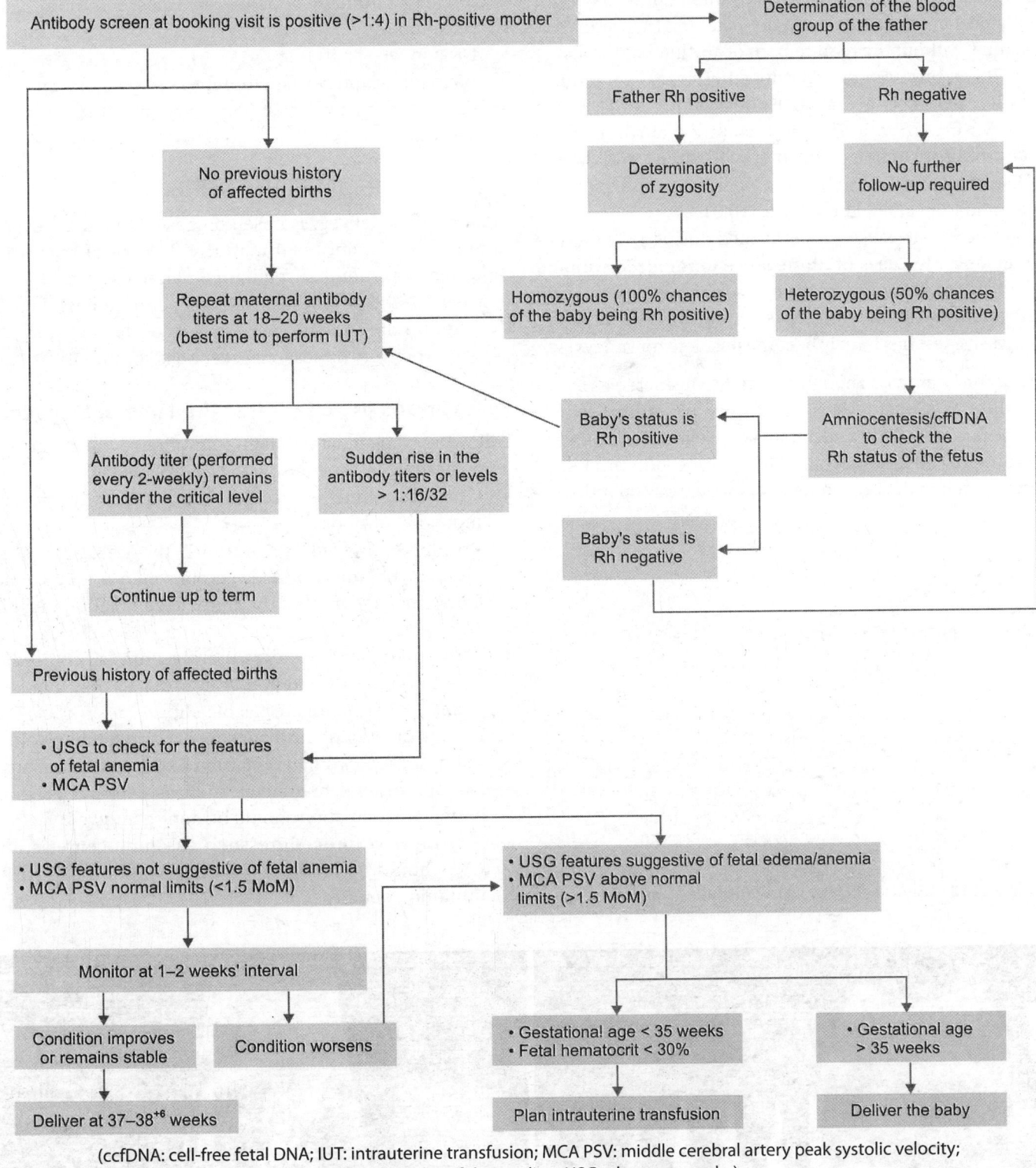

Flowchart 10.3: Antenatal management of immunized Rh-negative pregnancy.

(ccfDNA: cell-free fetal DNA; IUT: intrauterine transfusion; MCA PSV: middle cerebral artery peak systolic velocity; MoM: multiples of the median; USG: ultrasonography)

Though abnormally elevated MCA PSV **(Figs. 10.7A and B)** can be considered to have a high sensitivity (almost approaching 100%) in prediction of fetal anemia, it also has a false positive rate of approximately 12%.

Nowadays, previously used procedures such as serial amniocentesis for measuring delta OD 450 values and subsequently interpreting it with help of Liley's or Queenan curve have largely become obsolete due to the noninvasive nature of MCA PSV. The obstetricians nowadays are routinely using this method for predicting fetal anemia by observing an increase in the velocity of blood flow in the MCA in anemic fetuses in comparison to the normal ones [MCA PSV > 1.5 MoM on Mari's chart **(Table 10.7)**]. Specialized ultrasound machines available nowadays can calculate fetal hematocrit based on gestational age and MCA PSV value, without the requirement of any intervention.

- *PUBS or cordocentesis:* Cordocentesis, also sometimes called PUBS, is a diagnostic test which aims at the detection of fetal anomalies (e.g., chromosomal anomalies such as Down's syndrome, and blood disorders such as hemolytic anemia) through direct examination of fetal blood **(Fig. 10.8)**.

Cordocentesis is usually performed during 18–24 weeks of pregnancy. In cases of Rh-negative immunized women, the procedure of cordocentesis helps in estimating the fetal hemoglobin and hematocrit levels. As previously mentioned, this invasive test has largely become obsolete nowadays.

Risks of cordocentesis: Though generally considered as a safe procedure, cordocentesis is an invasive procedure, which must be performed after adequate counseling of the parents regarding its advantages and risks. Some potential side effects related to the procedure of cordocentesis include:

- There is a 1–2% risk of miscarriage
- Blood loss from the puncture site (most common)
- Infection
- Drop in fetal heart rate
- Premature rupture of membranes
- Fetal death rate of 5% (if performed prior to 24 weeks of gestation)

INTRAPARTUM MANAGEMENT

The timing of delivery is based on gestational age, severity of fetal anemia, and fetal maturity. In case of reassuring parameters on fetal surveillance, labor can be induced between 37 and 38 weeks. In this scenario, vaginal delivery can be attempted. However, in case of delivery prior to 34 weeks, delivery by cesarean section is common.

Precautions to be taken at the Time of Delivery

Following steps must be taken to minimize the chances of fetomaternal bleeding during the time of delivery:

- Cross-matched blood must be kept ready prior to induction of labor.
- Prophylactic ergometrine with the delivery of the anterior shoulder, routinely administered as a step under active management of the third stage of labor, must be withheld.
- If the manual removal of the placenta is required, it should be performed gently in order to minimize the chances of the fetomaternal bleeding.
- Rh-positive blood transfusion must be preferably avoided in Rh-negative women right from birth up to menopause.
- Any abdominal maneuver such as external version/abdominal palpation should be done gently.
- Any invasive procedure such as amniocentesis and CVS should be followed by administration of anti-Rh immunoglobulins.

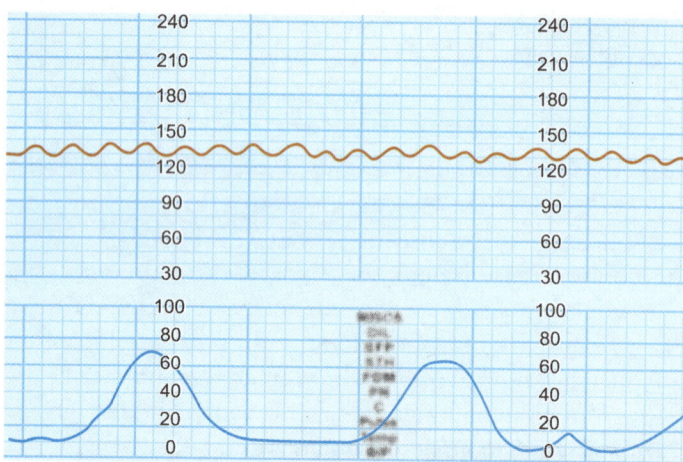

Fig. 10.6: Sinusoidal fetal heart rate pattern on CTG.

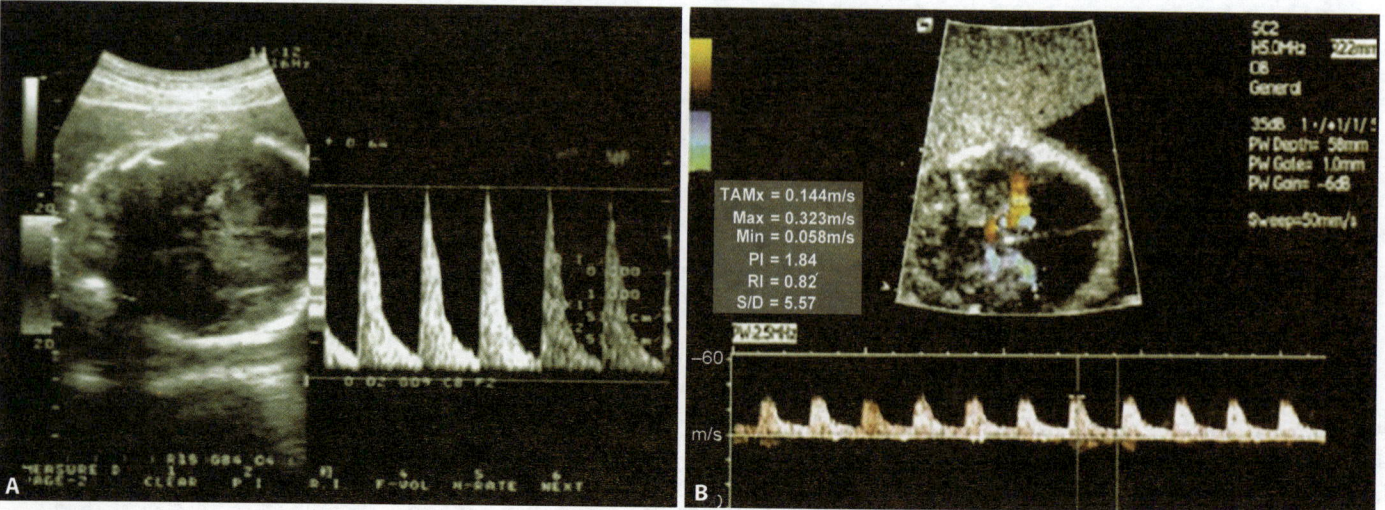

Figs. 10.7A and B: Doppler ultrasound study of MCA PSV to help predict fetal anemia. (A) MCA PSV Doppler waveforms in a severely anemic fetus at 22 weeks' gestation; (B) MCA PSV Doppler waveforms in case of a normal fetus.

TABLE 10.7: Mari's chart showing MCA PSV at gestational age 18–40 weeks.

Gestational age	Fetal MCA PSV	
	Median	1.5 MoM
18 weeks	23.2	34.8
20 weeks	25.5	38.2
22 weeks	27.9	41.9
24 weeks	30.7	46.0
26 weeks	33.6	50.4
28 weeks	36.9	55.4
30 weeks	40.5	60.7
32 weeks	44.4	66.6
34 weeks	48.7	73.1
36 weeks	53.5	80.2
38 weeks	58.7	88.0
40 weeks	64.4	96.6

(MCA PSV: middle cerebral artery peak systolic velocity; MoM: multiples of the median)

- The clinician should remain vigilant regarding the possibility for the occurrence of PPH since ergometrine is usually withheld.
- Umbilical cord clamping can be delayed.
- About 5–6 cm of cord length should be left intact with the fetus. This may prove useful for exchange transfusion, if required following the baby's birth.
- About 5 mL of cord blood should be collected and sent to the laboratory for tests such as complete blood count, ABO, and Rh typing; direct antiglobulin (Coombs) test; serum bilirubin levels (total and direct); peripheral smear; and reticulocyte count.
- At the time of cesarean section, all precautions should be taken to prevent any spillage of blood into the peritoneal cavity. As far as possible, manual removal of the placenta should not be done.
- A newborn with erythroblastosis should be attended to immediately by a pediatrician who must be prepared to perform an exchange transfusion at once, if required.
- In case preterm delivery is required, the mother must be administered an intramuscular dose of corticosteroids.

Timing of Delivery

Rh-Negative Nonimmunized Women

In Rh-negative nonimmunized women, the pregnancy must be allowed to continue up to term. However, the tendency to overrun the expected date of delivery must be curtailed.

Rh-Negative Immunized Women

As discussed previously, if there is no sign of fetal hemolytic disease on MCA PSV Doppler analysis, the pregnancy can continue up to 38–40 weeks. In case there is evidence of fetal hemolytic disease, early termination of pregnancy must be considered. If the period of gestation is 36 weeks or more, the labor must be induced. If the period of gestation is <36 weeks, cordocentesis may be done to determine fetal hemoglobin levels and hematocrit. If hematocrit is <30%, fetal intrauterine blood transfusion at 10–14 days' intervals, generally until 35–36 weeks' gestation, must be performed. Following the intrauterine blood transfusion, delivery is usually performed by 37–38 weeks of gestation.

TREATMENT OF FETAL ANEMIA

Treatment of the baby born with hemolytic anemia may require referral to fetal medicine specialist and comprises the following options:
- In utero transfusion, if fetal anemia is severe
- Exchange transfusion after birth

Some of the indications for referral to the fetal medicine specialist are tabulated in **Box 10.4**.

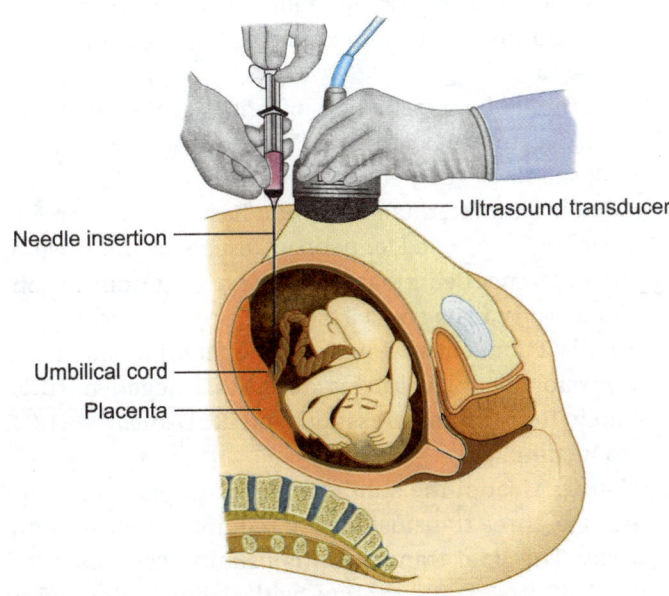

Fig. 10.8: Procedure of cordocentesis.

- Following the baby's birth, 100 μg (500 IU) of anti-D Ig must be administered to the mother in case the baby is Rh positive. Additional dose of anti-D Ig may be required in situations where a larger amount of FMH is suspected, e.g., abruptio placenta, manual removal of the placenta, ruptured uterus, multiple pregnancy, placenta previa, and abdominal trauma.
- Careful fetal monitoring needs to be performed during the time of labor.
- Delivery should be as nontraumatic as possible. The placenta should not be removed manually to avoid squeezing of fetal cells into the maternal circulation.

> **BOX 10.4:** Indications for referral to the fetal medicine specialist.
>
> - Raising antibody levels/titers
> - Titers above the critical/specific threshold (32 or more)
> - Ultrasound features of fetal anemia (MCA PSV >1.5 MoM or other signs of fetal anemia)
> - History of unexplained severe neonatal jaundice
> - History of neonatal anemia requiring exchange transfusion
> - If fetal hematocrit <30%, intrauterine transfusion may be required
>
> (MCA PSV: middle cerebral artery peak systolic velocity; MoM: multiple of median)

Fetal Intrauterine Blood Transfusion

There are two main techniques that are used to deliver intrauterine blood transfusion to a baby before birth. These include intraperitoneal transfusion and intravascular transfusion (IVT). Nowadays, IVT is preferred over intraperitoneal transfusion because it is associated with lower mortality and morbidity. Intrahepatic transfusion (into the baby's liver) or intracardiac transfusion (into the baby's heart) are also sometimes performed. A hematocrit of <30% (Hb = 8 g%) is an indication for in utero transfusion.

Intravascular Blood Transfusion

In this method, Rh-negative packed red cells of the blood group ABO type compatible with the baby, having the hematocrit of 80% that have been cross-matched with the mother, are usually transfused through the fetal umbilical vein.

- *Timing:* IVT is usually performed from 18 to 20 weeks of gestation.
- *Procedure:* IVT comprises the following steps:
    1. If fetal hematocrit is below 30%, IVT is initiated at the rate of 5–10 mL/minute.
    2. Transfusion is usually performed under ultrasound guidance to visualize the correct placement of the needle and to check for any abnormality in the fetal heart rate.
    3. IVT is performed in the umbilical vein at the site where the cord inserts into the placenta or baby's liver or into a free loop of cord. The most common site for performing IVT is the placental insertion of umbilical vein.
- *Amount of blood to be transfused:* One or more transfusions may be necessary to treat the episodes of anemia, hyperbilirubinemia, and bleeding. The amount of blood to be transfused (in mL) is calculated by multiplying number of weeks of gestation over 20 with 10. For example, at 34 weeks of gestation the amount of blood required to be transfused would be equal to (34 – 20) × 10 = 140 mL. The transfusion process can be repeated at weekly or 2-weekly intervals. Following the process of transfusion, fetal surveillance in the form of biweekly CTG and weekly ultrasound examinations to ensure fetal well-being must be performed.
- *Calculation of blood volume to be transfused:* Another formula for calculation of blood volume to be transfused is as follows:

Volume of blood transfused (mL) V =

$$\frac{C\text{ (final)} - C\text{ (initial)} \times \text{fetoplacental volume (FPV) (mL)}}{C\text{ (of the donor blood)}}$$

Where:
C = hematocrit
Fetoplacental volume refers to the volume of red cells required for IVT [FPV (mL) = 1.046 + estimated fetal weight (g) × 0.14] (where fetal weight is estimated using ultrasound).

The target hematocrit is aimed at 40–50%. An interval of 1–2 weeks is kept between the first and second IVTs.

- *Characteristics of the blood to be transfused:* The blood to be transfused must fulfill the following parameters:
    - It should be irradiated (to remove the WBCs, which could result in complications such as graft-versus-host reaction).
    - Blood must be fresh (not more than 72 hours old).
    - It should be cross-matched against the mother's blood.
    - It should be screened for infections such as hepatitis B, C, cytomegalovirus (CMV), and HIV.
    - It should have a hematocrit value of 75–85%.

Blood for intrauterine transfusion has the requirements similar to the blood used for neonatal exchange transfusion, the only difference being that in case of exchange transfusion, the blood used can be about 5 days old.

- *Aim:* IVT aims at maintaining the fetal hematocrit at a physiological level using adult RhD-negative RBCs, which help in suppressing fetal RhD-positive RBC production.
- *Timing:* Most of the studies have indicated that on an average, three transfusions are required in most of the cases. The final transfusion is usually recommended at 34–35 weeks of gestation, with delivery planned at 37–38 weeks. This management strategy, which helps in attaining pulmonary maturity, has been successful in eliminating the occurrence of hyaline membrane disease as well as the requirement of neonatal exchange transfusion for elevated levels of bilirubin.
- *Postprocedural precautions:* These include the following:
    - Mother is asked to keep a track of the count of fetal kicks.
    - Weekly ultrasound monitoring is done until the time of next transfusion.

Intraperitoneal Transfusion

With intraperitoneal transfusion, a needle is inserted through the mother's abdomen and uterus into the baby's peritoneal cavity under ultrasound guidance. RBCs injected into the baby's abdominal cavity are absorbed by the subdiaphragmatic lymphatics into the bloodstream. Rh-negative packed red cells of the blood group type O, having the hematocrit of 80% that have been cross-matched with the mother, are usually transfused.

Intraperitoneal transfusion is rarely used nowadays except in rare cases where due to high antibody titer, transfusion is required prior to 18 weeks of gestation. Options such as plasmapheresis and intravenous immunoglobulins may be useful in these cases. However, there is no definite evidence available to prove this.

Exchange Transfusion

Exchange transfusion is a potentially life-saving procedure that is done to counteract the effects of serious jaundice related to hemolytic anemia in a newborn child born to the mother with Rh incompatibility. This procedure helps in correcting neonatal anemia and congestive heart failure. It also helps in removing the circulatory antibodies. The procedure of exchange transfusion involves slow removal of the baby's blood and its replacement with fresh donor blood or plasma.

Early fetal anemia and hyperbilirubinemia are treated with top-up or exchange transfusion, whereas milder cases are treated using phototherapy. The use of recombinant erythropoietin has reduced the requirement for top-up transfusion.

- *Characteristics of the blood to be transfused:* The blood for exchange transfusion has requirements like the blood required for intrauterine transfusion, the only difference being that in case of intrauterine transfusion, the plasma is removed by the blood center to increase the hematocrit by 70–85%. The blood to be transfused for the purpose of exchange transfusion must fulfill the following parameters:
  - Blood must be ABO compatible with the baby. If ABO compatible blood is not available, O-negative blood can be used.
  - It should be RhD-negative whole blood with the specific volume.
  - Blood should be K negative as well as negative for antigens against which the woman may be having antibodies.
  - The blood should be cross-matched with the infant's serum.
  - It should be <5 days old (to ensure low supernatant potassium levels).
  - It should be CMV negative and irradiated (unless the risk of delaying transfusion while obtaining irradiated blood outweighs this).
  - It should be plasma-reduced rather than in saline–adenine–glucose–mannitol (SAGM) additive solution.
  - It should have a hematocrit of 0.50–0.60.
- *Small volume/top-up transfusion:* In case the volume of blood required to be transfused is much less than that required in cases of exchange transfusion, the following parameters need to be fulfilled:
  - Blood must be ABO compatible with the mother and the neonate.
  - It must be RhD negative.
  - It should be K negative and negative for corresponding antigens to which the mother has antibodies
  - It should be cross-match compatible.
  - It should be CMV negative.
  - It need not be irradiated unless the neonate had a previous intrauterine transfusion: In case the baby had a previous intrauterine transfusion, blood must be irradiated to prevent graft-versus-host disease.
  - Blood can be stored in SAGM (rather than being plasma-reduced).
  - It can be up to 35 days old.
- *Volume of the blood to be transfused:* The total volume of exchange should not exceed one adult unit of blood (450–500 mL). The volume of blood to be exchanged is calculated using the following formula:

$$\text{Volume exchanged (mL)} = \frac{\text{Blood volume (mL)} \times (\text{Hb desired} - \text{Hb initial})}{(\text{Hb Donor} - \text{Hb initial})}$$

where, blood volume = 70–90 mL/kg for term and 85–110 mL/kg for preterm infants.

The serum bilirubin concentration may rise by 2 hours after completion of the exchange transfusion. Therefore, the serum bilirubin concentration should be monitored at 2–4 hours' intervals after exchange. In case the serum bilirubin levels continue to remain elevated, phototherapy may be used.

- The infant may be fed after 2–4 hours following the procedure of exchange transfusion.

CARE OF THE NEONATE

- Regular clinical assessment of the neurobehavioral state of the neonate born to the Rh-immunized mother should be done. Such babies must also be regularly assessed for the development of jaundice and/or anemia by measuring their bilirubin, hemoglobin levels, and reticulocyte count. This needs to be done until 6 months of age or till reticulocytes are visualized in the fetal blood because intrauterine transfusion is likely to cause the bone marrow suppression. Such infants must therefore not be discharged early.
- Early breastfeeding must be encouraged because dehydration can increase the severity of jaundice.
- If the baby's bilirubin levels rise rapidly or are above the interventional threshold levels, phototherapy or exchange transfusion may be required.

COMPLICATIONS

Q. Discuss the complications likely to occur because of rhesus isoimmunization.

FETAL COMPLICATIONS

The various complications that can develop in the fetus or newborn baby due to Rh alloimmunization (previously known as isoimmunization) are shown in **Flowchart 10.4** and are also described below in detail.

Erythroblastosis Fetalis

Erythroblastosis fetalis, also known as hemolytic disease of the newborn, is an umbrella term used to denote various hemolytic disorders resulting due to Rh incompatibility.

Clinical manifestations of erythroblastosis fetalis include hydrops fetalis, icterus gravis neonatorum, and congenital anemia of the newborn. Erythroblastosis fetalis is a disease in the fetus or newborn caused by transplacental transmission of maternal antibodies, usually resulting from maternal and fetal blood group incompatibility **(Flowchart 10.5)**. Hemolysis produced due to Rh incompatibility may produce profound anemia, which may even result in fetal death in utero. As a compensatory mechanism to anemia, the fetal bone marrow starts producing immature erythroblasts into the fetal peripheral circulation, causing erythroblastosis fetalis. The overproduction of erythroblasts can produce enlargement of liver and spleen, resulting in development of hepatomegaly and splenomegaly, respectively.

Excessive destruction of RBCs results in excessive production of bilirubin, which is responsible for producing hyperbilirubinemia and jaundice. Low levels of jaundice are unlikely to cause any harm. However, if left untreated, uncontrollable hyperbilirubinemia leads to deposition of bilirubin in the brain, resulting in permanent damage and development of kernicterus, which can cause neurodevelopmental problems, deafness, speech problems, cerebral palsy, mental retardation, or motor and speech delays. Postnatal jaundice can be treated with phototherapy and exchange transfusion.

Hydrops Fetalis

Hydrops fetalis is a condition characterized by an accumulation of fluids within the baby's body in at least two body areas **(Fig. 10.9)**, resulting in development of ascites, pleural effusion, pericardial effusion, skin edema, etc. In many cases, it may also cause polyhydramnios and placental edema. Pleural effusion may interfere with the normal process of breathing, whereas pericardial effusion may be associated with congestive heart failure. Various mechanisms for the formation of fetal hydrops are listed in **Box 10.5**. Due to anemia, the fetal heart needs to pump out a greater

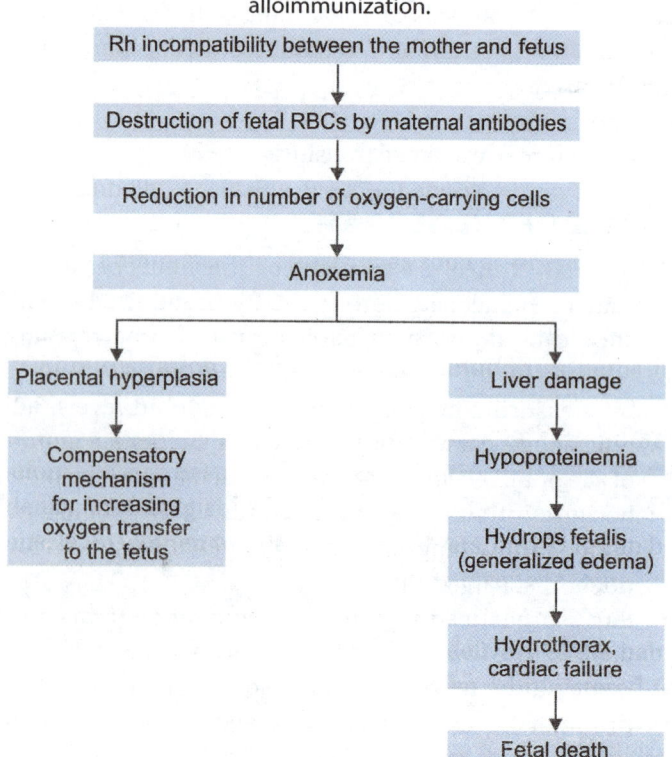

Flowchart 10.4: Various fetal complications arising from Rh alloimmunization.

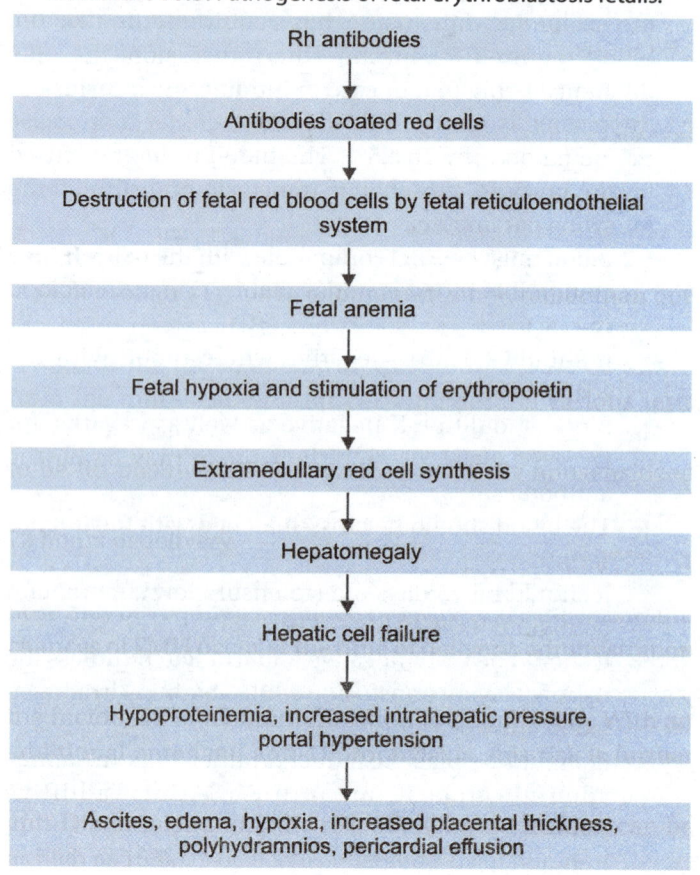

Flowchart 10.5: Pathogenesis of fetal erythroblastosis fetalis.

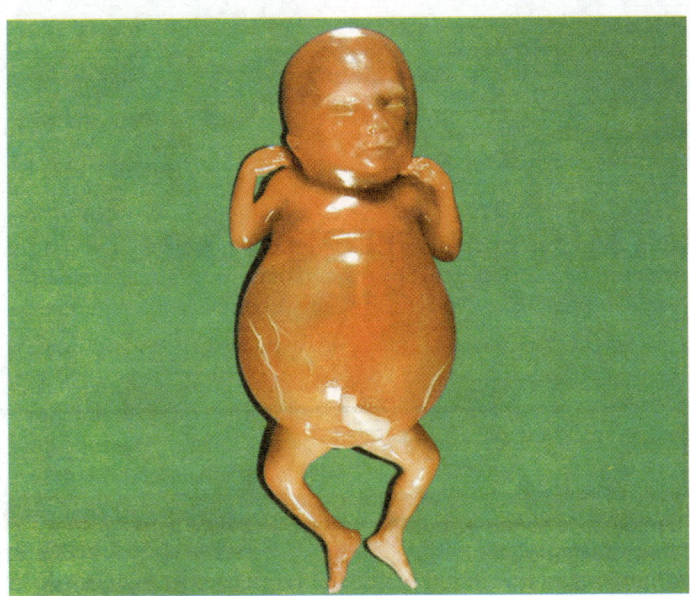

Fig. 10.9: Hydrops fetalis associated with fetal ascites and skin edema.

> **BOX 10.5:** Pathophysiological mechanisms responsible for development of fetal hydrops.
>
> - Reduced intravascular oncotic pressure resulting in interstitial fluid accumulation
> - Increased capillary hydrostatic pressure
> - Reduced lymphatic return
> - Elevation of central venous pressure
> - Elevations in the levels of aldosterone, renin, norepinephrine, and angiotensin I
> - Increase in the levels of atrial natriuretic peptide
> - Reduced nitric oxide production due to injury of fetal vascular endothelial cells

volume of blood to deliver the same amount of oxygen. Due to an increased demand for raised cardiac output, there occurs subsequent heart failure and edema. The fetus is particularly susceptible to interstitial fluid accumulation due to increased capillary permeability, hypoproteinemia, and obstruction to lymphatic return. Hydrops usually does not occur until there is a hemoglobin deficit of at least 7 g/dL below the mean gestational age. Other ultrasound features suggestive of fetal anemia include cardiomegaly, increased diameter of umbilical vein, enlargement of liver and spleen, and visualization of both sides of the bowel.

Recently, factors other than Rh alloimmunization have been found to be associated with development of fetal hydrops. The term nonimmune hydrops has been introduced to identify those cases of fetal hydrops which are caused by factors other than Rh alloimmunization. Some of the causes for nonimmune hydrops are listed in **Table 10.8**.

Maternal mirror syndrome: This is a rare complication of fetal hydrops, also known as the Ballantyne syndrome, which presents in the form of triple edema. There is a clinical triad of fetal hydrops, placentomegaly, and maternal edema. The syndrome has been named as such because the mother mirrors the hydropic fetus. Edema in the mother is related to preeclampsia. Fetal hydrops could be related to any of the causes, including Rh isoimmunization, twin-to-twin transfusion, congenital infection, chromosomal/structural anomalies, etc. This syndrome is also termed as pseudotoxemia because nearly 50% of the patients with mirror syndrome progress to develop hypertension and proteinuria.

TABLE 10.8: Causes of nonimmune hydrops.

Infectious causes	Genetic syndromes	Metabolic disorders	Chromosomal abnormalities
Infection with: • Parvovirus • Cytomegalovirus • Toxoplasmosis • Coxsackie virus type B	• Myotonic dystrophy (autosomal dominant) • Noonan syndrome (autosomal dominant with variable penetrance) • Sjögren's syndrome (uncertain inheritance) • Tuberous sclerosis (autosomal dominant)	• Glycogen-storage disease, type IV • Lysosomal storage diseases (Gaucher's disease, Niemann–Pick disease, etc.) • Hypothyroidism and hyperthyroidism	• Beckwith–Wiedemann syndrome (trisomy 11p15) • Cri-du-chat syndrome (chromosomes 4 and 5) • Down syndrome (trisomy 21) • Turner syndrome (45, X)
Intrathoracic tumors	**Abdominal tumors**	**Other conditions**	
• Pericardial teratoma • Rhabdomyoma • Mediastinal teratoma • Pulmonary fibrosarcoma • Leiomyosarcoma	• Metabolic nephroma • Polycystic kidneys • Neuroblastoma • Hepatoblastoma • Ovarian cyst	• Placental choriocarcinoma • Placental chorangioma • Cystic hygroma • Intussusception • Intracranial teratoma	

■ MATERNAL

Maternal complications such as history of recurrent miscarriages and intrauterine deaths can occur. Complications such as abortion and preterm labor are related to procedures such as fetal cord blood sampling.

EVIDENCE-BASED CLINICAL TRIALS

List of references can be scanned through QR code to enable the readers gain deeper insight of the subject by referring to the entire article or its abstract.

CHAPTER 11

Previous Cesarean Section

CASE STUDY

A 24-year-old G2P2L1 attended the booking antenatal clinic with a previous history of a cesarean section (CS) at term due to breech presentation. She is sure of her last menstrual period, and her period of gestation is 14 weeks both by dates and on abdominal examination.

INTRODUCTION

DEFINITION

> Q. Discuss in detail and critically evaluate the indications for cesarean delivery in modern obstetrics.

Cesarean section is the removal of a fetus from the uterus by abdominal and uterine incisions, after 28 weeks of pregnancy. If the removal of fetus is done before 28 weeks of pregnancy, the procedure is known as hysterotomy. Presently, there has been a considerable rise in the rate of cesarean delivery. Some of the common indications for cesarean delivery are described in **Box 11.1**. Pregnant women with a previous section may be offered either planned VBAC or ERCS. VBAC stands for vaginal birth after cesarean, which refers to vaginal birth following one or more cesarean births. On the other hand, ERCS stands for elective repeat cesarean section. More than 80% of women will be able to have a vaginal birth following a cesarean delivery. In the absence of any maternal or fetal complications, VBAC is the preferred mode of delivery because it is likely to be associated with a reduced maternal morbidity as well as reduced risk of complications in future pregnancies.

Trial of labor after CS (TOLAC) refers to a planned attempt for vaginal delivery in a woman with a previous history of cesarean delivery, irrespective of the outcome. This method is likely to help the woman achieve the goal of VBAC.

The rate of CS in India varies between 20 and 50%. The national average as per the national family health survey

BOX 11.1: Indications for a cesarean section.

Common indications:
- Failure to progress during labor or dystocia (18%)
- Nonreassuring fetal status (32%)
- Fetal malpresentation (19%)
- Suspected macrosomia (5,000 g in women without diabetes; 4,500 g in women with diabetes) (10%)
- Preeclampsia (10%)
- Maternal request (8%)

Less common indications:
- Abnormal placentation (e.g., placenta previa, vasa previa, and placenta accreta) (3%)
- Multiple pregnancy (with first fetus in noncephalic presentation)
- Fetal bleeding diathesis
- Cord presentation or cord prolapse
- Maternal infection (e.g., herpes simplex or HIV)

BOX 11.2: Indications not requiring a routine cesarean section.
- Preterm birth
- Twin pregnancy with first twin having a cephalic presentation
- Intrauterine growth restriction in the baby
- Infection with hepatitis B virus
- Infection with hepatitis C virus
- Recurrent genital herpes in the third trimester

(2015–2016) is 17–20%. As per the recommendation by the WHO, this rate must not be higher than 10–15%. Over the past few decades, there has been an alarming increase in the rate of CS around the world, including India. Efforts must be made to reduce unnecessary CS and at the same time, making sure that the women in need for CS have access to it.

Trial of labor after CS needs to be considered seriously because nearly 40% indication for CS in the present pregnancy is the history of previous CS. CS is associated with significant short-term and long-term risks. Some of the conditions where routine use of CS is not required are mentioned in **Box 11.2**. Factors which help reduce the likelihood of cesarean birth are enumerated in **Box 11.3**.

> **BOX 11.3:** Factors reducing the likelihood of cesarean birth.
>
> - Continuous support during labor from women with or without prior training
> - Induction of labor beyond 41 weeks
> - Use of partogram to monitor progress of labor in women with spontaneous labor having an uncomplicated singleton pregnancy at term
> - Involvement of consultant obstetricians in the decision-making process for cesarean delivery
> - In cases of abnormal FHR pattern, use of fetal blood sampling for detecting the cases of suspected fetal acidosis
>
> (FHR: fetal heart rate)

ROBSON'S TEN GROUP CLASSIFICATION SYSTEM FOR CESAREAN SECTION

Robson's ten group classification system (TGCS) **(Table 11.1)** is an excellent tool for auditing the rates of CS and must be introduced in every unit providing maternity care. This is a simple, robust, reproducible, and flexible tool, which allows audit of CS across all types of hospitals and populations. This tool has proved to be useful in reducing the rates of CS in units which have implemented this.

CESAREAN SECTION ON MATERNAL REQUEST

As per the ACOG (2019), maternal request for CS on its own is not an indication for CS. The healthcare provider needs to take into consideration her specific risk factors, such as age, BMI, accuracy of estimated gestational age, reproductive plans, and personal and cultural value. They also need to discuss and explore the specific reasons for this choice with the patient and her partner. The patient needs to be counseled that a plan for vaginal delivery is likely to be safe and appropriate in the absence of maternal or fetal indications for cesarean delivery. The woman should also be adequately informed about the risks and benefits of cesarean delivery. If the patient still decides to pursue cesarean delivery on maternal request, then in lieu of the high rates for repeat cesarean delivery, patients should be informed that the risks of complications such as placenta previa, placenta accreta spectrum, and gravid hysterectomy are likely to increase with each subsequent cesarean delivery.

If the healthcare provider feels that the woman is just being apprehensive and fearful of the normal vaginal delivery due to the pain involved, she needs to be adequately counseled. If the clinician feels that the woman's request is unreasonable, he/she can decline her request or may refer her for a second opinion.

HISTORY AND CLINICAL PRESENTATION

Detailed history regarding the reason for previous cesarean delivery needs to be taken.

TABLE 11.1: Robson's ten group classification system.

Group	Criteria	Subdivisions
I	Nulliparous women, singleton, cephalic presentation, at term in spontaneous labor	
II	Nulliparous women, singleton, cephalic presentation, at term, induced or cesarean section before labor	IIa: Labor induced IIb: Prelabor cesarean section
III	Multiparous women without uterine scar, single cephalic term pregnancy in spontaneous labor	
IV	Multiparous women without uterine scar, single cephalic term pregnancy, induced or cesarean section before labor	IVa: Labor induced IVb: Prelabor cesarean section
V	Multiparous women with at least one previous cesarean section, single cephalic pregnancy at term	Va: One previous cesarean section Vb: Two or more previous cesarean sections
VI	All nulliparous women with a single breech	
VII	All multiparous women with a single breech (including previous cesarean section)	
VIII	All women with multifetal gestation (including previous cesarean section)	
IX	All women with a single abnormal lie, transverse lie, or oblique (including previous cesarean section)	
X	All women with a singleton cephalic preterm pregnancy, <36 weeks (including previous cesarean section)	

The following questions regarding the previous CS need to be asked:
- What was the indication for the surgery?
- Was it for a repetitive or a nonrepetitive cause (e.g., if the indication for cesarean delivery is breech presentation, it is a nonrepetitive cause)? However, cephalopelvic disproportion (CPD) can be a repetitive cause requiring a repeat CS during future pregnancies.
- Was the CS elective one or an emergency surgery?
- Place where the previous surgery was performed
- The period of gestation at which the CS was performed and the skill of the obstetrician who had performed the surgery
- What was the type of the scar given (classical or the lower segment)?
- Were there any technical difficulties encountered during the procedure? Was there any lateral extension of the

uterine scar or uncontrolled bleeding during the surgery or any other complications at the time of surgery?
- Previous history of any other uterine surgery, especially myomectomy for myoma uterus, needs to be enquired. This is especially important as vaginal delivery following myomectomy may be complicated by uterine rupture.

GENERAL PHYSICAL EXAMINATION

- Patient must be considered high-risk, and frequent ANCs are required.
- Patient should be instructed to report to the clinician in case she experiences pain over the scar, reduced fetal movements, or bleeding per vaginum anytime during the pregnancy.

SPECIFIC SYSTEMIC EXAMINATION

Besides the routine obstetric abdominal examination (as described in Chapter 1), careful examination of the abdominal scar and elicitation of scar tenderness is important. The scar tenderness is palpated using the ulnar border of right hand in the region above the pubic symphysis for a few centimeters.

MANAGEMENT

In the past, management of the patient with a history of cesarean scar was considered as "once a cesarean, always a cesarean." This dictum has now been changed to "once a cesarean, always hospitalization." Since the management of cases with previous history of CS is still controversial, this dictum is also sometimes changed to "once a cesarean, always a controversy." Management options for the patient with previous history of cesarean delivery are presented in **Flowchart 11.1**.

INVESTIGATIONS

Routine ANC investigations include blood grouping (ABO and Rh typing), complete blood count, and ultrasound examination.

TREATMENT/OBSTETRIC MANAGEMENT

> **Q.** What should be the management option in the case described in the beginning of the chapter?
>
> **Q.** Write a long essay discussing the methods of reducing the rate of cesarean section.

There are two options for delivery in these patients:
1. Vaginal birth after cesarean (VBAC)
2. Elective repeat cesarean section (ERCS)

VAGINAL BIRTH AFTER CESAREAN DELIVERY

Women with a prior history of one or two uncomplicated lower segment transverse CS in an otherwise uncomplicated pregnancy at term, with no contraindication to vaginal birth, can be given the option of planned VBAC or ERCS. Women with a prior history of two uncomplicated low transverse CS in an otherwise uncomplicated pregnancy at term, with no contraindication for vaginal birth, need to be adequately counseled by a consultant obstetrician before being considered for VBAC.

Criteria for Vaginal Birth after Cesarean Section

The decision regarding VBAC must be individualized and taken only if the criteria for VBAC, enumerated in **Box 11.4**, are fulfilled. Predictors for a successful VBAC are enumerated in **Table 11.2**.

The decision for VBAC is usually taken after considering the following parameters:
- *Indication for the previous cesarean (recurrent or a nonrecurrent cause):* If the indication of previous CS was a nonrecurrent cause (e.g., fetal distress or nonprogress of labor), which may or may not recur in future pregnancies, the option of VBAC can be considered. However, if the indication for previous cesarean is a recurrent cause such as CPD, the option of ERCS would be more suitable.
- *Any associated obstetrical complications in the present pregnancy:* If the present pregnancy is associated with some other obstetrical indication for CS (e.g., grade III, IV placenta previa and breech presentation), the patient must be considered for ERCS.
- *Ultrasound estimated weight of the baby:* If the ultrasound estimated fetal weight is ≥4.0 kg, the option of ERCS should be considered due to the increased risk of shoulder dystocia and fetal injuries with vaginal deliveries.
- *Number of the previous sections:* According to recommendations by the RCOG (2015), women who have had two or more prior lower segment cesarean deliveries may be offered VBAC only once they have been counseled by a senior obstetrician. This should include explanation of the risk regarding uterine rupture and maternal morbidity. The likelihood of successful VBAC must be individualized based on her history (e.g., history of prior vaginal delivery). Clinician should especially be careful to ensure that her labor is conducted in a center having suitable expertise with the facilities for immediate surgical delivery, if required.
- *Strength of the scar as elicited from history and clinical examination:* If the scar appears to be healthy and strong as elicited from the history and clinical examination, the option of VBAC can be considered.
- *Informed consent of the patients:* If the clinician is satisfied after taking the patient's history and conducting a

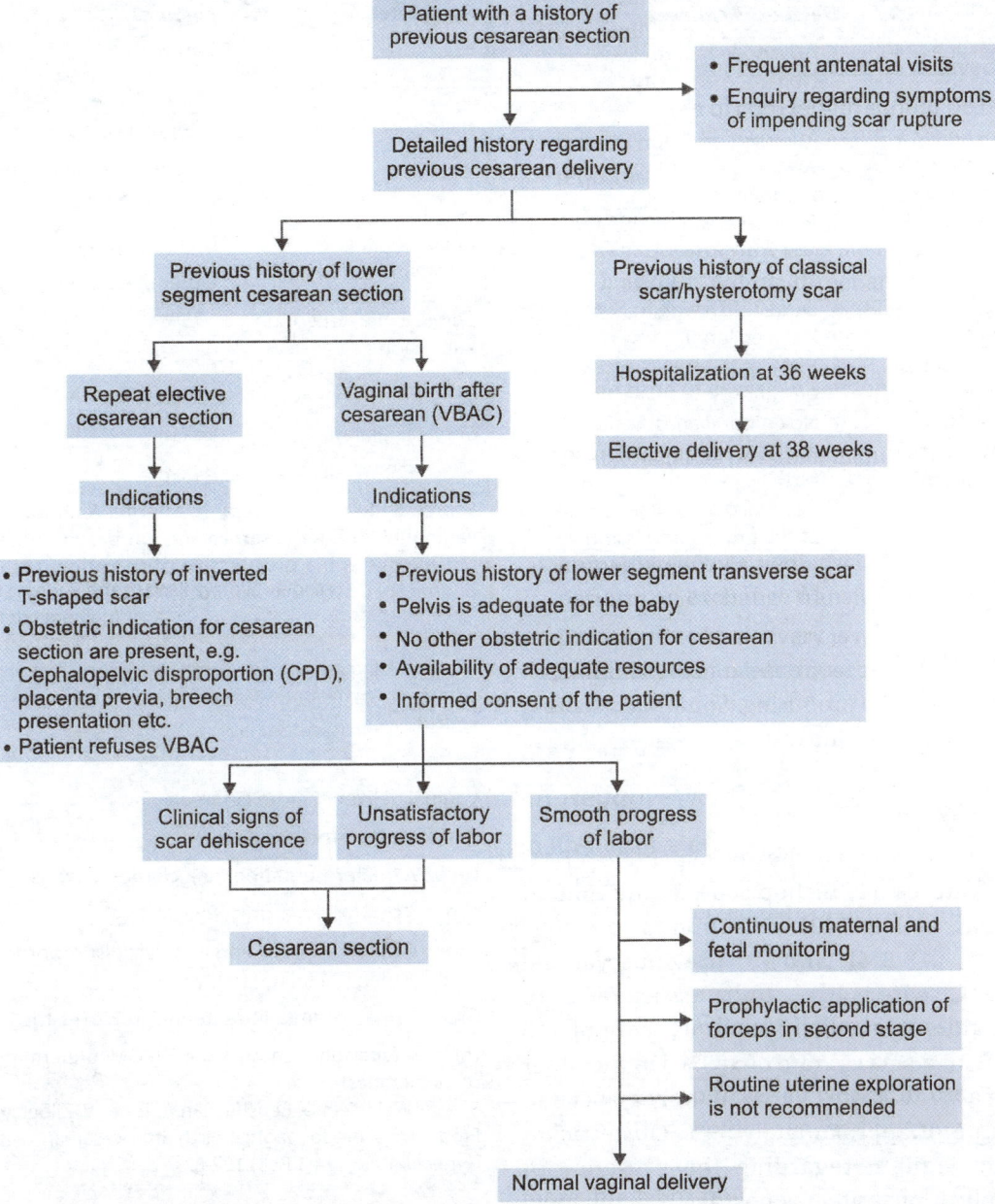

Flowchart 11.1: Management of a patient with a previous history of cesarean section.

BOX 11.4: Criteria for VBAC.

- Previous history of one uncomplicated lower segment transverse cesarean section (CS)
- Low transverse incision on the uterus
- Pelvis is adequate
- Patient is willing for VBAC
- Facilities for continuous fetal monitoring during labor are available
- No other contraindication for CS
- Previous history of vaginal birth, particularly VBAC
- VBAC should be undertaken in settings where facilities for emergency CS are present

(VBAC: vaginal birth after cesarean)

clinical examination that the patient appears to be a candidate for VBAC, this option must be discussed with the patient. VBAC should be undertaken only if the patient is herself satisfied with the decision and is willing to give an informed consent for the same.

- *Previous vaginal birth:* Previous history of vaginal birth, particularly previous VBAC, can be considered as the single best predictor for successful VBAC and is associated with a planned VBAC success rate of approximately 90%.

Prediction of Vaginal Birth after Cesarean Section

The VBAC calculator can be considered as a useful tool for predicting the success of women attempting VBAC and for counseling the patient for TOLAC, thereby helping in informed decision-making. Many models/tools for predicting the success rate of VBAC have been developed by several authors. However, further research is required

TABLE 11.2: Predictors for successful VBAC.	
Increased chances	Decreased chances
• Younger maternal age (<40 years) • Prior vaginal birth • Prior cesarean section for malpresentation, multiple gestation, placenta previa, nonreassuring fetal status • Greater maternal height • BMI < 30 kg/m^2 • Gestational age of <40 weeks • Infant birth weight < 4 kg • Spontaneous onset of labor • Vertex presentation • Fetal head engagement or presence at a lower station • Higher admission Bishop score	• Advanced maternal age • Nonwhite ethnicity • Short stature • Increased BMI or excessive weight gain during pregnancy • Prior cesarean section for arrest disorders • Maternal comorbidities • Larger birth weight (>4,000 g) • Induced labor • VBAC at or after 41 weeks of gestation • No epidural anesthesia • Previous preterm cesarean birth • Cervical dilatation of <4 cm at the time of admission • History of previous cesarean birth <2 years back

TABLE 11.3: Flamm and Geiger scoring system.		
Parameter	Findings	Points
Age	<40 years	2
	>40 years	0
History of vaginal delivery	After first cesarean delivery	2
	Before first cesarean delivery	1
	None	0
Indication for first cesarean section	Failure to progress	0
	Other reason	1
Cervical effacement on admission	>75%	2
	25–75%	1
	<25%	0
Cervical dilatation	>4 cm	1
	≤4 cm	0

Source: Sahu R, Chaudhary N, Sharma A. Prediction of successful vaginal birth after cesarean section based on Flamm and Geiger scoring system: a prospective observational study. Int J Reprod Contracept Obstet Gynecol. 2018;7(10):3998-4002.

to predict the VBAC success using these models, although initial results appeared to be promising. Some such scoring systems are given in the following text.

Schoorel Scoring System

Schoorel et al. (2014) created the retrospective VBAC score using five features: (1) Bishop score at the time of admission, (2) maternal age, (3) indication for previous cesarean delivery, (4) BMI, and (5) previous vaginal birth. Higher VBAC score is likely to be associated with a higher success rate. Women with a VBAC score of >16 were associated with a success rate of >85%. On the other hand, those with a VBAC score of 10 were only associated with a success rate of approximately 50%. Obstetrician needs to remain vigilant regarding the presence of underlying complications, such as postdated pregnancy, twin gestation, fetal macrosomia, antepartum stillbirth, or maternal age of 40 years or more, which act as relative contraindication for VBAC.

Maternal-fetal Medicine Unit VBAC Score Calculator

The maternal–fetal medicine unit (MFMU) is available free on internet and is easy to use. The parameters it takes into consideration include age, BMI, race, ethnicity, obstetric history (previous history of vaginal delivery), indication for previous CS, estimated gestational age at delivery, presence of hypertensive disease of pregnancy, cervical dilatation, station of fetal head, and labor spontaneous or induced.

A score of 60–70 is associated with higher chances for success and lower rupture rates.

TABLE 11.4: Weinstein scoring system for predicting VBAC.		
Factor	No	Yes
Bishop's score ≥ 4	0	4
Vaginal delivery before cesarean	0	2
Past indication for cesarean		
Group A (malpresentation, preeclampsia, twins)	0	6
Group B (APH, prematurity, PPROM)	0	5
Group C (fetal distress, cephalopelvic disproportion, cord accident, or failure to progress)	0	4
Group D (macrosomia, intrauterine growth restriction)	0	3

(APH: antepartum hemorrhage; PPROM: preterm premature rupture of membranes)
Source: Weinstein D, Benshushan A, Tanos V, Zilberstein R, Rojansky N. Predictive score for vaginal birth after cesarean section. Am J Obstet Gynecol. 1996;174(1 Pt 1):192-8.

Flamm and Geiger Scoring System

Higher VBAC score on Flamm and Geiger scoring system **(Table 11.3)** is likely to be associated with a higher success rate for VBAC. Most of the patients with total Flamm and Geiger score < 3 at the time of admission had emergency CS. On the other hand, most of the patients with score > 4 had successful VBAC. Total Flamm and Geiger scores of 4, 5, 6, and >8 were respectively associated with 53.3%, 75%, 85.7%, and 100% probabilities for successful VBAC.

Weinstein Scoring System for Predicting VBAC

Higher VBAC score on Weinstein scoring system **(Table 11.4)** is likely to be associated with a higher success rate for VBAC. Maximum score possible with this system is 12. If the total

Weinstein's score is 10, chances for VBAC are >85%, and with a score of 12, chances for successful VBAC can be >88%.

Advantages of Vaginal Birth after Cesarean Section

Vaginal birth after CS is associated with the following advantages:

- Prevention of surgery-related complications including death
- Prevention of blood loss
- Prevention of infection
- Prevention of injury to various organs including bowel, urinary bladder, etc.
- Prevention of thromboembolism
- Breastfeeding is generally easier after a vaginal birth.
- Vaginal birth is usually associated with reduced healthcare costs in comparison to cesarean births.
- VBAC is also associated with lower fetal mortality and morbidity in comparison to ERCS.

Contraindications for Vaginal Birth after Cesarean Section

Vaginal birth after cesarean is contraindicated in the presence of the conditions described in **Box 11.5**.

However, there may be exceptions in certain extreme circumstances (e.g., miscarriage and intrauterine fetal death) where the vaginal route (although risky) may not necessarily be contraindicated. The RCOG (2015) considers the previous history of three or more previous cesarean deliveries as a contraindication for VBAC. The ACOG also contemplates that the present evidence regarding the risk for women with prior history of more than two previous cesarean deliveries undergoing TOLAC is largely limited.

Also, presently there is insufficient information regarding the risk of uterine rupture in women with previous history of myomectomy or prior complex uterine surgery.

BOX 11.5: Contraindications for VBAC.

Absolute contraindications:
- Women with a history of previous uterine rupture
- Previous classical cesarean scar
- Women who have any absolute contraindication to vaginal birth, which is applicable irrespective of the presence or absence of a scar (e.g., major placenta previa)

Relative contraindications:
- Type of previous uterine incision (previous inverted T or J incisions, low vertical uterine incisions, or significant inadvertent uterine extension at the time of primary cesarean)
- Previous history of uterine surgery (e.g., hysteroscopic resection of uterine septum, laparoscopic or abdominal myomectomy, especially where the uterine cavity has been penetrated)
- Presence of underlying complications such as postdated pregnancy, twin gestation, fetal macrosomia, antepartum stillbirth, or maternal age of 40 years or more

---

VBAC in Twin Gestation

Regarding twin gestation, the ACOG has recommended that women with one previous cesarean delivery with a low transverse incision, who are otherwise suitable candidates for twin vaginal delivery, may be considered for TOLAC.

VBAC in Macrosomia

Regarding macrosomia, the ACOG states that suspected macrosomia alone should not prevent the obstetrician from considering the possibility of TOLAC. The RCOG, however, does not make specific recommendations and suggests that a cautious approach be adopted when considering planned VBAC in women with these circumstances, in the absence of definite evidence regarding the safety and efficacy of planned VBAC in such situations.

Unsuccessful Vaginal Birth after Cesarean Section

There are numerous other factors associated with a decreased likelihood of success at the time of planned VBAC and these are tabulated in **Table 11.2**.

Risk of Vaginal Birth after Cesarean Section

- If VBAC turns out to be unsuccessful, an emergency CS may be required.
- There is a risk of the scar dehiscence and rupture.
- There is an increased risk of maternal and perinatal mortalities in case of scar rupture.
- Failure of vaginal trial may end up in requirement for an emergency CS. It may also cause uterine rupture or pelvic floor dysfunction.

Counseling of Women for Vaginal Birth after Cesarean Section

All the women with a previous history of uncomplicated lower segment cesarean delivery, in an otherwise uncomplicated pregnancy at term, with no contraindication for vaginal birth, need to be counseled regarding both the delivery options because new evidence has now accumulated which shows that VBAC may not be as safe as was originally understood. These factors, together with fears for medicolegal litigations, have led to a recent decline in the rate of planned VBAC in the UK and North America. A final decision between the woman and her obstetrician regarding mode of birth should be established before the expected date of delivery (ideally by 36 weeks of gestation). Women considering the option for vaginal birth after a single previous cesarean should be informed that the chance of successful planned VBAC is approximately 70%. Women who want VBAC should be encouraged and supported. They should be counseled regarding the advantages and disadvantages of both the procedures. They should also be

> **BOX 11.6:** Points to be taken into consideration while counseling women with previous history of cesarean delivery.
>
> *Vaginal birth after cesarean (VBAC):*
> - Women should be made aware that successful VBAC is associated with the lowest rate of complications, and therefore, while choosing the mode of delivery it is important to estimate the success and failure rates of VBAC in each case
> - Trial of VBAC resulting in emergency cesarean delivery is associated with the greatest risk of adverse outcomes
> - Planned VBAC is associated with ~1 in 200 (0.5%) risk of uterine rupture
> - VBAC is associated with an extremely low absolute risk of birth-related perinatal deaths, which is comparable to that of nulliparous women in labor
> - The success rate of planned VBAC varies between 72 and 75%
> - Women with one or more previous vaginal births should be informed that the history of previous vaginal delivery, particularly previous VBAC, acts as the most important predictor for successful VBAC. This is associated with a planned VBAC success rate of 85–90%
>
> *Elective repeat cesarean section (ERCS):*
> - When a date for ERCS is being decided upon, a plan for the event of labor starting before the scheduled date should be documented in the patient's case notes
> - Women should be informed that ERCS is associated with a small increased risk of complications such as placenta previa, accreta, and/or pelvic adhesions in future pregnancies
> - The risk of perinatal death with ERCS is extremely low. However, there is a small increase in neonatal respiratory morbidity when ERCS is performed before 39^{+0} weeks of gestation

informed about the slightly increased chances of uterine rupture during VBAC in comparison with ERCS (about 1 per 10,000 risk of uterine rupture in cases with ERCS vs. 50 per 10,000 with VBAC). Though the occurrence of intrapartum fetal death is rare, it is slightly more in cases with VBAC compared with those with ERCS (about 10 per 10,000 for VBAC vs. 1 per 10,000 for ERCS).

Points to be taken into consideration while counseling women with previous history of cesarean delivery are listed in **Box 11.6**.

Advantages Conferred by Vaginal Birth after Cesarean Section

- VBAC helps in avoiding the potential future maternal consequences related to multiple cesarean deliveries.
- VBAC helps in avoidance of major abdominal surgery, which is associated with lower rates of complications such as hemorrhage and infection and a shorter recovery period.
- RCOG has reported that attempting VBAC helps in reducing the risk of the baby having respiratory problems after birth (risk of 2–3% with planned VBAC vs. 3–4% with ERCS).

Intrapartum Management

The following steps must be observed during the intrapartum period:
1. Blood should be sent for grouping, crossmatching, and complete blood count (including hemoglobin and hematocrit levels). One unit of blood should be arranged.
2. IV access to be established, and Ringer's lactate can be started.
3. Clinical monitoring of the mother for the signs of scar dehiscence needs to be done. This includes monitoring of vitals, especially the pulse rate and scar tenderness, which must be done every 15 minutes.
4. Careful monitoring of FHR, preferably using continuous external cardiotocograph. There is no role of intermittent auscultation in these cases.
5. Facilities for emergency CS should be available. The pediatrician, anesthetist, and operation theater staff must be informed well in advance, because they may be required at any time.
6. Although induction or augmentation of labor is not contraindicated in cases of TOLAC, it should be a consultant-led decision, which is preceded by careful obstetric assessment and appropriate maternal counseling. Regarding the use of prostaglandins for induction of labor, the ACOG recommends against the use of misoprostol [prostaglandin E1 (PGE_1)] for cervical ripening or labor induction in patients with a previous cesarean delivery or major uterine surgery. Regarding the use of dinoprostone [prostaglandin E2 (PGE_2)] for cervical ripening, the ACOG presently does not make any definitive recommendations regarding its use, in the absence of sufficient evidence. The ACOG supports the use of oxytocin infusion in patients undergoing TOLAC. It however avoids sequential use of prostaglandins and oxytocin for labor induction. The RCOG recommends that before using prostaglandins (both PGE_1 and PGE_2), women must be counseled regarding the higher risk of uterine rupture associated with their use. It recommends that the safe limit for prostaglandin dosage used for cervical priming in women with prior cesarean birth must not be exceeded. It also recommends that oxytocin augmentation should be titrated such that it should not exceed the maximum rate of contractions of four in 10 minutes, with the ideal contraction frequency being three to four in

10 minutes. The RCOG also recommends vigilant serial cervical assessments to be performed both in cases of augmented and nonaugmented labors to ensure adequate progress of labor.

7. Women should be informed that the risk of uterine rupture is increased by 2–3-folds while the risk of CS is increased by 1.5-folds in cases of induced and/or augmented labors (in the presence of a previous cesarean birth) in comparison with spontaneous labor. Women should also be informed that the risk of uterine rupture further increases when the labor is induced with the help of prostaglandins. The use of prostaglandins for induction of labor in women with previous history of CS must be best avoided. There should be careful serial cervical assessments, preferably by the same person, for both augmented and nonaugmented labors, to ensure that there is adequate cervicometric progress, thereby allowing the planned VBAC to continue.

The decision to induce, method chosen, decision to augment with oxytocin, time intervals for serial vaginal examination, selected parameters of monitoring progress, and advice on discontinuing VBAC should be discussed with the woman by a consultant obstetrician.

8. Oxytocin augmentation should be titrated such that it does not exceed the maximum rate of contractions of four in 10 minutes; the ideal contraction frequency would be three to four in 10 minutes.

9. When informing a woman about induction (prostaglandin or nonprostaglandin methods) and/or augmentation, clear information should be provided on all potential risks and benefits of such a decision and how this may impact on her long-term health. For example, women who are contemplating future pregnancies may accept the short-term additional risks associated with induction and/or augmentation in view of the reduced risk of serious complications in future pregnancies if they have a successful VBAC.

10. Epidural analgesia can be safely given at the time of labor.

11. Intrapartum monitoring regarding the progress of labor must be done using a partogram **(Fig. 11.1)**. This figure shows the modified WHO partogram as devised by the WHO previously. The WHO (2018) has devised a new labor monitoring device called the WHO labor care guide. Kindly refer to Chapter 2 for details.

12. Second stage of labor can be cut short by using prophylactic forceps or ventouse.

13. Routine uterine exploration following VBAC is not recommended.

If the patient shows signs of uterine rupture including tachycardia, hypotension, vaginal bleeding, etc., uterine exploration may be done. Laparotomy may be required if a uterine rent is found on uterine exploration.

The most important complication associated in a patient with previous history of CS is the possibility of scar rupture during future pregnancies, especially if given trial for vaginal delivery. Thus, it is the prime duty of the obstetrician to remain vigilant and at the earliest detect the signs related to impending scar rupture. Symptoms of impending scar rupture during the labor include the following:

- Dull suprapubic pain or severe abdominal pain, especially if persisting in between the uterine contractions
- Slight vaginal bleeding or hematuria
- Bladder tenesmus or frequent desire to pass urine
- Unexplained maternal tachycardia
- Maternal hypotension or shock
- Abnormal FHR pattern
- Scar tenderness
- Interruption of previously efficient uterine activity
- Severe abdominal pain, especially if persisting between contractions
- Chest pain or shoulder tip pain, or sudden onset of shortness of breath.

On vaginal examination, there may be a failure of normal descent of the presenting part, and the presenting part may remain high up. There also may be a sudden loss of station of the presenting part. None of the above-mentioned signs and symptoms is definite proof of the impending scar rupture. However, the presence of any of these symptoms must raise caution in the clinician's mind, and he/she must become more vigilant. The diagnosis of scar rupture is ultimately confirmed at the time of emergency cesarean delivery or postpartum laparotomy.

ELECTIVE REPEAT CESAREAN SECTION

> Q. Write a long essay on difficulties and complications faced by the obstetrician during ERCS. Also discuss its management.

For the physician, ERCS may offer a few advantages including convenience, saving of time, increased monetary compensation, and reduced fear of legal litigation in case of complications with VBAC. Though CS is safe, it is a major surgical intervention and would be therefore associated with some complications in comparison to normal vaginal delivery. Women with the history of one previous classical cesarean delivery are recommended to give birth by ERCS. The clinician must counsel the women regarding increased risks of complications such as cardiac arrests, thromboembolism, and major infections in comparison to those who deliver vaginally. However, the cesarean delivery does provide a few advantages in comparison to the normal vaginal delivery, some of which are listed in **Box 11.7**. CS has been found to have no effect on the incidence of complications such as hemorrhage, infection, genital tract injury, fecal incontinence, back pain, dyspareunia,

212 Complications of Pregnancy

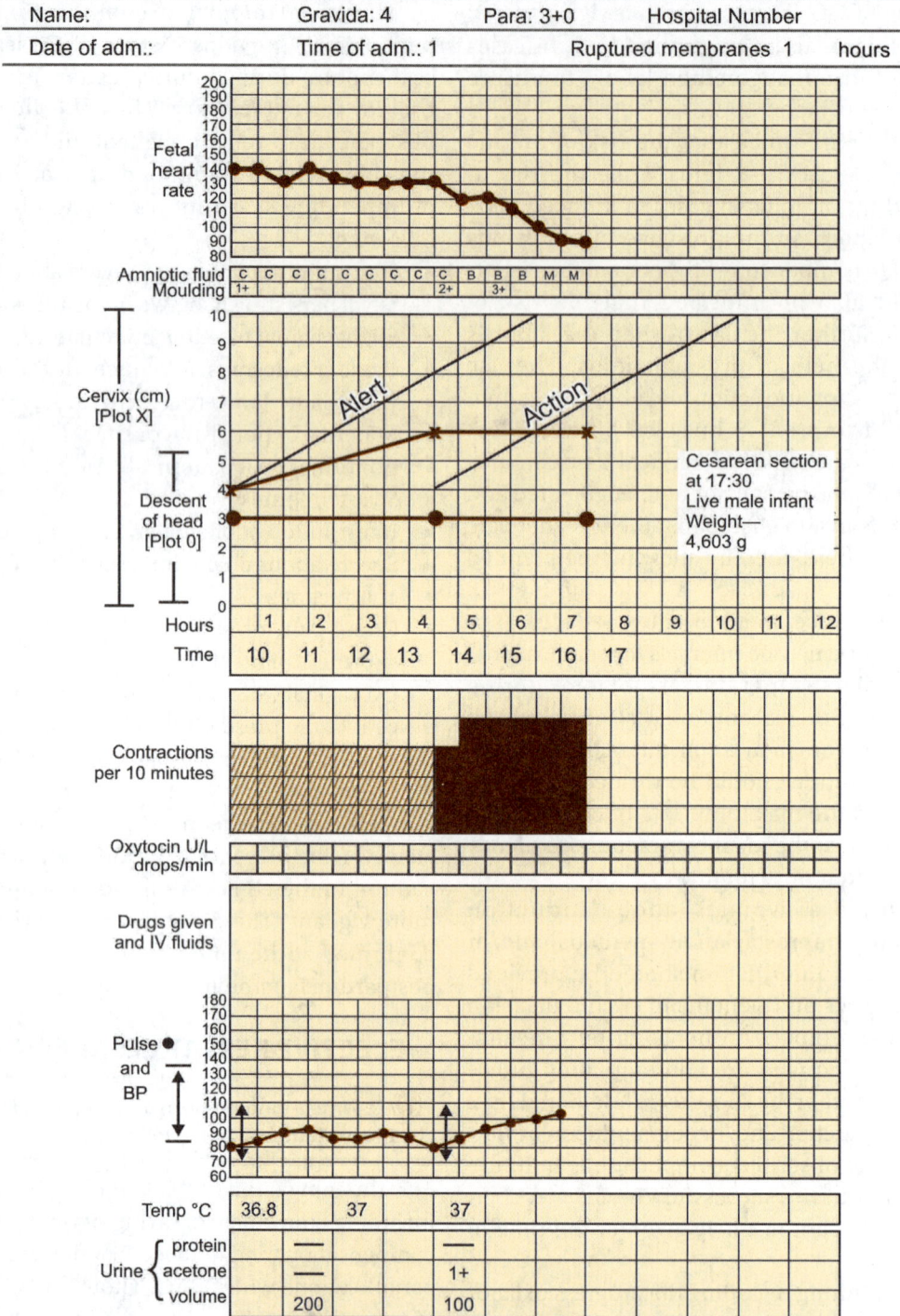

Fig. 11.1: Monitoring the progress of labor using a partogram.

> **BOX 11.7:** Advantages of cesarean delivery.
> - Reduced incidence of perineal pain
> - Reduced incidence of urinary incontinence
> - Reduced incidence of uterovaginal prolapse

Disadvantages of Cesarean Delivery

Cesarean delivery is associated with an increased risk of complications, enumerated in **Box 11.8**.

Timing for Cesarean Delivery

In case of previous history of classical scar, the woman must preferably be hospitalized at 36 weeks and posted for an elective CS at 38 weeks. In patients with previous history of lower segment uterine scar, the planned surgery

postnatal depression, neonatal mortality rate, intracranial hemorrhage, brachial plexus injuries, and cerebral palsy. Risks and benefits of planned VBAC versus ERCS from 39^{+0} weeks of gestation are listed in **Table 11.5**.

TABLE 11.5: Risks and benefits of planned VBAC versus ERCS from 39^{+0} weeks of gestation.

Benefits	Risks
Vaginal birth after cesarean (VBAC)	
• It is associated with the fewest complications • The absolute risk of birth-related perinatal death associated with VBAC is extremely low and comparable to the risk for nulliparous women in labor • Chances of VBAC being successful are 72–75% • If successful, VBAC is associated with a shorter duration of hospital stay and recovery period • It increases the likelihood of future vaginal births • Risk of maternal death with VBAC is lower than that with ERCS • It is associated with 2–3% risk of transient respiratory morbidity, which is lower than that with ERCS	• Greatest risk of adverse outcome occurs in a trial of VBAC, resulting in emergency cesarean delivery • Risk of uterine rupture associated with VBAC is ~0.5%. If occurs, it is associated with significant maternal morbidity and fetal morbidity/mortality • Risk of anal sphincter injury in women undergoing VBAC is 5% • It is associated with an increased risk of instrumental delivery • It is associated with an increased risk (0.08%) of hypoxic ischemic encephalopathy (HIE) • Associated with 4 per 10,000 (0.04%) risk of delivery-related perinatal death • The rates of hysterectomy, thromboembolic disease, transfusion, and endometritis do not differ significantly between planned VBAC and ERCS
Elective repeat cesarean section (ERCS)	
• May be possible to plan a known delivery date in selected patients • Practically avoids the risk of uterine rupture (actual risk is extremely low: less than 0.02%) • Associated with a reduced risk of pelvic organ prolapse and urinary incontinence • Offers the option for permanent sterilization if fertility is no longer desired • Less than 1 per 10,000 (<0.01%) risk of delivery-related perinatal death or HIE	• It is associated with a small increased risk of placenta previa and/or accreta in future pregnancies and of pelvic adhesions complicating any future abdominopelvic surgery • Risk of perinatal death with ERCS is extremely low, but there is a small increase in neonatal respiratory morbidity when ERCS is performed before 39^{+0} weeks of gestation • It is associated with a longer recovery period • Future pregnancies—likely to require cesarean delivery, increased risk of placenta previa or accreta, and adhesions with successive cesarean deliveries or abdominal surgery • Risk of maternal death with ERCS is higher than that with VBAC • Risk of transient respiratory morbidity of 4–5% (higher than that with VBAC)

BOX 11.8: Complications associated with cesarean delivery.

- Abdominal pain
- Injury to bladder, ureters, etc.
- Increased risk of ruptured uterus and maternal death
- Neonatal respiratory morbidity
- Hysterectomy
- Thromboembolic disease
- Increased duration of hospital stay
- Antepartum or intrapartum intrauterine deaths in future pregnancies
- Patients with a previous history of cesarean delivery are more prone to develop complications such as placenta previa and adherent placenta during future pregnancies

TABLE 11.6: National Confidential Enquiry into Patient Outcome and Death (NCEPOD) classification system for cesarean delivery on the basis of urgency.

Type	Category	Description
Unplanned CS	1	Immediate threat to the life of the woman or fetus
	2	Maternal or fetal compromise, which is not immediately life-threatening
Planned CS	3	No maternal or fetal compromise, but nevertheless early delivery is required
	4	Delivery timed to suit woman or staff

Source: Thool KN, Jain SM, Shivkumar PV, Jain MA, Podder MR. A clinical audit and confidential enquiry of cesarean section indications at rural tertiary health care center. Int J Reprod Contracept Obstet Gynecol. 2017;6:1478-83.

should be preferably done after 39 weeks. This is so as the risk of respiratory morbidity considerably increases in babies born by CS before 39 weeks of gestation. If the obstetrician is unsure about the exact period of gestation, it is best to wait for the onset of the uterine contractions or the rupture of membranes, whichever occurs earlier. However, an emergency CS may be required any time in cases of suspected or confirmed acute fetal compromise. In these cases, delivery should be accomplished as soon as possible, preferably within 30 minutes of the diagnosis of fetal distress.

Classification of Cesarean Delivery

Previously, CS had been classified as either elective or emergency procedure. Since the year 2000, a new system of categorization has been adopted throughout the UK, which groups the cesarean deliveries as "planned" and "unplanned" **(Table 11.6)**. Unplanned groups of cesarean deliveries belong to categories 1 and 2, where there is an immediate threat to the life of the mother or fetus (e.g., cord prolapse, prolonged bradycardia, pH < 7.20, and uterine rupture) or in cases where there is maternal or fetal compromise, which is not immediately life-threatening (e.g., failure to progress in labor, a patient booked as category 4 CS admitted in labor). In cases where there is an immediate threat to the life of either mother or fetus, a CS should be done as soon as possible, preferably within 30 minutes. In cases where there is no immediate threat to the mother or fetus, a CS should be performed as soon as possible, preferably within 75 minutes. Planned groups of cesarean deliveries belong to categories 3 and 4. These include cases where there is no maternal or fetal compromise, yet early delivery is required (e.g., failed induction with no maternal or fetal compromise, patient booked as category 4 CS presented with ruptured membranes, not in labor) or in cases where CS can be performed at a time to suit the woman and her maternity service (e.g., elective CS).

Preparations for an Elective Cesarean Section

- *Identification of anemia:* Since cesarean delivery is associated with the risk of blood loss, women posted for ERCS must be offered hemoglobin assessment before the surgery to identify those who have anemia.
- *Preoperative blood tests:* Although blood loss of >1,000 mL infrequently occurs after cesarean delivery, it may commonly occur in women having cesarean delivery for antepartum hemorrhage (both abruption and placenta previa) and uterine rupture. In such cases, the clinician should be prepared in anticipation of massive blood loss occurring at the time of surgery and should plan for blood transfusion services, well in advance. Such women must be offered the following tests prior to the surgery: grouping and saving of serum, cross-matching of blood, a clotting screen, and preoperative ultrasound for localization of placenta.
- *Antibiotic prophylaxis:* Prophylactic single-dose antibiotics in the form of first-generation cephalosporin (e.g., cefazolin) or ampicillin should be prescribed.
- *Thromboprophylaxis:* The risk for thromboembolism in these patients must be assessed as they may be confined to bed for long periods of time. Thromboprophylaxis in the form of graduated stockings, hydration, early mobilization, and low-molecular-weight heparin must be prescribed.
- *Prevention of aspiration pneumonitis:* Administration of anesthesia in women with full stomach is associated with the risk of aspiration pneumonitis. While the risk for aspiration pneumonitis is minimal in cases of ERCS, in which the patient is usually kept on an overnight fast, this may not be the scenario with emergency cesarean delivery, where the patient may be full stomach. In these cases, in order to reduce the risk of aspiration pneumonitis, the patient must be administered premedication with an antacid (sodium citrate 0.3%, 30 mL or magnesium trisilicate 300 mg) and H_2 receptor antagonists and/or proton pump inhibitors and antiemetics, all administered intravenously 1 hour before the surgery.
- *Urinary catheter:* It must be inserted in situ before the surgery in cases where regional anesthesia is planned because anesthetic block may interfere with normal bladder function, resulting in overdistension of the bladder. If bladder has not been previously catheterized, in all cases of CS, it should be catheterized as a routine before the surgery in order to prevent inadvertent injuries to the bladder at the time of surgery.
- *Prevention of hypotension:* IV ephedrine or phenylephrine should be used for management of hypotension encountered during the procedure. The operating table should have a lateral tilt of 15° because this helps in reducing the development of maternal hypotension.
- *Maternal position:* All obstetric patients undergoing CS should be positioned with left lateral tilt to avoid aortocaval compression. This can be accomplished by tilting the operating table to the left or placing a pillow or folded linen under the patient's right lower back.

Surgery for Cesarean Section

Anesthesia

Women who are having a cesarean delivery must preferably be offered regional anesthesia because it is safer and results in lower maternal and neonatal morbidity in comparison to general anesthesia. Women who are having a CS under regional anesthesia should be offered IV ephedrine or phenylephrine and volume preloading with crystalloids or colloids to reduce the risk of hypotension occurring at the time of surgery.

In case general anesthesia is used for unplanned cesarean delivery, it should comprise steps such as preoxygenation, cricoid pressure, and rapid sequence induction to reduce the risk of aspiration.

Preparation of the Skin

- The area around the proposed incision site must be washed with antiseptic soap solution (e.g., Savlon) and water.
- The woman's pubic hair must not be shaved as this may increase the risk of wound infection. The hair may be trimmed, if necessary.
- Routine cleaning of the patient's skin at the site of surgery must be done with antiseptic solution (e.g., Betadine) before surgery. Antiseptic skin cleansing before surgery is thought to reduce the risk of postoperative wound infections.

The antiseptic solution must be applied three times to the incision site using a high-level disinfected ring forceps and cotton or gauze swab. The surgeon must begin at the proposed incision site and move outward in a circular motion away from the site of incision site. In the end, the inner aspects of thighs and umbilicus must be swabbed.

- After reaching the edge of the sterile field, the previous swab must be discarded and new swab must be used.
- The surgeon must keep his/her arms and elbows high and surgical gown away from the surgical field.
- The woman must be draped immediately after the area of surgery has been adequately prepared, in order to avoid contamination.
- If the drape has a window, it should be placed directly over the incision site.

Type of Abdominal Skin Incision

A vertical or transverse incision can be given over the skin (Fig. 11.2).

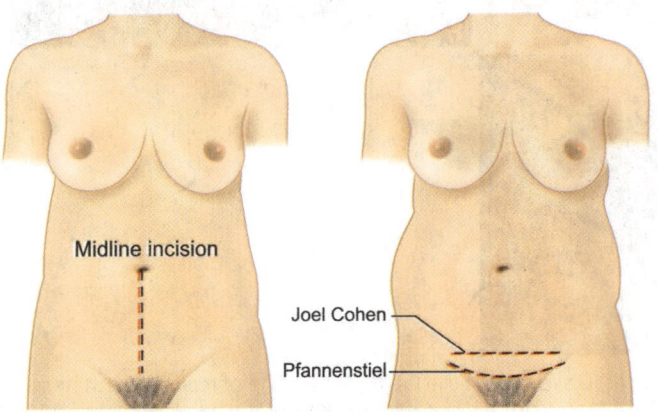

Fig. 11.2: Types of abdominal skin incision.

The vertical skin incision can be either in the midline or in the paramedian location, extending just above the pubic symphysis to just below the umbilicus **(Figs. 11.3A to C)**. Previously, vertical skin incision at the time of CS was favored as it was supposed to provide far more superior access to the surgical field in comparison to the transverse incision. Also, the vertical incision showed potential for extension at the time of surgery. However, it was associated with poor cosmetic results, an increased risk of wound dehiscence, and hernia formation. Therefore, nowadays, transverse incision is mainly favored due to better cosmetic effect, reduced postoperative pain, and improved patient recovery. Two types of transverse incisions are mainly used while performing CS: the sharp (Pfannenstiel) type and the blunt (Joel–Cohen) type.

Sharp Pfannenstiel Transverse Incision

In this type, a slightly curved, transverse skin incision passing through the external sheath of the recti muscles is given, about an inch above the pubic symphysis. The subsequent tissue layers are opened by using a sharp scalpel **(Figs. 11.4A to G)**.

Joel–Cohen Blunt Incision

In this type, a straight skin incision about 3 cm in size is given above the pubic symphysis, and the subsequent tissue layers are opened bluntly, without using a sharp scalpel. The initial cut is given only through the cutis. In the midline, which is free from large blood vessels, the cut is deepened to meet the fascia. A small transverse opening is made in the fascia with

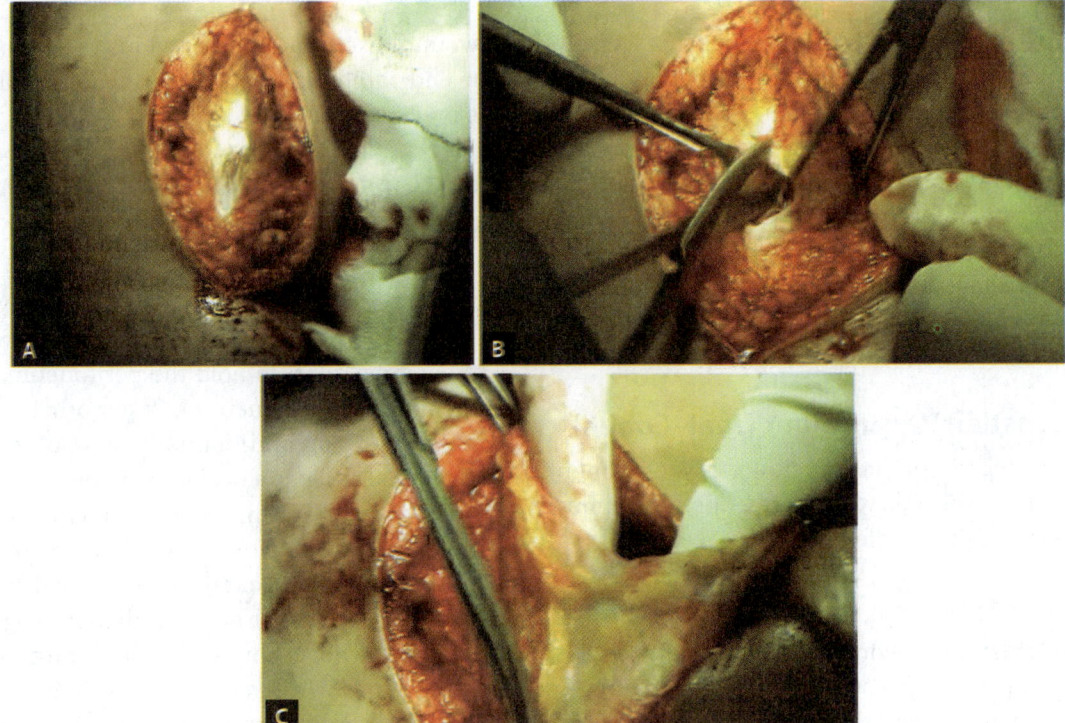

Figs. 11.3A to C: Vertical incision. (A) Vertical incision of skin and subcutaneous fat; (B) Fascial incision; (C) Peritoneal incision.

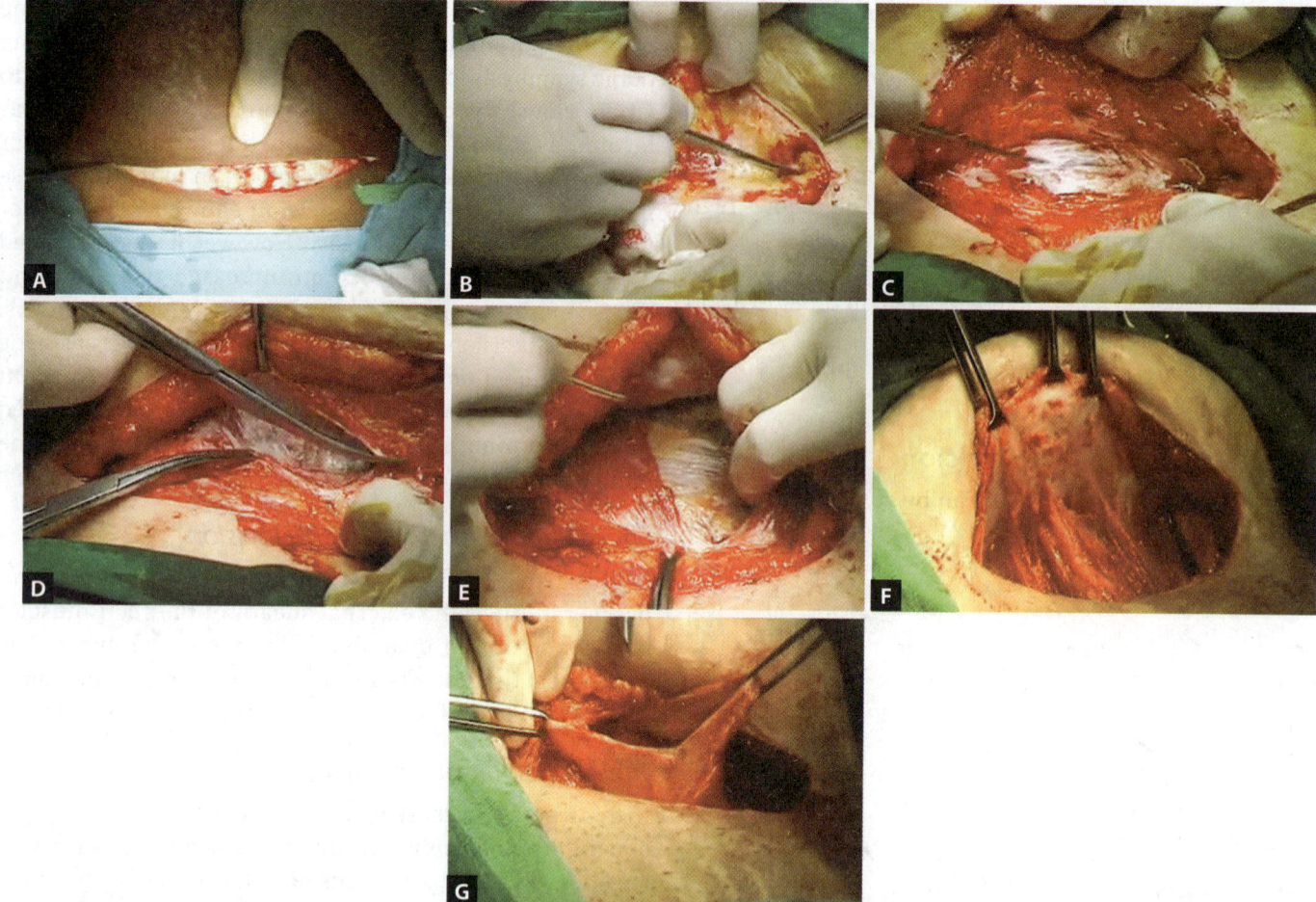

Figs. 11.4A to G: Pfannenstiel incision. (A) Giving a transverse skin incision; (B) Dissection of the fat; (C) Dissection of rectus sheath by giving an incision in the middle with help of a scalpel; (D) Extension of the rectus incision with help of scissors; (E) Separation of the rectus muscle from the rectus sheath; (F) Separation of the two recti muscles to visualize the parietal peritoneum; (G) Vertical incision of the peritoneum.

the scissors. The rest of the fascia is then opened transversely by pushing the slightly open tip of a pair of straight scissors, first in one direction and then in the other.

The fascia is stretched caudally and cranially using the index fingers to make room for the next step. The muscle and fat tissue are separated by applying manual bilateral skin traction using the index and middle fingers of both the surgeon and his assistant. The use of surgical knife must be avoided as far as possible and if required, the scissors can be used instead.

Sharp (Pfannenstiel) Versus Blunt (Joel–Cohen)

Presently, the transverse incision of choice is Joel-Cohen incision because it is associated with shorter operating times and reduced postoperative febrile morbidity.

Excision of Previous Scar

Excision of the existing previous scar must always be performed at the beginning of surgery by either giving an elliptical incision incorporating the scar or an incision over the previous scar, with the trimming of the fibrosed edges of the wound. Excision of the previous scar is usually difficult at the end of the surgery but must be done if it has not been done previously.

Dissecting through Different Layers of Abdomen until Uterus is Reached

- *Opening the peritoneum:* The transversalis fascia and peritoneal fat are dissected carefully to reach the underlying peritoneum. After placing two hemostats about 2 cm apart to hold the peritoneum, it is carefully opened. The peritoneum is superiorly incised up to the level of incision and inferiorly to a point just above the peritoneal reflection over the bladder.

  Once the parietal peritoneum has been opened, the uterus becomes visible. Before opening the peritoneum, its layers must be carefully examined to be sure that omentum, bowel, or bladder are not lying adjacent to it and they do not get injured while cutting the peritoneum.

- *Insertion of the Doyen's retractor:* Following the dissection of parietal peritoneum, the Doyen's retractor is inserted to expose the lower uterine segment **(Figs. 11.5A to C)**.

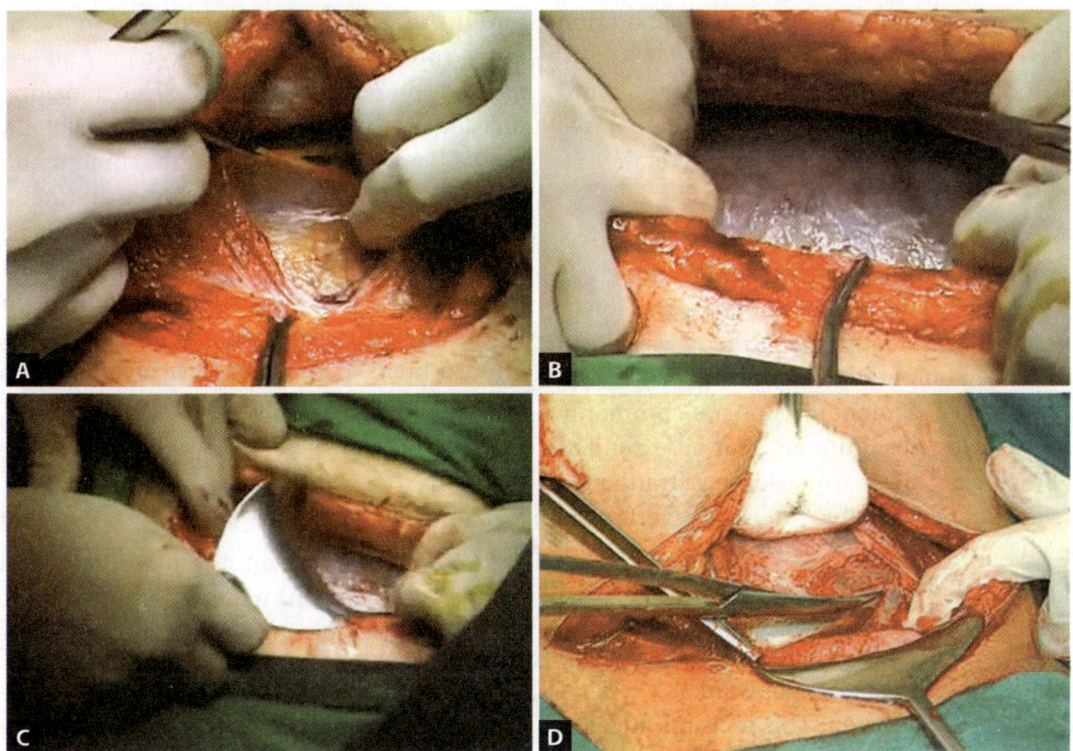

Figs. 11.5A to D: Steps of cesarean section until the separation of visceral peritoneum. (A) Opening the parietal peritoneum; (B) Visualization of uterus; (C) Insertion of Doyen's retractor; (D) Separating and cutting the visceral layer of peritoneum.

The loose fold of the uterovesical peritoneum over the lower uterine segment is then grasped with the help of forceps and incised transversely with the help of scissors **(Fig. 11.5 D)**. The underlying bladder is then separated by blunt dissection. Finally, the lower flap of peritoneum and the adjacent areolar tissue are also retracted by the Doyen's retractor to clear the lower uterine segment.

Types of Uterine Incision

Lower Segment Uterine Scar or the Upper Segment Uterine Scar

While in the past a vertical incision (classical) was commonly used, this was associated with high risk of scar rupture during future pregnancies. As a result, lower segment transverse incisions are nowadays preferred. The lower segment uterine scar is considered to be sounder than the upper segment due to the following reasons:

- Lower uterine segment is thinned out at the time of labor. As a result, the thin margins of the lower segment can be easily apposed at the time of uterine repair without leaving any pocket. In case of the classical scar, it may be difficult to oppose the thick muscle layer of the upper segment. Blood-filled pockets may be formed. This may be later replaced by fibrous tissues, resulting in the weakening of the scar.
- Lower segment usually remains inert in the postpartum period. On the other hand, the upper segment undergoes rapid contractions and retractions, resulting in the loosening of the uterine sutures. This can result in imperfect healing and further weakening of the uterine scar.
- When the uterus stretches in the future pregnancy, the stretch is along the line of the scar in the case of lower segment scar, whereas in cases of vertical scar, the uterus stretches in the direction perpendicular to the scar, thereby resulting in scar weakness.
- Chances of placental implantation in the area of the scar at the time of future pregnancy are highly unlikely in the case of lower segment scar. Whereas in case of classical scar, the placental tissue is quite likely to implant in the area of the scar at the time of future pregnancy. Penetration and invasion of the scar by placental trophoblasts are likely to produce further weakening of the scar.

As a result of the above-mentioned reasons, the lower segment scar is much stronger as compared to the upper segment scar and is unlikely to give way during subsequent pregnancies. Lower segment scar may rupture occasionally at the time of labor. On the other hand, upper segment scar is weak and may rupture both during the antenatal period and at the time of labor.

Indications for a Classical CS

Though nowadays classical incisions are rarely performed, they might be rarely done in cases where the lower segment is not easily accessible, e.g., bladder densely adherent to the lower segment; carcinoma cervix; the presence of an uterine myoma in the lower uterine segment; transverse lie of the fetus, with the shoulder impacted in the birth canal; and cases of placenta previa in which the placenta penetrates through the lower uterine segment (placenta percreta).

Variations in Lower Segment Incision

Presently, rather than performing a classical CS, the clinicians prefer to use some kind of variations in the lower segment uterine incision. Mostly, the surgeon is able to decide the exact incision only at the time of surgery.

Variations of the lower segment incision are commonly used in cases where there is requirement for an extended surgical field, in order to avoid scar extension, e.g., transverse lie with hand prolapse and large baby. Some of the variations include the following:

- *Inverted "T"-shaped incision*: This incision involves cutting upward from the middle of the transverse incision.
- *"J"-shaped or hockey-stick incision*: It involves extension of one end of the transverse incision upward.
- *"U"-shaped or trapdoor incision:* This incision involves extension of both ends of the transverse scar upward. Of all these various choices, the "T"-shaped scar is the worst choice due to its difficult repair, poor healing, and chances of scar rupture during subsequent pregnancies.

Blunt versus Sharp Uterine Incision

While making an incision in the uterus, a curvilinear mark of about 10 cm length is made by the scalpel, cutting partially through the myometrium. A short (3 cm) cut using the scalpel is made in the middle of this incision mark, reaching up to but not through the membranes. The rest of the incision can be completed either by stretching the incision using the two index fingers along both the sides of the incision mark **(Fig. 11.6A)** or using bandage scissors, to extend the incision on two sides **(Fig. 11.6B)**. The bandage scissor is introduced into the uterus over the two fingers in order to protect the fetus. In cases where the lower uterine segment is well-formed, blunt rather than sharp extension of the uterine incision is favored because this is associated with a reduced risk of blood loss, PPH, and the requirement of transfusion at the time of surgery. If the lower uterine segment is very thin, injury to the fetus can be avoided by using the handle of the scalpel or a hemostat (an artery forceps) to open the uterus. Delivery of the fetal head should be in the same way as during the normal vaginal delivery **(Figs. 11.7A to C)**. There is no need for routine use of forceps in order to deliver fetal head. Forceps should be used at cesarean only if there is difficulty while delivering the baby's head.

Placental Removal

At the time of cesarean, the placenta should be removed using controlled cord traction **(Fig. 11.7D)** and not manual removal as the former is associated with a reduced risk of endometritis.

Closure of the Uterine Incision

Single Layered or Double Layered Closure of Uterine Incision

Both single-layered and double-layered closure of uterine incision is being currently practiced. Though single-layered closure is associated with reduced operative time and reduced blood loss in the short term, the risk of the uterine rupture during subsequent pregnancies is increased.

The CAESAR (CAESARean section surgical techniques) trial, the largest RCT of CS surgical techniques undertaken till date, has not shown any significant differences in the various short-term outcomes such as length of hospital stay, preterm delivery, amnionitis, postpartum endometritis, placental abruption, PPH, blood transfusion, uterine dehiscence, etc. with single-versus-double-layered closure of the uterine

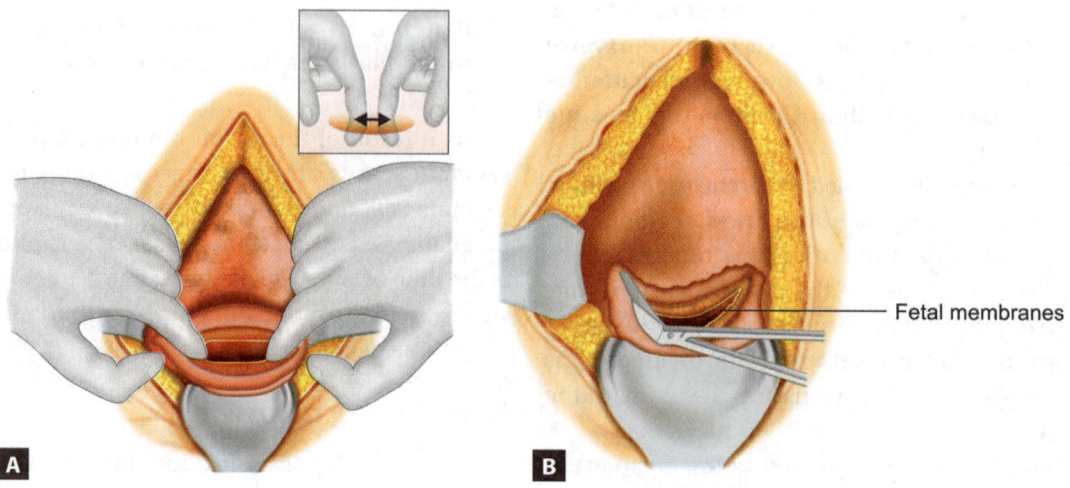

Figs. 11.6A and B: (A) Extension of the uterine incision by manual stretching using the index fingers; (B) Extension of the uterine incision with the help of scissors.

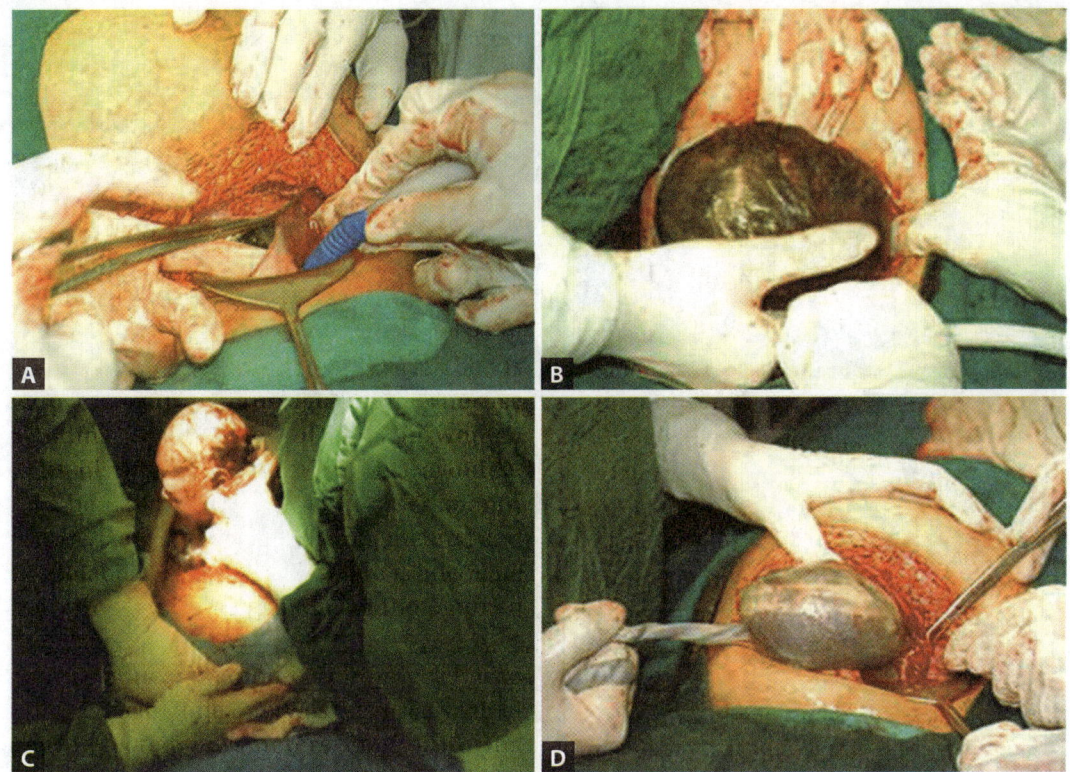

Figs. 11.7A to D: Steps of cesarean section until delivery of the baby and placenta. (A) Giving a uterine incision; (B) Delivery of fetal head; (C) Delivery of the rest of baby; (D) Delivery of the placenta.

incision. However, there are concerns related to the risk of uterine rupture in the future with the use of single-layered technique of closure.

Therefore, two-layered technique of closure is presently recommended until the results from the CAESAR follow-up trial become available. Currently, single layer closure of the uterine incision is best performed in research settings. The current recommendation by National Collaborating Centre for Women's and Children's Health (NCCWCH), 2011 and NICE is also to close the uterus in two layers **(Figs. 11.8A to D)**, as the safety and efficacy of closing uterus in a single layer presently remains uncertain.

Peritoneal Closure

The current recommendation by the RCOG is that neither the visceral nor the parietal peritoneum should be sutured at the time of CS as this reduces the operative time and the requirement for postoperative analgesia, and also improves maternal satisfaction.

Closure of Rectus Sheath

Closure of rectus sheath in cases of both vertical incision and Pfannenstiel incision is performed using continuous stitches. Since the strength of closure of rectus sheath is important for maintaining wound strength, some surgeons prefer to use continuous sutures, while locking each stitch. The angles must be secured using 1-0 Vicryl sutures. Method of closure of rectus sheath in case of Pfannenstiel and vertical incisions is respectively described in **Figures 11.9A and B and Figures 11.10 A and B**.

Closure of Subcutaneous Space

There is no need for the routine closure of the subcutaneous tissue space, unless there is more than 2 cm of subcutaneous fat because this practice has not been shown to reduce the incidence of wound infection.

Skin Closure

Obstetricians should be aware that presently the differences between the use of different suture materials and methods of skin closure at the time of CS are not certain. Skin closure can be performed either using subcutaneous, continuous repair absorbable or nonabsorbable stitches or using interrupted stitches with nonabsorbable sutures or staples. The use of staples is likely to be associated with similar outcomes in terms of wound infection, pain, and cosmetic results as compared to the use of sutures. The use of staples, however, is associated with an increased incidence of skin separation and requirement for reclosure if removed on day 3. In women who are at an increased risk of hematoma formation or infection, an interrupted method of closure can be adopted because with this method, there is an advantage of removal of one or two sutures to allow drainage when required.

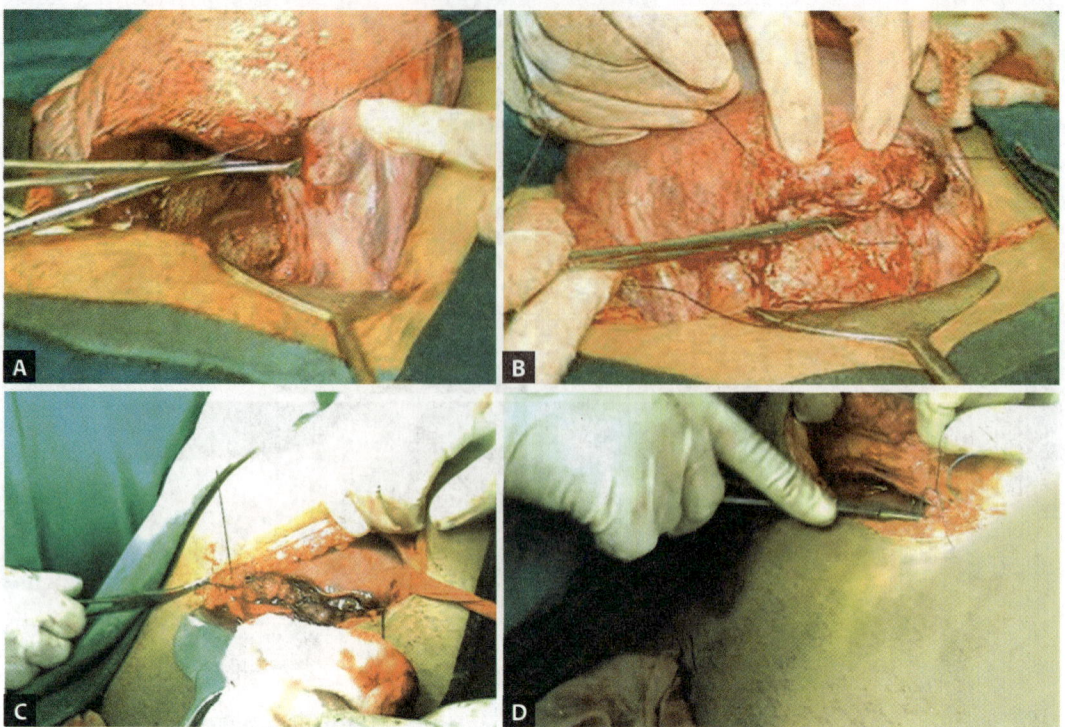

Figs. 11.8A to D: Steps of cesarean section involving closure of the uterine cavity and rectus sheath. (A) Holding the uterine angles using Allis forceps; (B) Stitching the uterine incision; (C) Uterine incision has been completely stitched; (D) Stitching the rectus sheath.

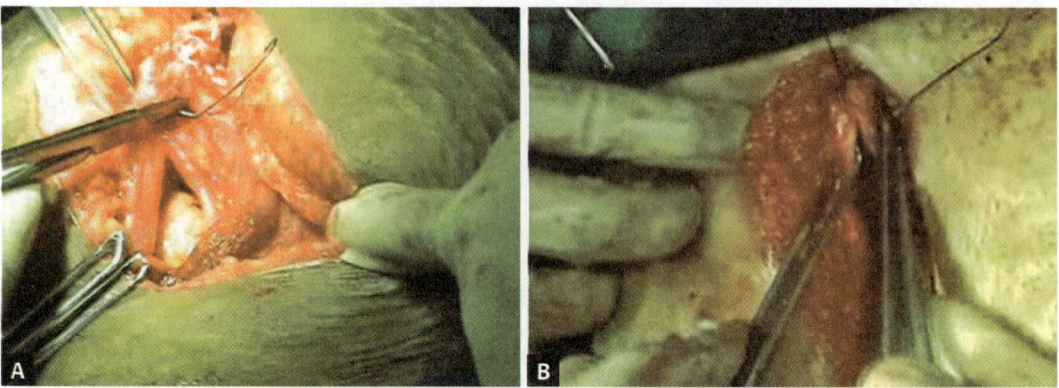

Figs. 11.9A and B: Closure of vertical incision: (A) Closure of peritoneum; (B) Closure of rectus sheath.

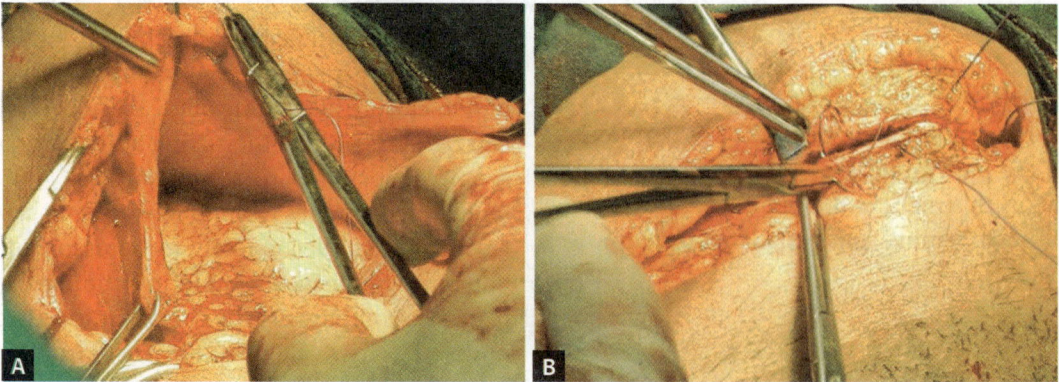

Figs. 11.10A and B: Closure of Pfannenstiel incision. (A) Closure of peritoneum; (B) Closure of rectus sheath.

Prophylactic Antibiotics with Cesarean Section

A single dose of prophylactic antibiotics in the dose of ampicillin 2 g IV or cefazolin 1 g IV must be offered to women prior to giving skin incision in order to reduce the risk of postoperative infections (NICE, 2011). According to the new NICE guidelines (2021), administration of antibiotics prior

> **BOX 11.9:** Summary of the essential steps in a cesarean delivery.
>
> - Use of a transverse lower abdominal incision (Joel–Cohen incision)
> - Use of blunt extension of the uterine incision
> - Manual removal of the placenta at the time of cesarean delivery must not be done
> - Controlled cord traction for removal of the placenta must be done
> - Routine use of forceps to deliver baby's head must not be employed
> - Uterine incision must be closed with two suture layers
> - Neither the visceral nor the parietal peritoneum needs to be sutured
> - Routine closure of subcutaneous space is not required unless the thickness of fat > 2 cm
> - Regular use of superficial wound drains is not required
> - Early skin-to-skin contact between the mother and baby must be encouraged

to the skin incision helps in reducing the risk of maternal infection in comparison to the administration of prophylactic antibiotics after skin incision. Also, this strategy is unlikely to have any effect on the baby.

Use of Uterotonics

Oxytocin 5 IU by slow IV injection should be used at the time of CS in order to encourage uterine contractions and reduce blood loss.

The various essential steps to be undertaken at the time of cesarean delivery are summarized in **Box 11.9**.

Measurement of Umbilical Artery pH

In cases of suspected fetal compromise, umbilical artery pH should be performed after all cesarean deliveries to help assess fetal well-being and guide ongoing care of the baby.

Thromboprophylaxis

Women having a cesarean delivery should be offered thromboprophylaxis because they are at an increased risk of venous thromboembolism. The various methods of prophylaxis may include graduated stockings, hydration, early mobilization, low-molecular-weight heparin, etc.

Immediate Postoperative Care

- After surgery is completed, the woman needs to be monitored in a recovery area.
- Monitoring of routine vital signs (blood pressure, temperature, breathing), urine output, vaginal bleeding, and uterine tonicity (to check if the uterus remains adequately contracted) needs to be done at hourly intervals for the first 4 hours. Thereafter, the monitoring needs to be done at every 4-hourly intervals for the first postoperative day at least. Adequate analgesia needs to be provided, initially through the IV line and later with oral medications.
- When the effects of anesthesia have worn off, about 4–8 hours after surgery, the woman may be transferred to the postpartum room.
- Following the baby's birth, umbilical artery pH should be measured in all cases of CS performed for suspected fetal compromise to help ensure the fetal well-being and care of the baby.

Pain Management after CS

Adequate postoperative pain control is important. A woman who is in severe pain may not recover well. However, excessive use of sedative drugs must be avoided as this may limit the patient's mobility, which is important to prevent thromboembolism.

Patient-controlled analgesia using opioid analgesics should be offered after CS as it is associated with higher rates of patient satisfaction. Women could be offered diamorphine (0.3–0.4 mg intrathecally) for intra- and postoperative analgesia. Nonsteroidal anti-inflammatory drugs may be used postoperatively as an adjunct to other analgesics because they help in reducing the requirement for opioids. Adding acetaminophen also increases the effects of other medications with very little additional adverse risk.

Analgesic rectal suppositories can also be used for providing relief from pain in women following CS.

Fluids and oral food after CS: As a general rule, about 3 L of fluids must be replaced by IV infusion during the first postoperative day, provided that the woman's urine output remains greater than 30 mL/h. If the urine output falls below 30 mL/h, the woman needs to be reassessed to evaluate the cause of oliguria. In uncomplicated cases, the urinary catheter can be removed by 12 hours postoperatively. IV fluids may need to be continued until she starts taking liquids orally. The clinician needs to remember that prolonged infusion of IV fluids can alter electrolyte balance. If the woman receives IV fluids for more than 48 hours, her electrolyte levels need to be monitored every 48 hours. Balanced electrolyte solution (e.g., potassium chloride 1.5 g in 1 L IV fluids) may be administered.

In case of uneventful surgery, early oral intake (preferably within 6 hours of surgery) is encouraged. If the surgery was uncomplicated, the woman may be given a light liquid diet in the evening after the surgery. If there were signs of infection or if the CS was for obstructed labor or uterine rupture, bowel sounds must be heard before prescribing oral liquids to the patient. In these cases, the woman can be given solid food, when she starts passing gas. Women who are recovering well and who do not have complications after the surgery can be advised to eat and drink, whenever they feel hungry or thirsty. The clinician must ensure that the woman is eating a regular diet before she is discharged from the hospital.

Ambulation after CS

The women must be encouraged to ambulate 6–8 hours following surgery. In case she finds it difficult to get up from the bed and walk, she can be asked to remain in bed and do simple limb exercises (e.g., leg elevation, foot dorsiflexion, and plantar flexion) and breathing exercises on the bed itself. Early ambulation enhances circulation, encourages early return of normal gastrointestinal function, and facilitates general well-being. Even in cases where complications were encountered at the time of surgery, mobilization must be preferably begun within 24 hours after the surgery.

Dressing and Wound Care

- The dressing must be kept on the wound for the first day after surgery so as to provide a protective barrier against infection. Thereafter, dressing is usually not required.
- If blood or fluid is observed to be leaking through the initial dressing, the dressing must not be changed. The amount of blood/fluid lost must be monitored.
- If bleeding increases or the blood stain covers half the dressing or more, the dressing must be removed and replaced with another sterile dressing. The dressing must be changed while using a sterile technique. The surgical wound also needs to be carefully inspected.

Urinary Catheter Removal after CS

The urinary bladder catheter should be removed once a woman is mobile after a regional anesthetic and not sooner than 12 hours after the last epidural "top-up" dose.

Length of Hospital Stay

The length of hospital stay is likely to be longer after a CS (an average of 3–4 days) in comparison to that after a vaginal birth (average 1–2 days). However, women who are recovering well and have not developed complications following cesarean may be offered early discharge (after 24 hours) and follow-up at home.

ALTERNATIVE TECHNIQUES FOR CESAREAN DELIVERY

In order to further reduce the operation time and complications associated with Joel–Cohen technique of cesarean delivery, several modifications of cesarean delivery have been introduced, some of which have been discussed next.

Misgav Ladach Technique

Misgav Ladach technique is a modified Joel–Cohen technique and is also known as Joel–Cohen–Stark technique. In this technique, the Joel–Cohen abdominal incision is used, and the uterus is also opened in a manner similar to the Joel–Cohen method. Following the manual removal of the placenta, the uterus is exteriorized. The myometrial incision is closed with one layer of locked continuous sutures. A second layer of sutures is placed only if required. The peritoneal layers (both visceral and peritoneal) are not sutured. The fascia is reapproximated with a continuous running stitch. The skin is closed with two or three mattress sutures. The skin edges between these sutures are approximated with the help of Allis forceps. Similar to the Joel–Cohen technique, the Misgav Ladach technique also favors minimization of sharp dissection. It has been shown that the use of Misgav Ladach technique is associated with fewer intraperitoneal adhesions at the time of repeat cesarean delivery.

Pelosi's Technique

Pelosi's technique can be described as a simple, least traumatic approach toward cesarean delivery. It is associated with short operating time, minimal instrumentation, reduced surgical dissection, and reduced rate of postoperative complications such as pain, blood loss, infection, and wound complications. In this technique, a Pfannenstiel abdominal incision is given. Electrocautery is used for transversely cutting the subcutaneous tissues and fascia. The rectus muscles are separated with the help of blunt dissection, using both the index fingers. The peritoneum is opened with blunt finger dissection, following which all the layers of the abdominal wall are stretched manually to the extent of the skin incision. The bladder is not reflected inferiorly. A small transverse incision is made over the lower uterine segment. It is extended laterally, curving upward with blunt finger dissection or scissors. The baby is delivered with external fundal pressure. Following the delivery of the baby, oxytocin is administered, and the placenta is removed after spontaneous separation. The uterus is massaged. The myometrial incision is closed with single layer of chromic catgut continuous locking sutures. Neither visceral nor parietal peritoneal layer is sutured. The fascia is closed with a continuous synthetic absorbable suture. If the subcutaneous layer is thick, interrupted 3-0 absorbable sutures are used for obliterating the dead space. The skin is closed with staples. Presently, there are no randomized trials comparing Pelosi's technique to other techniques.

Hemostatic Cesarean Section

Hemostatic CS is a new surgical technique used for managing pregnant women infected with HIV-1. The surgeon must adorn double gloves while performing CS in women who are HIV-positive. Hemostatic CS is a type of elective CS with technical modifications, which is used in all patients receiving antiretroviral treatment and in whom breast-feeding has been prohibited. The patient is scheduled for surgery at 38 weeks of gestation, while the patient is not in labor and membranes are intact. The technique involves management of lower uterine segment while maintaining the integrity of membranes. This helps in avoiding massive contact between maternal blood and the fetus. Thus, this technique helps in reducing the rate of vertical transmission to <2%.

Classical Cesarean Section

 Q. Write a short note on classical cesarean section.

Classical CS involves giving a vertical uterine incision. While in the past, a vertical incision (classical) was commonly used, this was associated with a high risk of scar rupture during future pregnancies. There are two types of vertical incisions: (1) low vertical (limited to the lower uterine segment) and (2) classical vertical (extending up to the uterine fundus). The low vertical incision appears to be as safe and strong as the low transverse incision. The classical incision is rarely performed at or near term because it is associated with a high rate of scar rupture in future pregnancies. As a result, lower segment transverse incisions are nowadays preferred.

Indications

Indications for considering a vertical uterine incision are as follows:
- Poorly developed lower uterine segment in settings where marked degree of intrauterine manipulation is anticipated (e.g., extremely preterm breech presentations, fetus in transverse lie where the back faces downward)
- Presence of pathology in the lower uterine segment due to which it may not be possible to give a transverse incision (e.g., large myoma, anterior placenta previa, or accreta)
- Densely adherent bladder
- Postmortem delivery

Strength of the Upper Segment Scar

The lower segment uterine scar is considered sounder than the upper segment scar due to the reasons previously described in the text.

Procedure

In case of a classical CS, the uterine incision is given vertically. The lower limit of the uterine incision is initiated as low as possible, usually above the level of bladder. The uterine incision is extended in the cephalad direction using bandage scissors, until the incision becomes large enough to facilitate delivery. Following the delivery of the baby and placenta, the uterine incision is closed in layers. A three-layered closure is usually used in case of classical incision due to an increased vascularity of the upper segment. The deeper layers are approximated using a layer of continuous 0 or no. 1 chromic catgut sutures. The outer layer is closed using figure-of-eight continuous sutures. The edges of the uterine serosa are approximated using continuous 2-0 chromic catgut sutures.

Avoiding a Classical Uterine Incision

A classical cesarean delivery is associated with a weaker scar in comparison to a transverse incision. Therefore, rather than performing a classical CS, the clinicians prefer to use some kind of variations in the lower segment uterine incision. Mostly, the surgeon is able to decide the exact incision only at the time of surgery. Variations of the lower segment incision are commonly used, in cases where there is a requirement for an extended surgical field, in order to avoid scar extension, transverse lie with hand prolapse and large baby, etc.

Some of the variations include the following:
- *Inverted T-shaped incision:* This incision involves cutting upward from the middle of the transverse incision.
- *J-shaped or hockey-stick incision:* This incision involves extension of one end of the transverse incision upward.

 COMPLICATIONS

Q. Write a long essay discussing the complications of cesarean delivery.

Q. Write a short essay on scar rupture following LSCS.

Q. Discuss the diagnosis and management of scar rupture in a G2P1L1 woman with previous history of cesarean section for breech presentation.

UTERINE RUPTURE

Approximately 15% of all deliveries in the United States occur in women with previous CS. In a patient with a previous CS, vaginal delivery may cause the previous uterine scar to separate. Disintegration of the scar, also known as scar rupture, is one of the most disastrous complications associated with VBAC. **Box 11.10** lists the clinical features associated with uterine scar rupture or impending scar rupture. The reported incidence of scar rupture for all pregnancies is 0.05%. The risk of scar rupture after vaginal delivery following one previous lower transverse segment CS on an average is estimated to be about 0.8–1%. However, the exact risk of scar rupture depends upon the type of uterine incision given at the time of previous CS **(Table 11.7)**. The weakest type of scar that may give way at the time of VBAC is the previous classical incision in the upper segment of the uterus, which is associated with almost 10% risk of development of scar rupture. Uterine rupture can result in complete extrusion of the fetus into the maternal abdominal cavity. In other cases, rupture is associated with fetal distress or severe hemorrhage from the rupture site. Factors which are likely to be associated with an increased risk of uterine rupture in women undergoing VBAC are listed in **Box 11.11**.

Types of Uterine Rupture

Uterine rupture is defined as a disruption of the uterine muscle extending to and involving the uterine serosa. At times, there may be disruption of the uterine muscle with extension to the bladder or broad ligament. Uterine rupture can be of two types: complete rupture and incomplete rupture.

Complete Rupture

Complete rupture describes a full-thickness defect of the uterine wall and serosa, resulting in direct communication between the uterine cavity and the peritoneal cavity **(Figs. 11.11A and B)**.

Incomplete Rupture

Incomplete rupture describes a defect of the uterine wall that is contained by the visceral peritoneum or broad ligament.

Incomplete rupture is also known as uterine dehiscence and can be described as partial disruption of the uterine muscle with the uterine serosa remaining intact.

The identification or suspicion of uterine rupture is a medical emergency and must be followed by an immediate and urgent response from the obstetrician. An emergency laparotomy is usually required to save the patient's life. Complete uterine rupture is very unlikely today. A complete rupture occurs in much less than 1% of women attempting VBAC. Incomplete rupture occurs in about 1–2% of the cases. There is no clear-cut predictive indicator for ruptured uterus. However, several factors which are indicative of a weak scar are mentioned in **Box 11.12**.

> **BOX 11.10:** Clinical features associated with uterine scar rupture or impending scar rupture.
>
> - Abnormal CTG trace
> - Dull suprapubic pain or severe abdominal pain, especially if persisting between contractions
> - Acute onset of scar tenderness
> - Abnormal vaginal bleeding
> - Hematuria
> - Cessation of previously efficient uterine activity
> - Unexplained maternal tachycardia, hypotension, fainting, or shock
> - Chest pain or shoulder tip pain or sudden onset of shortness of breath
> - Onset of unexpected antepartum hemorrhage or PPH
> - On vaginal examination, there may be loss of station of the presenting part
> - There may be a failure of normal descent of the presenting part, and the presenting part may remain high up on vaginal examination
> - Change in abdominal contour
> - Inability to pick up FHR at the old transducer site
> - Bladder tenesmus or frequent desire to pass urine
>
> (CTG: cardiotocography; FHR: fetal heart rate; PPH: postpartum hemorrhage)

TABLE 11.7: Risk of scar rupture based on the type of uterine scar given at the time of previous cesarean delivery.

Type of previous cesarean scar	Estimated risk of rupture (%)
Classical cesarean	4–9
T-shaped incision	4–9
Low vertical	1–7
Low-transverse incision	0.8–1

> **BOX 11.11:** Factors which are likely to be associated with an increased risk of uterine rupture in women undergoing VBAC.
>
> - Short interdelivery interval (<12 months since last delivery)
> - Postdated pregnancy
> - Maternal age of 40 years or more
> - Obesity
> - Lower prelabor Bishop score
> - Fetal macrosomia
> - Decreased ultrasonographic lower segment myometrial thickness

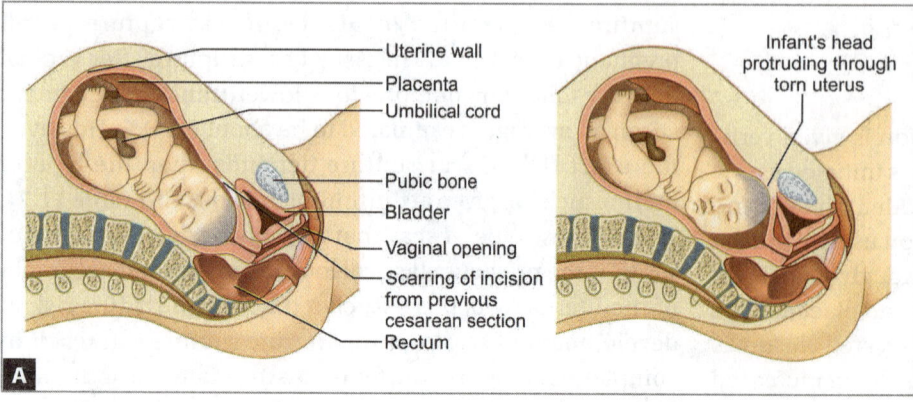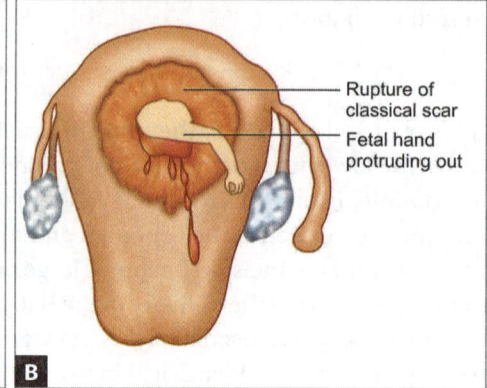

Figs. 11.11A and B: (A) Attempted VBAC associated with subsequent rupture of previous lower segment uterine scar; (B) Rupture of a previous classical uterine scar.

> **BOX 11.12:** Causes of a weak scar.
>
> - Improper hemostasis at the time of surgery
> - Imperfect coaptation of uterine margins at the time of surgery
> - Extension of the angles of uterine incision
> - Infection during healing
> - Placental implantation at the site of incision
> - Overdistension of the uterus

> **BOX 11.13:** Steps to be taken to reduce the amount of PPH.
>
> - Aortic compression can be applied to decrease bleeding
> - Administration of oxytocics (oxytocin, ergot alkaloids, carboprost, misoprostol, etc.)
> - Surgical options such as ligation of the hypogastric artery, uterine artery, or ovarian arteries

Management of Rupture Uterus

When uterine rupture is diagnosed or strongly suspected, surgery is necessary. While in the previous days, most cases of uterine rupture were managed with hysterectomy, nowadays most cases are managed by controlling the bleeding surgically and repairing the defect.

A decision must be made regarding whether to perform hysterectomy or repair the rupture site. If future fertility is desirable and the rent in the uterus appears to be reparable (straight-cut scar, rupture in the body of uterus; pelvic blood vessels are intact), repair of the rupture site must be performed. If future fertility is not desirable or the uterine rent appears to be irreparable (multiple rents with ragged margins, injury to the iliac vessels, etc.), hysterectomy should be performed. Typically, longitudinal tears, especially those in a lateral position, should be treated by hysterectomy, whereas low transverse tears may be repaired. A lower segment lateral rupture can cause transection of the uterine vessels. Therefore, the obstetrician must make special efforts to localize the site of bleeding, before placing clamps at the time of hysterectomy in order to avoid injury to the ureter and iliac vessels. Bladder rupture must also be ruled out at the time of laparotomy by clearly mobilizing and inspecting the bladder to ensure that it is intact.

Though steps must be taken to resuscitate the patient, surgery should not be delayed owing to hypovolemic shock because it may not be easily reversible until the hemorrhage from uterine rupture is controlled. Uterine rupture may be associated with massive PPH. Therefore, upon laparotomy, steps mentioned in **Box 11.13** can be taken to reduce the amount of bleeding. Due to the risk of rupture recurrence in a subsequent pregnancy, women with previously repaired uterine ruptures are advised not to attempt labor in the future. Ideally, a repeat CS should be performed prior to the onset of uterine contractions.

Assessment of Scar Integrity

In order to identify the previous cesarean scars, which are likely to give way during VBAC, the following investigations can be done:

- *Hysterogram:* Radiographic imaging of the uterus, which shows uterine defect in the lateral view
- *Ultrasound imaging:* Ultrasound examination for visualization of scar defects and measurement of scar thickness

TABLE 11.8: Risk of placenta previa and placenta accreta in subsequent pregnancies based on the number of previous cesarean deliveries.

Number of previous cesarean deliveries	Risk of placenta previa (%)	Risk of placenta accreta (%)
1	1	11–14
2	1.7	23–40
3 or more	2.8	Up to 67

Source: Gurol-Urganci I, Cromwell DA, Edozien LC, Smith GC, Onwere C, Mahmood TA, et al. Risk of placenta previa in second birth after first birth cesarean section: a population-based study and meta-analysis. BMC Pregnancy Childbirth. 2011;11:95.

- *Manual exploration:* Manual exploration of placenta to check scar integrity is especially useful in case of continuing PPH and other third-stage problems.

Ultrasound Imaging for Visualization of Scar Defects and Measurement of Scar Thickness

Ultrasound measurement of scar thickness at 37 weeks of gestation is based on the fact that the risk of a defective scar is directly related to the degree of thinning of the lower uterine segment at around 37 weeks of pregnancy. According to the largest study by Rozenberg et al. (1996), cutoff value of 3.5 mm on ultrasound measurement of scar thickness at 36 weeks was observed to show negative predictive value of 99.3% for scar rupture. The high negative predictive value of this method may encourage the obstetricians to offer a trial of labor to patients with a thickness value of 3.5 mm or greater. Different studies show different cutoff values for estimating the strength of the scar. As per the meta-analysis by Kok et al. (2013), presently there is no clear-cut value of scar thickness to indicate the strength of the scar. Nevertheless, the use of sonographic antenatal lower uterine scar thickness measurement is recommended for prediction of a uterine defect during trial of labor. Transvaginal ultrasound seems to be more accurate than transabdominal ultrasound, yet it is not commonly used.

PLACENTA PREVIA/ADHERENT PLACENTA

The risk of having complications such as placenta previa and adherent placenta increases with the number of previous cesarean deliveries **(Table 11.8)**. Therefore, women who plan to have multiple (e.g., 3 or more) pregnancies in the future should be counseled that opting for ERCS may result in greater surgical risks for future pregnancies due to the risk of complications, such as placenta previa, placenta accreta, and hysterectomy.

INFECTION

Infection is a complication which can commonly develop after CS. Endometritis or infection of the endometrial cavity must be suspected if there is excessive vaginal bleeding/discharge following the surgery. Infection of the urinary tract can result in symptoms such as dysuria, increased urinary frequency, and pyuria.

TRAUMA TO THE URINARY TRACT

Trauma to the urinary tract can occur during cesarean surgery and if not appropriately handled can result in the development of urinary tract fistula.

THROMBOEMBOLISM

Thromboembolism must be suspected if the patient develops cough, swollen calf muscles, or positive Homan's sign. A positive Homan's sign is associated with deep vein thrombosis and is said to be present when passive dorsiflexion of the ankle by the examiner elicits sharp pain in the patient's calf.

EVIDENCE-BASED CLINICAL TRIALS

List of references can be scanned through QR code to enable the readers gain deeper insight of the subject by referring to the entire article or its abstract.

CHAPTER 12

Hydatidiform Mole

CASE STUDY

A 20-year-old primigravida patient presented with bleeding at 9 weeks of gestation. Per vaginal examination revealed a bulky soft uterus, and the urine pregnancy test was positive. Ultrasound examination showed an ill-defined gestational sac with absent cardiac pulsations and a few small cisterns in the region of placenta. A possible diagnosis of missed abortion was made. However, possibility of a partial mole also could not be ruled out. Serum beta human chorionic gonadotropin (β-hCG) levels were found to be 125,000 mIU/mL at the time of initial visit, and it increased to 138,000 mIU/mL after 48 hours. The suspicion of molar gestation became stronger and suction evacuation was performed. The evacuated products were sent for histopathological examination, which confirmed the diagnosis of partial hydatidiform mole (PHM).

INTRODUCTION

Q. What is gestational trophoblastic disease? Also briefly describe the differences between complete and partial mole.

Hydatidiform mole (H.mole) belongs to a spectrum of diseases known as gestational trophoblastic disease (GTD), resulting from overproduction of the chorionic tissue, which is normally supposed to develop into the placenta. H. mole can be considered as a neoplasm of trophoblastic tissue and involves both syncytiotrophoblast and cytotrophoblast. H. moles are nonviable and genetically abnormal conceptions, showing excessive expression of paternal genes. In this condition, the placental tissues develop into an abnormal mass. There also occurs edema or hydropic degeneration of the connective tissue stroma of the villi, leading to their distension and formation of vesicles **(Figs. 12.1A and B)**. Disappearance of blood vessels from the

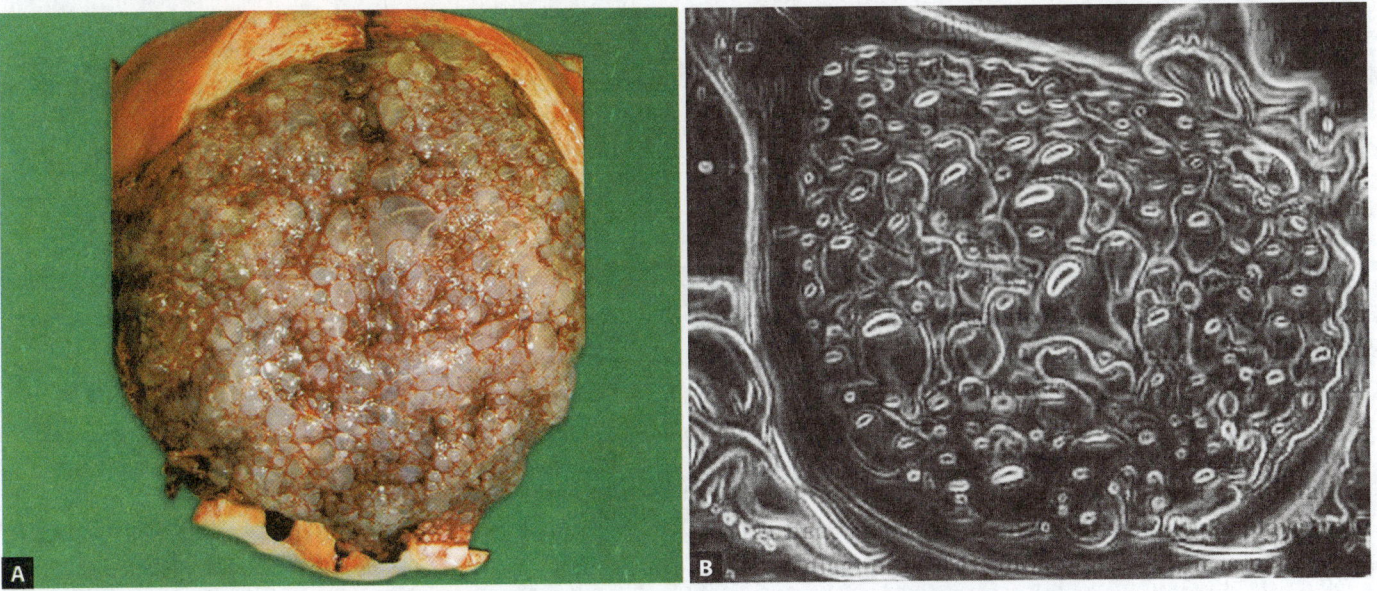

Figs. 12.1A and B: (A) Clinical specimen of complete hydatidiform mole; (B) Computerized generation of the image showing an artist's interpretation of H. mole.

villi is often responsible for avascularity of the villi, resulting in an early death of the embryo. Often, there is no fetal mass at all. These changes are accompanied with excessive secretion of hormones such as hCG, chorionic thyrotrophin, and progesterone. On the other hand, estrogen production is often on the lower side. However sometimes, partial moles may show the presence of fetal tissue. This disease can occur even during or after an intrauterine or ectopic pregnancy. GTD represents a spectrum of premalignant and malignant diseases (Box 12.1) including potentially benign entities such as complete hydatidiform mole (CHM) and PHM, and potentially malignant entities which are collectively known as gestational trophoblastic neoplasia (GTN). This may include entities such as invasive mole, choriocarcinoma, and placental site trophoblastic tumor (PSTT). GTN is characterized by the persistence of GTD, most commonly defined as a persistent elevation of β-hCG (even after 8–10 months following suction evacuation). The difference between CHM and PHM is listed in Table 12.1.

PATHOPHYSIOLOGY OF COMPLETE AND PARTIAL MOLE

> **Q. Discuss in detail the pathogenesis of molar gestation.**

The normal process of fertilization in which a sperm (containing 23 chromosomes) fertilizes an ovum (containing 23 chromosomes) resulting in the formation of a diploid zygote (containing 46 chromosomes) is shown in **Figure 12.2A**. A H. mole is an abnormal pregnancy in which placental villi become edematous (hydropic) and start proliferating. During the formation of H. mole, firstly there is an edema of the whole central core, causing the villus to develop into a rounded cyst-like structure filled with watery fluid. The entire embryonic chorionic tissue gets converted into grape-like structures in which each vesicle is connected to each other with the help of fine stalk-like structures (**Fig. 12.3**). Both CHMs and PHMs overexpress paternal genes. CHMs are usually diploid, with all chromosomes being derived from the father by means of either monospermic or dispermic fertilization. Monospermic fertilization results from fertilization of a sperm with an anucleate oocyte (**Fig. 12.2B**). The genetic material is duplicated, resulting in a 46XX karyotype, because 46YY zygotes are incapable of developing independently. Rarely, CHM can also be produced due to dispermic fertilization in which there is fertilization of two different sperms with an anucleate oocyte. Dispermic fertilization may result in either a 46XX or a 46XY karyotype. A 46XX karyotype is found in 90% of CHMs. PHMs on the other hand are usually triploid, formed as a result of dispermic fertilization of two different sperms with an ovum (**Fig. 12.2C**). As a result, partial moles usually show a triploid karyotype having two sets of paternal chromosomes and one set of maternal chromosomes (69XXX, 69XXY, or 69XYY). About 10% of PHMs have tetraploid or higher karyotypes consisting of multiple sets of paternal chromosomes combined with one set of maternal chromosomes (**Figs. 12.2A to C**).

Normal Anatomy

As the blastocyst (early embryo) reaches 58-celled stage at about fourth to fifth day of fertilization, it gets transformed into two types of cells: trophectoderm, which gives rise to trophoblast cells that serve as the precursor for placenta, and an inner cell mass, which forms the embryo proper. The early trophoblastic cells help in transferring nutrients between the maternal endometrium and the embryo. The trophoblast eventually develops into the functional part of the placenta and serves as a surface for the exchange of oxygen and nutrients. By the eighth day following fertilization, the trophoblast gets divided into two layers: the syncytiotrophoblast and the cytotrophoblast (**Fig. 12.4**). Proliferation of syncytiotrophoblast accounts for the marked β-hCG elevation seen in H. mole.

> **BOX 12.1:** Classification of gestational trophoblastic disease.
>
> *Benign forms (90%)*
> - Complete hydatidiform mole
> - Partial hydatidiform mole
>
> *Malignant forms (10%)*
> - Invasive mole
> - Choriocarcinoma
> - Placental site trophoblastic tumor
> - Epithelioid trophoblastic tumor

TABLE 12.1: Comparison between complete and partial moles.

Parameter under consideration	Complete mole	Partial mole
Cytogenetic studies	46XX karyotype	Triploid karyotype 69XXY
Pathophysiology	Duplication of the haploid sperm following fertilization of an "empty" ovum or dispermic fertilization of an "empty" ovum	These contain two sets of paternal haploid genes and one set of maternal haploid genes. They usually occur following dispermic fertilization of an ovum
Histopathological analysis	There is no evidence of fetal tissue	There may be evidence of fetal tissue or red blood vessels
Invasive potential and propensity for malignant transformation	Persistent trophoblastic disease following uterine evacuation may develop in about 15% cases with a complete mole	Persistent trophoblastic disease may develop in <5% cases of partial mole

Hydatidiform Mole

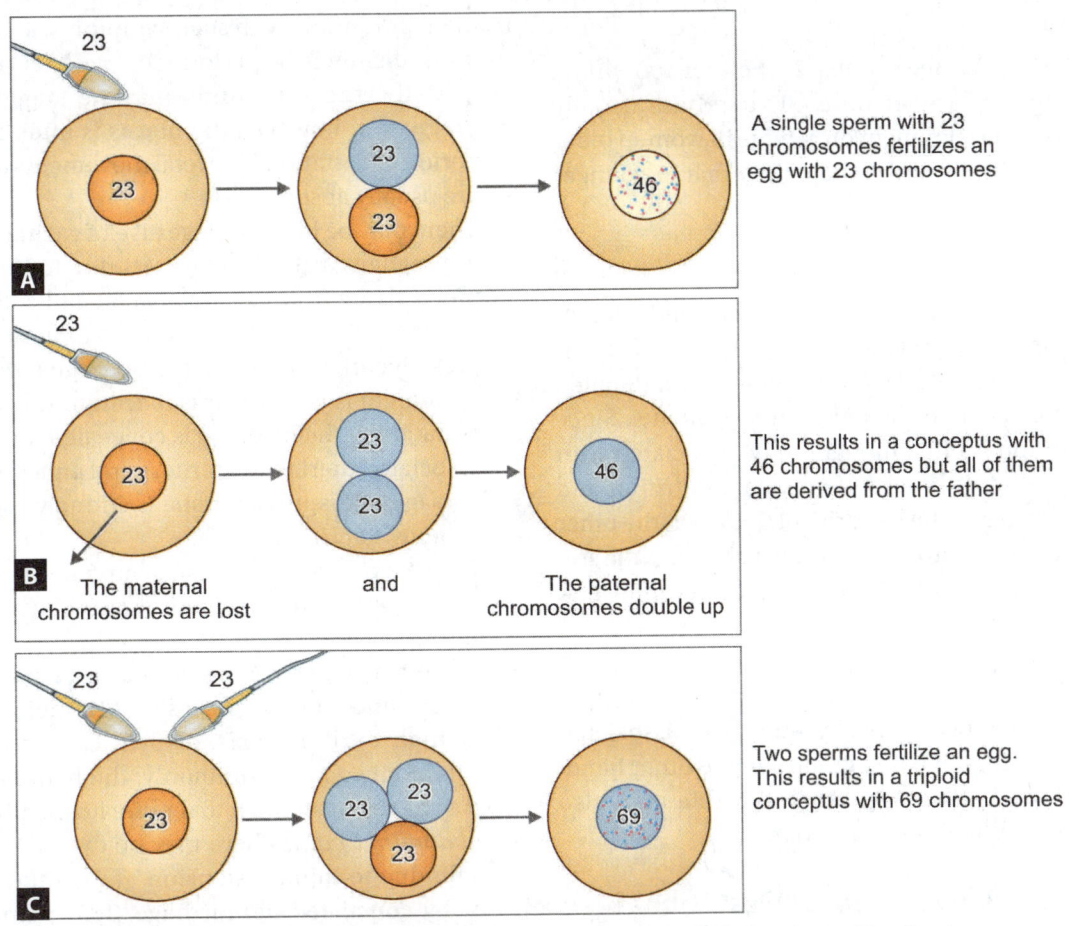

Figs. 12.2A to C: Pathophysiology of molar gestation. (A) Normal process of fertilization; (B) Complete hydatidiform mole; (C) Partial hydatidiform mole.

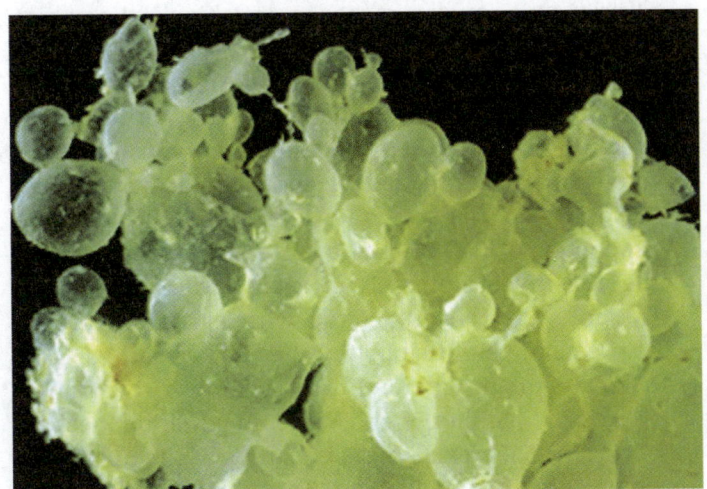

Fig. 12.3: Magnified view showing vesicular structures.

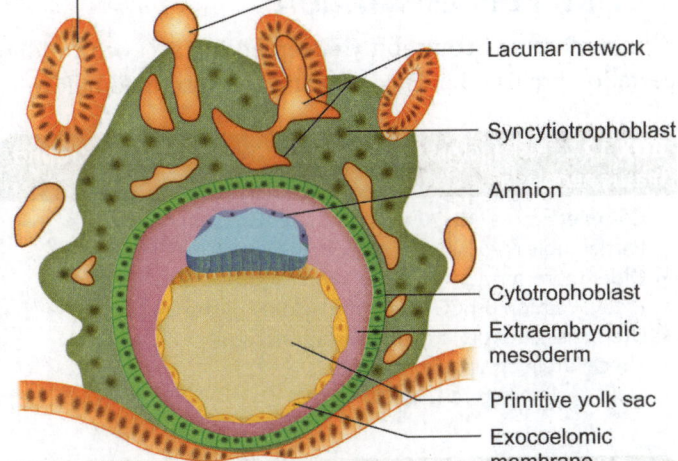

Fig. 12.4: Blastocyst and trophoblast at the time of implantation.

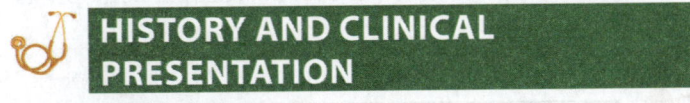

HISTORY AND CLINICAL PRESENTATION

RISK FACTORS

Factors which may be associated with an increased risk for CHM and need to be elicited while taking history are described in the following text.

Race and Ethnicity

Though the exact reasons are not known, the Asian populations are affected more in comparison to other ethnic groups. In many Asian countries, the rates may be as high as 8–10 cases per 1,000 population. On the other hand, in the US, H. mole may occur in 1 per 1,000–2,000 pregnancies.

Maternal Age

Mothers in extremes of age groups, i.e., either too young (<20 years) or too old (older than 40 years) are usually affected. The risk of development of H. mole in women older than 40 years is about five times more than that in younger women.

Faulty Diet

Inadequate diet deficient in proteins, folic acid, and vitamin A, and containing excessive amounts of fats, has also been found to be associated with H. mole. Therefore, a detailed dietary history needs to be elicited in these patients. Since inadequate nutrition is often thought to be associated with pathogenesis of H. mole, intake of adequate nutrition and well-balanced diet may reduce the risk of CHM. On the other hand, partial mole is reported to be associated with the use of oral contraceptives, history of irregular menstruation, and not with dietary factors.

Blood Group

Hydatidiform mole has been typically found to be associated with individuals having AB blood group. On the other hand, a woman with blood group A, partnered with a man also having blood group A, is at the lowest risk.

Risk Factors for Development of Gestational Trophoblastic Neoplasia

Risk factors for development of GTN are listed in **Box 12.2**.

CLINICAL PRESENTATION

Clinical features commonly observed in cases with molar gestation are listed in **Box 12.3** and are described below. In a patient presenting with such symptoms, a urine pregnancy test must definitely be performed.

- Initially, the symptoms may be suggestive of early pregnancy; however, the uterus is often larger than the period of gestation. The fetal movements and heart tones are usually absent.
- There may be history suggestive of vaginal bleeding early in pregnancy. Bleeding occurs due to the separation of molar tissue from decidua. Vaginal bleeding is the most common clinical presentation of molar pregnancy. The presence of "prune juice" discharge (brownish watery discharge) is a characteristic feature suggestive of molar gestation. If the bleeding is concealed, there may also be associated uterine tenderness and enlargement.
- Passage of grape-like tissue is strongly suggestive of the diagnosis of H. mole.
- The second most common symptom of molar gestation is excessive uterine enlargement in relation to the gestational age.
- There may be excessive nausea and vomiting. Excessive nausea and vomiting in cases of H. mole may be related to high serum levels of β-hCG. Hyperemesis may commonly occur. Commonly, the nausea and vomiting may be severe enough to require hospitalization.
- *Abdominal pain:* There may be dull-aching abdominal pain due to rapid distension of the uterus by the mole or by concealed hemorrhage. This pain may become colicky in nature when the patient starts expelling the vesicular structures. A perforating mole may produce abdominal pain, which is sudden and severe by nature. Ovarian pain could be related to stretching of the ovarian capsule caused by the presence of theca lutein cysts or as a result of torsion of the ovarian cystic mass.
- There may be symptoms suggestive of hyperthyroidism including tachycardia, restlessness, nervousness, heat intolerance, unexplained weight loss, diarrhea, tremors in hands, etc. Hyperthyroidism could be related to the production of TSH by the trophoblastic tissues or due to the similarity of alpha subunits of hCG with that of TSH.
- H. mole may be associated with early appearance of preeclampsia (usually by the first or early second trimester of pregnancy). This symptom is strongly suggestive of either H. mole or twin gestation, because occurrence of preeclampsia is extremely rare during this time period in normal pregnancies.
- Metastasis to the lungs (in cases of malignant moles) may result in symptoms such as dyspnea, cough, hemoptysis, and chest pain.

> **BOX 12.2:** Risk factors for development of gestational trophoblastic neoplasia.
>
> - Complete mole (15–20% risk of malignant sequel)
> - Partial mole (1–5% risk of malignant sequel)
> - Older maternal age
> - Preevacuation β-hCG levels of >100,000 mIU/mL
> - Uterine size that is large for gestational age
> - Theca lutein cysts (>6 cm in size)
> - Slow decline in β-hCG levels

> **BOX 12.3:** Clinical signs and symptoms in molar gestation.
>
> - Irregular vaginal bleeding
> - Hyperemesis
> - Exaggeration of the normal early pregnancy symptoms and signs (related to excessive beta human chorionic gonadotropin production)
> - Excessive uterine enlargement
> - Abdominal pain
> - Early failed pregnancy
> - Rarely, symptoms such as hyperthyroidism, early onset preeclampsia, or abdominal distension (due to theca lutein cysts)

GENERAL PHYSICAL EXAMINATION

- *Signs suggestive of preeclampsia:* Signs including high blood pressure, proteinuria, and swelling in ankles, feet, and legs may be observed.

- *Signs suggestive of hyperthyroidism:* Signs including warm, moist skin, heat intolerance, restlessness, tremors in hands, etc. may be observed.
- *Signs suggestive of early pregnancy:* These may include signs such as amenorrhea, positive pregnancy test, and breast changes suggestive of pregnancy.
- *Extreme pallor:* The patient may appear extremely pale. The pallor may be disproportionate to the amount of blood loss due to concealed hemorrhage.

SPECIFIC SYSTEMIC EXAMINATION

ABDOMINAL EXAMINATION

On abdominal examination, the uterine size is usually abnormal in relation to the period of gestation. In most of the cases of CHM the uterine size may be larger than the period of gestation, whereas in cases of PHM the uterine size may be smaller in relation to the period of gestation. The uterus may appear doughy in consistency due to lack of fetal parts and amniotic fluid. Fetal movements and fetal heart sounds are absent. Fetal parts are usually not palpable. External ballottement is absent.

VAGINAL EXAMINATION

There may be some vaginal bleeding or passage of grape-like vesicles. Internal ballottement cannot be elicited due to lack of fetus. Unilateral or bilateral enlargement of the ovaries in the form of theca lutein cysts may be palpable.

DIFFERENTIAL DIAGNOSIS

PREGNANCY-RELATED DISORDERS

Symptoms related to molar gestation may require differentiation from various pregnancy-related disorders such as hyperemesis gravidarum, hypertension (preeclampsia), and hyperthyroidism.

ANEMBRYONIC GESTATION

Anembryonic gestation, specifically the blighted ovum, can present with clinical and sonographic findings similar to that of H. mole. Blighted ovum implies developmental arrest of the preembryonic cells or embryonic disk before the formation of a live embryo. As a result, the gestational sac is empty and does not contain the embryo. In most of the cases, blighted ovum results from a chromosomal abnormality (trisomy 16 or 22). Although blighted ova may sonographically and pathologically mimic CHMs, they are genetically distinct from it. All blighted ova have maternal and paternal chromosomes, whereas all CHMs have only paternal chromosomes.

THREATENED ABORTION

Hydatidiform mole may commonly mimic threatened abortion as both the conditions are associated with vaginal bleeding and similar sonographic findings.

PRESENCE OF FIBROID OR AN OVARIAN TUMOR WITH PREGNANCY

These conditions are sometimes confused with H. mole as they may cause the uterine size to be larger in relation to the period of gestation.

MULTIPLE GESTATION

Complete hydatidiform mole may sometimes be confused with H. mole as both the conditions may be associated with early onset of preeclampsia before 20 weeks.

ULTRASONOGRAPHIC DIFFERENTIAL DIAGNOSIS

The ultrasonographic differential diagnosis is tabulated in the **Table 12.2**.

MANAGEMENT

Management plan for patients with H. mole is shown in **Flowchart 12.1**. The initial management plan in patients with molar gestation comprises the following steps:

1. Stabilize the patient (maintenance of airway, breathing, and circulation)
2. Blood transfusion in the presence of anemia
3. Correction of any underlying coagulopathy
4. Treatment of hypertension or extreme symptoms of hyperthyroidism (thyroid storm), if present.

INVESTIGATIONS

Ultrasound examination helps in establishing the diagnosis prior to evacuation; however, the definitive diagnosis is made only following the histological examination of the products of conception.

COMPLETE BLOOD COUNT, BLOOD GROUPING, AND CROSSMATCHING

Determination of hematocrit and hemoglobin levels help in estimating the degree of anemia. Blood grouping and crossmatching are required as blood transfusion may be required in case of severe maternal anemia.

PLATELET COUNT AND COAGULATION PROFILE

Measurement of platelet count and various coagulation parameters (bleeding time, clotting time, etc.) help in detecting the presence of any underlying coagulopathy.

TABLE 12.2: Ultrasound-mediated differential diagnosis.

Diagnosis	Ultrasound features	Differentiating features
Hydropic degeneration of placenta	There may be marked swelling of the villi, showing resemblance to the molar tissue. There may be presence of vesicles, cysts, fetal remains, and an abnormal placenta	β-hCG levels are generally lower in comparison to molar gestation
Complete mole with coexistent fetus	Presence of echogenic intrauterine tissue that is interspersed with numerous punctuated sonolucencies	In cases of live fetus, β-hCG levels are within the normal range
Leiomyoma of uterus	Areas of hyaline degeneration in a leiomyoma can mimic the appearance of hemorrhage within mole	• Whorled internal consistency of a leiomyoma is markedly different than vesicular pattern in molar gestation • Leiomyoma lacks the cystic appearance of a mole
Retained products of conception	• There are tissues of mixed echogenicity • No gestational sac is present • There is an absence of the vesicular pattern	Low levels of β-hCG
Choriocarcinoma	• No villi are present • There is a well-circumscribed echogenic lesion in myometrium	Abnormally high β-hCG levels
Missed abortion	Echo-refringent and nonhomogeneous chorionic tissue remains present inside the uterine cavity	Low or negative β-hCG levels
Ectopic pregnancy	Presence of pseudovesicles and a pseudosac	The combined use of quantitative determinations of hCG and vaginal ultrasound may help establish the diagnosis
Blighted ovum	• There is perfect interior delimitation of the embryonic sac • There is no evidence of any embryo	Low levels of β-hCG

BETA HUMAN CHORIONIC GONADOTROPIN LEVELS

Beta human chorionic gonadotropin is secreted by active trophoblastic tissues of the placenta and is detected in the blood 7–9 days following ovulation. In normal gestation, a concentration of 100 mIU/mL is reached 2 days after the date of expected menses. Peak levels of hCG (approximately 100,000 mIU/mL) are attained by 10 weeks of gestation. Normal serum β-hCG levels during pregnancy depending on the period of gestation are tabulated in **Table 12.3**. The rate of hCG rise during normal pregnancy is as follows:

- When β-hCG levels are below 1,200 IU/L, its concentration doubles every 48–72 hours.
- When β-hCG levels are between 1,200 and 6,000 IU/L, its concentration doubles every 72–96 hours.
- When β-hCG levels are above 6,000 IU/L, its concentration doubles every 4 days.

Estimation of β-hCG levels may be helpful in diagnosing molar pregnancies. In molar gestation, β-hCG levels in both serum and urine are raised. While in normal pregnancy, urine pregnancy test is positive in dilutions up to 1/100, in cases of molar gestation, this test is positive in high dilution; positive test in a dilution of 1/200 is highly suggestive, whereas a positive test in a dilution of 1/500 is surely diagnostic of molar gestation. Serum β-hCG levels greater than two multiples of the median are also indicative of molar gestation. In cases of complete mole, serum β-hCG levels may be more than 100,000 mIU/mL.

SERUM INHIBIN A AND ACTIVIN A LEVELS

Serum levels of both inhibin A and activin A have been found to be increased by several folds in molar pregnancies in comparison to normal pregnancies. However presently, measurement of β-hCG levels forms the standard of care in patients with molar gestation.

CYTOFLOWMETRY

Cytoflowmetry involves study of deoxyribonucleic acid (DNA) content of curetted material. This investigation is sometimes required for confirmation of diagnosis, especially when there is confusion related to the diagnosis. Otherwise, this investigation is mainly used for scientific reports and research purposes.

ULTRASOUND OF THE PELVIS

Sonography is the imaging investigation of choice to confirm the diagnosis of H. mole.

Sonographic examination is not only helpful in establishing the initial diagnosis but also helps in assessing the response to treatment regimens, determining the degree of invasion in malignant forms of GTN, determining the disease recurrence in malignant forms of GTN, and evaluating liver metastasis. Both transabdominal and transvaginal imaging must be performed using transducers with the highest ultrasound frequency possible. The specificity of ultrasound examination in the diagnosis of complete molar pregnancy may be increased if the sonographic findings are

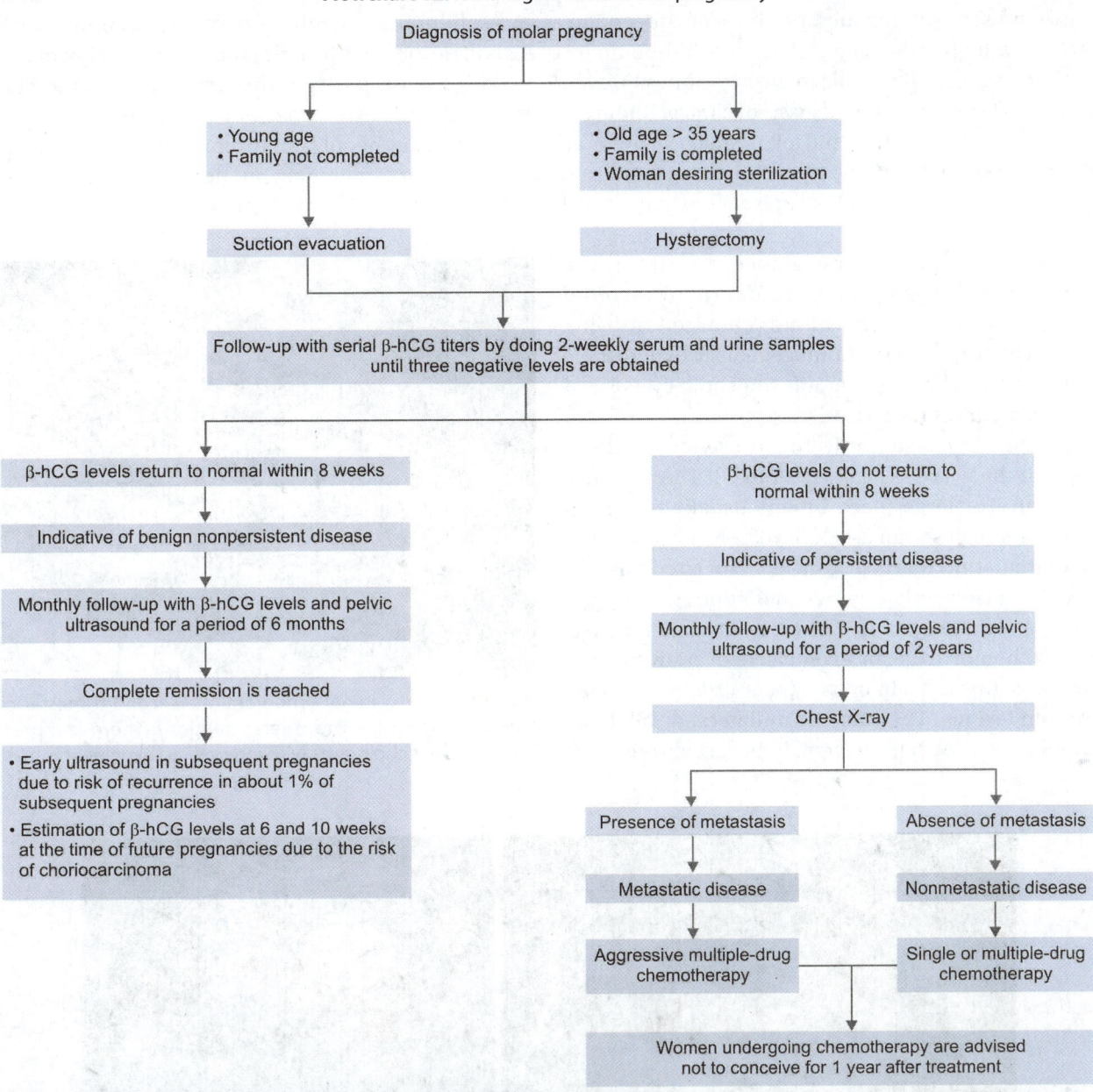

Flowchart 12.1: Management of molar pregnancy.

TABLE 12.3: Measurement of serum β-hCG levels in normal pregnancy.		
Period of gestation (from the date of conception)	**Period of gestation (from last menstrual period)**	**Serum β-hCG levels (IU/L)**
7 days	3 weeks	0–5
14 days	28 days	3–426
21 days	35 days	18–7,340
28 days	42 days	1,080–56,500
35–42 days	49–56 days	7,650–229,000
43–64 days	57–78 days	25,700–288,200
57–78 days	79–100 days	13,300–253,000
17–24 weeks	Second trimester	4,060–65,400
After several days postpartum	–	Nonpregnant levels

interpreted in correlation with the β-hCG levels. While the sonographic picture of both H. mole and missed abortion may appear similar, a complete mole is usually associated with higher serum levels of β-hCG in comparison with the cases of missed abortion.

Complete Mole

> Q. Write a short note on theca lutein cysts.

On ultrasound examination, the following features are observed:
- Early complete molar pregnancies are commonly misdiagnosed as cases of missed miscarriage or anembryonic pregnancy (blighted ovum) on ultrasound examination. There may be presence of a gestational sac

without an embryo. Additionally, second trimester CHM can be confused with retained products of conception. Therefore, a high index of suspicion should be maintained for diagnosis of H. mole in the first trimester, even when it is not suspected on the basis of clinical findings.

Characteristic vesicular pattern, also known as "snowstorm appearance" may be present due to generalized swelling of the chorionic villi and the presence of many small cystic spaces.

The typical sonographic appearance of CHM in the second and third trimesters on modern ultrasound equipment is the presence of an enlarged uterine endometrial cavity containing homogeneously hyperechoic endometrial mass with innumerable anechoic cysts sized 1–30 mm **(Figs. 12.5 and 12.6)**.

Ultrasound may also show the presence of theca lutein cysts in the ovaries **(Figs. 12.7A to C)**. The presence of bilateral and/or large theca luteins usually occurs in association with high serum β-hCG levels of >100,000 mIU/mL. High circulating levels of β-hCG associated with H. mole usually cause ovarian hyperstimulation, resulting in the formation of these cysts. In rare cases, theca lutein cysts may rupture, hemorrhage, or even cause ovarian torsion. On sonograms, theca lutein cysts appear as large, septate, cystic ovarian lesions. They may be unilateral or bilateral, and at times may be extremely large. If the lesions are large, transvaginal scanning may be of little use. In these cases, transabdominal scanning may be required for complete visualization of the enlarged ovaries. However, before making the diagnosis of theca lutein cysts, the radiologist must exclude the possibility of a preexisting or concomitant cystic ovarian neoplasm. A repeat sonographic evaluation must be done following suction evacuation after serum β-hCG levels have normalized.

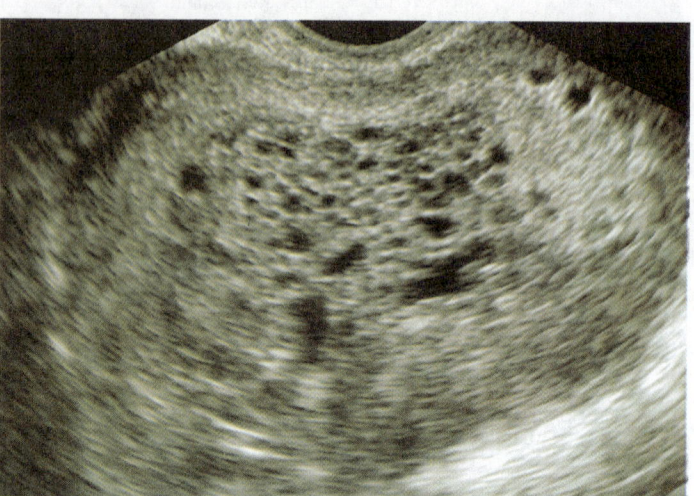

Fig. 12.5: Transvaginal sonogram of a second trimester complete hydatidiform mole (transverse section). There is a presence of numerous anechoic cysts with intervening hyperechoic material.

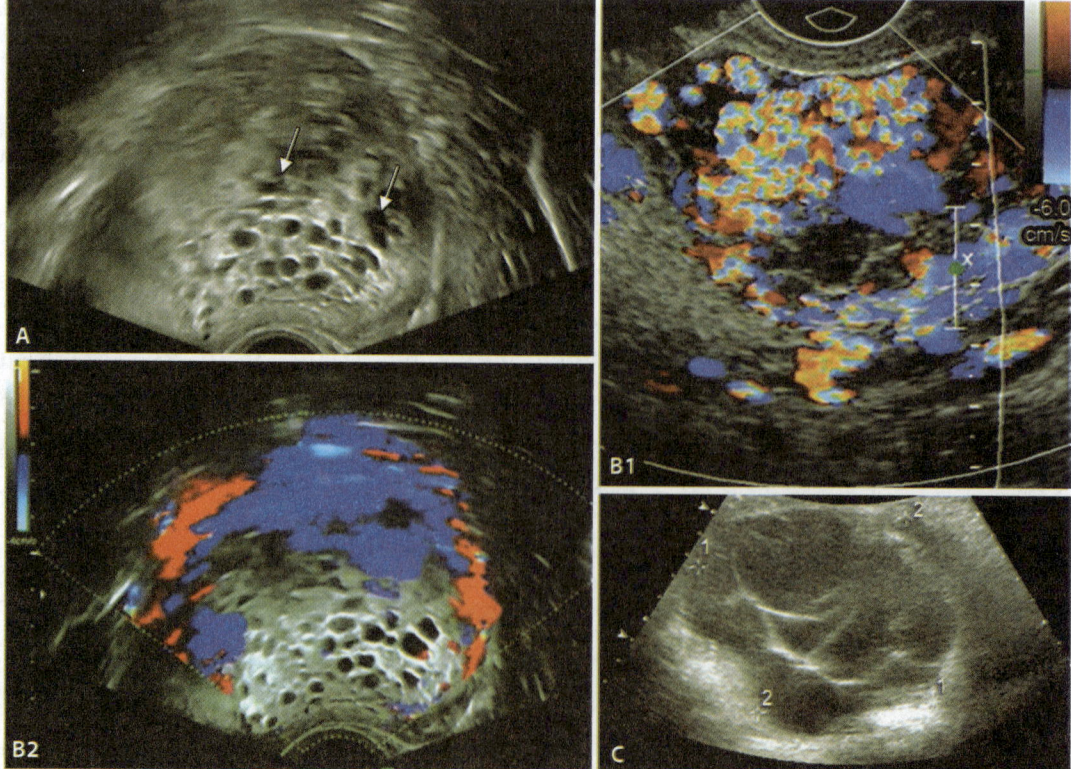

Figs. 12.6A to C: Ultrasound appearance of hydatidiform mole in a 20-year-old primigravida patient presenting with bleeding at 9 weeks gestation. (A) Cluster of grape appearance on TVS (white arrows); (B1 and B2) Doppler ultrasound showing highly vascularized tissues; (C) Left-sided ovary with theca lutein cyst (size of the left ovary is about 10.58 cm × 9.65 cm).

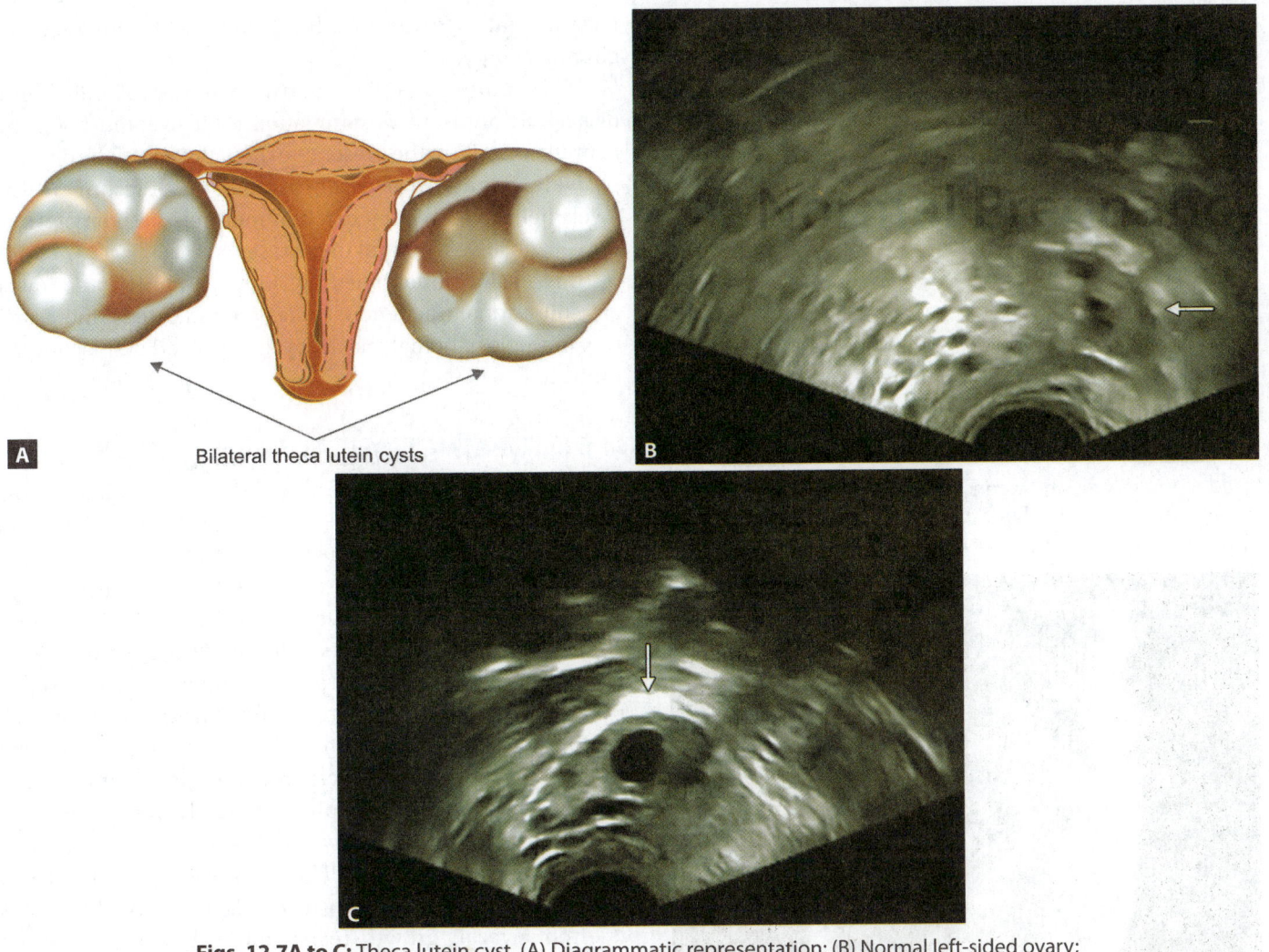

Figs. 12.7A to C: Theca lutein cyst. (A) Diagrammatic representation; (B) Normal left-sided ovary; (C) Right-sided ovary with theca lutein cyst (indicated by the arrow).

Being hormone dependent, theca lutein cysts regress within 8–12 weeks after the evacuation of H. mole in most patients. Therefore, they are not removed surgically unless they develop a complication such as ovarian torsion or rupture.

Partial Mole

- In cases of PHM, the ultrasound findings include: a large placenta, cystic spaces within the placenta, an empty gestational sac, or the sac containing amorphous echoes or growth-retarded fetus.
- Another sonographic finding which is significantly associated with the diagnosis of partial hydatidiform is the increase in ratio of transverse to anterior–posterior dimension of the gestational sac to a value >1.5.

DOPPLER ULTRASONOGRAPHY

Doppler ultrasound has no well-defined role in the evaluation of H. mole. The presence of cystic vascular spaces showing high-velocity, low-impedance flow on Doppler ultrasound is characteristic of invasive disease. Doppler ultrasonography also has a role in monitoring the response of the disease following chemotherapy. Regression of cystic vascular masses following chemotherapy is indicative of successful treatment.

CHEST X-RAY

The lungs are the most common site for metastasis in case of malignant GTD and may show the presence of distinct nodules or cannon ball appearance **(Fig. 12.8)**. Other radiographic patterns which can be produced on the X-ray include an alveolar or snowstorm pattern, pleural effusion, and an embolic pattern caused by pulmonary arterial occlusion. Metastasis to lungs is often associated with symptoms such as dyspnea, cough, hemoptysis, and chest pain. A suspicion of pulmonary metastasis on chest X-ray must be followed by a CT or MRI examination of both head and abdomen. At present, MRI plays no role in the diagnosis of H. mole; however, it is beneficial in diagnosing the metastatic disease **(Fig. 12.9)**. MRI is also used for characterizing the degree of myometrial and/or

236 Complications of Pregnancy

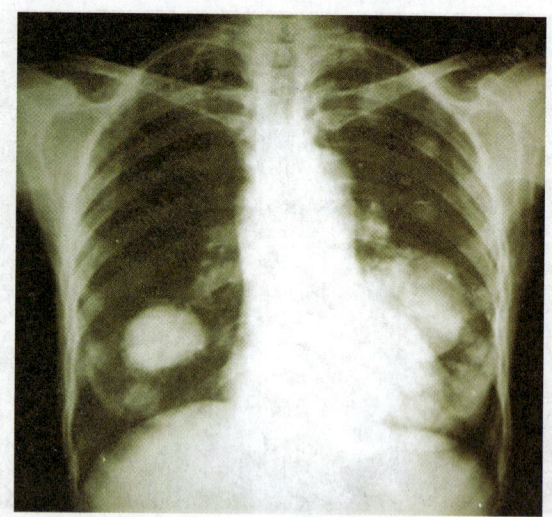

Fig. 12.8: Chest X-ray showing a cannonball appearance, in which there are multiple, well-defined, pulmonary nodules of varied sizes suggestive of pulmonary metastasis.

parametrial invasion and for assessing the response to chemotherapy.

If abdominal CT shows any evidence of metastatic disease, an ultrasound examination of the liver must be done in order to confirm the presence of hepatic metastatic disease.

Determination of cerebrospinal fluid/serum β-hCG levels helps in detecting cerebral metastasis. Titers of >1:60 are diagnostic of cerebral metastases.

If gastrointestinal bleeding is present, upper and lower gastrointestinal tract endoscopies are indicated, whereas in the presence of hematuria, IV pyelogram and cystoscopy are indicated.

HISTOPATHOLOGICAL EXAMINATION

The diagnosis of H. mole is confirmed by histological examination. Therefore, all products of conception from nonviable pregnancies must be submitted for routine pathological evaluation to exclude the presence of trophoblastic neoplasia. On pathologic evaluation, both CHMs and PHMs demonstrate swollen chorionic villi having a grape-like appearance, along with the presence of hyperplastic trophoblastic tissue **(Figs. 12.10A and B)**. Ploidy status and immunohistochemistry staining for P57 of these evacuated products may help in distinguishing partial mole from a complete mole. Though complete mole does not contain any fetal tissue, fetal tissue may sometimes be present in PHM. However, this fetal tissue is usually nonviable. Even if fetal tissue is viable, fetus is often severely growth-restricted or may have multiple anomalies.

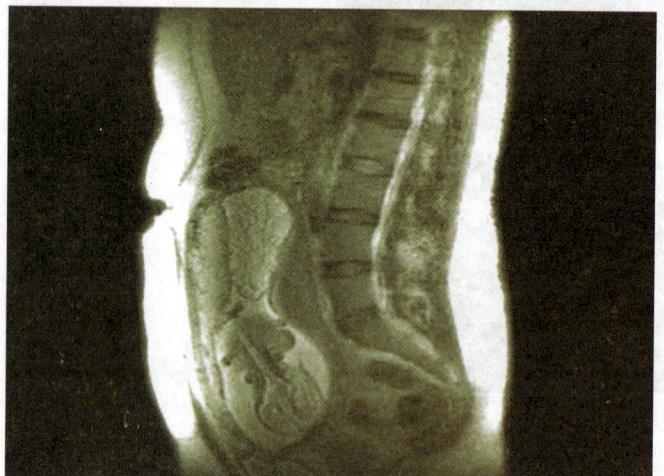

Fig. 12.9: Sagittal T2-weighted MRI showing the presence of high signal intensity heterogeneous material filling the uterine cavity (histopathological examination revealed complete molar pregnancy).

DIAGNOSIS OF GESTATIONAL TROPHOBLASTIC NEOPLASIA

Criteria for the diagnosis of GTN are mentioned in **Box 12.4**.

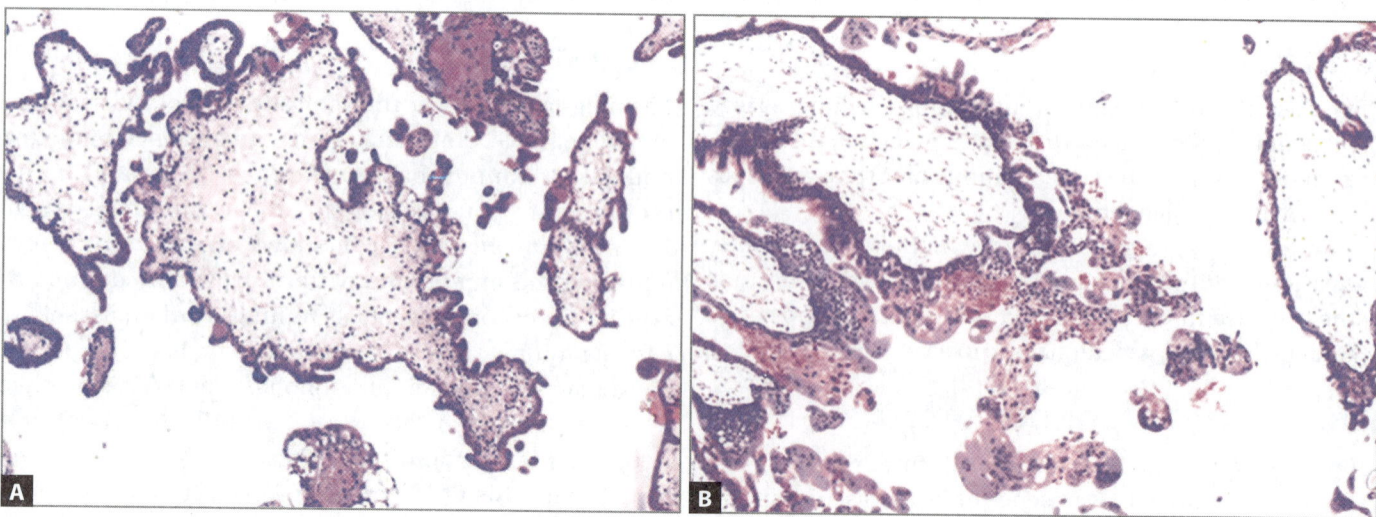

Figs. 12.10A and B: Histopathological examination. (A) Histopathological slide of complete hydatidiform mole showing diffuse trophoblastic hyperplasia; (B) Histopathological slide of partial hydatidiform mole showing focal trophoblastic hyperplasia and the presence of fetal tissue.

> **BOX 12.4:** Criteria for diagnosis of gestational trophoblastic neoplasia (GTN).
>
> - Plateau of β-hCG levels (±10%) for four measurements during a period of 3 weeks or longer (day 1, 7, 14, and 21)
> - Rise of β-hCG levels > 10% during 3-weekly consecutive measurements or longer during a period of 2 weeks or more (days 1, 7, and 14)
> - Serum β-hCG levels remain detectable for a period of 6 months or more
> - Histological criteria for choriocarcinoma

TREATMENT/OBSTETRIC MANAGEMENT

> **Q.** What should be the next step of management in the patient described in the case presentation at the beginning of this chapter?

The two main treatment options in case of H. mole are suction evacuation and hysterectomy. Hysterotomy may be sometimes required for evacuation of a large mole in order to minimize and facilitate control of bleeding.

TREATMENT OF BENIGN DISEASE

Treatment by Suction Evacuation

In case of complete absence of fetal parts, evacuation of the uterine contents is carried out by means of suction evacuation, irrespective of the uterine size. Due to the lack of fetal parts, a suction catheter, up to a maximum size of 12 mm, is usually sufficient to evacuate all complete molar pregnancies. A uterus of size up to 20 weeks can be readily evacuated. In case of partial mole with the presence of fetal parts, medical method of evacuation (oxytocic agents) can be used. The use of oxytocic agents must be avoided in cases of complete mole because of the potential of trophoblastic tissue to embolize and disseminate itself through the venous system. Presently, there is limited data related to the management of molar pregnancies with mifepristone and misoprostol. Therefore presently, the use of these agents in cases of molar pregnancies should be avoided as far as possible.

Prior to suction evacuation, an IV line must be set up. Blood should be crossmatched and kept available. Cervical dilatation is usually not required as the cervix is soft and readily permits the entry of a suction cannula. Prolonged cervical preparation with prostaglandins is not usually required and should be avoided wherever possible to reduce the risk of embolization of trophoblastic cells. Passage of uterine sound prior to the evacuation is avoided as this may cause uterine perforation. The tip of the suction cannula must be inserted just beyond the internal os. If the uterus is larger than 12 weeks in size, one hand must be placed on the fundus and the uterus should be massaged with the other in order to stimulate uterine contractions, thereby reducing the risk of uterine perforation.

Routine curettage following suction evacuation is not recommended. Sharp curettage should be avoided due to the possible risk of uterine perforation. Usually, repeat evacuation is not required as the initial evacuation is able to remove most of the molar material and cause the involution of residual tissues. Sometimes when a large amount of molar material is left behind in the uterine cavity at the time of first evacuation, further evacuation within the next few days may help in reducing symptoms and prevent the need for future chemotherapy. However, if little residual material is left after the initial procedure, the RCOG (2004) recommends that no further evacuation for persistent disease is required. Anti-D immunoglobulins (50 μg) must be administered to Rh-negative mothers.

There has been some debate regarding the use of oxytocin during and after the evacuation procedure. Some investigators have expressed concern that the use of oxytocin may promote metastasis of trophoblastic tissue. However, presently there is no good evidence to show that uterine stimulation during evacuation increases the risk of persistent tumor.

Administration of IV oxytocin helps in increasing myometrial tone and facilitating contraction, thereby reducing the total blood loss. The RCOG (2004) has recommended that where possible, oxytocin infusions must only be commenced once evacuation has been completed. If the woman is experiencing significant hemorrhage prior to suction evacuation, the use of oxytocin helps in controlling the amount of bleeding.

The medical termination of complete molar pregnancies, including cervical preparation with prostanoids (prostaglandin E2) prior to suction evacuation in cases with hydatidiform moles, is discouraged. This is so as the prostaglandins may induce uterine contractions, thereby causing trophoblastic embolization to the pulmonary vasculature and disseminated disease. The RCOG (2004) has recommended that prostaglandin analogs should be used in cases where oxytocin is ineffective in controlling uterine hemorrhage. In partial molar pregnancies where suction curettage cannot be used due to the presence of fetal parts, the use of medical termination serves as a useful alternative.

Follow-up with β-hCG Levels Following Suction Evacuation

Patients with both complete and partial molar pregnancies should be monitored with serial β-hCG measurements after evacuation to ensure that complete sustained remission has been achieved. The plan for follow-up in cases of GTD is summarized in **Box 12.5**. Serial assays of serum and urine β-hCG levels should be carried out on 2-weekly basis until three negative levels are obtained. In benign disease, hCG

> **BOX 12.5:** Plan of follow-up in cases of gestational trophoblastic disease.
>
> - Follow-up after GTD needs to be individualized for each case
> - *Serum β-hCG levels have come back to normal within 8 weeks of the pregnancy event:* Follow-up would be for 6 months from the date of uterine evacuation
> - *Serum β-hCG levels have not come back to normal within 8 weeks of the pregnancy:* Follow-up will be for 6 months from the date of normalization of the hCG levels
> - Irrespective of the outcomes of future pregnancy, β-hCG levels must be measured 6–8 weeks after the end of the pregnancy to exclude disease recurrence

concentrations spontaneously return to normal by 8 weeks following evacuation of molar pregnancy. In these cases, regular follow-up in the form of pelvic examination and urine β-hCG titers at monthly intervals needs to be done for a period of 6 months. However, women who have the malignant form of trophoblastic disease may show β-hCG titers, which either plateau or rise and remain elevated beyond 8 weeks. Such patients should have monthly follow-up in the form of pelvic examination and urine β-hCG titers for at least 2 years. A chest X-ray is indicated to rule out metastatic disease if the β-hCG levels rise. If β-hCG levels remain elevated, it is also important to rule out the occurrence of a new conception.

Since persistent GTN may develop after a molar pregnancy, nonmolar pregnancy, or even following live birth, women with persistent abnormal vaginal bleeding after a nonmolar pregnancy should undergo serial determination of β-hCG levels to exclude persistent GTN.

Possibility of persistent GTN should also be considered in any woman developing acute respiratory or neurological symptoms after any pregnancy.

Contraceptive measures should be instituted, and the patient is advised to avoid pregnancy until hCG values have remained normal for 6 months. An early ultrasound should be performed in all subsequent pregnancies because H. mole may recur in about 1% of subsequent pregnancies.

Estimations of β-hCG levels must be done at 6 and 10 weeks after any future pregnancy due to a small increase in the risk of development of choriocarcinoma in such patients.

Ruling Out the Presence of Persistent Disease

Following suction evacuation, the patient needs to be investigated to rule out the presence of persistent GTD. For this, serial determination of β-hCG levels needs to be done. Measurement of three consecutive negative levels helps in ensuring that complete sustained remission has been achieved. Following evacuation, serial assays of serum and urine β-hCG levels should be carried out on 2-weekly basis for at least 8 weeks.

In benign disease, β-hCG concentrations spontaneously return to normal by 8 weeks following evacuation of molar pregnancy. In these cases, regular follow-up in the form of pelvic examination and urine β-hCG titers at monthly interval needs to be carried for a period of 6 months. However, women who have the persistent form of GTN may show plateauing or rising β-hCG titers, which usually remain elevated beyond 8 weeks. Such patients should have monthly follow-up in the form of pelvic examination and urine β-hCG titers for at least 2 years.

Hysterectomy with Mole in Situ

Hysterectomy may serve as an option in the following cases:
- Elderly multiparous women (age > 40 years) who do not wish to become pregnant in the future
- Those women with H. mole desiring sterilization
- Those with severe infection or uncontrolled bleeding
- Patients with nonmetastatic persistent disease who have completed childbearing or are not concerned about preserving fertility

If theca lutein cysts are present, they must be left as it is at the time of surgery or at the most, they can be aspirated in order to reduce their size. The ovaries must be conserved. At the time of surgery, it is important to inform the patient that since hysterectomy does not prevent metastatic disease, follow-up with β-hCG levels is essential even after surgery. Hysterectomy however does eliminate the complications related to local invasion.

Chemotherapy Following Evacuation

Women who undergo chemotherapy following evacuation are advised not to conceive for 1 year after completion of treatment. OCPs or any other acceptable method of contraception can be used. Some indications for chemotherapy [as recommended by the Society of Obstetricians and Gynecologists of Canada, (2002)], following evacuation of molar gestation, are as follows:
- Abnormal β-hCG regression pattern (a 10% or greater rise in hCG levels or plateauing of hCG levels comprising three stable values over 2 weeks)
- Histological diagnosis of choriocarcinoma or PSTT
- Presence of metastases in brain, liver, gastrointestinal tract, lungs, or vulvar or vaginal walls
- High hCG levels (>20,000 mIU/mL more than 4 weeks postevacuation).
- Persistently elevated hCG levels 6 months postevacuation

Contraception and Hormone Replacement Therapy in Patients with Hydatidiform Mole

Hormone replacement therapy may be used safely once hCG levels have returned to normal. The RCOG recognizes that the combined oral contraceptive therapy and HRT is safe to use after hCG concentrations have returned to normal.

Management Plan in Twin Gestation with One Viable Fetus and Other Pregnancy Molar

In cases of twin gestation, where there is one viable fetus and the other pregnancy is molar, the pregnancy should be allowed to proceed if the mother wishes, following appropriate counseling regarding the increased risk of perinatal morbidity and mortality. There is nearly 40% risk of early fetal loss and 36% risk of premature delivery. Moreover, there is an increased risk of developing complications such as pulmonary embolism and preeclampsia. There is no increased risk of developing persistent GTN after such a twin pregnancy, and outcome after chemotherapy is similar to that of singleton pregnancy. Prenatal invasive testing for fetal karyotype may be considered in cases where it is uncertain if the pregnancy is a complete mole or a partial one with a coexisting normal twin. Prenatal invasive testing may also be required in cases of placental abnormalities such as mesenchymal hyperplasia of the placenta.

TREATMENT OF PERSISTENT DISEASE

> Q. Write a long essay regarding treatment options in patients with persistent disease?

Any woman experiencing persistent or irregular vaginal bleeding following a pregnancy event (miscarriage, therapeutic termination of pregnancy, or following the baby's delivery) is at risk of developing GTN. Symptoms due to metastatic disease such as dyspnea or abnormal

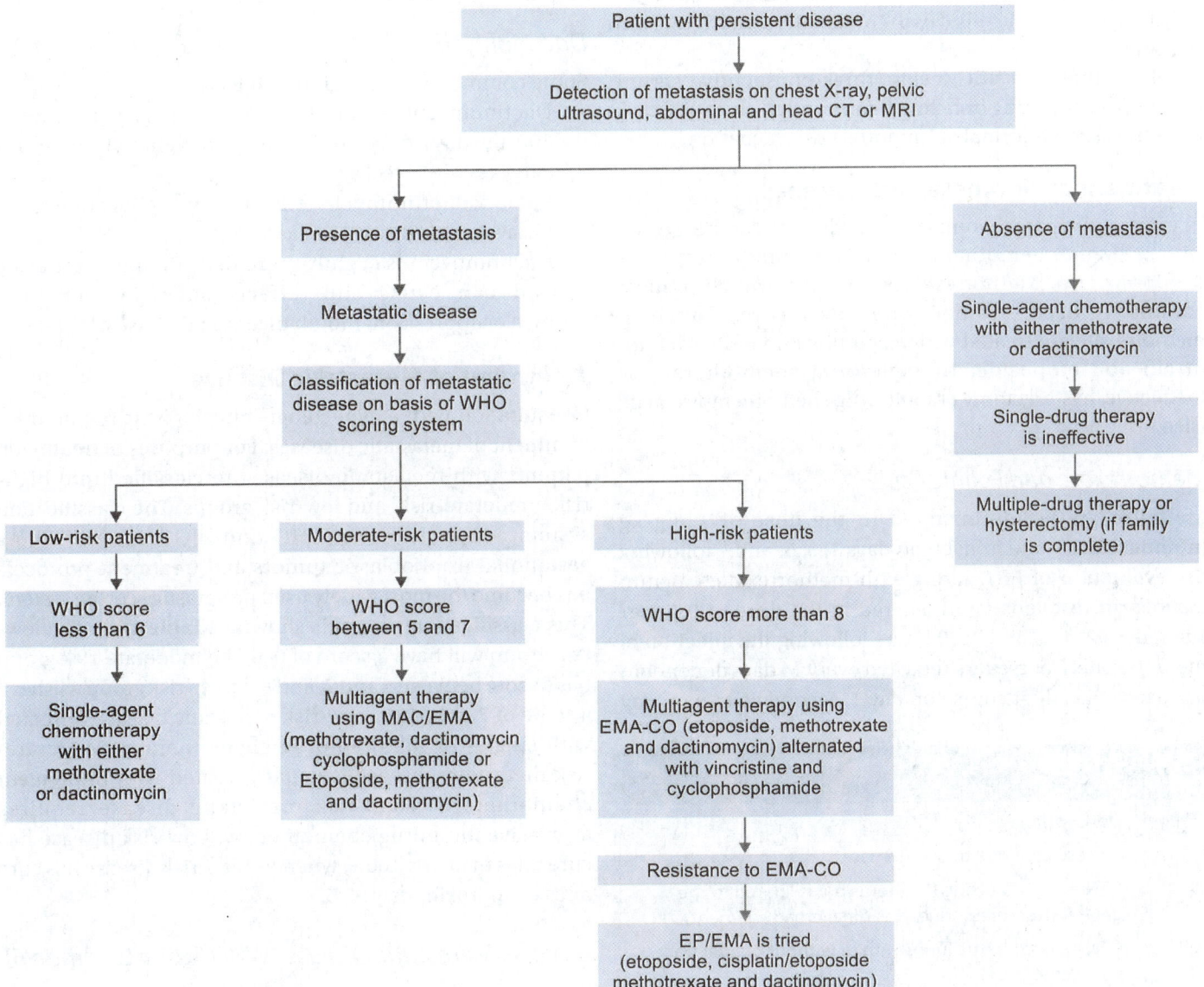

Flowchart 12.2: Management of persistent disease.

(CT: computed tomography; MRI: magnetic resonance imaging; WHO: World Health Organization)

neurological symptoms can occur rarely. The management plan for the treatment of persistent disease is shown in **Flowchart 12.2**. In these cases, it is important to measure β-hCG levels. If the β-hCG level does not normalize within 8–10 weeks, the disease is classified as persistent.

In these cases, chest X-ray and CT scan of brain, chest, abdomen, and pelvis need to be done. If metastasis is detected on these investigations, the disease is classified as metastatic. The FIGO staging of malignant disease is shown in **Table 12.4**. If no metastasis is detected, the disease is classified as nonmetastatic. If the chest X-ray is clear, diagnosis of a nonmetastatic tumor is made. The metastatic disease can spread through the bloodstream to lungs (80%), vagina (30%), pelvis (20%), brain (10%), and liver (10%). Metastasis to the vagina can occur in the fornices or suburethrally. If pulmonary metastases are present, CT scans of the brain and abdomen are also indicated. Persistent disease is usually treated with chemotherapy. Indications for chemotherapy are as follows:

- Serum β-hCG > 20,000 IU/L at greater than 4 weeks
- Rising β-hCG levels (two consecutive rising serum samples)
- Plateauing of β-hCG levels (three consecutive serum samples not rising or falling significantly)
- β-hCG still abnormal at 6 months postevacuation.

Treatment of Nonmetastatic Disease

In most of the cases, nonmetastatic disease can be treated with a single chemotherapeutic drug (methotrexate or dactinomycin). Methotrexate is the drug which is most commonly used. Women who develop resistance to methotrexate are treated with a combination of IV dactinomycin and etoposide. If single-drug chemotherapy is ineffective, hysterectomy or multidrug chemotherapy can be tried.

Methotrexate and Folinic Acid

Methotrexate is administered in the dose of 1 mg/kg intramuscularly and is given on days 1, 3, 5, and 7 following the evaluation of LFT. Along with methotrexate, calcium leucovorin rescue is administered in the dose of 0.1 mg/kg on days 2, 4, 6, and 8, 30 hours following the injection of methotrexate. Courses are repeated every 14 days dependent on toxicity, i.e., first course on day 1, second course on day 15, third course on day 29, and so on. An adequate response to chemotherapy is defined as fall in the-hCG levels by 1 log after a course of chemotherapy. If the response to 1 mg/kg dose is inadequate, the dose is increased to 1.5 mg/kg for each of the 4 treatment days. If even then the response after two consecutive courses of methotrexate-folic acid is inadequate, the patient is considered resistant to methotrexate. In these cases, patients may be administered the alternative drug dactinomycin. While on chemotherapy, monitoring of the patient is done with the help of 2-weekly β-hCG levels, hemogram, and LFT. Chemotherapy is continued until the patient gets three consecutive normal values for β-hCG. Following this, the follow-up is done every month for consecutive 24 months or 2 years. Two–three consolidation cycles may be required even if the β-hCG levels come back to normal.

Methotrexate can produce side effects such as mouth ulcers and soreness in the eyes. These can be treated using mouthwash, hypromellose eye drops, and folinic acid.

Dactinomycin

Some commonly used regimens include:
- Dactinomycin in the dose of 9–13 μg/kg (maximum 500 μg/day) is administered intravenously daily for 5 days every 2 weeks.
- Pulsed dactinomycin 1.25 mg/m² is administered intravenously every 2 weeks.
- Dactinomycin is slightly more toxic than methotrexate and can cause side effects such as hair loss, myelosuppression, mouth ulcers, and nausea.

Treatment of Metastatic Disease

Consultation with a gynecologic oncologist is required for treatment of metastatic diseases. For purposes of treatment, patients with metastatic disease are classified into high-risk, moderate-risk, and low-risk groups. The classification system adopted by the WHO and FIGO for classifying gestational trophoblastic tumors and treatment protocols has become the most widely used prognostic scoring system. This classification system is shown in **Table 12.5**. The low-risk group will have a score of 0–6, the moderate-risk group has a score between 5 and 7, and the high-risk group will have a score of 7 or higher. Low-risk metastatic disease is treated with single- or multiple-drug chemotherapy. Moderate-risk metastatic disease is usually treated with multiagent chemotherapy. High-risk metastatic disease requires aggressive multidrug chemotherapy. Low-risk disease has cure rates of nearly 100%, whereas high-risk disease has cure rates of approximately 95%.

Low-risk Metastatic Disease (WHO Score: Less than 6)

Women belonging to low risk, i.e., scoring 6 or less on the classification system **(Table 12.5)**, must receive IM

TABLE 12.4: FIGO staging of gestational trophoblastic neoplasia (GTN).

Stage	Description
I	Disease confined to the uterus
II	GTN extends outside the uterus but is limited to the genital structures (adnexa, vagina, broad ligament)
III	GTN extends to the lungs with or without genital tract involvement
IV	All other metastatic sites

TABLE 12.5: The classification system by the WHO and FIGO for classifying gestational trophoblastic tumors and treatment protocols.

Risk factor	Risk score			
	0	1	2	4
Age (years)	<40	≥40	–	–
Antecedent pregnancy	Mole	Abortion	Term	–
Interval (end of antecedent pregnancy to chemotherapy) in months	<4	4–6	7–13	>13
Human chorionic gonadotropin (IU/L)	$<10^3$	10^3–10^4	10^4–10^5	$>10^5$
Number of metastases	0	1–4	5–8	>8
Site of metastasis	Lung	Spleen, kidney	Gastrointestinal tract	Brain, liver
Largest tumor mass	–	3–5 cm	>5 cm	–
Previous chemotherapy	–	–	Single drug	≥2 drugs

methotrexate. Methotrexate is administered intramuscularly, alternating daily with folinic acid for 1 week followed by 6 rest days. Women who develop resistance to methotrexate are treated with a combination of IV dactinomycin and etoposide. The dosage and treatment schedule for methotrexate and dactinomycin is same as that for patients with nonmetastatic disease and has already been discussed.

Chemotherapy is changed from methotrexate to dactinomycin if the hCG level plateaus (implying resistance to methotrexate) or if toxicity to methotrexate precludes adequate chemotherapy. With the development of metastases or an elevation in β-hCG titers, combination chemotherapy should be started. Treatment is continued for one to two courses past the first normal hCG levels.

Moderate-risk Patients (WHO Score: 5–7)

Traditionally, moderate-risk patients (WHO score of 5–7) have been treated with multi-agent chemotherapy. The most commonly used combination chemotherapy includes: MAC-based combination (methotrexate, dactinomycin, cyclophosphamide, or chlorambucil) or EMA (etoposide, methotrexate, and dactinomycin). The Charing Cross group (UK) has been recently treating moderate-risk patients with methotrexate and folinic acid, similar to low-risk patients.

High-risk Patients (WHO Score: 8 or Greater)

Women with high-risk GTN or chemoresistant GTN (resistant to methotrexate and actinomycin D) usually require combination chemotherapy with selective use of surgery and radiotherapy. This group may include patients with metastases to the brain, liver, and gastrointestinal tract. Complications such as massive bleeding may occur early in the disease. The standard chemotherapy regimen in high-risk group is EMA/CO **(Box 12.6)** in which the drugs such as etoposide, dactinomycin, and methotrexate are alternated at weekly intervals with vincristine and cyclophosphamide. The commonly used regimen for resistant disease is EP/EMA **(Box 12.7)**, which includes drugs such as etoposide,

> **BOX 12.6:** EMA/CO regimen for high-risk patients with gestational trophoblastic disease.
>
> *Regimen 1 (EMA)*
>
> *Week 1–day 1:*
> - Actinomycin D 0.5 mg IV bolus
> - Etoposide 100 mg/m² IV in 500 mL normal saline over 30 minutes
> - Methotrexate 300 mg/m² IV in 1 L normal saline over 12 hours
>
> *Day 2:*
> - Actinomycin D 0.5 mg IV bolus
> - Etoposide 100 mg/m² IV in 500 mL normal saline over 30 minutes
> - Folinic acid 15 mg IM 12-hourly × 4 doses starting 24 hours after commencing methotrexate
>
> *Regimen 2 (CO)*
>
> *Week 2–day 1:*
> - Vincristine (oncovin) 1.4 mg/m² IV bolus (maximum 2 mg)
> - Cyclophosphamide 600 mg/m² IV in 500 mL normal saline over 30 minutes

> **BOX 12.7:** EP/EMA regime for patients with disease resistant to EMA/CO.
>
> *Regimen 1 (EP)*
>
> *Week 1–day 1:*
> - Etoposide 150 mg/m² IV in 500 mL normal saline over 30 minutes
> - Cisplatin 25 mg/m² IV over 4 hours
>
> *Regimen 2 (EMA)*
>
> *Week 2–day 1:*
> - Etoposide 100 mg/m² IV over 30 minutes
> - Methotrexate 300 mg/m² IV over 24 hours
> - Actinomycin D 0.5 mg IV bolus
>
> *Day 2:*
> - Folinic acid 15 mg PO 12-hourly for four doses (to start 24 hours after starting methotrexate)

cisplatin, methotrexate, and dactinomycin. There are few reports of treatment with the newer anticancer agents such as paclitaxel, employment of granulocyte colony-stimulating factor and high-dose chemotherapy with autologous bone

> **BOX 12.8:** Indications for surgery.
> - Pelvic sepsis
> - Pelvic hemorrhage/acute bleeding
> - Placental site trophoblastic tumor
> - Intraperitoneal hemorrhage
> - Age > 40 years
> - Extensive metastasis to brain/liver, etc.

marrow support. Chemotherapy drugs such as cisplatin, vinblastine, and bleomycin may also prove to be effective as second-line therapeutic agents. Regimens 1 and 2 are alternated each week. High-risk GTN can also be treated with paclitaxel/cisplatin alternating with paclitaxel/etoposide (TP/TE).

Chemotherapy is continued until the patient gets three consecutive normal values for β-hCG. Three further consolidation cycles may be required once β-hCG levels come back to normal. Subsequently, the follow-up is done every month for 1 year and 3-monthly for 2 years.

Contraception

Women with GTN who have successfully completed chemotherapy are advised to delay pregnancy for 1 year because most relapses are likely to occur during this period. Also, methotrexate may persist in human tissues for several months. During this period, they are advised to use a contraceptive method. Any form of contraception including the combined hormonal contraception or progestogen-based injectables can be used. The use of IUCDs is avoided as it may cause bleeding/perforation, etc. Nevertheless, women who conceive within 1 year postchemotherapy for GTN may be reassured of favorable outcomes.

Surgery

While chemotherapy is effective in most of the cases, surgery may be required rarely in some circumstances **(Box 12.8)**.

Poor Prognostic Factors

Poor prognostic factors for the disease include the following:
- Disease has spread to the liver or brain.
- Serum β-hCG level is >40,000 mIU/mL at the time the treatment begins.
- The patient had received chemotherapy in the past.
- Symptoms had been present for more than 4 months before starting chemotherapy treatment.
- Choriocarcinoma occurred after a pregnancy that resulted in the birth of a child.

Long-term Outcome

The women who receive chemotherapy for GTN are likely to experience an earlier menopause. Menopause is advanced by 1 year on an average amongst women receiving single-agent chemotherapy and by 3 years amongst women receiving multiagent chemotherapy. Women with high-risk GTN who require multiagent chemotherapy, including etoposide, should also be counseled regarding increased risk of developing secondary cancers such as acute myeloid leukemia, melanoma, and breast cancer.

COMPLICATIONS

Benign forms of H. mole can result in complications such as uterine infection, sepsis, hemorrhagic shock, and preeclampsia, which may occur during early pregnancy. Recurrence of molar gestation may occur in 1–2% cases. Excessive vaginal bleeding can be associated with molar pregnancy. However, routine use of oxytocin infusion must be avoided due to theoretical concerns related to embolization of trophoblastic tissue. Nevertheless, in order to control life-threatening bleeding, oxytocic infusions may be used. Infection can commonly occur due to the absence of the amniotic sac and due to the large surface area left after expulsion or evacuation of the mole.

Gestational trophoblastic disease does not impair fertility or predispose to prenatal or perinatal complications (e.g., congenital malformations and spontaneous abortions). The most important complication related to GTD is the development of GTN, which includes conditions such as invasive mole, choriocarcinoma, and PSTT. All of these may metastasize and are potentially fatal if left untreated.

INVASIVE MOLE

Invasive mole (chorioadenoma destruens) is a histologically benign condition resulting due to the invasion of abnormal trophoblasts into myometrium. It may also develop due to embolization of molar tissue through pelvic venous plexus. Approximately 15% of patients with invasive mole may develop metastases, lodging most commonly in the vagina and lungs.

GESTATIONAL CHORIOCARCINOMA

Also known as chorioblastoma, trophoblastic tumor, chorioepithelioma, or GTN, gestational choriocarcinoma is a widely metastatic tumor composed of malignant trophoblastic cells, which arises from trophoblastic tissue of term pregnancies, as well as from ectopic gestation, and spontaneous or induced abortions.

Choriocarcinoma is a highly invasive tumor, which metastasizes early and is often widespread at the time of diagnosis. Lungs are the most common sites for metastases and are present in almost all patients with extrauterine disease. Other sites of metastasis include brain, liver, vagina, kidney, and intestines.

PLACENTAL SITE TROPHOBLASTIC TUMOR

Placental site trophoblastic tumor is a rare manifestation of gestational trophoblastic tumor, which develops at placental implantation site. These tumors usually originate from the intermediate trophoblastic cells. They may present with a wide spectrum of clinical behavior, ranging from a self-limited state to persistent disease to a highly aggressive metastatic neoplasm, showing metastases to the lung, liver, peritoneal cavity, brain, etc. Due to the lack of syncytiotrophoblastic tissue, levels of serum hCG are only modestly elevated in PSTTs. Therefore, measurement of levels of human placental lactogen (hPL) is more likely to be useful in these cases. They may complicate any type of pregnancy and may be diagnosed following a dilatation and evacuation procedure either for missed abortion or for a H. mole. They have also been described following term pregnancies. PSTT is relatively resistant to chemotherapy but responds well to surgery (hysterectomy) if the disease is localized. However, in cases of advanced disease, chemotherapy with the EMA/CO protocol is usually used.

EVIDENCE-BASED CLINICAL TRIALS

List of references can be scanned through QR code to enable the readers gain deeper insight of the subject by referring to the entire article or its abstract.

CHAPTER 13

Bad Obstetric History

CASE STUDY

A 32-year-old woman G4P0A3L0 with previous history of three miscarriages all in the first trimester presented with 14 completed weeks of gestation for regular antenatal care check-up.

INTRODUCTION

The above-described case symptoms are suggestive of bad obstetric history (BOH). The term BOH is used in those patients in whom the obstetric future is likely to be modified by the nature of previous disaster.

WHO has defined BOH as previous unfavorable fetal outcome in terms of two or more consecutive spontaneous miscarriages, early neonatal deaths, stillbirths, intrauterine fetal deaths, intrauterine growth restriction, congenital anomalies, etc. This chapter would specifically focus on recurrent miscarriage as a cause of BOH.

DEFINITION

> Q. Write a short note on recurrent early pregnancy loss.

Miscarriage can be defined as expulsion of fetus or embryo before a particular gestational age (usually taken as 20 weeks of gestation), when the fetus becomes capable of independent survival or before attaining a weight of 500 g (WHO, 2006). This is the definition followed by most of the centers in India.

Definitions of some commonly used terminology related with pregnancy loss are described in **Table 13.1**.

Royal College of Obstetricians and Gynaecologists (RCOG, 2011) has defined recurrent miscarriage as the clinically recognized consecutive loss of three or more pregnancies with the same partner before 24 weeks of gestation. Due to advances in neonatal care, a small number of babies are also able to survive before 24 weeks of gestation. RCOG is the only authority which uses the term "consecutive" in its definition.

TABLE 13.1: Definition of some commonly used terminology related with pregnancy loss.

Terminology	Definition
Early miscarriage	Pregnancy loss at ≤ 12 weeks
Late miscarriage	Pregnancy loss between 12 and 20 weeks
Blighted ovum	Anembryonic pregnancy
Embryonic loss	Miscarriage at ≤ 8th gestational week
Fetal loss	Miscarriage between 9 and 20 weeks
Stillbirth	Pregnancy loss at ≥ 20th week

On the other hand, European Society of Human Reproduction and Embryology (2017) have defined recurrent miscarriage as two or more pregnancy losses before the fetus reaches 24 weeks of gestation. If identified, ectopic and molar pregnancies or implantation failure should not be included in this definition.

The practice committee of the American Society for Reproductive Medicine (ASRM, 2008) has defined recurrent miscarriage as two or more pregnancy losses, consecutive or otherwise (up to 20 weeks' gestation). They have suggested that investigations must be initiated following two miscarriages and a thorough evaluation be performed after three. Prevalence of recurrent pregnancy loss varies between 1 and 5%. If the definition of three or more pregnancy losses is considered, the incidence of recurrent pregnancy loss is 1%, whereas if we consider the definition of two or more pregnancy losses, the incidence is approximately 5%.

The clinician should start investigating the woman presenting with a history of recurrent abortions in the following cases:
- More than or equal to two abortions
- Unexpected fetal death after 16 weeks
- Severe IUGR
- Severe preeclampsia/eclampsia before 34 weeks.

Bad obstetric history could be related to recurrent miscarriage or a history of previous unfavorable fetal outcome in terms of two or more consecutive spontaneous abortions, early neonatal deaths, stillbirths, intrauterine fetal deaths, congenital anomalies, etc. Clinical investigations can be initiated after two consecutive spontaneous miscarriages, especially if the fetal heart activity had been previously present; when the woman is older than 35 years of age or when the couple has difficulty conceiving. Miscarriage can be considered as primary, when there is no previous history of live birth and considered as secondary when fetal loss occurs following a successful pregnancy.

BOX 13.1: Causes of recurrent pregnancy loss.

- *Genetic* (2–5%)
  - Chromosomal abnormalities/aneuploidy in the embryo or fetus
  - Parental chromosomal abnormalities
- *Anatomic* (12–16%)
  - Congenital uterine malformations (e.g., unicornuate uterus, uterine didelphys, septate uterus, etc.)
  - Leiomyomas: Submucous
  - Intrauterine adhesions
- *Immunologic*
  - Autoimmune: SLE and APLA (12–15%)
  - Alloimmune: Abnormal maternal response to fetal or placental antigens (due to maternal cytotoxic antibodies, absent maternal blocking antibodies and/or disturbances in the natural killer cell function and distribution)
- *Inherited thrombophilias* (mutation in prothrombin gene, hyperhomocysteinemia, deficiencies in antithrombin III, protein S, C, etc.). These cause microthrombi/thrombosis/infarction of the placental vessels
- *Endocrine* (17–20%)
  - Thyroid disease, diabetes, PCOS, and luteal phase deficiency
- *Infectious causes* (0.5–5%)
  - Chlamydia, Ureaplasma, Mycoplasma, toxoplasmosis, Listeria, Campylobacter, Herpes, Cytomegalovirus, bacterial vaginosis
- *Environmental*
  - Smoking, alcohol, and heavy coffee consumption
- *Unexplained* (40–50%)

(APLA: antiphospholipid antibody; PCOS: polycystic ovarian syndrome; SLE: systemic lupus erythematosus)

ETIOLOGY

Q. Discuss the etiology of RPL. How will you manage and diagnose the case of cervical incompetence?

Q. Discuss at length the etiology and management of recurrent abortions.

Q. With the help of a long essay, evaluate the causes of recurrent pregnancy loss and the suggestive preventive measures.

Some important causes of BOH include genetic causes, abnormal maternal immune response, abnormal hormonal response, maternal infection and anatomical factors. BOH could also be because of environmental factors—radiation exposure, occupational hazards, addictions and habits. Each of these is discussed next in detail. It is important to exclude each of these factors by taking the relevant history. The etiology of recurrent abortion is described in **Box 13.1 and Figure 13.1**. Prognostic factors for RPL include the following:

- *Maternal age:* Pregnancy loss is lowest in women aged 20–35 years. However, the rate of pregnancy loss rapidly increases after the maternal age of 40 years. Paternal age is also an important factor as father's age >40 years is associated with approximately 23% increased risk.
- *Number of previous miscarriages:* Higher number of previous miscarriages is associated with a poorer prognosis.

Genetic Causes

Q. With help of a long essay discuss the role of genetic factors in recurrent pregnancy loss.

Presence of chromosomal abnormality in either of the parents is responsible for a high proportion of early first

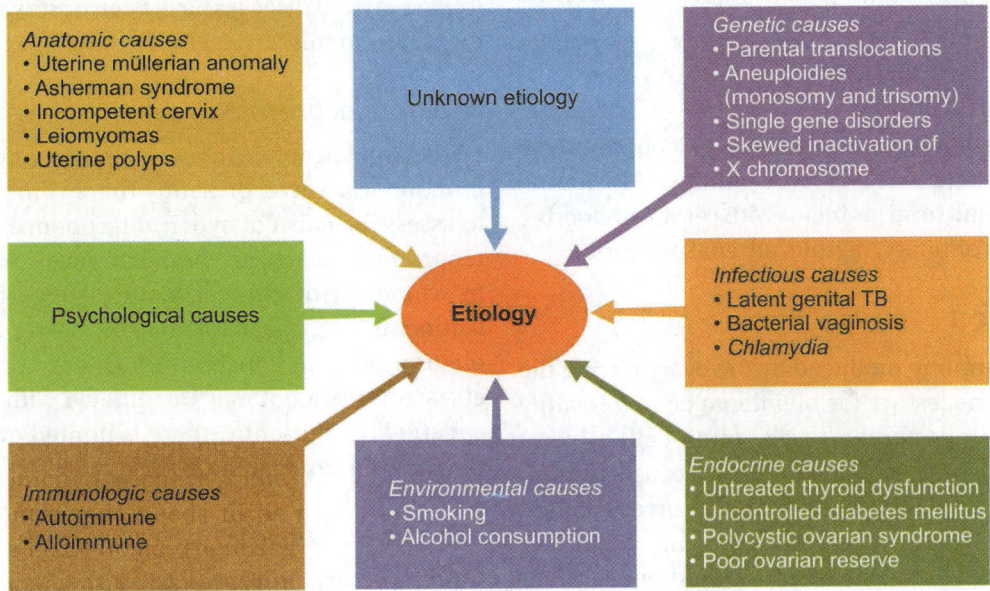

Fig. 13.1: Causes of recurrent miscarriage.

trimester miscarriages. All couples with a history of recurrent miscarriage should have peripheral blood karyotyping performed. Chromosomal abnormalities of the conceptus account for more than half of sporadic (pre) embryonic losses and in many cases, a visible embryo never forms. The most common types of parental chromosomal abnormalities are balanced reciprocal or Robertsonian translocations. These are commonly associated with advanced maternal age and premature ovarian failure.

Single gene defects and skewed inactivation of X chromosome are other emerging causes of recurrent miscarriage. As the number of miscarriages increases, the possibility of the miscarriage due to the presence of chromosomal abnormality decreases and the chance of miscarriage due to the presence of recurring maternal cause increases. Genetic factors are the most important causes for the sporadic miscarriage. If an abnormal parental karyotype is identified, the patient in any case must be referred to a clinical geneticist and offered genetic counseling, familial chromosomal studies and appropriate prenatal diagnosis in future pregnancies. In all couples with a previous history of recurrent miscarriage, cytogenetic analysis of the products of conception should be performed if the next pregnancy fails.

Approximately 50–70% of genetic pregnancy losses are due to chromosomal aneuploidies, the most common among which are monosomy X, other autosomal trisomies such as trisomy 16, 13, 18, and 21.

Factor V Leiden (FVL) and prothrombin G20210A mutations are common genetic mutations that predispose the carriers to develop venous thromboembolism. FVL is the most common cause of primary and recurrent venous thromboembolism in pregnancy. FVL carriage has also consistently been shown to increase the risk of early onset gestational hypertension, HELLP (hemolysis, elevated liver enzymes, and low platelets) syndrome, severe placental abruption and fetal growth retardation.

Hormonal Causes

Hormonal factors have been proposed to contribute to recurrent miscarriage in 17–20% of patients. Hormonal aberrations may result from problems with certain endocrine glands, such as the pituitary, thyroid, adrenal or ovaries.

Luteal Phase Defect

Progesterone, a hormone produced by the ovary during the secretory stage, is necessary for maintenance of a healthy pregnancy. Low progesterone levels, often called luteal phase defect (LPD), has been thought to be a cause of spontaneous abortions. LPD has been found to be associated with poor follicular phase oocyte development, which may result in disordered estrogen secretion and subsequent dysfunction of the corpus luteum.

Polycystic Ovary Syndrome

Polycystic ovary syndrome has been considered as a cause of a variety of menstrual disorders ranging from amenorrhea to dysfunctional uterine bleeding, hirsutism and infertility. Hypersecretion of luteinizing hormone (LH) in polycystic ovarian syndrome (PCOS), resulting in the elevation of LH:FSH ratio, is thought to be responsible for causing recurrent miscarriages.

All women with PCOS may not be necessarily at a high risk of recurrent miscarriage. Polycystic ovarian morphology is a classical feature of PCOS. Though the prevalence of PCOS is significantly higher among women with recurrent miscarriage in comparison with the general population, polycystic ovarian morphology by itself is not a predictor for an increased risk of future pregnancy loss among ovulatory women with a history of recurrent miscarriage who conceive spontaneously.

Hypothyroidism

Maternal hypothyroidism may place the mother at an increased risk of adverse obstetrical outcomes. Thyroid disease may cause ovulatory dysfunction and LPDs. Treated thyroid dysfunction, however, is not a risk factor for recurrent miscarriage. Untreated hypothyroidism, on the other hand can result in an increased risk for preeclampsia, placental abruption, miscarriage and perinatal mortality. Maternal hypothyroidism in the second trimester has been found to be associated with an increased rate of fetal death after 16 weeks of gestation.

Diabetes Mellitus

Women with diabetes who have high hemoglobin A1c (glycosylated hemoglobin) levels in the first trimester are at an increased risk of miscarriage and fetal malformations.

However, neither well controlled diabetes mellitus nor treated thyroid diseases have been observed to be risk factors for recurrent miscarriage.

Hyperprolactinemia

Hyperprolactinemia may adversely affect corpus luteal function. However, presently there is insufficient evidence to assess the effect of hyperprolactinemia as a risk factor for recurrent miscarriage. Prolactin levels must be measured in women with clinical history suggestive of hyperprolactinemia (e.g., galactorrhea, or history of amenorrhea or oliguria prior to conception). In case prolactin levels are elevated, treatment may be initiated with bromocriptine or cabergoline. Presently, there is limited evidence related to the safety of cabergoline in pregnancy.

Infectious Causes

Infections are thought to be responsible for a minor proportion (0.5–5%) of cases of recurrent miscarriage.

The role of infection in recurrent miscarriage is unclear. An infection can be implicated in the etiology of repeated pregnancy loss, only if it is capable of persisting in the genital tract, without being detected early or without causing sufficient symptoms, which could disturb the women. TORCH group of infections such as *Toxoplasma gondii*, rubella virus, and cytomegalovirus infections do not fulfill these criteria and are no longer considered to be responsible for recurrent miscarriages. The RCOG recommends that routine TORCH screening in cases of recurrent miscarriages should be abandoned. Other infectious organisms that have been implicated in the causation of recurrent miscarriages include *L. monocytogenes, M. hominis*, Herpes simplex virus, *C. trachomatis, Ureaplasma spp.*, etc.

Bacterial vaginosis has also been found to be strongly associated with late miscarriage, preterm rupture of membranes and preterm labor. The standard antibiotic regime recommended for treatment of bacterial vaginosis in pregnancy is metronidazole 400 mg 12 hourly for 5–7 days. In order to reduce systemic side effects, intravaginal 2% clindamycin cream or 0.75% metronidazole gel may also be used. Single dose therapy in the form of 2 g metronidazole or tinidazole 2 g has also been found to be effective in pregnancy. Long-term treatment with probiotics may play a role in re-establishing normal vaginal flora.

Syphilis, a sexually transmitted disease, has been implicated as the cause for second trimester miscarriages, stillbirths, preterm labor, growth retardation, neonatal infections, etc.

Chronic endometritis may be due to organisms such as *Chlamydia, Mycobacterium tuberculosis*, etc. Low virulence organisms associated with bacterial vaginosis may also result in infertility and unexplained miscarriages. PCR-based testing for *M. tuberculosis* and *Chlamydia* can be performed on endometrial aspirates. Hysteroscopic diagnosis using chromohysteroscopy with methylene blue has been suggested as a diagnostic procedure.

Anatomical Causes

Anatomical defects of the reproductive system could be one of the most common causes of BOH. Uterine malformations, either congenital or acquired, could be responsible for approximately 12–16% cases of recurrent miscarriage. History of uterine malformations is often associated with late miscarriages. Congenital uterine anomalies include Müllerian duct abnormalities, presence of uterine septum and uterine/cervical anomalies **(Fig. 13.1)**. Acquired uterine anomalies leading to fetal loss include leiomyomas and endometriosis.

Uterine abnormalities could result in impaired vascularization of pregnancy and limited space for the growing fetus due to distortion of the uterine cavity. Hysterosalpingography (HSG) helps in diagnosing uterine anomalies. However, the routine use of HSG as a screening test for uterine anomalies in women with recurrent miscarriage is questionable.

TABLE 13.2: American Fertility Society classification of Müllerian anomalies.

Classification	Anomaly
Class I	Segmental Müllerian agenesis-hypoplasia A. Vaginal B. Cervical C. Fundal D. Tubal E. Combined anomalies
Class II	Unicornuate A. Communicating B. Noncommunicating C. No cavity D. No horn
Class III	Didelphys
Class IV	Bicornuate A. Complete (division down to internal os) B. Partial
Class V	Septate A. Complete (septum to the internal os) B. Partial
Class VI	Arcuate
Class VII	Diethylstilbestrol related

Uterine Malformations

Müllerian anomalies could result in an abnormal or irregularly shaped uterus, which could result in improper implantation and/or growth of the embryo, thereby resulting in recurrent miscarriages. The various Müllerian anomalies, which can be implicated as a cause of recurrent miscarriage, include septate uterus (50–60%), unicornuate uterus (34–44%), uterus didelphys, etc. The classification of the Müllerian anomalies by the American Fertility Society is shown in **Table 13.2** and **Figure 13.2**. Presence of a uterine anomaly such as uterine septum is a potentially treatable cause for recurrent miscarriage or infertility. However, not all patients with uterine anomalies experience repeated pregnancy losses. For example, patients with bicornuate uterus and uterus didelphys are not associated with recurrent miscarriage. It is yet not explained why some patients with uterine anomalies have normal reproductive function, while others experience recurrent miscarriages. Three-dimensional ultrasound is mandatory for the diagnosis of anatomical uterine anomalies.

Uterine septum: Presence of a uterine septum results in repeated pregnancy losses due to the following factors:
- Reduced intrauterine space for fetal growth
- Placental implantation on a poorly vascularized uterine septum

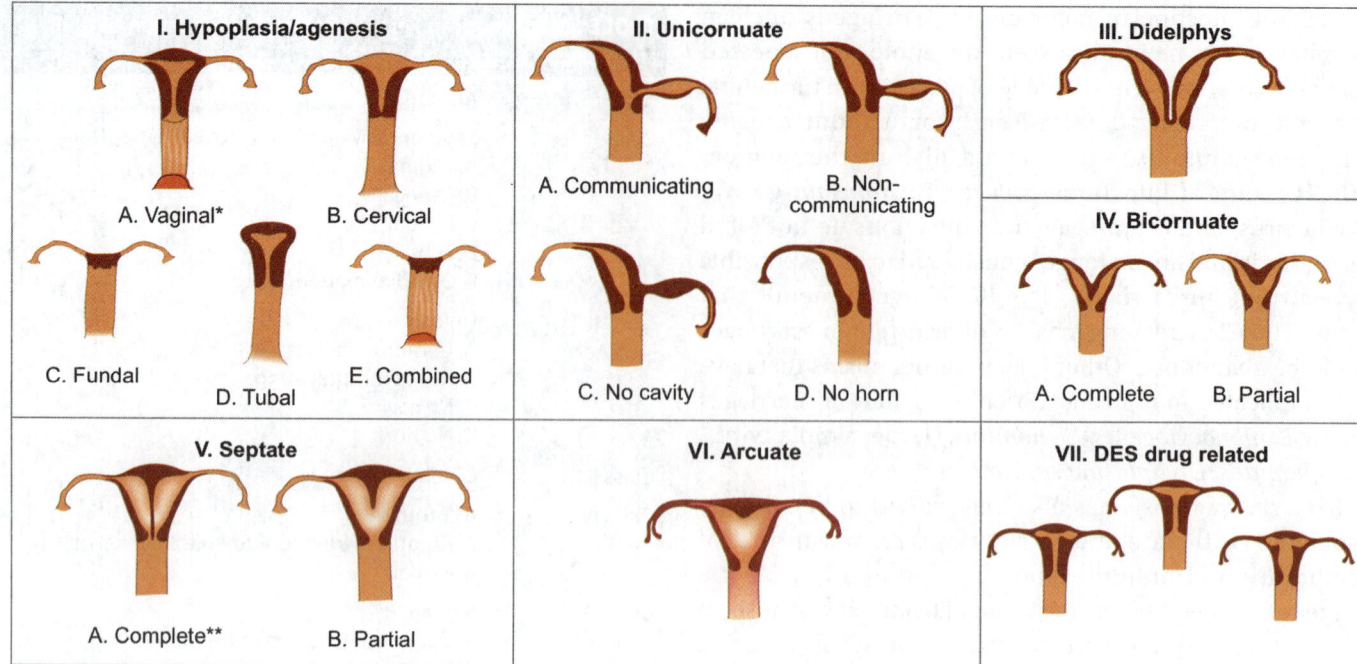

Fig. 13.2: Classification of the uterine anomalies by the American Society for Reproductive Medicine (1998).
*Uterus may be normal or take a variety of abnormal forms.
**May have two distinct cervices.
Source: The American Fertility Society classifications of adnexal adhesions, distal tubal occlusion, tubal occlusion secondary to tubal ligation, tubal pregnancies, Müllerian anomalies and intrauterine adhesions. Fertil Steril.1988;49(6):944-55.

- Associated cervical incompetence, luteal phase insufficiency and distortion of the uterine milieu.

Removal of uterine septum or metroplasty is best performed using operative hysteroscopy **(Figs. 13.3A to D)**. Patients with septate uterus are likely to show an improved pregnancy outcome following hysteroscopic septum resection.

Asherman's Syndrome

In addition to Müllerian anomalies, an acquired anatomical cause of recurrent abortions is Asherman's syndrome, which is characterized by development of intrauterine adhesions, occurring in women who have had several dilatation and curettage procedures. The pathogenesis of intrauterine adhesions and Asherman's syndrome is most often related to endometrial trauma. These adhesions may cause amenorrhea, repeated miscarriages and infertility. Diagnosis of Asherman's syndrome can be reached by doing tests such as hysteroscopy and transvaginal ultrasound examination.

Treatment involves hysteroscopic surgery to cut and remove the adhesions or scar tissue **(Figs. 13.4A to D)**. After the removal of scar tissue, the uterine cavity must be kept open. Over the years, many surgical adjuncts have been tested in an attempt to prevent the reformation of adhesions. Some of these surgical adjuncts include, intrauterine devices (inert), intrauterine Foley catheters, antiadhesion barriers, amnion grafts, hormonal therapy, antibiotic therapy, etc.

Postoperative evaluation for reformation of adhesion in form of HSG or hysteroscopy should be considered mandatory.

Uterine Fibroids

Uterine fibroids, most commonly those which are submucosal may distort the endometrial cavity, thereby resulting in recurrent pregnancy losses. No association with recurrent miscarriage could be established for either intramural or submucosal fibroids. Presently, there is insufficient evidence regarding the removal of fibroids for management of cases of recurrent miscarriages and the guidelines do not recommend this.

Endometrial Polyps

Endometrial polyps are frequently associated with infertility. Most experts feel that polypectomy should be performed with hysteroscopic guidance. Polypectomy can be performed by grasping and avulsing the stalk with ring forceps or sharply severing the base with electrosurgical instruments.

Cervical Incompetence

> **Q.** Write a long essay discussing the diagnosis of cervical incompetence. Also, discuss the role of cervical encerclage in modern obstetrics.
>
> **Q.** With help of a long essay, discuss the diagnosis and management of cervical incompetence in pregnancy.

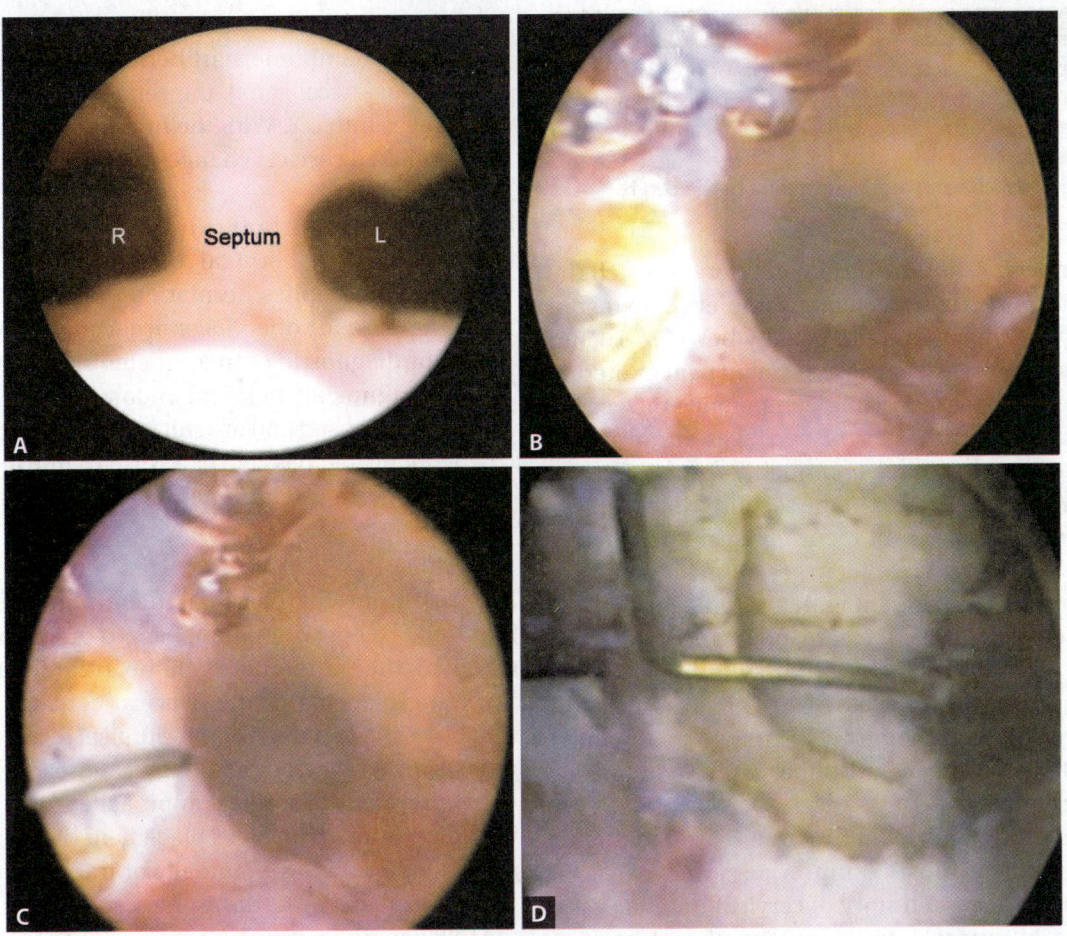

Figs. 13.3A to D: Resection of uterine septum. (A) Hysteroscopic visualization of uterine septum; (B) Septum before the resectoscope loop touched it; (C and D) Resectoscope loop transecting the uterine septum.

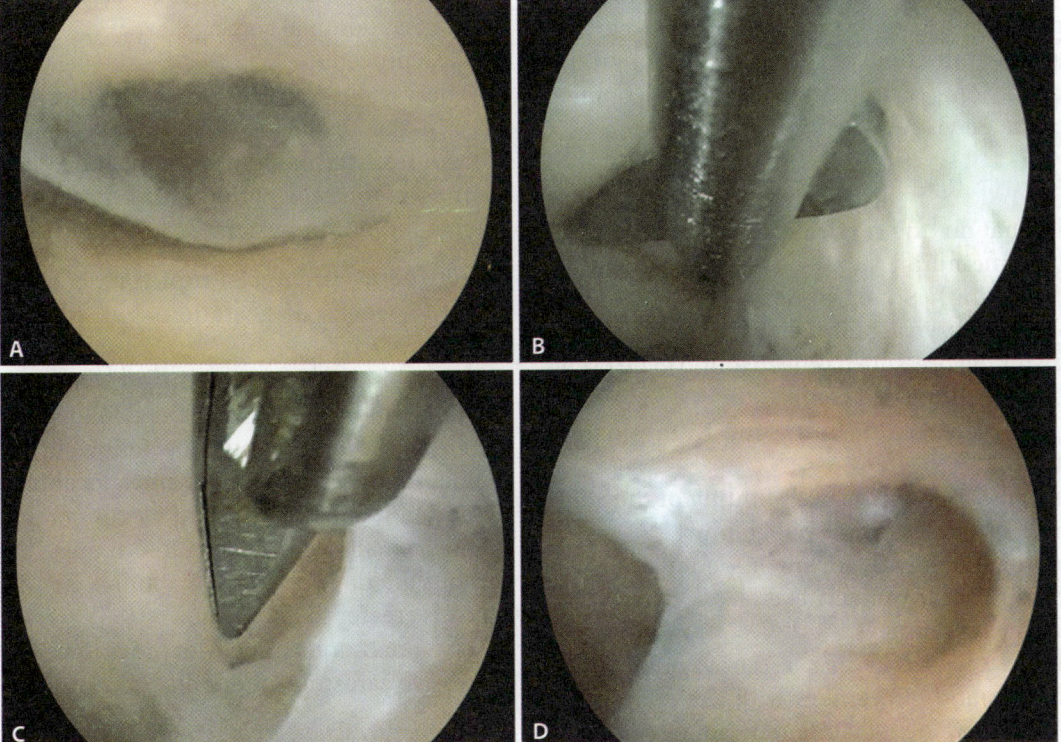

Figs. 13.4A to D: (A) Visualization of intrauterine adhesions at the time of hysteroscopic examination; (B and C) Resection of the intrauterine adhesion using a hysteroscopic scissors; (D) View of the uterus following the completion of resection.

> **BOX 13.2:** Risk factors for development of cervical incompetence.
>
> - Diagnosis of cervical incompetence in a previous pregnancy
> - Previous history of preterm premature rupture of membranes
> - History of diethylstilbestrol exposure, which can cause anatomical defects in uterus and cervix
> - History of previously having received trauma to the cervix

Cervical incompetence is a medical condition in which the pregnant woman's cervix starts dilating and effacing before her pregnancy has reached term, usually between 16 and 28 weeks of gestation, without any associated pain or uterine contractions. As a result, cervical incompetence may cause the second and third trimester miscarriages and preterm births. Cervical incompetence is probably responsible for causing 20–25% of miscarriages in the second trimester.

The woman gives history of recurrent second trimester pregnancy losses, occurring earlier in gestation in successive pregnancies and usually present with a significant cervical dilatation of 2 cm or more in the early pregnancy. However, usually there is absence of any other symptoms. In the second trimester, cervix may dilate up to 4 cm in association with active uterine contractions. This may be associated with rupture of the membranes resulting in the spontaneous expulsion of the fetus.

Cervical incompetence could be due to congenital or acquired causes. The most common acquired cause of cervical incompetence is a history of cervical trauma or the previous history of cervical lacerations. Therefore, history of any cervical procedure including cervical conization, loop electrosurgical excision procedure (LEEP), instrumental vaginal delivery or forceful cervical dilatation during previous miscarriage needs to be elicited. History of any cervical cerclage performed at the time of previous pregnancy also needs to be elicited. Some of the risk factors for development of cervical incompetence are listed in **Box 13.2**.

Diagnosis

On clinical examination, the cervical canal may be dilated and effaced. Fetal membranes may be visible through the cervical os (funneling). Sonographic serial evaluation (every 2 weeks) of the cervix for funneling and shortening in response to transfundal pressure has been found to be useful in the evaluation of incompetent cervix.

Other findings observed on ultrasound examination include the following:
- Cervical length <25 mm. However, finding of the short cervical length on transvaginal sonography (TVS) is not a confirmed diagnostic test for incompetent cervix. It could also be due to early preterm labor.
- Protrusion of the membranes.
- Presence of the fetal parts in the cervix or vagina.
- Cervical dilation and effacement with the changes in form of T, Y, V, U (can be remembered using the mnemonic "Trust Your Vaginal Ultrasound") **(Figs. 13.5A and B)**. T-shaped cervix on ultrasound examination points toward a normal cervix. As the internal cervical os opens and the membrane start herniating into the upper part of endocervical canal, the cervical shape on ultrasound changes into a Y. With the further progression of above-mentioned cervical changes, Y shape changes into V and then into U.
- Another important finding on TVS examination suggestive of cervical incompetence is funneling. Funneling implies herniation of fetal membranes into the upper part of endocervical canal. However, this too is not diagnostic of incompetent os. Some of the tests for diagnosing cervical incompetence, which were previously used and are still used at some places, include the following: passage of a No. 8 (8 mm) Hegar's dilator, traction using an intrauterine Foley's catheter, etc.

Treatment

No treatment for cervical incompetence is generally required, except when it appears to threaten a pregnancy. Cervical incompetence can be treated using surgery involving placement of a cervical cerclage suture which reinforces the cervical muscle. Surgical repair of the cervix is done using a vaginal or abdominal approach.

At present, the surgical approaches form the treatment of choice. Surgery involves placement of a cervical cerclage suture, either transabdominally or transvaginally. Different types of surgical procedures that can be performed include the following:
- McDonald procedure
- Shirodkar operation
- Wurms procedure (Hefner cerclage)
- Transabdominal cerclage
- Lash procedure

The various surgical procedures have been explained later in the text. Out of the above-mentioned surgical procedures, McDonald procedure and Shirodkar procedure are most commonly performed. Cerclage could be either an emergency or prophylactic.

Prophylactic cerclage: Prophylactic cerclage is placed at 12–16 weeks of gestation, but antibiotics are given perioperatively.

Sexual intercourse, prolonged standing (> 90 minutes) and heavy lifting are to be avoided following cerclage.

These patients should be followed up with periodic vaginal sonography to assess stitch locations and funneling. No additional restrictions are recommended as long as the stitches remain within the middle or upper third of the cervix without the development of a funnel and the length of the cervix is greater than 25 mm.

If vaginal surgery does not prove to be successful despite aggressive care, transabdominal cerclage can be tried.

Emergency/rescue cerclage: Emergency or rescue cerclage is used in cases of patients with acute presentation of incompetent cervix. Placement of emergency cerclage

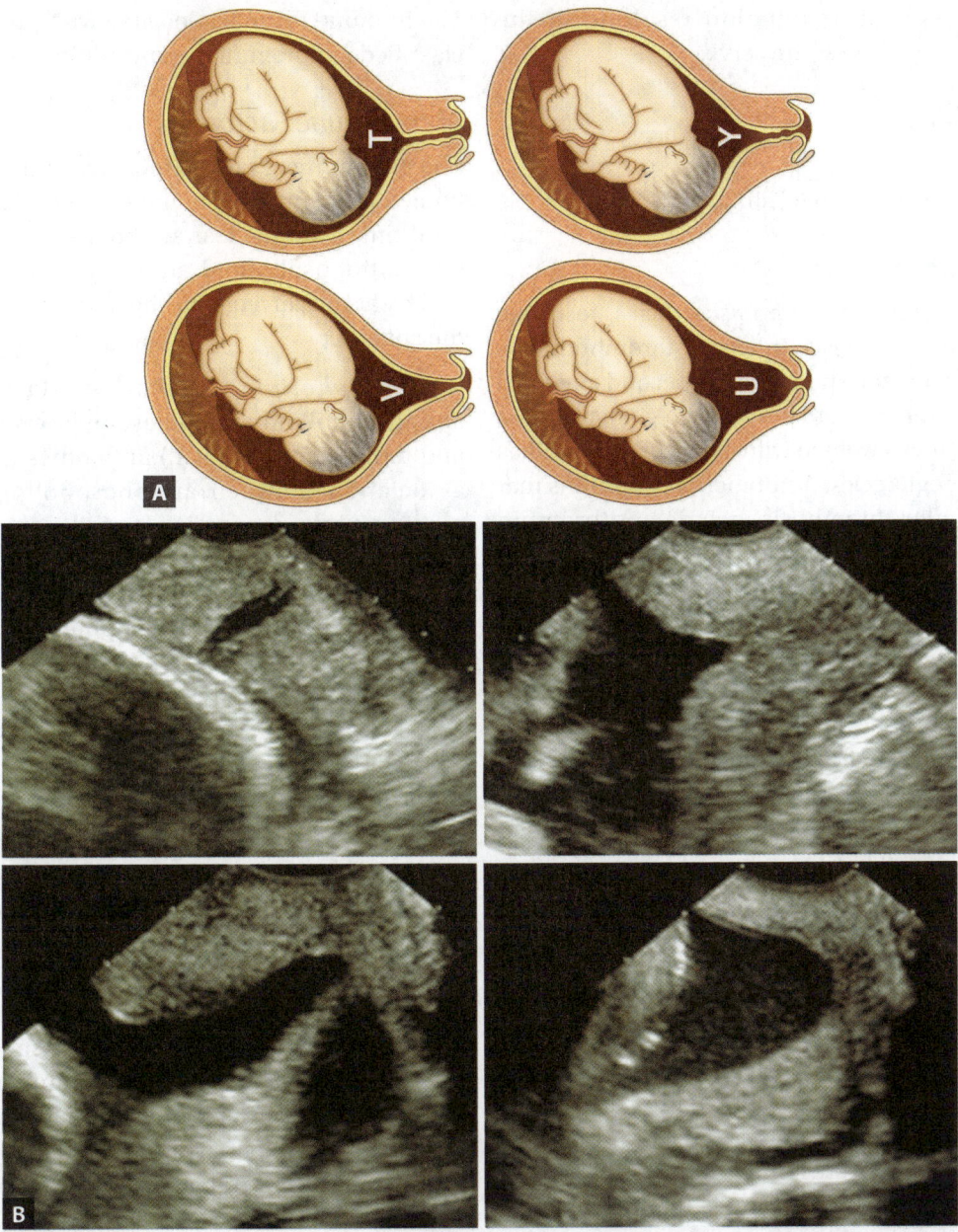

Figs. 13.5A and B: Changes in cervix related to cervical incompetence. (A) Anatomical changes in the endocervical canal associated with cervical incompetence; (B) Ultrasound changes in endocervical canal with cervical incompetence.

is both difficult and controversial. This surgery must be undertaken when there is still 10–15 mm or more of cervical canal left.

Patient must be admitted for at least 24 hours prior to the surgery. Perioperative treatment with indomethacin and antibiotics must be administered before placing the cerclage. Patient must be observed for 2–4 days postoperatively. The cerclage is rarely performed after 24–25 weeks of pregnancy. The cerclage is normally removed at 37 weeks or at the onset of the labor.

Indications for Cerclage

Indications for cerclage are as follows:
- History compatible with incompetent cervix
- Sonogram demonstrating funneling
- Clinical evidence of extensive obstetric trauma to the cervix.

Contraindications for Cerclage

- Uterine contractions/bleeding
- Chorioamnionitis
- Premature rupture of membranes
- Cervical dilatation of >4 cm
- Polyhydramnios
- Fetal anomaly incompatible with life.

Risks of Cerclage

- Premature rupture of the membranes
- Chorioamnionitis
- Preterm labor

- Cervical laceration or amputation resulting in the formation of scar tissue over the cervix
- Bladder injury
- Maternal hemorrhage
- Cervical dystocia
- Uterine rupture, vesicovaginal fistula.

Inherited Thrombophilias

This can cause both early and late miscarriages, resulting due to intravascular thrombosis. Inherited thrombophilias have shown a stronger association with late second and third trimester losses in comparison to the early pregnancy losses. It is also known that many women with these thrombophilias may have normal pregnancies. A number of conditions that predispose to vascular thrombosis include antithrombin III deficiency, protein C deficiency, protein S deficiency, FVL gene mutation, prothrombin G20210A mutation and hyperhomocysteinemia. Proteins C and S are the natural inhibitors of coagulation. Systemic thrombosis has been implicated as a cause of recurrent miscarriage and numerous pregnancy related complications including preeclampsia, abruption placenta, placental infarction, intrauterine growth retardation, intrauterine death, etc. On the other hand, RCOG (2011) recommends screening of all pregnant women with recurrent pregnancy loss for inherited thrombophilias including FVL mutation, factor II (prothrombin) gene mutation and protein C and S deficiency. The ACOG recommends inherited thrombophilia screening only for unexplained second trimester or third trimester losses.

Treatment of these thrombophilias usually requires continuation of heparin therapy throughout pregnancy. The presumed mechanism of late pregnancy losses due to these inherited thrombophilias is the thrombosis of uteroplacental circulation. Presently, there is absence of a randomized trial to justify routine screening for FVL mutation. Currently, there is no test that can reliably discriminate those women with recurrent miscarriage and FVL mutation who are destined to miscarry from those who are destined to have a successful pregnancy. However, due to the fact that this mutation is associated with poor pregnancy outcome and maternal risks during pregnancy, the practice of routine screening for FVL and offering thromboprophylaxis to those with FVL mutation and evidence of placental thrombosis, is completely justified.

Immune Causes

> Q. Write a short note discussing the immunological factors causing habitual abortion and its management.
>
> Q. Discuss in detail immunomodulation in pregnancy and its role in recurrent miscarriage and its management
>
> Q. Write a short note on immunology of recurrent abortion.

The immune factors associated with pregnancy loss can be classified as autoimmune and alloimmune factors.

Autoimmune Factors

The autoimmune factors include the synthesis of autoantibodies, e.g., antiphospholipid antibodies (antiphospholipid syndrome), antinuclear antibodies, antithyroid antibodies, etc. Antiphospholipid antibody syndrome as a cause of recurrent miscarriage has been described in detail later in the chapter.

Antiphospholipid antibodies: The main types of antiphospholipid antibodies are lupus anticoagulant (LA) and anticardiolipin (aCL) antibodies (IgG and IgM). The association between antiphospholipid antibodies and recurrent miscarriage is referred to as antiphospholipid syndrome. Presence of antiphospholipid antibodies in the blood may result in an increase in the blood viscosity. This may result in the development of thrombosis inside the placental blood vessels, which may be responsible for producing placental insufficiency and/or miscarriage (**Fig. 13.6**).

Alloimmune Factors

Under normal circumstances, the maternal immune system recognizes implanting embryo as foreign body and produces "blocking antibodies", thereby protecting embryo from rejection. These blocking antibodies coat the placental cells, thereby preventing their destruction by maternal lymphocytes. In recurrent miscarriages, there is absence of these blocking antibodies due to failure of recognition of cross-reactive antigens of trophoblast lymphocyte by the mother (**Fig. 13.7**). Level of natural killer cells is also increased amongst women with recurrent pregnancy loss. Alloimmune traits such as immunologic differences

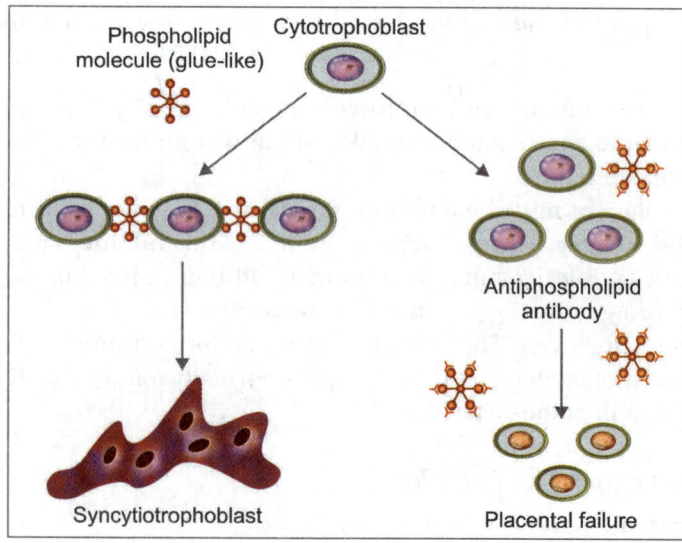

Fig. 13.6: Antiphospholipid antibody (APLA) syndrome as a cause of miscarriage.

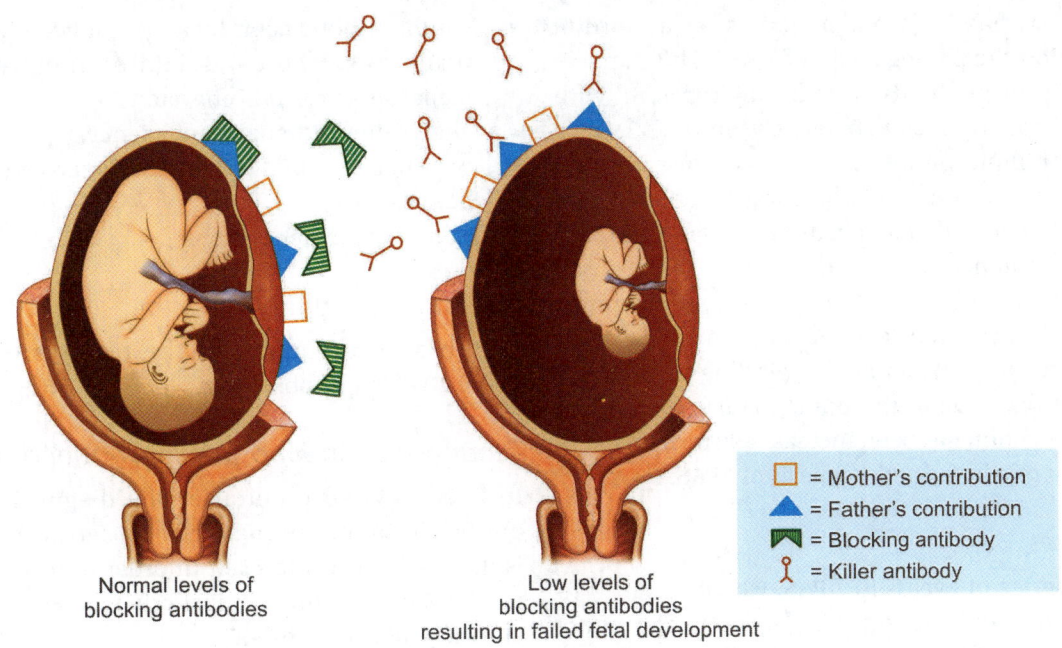

Fig. 13.7: Absence of blocking antibodies as a cause of miscarriage.

between reproductive partners have been proposed as the factor responsible for this. HLA-G antigen incompatibility among couples was also thought to be responsible for causing recurrent pregnancy losses. However, presently, there is no evidence to prove this. Therefore, tests for HLA type and antipaternal cytotoxic antibody are not routinely recommended in cases with recurrent miscarriages.

Antiphospholipid Antibody Syndrome

Antiphospholipid antibody syndrome (APAS), also known as Hughes syndrome is an autoimmune condition that may manifest with recurrent fetal loss, thrombosis (both arterial and venous) and/or autoimmune thrombocytopenia. APAS has emerged as the most important treatable cause of recurrent miscarriage, early onset preeclampsia, preterm labor, low birth weight babies and intrauterine growth restriction. There are three primary classes of antibodies associated with the APAS:

1. Anticardiolipin antibodies (directed against membrane anionic phospholipids)
2. The lupus anticoagulant
3. Antibodies directed against specific molecules including a molecule known as beta-2 glycoprotein I.

Based on the presence or absence of an underlying autoimmune disorder, such as systemic lupus erythematosus, APAS may be classified into two, primary and secondary. If the patient has an underlying autoimmune disorder, the patient is said to have secondary APAS. If the patient has no known underlying autoimmune disorder, it is termed as primary APAS. Adverse pregnancy outcomes in association with APAS include the following:

- Three or more consecutive miscarriages before 10 weeks of gestation
- One or more morphologically normal fetal deaths after the 10th week of gestation
- One or more preterm births before the 34th week of gestation due to severe preeclampsia, eclampsia or placental insufficiency.
- Women with recurrent miscarriage associated with high levels of antiphospholipid antibodies are at a high risk of complications during the three trimesters including repeated miscarriage, preeclampsia, fetal growth restriction and preterm birth.

Pathophysiology of the Antiphospholipid Antibody Syndrome

> Q. Write a long essay discussing the role of APLA in adverse pregnancy outcomes.
>
> Q. Write a long essay on APLA syndrome.

The APAS is an autoimmune phenomenon. This disease causes miscarriage by forming antibodies against the body's own tissues and placenta, resulting in thrombosis of vessels and placental infraction **(Fig. 13.6)**. The uteroplacental blood flow reduction results in intrauterine growth retardation, oligohydramnios, and fetal hypoxia, all of which lead to fetal demise.

The exact mechanism by which the antiphospholipid and anticardiolipin (aCL) antibodies induce thrombophilic state is not known. In APAS, the homeostatic regulation of blood coagulation is altered. However, the mechanisms of thrombosis have yet not been defined. For women with known APAS, it is recommended that prepregnancy counseling is given to the woman and that she be monitored closely from the beginning of the pregnancy. Defect in cellular apoptosis has been postulated as an important hypothesis behind the pathogenesis of APAS. This exposes the membrane phospholipids so that they can bind with various plasma proteins, such as beta-2 glycoprotein I. Once bound, a phospholipid-protein complex is formed, which subsequently becomes the target of autoantibodies. There may be production of antibodies against coagulation factors, including prothrombin, protein C, protein S and annexins.

Activation of platelets further enhances adherence capacity of endothelial surface. Activation of vascular endothelium, in turn, facilitates the binding of platelets and monocytes resulting in the damage related to APAS. Complement activation has been increasingly recognized to play a significant role in the pathogenesis of APAS.

Clinical Features

Clinically, the series of events in APAS, which can lead to hypercoagulability and recurrent thrombosis can affect virtually any organ system, as shown in the **Table 13.3**.

Thus, history of any of the following should raise the suspicion for APAS in obstetrician's mind:

- Thrombosis [e.g., deep vein thrombosis (DVT), myocardial infarction, transient ischemic attack, cerebrovascular accident, etc.]. This is especially important if the episodes are recurrent, occur at an earlier age, or in the absence of other known risk factors.
- History of recurrent miscarriages (especially late trimester) or premature birth.
- History of heart murmur or cardiac valvular vegetations.
- History of hematologic abnormalities, such as thrombocytopenia or hemolytic anemia.
- History of nephropathy.
- Nonthrombotic neurologic symptoms, such as migraine, headaches, chorea, seizures, transverse myelitis, Guillain-Barré syndrome, etc.
- Unexplained adrenal insufficiency.
- Avascular necrosis of bone in the absence of other risk factors.
- Pulmonary hypertension.

Physical Examination

On physical examination, the features enumerated in **Table 13.4** can be observed.

Diagnosis of Antiphospholipid Antibody Syndrome

In 2006, revised criteria for the diagnosis of APS were published in an international consensus statement. This is described in **Table 13.5**. In order to reach the diagnosis of APAS, at least one clinical criterion and one laboratory criterion must be present.

Investigations

The following laboratory tests should be considered in a patient suspected of having APS:

- aCL antibodies (IgG, IgM)
- Anti-beta-2-glycoprotein I antibodies (IgG, IgM)
- Prolongation of the following clotting assays due to the presence of LA:
  - Kaolin clotting time (KCT)
  - Dilute Russell viper venom time (DRVVT)
  - Activated partial thromboplastin time (APTT)

TABLE 13.3: Clinical features of APAS depending on the organ system affected.

Organ system affected	Symptom
Peripheral venous system	Deep venous thrombosis
Central nervous system	Cerebrovascular accident, stroke, etc.
Hematologic system	Thrombocytopenia, hemolytic anemia
Effect on pregnancy	Recurrent pregnancy losses, IUGR, preeclampsia, etc.
Pulmonary system	Pulmonary embolism, pulmonary hypertension
Dermatologic effect	Livedo reticularis, purpura, infarcts, ulceration
Cardiovascular system	Libman–Sacks valvulopathy, myocardial infarction
Ocular effects	Amaurosis, retinal thrombosis
Adrenal system	Infarction, hemorrhage, etc.
Musculoskeletal	Avascular necrosis of bone

TABLE 13.4: Physical features of APAS observed on clinical examination.

Cutaneous lesions	Venous thrombosis	Arterial thrombosis
• Livedo reticularis • Superficial thrombophlebitis • Leg ulcers • Painful purpura • Splinter hemorrhages	• Leg swelling (deep vein thrombosis) • Ascites (Budd-Chiari syndrome) • Tachypnea (pulmonary embolism) • Peripheral edema (renal vein thrombosis) • Abnormal funduscopic examination results indicate thrombosis of retinal vein	• Abnormal results on neurological examination • Digital ulcers, gangrene of distal extremities • Signs of myocardial infarction • Heart murmurs (frequently indicative of aortic or mitral insufficiency and Libman–Sacks endocarditis • Abnormal funduscopic examination results indicating retinal artery occlusion

TABLE 13.5: Revised Sapporo's classification criteria for the antiphospholipid syndrome.

Clinical criteria	
Vascular thrombosis	One or more clinical episodes of arterial, venous, or small vessel thrombosis in any tissue or organ confirmed by findings from imaging studies, Doppler studies, or histopathology (for histopathologic confirmation, thrombosis should be present without significant evidence of inflammation in the vessel wall) or presence of pregnancy morbidity
Pregnancy morbidity (poor obstetric history)	Unexplained death of a morphologically normal fetus at or beyond 10 weeks. One or more premature deliveries before 34 weeks of gestation because of severe preeclampsia/eclampsia or severe IUGR. Three or more unexplained consecutive abortions before 10 weeks of gestation (this is controversial, if no fetal heart has been seen, as some believe that very early abortion is not caused by APAS)
Paraclinical/laboratory criteria	
<ul><li>The presence of lupus anticoagulant in plasma on two or more occasions at least 12 weeks apart</li><li>Presence of moderate to high levels of anticardiolipin (IgG or IgM) in serum or plasma (i.e. > 40 IgG phospholipid units (GPL)/mL or IgM phospholipid units (MPL)/mL or > 99th percentile) on two or more occasions at least 12 weeks apart</li><li>Presence of moderate to high levels of anti-beta-2 glycoprotein I antibodies (IgG or IgM) in serum or plasma (> 99th percentile) on two or more occasions at least 12 weeks apart</li></ul>	

- Serologic test for syphilis (false-positive result)
- *Complete blood count (thrombocytopenia, hemolytic anemia):* Thrombocytopenia is fairly common in persons with APS.

Lupus anticoagulant (LA): It is directed against plasma coagulation molecules, thereby prolonging the in vitro clotting times of plasma by interfering with assembly of components of the coagulation cascade on a phospholipid template. In vitro, presence of this antibody therefore results in the prolongation of clotting assays, such as APTT, KCT and DRVVT. The presence of LA is confirmed by mixing normal platelet poor plasma with the patient's plasma. If a clotting factor is deficient, the addition of normal plasma corrects the prolonged clotting time.

Anticardiolipin antibodies: aCL antibodies react primarily with membrane phospholipids, such as cardiolipin and phosphatidylserine. There are three known isotypes of aCL, i.e., IgG, IgM, and IgA. Of these three isotypes of aCL, the values of IgG most strongly correlate with the occurrence of thrombotic events. Cardiolipin is the dominant antigen used in most serologic tests for syphilis; consequently, these patients may have a false-positive test result for syphilis.

Cut-off levels for IgG aCL [in IgG phospholipid (GPL) units] and IgM aCL [in IgM phospholipids (MPL) units] have been presented in guidelines issued by the Association of Clinical Pathologists, with negative results defined as <5 GPL units and <3 MPL units, low positive results defined as values <15 GPL units and <6 MPL units, medium levels defined as 15–80 GPL units and 6–50 MPL units and high levels defined as <80 GPL units or <50 MPL units. In detection of LA, the DRVVT test is more sensitive and specific than either the APTT or the KCT tests. Anticardiolipin antibodies are detected using a standardized enzyme-linked immunosorbent assay (ELISA).

Seronegative APLA: APLA can be defined as seronegative if the clinical criteria are fulfilled, but the serological criteria are persistently negative on at least two occasions. In these cases, the diagnosis is based on exclusion.

Imaging Studies

- Imaging studies are helpful for confirming a thrombotic event, e.g., the use of CT scanning or MRI of the brain (cerebrovascular attack), chest (pulmonary embolism), or abdomen (Budd-Chiari syndrome).
- Doppler ultrasound studies are recommended for possible detection of DVT.
- Two-dimensional echocardiography may help demonstrate an asymptomatic valve thickening, vegetations or valvular insufficiency. Aortic or mitral insufficiency is the most common valvular defect found in persons with Libman–Sacks endocarditis.

Classification of Antiphospholipid Syndrome

- *Definite or classic APS:* This category includes patients with LA or medium-to-high levels of IgG or IgM aCL antibodies and those with fetal death, recurrent prembryonic or embryonic pregnancy loss, thrombosis, or neonatal death after delivery due to severe preeclampsia or fetal distress.
- *Familial APS:* There is some evidence that familial APS shows dominant or codominant inheritance.

Environmental Factors

These factors become important because these are modifiable and hence can be controlled. Exposure to noxious or toxic substances is supposed to result in miscarriages. Various environmental factors, exposure to which is supposed to result in spontaneous miscarriages include the following:

- Cigarettes
- *Alcohol and caffeine:* Consuming 3 or more cups of coffee every day is likely to increase the risk of recurrent miscarriage. Also consuming large amounts of alcohol: more than 3 drinks per week in the first trimester or more than 5 drinks per week throughout pregnancy (amounting to 6 pints of beer or 10 glasses of wine) is

likely to be associated with an increased risk of recurrent miscarriage.
- Antiprogestogens
- Antineoplastic agents
- Anesthetic gases
- Petroleum products
  - Ionizing radiation
- Exposure to organic solvents, environmental toxins (heavy metals)
- *Exposure to diethylstilbestrol (DES):* Exposure to DES can cause complex congenital anomalies, including uterine hypoplasia, or T-shaped uterus, cervical weakness and vaginal changes. DES is a synthetic estrogen compound which was administered to some pregnant women during the 1950s and 1960s. Exposure of a pregnant woman to DES is supposed to cause uterine malformations in the developing female fetus.
- *Obesity:* Obesity serves as an independent risk factor for poor oocyte and embryo quality and thus may be associated with recurrent miscarriage. For Asian women BMI in the range 23–27.5 is considered as overweight and >27.5 is considered as obese.
- *Stress:* Though it is not a direct cause, stress may be often associated with recurrent miscarriage.

Unexplained Cases of Recurrent Miscarriage
In nearly 50% of the cases with recurrent miscarriage, no cause can be identified, despite careful investigations.

HISTORY AND CLINICAL PRESENTATION

RISK FACTORS
Detailed history from both the partners needs to be taken. The different risk factors for recurrent miscarriages need to be elicited as follows:

Maternal age: Maternal age is an important risk factor for a further miscarriage. Advanced maternal age adversely affects ovarian function, giving rise to a decline in the number of good quality oocytes.

History of specific medical illness: It is important to elicit the history of specific medical illnesses such as diabetes, thyroid disease **(Boxes 13.3 and 13.4)**, etc.

History suggestive of infectious disease: TORCH infections and infections by other microorganisms (*Neisseria gonorrhoeae, Chlamydia, Mycoplasma,* etc.) have been implicated as a cause of recurrent miscarriages. It is important to take the history of an infective illness in the past especially that was associated with fever and rashes.

History of exposure to environmental toxins: The obstetrician needs to elicit history of exposure to environmental toxins

BOX 13.3: Symptoms suggestive of hyperthyroidism.
- Palpitations, nervousness, breathlessness
- Heat intolerance
- Insomnia
- Increased bowel movements
- Light or absent menstrual periods
- Tachycardia
- Tremors in hands
- Weight loss
- Muscle weakness
- Warm moist skin
- Hair loss

BOX 13.4: Symptoms suggestive of hypothyroidism.
- Weight gain or increased difficulty in losing weight
- Fatigue, weakness
- Hair loss, coarse, dry hair; dry, rough, pale skin
- Reduced thermogenesis resulting in cold intolerance
- Muscle cramps and frequent muscle aches
- Constipation
- Memory loss
- Husky, low-pitched and coarse voice
- Abnormal menstrual cycles, decreased libido
- Depression, irritability
- Pitting edema in the lower extremities

(e.g., history of smoking, drinking alcohol, exposure to radiations, DES, etc.).

History suggestive of previous episodes of thrombosis: Symptoms suggestive of DVT include sudden unilateral swelling of an extremity; presence of pain or aching of an extremity, etc. This would help in ruling out thrombophilia as the cause for recurrent miscarriage.

History suggestive of APAS: Signs and symptoms suggestive of APAS have been enumerated in **Table 13.3**.

Family history related to the presence of genetic disorders: Stepwise genetic evaluation of couples with recurrent miscarriage comprises the following:
- Detailed medical, antenatal, and family history especially about history of mental retardation, learning disabilities, progressive muscle weakness, early cataracts, infertility, stillbirth, recurrent miscarriage, and coagulation disorders needs to be taken in order to ascertain the genetic etiology
- A three-generation pedigree chart must be made
- Enquiry must be made regarding the history of consanguinity

History of previous miscarriages: This is an independent risk factor for further miscarriages. Timing for previous miscarriage is also important. Since the causes for early and late pregnancy losses are different, it is important for the clinician to ask the time of previous pregnancy losses. Early miscarriage can be defined as pregnancy loss at ≤12 weeks.

GENERAL PHYSICAL EXAMINATION

General physical examination should be done with the aim of detecting the causes for recurrent miscarriage, including PCOS (hirsutism and hyperandrogenism), diabetes, prolactin disorders (galactorrhea), and thyroid disorders (thyroid enlargement). Pedal edema, though a feature of hypothyroidism, is a common finding in normal pregnancy; therefore if thyroid disorder is suspected, investigations for thyroid function test must be carried out.

SPECIFIC SYSTEMIC EXAMINATION

EXAMINATION OF EXTERNAL GENITALIA

Examination of external genitalia is important to detect the presence of blisters, sores, chancres, etc., which could be associated with genital tract infection. Infections of the genital tract could be associated with the presence of abnormal vaginal discharge.

Herpes viral infection: This is associated with presence of multiple ulcers on the external genitalia.

Syphilis: Primary syphilis infection is associated with the presence of a painless sore on external genitalia, which are usually painless, firm, oval and round. Swelling of the glands in the groin may occur but is usually nontender.

ABDOMINAL EXAMINATION

Abdominal examination as described in Chapter 1 needs to be carried out.

PELVIC EXAMINATION

Pelvic examination should be done to look for signs of infection, cervical anatomy, uterine size and shape (uterine leiomyomas, uterine malformations such as bicornuate uterus, septate uterus, etc.).

MANAGEMENT

> Q. A 30 year-old woman with previous history of pregnancy loss at 3 months of gestation has come to you for advice. Write a long essay on the response you would give her.
>
> Q. Write a long essay on the management of recurrent pregnancy loss.
>
> Q. How would you investigate and manage a case of recurrent pregnancy loss.
>
> Q. Write a long essay discussing the causes, diagnosis and management of RPL.

Management comprising of investigations and definitive obstetric management is discussed next and is also described in **Flowchart 13.1**.

INVESTIGATIONS

Various investigations required for a case of BOH need to be decided based on the patient's history and examination.

PARENTAL KARYOTYPE

All couples with a history of recurrent miscarriages should have peripheral blood karyotyping and cytogenetic analysis of the products of conception.

THYROID FUNCTION TEST

Tests for thyroid function include tests for thyroid hormones (T3, T4 and TSH) and detection of antibodies (antithyroid antibodies). Measurement of TSH levels in the second trimester is a sensitive indicator of thyroid function.

SERUM PROLACTIN LEVELS

Normal serum prolactin levels in nonpregnant women vary from 2 to 29 ng/mL. During pregnancy, the prolactin levels normally increase and may lie in the range of 10–209 ng/mL.

Hyperprolactinemia has been reported as an important cause for recurrent miscarriage. Treatment with bromocriptine has been found to significantly reduce the rate of miscarriage.

BLOOD GLUCOSE LEVELS

Blood sugar levels (both fasting and postprandial) need to be carried out. For ruling out diabetes mellitus and gestational diabetes, tests such as oral glucose tolerance test (OGTT) and glucose challenge test (GCT) also need to be carried out respectively (Chapter 19).

BLOOD GROUPING

ABO and Rh typing of both the parents must be done as Rh isoimmunization is an important cause for repeated pregnancy losses (Chapter 10).

VDRL TORCH TEST

The most common tests for detection of syphilis using nonspecific antibodies are rapid plasma reagin (RPR) and venereal disease research laboratory (VDRL) tests.

HIGH VAGINAL SWAB

High vaginal swab helps in detection of infections such as Chlamydia, bacterial vaginosis, etc.

TESTING FOR ANTIPHOSPHOLIPID ANTIBODY SYNDROME

> Q. Discuss briefly the antiphospholipid syndrome.
>
> Q. Write a long essay on screening for APLA syndrome.

Flowchart 13.1: Evaluation of a patient with recurrent miscarriage.

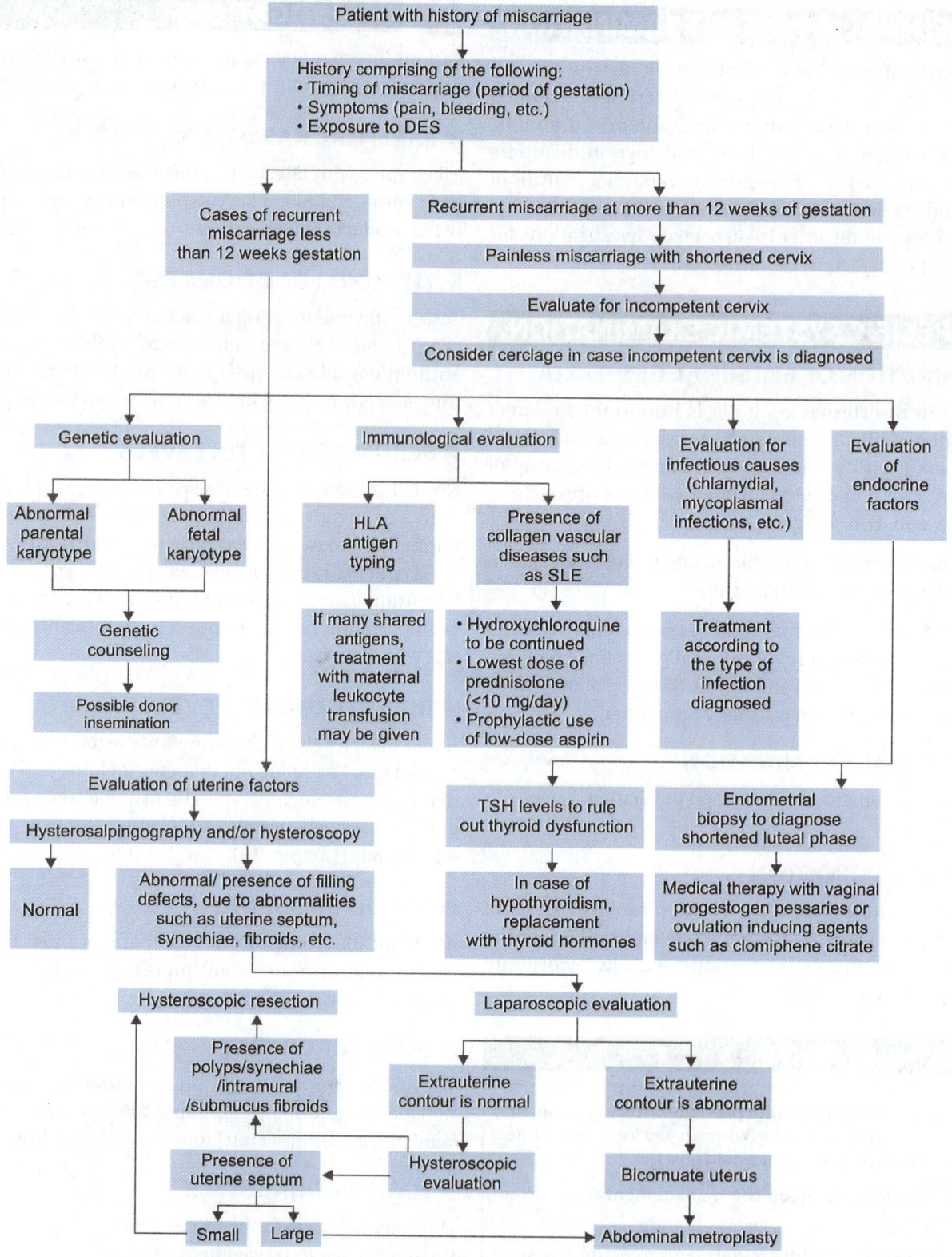

(DES: diethylstilbestrol; HLA: human leukocyte antigen; SLE: systemic lupus erythematosus; TORCH: toxoplasmosis, rubella, cytomegalovirus, herpes simplex and HIV; TSH: thyroid stimulating hormone)

Testing for Lupus Anticoagulant or Anticardiolipin Antibodies

For the diagnosis of APAS, it is mandatory that the patient should have two positive tests at least 6 weeks apart for either LA or aCL antibodies of IgG and/or IgM class (present in medium or high titer, see **Table 13.5**).

SONOHYSTEROGRAPHY

Sonohysterography is a new technique which helps in imaging of the uterine cavity in order to better diagnose the uterine anomalies. In this technique, sterile saline solution is infused inside the uterine cavity with help of a plastic catheter in conjunction with transvaginal ultrasound.

The saline infusion distends the uterine cavity and provides an excellent contrast to the endometrial lining, providing improved visualization of uterine and endometrial pathology.

Sonohysterography therefore acts as a sensitive and specific screening tool for evaluating the uterine cavity and it could be an accurate alternative to HSG in screening for uterine abnormalities.

HYSTEROSALPINGOGRAPHY

Hysterosalpingography is a procedure which involves taking X-ray of the pelvis following the instillation of radiopaque contrast agent. This technique is not more sensitive than either ultrasound examination or sonohysterography. HSG helps in delineating the shape of the uterine cavity and in confirming the patency of the fallopian tubes (**Fig. 13.8A**). HSG also helps in diagnosing causes of recurrent miscarriage including uterine malformations, cervical incompetence, Asherman's syndrome (**Fig. 13.8B**), etc. For the true assessment of the deformity, HSG must be taken at right angles to the axis of uterus. Sometimes, it may not be possible to differentiate a septate uterus (**Fig. 13.8C**) from a bircornuate uterus (**Fig. 13.8 D**) by HSG alone. Septate uterus may be differentiated from bicornuate uterus on the basis of the angle between the uterine cavities. In case of

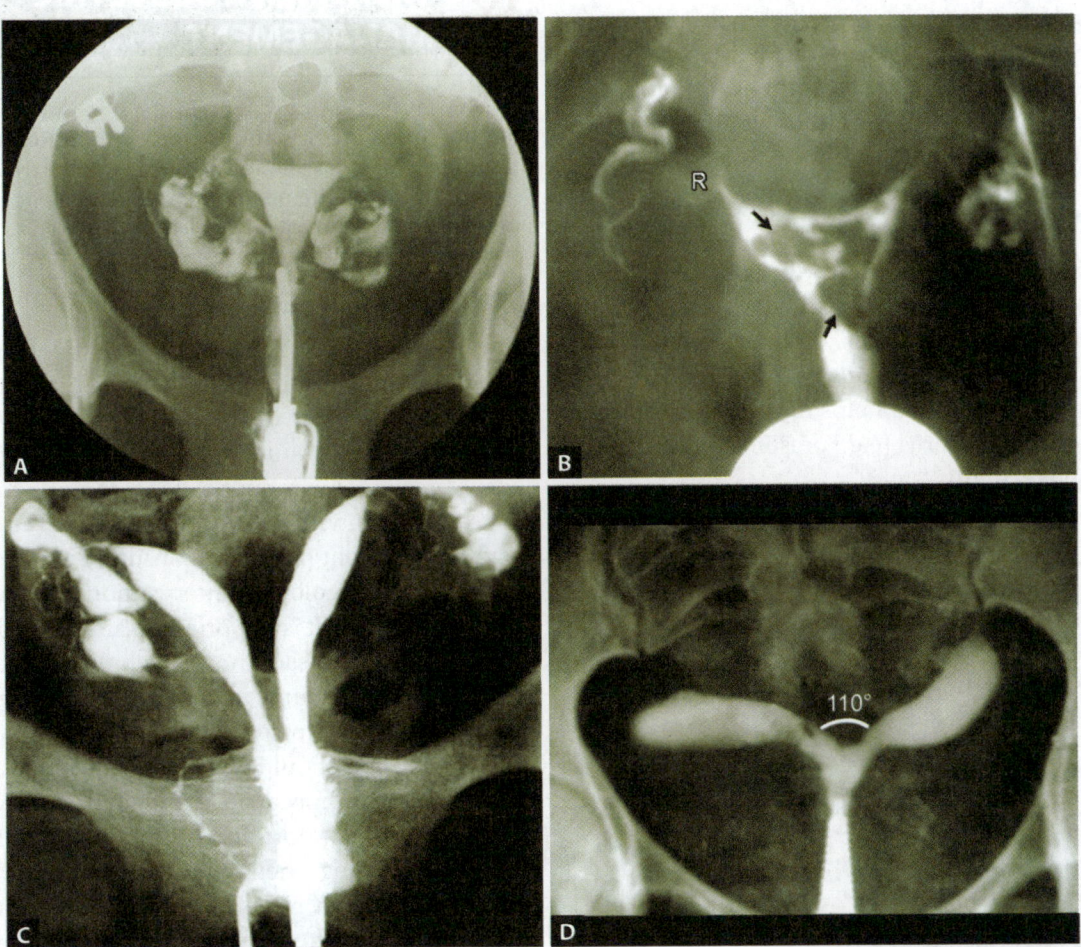

Figs. 13.8A to D: Use of hysterosalpingography (HSG) for diagnosis of uterine abnormalities. (A) Normal hysterosalpingogram showing smooth triangular uterine cavity, with the dye spilling from the ends of both tubes; (B) Hysterosalpingogram revealing irregular filling defects in the endometrium suggestive of endometrial adhesions (arrows represent adhesions). The patient was diagnosed to be suffering from Asherman's syndrome on hysteroscopy on which resection of the intrauterine adhesions was done; (C) HSG showing presence of uterine septum, which was confirmed on hysteroscopy; (D) Hysterosalpingogram showing a single cervical canal and a possible duplication of the uterine horns. It was difficult to differentiate between bicornuate uterus and septate uterus on ultrasound alone. Since an angle of greater than 105° was found to be separating the two uterine horns, the diagnosis of bicornuate uterus was made.

septate uterus, this angle is usually <75°. If this angle is ≥105°, diagnosis of a bicornuate uterus is usually made. Angles between 75° and 105° are more likely to be due to septate uterus, but an ultrasound examination or a laparoscopy may be required to confirm the diagnosis. The external uterine configuration is better assessed with help of laparoscopy. If the uterine fundal contour can be visualized, the diagnosis of septate uterus can be made. Uterus didelphys, another Müllerian duct anomaly, which closely resembles bicornuate uterus can be differentiated from it on the basis of the number of cervical canals present. In cases of uterus didelphys, two cervical canals are present but only one is seen in cases of bicornuate uterus.

ULTRASOUND EXAMINATION

All women with recurrent miscarriage should undergo an ultrasound examination for assessment of uterine anatomy and morphology **(Fig. 13.9)**. Ultrasound, especially a vaginal scan helps in detection of abnormalities inside the uterus (uterine septa, intrauterine adhesions, submucosal adhesions, leiomyomas), testing the ovarian reserve and making diagnosis of polycystic ovaries. With the advent of three-dimensional ultrasound examination, the requirement for diagnostic hysteroscopy and laparoscopy has considerably reduced.

HYSTEROSCOPY

Hysteroscopic examination helps in visualization of the interior of the uterine cavity (presence of structural uterine anomalies, e.g., adhesions, uterine septa, etc.), the endometrial lining and shape of the uterus.

Laparoscopic examination helps in the visualization of external surface of the uterus (e.g., presence of bicornuate uterus, unicornuate uterus, etc.).

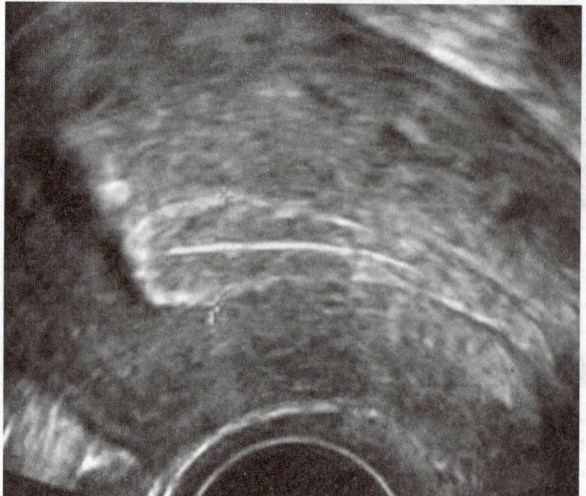

Fig. 13.9: Transvaginal ultrasound image of a uterus in a 32-year-old woman, with a normal endometrial lining that is 11.2 mm showing the normal "triple stripe" appearance.

THROMBOPHILIA SCREENING

This includes screening for FVL, prothrombin G20210A mutation and thrombophilia screening.

TEST FOR CERVICAL INCOMPETENCE

Ultrasonography

Ultrasound examination for diagnosing the cases of cervical incompetence has been described previously in the text.

Passage of No. 6–8 Hegar's Dilator

If the clinician is able to pass No. 6–8 Hegar's dilator through the internal os without any pain or resistance especially in the premenstrual period, this test is indicative of cervical incompetence.

Also, there is absence of a snapping sound as the Hegar's dilator is suddenly withdrawn out of cervical canal in cases of cervical incompetence.

℞ TREATMENT/OBSTETRIC MANAGEMENT

> **Q.** In the case described in the beginning of the chapter, all the initial investigations were within normal limits and a diagnosis of unexplained recurrent miscarriage was made. What should be the next line of management in women with unexplained recurrent miscarriage?

UNEXPLAINED ABORTION

Unexplained RPL is a diagnosis of exclusion. About 40–50% of the total cases of recurrent miscarriage remain unexplained despite detailed investigations. In these cases, women can be reassured that the prognosis for a successful future pregnancy with supportive care alone is approximately 75%. Women with unexplained recurrent miscarriage have an excellent prognosis for future pregnancy outcome without pharmacological intervention, if offered supportive care (TLC) alone. It is important to alleviate patient's anxiety and to provide reassurance, psychological support or TLC especially by the family and the partner. However, presently there are no randomized controlled trials in support of TLC. All obstetricians should be aware of the psychological sequel associated with miscarriage and should provide adequate psychological support and follow-up, as well as access to formal counseling when required.

These women should be advised to attend the RPL evaluation clinics for weekly check-up and ultrasound-aided evaluation to reassure the patient. The woman should also be started on progesterone supplements from the midluteal phase, which should be preferably continued until 28 weeks. Synthetic progesterone preparation such as dydrogesterone is thought to be more effective. Low-dose aspirin may be administered periconceptionally in these cases.

Hydroxychloroquine 400 mg acts as an immunomodulator in these cases.

GENETIC COUNSELING

Genetic abnormalities require referral to a clinical geneticist. In case of detection of a chromosomal anomaly, genetic counseling, familial chromosomal studies, and appropriate prenatal diagnosis in future pregnancies gives the couple a good prognosis for future pregnancies. These couples should also be offered the options of preimplantation genetic diagnosis, IVF, donor gametes, adoption, etc. Preimplantation genetic diagnosis or prenatal diagnosis (amniocentesis and chorionic villus sampling) helps in identifying embryos having or not having chromosomal abnormalities. Various IVF procedures which can be considered in different cases of recurrent miscarriage are enlisted in **Table 13.6**.

ROUTINE PROGESTOGEN OR hCG SUPPLEMENTATION

> **Q. Discuss briefly the role of hCG in repeated pregnancy wastage.**

There is presently insufficient evidence to evaluate the effect of progesterone or hCG supplementation in pregnancy to prevent a miscarriage. The present evidence regarding the use of both progesterone and hCG for treatment of recurrent pregnancy losses has presented with conflicting results. Furthermore, the presence of low progesterone levels may indicate a pregnancy that has already failed. Use of exogenous supplementation with progesterone or hCG can be recommended only if well designed randomized controlled trials in future are able to prove the efficacy of these strategies. However, despite of lack of good quality evidence, supplementation with progestogens and hCG is commonly being used in clinical practice.

CONTROL OF DIABETES AND THYROID DYSFUNCTION

Prepregnancy glycemic control is particularly important for women with overt diabetes mellitus. Replacement with thyroid hormone analogs may be required in hypothyroid women. As per the guidelines by FOGSI and Indian Thyroid Association, hypothyroidism must be treated in case the TSH values are >2.5 mIU/L in the first trimester and >3 mIU/L in the second and third trimester. On the other hand, as per the recommendations by American thyroid Association, treatment for hypothyroidism in cases of recurrent miscarriage must be initiated when TSH levels are >4 mIU/L.

OPERATIVE HYSTEROSCOPY

Operative hysteroscopy can help in treatment of the following anomalies:
- Removal of submucous leiomyomas
- Resection of intrauterine adhesions
- Resection of intrauterine septa.

TREATMENT OF LUTEAL PHASE DEFECTS

Treatment of LPD is done using micronized progesterone in the dosage of 100 mg daily. Progesterone supplementation must continue until 10–12 weeks following gestation.

ANTIPHOSPHOLIPID ANTIBODY SYNDROME

> **Q. Discuss diagnosis and management of RPL due to APLA syndrome.**
>
> **Q. Write a short essay discussing the management of APLA syndrome in pregnancy with recurrent fetal loss.**

Principles of management are enumerated in **Box 13.5** and are described in detail here. The prophylactic measures comprise elimination of various risk factors, such as oral contraceptives, smoking, hypertension or hyperlipidemia.

Prevention of Thrombosis

Patients with recurrent pregnancy loss must be administered a prophylactic dose of subcutaneous heparin [preferably low

TABLE 13.6: Indications for in vitro fertilization in cases of recurrent miscarriage.

Indication	IVF procedure
Balanced chromosomal translocation and advanced maternal age	IVF with donor oocytes
Premature ovarian failure	IVF with donor oocytes
Male factors (i.e., reduced capacitation or reduced fertilization potential) responsible for reduced fertility	Intracytoplasmic sperm injection (ICSI)
Uncorrectable uterine factors	Surrogate mother
Recurrent implantation failure	Blastocyst culture with assisted hatching
Immunological causes	IVF with multiple embryo replacement
Patients undergoing preimplantation genetic screening	Selection, and intrauterine transfer of normal embryos
Irreversible endometrial damage (e.g., Asherman's syndrome)	IVF with surrogacy

BOX 13.5: Principles of management in cases of APAS.
- Prevention of thrombosis (thromboprophylaxis)
- Antenatal maternal and fetal surveillance
- Peripartum care
- Postpartum prophylaxis

molecular weight heparin (LMWH) because it is associated with fewer side-effects] and low dose aspirin. Unfractionated heparin (UFH) is administered in prophylactic doses of 5,000 IU twice daily. Since long-term use of heparin can cause osteoporosis, patients who require heparin administration throughout pregnancy should also receive calcium and vitamin D supplementation and advised to do skeletal weight bearing exercises. Another dreaded immune-mediated complication of heparin is heparin-induced thrombocytopenia, which necessitates stopping heparin immediately. Thus, platelet counts must be measured 1 week after commencement of therapy and monthly thereafter in all patients on heparin therapy. Therapy is usually withheld at the time of delivery and is restarted after delivery, continuing for 6–12 weeks postpartum. Most obstetricians prefer to avoid the use of warfarin (coumadin) during pregnancy as it can cross the placental barrier and produce teratogenic changes in the fetus. LMWH in comparison to UFH has fewer complications and is being more frequently used in pregnancy. LMWH inhibits factor Xa and in addition has an anticoagulant effect through its action on antithrombin III and factor IIa. Thus, bleeding complications with LMWH are few with little alteration of PT and APTT.

- Aspirin helps in improving pregnancy outcome by inhibiting thrombosis and preventing damage to trophoblast. ACOG recommends the use of low dose aspirin in the dosage of 150 mg daily (two 81 mg tablets available in the US).
- A Cochrane review by Hamulyák et al. (2020) has shown that the combination treatment comprising aspirin plus unfractionated heparin is likely to result in a significant increase in the rate of live births among women with APS. However, more research is required in this area to further assess the potential risks and benefits of this treatment strategy, especially among women with APAS and recurrent pregnancy loss.
- Some researchers have examined the use of combination comprising of aspirin and prednisone during pregnancy. Most of the studies suggest that complications associated with prednisone use usually outweigh the benefits associated.

Thus, prednisone must not be used in addition to aspirin. In patients for whom the treatment with aspirin and heparin is not successful, intravenous immunoglobulins can be used. At this time, the studies suggest this may be helpful in refractory cases but is not recommended for use on a routine basis.
- In patients with SLE, hydroxychloroquine, which may have intrinsic antithrombotic properties, can be considered.
- Consultations with specialists such as rheumatologist, hematologist, neurologist, cardiologist, pulmonologist, hepatologist, ophthalmologist, etc., may be required depending on clinical presentation.
- Women with aPL antibodies who experience recurrent miscarriages may have favorable prognoses in subsequent pregnancies, if treated with aspirin and heparin.
- The patient must be educated about anticoagulation therapy and explained the importance of planned pregnancies so that long-term warfarin can be switched to aspirin and heparin before pregnancy is attempted. Thromboprophylaxis regimes in cases of APAS are described in **Table 13.7**.

Antenatal Maternal and Fetal Surveillance

Due to a high frequency of pregnancy complications especially preeclampsia and intrauterine growth restriction, despite treatment, the obstetrician should introduce appropriate surveillance starting right from 32 weeks of gestation. This must comprise the following steps:

- *A complete profile of antiphospholipid antibodies:* If this has been done in preconception period, these tests need not be repeated during pregnancy
- Frequent antenatal visits, at least every 2–4 weeks before third trimester and every 1–2 weeks thereafter
- Close maternal and fetal surveillance in form of monitoring of maternal blood pressure, proteinuria, and other features of preeclampsia
- Obstetric ultrasound to assess fetal growth and amniotic fluid volume
- Uterine and umbilical artery Doppler to detect fetal growth restriction and if detected, appropriate fetal surveillance may be required

TABLE 13.7: Thromboprophylaxis regimes in cases of APAS.

Situation	Treatment regimen
Antiphospholipid syndrome without previous thrombosis and recurrent early miscarriage	LDA alone or LDA + unfractionated heparin 5,000–7,500 IU SC every 12 h or LMWH in usual prophylactic doses
Antiphospholipid syndrome without previous thrombosis and fetal death (> 10 weeks gestation) or previous early delivery (< 34 weeks gestation)	LDA + unfractionated heparin, 5,000–10,000 IU SC every 12 h (mid-interval APTT 15 times control) or LMWH in prophylactic doses
Antiphospholipid syndrome with thrombosis	LDA + unfractionated heparin, 7,500–10,000 IU SC every 8–12 h (APTT in therapeutic range) or LMWH (therapeutic dose: for twice-daily administration, the therapeutic range is 0.6–1.0 IU/mL and with once daily administration, the range is 1.0–2.0 IU/mL)*

*Prophylactic dose of LMWH is usually half of the therapeutic dose (APTT: activated partial thromboplastin time; LDA: low-dose aspirin; LMWH: low molecular weight heparin; SC: subcutaneous)

Termination of pregnancy must be considered at 37 completed weeks of gestation

Peripartum Care

This comprises the following steps:
- Low-to-moderate risk patients on LMWH can be changed over to UFH at 36–37 weeks of gestation
- Heparin should be discontinued once patients go into labor.
- In patients undergoing induction of labor or elective cesarean delivery, heparin must be discontinued 12–24 hours before the procedure.
- In most of the cases, heparin infusion is restarted 6–8 hours following delivery

Postpartum Prophylaxis

Antithrombotic coverage during the postpartum period is recommended in all women with APS, with or without previous episode of thrombosis.
- In low-risk women, prophylactic dose of heparin or LMWH is continued for 4–6 weeks after delivery, although warfarin can also be used as an option.
- Breastfeeding women may be administered the combination of heparin and warfarin. If warfarin therapy is instituted, the patient must be instructed to avoid excessive consumption of foods that contain vitamin K.

■ CERVICAL INCOMPETENCE

> Q. Discuss brief about McDonald cervical cerclage.
>
> Q. Discuss at length management of cervical incompetence.
>
> Q. Write a long essay discussing the recent trends in the management of cervical incompetence.

Various surgical procedures for cervical incompetence are described as follows:

McDonald Procedure

In McDonald procedure, a 5 mm band of permanent purse string suture using 4–5 bites is placed high on the cervix (Fig. 13.10). It is usually removed at 37 weeks, unless there is a reason (e.g., infection, preterm labor, preterm rupture of membrane, etc.) for an earlier removal.

In McDonald procedure, no bladder dissection is required. The advantages of McDonald procedure over Shirodkar procedure include the following:
- Simplicity of the procedure (does not involve bladder dissection or complete burial of the sutures)
- Ease of removal at the time of delivery
- The stitch can also be applied when the cervix is effaced or the fetal membranes are bulging.
- The disadvantage of the procedure is the occurrence of excessive vaginal discharge with the exposed suture material.

Shirodkar Technique (Figs. 13.11A to G)

In Shirodkar procedure, a permanent purse string suture which would remain intact for life is applied. Therefore, the patient is delivered by a cesarean section. The suture is placed submucosally as close to the internal os as possible by giving incisions both over the mucosa on the anterior and posterior aspects of the cervix. This is followed by dissection and separation of the bladder and the rectum from both anterior and posterior surface of the cervix respectively. Though the original Shirodkar procedure involved the dissection of both bladder and rectal mucosa, the Shirodkar procedure performed nowadays mainly

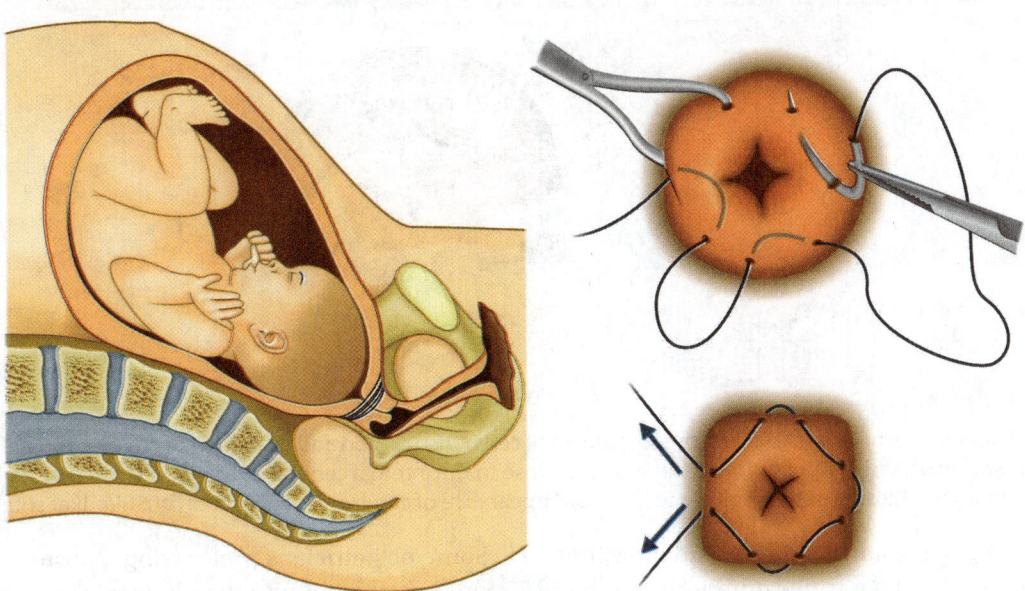

Fig. 13.10: McDonald procedure.

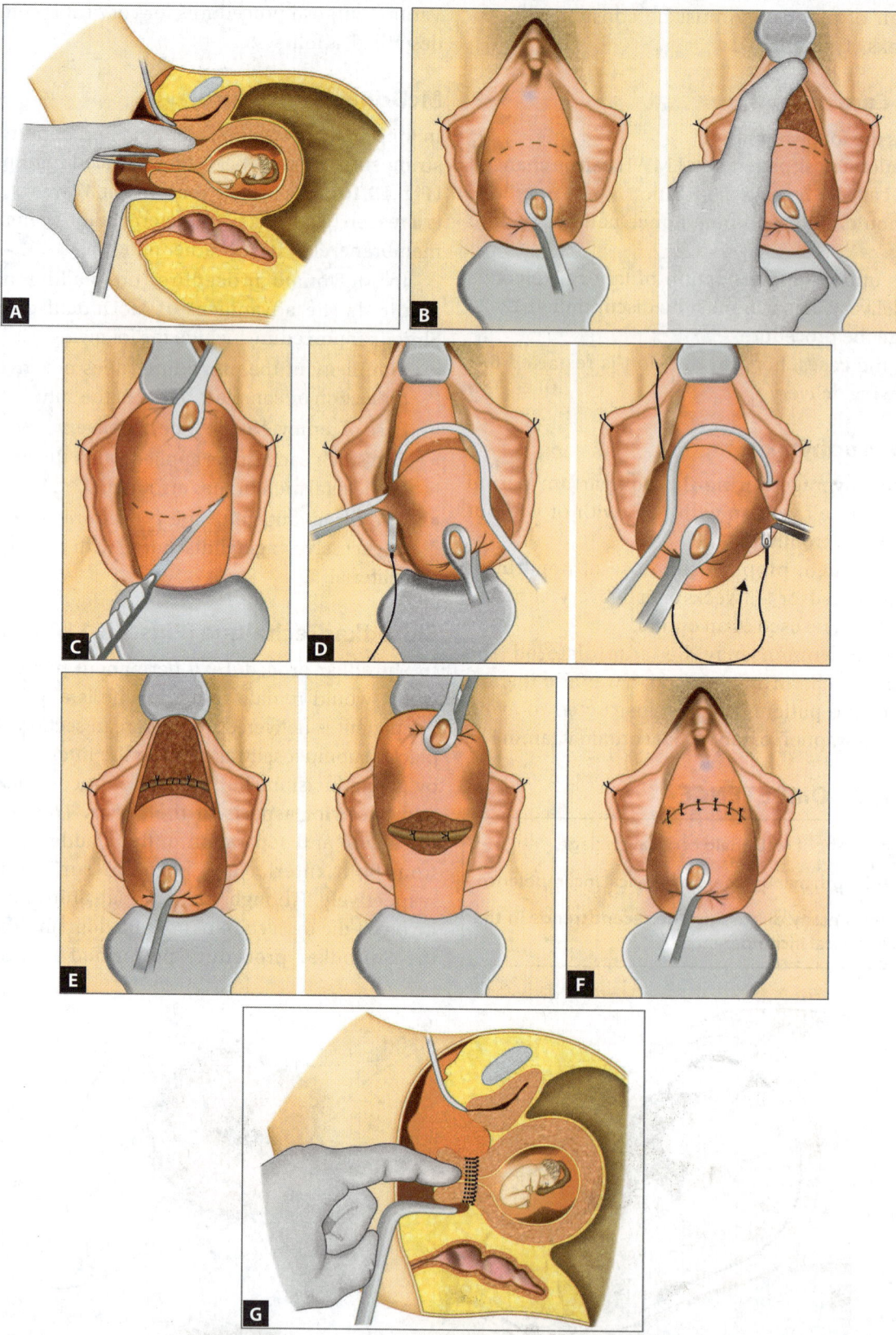

Figs. 13.11A to G: Shirodkar technique. (A) Pulling the anterior lip of cervix; (B) Incision and dissection of anterior vaginal mucosa; (C) Incision of posterior vaginal wall mucosa; (D) Application of the suture as close to the internal cervical os as possible; (E) Sutures have been tied both anteriorly and posteriorly; (F) Closure of the vaginal mucosa; (G) Appearance of cervix after application of Shirodkar stitch.

involves the opening of the anterior fornix and dissection of the adjacent bladder. The knot is tied anteriorly and buried by suturing the mucosal opening in the anterior fornix.

Some obstetricians prefer tying a posterior knot in order to prevent erosion into the bladder. This procedure is usually performed under spinal or epidural anesthesia. Initially, both Shirodkar and the McDonald started suturing with the catgut, but eventually Shirodkar turned to fascia lata and McDonald turned to silk. Presently, mersilene tape is used as an appropriate suture material. Both the procedures have been found to be equally effective. However, it is generally easier to perform McDonald suture as no bladder dissection is involved.

Wurm's Procedure

It is also known as Hefner's cerclage, it is done by application of U or mattress sutures **(Fig. 13.12)** and is of benefit when minimal amount of length of cervical canal is left.

Transabdominal Cerclage

If either of the cervical procedures fails, transabdominal cerclage is used. The indications for transabdominal cerclage include the following: traumatic cervical lacerations, congenital shortening of the cervix, previous failed vaginal cerclage and advanced cervical effacement. The original intention with transabdominal approach was that the suture was inserted between pregnancies or in the early pregnancy and left in situ for the rest of the life. The delivery was undertaken by cesarean section during each pregnancy. As a result, the major disadvantage associated with transabdominal cerclage is the requirement of two abdominal procedures: one to place the suture and other for cesarean delivery.

Also, since the surgery is performed in a highly vascular area of the cervix, which is adjacent to the uterus, it is associated with a high rate of complications. The procedure of transabdominal cerclage comprises the following steps:

- A midline or Pfannenstiel incision is given over the abdominal wall.
- The vesicouterine fold of the peritoneum is divided.
- Bladder is reflected caudally.
- Uterine vessels are identified and a mersilene tape suture is passed through the broad ligament below the uterine vessels in the potential free space between the uterine vessels and the ureter.
- The suture is tied either anteriorly or posteriorly and the bladder is replaced.

Lash Procedure

This surgical procedure is usually performed in nonpregnant woman. It is usually performed for an anatomical defect in cervix resulting from cervical trauma. In this surgery, the cervical mucosa is opened anteriorly, bladder reflected and the cervical defect repaired with interrupted transverse sutures before closing the vaginal mucosa.

■ INHERITED THROMBOPHILIAS

Antithrombotic therapy with heparin (5,000 IU subcutaneously) or LMWH (subcutaneously) once daily has been found to be effective. Antithrombotic therapy is usually administered up to 34 weeks of gestation.

■ POLYCYSTIC OVARIAN SYNDROME

Treatment of PCOS involves weight reduction, use of insulin sensitizing agents (metformin) and ovulation induction with clomiphene citrate.

■ INFECTIONS

For cases in which an infectious organism has been identified, appropriate antibiotics should be administered, e.g., penicillin (syphilis); ganciclovir (cytomegalovirus); acyclovir (genital herpes); pyrimethamine and sulfadiazine (toxoplasmosis).

Post-treatment cultures must be done in order to verify eradication of the infectious agent before the patient is advised to attempt conception.

EVIDENCE-BASED CLINICAL TRIALS

List of references can be scanned through QR code to enable the readers gain deeper insight of the subject by referring to the entire article or its abstract.

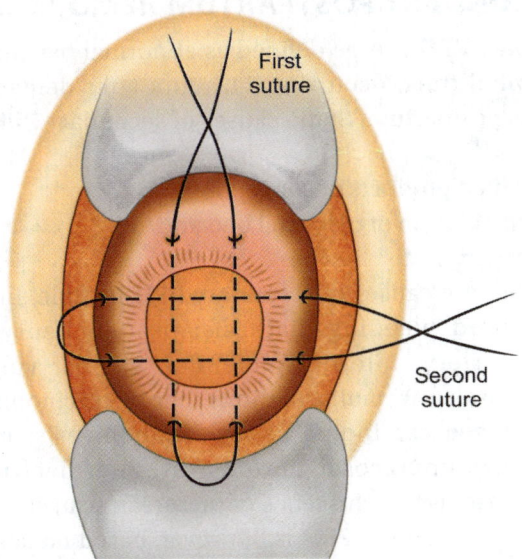

Fig. 13.12: Application of Wurm's stitch.

CHAPTER 14

Postpartum Hemorrhage

CASE STUDY

A 30-year-old G4P3L3 patient had a normal vaginal delivery in the morning at the hospital. A live healthy baby weighing 4.5 kg was delivered. The woman was transferred to the postpartum ward after 3–4 hours of delivery. At the time of transfer the patient was stable, her uterus was well contracted on per abdominal examination and slight amount of vaginal bleeding was present. However, she had to be shifted to the emergency ward in evening in the state of shock due to excessive bleeding.

INTRODUCTION

The above-mentioned case scenario is suggestive of postpartum hemorrhage (PPH). PPH can be considered as a major obstetric emergency and a leading cause of maternal mortality and morbidity. Some amount of blood loss can occur normally during the process of childbirth. Approximate blood loss at the time of normal vaginal delivery is considered to be 250 mL. Incidence of PPH in Indian scenario following vaginal delivery is 4%, whereas that following cesarean delivery is 6%. PPH accounts for nearly 30% of maternal deaths in India.

According to WHO, 2012, PPH can be defined as blood loss of 500 mL or more per vaginum during the first 24 hours after delivery (irrespective of the route of delivery). Severe PPH can be defined as the blood loss of 1,000 mL or more during the first 24 hours after delivery. Blood loss in the excess of 1,000 mL can be considered as being physiologically significant and can cause hemodynamic instability. The WHO has classified PPH into two—(1) primary PPH and (2) secondary PPH.

American Congress of Obstetricians and Gynecologists (2017) has defined PPH as a cumulative blood loss of 1,000 mL or more blood loss accompanied by signs and symptoms of hypovolemia within 24 hours after the delivery, irrespective of the route of delivery.

As per RCOG (2016), minor PPH is defined as blood loss varying between 500 and 1,000 mL, whereas major PPH is >1,000 mL. Major PPH can be further classified as moderate (varying between 1,001 and 2,000 mL) or severe (>2,000 mL).

The International Expert Panel has defined PPH as active bleeding >1,000 mL within 24 hours following birth, which continues despite the use of initial measures (including the use of first-line uterotonic agents and uterine massage).

According to SOGC (2018), PPH is defined as any amount of bleeding which is likely to threaten the patient's hemodynamic stability.

PRIMARY POSTPARTUM HEMORRHAGE

Primary PPH can be defined as blood loss, estimated to be >500 mL, occurring from the genital tract, within 24 hours of delivery. Primary PPH can be considered as the most common cause for obstetric hemorrhage.

SECONDARY POSTPARTUM HEMORRHAGE

Secondary PPH can be defined as abnormal bleeding from the genital tract, occurring 24 hours after delivery until 6 weeks postpartum. Some causes of secondary PPH are as follows:
- Retained products of conception
- Subinvolution of placental bed and/or
- Infection

Some rare causes of secondary PPH include, inherited or acquired bleeding diathesis; pseudoaneurysms of uterine artery, internal pudendal, vagina, vulvar, or labial vessels; AV malformations, choriocarcinomas, and undiagnosed carcinoma cervix; adenomyosis; infected polyps or submucosal fibroids; uterine diverticulum; hypoestrogenism; dehiscence of caesarean scar, etc.

This definition of PPH is, however, based on subjective observations because it may be difficult to accurately assess the amount of blood loss. Some of the parameters, which can help in assessing the blood loss include the following:
- *Hemodynamic stability of the patient:* Is the patient stable or unstable based on hemodynamic parameters (pulse, blood pressure, etc.)?

- *Change in the patient's hematocrit:* A rapid decline in the patient's hematocrit of ≥10% between the time of admission and the postpartum period.
- Does the patient require a transfusion of red blood cells?

ESTIMATION OF BLOOD LOSS POSTPARTUM

It is difficult to assess the exact amount of blood loss during and after delivery. The most practical technique for assessing the blood loss is the direct volumetric method, in which the approximate blood volume is measured from the basins and sponges. This method seems best suited for vaginal deliveries and is the only one still in use. Some other methods for estimating the blood loss are as follows:
- Collection of blood into blood pans and plastic bags
- Use of calibrated drapes and receptacles at the time of delivery to estimate the blood loss.
- Weighing the sponges soaked in blood and calculating the change in weight of the dry and soaked sponges.
- *Acid/alkali hematin method:* The collected blood is converted into hematin and the amount is determined by calorimetric readings.

The blood loss estimated through these methods is usually one-third of the actual amount because these methods do not estimate the insensible losses.

CAUSES OF POSTPARTUM HEMORRHAGE

The previously used mnemonic "4 Ts" (**T**one, **T**rauma, **T**issue, and **T**hrombin), which helped in describing the four important causes of PPH, are enumerated in **Box 14.1**. This mnemonic has now been changed to "6Ts", where the fifth and sixth Ts, respectively stand for **T**heatre and **T**raining. Lack of training and lack of theatre (surgical management) are important causes for PPH.

ATONIC UTERUS

Uterine atony is one of the most important causes for PPH, responsible for nearly 90% cases. Uterine atony refers to the failure of the uterine muscle to contract normally following delivery of the baby and placenta (**Fig. 14.1**). Separation of the placenta from the wall of the uterus results in shearing off of the maternal blood vessels, which supply blood to the placenta. Under normal circumstances, the contraction of the uterine musculature causes compression of these blood vessels. However, the bleeding would continue to occur if the uterine musculature does not effectively contract.

Causes of Atonic Uterus

Risk factors for development of uterine atony are as follows:
- Overdistention of uterus
- Induction of labor
- Prolonged/precipitate labor
- Anesthesia (halogenated drugs like halothane) and analgesia
- Tocolytics
- Grand multiparity
- Mismanagement of third stage of labor
- Full bladder
- Antepartum hemorrhage (placenta previa, abruption placenta, couvelaire uterus, etc.)
- Prolonged labor
- Fibroids (by causing uterine distension and reduced uterine contractility)
- Fundal implantation of placenta
- Short umbilical cord
- Chorioamnionitis
- Polyhydramnios
- Fetal macrosomia
- Dystocia

Traumatic Causes for Postpartum Hemorrhage

The various traumatic causes for PPH are as follows:
- Large episiotomy and extensions
- Tears and lacerations of perineum, vagina or cervix

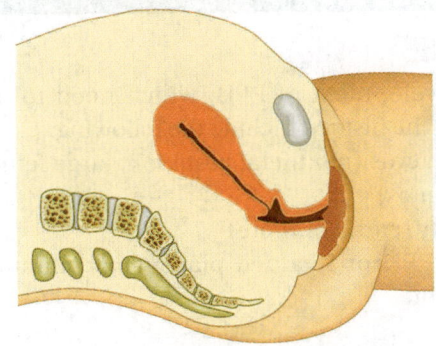

Normal postpartum patient with contracted uterus preventing hemorrhage

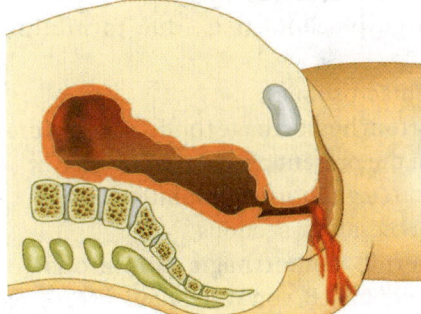

Uterine atony allows hemorrhage to flow through the uterus

Fig. 14.1: Mechanism of bleeding in an atonic uterus.

> **BOX 14.1:** Causes of postpartum hemorrhage.
>
> - *Tone:* Atonic uterus
> - *Trauma:* Cervical, vaginal and perineal lacerations, pelvic hematomas, uterine inversion, and ruptured uterus
> - *Tissue:* Retained tissue (placental fragments), invasive placenta
> - *Thrombin:* Coagulopathies
> - *Theater:* Surgical methods for controlling PPH may be required if there is a failure of medical or conservative methods. Lack of theater is a cause for PPH
> - *Training:* Attending PPH drills, training of self and colleagues. Lack of training is a cause of PPH

- Pelvic hematomas and uterine inversion
- Ruptured uterus

Tissue—Retained Tissue (Placental Fragments), Invasive Placenta

Postpartum hemorrhage can commonly occur if retained bits of placental tissue or blood clot remain inside the uterine cavity and are not expelled out. Invasive placenta refers to abnormal adherence of the placenta to the uterine wall due to invasion of the uterine wall by the placental trophoblasts. Adherent placenta can be of three types: (1) placenta accreta; (2) placenta increta, and (3) placenta percreta. These would be described later in the chapter.

Thrombin—Coagulopathies

Abnormalities of the coagulation pathway (both intrinsic and extrinsic) can also commonly result in PPH. Abnormalities of coagulation may occur in cases of preeclampsia, inherited deficiency of clotting factors, (e.g., von Willebrand factor deficiency, hemophilia etc.), severe infection, amniotic fluid embolism, etc.

Theater

Lack of facilities for surgical management of PPH in case medical or conservative management of PPH fails.

Training

Lack of adequate training facilities for doctors acts as another causative factor for PPH.

HISTORY AND CLINICAL PRESENTATION

RISK FACTORS

Risk factors for development of PPH, which need to be elicited while taking the history, include the following:
- Overdistended uterus (multifetal gestation, large fetus, and polyhydramnios)
- Grand multiparity (para 4 or more)
- Past history of PPH or retained placenta or manual removal of placenta
- Prolonged labor
- Operative delivery (use of forceps, ventouse, etc.)
- Delivery of a large placenta (e.g., due to multifetal gestation)
- Episiotomy, fetal macrosomia
- History of antepartum hemorrhage (both placenta previa and abruption) in the present pregnancy
- History of infection (e.g., chorioamnionitis)
- Previous history of cesarean sections
- Preexisting maternal hemorrhagic conditions (e.g., hemophilia A, hemophilia B, von Willebrand disease, etc.).

The obstetrician needs to enquire about the woman's personal or family history of bleeding, including bleeding with minor trauma, medications, postsurgical bleeding, and tooth extractions. History of excessive bleeding from various sites including menorrhagia, epistaxis, hematuria, etc. also needs to be taken.

Risk Factors during Labor

The presence of following risk factors at the time of labor must prompt extravigilance among clinical staff regarding the early detection and management of PPH in these cases. Some of these factors include:
- Delivery by emergency cesarean section
- Delivery by elective cesarean section
- Retained placenta
- Mediolateral episiotomy
- Prolonged labor (>12 hours)
- Delivery of a big baby (>4 kg)
- Operative vaginal delivery
- Pyrexia in the intrapartum period

GENERAL PHYSICAL EXAMINATION

Though a case of PPH is unlikely to be given as a clinical case during examinations, it is being discussed in detail because it is an obstetrical emergency which is commonly encountered in obstetric practice. Therefore every obstetrician must be well prepared to deal with this potentially life-threatening emergency.

SIGNS AND SYMPTOMS

Vital signs are highly unreliable indicators of the severity of bleeding. Mild-to-moderate degree of blood loss of 500–1,000 mL (10–15%) is unlikely to affect the vital signs like pulse, blood pressure, etc. However, severe degrees of blood loss are likely to produce signs and symptoms as described in **Table 14.1**. Blood loss exceeding 30% of blood volume or more may be associated with a positive tilt test.

Tilt Test

An increase in heart rate of >10 beats/min and/or decrease in diastolic blood pressure of >10 mm Hg when the patient is tilted from supine to a semirecumbent body position (45° from the horizontal) can be described as a positive tilt test.

SPECIFIC SYSTEMIC EXAMINATION

ABDOMINAL EXAMINATION

The uterus must be palpated per abdominally to assess if it is well contracted or not. If the uterus appears to be well contracted and hardened, PPH due to uterine atonicity can be ruled out. In these cases, the most important cause of PPH could be trauma to the genital tract or retained tissue fragments inside the uterine cavity.

Postpartum Hemorrhage

TABLE 14.1: Changes in vital signs with increasing amount of blood loss.

Blood loss (% blood volume)	Pulse rate	Systolic blood pressure (mm Hg)	Degree of shock	Symptoms
10–15% (500–1,000 mL)	Normal	Normal	Compensated	Postural hypotension, palpitations, dizziness
15–25% (1,000–1,500 mL)	Slight increase (80–100 beats/min)	Slight fall (80–100)	Mild	Thirst, weakness
25–35% (1,500–2,000 mL)	Marked increase (100–120 beats/min)	Moderate fall (60–80)	Moderate	Pallor, oliguria, confusion
>40% (2,000–3,000 mL)*	Highly marked tachycardia	Marked fall (40–60)	Severe	Anuria, air hunger, coma, death

*A blood loss of > 2.5 L is likely to be associated with 50% mortality rate if not urgently managed.

PER SPECULUM EXAMINATION

Vagina must be inspected in good light to visualize any tears or lacerations, which could be responsible for bleeding. If the patient is not cooperative and vaginal injury is being suspected as a cause of PPH, a thorough examination of the lower genital tract under general anesthesia may be required. A per speculum examination of the cervix (**Fig. 14.2**) may also be carried out to rule out the presence of cervical and vaginal tears.

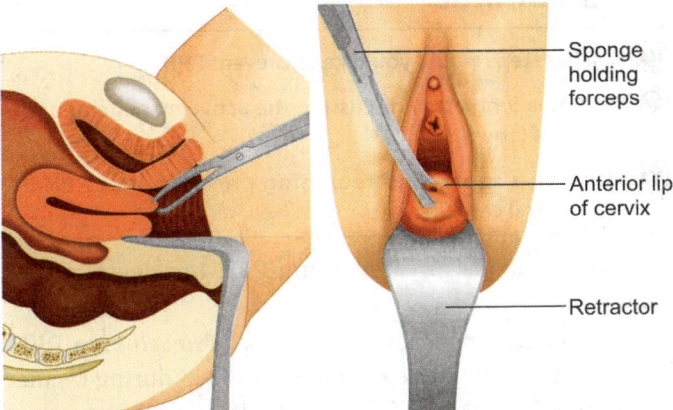

Fig. 14.2: Per speculum examination of cervix.

DIFFERENTIAL DIAGNOSIS

As described in **Box 14.1**, various reasons for PPH could be uterine atonicity, trauma, retained tissue, coagulation abnormalities, lack of surgical facilities for management of PPH, or lack of appropriate training.

The obstetrician needs to find out the exact cause of PPH through history, clinical examination, and diagnosis.

Various coagulation abnormalities which could be responsible for producing PPH are enumerated in **Box 14.2**.

BOX 14.2: Coagulation abnormalities resulting in postpartum hemorrhage.

- Drugs (e.g., aspirin, heparin, warfarin, alcohol, and chemotherapy)
- Liver disease
- Severe vitamin K deficiency
- Disseminated intravascular coagulation
- von Willebrand disease
- Hemophilia
- Idiopathic thrombocytopenic purpura
- Heparin induced thrombocytopenia

MANAGEMENT

Management comprising of investigations and definitive obstetric management is discussed next.

INVESTIGATIONS

The following investigations need to be done in cases of PPH:
- Complete blood count with peripheral smear
- *Coagulation profile:* Platelet count, prothrombin time (PT) (evaluates extrinsic pathway—factors X, VII, V, II, and I); activated partial thromboplastin time (APTT) (evaluates intrinsic pathway—XII, XI, IX, VIII, V, II, and I); thrombin time (measures ability of thrombin to transform fibrinogen into fibrin), bleeding time (evaluates platelet function and capillary integrity)
- Urinalysis (for hematuria)
- High vaginal swab, to rule out infection (especially gonorrhea, *Chlamydia*, etc.)
- *Transabdominal or transvaginal ultrasound:* Ultrasound examination may especially be required if retained products of conception (POCs) are suspected. Presence of a normal endometrial stripe on transvaginal sonography almost always helps in ruling out the presence of retained placental fragments.

TREATMENT/OBSTETRIC MANAGEMENT

Q. What are the advantages and disadvantages of the use of active management of labor as a routine?

Q. Discuss in detail the active management of third stage of labor.

Active management of third stage of labor is associated with clinically significant reduction in the amount of estimated postpartum blood loss, improvement in postpartum hemoglobin levels, and reduction in requirement for blood transfusion.

However, active management of labor is also associated with some disadvantages including an increased incidence of nausea, vomiting, headache, postpartum hypertension, retained placenta, and secondary PPH.

Since PPH can present as a major obstetrical emergency, more important than managing PPH is preventing PPH from occurring in the first place.

PREVENTION OF POSTPARTUM HEMORRHAGE

Q. What steps would you take to prevent PPH?

Q. Write a long essay discussing the active management of third stage of labor.

Q. Write a short note regarding prevention of PPH in primary referral cases.

Some of the steps for preventing PPH are described as follows:

- *Identification of cases at high risk of developing PPH:* Such cases should be carefully assessed during regular antenatal checkups. All women with significant risk of PPH should be managed at a hospital equipped with intensive care facilities and access to specialist services. Such patients are the ideal candidates for monitoring of obstetric/maternal early warning or MEWS score **(Table 14.2)**.

  Identification of abnormal physiological parameters may help identify pregnant women at risk of deterioration, thereby facilitating early intervention, which is likely to result in a considerable reduction in maternal morbidity and mortality. Triggers in MEWS include conditions such as cardiovascular disease, sepsis, thromboembolic disease, hemorrhage, preeclampsia, etc.

- *Diagnosis and management of anemia:* Since anemia is an important risk factor contributing to the mortality and morbidity related to PPH, it should be diagnosed and treated as soon as possible in the antenatal period itself.

- *Active management of third stage of labor:* The most important step which must be routinely used in the third stage for prevention of PPH is the active management of third stage of labor. Active management of labor comprises the following steps:
  - Administering a uterotonic drug, usually 0.25 mg of methergine or ergometrine 0.2 mg soon after the delivery of the anterior shoulder and/or oxytocin 5 IU to be diluted in 5 mL of normal saline to be administered IV bolus over 5 seconds at the delivery of anterior shoulder or within 1 minute of the birth of the baby.

TABLE 14.2: Maternal Early Warning Score.

Physiological parameter	Normal	Yellow zone	Red zone
Respiratory rate (per minute)	10–20 breaths per minute	21–30 breaths per minute	<10 or >30 breaths per minute
O$_2$ saturation	96–100%		<96%
Temperature	36–37.4°C	35–36°C or 37.5–38°C	<35°C or > 38°C
Systolic BP (mmHg)	100–139 mm Hg	150–180 mm Hg or 90–100 mm Hg	>180 mm Hg or <90 mm Hg
Diastolic BP (mmHg)	50–89 mm Hg	90–100 mm Hg	>100 mm Hg
Heart rate (per minute)	50–99 BPM	100–120 or 40–50 BPM	>120 BPM or < 40 BPM
Neurological response	Alert	Response to voice	Unresponsive, response to pain

(BPM: beats per minute)
Source: Nair S, Spring A, Dockrell L, Colgain SM. Irish Maternal Early Warning Score. Ir J Med Sci. 2020;189:229-35. DOI.org/10.1007/s11845-019-02028-1
1 yellow alert: Repeat observations in 30 minutes; 2 yellow alerts or 1 red alert: Call the obstetrician and repeat observations in 30 minutes; Greater than 2 yellow alerts or ≥ 2 red alerts: Immediate review by obstetrician and repeat observations in 15 minutes or continuous monitoring.

TABLE 14.3: Fourth stage stamp.

Time of delivery	0 h	1 h	1.5 h	2 h
BP				
Pulse				
Uterine fundus				
Amount of bleeding				

  - Clamping the cord as soon as it stops pulsating.
  - Uterine massage (would be described later)
  - Controlled cord traction or Brandt-Andrews maneuver (would be described in detail later)

- *Fourth stage of labor:* Women must be closely observed during the fourth stage which are the golden 2 hours following the delivery of placenta during which maternal hemostatic stabilization occurs. Various complications may be observed during this stage. Fourth stage stamp **(Table 14.3)** is a chart on which various maternal parameters are plotted during the fourth stage of labor.

- *Controlled cord traction:* The procedure of controlled cord traction is shown in **Figure 14.3** and comprises the following steps:
  - The cord must be clamped as close to the perineum as possible.
  - The clinician must look for the signs of placental separation.

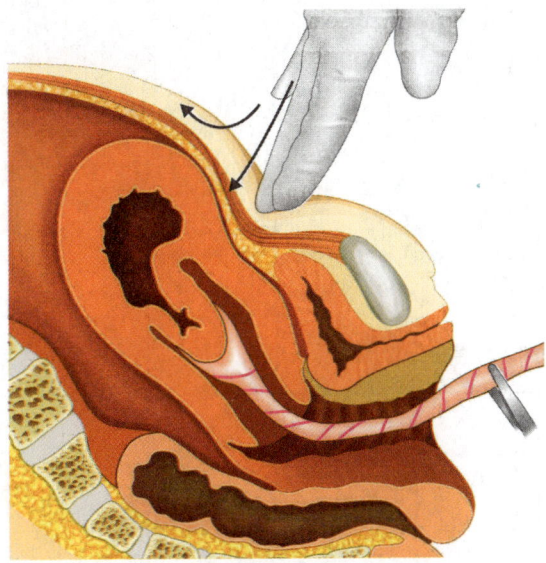

Fig. 14.3: Controlled cord traction.

- Some of the signs of placental separation are as follows:
  - Appearance of a suprapubic bulge due to hardening and contraction of uterus. This is usually the first sign to appear.
  - Sudden gush of blood
  - A rise in the height of the uterus (as observed over the abdomen) due to the passage of placenta to the lower uterine segment.
  - Irreversible cord lengthening.
- Once these above-mentioned signs occur, the clinician must hold the cord with the right hand and place the left hand over the mother's abdomen just above the pubic bone.
- The clinician must apply slight tension on the cord with right hand in downward and backward direction. At the same time the uterus must be stabilized by applying counter pressure in upward and backward direction during the controlled traction with the left hand.
- The mother should be encouraged to push with the uterine contractions.
- The cord should never be pulled without applying counter traction above the pubic bone.
- As the placenta delivers, it should be held in two hands and gently turned, until the membranes are twisted and stripped off intact from the uterine wall.
- If the membranes tear, gentle examination of the upper vagina and cervix must be carried out to look for torn bits of membrane. These if present, can be removed with the help of a sponge forceps.
- The entire placenta and membranes must be examined carefully to look for any missing lobe/membrane bit.

MANAGEMENT OF POSTPARTUM HEMORRHAGE

> Q. Write a long essay discussing the management in a multiparous woman who goes into shock with tachycardia and low blood pressure, a few hours after a term delivery.

> Q. Write a long essay discussing the etiology and management of PPH.
>
> Q. With help of a long essay discuss the prevention and management of PPH.
>
> Q. Write a long essay discussing the management of intractable PPH.
>
> Q. With help of a long essay discussing the management of atonic PPH.
>
> Q. Evaluate in detail the methods of controlling severe atonic PPH
>
> Q. Discuss in brief management of atonic PPH.
>
> Q. What could have been the likely cause of shock in the case study mentioned in the beginning of the chapter?
>
> **Ans:** The case scenario mentioned in the beginning of the chapter is suggestive of PPH. Since uterus was well contracted at the time of shifting the patient to the postpartum ward, atonic uterus as a cause of PPH can be ruled out. The history of delivery of a large sized baby (weight ≥ 4 kg) points toward an increased likelihood of trauma to the vagina and cervix. Small cervical or vaginal lacerations can also be associated with slight vaginal bleeding. Such traumatic injuries, if left unattended can result in significant amount of blood loss over a period of time.
>
> Q. What should be the further line of management in this case?
>
> **Ans.** The first priority should be toward the maternal resuscitation. While resuscitating the patients (steps have already been described in the text), as per abdominal examination should be simultaneously performed to check the uterine tonicity. If the uterus is found to be well contracted, arrangements for a proper vaginal inspection and examination should be made as soon as possible. The vagina and cervix, both should be thoroughly inspected. Any tear, injury or laceration in the genital tract should be appropriately handled and repaired.

Management of a patient with PPH is shown in **Flowchart 14.1**. According to the guidelines by the Scottish Executive Committee of the RCOG, the immediate management in case with PPH comprises of the steps enumerated in **Box 14.3** and is described next. All of these steps are required to be undertaken simultaneously. Management of PPH shall be described mainly under three headings: (1) medical, (2) surgical, and (3) conservative. Before deciding the mode of treatment, the parameters, which need to be taken under consideration, include the acuity of a patient's condition and her wishes to preserve her future fertility. Some initial steps involved in the management of PPH are described next:

Communication

If the perceived blood loss is 500–1,000 mL and there are no signs of clinical shock, basic measures like typing and crossmatching 2 units of blood, carrying out a coagulation profile, establishing intravenous access, and monitoring clinical parameters should suffice.

Flowchart 14.1: Management of postpartum hemorrhage.

```
Postpartum hemorrhage
        │
        ▼
Immediate management
 • Call for help
 • Evaluation of ABC (Airway, Breathing and Circulation)
 • Send blood for typing and crossmatching
 • Establishment of IV access
 • Infusion of crystalloids, consider blood transfusion
 • Administer oxygen via facial mask
        │
        ▼
  Placenta has delivered
    ┌────┴────┐
   Yes        No
    │          │
Abdominal   Manual exploration
palpation   of uterus
```

Placenta delivered = Yes → Abdominal palpation:
- Uterus soft and flabby (atonic PPH) → Oxytocics, fundal massage → Uterus still remains atonic → Bimanual uterine compression, Uterine tamponade → Uterus atonic → Consider surgical procedures: Uterine artery/ovarian artery ligation, Internal iliac artery ligation, B-lynch brace sutures, Angiographic embolization → Nothing works → Hysterectomy
- Uterus hard and contracted → Explore the cervix, vagina and vulva:
  - Vaginal or vulval hematoma → Up to 4 cm and stable → Ice packs and observation; 4 cm or larger and expanding → Incise, drain and pack
  - Vaginal or cervical tears → Repair
  - No lesions → Manual exploration of uterus

Placenta delivered = No → Manual exploration of uterus:
- Uterus soft and flabby (atonic PPH) → Manual extraction of placenta, Use of oxytocics, Fundal massage
- Uterus hard and contracted → Possibility of placenta accreta
  - Future fertility desirable → Conservative management
  - Future fertility not desirable → Urgent hysterectomy

Manual exploration of uterus findings:
- Retained placental bits or clots → Remove
- Uterine rupture → Resuscitation/urgent laparotomy
- Uterine inversion → Resuscitation/replace uterus
- No cause found → Seek consultant advice, observations, stabilize mother, repeat algorithm

(IV: intravenous; PPH: postpartum hemorrhage)

BOX 14.3: Steps involved in the immediate management of patients with postpartum hemorrhage.

- Communicate (call for help)
- *Resuscitation of the patient* (ABC: Airway, breathing, and circulation)
- Monitoring the patient and carrying out certain investigations
- Treating the underlying cause of bleeding

However, loss of >1,000 mL or any signs of shock should fully alert the clinical team. Since severe PPH can often develop into a life-threatening emergency, the following people must be urgently called and alerted: experienced midwife and other nursing staff; senior obstetrician and/or consultant; senior anesthetic and/or consultant; blood bank staff; hematologist; blood transfusion services, operation theater staff, etc.

Resuscitation

Patient resuscitation must be done to assess airway, breathing and circulation (ABC). Since excessive bleeding can result in the development of hypovolemic shock, immediate intravenous access using two wide bore cannula (14–16 Gauge) must be established. The foot end of the patient's bed must be elevated or the head can be tilted down in order to facilitate circulation. Oxygen must be administered with the help of a face mask. The patient must be kept warm and dry.

Hemodynamic resuscitation must involve the following in the order of priority:
- Restoration of blood volume
- Restoration of hemoglobin concentration
- Restoration of coagulation

Restoration of Blood Volume

Crystalloids (e.g., Hartmann's solution, normal saline, etc.) must be intravenously transfused. Normal saline is the safe initial fluid. If urine output is not maintained to at least 30 mL/h, central venous pressure (CVP) line must be placed. If despite of adequate CVP, urine output remains inadequate or the left ventricular function appears compromised, a Swan-Ganz catheter must be placed.

Restoration of Hemoglobin Concentration

If the patient is suffering from excessive blood loss or severe hypovolemic shock, blood transfusion may be required. In emergency, if the patient's own blood group is not available, O-negative blood may be used. Whole blood is frequently used for rapid correction of volume loss because of its ready availability, but component therapy is ideal.

Restoration of Coagulation

Transfusion of FFP may be considered if PT/APTT is >1.5 times normal. Cryoprecipitate may be administered if fibrinogen levels are <1 g/L. Platelet concentrates may be administered in case of low platelet count. If clinically indicated (in presence of coagulation abnormalities), up to 1 L of FFP and 10 units of cryoprecipitate can be transfused.

Calculation of Shock Index

Shock index (SI) is calculated by dividing heart rate by systolic blood pressure. This has been suggested as a marker for predicting the severity of hypovolemic shock. The accepted value varies between 0.5 and 0.6. SI can be divided into four groups:
1. *SI of <0.6:* No shock
2. *SI ≥0.6 to <1.0:* Mild shock
3. *SI ≥1.0 to <1.4:* Moderate shock
4. *SI ≥1.4:* Severe shock

SI ≥1.4 is associated with an increased mortality and morbidity.

Patient Monitoring and Investigations

The investigations that need to be carried out have already been described before, whereas the parameters that need to be monitored are described below in **Box 14.4**.

> **BOX 14.4:** Parameters to be monitored in patients with postpartum hemorrhage.
> - Continuous pulse/BP monitoring in cases of severe PPH with shock. In moderate cases of PPH, monitoring can be done at 15–30 minutes intervals depending upon the patient's condition
> - Electrocardiography/pulse oximetry, especially in cases of severe PPH
> - Amount of vaginal bleeding (to be assessed at every 15–30 minutes intervals)
> - Uterine tone to be assessed at 15–30 minutes intervals depending upon the patient's condition
> - Hourly monitoring of urine output (must be at least 30 mL/h)
> - Central venous pressure (CVP) monitoring (if urine output is inadequate)
> - Swan Ganz catheter (if urine output remains inadequate despite an adequate CVP)

Treating the Cause of Bleeding

Once the maternal condition has stabilized, the cause of PPH must be identified and treated. The further management must be decided based on the fact whether placenta has delivered or not. If the placenta has delivered, PPH could be due to uterine atonicity, uterine trauma, retained placental tissue, coagulation disorder, etc. Both these conditions are described as follows.

Placenta has Delivered

If the placenta has delivered, the main thing the clinician needs to see is whether the uterus has contracted or not.

Uterus well contracted: If the uterus contracts but the bleeding continues despite a well-contracted uterus, the clinician must look for other causes including traumatic causes and coagulation abnormalities. The following steps need to be taken:
- Inspection of the placenta and lower genital tract needs to be carried out to ascertain the origin of bleeding. This is especially important in cases in which the uterus appears to be firm and well contracted. There could be a missing placental cotyledon on inspection of placenta, which suggests that PPH could probably be due to retained placental bits inside the uterine cavity. If inspection of the lower genital tract reveals laceration, tear or injury on the cervix, vagina, it needs to be repaired as soon as possible in order to stop the bleeding.
- The woman must be positioned in lithotomy with adequate anesthesia/analgesia so as to ensure the proper examination of lower genital tract.
- The obstetrician must ensure that appropriate lighting, assistance, and instruments are available in order to provide adequate exposure of the genital tract.
- It may be necessary to take the woman to theater to examine under anesthesia, if proper visualization of lower genital tract does not appear to be possible.
- The vulva, vagina, cervix, and perineum must be inspected for trauma. In patients with previous history of lower segment cesarean section, the possibility of

uterine scar rupture must be kept in mind and manual exploration of the scar must be done. Speculum examination will allow visualization of cervix and lower genital tract to exclude lacerations. If clot is visible within the cervical os, it may be removed with a sponge holding forceps.
- Any injury if found, must be adequately sutured and repaired.
- If infection is suspected, combinations of broad spectrum antibiotics, e.g., amoxicillin, gentamicin and metronidazole, can be given.
- In case no trauma to the lower genital tract is found, the obstetrician must suspect the presence of coagulation abnormalities. In such cases, the obstetrician must send a complete coagulation profile, if it had not been sent earlier.

The following investigations need to be done: PT, APPT, and levels of D-dimer, fibrinogen, and fibrinogen degradation products. Possibility of DIC should be kept in mind, especially if the woman has a history of abruption placenta, intrauterine death, etc. Consultation with a hematologist may be required if DIC is suspected.

Uterus is atonic: If the placenta has delivered, but the uterus is not hard and contracted, instead appears to be atonic and flabby, the PPH is of atonic type. In this case, the following steps need to be carried out:
- The urinary bladder must be emptied.
- The uterine cavity must be explored for any retained placental bits.
- The vagina and cervix must be still inspected for presence of lacerations and tears (traumatic PPH is commonly present in association with atonic PPH).
- Repeat administration of uterotonics
- Bimanual uterine massage

Bimanual uterine massage: If the clinician finds the uterus to be soft upon bimanual examination, a bimanual uterine massage must be performed to contract the myometrial muscles. The maneuver involves the massage of the posterior aspect of the uterus with the abdominal hand and that of the anterior aspect of the uterus with the vaginal hand and comprises the following steps (Fig. 14.4):
- One of the clinician's hands is formed into a fist and placed inside the vagina, with the back of the hand directed posteriorly and knuckles in the anterior fornix so as to push against the body of the uterus (Fig. 14.4). The other hand compresses the fundus from above through the abdominal wall. The fundus of the uterus must be immediately massaged, until uterus is well contracted.
- Uterus must be massaged every 15 minutes during the first 2 hours. If this maneuver controls the bleeding, the clinician must maintain this compression for at least 30 minutes.

MEDICAL MANAGEMENT OF ATONIC UTERUS

Q. Discuss the role of medical methods in the management of atonic PPH.

Medical management of PPH includes use of uterotonic agents such as oxytocin (syntocinon), ergot alkaloids (methyl ergometrine), prostaglandin analogs (misoprostol), and recombinant factor VIIa **(Table 14.4)**.

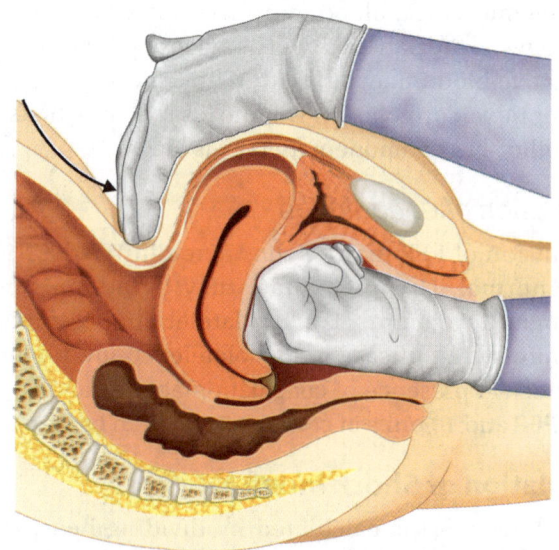

Fig. 14.4: Bimanual uterine compression.

Drug	Dosage	Side effects	Contraindications
Oxytocin	20 IU in 1 L of saline may be infused intravenously at a rate of 125 mL/h	Water intoxication and nausea at high dosage	Nil
Methylergometrine (methergine)	0.25 mg intramuscularly or intravenously	Nausea, vomiting, hypertension, retained placenta, if given before placental separation occurs	Hypertension, and heart disease
Carboprost (15-methyl PGF2α)	250 µg given as intramuscular injection every 15 minutes for a maximum of eight doses	Diarrhea, vomiting, flushing, pyrexia, hypertension, bronchoconstriction, etc.	Significant pulmonary, cardiac, hepatic, or renal disease
Misoprostol	600–1,000 µg per rectally or orally. Dose and frequency has yet not been standardized	Diarrhea, pyrexia (> 40°C)	Significant pulmonary, cardiac, hepatic, or renal disease

TABLE 14.4: Various oxytocics used for controlling postpartum hemorrhage.

Oxytocin

Oxytocin is a nonapeptide, released by the posterior pituitary. Oxytocin stimulates the upper segment of the myometrium to contract rhythmically. This causes constriction of spiral vessels which helps in reducing the blood flow through the uterus. The lower segment remains relaxed. Oxytocin (syntocinon) is an effective first line treatment for PPH. The preparations available are synthetic oxytocin ampule containing 2, 5, and 10 IU/mL. It needs to be stored in a refrigerator at 2–6°C. It can be injected 10 IU IM or as a bolus, or 20 IU in 500 mL of saline may be infused at a rate of 250 mL per hour (60 drops per minute) over 2 hours. As much as 500 mL can be infused over 10 minutes without complications. For a sustained effect, continuous infusion of oxytocin is usually preferred. Its effect subsides completely within an hour of cessation of therapy. In cases of circulatory collapse, 10 units may be administered intramyometrially. Intravenous route is favored over the intramuscular route, which is very painful. Oxytocin is the preferred uterotonic and is recommended as the first-line drug in active management of third stage of labor due to its short half-life and good intensity of action. Also, its action can be quickly terminated and it does not cause contraction of the lower segment. Therefore, it does not cause entrapment of the placenta. Moreover, it can be used safely in women with cardiac disease and hypertension where ergometrine is contraindicated.

Some adverse effects of oxytocin include water intoxication, due to its antidiuretic hormone (ADH) like action when used in high doses (30–40 mIU/min). Water intoxication is manifested by symptoms of hyponatremia such as confusion, coma, convulsions, congestive cardiac failure, and death. This can be prevented by avoiding high doses of oxytocin. Bolus intravenous injection should be avoided in patients with PPH where patient is hypovolemic or in patients with heart disease because of the risk of development of hypotension. Occasionally, oxytocin may also produce anginal pain.

Ergot Alkaloids (Ergometrine and Methylergometrine)

> Q. Write a short note discussing the advantages and disadvantages of methergine in the third stage of labor.

Ergotamine is an alkaloid isolated from a fungus *Claviceps purpurea*, which commonly occurs in cereals like rye, wheat, etc. Methylergometrine is a semisynthetic product derived from lysergic acid. Both methylergonovine (methergine) and ergometrine cause generalized smooth muscle contraction. As a result, the upper and lower segments of the uterus contract tetanically and pass into a state of spasm without any relaxation in between.

Ergometrine (ergonovine) is available in ampules of 0.25 mg and 0.5 mg and tablets of 0.5 mg and 1 mg. Methergine is available in ampules of 0.2 mg and tablets of 0.5 mg and 1 mg.

A typical dose of methylergonovine, 0.2 mg administered intramuscularly, may be repeated as required at intervals of 2–4 hours. The dose of ergometrine is 0.25 mg IM which can be repeated every 5 minutes up to a maximum dose of 1.25 mg. The onset of action on the uterus after oral administration is 15 minutes, after IM injection is 5 minutes and after intravenous injection is almost immediate. It can be administered directly in the uterine muscle, if necessary. The total dose of ergometrine in 24 hours must not exceed 1,000 μg. Ergot alkaloids are sometimes used orally in a dose of 0.125 mg TDS for a maximum of 7 days to help in uterine involution in secondary PPH.

Since the stimulant action of ergometrine also involves the lower segment of the uterus along with the upper segment, this can occasionally result in the entrapment of the separated placenta. Its use can result in adverse effects such as vomiting, elevation of blood pressure, and pain after birth requiring analgesia. It can inhibit lactation if higher doses are used for many days postpartum, as it inhibits prolactin release (dopaminergic action). Its prolonged use may lead to gangrene of the toes due to its vasoconstrictive effect. Moreover, ergometrine should be used with caution in the following cases:

- *Suspected multifetal pregnancy:* Administration of ergometrine with the delivery of the first baby can result in the entrapment of second baby due to tetanic contractions of the uterus.
- *Organic cardiac disease in the mother:* It may cause sudden sequestration of the uterine blood into the general circulation causing overloading of the right heart resulting in pulmonary edema.
- *Severe preeclampsia and eclampsia:* Injection of ergometrine in these cases can result in a sudden rise in blood pressure.
- *Rh-negative mothers:* Injection of ergometrine can result in fetomaternal hemorrhage.

Carbetocin

Carbetocin is a new, synthetic, long-acting analog of oxytocin having a rapid onset of action. It is an oxytocin receptor agonist and exerts its action on oxytocin receptors of myoepithelial cells. It can be administered IV or IM and each ampule contains 100 μg of carbetocin which is administered slowly over 1 minute. The onset of action is within 2 minutes and lasts for approximately 1 hour. A single injection of carbetocin is equivalent to 8 hours of oxytocin infusion.

Syntometrine

Syntometrine is a combination of ergometrine 0.5 mg and oxytocin 5 IU which is administered via intramuscular route. It is the agent of choice for prophylaxis in the third stage of labor. It is likely to have an efficacy similar to that of oxytocin in the prevention of PPH. However, it has more side effects especially vomiting in comparison to oxytocin. In case of atonic PPH, syntometrine one ampule may be administered intramuscularly if it had not been previously given. Caution should be observed in hypertensive women. In these women, it is more suitable to use prostaglandins.

Prostaglandins (PGF2α)

Amongst the various prostaglandins (PGE2, PGF2, and PGI2), which were first isolated from the seminal fluid in 1935, PGF2α acts predominantly on the myometrium, while PGE2 acts mainly on the cervix due to its collagenolytic property. Prostaglandins F2α enhance uterine contractility and cause vasoconstriction. The prostaglandin most commonly used for controlling PPH is 15-methyl prostaglandin F2α, or carboprost (containing 2.5 mg/10 mL vial). Hemabate is carboprost tromethamine available as 250 μg/mL sterile solution suitable for intramuscular use.

Carboprost is usually administered intramuscularly in a dose of 0.25 mg; this dose can be repeated every 15–90 minutes for a total dose of 2 mg or a maximum of eight doses. In severe cases of PPH, carboprost can also be administered intramyometrially. Carboprost has been proven to control hemorrhage in up to 84–96% of patients. Its use will often obviate the requirement for surgical intervention in a case of atonic PPH. Carboprost should be used with caution in patients with asthma, hypertension, hepatic, or renal diseases. Side effects associated with its use include nausea, vomiting, diarrhea, hypertension, headache, flushing, bronchoconstriction, and pyrexia. It is contraindicated in patients with cardiovascular, renal, pulmonary, or hepatic dysfunction.

It has been shown that prostaglandins are not preferable over conventional uterotonics like oxytocin for the management of third stage of labor and the prevention of PPH. However, if PPH occurs after administration of oxytocin, administration of parental prostaglandins serves an effective form of treatment.

Misoprostol

Misoprostol is another prostaglandin that increases uterine tone and decreases postpartum bleeding. Misoprostol is effective in the treatment of PPH, but side effects such as diarrhea, fever, and shivering may limit its use. It can be administered sublingually, orally, vaginally, and rectally. Doses range from 600 μg to 1,000 μg. The dose recommended by FIGO (2017) for prevention of PPH is a single dose of 600 μg misoprostol administered orally immediately after delivery of the newborn. For treatment of PPH, FIGO (2017) recommends a single dose of 800 μg misoprostol, to be administered sublingually immediately after PPH is diagnosed and if 40 IU IV oxytocin is not immediately available. This dose must be administered irrespective of the prophylactic measures which had been previously taken. Misoprostol can also be rapidly absorbed by the sublingual, vaginal, and rectal routes. Prophylactic administration for active management of third stage of labor is 600 μg sublingually or vaginally. The vaginal route is more potent and side effects are fewer compared to the sublingual route. However, the vaginal route could be inappropriate in patients with heavy bleeding. In such cases, 600 μg can be administered sublingually or 800–1,000 μg can be given rectally.

Although misoprostol is widely used in the treatment of PPH, it is presently not approved by the US Food and Drug Administration for this indication. Misoprostol, however, is safe, inexpensive, is stable at room temperature, has a long shelf life and is easily storable. Therefore it has a high potential of usefulness in developing countries. Its administration also reduces the incidence of PPH in the home birth setting.

There is evidence that misoprostol does not provide any additional benefits when used in combination with another uterotonic drug like oxytocin. Moreover, oxytocin is still the drug of choice for prevention of PPH as it is less expensive than misoprostol and is associated with fewer side effects. Misoprostol can commonly cause side effects such as maternal pyrexia and shivering. In rare cases, misoprostol can cause uterine tachyphylaxis which can lead to uterine tetanus and the risk of uterine rupture. Its use is contraindicated in patients with a uterine scar and hypersensitivity to the drug.

Antifibrinolytics (Tranexamic Acid)

Antifibrinolytics are drugs which inhibit plasminogen activation thereby inhibiting fibrinolysis and preventing clot dissolution. Tranexamic acid, an antifibrinolytic drug, is a competitive inhibitor of plasminogen activation. It can be used in prevention and treatment of PPH. Since tranexamic acid has a very high affinity for the lysine binding sites of plasminogen, it blocks these sites and prevents binding of activated plasminogen to the fibrin surface, thereby exerting its antifibrinolytic effect. Placental bleeding appears to result from structural weakness and vascular defects in uteroplacental blood vessels. Tranexamic acid retards this process by preventing clot lysis. Its side effects are nausea, vomiting, diarrhea, headache, giddiness, thrombophlebitis of the injected vein, and disturbances in color vision. It is available in 500 mg/5 mL ampule for IV use and 500 mg oral tablets. It is administered in the dosage of 1 g by slow IV injection (within 3 hours of delivery), repeated three to four times per day. As per a large, international, randomized, placebo-controlled trial (WOMAN trial, 2010) regarding the use of tranexamic acid in the management of primary PPH, tranexamic acid may be administered during the third stage of labor in addition to other medications routinely used for the prevention of PPH.

Recombinant Factor VIIa (Novoseven)

If even surgical intervention and attempts to correct coagulopathies fail to control bleeding, recombinant factor VIIa may be used in cases of severe PPH. Recombinant factor VIIa acts by activating factor X on the surface of activated platelets with consequent "thrombin burst" which causes the conversion of prothrombin to thrombin and local formation of stable fibrin clot that may help control bleeding. Novoseven is unlikely to work if the platelet count is $< 50 \times 10^9/L$, fibrinogen is <0.5 g/L and the pH is <7.2. Initial dose would be 90 µg/kg. More Novoseven can be given after 1–2 hours in a dose of 120 µg/kg, but if bleeding persists after two doses, further Novoseven is unlikely to be of benefit. Tranexamic acid is useful in addition to Novoseven in order to stabilize the clot. Presently, there are no published randomized trials regarding the role of recombinant FVIIa in cases of PPH, even though trials are ongoing in Belgium and Switzerland.

Vasopressin

Arginine vasopressin, commonly known as vasopressin or ADH, is a posterior pituitary hormone which is very similar in structure to oxytocin. It can be administered orally, intranasally, or via IM or IV routes for emergency control of PPH in cases where no other medical treatment seems to work. One milliliter (5 IU) of vasopressin is diluted in 19 mL of normal saline and is injected subendometrially. Its onset of action is almost immediate and lasts for 2–8 hours. Its side effects include headache, hyponatremia, seizures, etc.

Transfusion Support in Severe Postpartum Hemorrhage

Most of the morbidity and mortality associated with PPH usually occurs at hemoglobin level < 5 g/dL. Theoretically, whole blood is the ideal replacement therapy for massive hemorrhage. The transfusion protocol varies from hospital to hospital. Most recent transfusion protocol in case of massive hemorrhage supports using a ratio of 1:1:1 of packed red cells, free frozen plasma (FFP), and platelet concentrates.

NONSURGICAL/CONSERVATIVE MANAGEMENT

When uterotonics fail to cause hemorrhage control, packing or tamponade of the uterine cavity can be considered as a form of conservative management. This may prove effective in controlling PPH due to uterine atony, placenta accreta, and placenta previa. However, packing should be initiated only after excluding genital tract lacerations. Some methods for conservative management are described next.

Transvaginal Uterine Artery Clamp

Transvaginal uterine artery clamp (TVUAC) is likely to be a safe and effective method for controlling PPH, especially in the low-resource settings. Its use is likely to reduce the requirement of surgical interventions for controlling PPH and is likely to act as an adjunct to medical methods for controlling PPH.

Procedure: Hold both the lips of the cervix with sponge holding forceps. Apply TVUAC with open blades at 3 and 9o' clock position of the cervix and push it upward for 2 cm till you meet the resistance of fornix (**Figs. 14.5A to C**). This is likely to take care of the uterine artery as well as the descending cervical branch, thereby immediately controlling the bleeding.

Suction Cannula

Two innovative approaches used in the Indian scenario for controlling PPH include the SR suction cannula (**Fig. 14.6**) and Panicker's vacuum suction cannula. In both the approaches, vacuum retraction is created with help of negative pressure within the uterine cavity using a cannula made up of stainless steel, which is available in various sizes. This helps in shrinking the uterus which can assist the natural process physiological process of retraction and contraction, thereby preventing the atonic uterus from bleeding.

Procedure: The uterine retraction vacuum system developed by Dr Samartha Ram H uses the SR suction cannula. This cannula, which is 21 cm long must be inserted into the uterus till the fundus, making sure that all the holes of the cannula lie within the uterine cavity. Following this, the cannula must be connected to the suction machine and pressure up to 600–800 mm Hg for 15 minutes, every hourly for 3 hours. The cannula is left in situ until the bleeding is controlled, even up to as long as 24 hours. An adverse effect of this method is that the tissue may sometimes get trapped in the holes present on this cannula. This may result in injury at the time of removal of cannula. This can be avoided by gentle separation of these adhesions with finger manipulations at the time of removal.

Uterine Tamponade

This method aims at increasing intrauterine pressure greater than systemic arterial pressure in order to control uterine bleeding. The word "tamponade" is derived from a French word meaning tampon, which implies insertion of a plug, a bung or a stopper into an open wound or a body cavity to stop the flow of blood. Uterine tamponade can be considered as a simple, cheap, rapidly acting, conservative, and emergency lifesaving procedure. It does not require special expertise, so can be used effectively even by people with limited medical expertise or in situations where other options are not available or when PPH does not respond to the conventional pharmacologic measures. This method, however, carries the potential risk of infection and trauma. It may also conceal the bleeding and give a false sense of security. Uterine tamponade can be achieved in two ways:

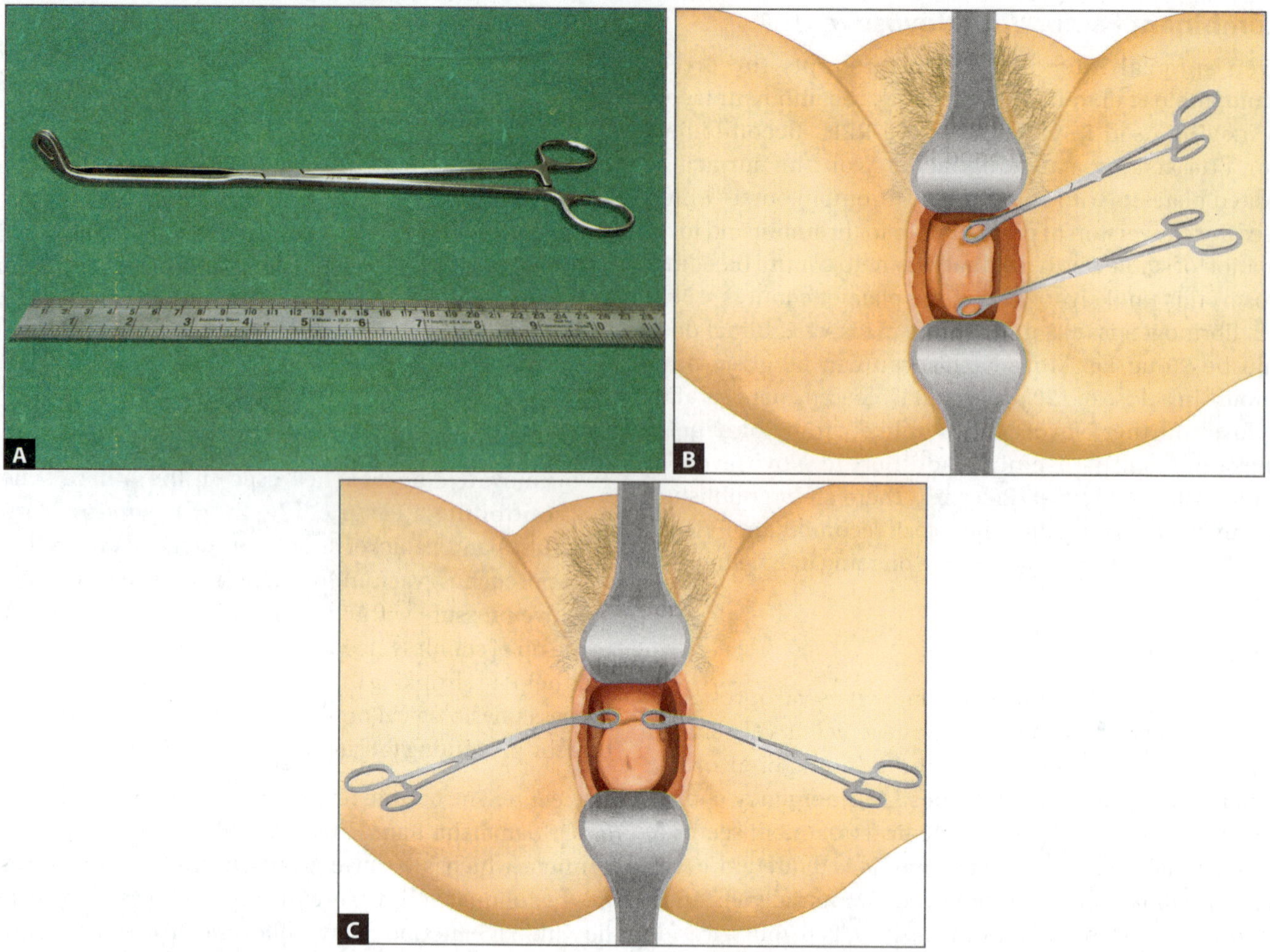

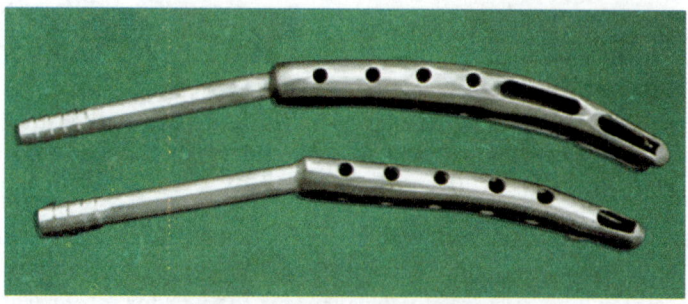

Figs. 14.5A to C: Application of transvaginal uterine artery clamp. (A) Transvaginal uterine artery clamp; (B) Holding the cervical lips using sponge forceps; (C) Application of TVUAC over the uterine arteries of both the sides.

Fig. 14.6: SR suction cannulas for prevention of atonic PPH after delivery.

1. *Balloon tamponade:* Balloon tamponade can be achieved by using a Foley catheter, a Sengstaken-Blakemore tube, a Rusch urological catheter (which has a larger volume balloon than a Foley's catheter), or an SOS Bakri tamponade balloon **(Figs. 14.7A to E)**. A Foley's catheter with a balloon of 30 mL (which may be inflated up to 100 mL) is quite effective in controlling postpartum bleeding. However, the shape of the balloon may not correspond to that of elongated uterine cavity. Despite this, insertion of a Foley's catheter is especially useful in cases where cervical lacerations that have been repaired, continue to bleed. When a Sengstaken-Blakemore tube is used, it must be left inflated for 24 hours and then deflated. Sengstaken-Blakemore tube is a three-way catheter tube with stomach and esophageal balloon components **(Fig. 14.7B)**. However, the Sengstaken-Blakemore tube was originally designed to control bleeding from the esophageal varices and not that from the uterine cavity. The recently available SOS Bakri tamponade balloon **(Figs. 14.7D and E)**, made up from silicon and no latex, has been specifically designed to deal with PPH. The Bakri balloon catheter helps in temporary control of PPH, potentially avoiding a hysterectomy. The balloon portion of the catheter is inserted past the cervical canal and internal ostium into the uterine cavity under ultrasound guidance.

At cesarean delivery, the tamponade balloon can be passed via the cesarean incision into the uterine cavity with the inflation port passing into the vagina via the cervix. An assistant pulls the shaft of the balloon through the vaginal canal until the deflated balloon base comes into contact with the internal cervical os. The uterine incision is closed in the usual fashion, taking care to avoid

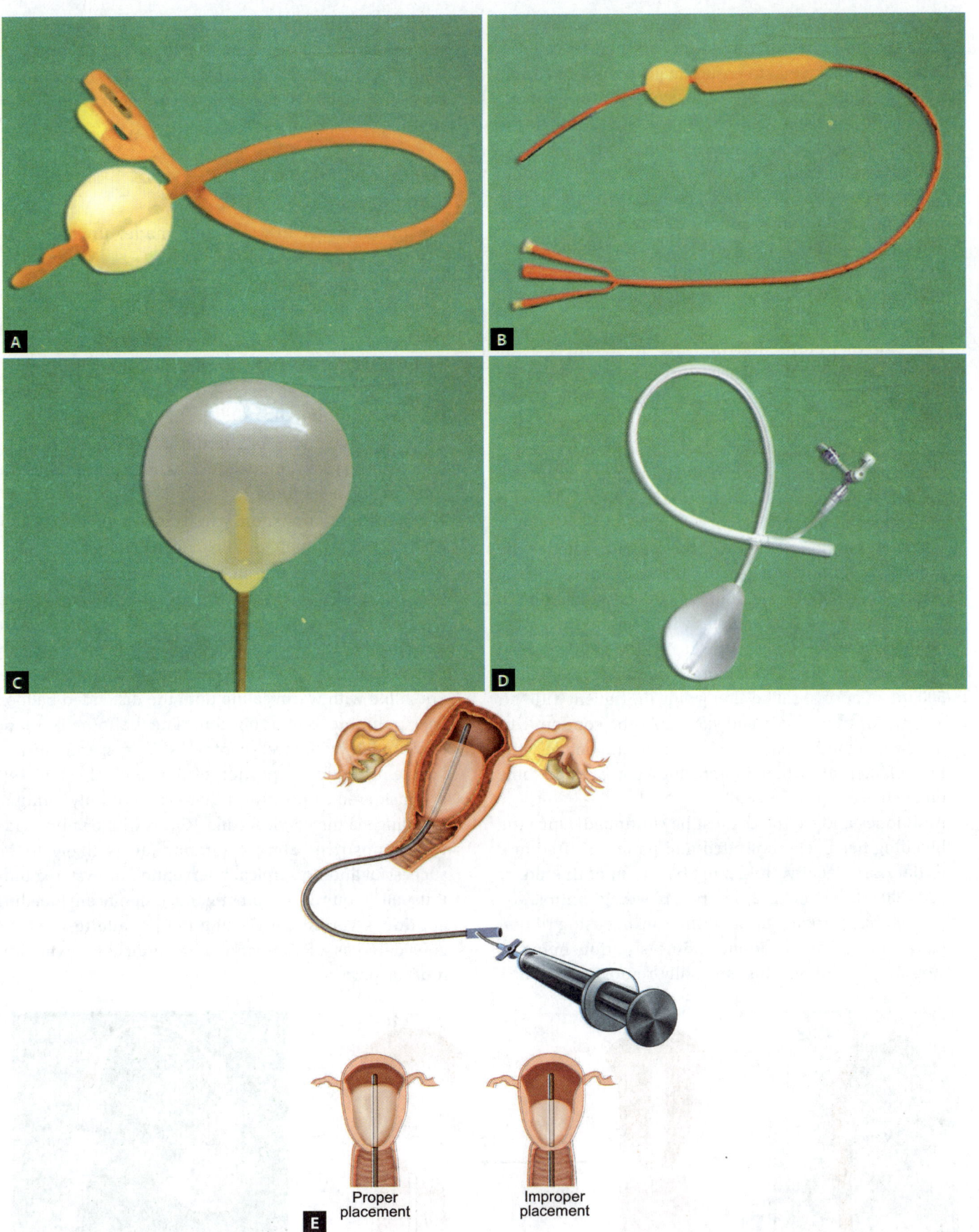

Figs. 14.7A to E: Different types of devices used for uterine tamponade. (A) Foley's catheter; (B) Sengstaken–Blakemore tube; (C) Rusch hydrostatic urological balloon; (D and E) SOS Bakri tamponade balloon.

puncturing the balloon while suturing. A gauze pack soaked with iodine or antibiotics can then be inserted into the vaginal canal to ensure maintenance of correct placement of the balloon and maximize the tamponade effect. The balloon is then inflated with sterile fluid to the desired volume for tamponade effect.

2. *Condom tamponade (condom catheter):* Use of condom tamponade **(Figs. 14.8A to C)** is likely to be helpful in reducing the mortality and morbidity associated with PPH. This method is likely to serve as an efficient, cost-effective, easily available procedure, not requiring high levels of skills, which is particularly likely to prove useful in low-resource settings.

   Procedure: Before starting the procedure, it is recommended to have all necessary equipment in a PPH box, which contains: sterile pair of gloves, one plastic tubing, IV fluids, condom, suture or sterile string, clamp, a pair of scissors, and Sim's speculum. After wearing a sterile pair of gloves, a sterile condom is inserted over a sterile No 14 Nelaton's catheter or a Ryle's tube. The end of catheter should project for a length of at least 4 inch inside the condom. The end of the catheter is tied to the mouth of condom with help of silk. An additional plastic catheter can be used for draining out collected blood in the uterine cavity. The catheter with condom must then be inserted inside the uterine cavity and gently guided toward the fundus. Condom must be inflated with 300–500 mL of normal saline after giving the patient a 15° tilt and packing the cervix and vagina. As the condom gets filled with fluid it expands and acts as a tamponade at the level of internal os, thereby applying a compressive force on the bleeding uterine walls.

   Antibiotics and oxytocics must be continued. Once the bleeding has been controlled and patient shifted to a tertiary care facility, fluid must be let out at the rate of 100–300 mL/h after 12–24 hours of bleeding control.

3. *Intrauterine packing:* Intrauterine packing using ribbon gauze soaked in povidone-iodine solution helps in stopping bleeding. This is usually removed 24 hours later. Though this method can help stop bleeding, it has a potential to cause infection. Due to the risk of concealed hemorrhage and infection, this procedure is not routinely practiced but can be lifesaving in emergency situations if nothing else is available.

Prerequisites for Application of Uterine Tamponade

Before initiation of uterine tamponade, the following prerequisites should be ensured:

- Bladder should be emptied
- Uterine cavity explored to rule out retained tissue and clots
- All medical methods should have been applied.
- All lacerations and tears should have been properly explored and sutured.
- Proper arrangements for anesthesia and surgery must be kept ready in case tamponade does not work and surgical intervention is required.
- If it is required, transport arrangements should be kept ready to refer woman to a higher center.
- Before initiation of uterine tamponade, tamponade test can be done to assess the effectiveness of tamponade. Originally in this test, a Sengstaken–Blakemore esophageal catheter was inserted into the uterine cavity via the cervix, using ultrasound guidance when possible, and filled with warm saline until the distended balloon was palpable per abdomen. The balloon is to be surrounded by the well-contracted uterus, and must be visible at the lower portion of the cervical canal. Test is considered as positive if there is no or only minimal bleeding via the cervical canal. Cases where tamponade test is positive, uterine tamponade is likely to be successful and no surgical intervention or hysterectomy is usually required. On other hand, if significant bleeding continues via the cervix, the tamponade test can be considered as a failure and other surgical interventions must be performed.

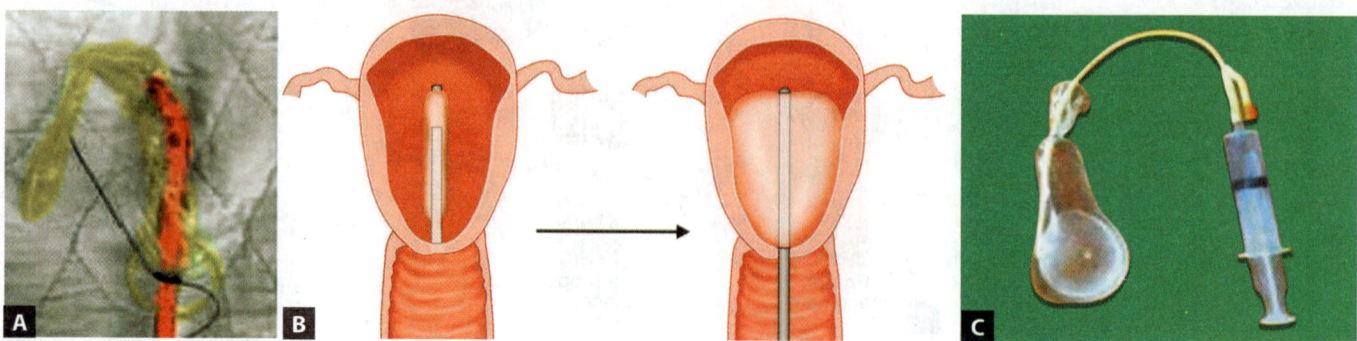

Figs. 14.8A to C: Assembly and insertion of a condom catheter for uterine tamponade. (A) The condom is tied to the catheter; (B) Insertion of the catheter inside the uterine cavity followed by its inflation; (C) A condom catheter being inflated with normal saline outside the uterine cavity.

Postoperative Care

Postoperative care after successful uterine tamponade comprises the following steps:
1. Close monitoring of these patients for vital signs, fluid input/output, fundal height, and vaginal blood loss
2. Continued oxytocin infusion may be required to keep the uterus contracted over 12–24 hours
3. Administration of prophylactic broad-spectrum antibiotic cover is necessary to prevent serious infections.
4. The tamponade balloons or uterine packs must be left inside the uterine cavity for an average time period of 8–48 hours.
5. A graduated deflation of the balloon must be done at every 6-hourly interval (letting out 50 mL of saline) to reduce the potential risk of further bleeding. Deflation should be initiated only once the patient stabilizes. Reinflation to the previous level may be required if bleeding reoccurs while deflating. If bleeding is not controlled within 15 minutes of initial insertion of catheter, the procedure must be abandoned and surgical intervention must be initiated immediately.

TIMELY REFERRAL

In case medical or conservative management is unable to control the blood loss, appropriate referral to facilities offering surgical management may be required in case adequate facilities are not available at the initial place. At the time of transfer, she should have a nonpneumatic antishock garment, condom tamponade, Bakri balloon and oxytocics in the ambulance, facilities for ALS (advanced life support) and an accompanying doctor.

BLOOD TRANSFUSION

If bleeding persists despite initial management, transfusion of blood and blood products may be required:
- 1 liter of blood requires replacement with 4-5 L of crystalloids. This includes up to 2 L of Hartmann's solution.
- Ideally cross-matched blood should be transfused. However, if that is not possible, O-negative blood may be used.
- 4 units of FFP must be transfused for every 4 units of packed cells transfused in order to prevent coagulopathy.
- Activation of massive transfusion protocol with viscoelastic testing, such as ROTEM (rotational thromboelastometry) may be useful in cases of massive hemorrhage. Massive transfusion protocol refers to rapid administration of large amounts of blood products (at least 6 units of packed red blood cells (PRBC's) in a fixed ratio, (PRBCs: cryoprecipitate/FFP: platelets = 1:1:1) for management of massive hemorrhagic shock. Candidates for massive transfusion protocol include patients with actual or anticipated blood requirement of 4 units RBCs in <4 hours along with hemodynamic instability with or without anticipated ongoing bleeding due to obstetric hemorrhage. ROTEM can be performed to detect and treat any abnormality that may develop during hemorrhage, e.g., low fibrinogen or platelet levels, hyperfibrinolysis, or coagulation factor deficiency. ROTEM provides quick global assessment of clotting and can further guide resuscitation to help fight specific derangements of physiologic coagulation.
- The transfusion of PRBCs, platelets, and cryoprecipitate/FFP must be continued until the transfusion targets mentioned in **Box 14.5** are achieved. Coagulation profile must be checked every 2-hourly. Emergency crash cart with all the things for a peripartum hysterectomy must be kept ready including all the equipment, medications, and instruments.

MASSIVE PPH

In case of massive PPH, medical and conservative methods are unable to control the bleeding. In these cases, the clinician would be required to resort to the surgical methods for controlling bleeding, mainly with help of laparotomy. Massive PPH is defined by criteria listed in **Box 14.6**. Before proceeding for laparotomy, clinician needs to check the patient's coagulation profile as well as recheck for signs of trauma.

SURGICAL OPTIONS FOR TREATMENT OF ATONIC UTERUS

> **Q.** Write a short note discussing the surgical management of PPH.
>
> **Q.** Discuss briefly surgical and radiological management of PPH.

If all the above-described conservative measures fail to control PPH, laparotomy may be required to save the

---

BOX 14.5: Transfusion targets which need to be achieved during transfusion.

- Hb > 7.5 g%
- Platelet count > 50,000/mm^3
- Fibrinogen levels > 300 mg/dL
- Prothrombin time < 1.5 times the control value
- APTT < 1.5 times the control value

BOX 14.6: Criteria for defining massive PPH.

- Rule of thirty
  - Fall in systolic blood pressure by 30 mm Hg
  - Rise in heart rate by 30 breaths/min
  - Increase in respiratory rate to 30 breaths/min
  - Drop in hematocrit by 30%
  - Decrease in urine output to < 30 mL/h
- Blood loss of > 2 L
- Blood loss of > 30% of blood volume
- Blood loss of > 125 mL/min after birth
- Gradual blood loss of > 125 mL/h over >12 hours

mother's life. Surgical hemostasis must be initiated as soon as possible in order to save the patient's life. Though there are different surgical options available, the surgical option of choice to be used in a particular patient depends upon the following factors:

- Extent and cause of hemorrhage
- General condition of patient
- Desirability for future reproduction
- Experience and skill of the obstetrician-incharge

Available Surgical Options

If the above-described conservative and medical therapeutic options are unable to control the bleeding, the obstetrician may have to resort to surgery as the last therapeutic option.

Application of aortal compression at the time of surgery must be considered. Various surgical options that are now available to control PPH are described below:

- *Brace sutures of uterus:* B-Lynch suture and its modifications such as Cho sutures, Hayman suturing, etc.
- Uterine artery or utero-ovarian artery ligation
- Bilateral ligation of internal iliac (hypogastric arteries)
- Angiographic embolization
- Hysterectomy

Hysterectomy should be considered the option of last resort in the management of PPH secondary to uterine causes. If a hysterectomy is considered, a supracervical or subtotal hysterectomy must be preferred over total hysterectomy, because supracervical hysterectomy can be considered as a quicker, simpler, and safer procedure, which is associated with less blood loss in comparison to a total hysterectomy. Before describing each surgery in detail, it is important to describe blood supply to the pelvis.

Blood Supply to the Female Pelvis

Discussion of the blood vessels supplying the pelvis and the uterus is important because the surgical methods for controlling PPH aim at controlling the blood supply to the uterus by ligation of some of these vessels. Blood supply to the pelvis and uterus are shown in **Figures 14.9A and B**, respectively.

The blood supply to the pelvic structures is mainly by the common iliac vessels, which give rise to internal iliac and external iliac arteries. The internal iliac artery (formerly known as the hypogastric artery) has an anterior division and a posterior division. Anterior division gives rise to five visceral branches and three parietal branches. The visceral branches are: uterine, superior vesical, middle hemorrhoidal, inferior hemorrhoidal, and vaginal arteries, whereas the parietal branches are obturator artery, inferior gluteal, and internal pudendal arteries. The posterior division on the other hand gives rise to the following branches—collateral branches to the pelvis, iliolumbar, lateral sacral, and superior gluteal arteries.

The blood supply to the uterus is mainly via the uterine and ovarian vessels. The ovarian arteries are direct branches of the aorta beneath the renal arteries. The uterine artery is the branch of internal iliac vessel. Uterine artery assumes important role at the time of pregnancy because it supplies maternal circulation to the placenta during this time. The uterine artery passes inferiorly from its origin into the pelvic fascia. It runs medially in the base of broad ligament to reach the uterus. It then reaches the junction of the body and cervix of the uterus (internal os) by passing superiorly. While taking such a course, the uterine artery passes above the ureter at right angles. It then ascends along the lateral margin of the uterus within the broad ligament. It continues to move along the lower border of the fallopian tubes where it ends by anastomosing with the ovarian artery which is a direct branch

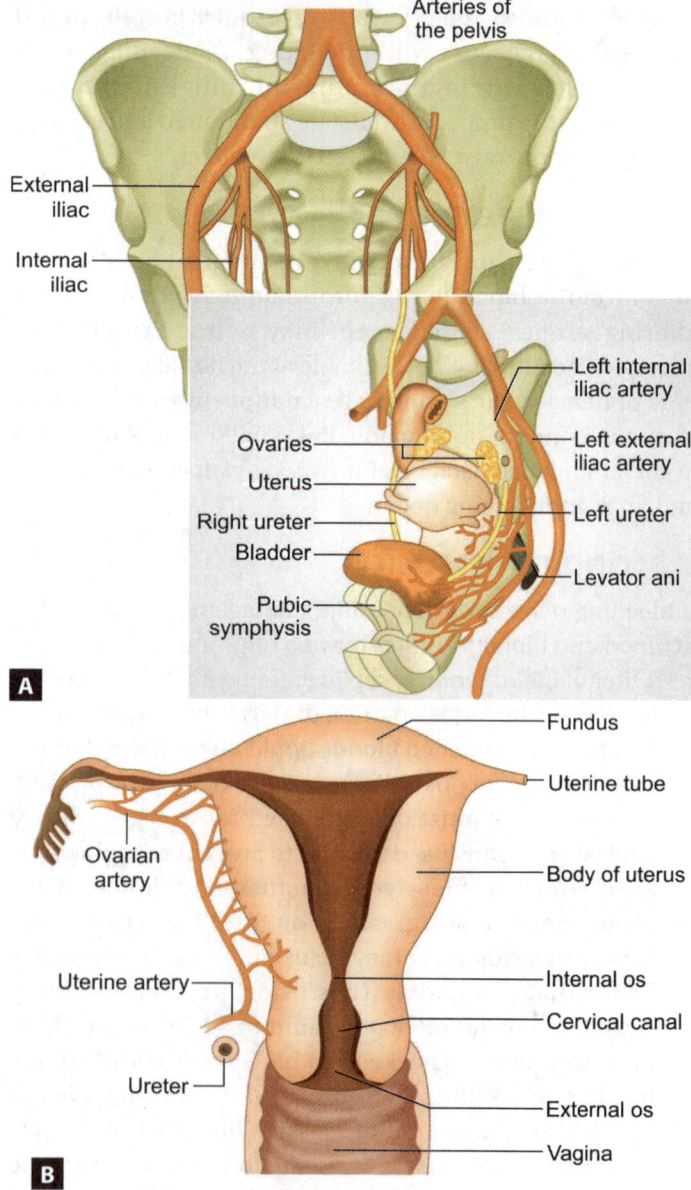

Figs. 14.9A and B: Anatomical view of pelvic blood vessels. (A) Front view of the pelvis showing the blood supply; (B) Blood supply to the uterus.

from the abdominal aorta. The uterine artery also gives off a small descending branch that supplies the cervix and the vagina. The uterine vein follows the uterine artery all along its course and ultimately drains into the internal iliac vein.

Blood supply to anterior and posterior walls is provided by the arcuate arteries, which run circumferentially around the uterus. The arcuate arteries give rise to the radial arteries which enter the endometrium. The ultimate branches of uterine artery, which connect maternal circulation to the endometrium, are the spiral and the basal arteries.

TYPES OF SURGICAL OPTIONS

Hemostatic Compression Sutures

B-Lynch Compression Sutures

Compression sutures can be considered as the best form of surgical approach for controlling PPH as it helps in preserving the anatomical integrity of the uterus. Uterine bracing suture (the B-Lynch suture), has now become the preferred surgical technique to control PPH.

This procedure was first performed and described by Mr Christopher B-Lynch during the management of a patient with a massive PPH in November 1989. The B-Lynch suture may be beneficial in cases of bleeding related to placenta accreta, percreta, and increta. Data suggests that brace suturing can negate the requirement for hysterectomy in up to 80% of cases of PPH. This technique is safe, effective, and helps in retaining future fertility. These brace like sutures control bleeding by causing hemostatic compression of the uterine fundus and lower uterine segment by opposing the anterior and posterior walls. Prior to application of these sutures, an incision is required in the lower uterine segment and bladder needs to be pushed below by 5 cm. In this method, anterior and posterior uterine walls are compressed with help of absorbable sutures, No. 2 chromic or No. 1 Vicryl. Although originally described using No. 2 chromic catgut, monocryl suture (code WC3709) is commonly used nowadays in clinical settings. These sutures are secured vertically around the anterior and posterior uterine walls giving appearance of suspenders. The sutures are first anchored in the anterior aspect of lower uterine segment, passed over the uterine fundus, anchored in the posterior aspect of the lower uterine segment, then again brought back anteriorly passing over the fundus of the uterus. These sutures are finally anchored near the entrance point on the anterior aspect of the lower uterine segment (**Figs. 14.10 to 14.12**). Simultaneously, the uterus is also massaged and manually compressed in order to reduce its size.

This method has been found to be safe and effective, and there have been reports of successful pregnancy following its use. Before using the B-Lynch suture, the following test must be performed to assess the effectiveness of these sutures.

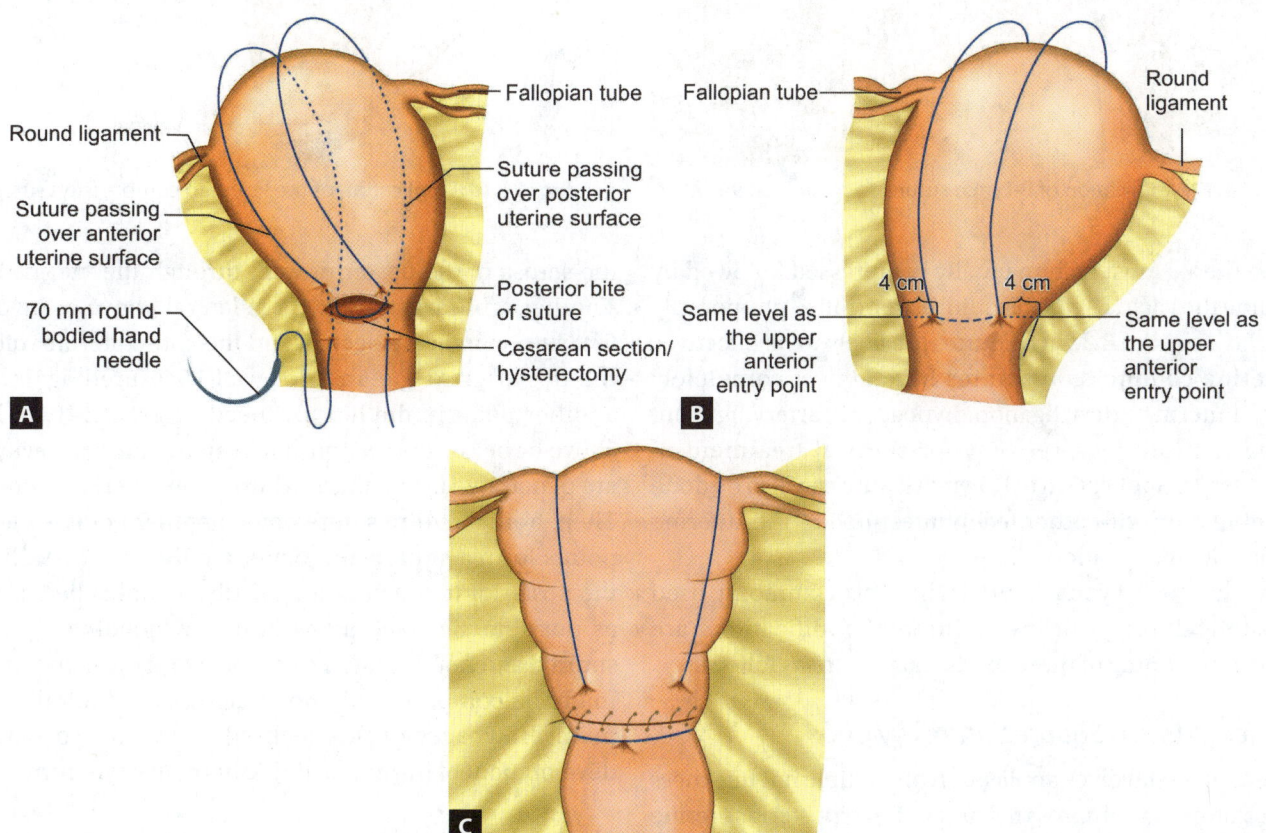

Figs. 14.10A to C: Technique of applying B-Lynch sutures.
Source: B-Lynch C, Coker A, Lawal AH, Abu J, Cowen MJ. The B-Lynch surgical technique for the control of massive postpartum hemorrhage: An alternative to hysterectomy? Five cases reported. Br J Obstet Gynaecol. 1997;104(3):3725.

284 Complications of Pregnancy

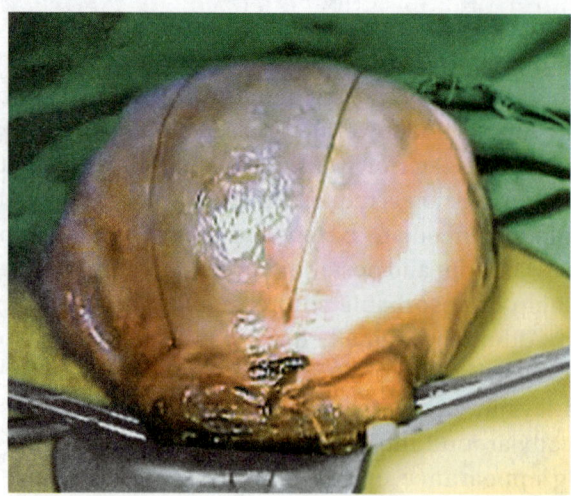

Fig. 14.11: B-Lynch suture.

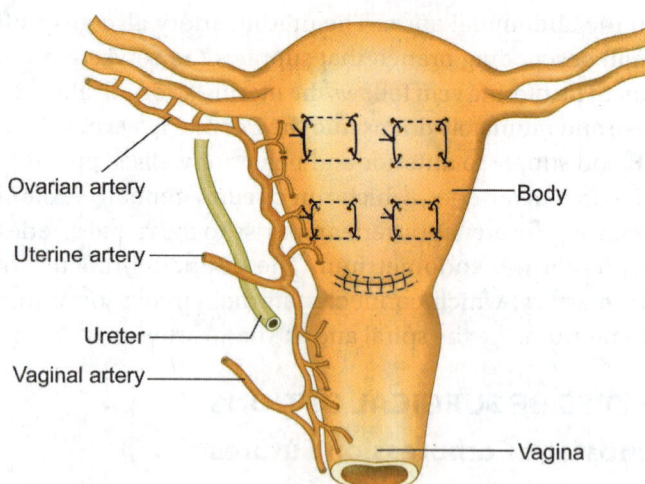

Fig. 14.13: Cho multiple square sutures compressing anterior to posterior uterine walls.

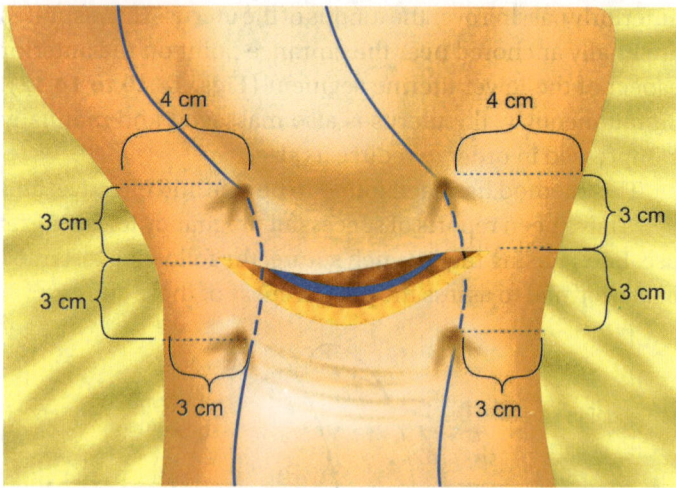

Fig. 14.12: Application of B-Lynch sutures, a magnified view.

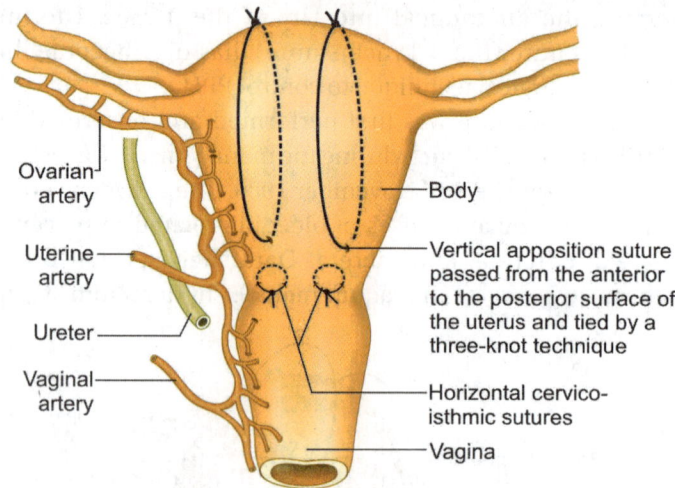

Fig. 14.14: Application of the Hayman compression suture.

The uterus must be bimanually compressed followed by swabbing the vagina. If the bleeding is controlled temporarily in this fashion, the B-Lynch sutures are likely to be effective.

Uterine compression sutures have almost completely replaced uterine artery ligation, hypogastric artery ligation, and postpartum hysterectomy for surgical treatment of atonic uterus. Application of B-Lynch suture can also be done in combination with other techniques such as intrauterine balloons or embolization.

Though the B-Lynch suture is the most commonly used hemostatic suture worldwide, newer modifications are gaining favor. Some of these modifications are as follows:

Modified B-Lynch Square Sutures by Cho

This technique involves application of multiple full thickness square sutures to compress the anterior and posterior uterine walls **(Fig. 14.13)**. This technique involves selection of an arbitrary point in the heavily bleeding area and then suturing the entire uterine wall from the serosa of the anterior wall to the serosa of the posterior wall, through the uterine cavity. Another arbitrary point 2–3 cm lateral above or below the first suture point is selected, and the entire uterine wall from the posterior to the anterior wall is sutured again. From another point in the heavily bleeding area, 2–3 cm lateral above or below the second suture point, uterine cavity walls are penetrated again, this time from the anterior to posterior. Then, from the third suture point, another point is set so the points form a square and penetrate the uterine walls from the posterior to the anterior. Finally, a knot is tied as tightly as possible. Selected areas of heavy bleeding are square sutured and not the entire cavity, because the blood drainage might be compromised and compression diminished. The main drawbacks of this technique are the possibility of development of pyometra and Asherman's syndrome.

Hayman Technique

In this technique, two vertical compression sutures are placed and tied over the uterine fundus **(Fig. 14.14)**. Since the technique does not require opening of the uterine cavity, it is quicker to perform. Also, two separate sutures are likely to result in more tension and chances of slippage are also fewer.

However, this does not allow for exploration of the uterine cavity under direct vision. As a result, there is no potential for spontaneous drainage of blood and debris. Therefore, this technique is associated with potential for development of complications such as hematometra, pyometra, and Asherman's syndrome.

An add-on to Hayman's technique is the application of horizontal cervicoisthmic stitches without obliterating the cervical canal along with the vertical apposition sutures on the upper segment as previously mentioned. This may especially be useful if the placental insertion was in the lower segment.

The Pereira Technique

Pereira from Portugal advocated the insertion of a series of longitudinal and transverse sutures around the uterus **(Fig. 14.15)**. Two or three transverse circular sutures were placed first, starting in the anterior aspect of the uterus, crossing the broad ligament toward the posterior aspect of the uterus then crossing the opposite broad ligament toward the anterior aspect and tying the suture over the anterior aspect of the uterus. The number of bites taken varied from case to case depending on the size of the uterus. Whenever the suture crossed the broad ligament, it was important to select an avascular area and ensure that the fallopian tube, the utero-ovarian ligament, and the round ligament were not included in the suture. The last transverse circular suture in the lower uterine segment served as an anchor for two or three longitudinal sutures. Each longitudinal suture started on the dorsal side of the uterus using a knot to fix it to the lowest circular suture and ended on the ventral side using another knot attached to the lowest transverse suture.

None of the sutures penetrated the endometrial cavity.

The Ouahba's Technique

This Ouahba's technique involves placement of four sutures—two transverse and two near the horns **(Fig. 14.16)**. Uterine compression created by this technique is sufficient for stopping bleeding in approximately 95% of women.

Modified U-Suturing Technique by Hackethal

This technique involves placement of approximately 6–16 horizontal interrupted sutures **(Figs. 14.17A to C)** starting at the fundus and ending at the cervix.

Hypogastric Artery Ligation

Hypogastric artery or internal iliac artery ligation is rarely used nowadays because the success rate of this procedure is less than that of uterine artery ligation (40–75%) and is mainly likely to be useful in cases of traumatic PPH. Moreover, tissue edema and hematoma may make the procedure difficult.

Indications

Internal iliac ligation is useful in the following circumstances:
- There is obstetrical traumatic injury, which has not involved the uterus.
- There is a hematoma formation at the ligation site after uterine artery ligation.
- Uterine artery ligation has failed to achieve hemostasis.

Procedure

The technique of ligation of anterior division of internal iliac artery **(Fig. 14.18)** was first propounded by Dr Howard Kelly in 1894 and comprises of the following steps **(Figs. 14.19A to C)**:
- The hypogastric artery (internal iliac artery) is exposed by ligating and cutting the round ligament. The peritoneum over the pelvic sidewall, cephalad and

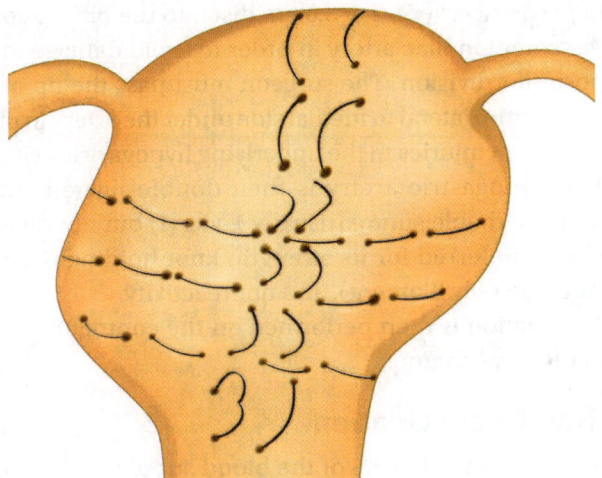

Fig. 14.15: The Pereira technique—placement of longitudinal and transverse sutures around the uterus.

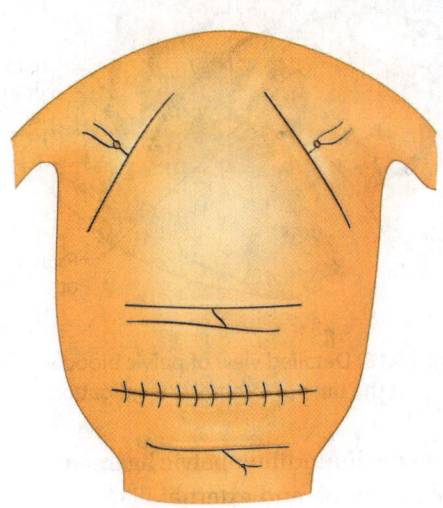

Fig. 14.16: Application of the four suture Ouahba technique.

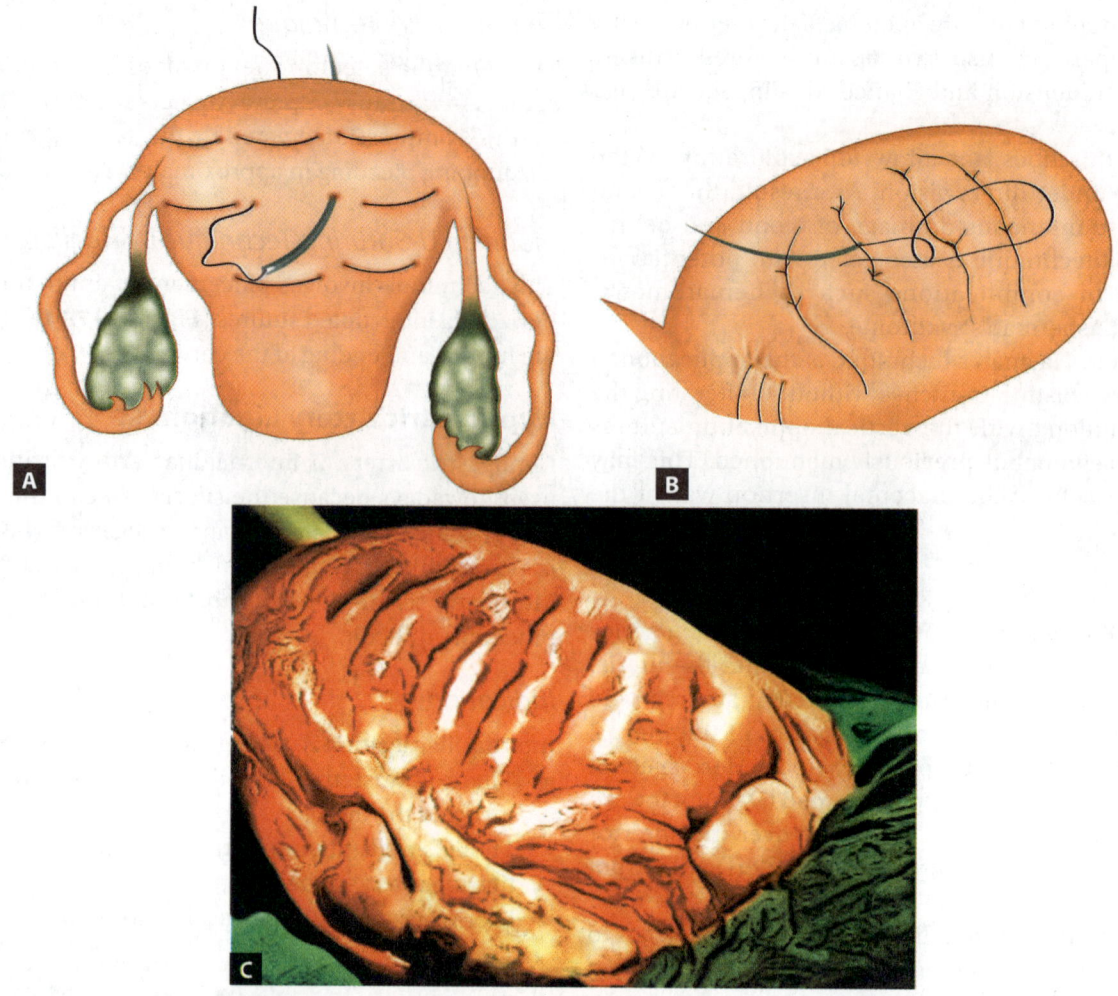

Figs. 14.17A to C: Modified U-suturing technique—demonstrating placement of horizontal interrupted suture. (A) Posterior view of the uterus showing the U-suturing technique; (B) Anterior view of the uterus showing the U-suturing technique; (C) Intraoperative position showing the uterus after U-suturing (computerized generation of the image).

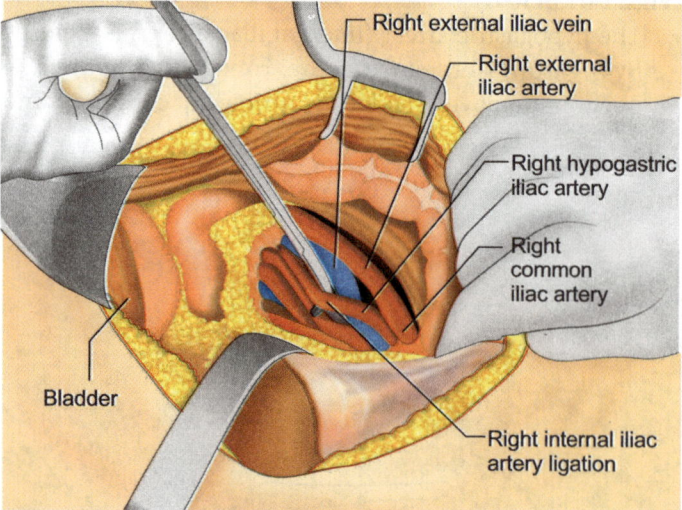

Fig. 14.18: Detailed view of pelvic blood vessels at the time of internal artery ligation.

parallel to the infundibulopelvic ligament is incised. The common, internal, and external iliac arteries must then be identified clearly.

- The common iliac artery is dissected until the bifurcation of external and internal iliac arteries. The areolar sheath over the internal iliac artery is incised longitudinally.
- A blunt-tipped, right-angled artery forceps, usually Mixter's artery forceps is gently placed around the hypogastric artery, 2.5–3.0 cm distal to the bifurcation of the common iliac artery in order to avoid damage to the posterior division. The surgeon must pass the tip of the clamp from lateral to medial side under the artery in order to prevent injuries to the underlying hypogastric vein.
- The hypogastric artery is then double-ligated with a nonabsorbable suture (usually 1-vicryl) but not divided. Silk is preferred for its strength, knot holding property (braided poly filament), and nonreactivity.
- The ligation is then performed on the contralateral side in the same manner.

Uterine Artery Ligation

Since approximately 90% of the blood supply to the uterus is via the uterine artery, ligation of this vessel through the uterine wall at the level of cervical isthmus above the bladder

Postpartum Hemorrhage

flap is likely to control the amount of bleeding. Uterine artery ligation should be attempted before considering internal iliac artery ligation. Ligation of uterine artery is likely to control bleeding in nearly 80% cases of PPH. Step-wise uterine artery ligation as devised by Abdrabbo is as follows:
- Unilateral uterine vessel ligation
- Bilateral uterine vessel ligation
- Right low uterine vessel ligation
- Left low uterine vessel ligation
- Unilateral utero-ovarian vessel ligation
- Bilateral utero-ovarian vessel ligation

This technique entails above-mentioned successive steps so if the bleeding is not controlled by one step, the next successive step is taken until the bleeding is controlled **(Fig. 14.20)**.

Procedure

The initial technique of uterine vessel ligation as described by O'Leary is as follows:
- The broad ligament is stretched laterally to accentuate the uterine vessels. The uterine vessels are delineated better by placing a hand behind the respective broad ligament and the lateral wall of uterus.
- The curved needle is passed through the full thickness of myometrium from anterior to posterior wall. The operator's hand placed behind the respective broad ligament prevents the needle from inadvertently pricking the bowel behind. The needle is then turned laterally and is brought to the front by piercing a clear area in the broad ligament lateral to the uterine vessels.
- The ligature is then tied to obliterate the blood vessel as well as to firmly anchor the vessel bundle to the lateral wall of the uterus. Synthetic absorbable material is preferred for ligating the vessels because they produce lesser inflammatory reaction while getting absorbed.

Vascular studies have confirmed that approximately 5–10% ovaries get their entire blood supply from the uterine vessels and do not get any blood from the ovarian vessels. As the uterine artery is an end artery, its obliteration in these 5–10% women may result in a premature cessation of ovarian function on the side on which the uterine vessel is ligated.

Uterine Artery Embolization

While some obstetricians use embolization only in cases where both medical and surgical management have failed, others believe that embolization should be used once patients fail medical or conservative management. Technically, an angiogram and embolization performed in a patient with PPH are similar to the pelvic embolization procedures performed for other indications. In this procedure, unilateral femoral access is typically achieved and the uterine arteries are then selectively catheterized and imaged, following which embolization of both uterine

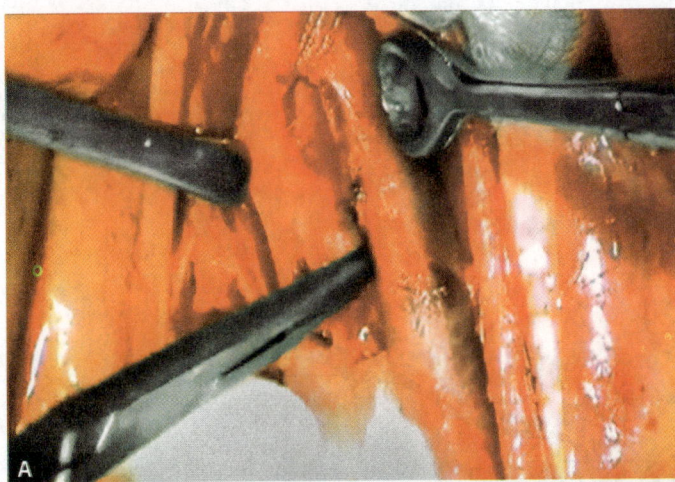
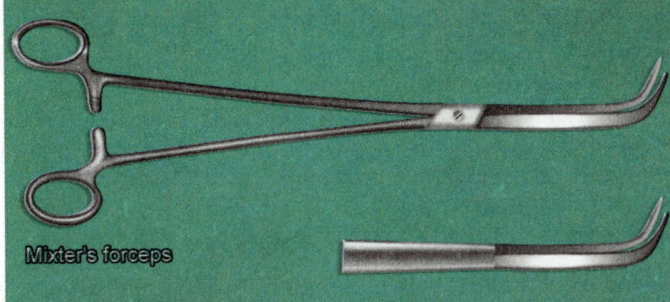
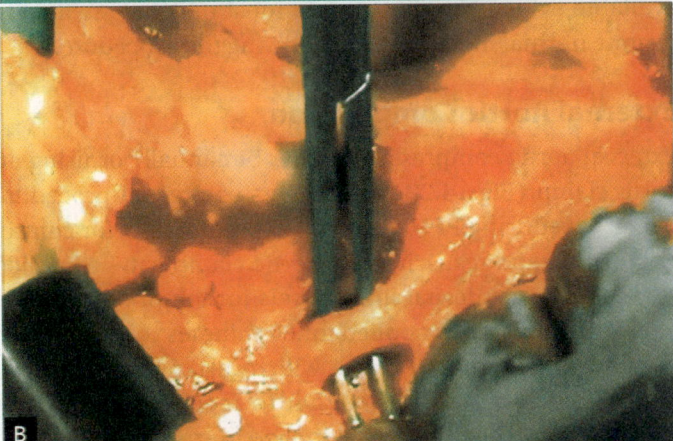
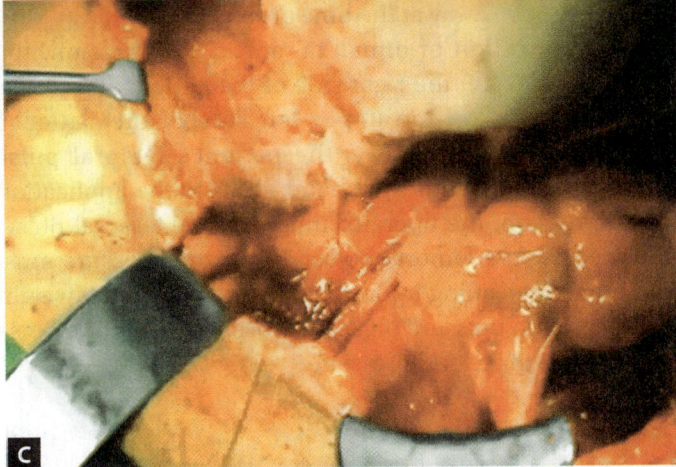

Figs. 14.19A to C: Process of internal iliac artery ligation. (A) Dissection of the retroperitoneal tissues to identify the internal iliac artery; (B) Mixter's forceps and placement of Mixter's forceps around the internal iliac artery; (C) The ligation of internal iliac artery.

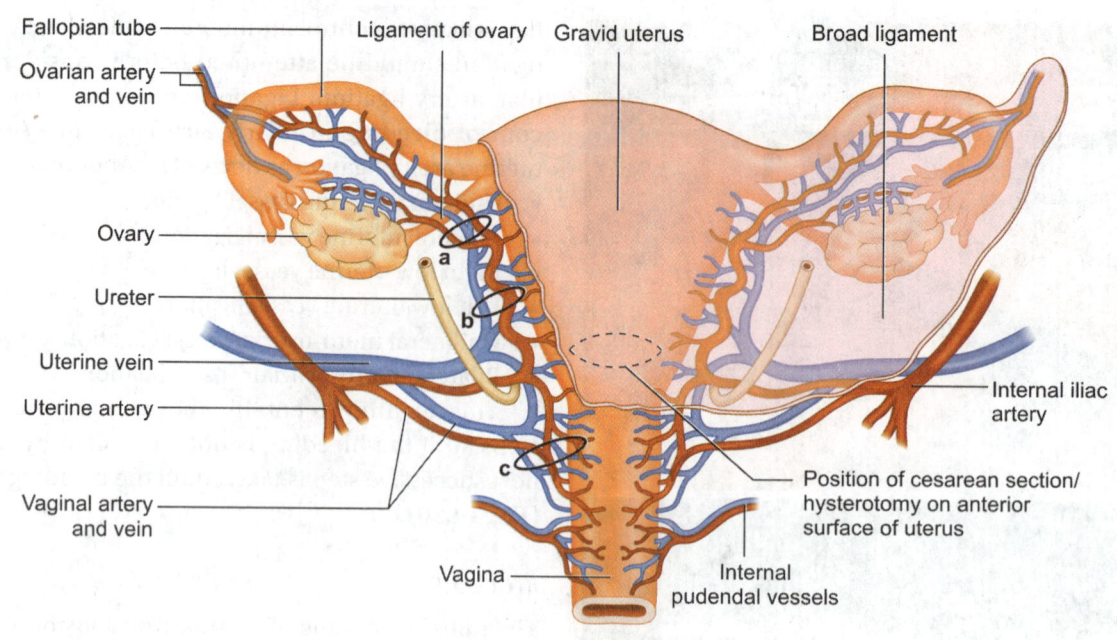

Fig. 14.20: Placement of ligatures in the process of stepwise devascularization.
(A: utero-ovarian vessel; B: uterine vessel; C: low uterine vessel)

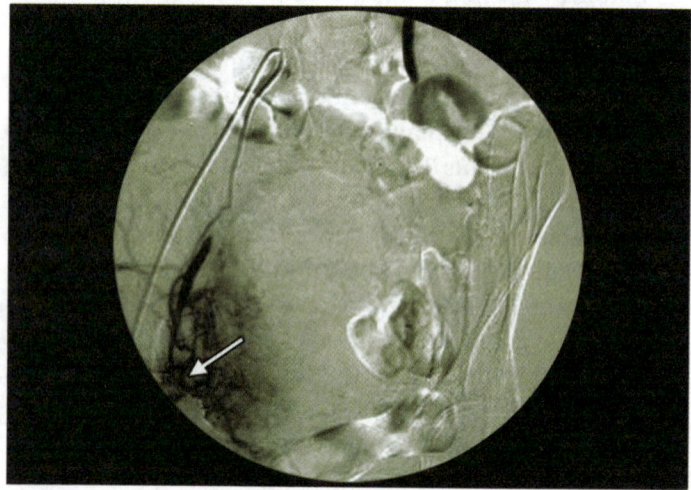

Fig. 14.21: Reduced blood flow in the right uterine artery after embolization (indicated by arrow).

arteries is then performed through internal iliac vessels. The embolizing agent most commonly used is gelatin foam or polyvinyl alcohol, which is injected until stasis of flow in the target artery is achieved **(Fig. 14.21)**. This method has been found to be particularly useful in cases of retroperitoneal hematomas where surgery may be difficult. Success rate of up to 95% has been reported with this method.

Though this method has been found to be generally safe, cases of secondary amenorrhea have been reported following this method due to necrosis of the uterine wall and obliteration of the cavity. Perforation of internal iliac artery during the embolization procedure has also been reported in some cases. While there is no definite answer to the question that whether the patients undergoing embolization procedure are able to retain their fertility or not, the presently available evidence indicates that most patients are able to resume normal menstruation following the procedure.

External Aortic Compression

External aortic compression, either bimanually or using an aortic clamp, **(Figs. 4.22A and B)** is an emergency procedure aimed at reducing PPH, thereby permitting time for control of bleeding and resuscitation. Aortic clamp can be applied to the aorta or internal iliac vessels for temporary control of bleeding. It can be applied for 30 minutes to 1 hour. This instrument has smooth blades with a gap of 2 mm between the blades. It has a long ratchet to regulate the force of compression. They should be applied in such a way that the blades don't slip away at the time of surgery.

For application of bimanual aortic compression, the operator stands on the right side of the patient and places his/her left fist on the upper left side of the patient's umbilicus. Simultaneously, the patient's femoral pulse must be palpated with right hand. Prior to the application of compression, the operator must feel the femoral pulse. Upon feeling the femoral pulse, downward pressure must be applied by leaning upon the patient, using body weight to increase the pressure on aorta. Absence of femoral pulse confirms adequate compression.

Obstetric Hysterectomy

Sometimes, removal of the uterus or obstetric hysterectomy may be the only option left to save the patient's life. Decision to remove the uterus may be easily taken in a multiparous woman who has completed her family. However, this may

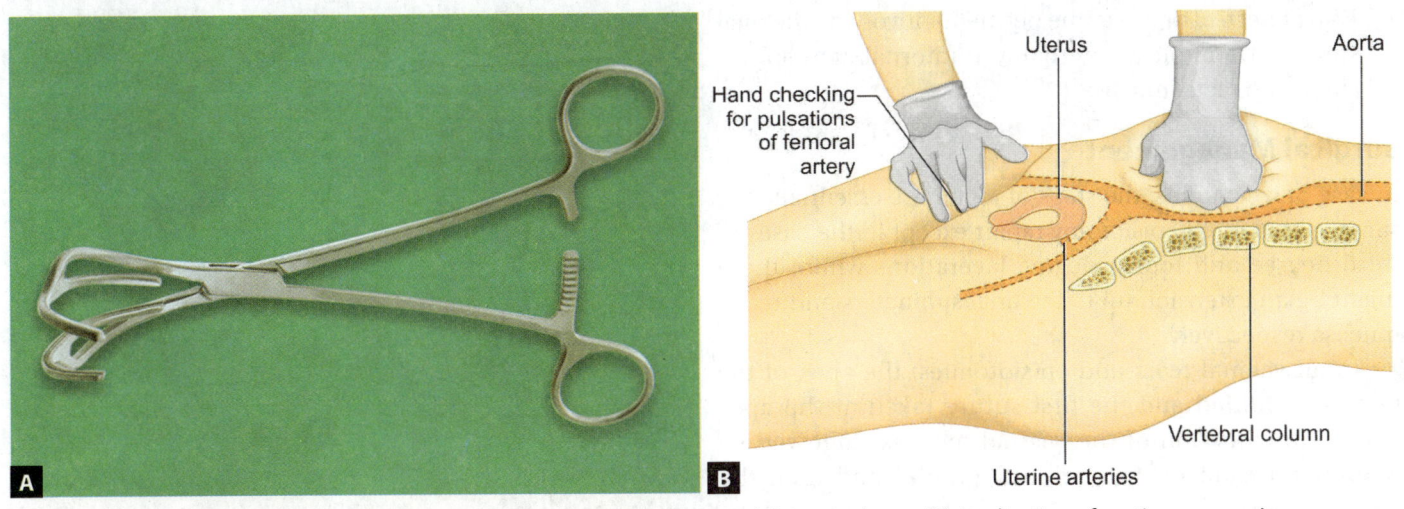

Figs. 14.22A and B: Application of external aortic compression. (A) Aortic clamp; (B) Application of aortic compression.

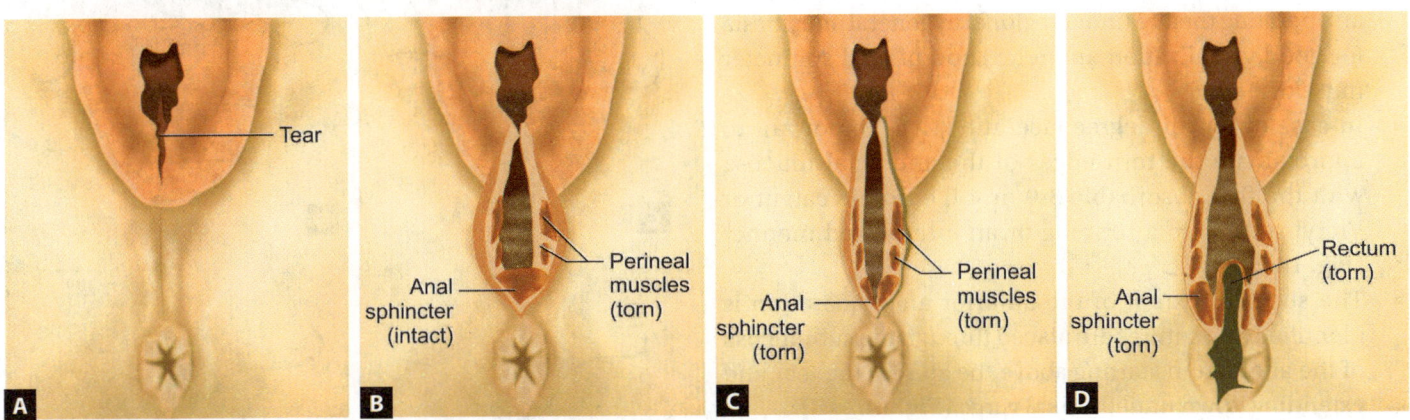

Figs. 14.23A to D: Degrees of perineal tear. (A) First degree perineal tear; (B) Second degree perineal tear; (C) Third degree perineal tear; (D) Fourth degree perineal tear.

be a difficult patient in case of a primigravida who may have delivered her first child. Nevertheless, clinician must make a timely decision in order to save the woman's life. However, once the decision is made, the surgery must be quickly performed, preferably by a senior anesthetist and a senior obstetrician. Clamp-cut-and-drop technique must be followed at the time of clamping the pedicles. Ligation of the pedicle stumps can be done later. Preferably double or triple ligation of the pedicle stumps must be performed. Localization of the cervix may be difficult in case of an atonic uterus. Therefore, subtotal hysterectomy must be undertaken. However, in case of rupture uterus or colporrhexis extending to lower uterine segment, total hysterectomy must be done. In these cases, the anterior leaf of broad ligament must be explored to look for any hematoma. In case of bleeding from the vault, a wide-bore drain (urobag or a pelvic pressure pack) can be left with the tip in the pelvis in selected cases.

In case of rupture uterus, with the tear extending downward into the vagina, the bleeding from the vagina may be tackled from below. Posthysterectomy, once the patient has stabilized, she should be put in a lithotomy position and her vagina must be explored.

REPAIR OF VAGINAL AND PERINEAL INJURIES

The perineal and vaginal injury commonly occurs during the process of childbirth and is an important cause of PPH. Since traumatic injury to the genital tract is an important cause of PPH, careful examination of the external genitalia, vulva, perineum, vagina, and cervix needs to be carried out in good light to rule out any tears or injuries. In case any tears or lacerations are present, these need to be repaired. Perineal injury can be classified into the following degrees **(Figs. 14.23A to D):**

- *First degree:* Injury to the vaginal mucosa not involving the perineal muscles
- *Second degree:* Injury to the perineum involving the perineal muscles, but not the anal sphincters
- *Third degree:* Injury to the perineum involving the anal sphincter complex (external and internal anal sphincter):
  - 3a: <50% of external anal sphincter is torn.
  - 3b: >50% of external anal sphincter is torn.
  - 3c: Internal anal sphincter also gets involved.

- *Fourth degree:* Injury to the perineum involving the anal sphincter complex (external and internal anal sphincters) and rectal mucosa.

Surgical Management

In case of lacerations, the steps of repair are essentially the same as that of an episiotomy repair except in the cases of third-degree and fourth-degree lacerations where there might be an extension up to the anal sphincters and rectal mucosa respectively.

In all vaginal tears and episiotomies, the apex of the tear is identified and the first suture taken at the apex with approximation of the vaginal mucosa, followed by reapproximation of the perineal muscles and then the perineal skin.

- Repair of third- or fourth-degree tear should be done in an operating theatre under regional or general anesthesia for good visualization and relaxation of anal sphincter muscles.
- In case of fourth-degree laceration, it is important to approximate the torn edges of the anorectal mucosa with the fine absorbable 3-0 or 4-0 chromic catgut or Vicryl sutures in a running or an interrupted manner **(Fig. 14.24A)**.
- The superior extent of the anterior anal laceration is identified and sutures are placed through the submucosa of the anorectum starting above the apex of the tear and extending down until the anal verge **(Fig. 14.24B)**.
- Finally, the torn edges of the anal sphincter are isolated, approximated, and sutured together with three or four interrupted stitches using 3-0 polydioxanone (PDS) or 2-0 polyglactin (Vicryl).
- Following the repair of internal anal sphincters, the torn edges of external anal sphincters are identified and grasped with Allis clamp because if not grasped together, these have a tendency to retract. The repair of these sphincters can be performed either using end-to-end repair **(Figs. 14.24C to F)** or the overlap method using a 3-0 PDS **(Fig. 14.25)**.
- In evaluating the optimal technique of external anal sphincter repair, comparing the overlap method with end-to-end anastomosis, the overlap primary repair appears to be associated with a reduced risk for complications such as fecal urgency, etc. However, presently there is no published study confirming the same.
- Following the repair of the external anal sphincter, repair of the vaginal mucosa, perineal muscles, and perineal skin is similar to that of second-degree tear.
- At the completion of the repair, it is important to ensure that there is no active bleeding and rectal examination is performed to ensure that repair is intact.
- Bladder catheterization for 24–48 hours is helpful in cases of third- and fourth-degree perineal injury.

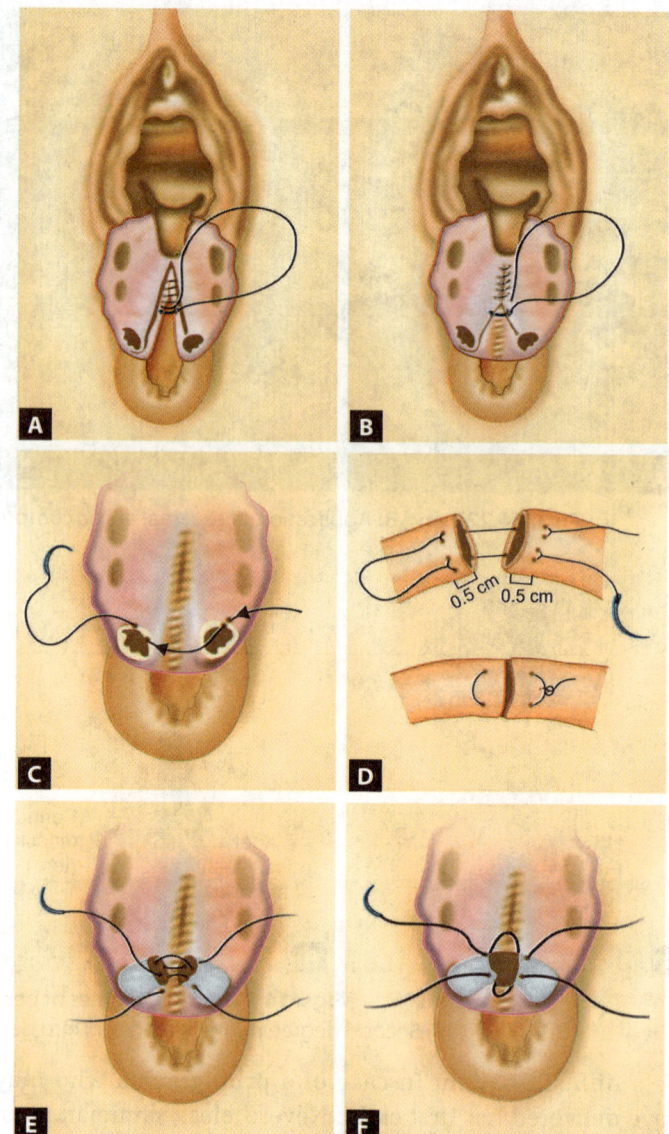

Figs. 14.24A to F: Repair of anal sphincters. (A) Approximation of anorectal mucosa and submucosa using continuous sutures; (B) Second layer of sutures placed through the rectal muscularis; (C) End-to-end approximation of the external anal sphincter. Sutures being placed through the posterior wall of external anal sphincters (these would be tied in the end); (D) Close-up view of the external anal sphincters showing end-to-end approximation; (E) End-to-end sutures taken through the interior of external anal sphincter (shown in whitish blue); (F) Approximation of the anterior wall of external anal sphincter.

- In anterior vaginal wall tears with periurethral extensions, it is important to insert a urinary catheter before starting the repair to avoid any unintentional damage to the urethra.

Postrepair Care

If infection is suspected, combinations of broad-spectrum antibiotics can be administered.

- Application of an ice-pack or regular use of a warm sitz bath over the stitches may help in reducing pain and inflammation over the site of incision.

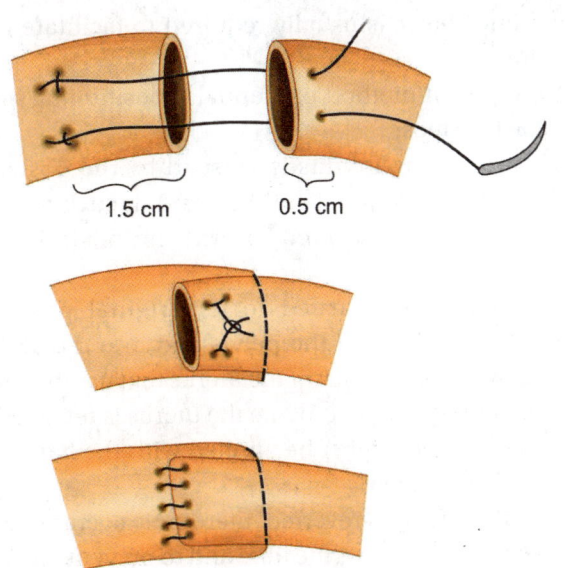

Fig. 14.25: Overlap method of suturing the anal sphincters.

- The woman should be advised to maintain perineal toilet with water only after bladder or bowel motion and to avoid the use of antiseptic solutions like betadine or Dettol.
- The patient must be advised to ambulate around as much as possible and regularly perform pelvic floor exercises once the tear has healed.
- Use of pain killers, such as paracetamol, may help in providing pain relief.
- Immediately following the surgery, the patient must be advised to take liquid diet for a day and then gradually convert to low-residue diet over few days.
- Vaginal or rectal examination and sexual intercourse must be avoided for at least 2 weeks following the repair.
- In case of fourth-degree tears where the injury has extended until the rectal mucosa, the patient should be prescribed stool softeners (lactulose 15 mL twice a day) and bulking agents (fiber) for about a week or two.

HEMATOMAS

Vulvar or vaginal hematomas may occur due to the following:
- Vaginal or perineal lacerations
- Cervical tears
- Broad ligament hematomas (incomplete rupture uterus)
- Rupture uterus

Based on the relationship of location of hematoma in relation to the levator ani muscle, vulvovaginal hematomas can be classified as follows:
- *Infralevator hematoma:* Hematomas lying below the pelvic diaphragm.
- *Supralevator hematoma:* Vulvovaginal hematomas lying above the pelvic diaphragm. This type of hematoma may end up becoming broad ligament hematoma.

Management

- If hematoma is <3 cm, and not enlarging, it can be left as it is. On the other hand, if the hematoma is >3 cm in size and enlarging, it must be evacuated. The bleeder must be identified and sutured with figure of eight stitches.
- Following this vagina can be packed and continuous bladder drainage be initiated followed by the administration of antibiotics.
- In case of supralevator or broad ligament hematomas, internal iliac artery ligation may be done. If the patient is stable, uterine artery embolization may also be considered.

Steps to Prevent Formation of Hematomas

- At the time of stitching episiotomy, suturing of vaginal mucosa should be started just above the apex.
- Submucosal tunneling should be noted and if present must be closed at the time of stitching the episiotomy.
- In order to accurately identify the bleeder, stitching of episiotomy must be done under good illumination, using proper instruments.
- If the patient is uncooperative or it is becoming difficult to identify the bleeders, the procedure must be preferably performed under anesthesia.
- Vaginal mucosa must be sutured using continuous stitches.
- Muscle bleeders must be caught and ligated separately. No dead space must be left.
- Episiotomy must be administered only at the time of crowning of fetal head over perineum or climbing of breech over perineum following infiltration with local anesthesia. At this time, episiotomy should be given at an angle of 60° so that following the baby's delivery, it may get converted to 45°. A liberal episiotomy should be administered in case of big baby, breech and shoulder dystocia to prevent extensions.

UTERINE INVERSION

> Q. Write a short note discussing acute inversion of uterus.
> Q. Write a short note on postpartum inversion of uterus.

Uterine inversion is rare but may be sometimes present in the third stage of labor, occurring in 0.05% of deliveries. In this condition, the uterus is turned inside out, either partially or completely. The inverted uterus usually appears as a bluish-gray mass protruding from the vagina. The practices of applying undue fundal pressure, undue cord traction, and Crede's expression of placenta have been thought to be the causative factors. Active management of the third stage of labor may help reduce the incidence of uterine inversion.

Diagnosis

Abdominal examination may show dimpling of the uterine fundus. Bimanual examination helps in

confirming the diagnosis. The degrees of uterine inversion (**Figs. 14.26A to C**) are as follows:
- *First degree*: Dimpling of the uterine fundus which remains well above the level of internal os.
- *Second degree*: Uterine fundus passes through the cervix, but lies insides the vagina
- *Third degree (complete)*: The uterus protrudes completely out of the vaginal introitus. The uterine endometrium with or without the attached placenta may be visible.

In terms of onset of the inversion, it can be classified as acute, subacute, and chronic. Often, the degree of shock is disproportionate to the amount of bleeding.

Treatment

The mainstay of treatment is urgent manual replacement of the uterus, preferably under general anesthesia. The placenta often is still attached to the uterus and it should be left in place until after reduction. Every attempt should be made to replace the uterus quickly. Acute inversion can be managed with manual reposition (Johnson's method) or hydrostatic replacement (O'Sullivan's method). Tocolysis or general anesthesia is usually required to facilitate uterine reposition.

The Johnson method of manual repositioning involves the following steps:
- The protruding fundus is grasped by the obstetrician with the help of palms of the hand in such a way that the fingers are directed toward the posterior fornix (**Fig. 14.27A**).
- The uterus is returned to its original position by lifting it up through the pelvis and into the abdomen (**Fig. 14.27B**). The part of the uterus that has inverted last must be replaced first. While the uterus is returned back, counter support must be applied with the hand placed over the abdomen.
- Once the uterus is reverted, uterotonic agents should be given to promote uterine tone and to prevent recurrence.
- Additionally, after the replacement, the hand should remain inside the uterine cavity until the uterotonic agents have taken their effect (**Fig. 14.27C**).

THE PLACENTA HAS YET NOT DELIVERED

Nonadherent Placenta

The mean time from delivery until placental expulsion is 8–9 minutes. Longer intervals are associated with an increased risk of PPH, with rates doubling after 10 minutes. The following steps can be taken to facilitate the placental delivery:
- A maternal uterine massage must be performed to expel any clots.
- The dose of oxytocics can be repeated, e.g., syntocinon 10 IU intravenous or 10 IU intramuscular. Ergometrine/syntometrine must be avoided for retained placenta because they may cause tonic uterine contraction, which may delay expulsion.
- The urinary bladder must be emptied by catheterizing, if it has previously not been done.

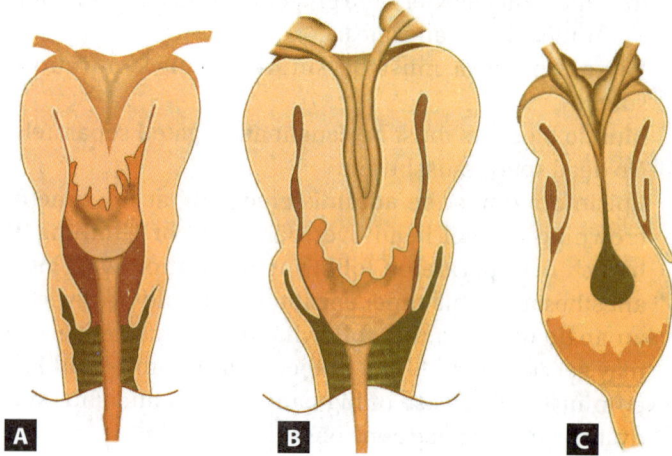

Figs. 14.26A to C: Degrees of uterine inversion. (A) First degree; (B) Second degree; and (C) Third degree.

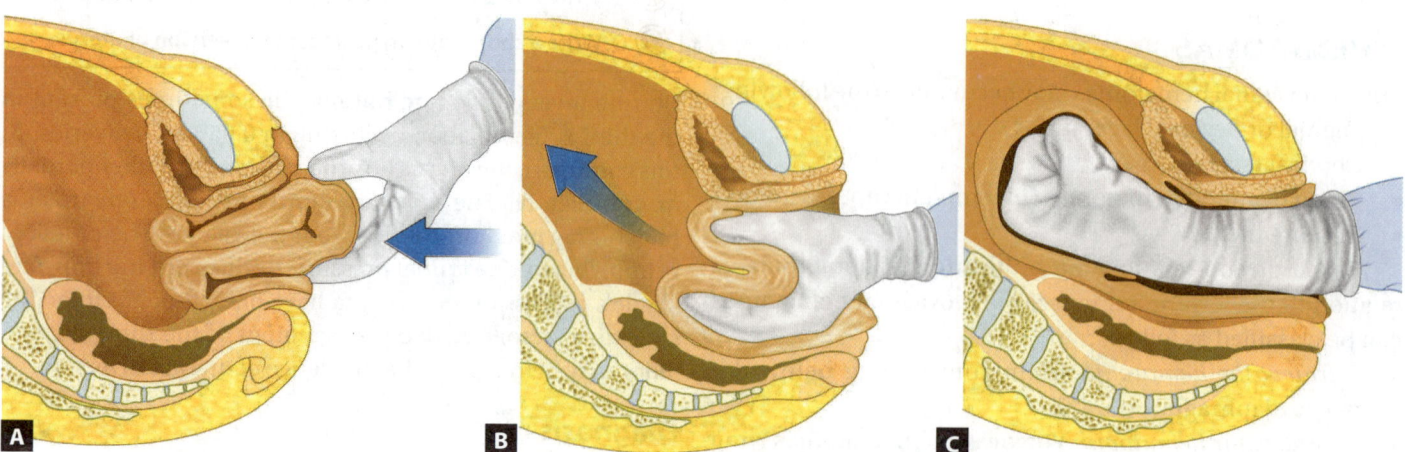

Figs. 14.27A to C: Johnson's method of manual repositioning. (A) Grasping the protruding fundus; (B) Gentle repositioning of the uterus; and (C) The clinician's hand must remain inside the uterine cavity, until the uterus has contracted.

- Controlled cord traction must be repeated to deliver the placenta.
- If possible a portable ultrasound scan must be done to see if the placenta is still in the upper segment or whether it has separated and is in the lower segment of the uterus.
- If the placenta appears to be trapped in the lower uterine segment, a vaginal examination must be performed to remove the placenta and other clots.
- Injection to the umbilical vein with 20 mL solution of 0.9% saline and 20 units of oxytocin significantly helps in reducing the need for manual removal of the placenta in comparison with injection of saline alone.
- If the placenta does not deliver even within 30 minutes of the delivery of the baby, the patient must be taken to the OT for manual exploration of placenta under general anesthesia. Further clinical management depends on whether or not a distinct cleavage plane between the placenta and the uterine wall can be located or not. If a distinct cleavage plane between the placenta and the uterine wall can be located, management options include manual removal of the placenta, using appropriate analgesia.

Manual Removal of Placenta (Fig. 14.28)

The procedure must be performed under anesthesia after taking adequate aseptic precautions. The patient must be placed in lithotomy position and bladder must be catheterized.

Abdomen should be stabilized with one hand placed over the abdomen, while the other hand, smeared with antibiotics is introduced inside the vagina in a cone-shaped manner.

It is then passed into the uterine cavity along the umbilical cord. As the placental margin is reached, the ulnar border of the hand is used to gradually separate the placenta from the uterine wall. The placental tissue is gradually separated by using the sideways slicing movements of the fingers. Once the placenta has separated, it can be grasped with the entire hand and gradually taken out. The abdominal hand helps in stabilizing the fundus and helps in guiding the movements of the fingers inside the uterine cavity until the placenta has completely separated.

Adherent Placenta

If a distinct cleavage plane between the placenta and the uterine wall cannot be located and if the tissue plane between the uterine wall and placenta cannot be developed through blunt dissection with the edge of the gloved hand, diagnosis of invasive placenta should be considered.

Invasive placenta can be a life-threatening condition. The incidence has increased from 0.003% to 0.04% of deliveries since 1950s; this increase is likely as a result of an increase in cesarean section rates. Adherent placenta can be classified into three: (1) placenta accreta, (2) placenta increta, and (3) placenta percreta. **Table 14.5** describes these different types of placentas based on their depth of myometrial invasion. In placenta accreta, the abnormally firm attachment of the placenta to the uterine wall prevents the placenta from separating normally after delivery. The retained placenta interferes with uterine contraction that is necessary to control bleeding after delivery, thereby resulting in PPH. Several risk factors for placenta accreta have been identified. Among these, the most important one appears to be placenta previa **(Chapter 8)**.

In patients with placenta previa, the incidence of placenta accreta appears to correlate with the number of previous cesarean sections. Maternal age > 35 and placental location overlying the previous uterine scar also increases the risk of accreta. Other reported risk factors include multiple previous pregnancies, previous uterine surgery, and previous D&C. In a patient with a previous cesarean section and a placenta previa, the risk of placenta accreta is dependent upon the number of previous cesarean sections as follows:

- Woman with previous one cesarean section has 14% risk of placenta accreta.
- Woman with previous two cesarean sections has a 24% risk of placenta accreta.
- Woman with previous three cesarean sections has 44% risk of placenta accreta.

Management of an Adherent Placenta

Conservative Management

- In case of densely adherent placenta, the clinician must not try to remove any nonadherent portions of the placenta.

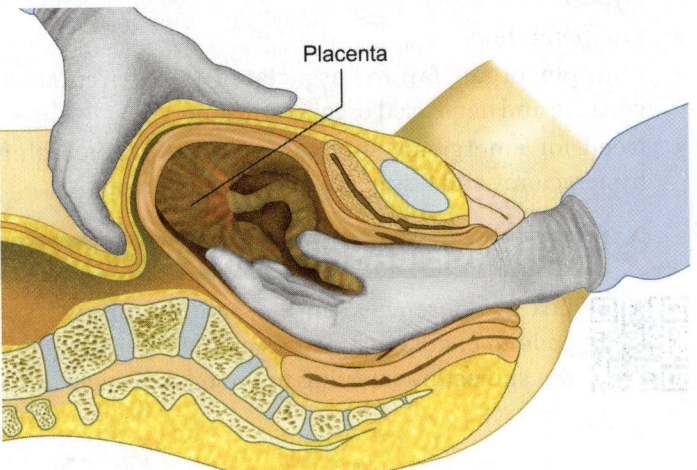

Fig. 14.28: Manual removal of the placenta.

TABLE 14.5: Types of adherent placentas.	
Classification	**Description**
Placenta accreta	Placenta adheres to the myometrium
Placenta increta	Placenta invades the myometrium
Placenta percreta	Placenta penetrates the myometrium to or beyond the serosa

- The cord can be trimmed.
- The patient's vital signs and amount of bleeding should be closely observed.
- Antibiotics should be administered.
- In the woman who is stable, hysterectomy may be avoided by the use of methotrexate.

Surgical Management

If the bleeding remains uncontrolled despite of using conservative management, the following surgical options can be used:
- Uterine artery embolization
- Low and high bilateral uterine vessel ligation
- Ligation of internal iliac arteries

If the above-mentioned surgical options are unable to control the hemorrhage, hysterectomy is the only choice left to save the woman's life.

SECONDARY POSTPARTUM HEMORRHAGE

> Q. Write a short note discussing the causes and management of secondary PPH.
>
> Q. Discuss the management of secondary PPH.
>
> Q. Enumerate the causes, diagnosis, and management of secondary PPH.

The most common cause for secondary PPH is retained tissue fragments inside the uterine cavity. Diagnosis of retained POCs is mainly done using color Doppler ultrasound. High-velocity, low-resistance arterial flow in the echogenic intracavitary material on spectral and color flow Doppler is the most important feature, pointing to the diagnosis of retained POCs. On the other hand, lack of vascularity on color flow Doppler is consistent with the diagnosis of a blood clot.

Subinvolution of the placental site may be another cause of secondary PPH. This diagnosis may be suspected when hyperechoic tortuous vessels are observed along the inner third of myometrium. In these cases, pulsed wave Doppler sonography shows increased peak systolic velocity (PSV) > 0.83 m/s third day postpartum, falling to 0.10 m/s after 6 weeks along with a low-resistance waveform.

Treatment of secondary PPH is shown in **Flowchart 14.2** and involves the following:
- Stabilization of the patient, blood may be transfused if required.
- Administration of antibiotics
- Ultrasound examination for detection of remnant bits of placenta inside the uterine cavity
- Removal of placental remnants
- Curettage of the uterus, preferably under general anesthesia.

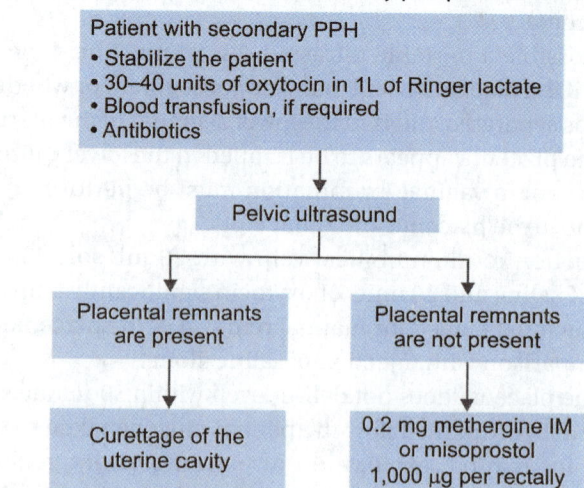

Flowchart 14.2: Treatment of secondary postpartum hemorrhage.

COMPLICATIONS

Postpartum hemorrhage is one of the important causes for maternal morbidity and mortality. Some of the complications related to PPH include the following:
- Blood loss occurring due to PPH can result in the development of orthostatic hypotension, anemia, and fatigue. Moreover, postpartum anemia increases the risk of postpartum depression. Severe cases of PPH can result in the development of shock, DIC, septicemia, occult myocardial ischemia, dilutional coagulopathy, and even death.
- Renal failure
- Puerperal sepsis
- In severe cases, hemorrhagic shock may result in anterior pituitary ischemia or postpartum pituitary necrosis, also known as Sheehan's syndrome, which may cause failure of lactation.
- Blood transfusion reaction
- Thromboembolism
- Hypovolemic shock
- Puerperal shock
- Multiple organ failure associated with circulatory collapse and decreased organ perfusion
- Need for emergency surgical intervention including hysterectomy and loss of childbearing potential.

EVIDENCE-BASED CLINICAL TRIALS

List of references can be scanned through QR code to enable the readers gain deeper insight of the subject by referring to the entire article or its abstract.

TABLE 15.3: Differences between symmetric and asymmetric IUGR.

Symmetric IUGR	Asymmetric IUGR
Growth is affected before 16 weeks of gestation	Fetal growth is affected later in gestation
Fetus is proportionately small	Fetus is disproportionately small
Cell hyperplasia is affected	Cellular hypertrophy is mainly affected
Causes of symmetric IUGR mainly include congenital abnormalities, chromosomal aberrations, intrauterine infections, etc.	Causes of asymmetric IUGR include hypertension, anemia, heart disease, accidental hemorrhage, etc.
Pathological process is intrinsic to the fetus	Pathological process is extrinsic to the fetus
Such neonates are small in all parameters	Head circumference is not as much affected as is AC
Catchup growth occurs poorly after birth	Catchup growth occurs reasonably well after birth
Neonatal prognosis is usually poor	Neonatal prognosis is usually good
Ponderal index is normal	Ponderal index is low
HC/AC and FL/AC ratios are normal. In normal pregnancies, FL/AC is 22 for all gestational ages from 21 weeks onward. Also, HC/AC at <32 weeks of normal gestation is >1, between 32 and 34 weeks of gestation is 1, at >34 weeks of gestation is <1	These ratios are elevated. HC and FL remain unaffected, whereas AC is reduced. As a result, HC/AC and FL/AC are elevated
Also termed as type II (low-profile IUGR)	Also termed as type I (late-flattening IUGR)
Less common: Usually responsible for 20% cases of IUGR	*More common:* Usually responsible for 80% cases of IUGR

(AC: abdominal circumference; FL: femur length; HC: head circumference; IUGR: Intrauterine growth restriction)

TABLE 15.4: Differences between early and late-onset IUGR.

Characteristics	Early-onset IUGR	Late-onset IUGR
Time of onset	Detected before 32 weeks of gestation	Detected after 32 weeks of gestation
Prevalence	30%	70%
Etiology	Usually due to fetal abnormalities, fetal infection, and severe uteroplacental dysfunction	Usually due to uteroplacental dysfunction
Placental histopathology	Poor placental implantation, spiral artery abnormalities, maternal vascular malperfusion	*Less specific placental findings:* Mainly altered diffusion
Maternal cardiovascular hemodynamic status	Low cardiac output, high peripheral vascular resistance	Less marked cardiovascular findings
Main challenge	Management	Diagnosis
Hypoxia	Present	May be present or absent
Placental disease	• Severe • High association with preeclampsia	• Mild • Low association with preeclampsia
Doppler findings	Spectrum of Doppler abnormalities in umbilical artery, middle cerebral artery, and ductus venosus	Redistribution of blood flow in middle cerebral artery
Ultrasound findings	Fetus may be very small	Fetus may not be necessarily very small
Fetal maturity	Immature with high tolerance of hypoxia	Mature with low tolerance toward hypoxia
Morbidity and mortality	High	Low (but common cause of late stillbirth)

TABLE 15.5: Delphi consensus criteria for fetal growth restriction.

Early fetal growth restriction Gestational age ≤ 32 weeks	Late fetal growth restriction Gestational age > 32 weeks
AC or EFW < 3rd percentile or *Umbilical artery:* AEDF	AC or EFW < 3rd percentile
Or two out of three criteria below:	
1. AC or EFW < 10th centile 2. *Uterine artery:* PI > 95th centile and/or 3. *Umbilical artery:* PI > 95th centile	1. AC or EFW < 10th centile 2. AC or EFW drop > 2 quartiles on the growth chart* 3. CPR < 5th centile or umbilical artery PI > 95th centile

Note: *Percentiles are not individualized; individual measurement of the fetus should be analyzed in each case of low percentile.
(AC: abdominal circumference; AEDF: absent end-diastolic flow; CPR: cerebroplacental ratio; EFW: estimated fetal weight; PI: pulsatility index)

TABLE 15.6: Etiology of IUGR.

Maternal factors	Fetal factors	Placental factors
• Constitutionally small mothers • Maternal undernutrition • Tobacco smoking, excessive alcohol intake, drug abuse during pregnancy, etc. • Chronic placental insufficiency due to preeclampsia, chronic hypertension, renal disease, connective tissue disorders, gestational diabetes, etc. • Maternal consumption of drugs including hydantoin, coumarin, etc. • Maternal hypoxia (pulmonary diseases, cyanotic congenital heart disease, etc.) • Endocrine disorders (e.g., diabetic nephropathy, hyperthyroidism, and Addison's disease)	• *Multiple pregnancy:* TTTS, inborn errors of metabolism • Congenital malformations (congenital heart disease, renal agenesis, etc.) • Chromosomal abnormalities (trisomy 21, 13, 18, 16, etc.) • Intrauterine fetal infections (rubella, CMV, herpes, toxoplasmosis, tuberculosis, syphilis, etc.) • Genetic syndromes	*Uteroplacental insufficiency:* • Unexplained • Essential hypertension • Preeclampsia • Chronic renal disease • Elevated maternal AFP *Fetoplacental insufficiency:* • Single umbilical artery • Velamentous insertion of cord • Placental hemangioma *Abnormal placentation:* • Abruptio placentae • Placenta previa • Placenta accreta *Placental abnormalities:* • Placental thrombosis • Placental infection and chorioamnionitis, placental cysts, etc.

(AFP: alpha-fetoprotein; CMV: cytomegalovirus; TTTS: twin-to-twin transfusion syndrome)

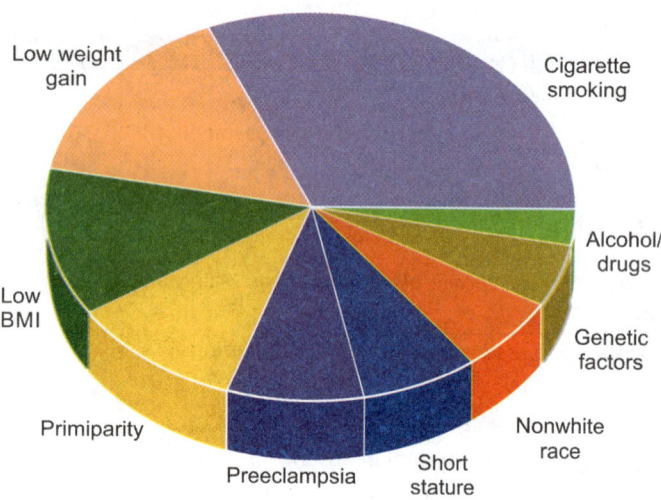

Fig. 15.3: Causes of IUGR.

or velamentous cord insertion, placenta previa, placenta abruption, etc., may also be sometimes responsible.

PATHOGENESIS

Q. With the help of a long essay, discuss the types and pathophysiology of FGR.

Trophoblastic invasion of the spiral arterioles is a continuous process responsible for placental adaptation occurring at the time of normal pregnancy. This has been described in detail in Chapter 18 (Preeclampsia). Due to this invasion the spiral arterioles lose their musculoskeletal layer, which is subsequently replaced by fibrin matrix. This results in loss of elasticity and tone, causing the development of low-resistance, high-flow circulation. The first wave of trophoblastic invasion occurs between 6 and 12 weeks and involves the intradecidual segments of spiral vessels. The second wave of trophoblastic invasion occurs between 16 and 18 weeks and involves intramyometrial segments of spiral arterioles. This causes reduced vascular resistance and lower responsiveness to local vasoconstrictive agents. Failure of trophoblastic invasion is a major factor implicated behind the pathogenesis of FGR.

HISTORY AND CLINICAL PRESENTATION

Proper history-taking is of prime importance in cases of IUGR to elicit the exact cause of IUGR. As previously mentioned, various maternal, fetal, and placental etiological factors are associated with IUGR. It is important to elicit each of these maternal factors while taking history:

- History of maternal malnutrition, chronic illness, drug abuse, bleeding, etc.
- Past history of giving birth to IUGR fetuses
- Low maternal weight gain during the antenatal visits
- History of reduced fetal movements
- Previous history of any medical disorder (e.g., essential hypertension and chronic renal disease)
- History of poor nutrition (taking a detailed nutritional history is important in these cases)
- *Constitutionally small mothers:* They may give birth to small-sized babies.
- Low maternal weight, especially a low body
- *Tobacco smoking:* Poor placental function is uncommon in a healthy woman who does not smoke.
- Excessive alcohol intake
- Strenuous physical work
- Poor socioeconomic conditions

Intrauterine Growth Restriction

TABLE 15.7: Reassigning EDD and GA based on the discrepancy between LMP-based EDD and USG-based EDD.

Gestational age (weeks + days) based on the first day of LMP	Difference in LMP-based and ultrasound-based GA when LMP-based EDD must be changed to USG-based EDD (days)
$\leq 8^{+6}$	5
9^{+0}–13^{+6}	7
14^{+0}–15^{+6}	7
16^{+0}–21^{+6}	10
22^{+0}–27^{+6}	14
$\geq 28^{+0}$	21

(EDD: estimated due date; GA: gestational age; LMP: last menstrual period; USG: ultrasonography)

TABLE 15.8: Risk factors for SGA fetuses.

Major risk factors	Minor risk factors
Maternal factors	
• Maternal age > 40 years • Smoker: ≥11 cigarettes per day • Maternal cocaine abuse • Daily vigorous exercises	• Maternal age < 40 years and ≥35 years • Smoker: 1–10 cigarettes per day • BMI < 20 kg/m² and >25 kg/m² • IVF singleton pregnancy • Low fruit intake prior to pregnancy • Nulliparity
Previous pregnancy history	
• Previous history of SGA baby • Previous stillbirth	• Preeclampsia • Pregnancy interval of <6 months and ≥60 months
Maternal medical history	
• Maternal SGA • Chronic hypertension • Diabetes with vascular disease • Renal impairment • Antiphospholipid syndrome	
Paternal medical history	
Paternal SGA	
Complications associated with current pregnancy	
• Heavy bleeding such as menses in cases of threatened abortion • Ultrasound appearance of echogenic bowel • Preeclampsia • Severe pregnancy-induced hypertension • Unexplained APH • Down syndrome marker: PAPP-A < 0.4 MoM	• Mild pregnancy-induced hypertension • Placental abruption • Caffeine ≥ 300 mg/day in third trimester

(APH: antepartum hemorrhage; BMI: body mass index; IVF: in vitro fertilization; MoM: multiples of median; PAPP-A: pregnancy-associated plasma protein-A; SGA: small for gestational age)

- Preeclampsia and chronic hypertension
- Poor maternal weight gain is of very little value in diagnosing IUGR.
- Maternal anemia, especially sickle cell anemia

The following fetal factors need to be elicited at the time of taking history:

- Multiple pregnancy
- Chromosomal abnormalities, e.g., trisomy 21
- Severe congenital malformations
- Chronic intrauterine infection, e.g., congenital syphilis, TORCH infections [especially rubella and cytomegalovirus (CMV)], viral, bacterial, protozoal, and spirochetal infections. CMV infection causes cytolysis, thereby resulting in loss of cells, whereas rubella results in vascular insufficiency by causing endothelial damage. Hepatitis A and B are associated with preterm delivery, whereas listeriosis, tuberculosis, and syphilis can cause FGR.

Accurate estimation of gestational age is the first prerequisite before making a diagnosis of IUGR. Therefore, accurate estimation of LMP needs to be done at the time of taking history. In case of discrepancy between the gestational age calculated by LMP/estimated due date (EDD) and that by ultrasound, the parameters mentioned in **Table 15.7** need to be followed.

RISK FACTORS

Various risk factors which may be responsible for causing IUGR have been mentioned in **Table 15.8**.

GENERAL PHYSICAL EXAMINATION

There may be no specific findings on general physical examination.

The woman may be constitutionally small and may have a low BMI. She may be showing signs of poor nutritional status such as anemia and chronic malnutrition. However, the use of repeated maternal weight checkups has not been proven to be a good predictor of IUGR.

SPECIFIC SYSTEMIC EXAMINATION

ABDOMINAL EXAMINATION

Approximate size of the fetus can be estimated on abdominal examination. Palpation of fetal head gives an estimation of fetal size and maturity. The diagnostic accuracy of abdominal palpation in predicting IUGR is limited. Thus, abdominal palpation itself should not be used for diagnosing IUGR. Instead, it should be used in combination with ultrasound parameters for diagnosing IUGR. The following findings may be observed on clinical examination:

- Failure to gain maternal weight

- Pregnant uterus feels small.
- SFH less than the period of amenorrhea by 3 cm
- Slow static growth on serial measurement of SFH on a customized chart
- Single SFH < 10th centile in a customized chart
- Presence of reduced liquor

Estimation of Symphysis–Fundus Height

Symphysis–fundus height is measured in centimeters from the upper edge of the symphysis pubis to the top of the fundus of the uterus. If the uterus is deviated toward one side, it should be stabilized in the middle using one hand, before taking measurement. While taking the measurement, the readings of the measurement tape should be facing the patient's abdomen and not the examiner in order to prevent the measurement bias. After 24 weeks of gestation, SFH corresponds to the period of gestation. A lag of 4 cm or more is suggestive of FGR. Ideally the SFH in centimeters should be plotted against the gestational age on the symphysis–fundus (S-F) growth curve **(Fig. 15.4)**. A customized fundal height chart, which is adjusted for various maternal variables including, height, weight, parity, ethnicity, etc., helps in improving the accuracy of SFH in predicting SGA fetus.

These charts may not be useful after 36 weeks of gestation. Due to the descent of the presenting part into the pelvis from 36 weeks of gestation onward, measurement of the SFH would no longer be accurate. At this time, even a reduction in the SFH may be observed.

The S-F growth curve compares the SFH with the period of gestation. The growth curve should preferably form part of the antenatal card. The middle line of the growth curve represents the 50th centile, whereas the upper and lower lines represent the 90th and 10th centiles, respectively. If intrauterine growth is normal, the SFH will fall between the 10th and 90th centiles. If IUGR is present, the SFH and the expected baby's weight would fall below the 10th centile.

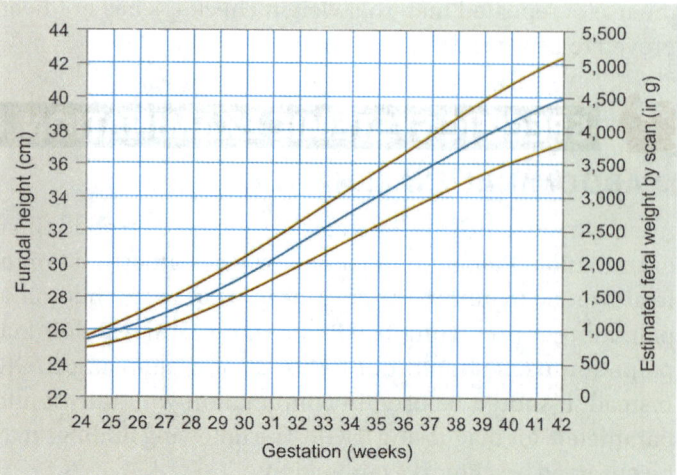

Fig. 15.4: Symphysis–fundus growth curves.

Growth restriction is also suggested when three successive measurements of fetal weight "plateau" at approximately the same level, without necessarily crossing below the 10th centile. Growth restriction is considered as severe when the discrepancy between the actual duration of pregnancy and that suggested by plotting SFH is 4 weeks or more.

If the baby's weight falls above the 90th centile, it points toward a macrosomic baby (see Chapter 19).

Like abdominal palpation, measurement of SFH is also associated with limited diagnostic accuracy in predicting a baby which would be affected by IUGR. Measurement of SFH is associated with low rates of sensitivity, high false-positive rates, and significant intra- and interobserver variations.

MANAGEMENT

Q. Write a long essay discussing the diagnosis and management of IUGR.

Q. With the help of a long essay, discuss management of pregnancy with IUGR.

Q. What should be the management of the patient described at the beginning of this chapter?
Ans. This appears to be a case of late-onset IUGR. The woman should be advised to come for regular antenatal visits at weekly intervals. She should be given a daily fetal movement count (DFMC) chart and instructed to record her fetal movements every day on that chart. She must be instructed to bring the chart with her at time of each antenatal visit. She must be advised to report immediately for checkup if at any time she perceived reduced fetal movements. Other tests for fetal surveillance in this case include biweekly NST, weekly BPP, monthly fetal ultrasound biometry, and Doppler analysis at every 2–3 weeks. Even if no abnormality is detected, there is little point in continuing pregnancy beyond 37 completed weeks of gestation. Labor must be induced at 37 completed weeks of gestation.

Q. The same patient presented again at 34 weeks with complaints of reduced fetal movements since last 10 days. However, she did not come immediately for checkup earlier due to some personal circumstances. Doppler analysis of umbilical arteries showed absent end diastolic blood flow. The pulsatility index of middle cerebral artery (MCA) was reduced. What is the next step of management of this case?
Ans. The fetus in this case appears to be in compromised state in view of reduced fetal movements and reduced amniotic fluid liquor. Doppler analysis of fetal vessels showing absent end-diastolic blood flow in umbilical arteries confirms the compromised state of the fetus. The pulsatility index (PI) of middle cerebral artery (MCA) is reduced, showing redistribution of blood to the fetal brain, indicating fetal distress. The possibility of fetal distress or fetal death appears to be likely. Therefore, decision should be made to immediately deliver the baby. In case of an unfavorable cervix, a cesarean section may be required.

Management comprising investigations and definitive obstetric management is discussed below. The initial workup plan in a patient with IUGR is described in **Flowchart 15.1**.

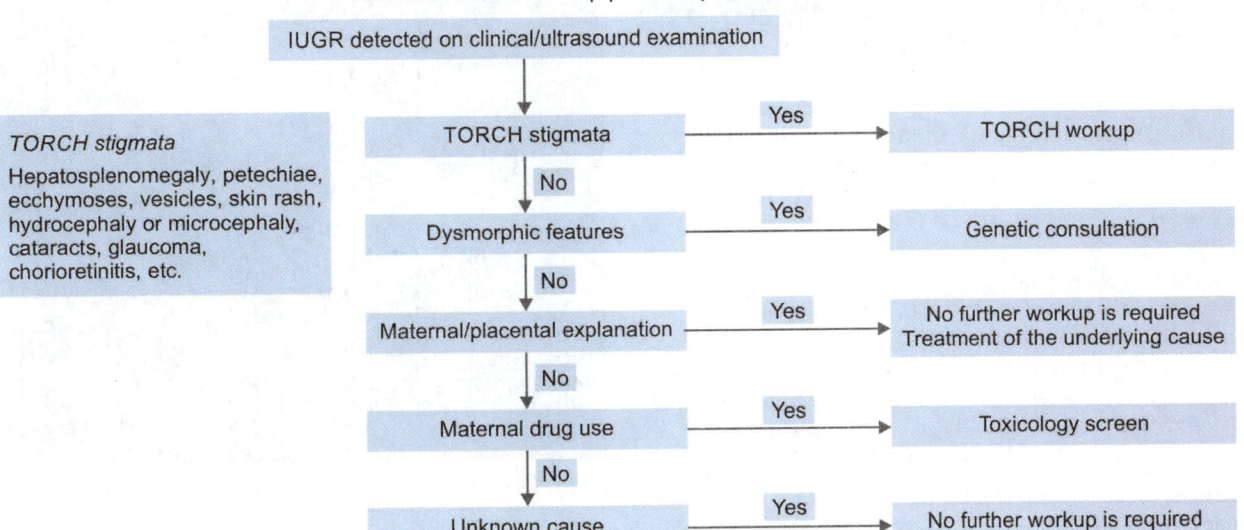

Flowchart 15.1: Workup plan in a patient with IUGR.

BOX 15.1: Ultrasound findings in an early-onset IUGR at 34 weeks.

Biometry
- EFW: 2,300 g (<10th percentile)
- HC/AC ratio: 1.35 (normal < 1.2)
- AFI: 7 cm (normal 10–20 cm)

Doppler ultrasound
- *Uterine artery:* Bilateral early diastolic notch
- Left uterine artery PI 1.97; right uterine artery PI 1.65
- *Umbilical artery:* Absent end-diastolic flow in both
- Smooth umbilical venous cord flow (peak velocity of 16 cm/s)
- MCA PI 1.12 (redistribution)
- *Ductus venosus:* Positive A wave 32 cm/s (normal)
- *BPP score:* 8/8 (normal)
- *Anatomic evaluation:* Short femurs, mildly echogenic bowel

(AC: abdominal circumference; AFI: amniotic fluid index; BPP: biophysical profile; EFW: estimated fetal weight; HC: head circumference; MCA: middle cerebral artery; PI: pulsatility index)

Box 15.1 enlists the ultrasound findings in an early-onset IUGR at 34 weeks.

INVESTIGATIONS

A distinction needs to be made between biometric tests (which help in measuring fetal size and gestational age) and biophysical tests (which help in assessing fetal well-being).

Biophysical tests are not important in measuring fetal growth but provide an important measure of fetal well-being. Various biometric and biophysical investigations for diagnosing IUGR are listed in **Table 15.9**. Each of these investigations would be described below in detail.

B-MODE IMAGING

Estimation of gestational age can be accurately done using ultrasound biometry. Besides the accurate dating of fetal gestation, ultrasound examination is also important for excluding serious congenital abnormalities in the fetus, estimating the amount of liquor, and ruling out multifetal gestation. The various ultrasound measurements and parameters which help in accurately predicting the gestational age are described below. Out of all these parameters, AC is considered to be the most accurate in predicting FGR.

According to the RCOG (2014), the fetal AC and expected fetal weight are the most accurate parameters determined using B-mode imaging used for predicting IUGR. Measurement of growth velocity using various ultrasound parameters is also useful in predicting FGR. For measurement of growth velocity, the interval between two individual scans must be about 3–4 weeks. Reduced growth velocity is defined as a fall of >50th percentile of AC or EFW. Ratio measurements [head circumference (HC)/AC or femur length (FL)/AC] are poorer than both AC and estimated birth weight in predicting FGR.

Crown-Rump Length

Crown-rump length (CRL) is an ultrasonic measurement, which is made earliest in pregnancy, when the gestational age is between 7 and 13 weeks (**Fig. 15.5**). The measurement of CRL of the fetus gives most accurate measurement of the gestational age. Early in pregnancy, the accuracy of determining gestational age through CRL measurement is within ±4 days, but later in pregnancy due to different growth rates of the fetus, the accuracy of determining gestational age with the help of ultrasound is less. In that situation, other parameters can be used in addition to CRL.

Biparietal Diameter

Biparietal diameter (BPD) is the distance between the two sides of the head. BPD can be measured at the level of the plane defined by the frontal horns of the lateral ventricles

302 Complications of Pregnancy

TABLE 15.9: Investigations for diagnosing IUGR.	
Biometric tests	**Biophysical tests**

• *Ultrasound biometry:*
  – AC
  – Ultrasound-estimated fetal weight
• *Invasive tests:*
  – Karyotyping
  – Screening for congenital infections
	• NST
	• BPP, amniotic fluid volume
	• Ultrasound Doppler flow velocimetry
	  – Umbilical artery:
	    - S/D ratio
	    - Resistance index
	    - Pulsatility index
	  – Middle cerebral artery
	  – Venous Doppler
	    - Reversal of blood flow in IVC, DV, and UV at the end of diastole
	• Fetal CTG

(AC: abdominal circumference; BPP: biophysical profile; CTG: cardiotocography; DV: ductus venosus; IVC: inferior vena cava; NST: nonstress test; S/D: systolic/diastolic; UV: umbilical vein)

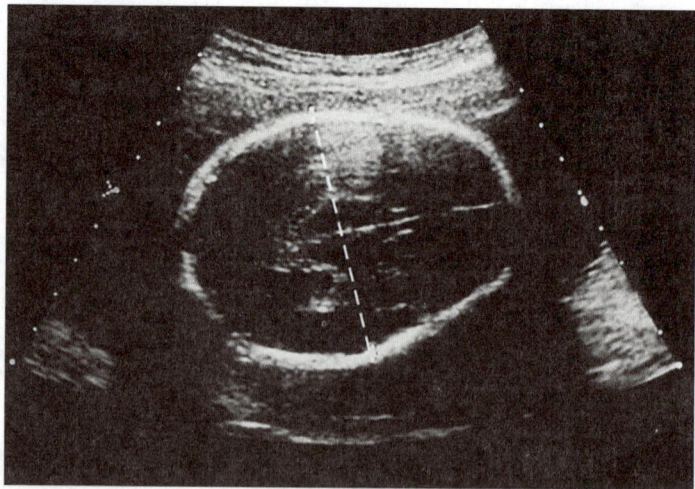

Fig. 15.6: Ultrasound measurement of biparietal diameter (BPD).

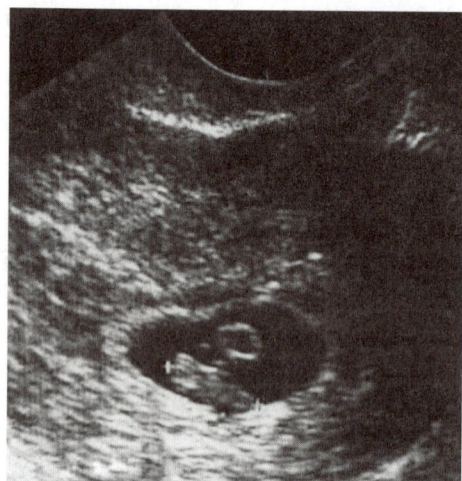

Fig. 15.5: Ultrasound measurement of CRL.

and the cavum septum pellucidum anteriorly, falx cerebri in the midline, the thalami symmetrically positioned on either side of the falx in the center and occipital horns of the lateral ventricles, Sylvian fissure, cisterna magna, and the insula posteriorly **(Fig. 15.6)**. Septum pellucidum can be visualized at one-third of the fronto-occipital distance. The measurement of BPD is taken from outer table of the proximal skull to the inner table of the distal skull with the septum cavum perpendicular to the ultrasound beam. BPD is usually measured after 13 weeks of pregnancy for dating of pregnancy. It increases from about 2.4 cm at 13 weeks to about 9.5 cm at term. Different babies of the same weight can have different head size; therefore, dating in the later part of pregnancy is generally considered unreliable.

The BPD remains the standard against which other parameters of gestational age assessment are compared. At 20 weeks of gestation, accuracy of BPD is within 1 week. It can be smaller (and sometimes much smaller than is expected) in fetuses with flatter heads. If the head really looks flat on the scan, the corrected BPD (in which the head area or circumference has been taken into consideration) is used. If the value of corrected BPD is within the normal range, then most likely the discrepancy is due to a flat head. The obstetrician must monitor the growth of the fetal head with the HC from then onward. The cephalic index (CI) will also be useful.

Corrected BPD

Corrected BPD can be calculated using the following formula:

$$\text{Corrected BPD} = \left(\frac{\text{BPD} \times \text{OFD}}{1.265} \right)^{1/2}$$

where, OFD = Occipitofrontal diameter.

The shape of fetal head can also be obtained by calculating the CI as follows:

$$\text{CI (\%)} = \frac{\text{BPD (outer to inner)}}{\text{OFD (outer to outer)}} \times 100$$

Cephalic index of <74% represents dolichocephaly (long-headed), whereas that of >83% represents brachycephaly (short-headed).

Occipitofrontal diameter is measured in the same plane as the BPD. However, instead of taking measurement from outer table to inner table, the measurement is taken from outer table of proximal skull to outer table of the distal skull.

Abdominal Circumference

Abdominal circumference is a measure of fetal abdominal girth. The AC is measured in an axial plane at the level of the stomach and the bifurcation of the main portal vein into the right and left branches **(Fig. 15.7)**. While measuring the AC, the radiologist must be careful about keeping the section

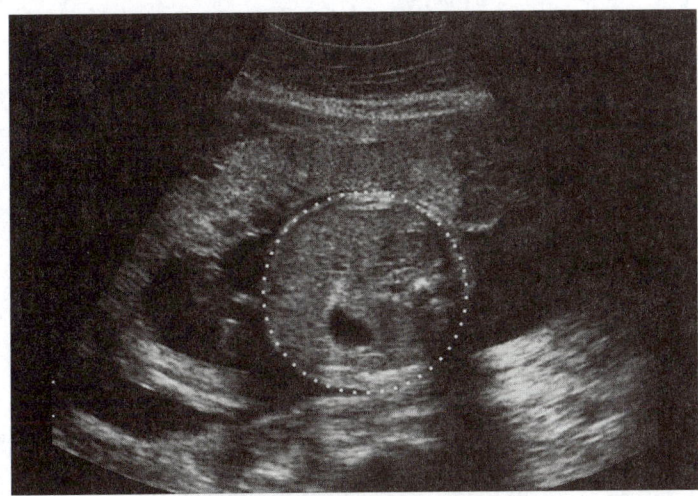

Fig. 15.7: Ultrasound measurement of abdominal circumference (AC).

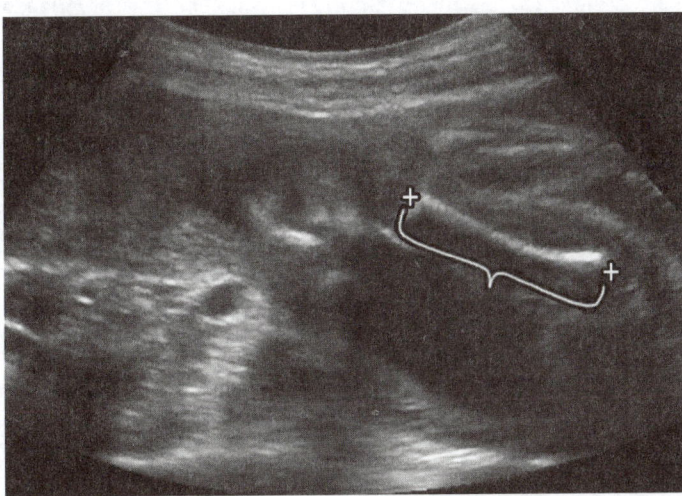

Fig. 15.8: Femoral length measurement on transvaginal sonography.

as round as possible and not letting it get deformed by the pressure from the probe.

Femur Length

Femur length is the length of femoral diaphysis, the longest bone in the body, and represents the longitudinal growth of the fetus. It is measured from the origin of the shaft to the distal end of the shaft, i.e., from greater trochanter to lateral femoral condyle **(Fig. 15.8)**. The femoral diaphysis should be horizontal, showing a homogeneous echogenicity.

The femoral head and distal femoral epiphysis present after 32 weeks are not included in the measurements. Its usefulness is similar to the BPD. Besides telling about the longitudinal growth of the fetus, measuring the FL also helps in excluding dwarfism in the fetus. The ultrasound ratio of AC/FL is an important measure of IUGR. The use of FL in dating is similar to the BPD and is not superior unless a good plane for the BPD cannot be obtained or that the head has an abnormal shape.

Fetal Ponderal Index

Fetal ponderal index (FPI) is another ultrasound-measured fetal index which is used for diagnosing IUGR. FPI is calculated with the help of the formula as described below:

$$FPI = \frac{\text{Estimated fetal weight}}{(\text{Femur length})^3}$$

ULTRASOUND-ESTIMATED FETAL WEIGHT

Some of the commonly used formulas for estimating fetal weight using various ultrasound parameters are described in **Table 15.10**. In clinical practice, estimation of fetal weight is usually based on Hadlock's formula.

TABLE 15.10: Ultrasound-based estimation of fetal weight.

Shepard's formula	Log10EFW = 1.2508 + (0.166 × BPD) + (0.046 × AC) − (0.002646 × AC × BPD)
Aoki's formula	EFW = (1.25647 × BPD3) + (3.50665 × FAA × FL) + 6.3
Hadlock's formula	Log10EFW = 1.3596 − 0.00386 (AC × FL) + 0.0064 (HC) + 0.00061 (BPD × AC) + 0.0425 (AC) + 0.174 (FL)

[AC: abdominal circumference (cm); BPD: biparietal diameter (cm); EFW: estimated fetal weight (g); FAA: fetal abdominal area (cm^2); FL: femur length (cm); HC: head circumference (cm)]

MEASURES OF FETAL SURVEILLANCE/ BIOPHYSICAL TESTS

Fetal surveillance measures include the biophysical tests which aim at identifying the fetus with IUGR before it becomes acidotic. Some of these measures have been enumerated in **Flowchart 15.2** and would be described below in detail.

Fetal surveillance is of utmost importance in cases of IUGR. The patient must be instructed to maintain a daily count of number of fetal movements she experiences. NST should be done biweekly. If NST is abnormal, BPP must be performed on weekly basis. Ultrasound for measuring fetal growth velocity must be carried out on bimonthly basis. Frequency of Doppler monitoring in IUGR fetuses need not be more than once every fortnightly.

ULTRASOUND DOPPLER FLOW VELOCIMETRY

> **Q.** Write a long essay on the role of Doppler in IUGR.

The evaluation of fetal well-being by Doppler velocimetry in cases of IUGR is of great importance as it is very useful in detecting those IUGR fetuses that are at high risk because of hypoxemia. Several Doppler studies which were initially

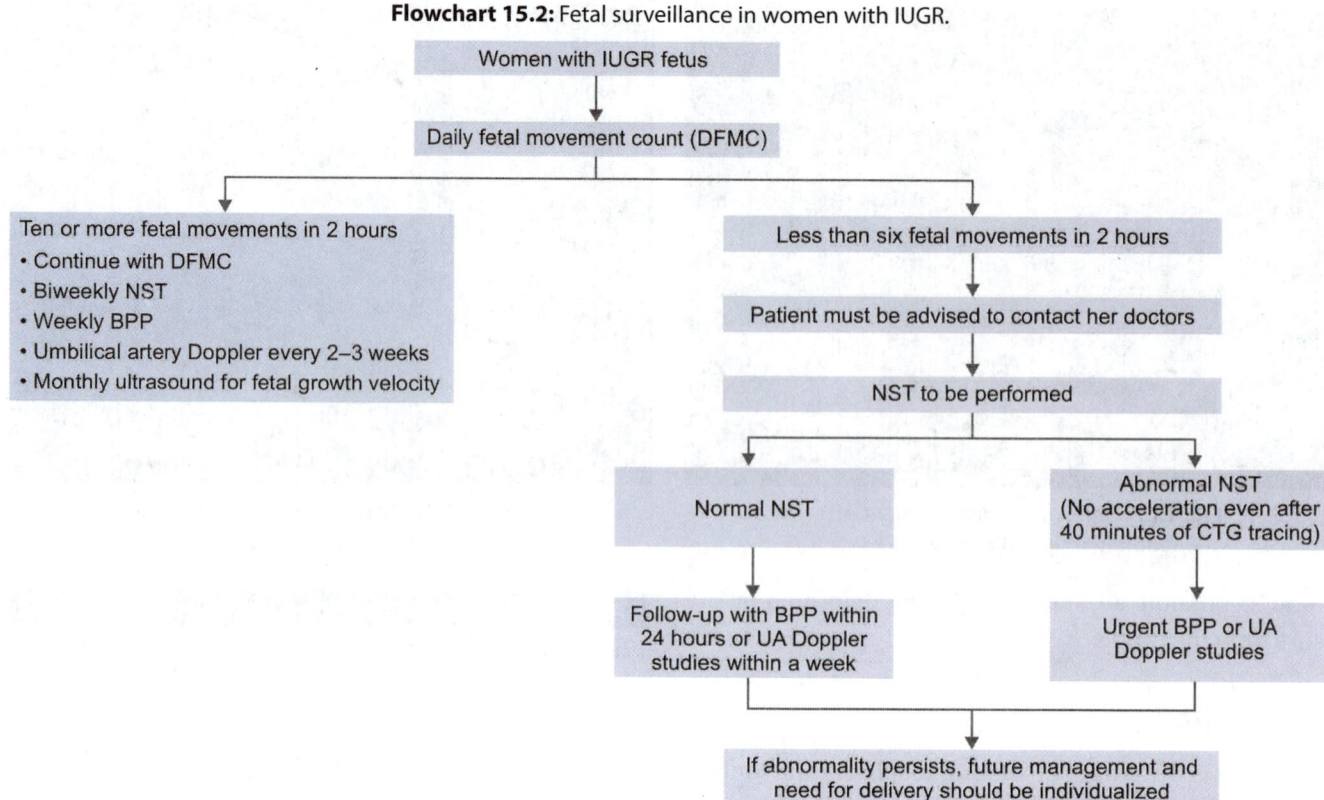

(BPP: biophysical profile; CTG: cardiotocography; IUGR: intrauterine growth restriction; NST: nonstress test; UA: umbilical artery)

TABLE 15.11: Summary of Doppler studies.	
Type of Doppler study	**Assessment**
Uterine artery and umbilical artery	Assessment of uteroplacental function
Middle cerebral artery	Assessment of fetal adaptation to hypoxia
Ductus venosus	Fetal cardiac status

performed on fetal arteries (umbilical arteries, uterine arteries, MCAs, etc.) and recently on the fetal venous system [ductus venosus (DV)] provide valuable information for the clinicians concerning the optimal time of delivery. The various types of indices which provide information regarding the amount of blood flow in various vessels are described in **Table 15.11** and **Figures 15.9A and B**.

Changes Occurring in Various Doppler Velocity Waveforms in Intrauterine Growth-restricted Fetuses

Umbilical artery Doppler serves as the primary surveillance tool for management of IUGR fetuses. The Doppler measurements from umbilical artery, uterine artery, MCA, and DV are important for diagnosing placental insufficiency. The major Doppler detectable modifications in the fetal circulation associated with IUGR and fetal hypoxemia include increased resistance in the umbilical artery, fetal peripheral vessels, and maternal uterine vessels, in association with decreased resistance in the fetal cerebral vessels **(Flowchart 15.3)**.

Uterine Artery Doppler

The uterine artery Doppler is indicative of uteroplacental circulation by showing the presence or absence of resistance to the blood flow. In normal pregnancy, both uterine artery in the placental bed and fetal umbilical artery circulations exhibit high diastolic flow velocities caused by low resistance **(Fig. 15.10)**. With advancing gestational age, there occurs trophoblastic invasion of the uterine spiral arteries, causing its dilatation and fall in the resistance to the blood flow. Uterine blood flow in a nonpregnant woman is about 50 mL/min and increases to 700 mL/min in the third trimester. Therefore, diastolic component in early pregnancy comprising low peak flow velocity and early diastolic notch is transformed into one with high peak flow velocity and no diastolic notch by midgestation, and PI value < 1.2. Abnormal uterine artery Doppler studies characterized by reduced diastolic flow suggest a maternal cause for IUGR. Increased resistance to the blood flow in uterine vessels, resulting in reduced diastolic flow, causes increased systolic/diastolic (S/D) ratio of flow velocities in uterine vessels. PI > 1.45 with bilateral diastolic notches is suggestive of clinically significant uteroplacental vascular ischemia **(Figs. 15.11A and B)**.

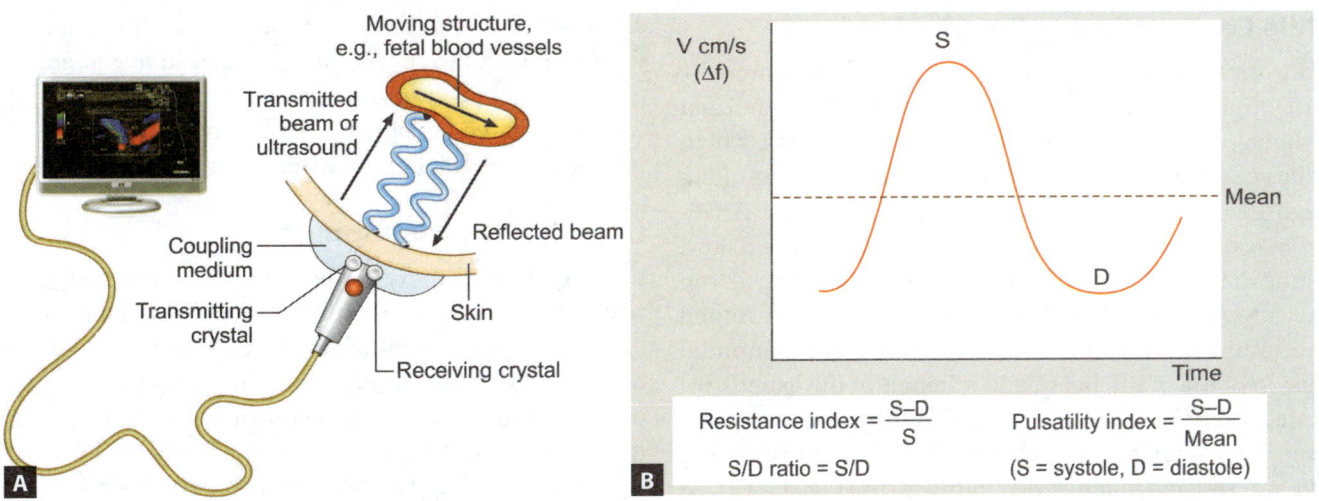

Figs. 15.9A and B: Doppler ultrasound. (A) Principle of Doppler ultrasound; (B) Description of various Doppler indices.

Resistance index = $\frac{S-D}{S}$ Pulsatility index = $\frac{S-D}{Mean}$

S/D ratio = S/D   (S = systole, D = diastole)

Flowchart 15.3: Changes occurring in various Doppler velocity waveforms in IUGR fetuses.

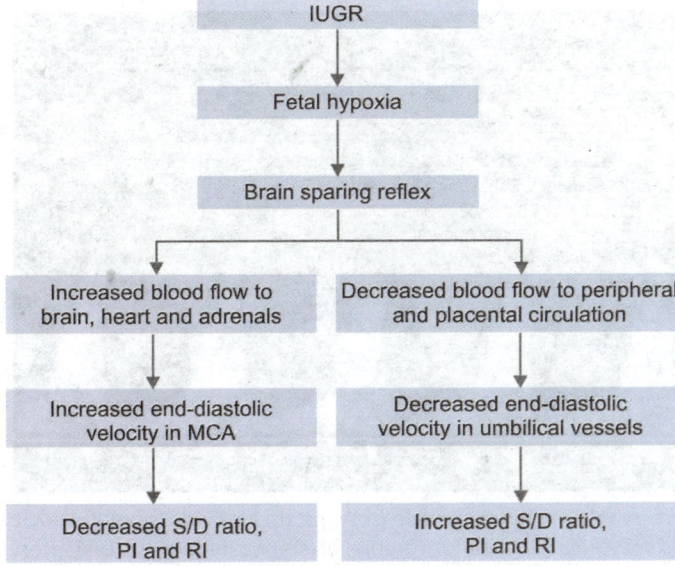

(MCA: middle cerebral artery; PI: pulsatility index; RI: resistance index; S/D: systolic/diastolic)

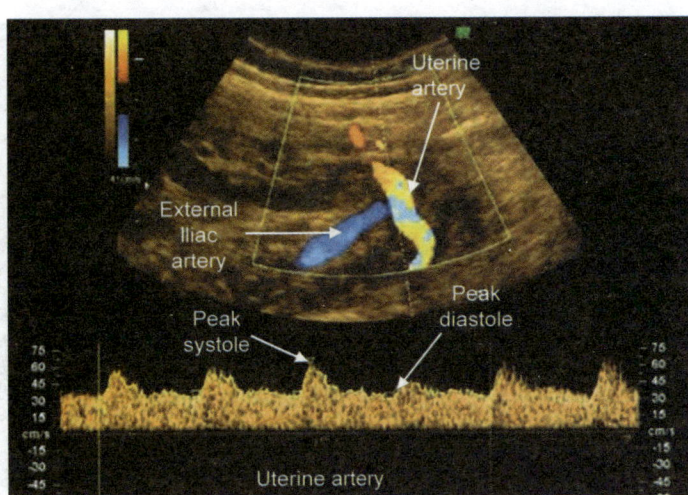

Fig. 15.10: Normal uterine artery Doppler analysis at 22 weeks' gestation.

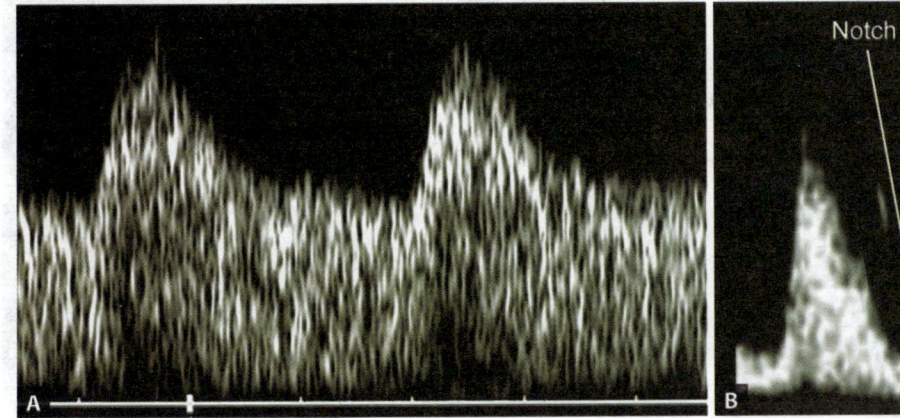

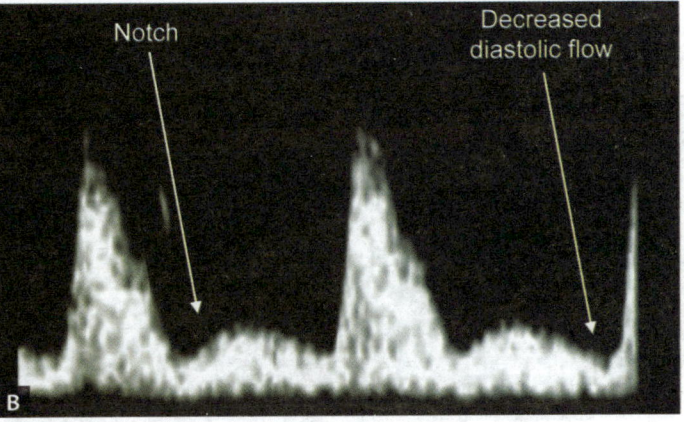

Figs. 15.11A and B: Uterine artery blood flow patterns. (A) Normal uterine artery blood flow; (B) Abnormal uterine artery Doppler waveforms with decreased diastolic flow and early diastolic notching.

Middle Cerebral Artery Doppler Studies

Middle cerebral artery can be easily demonstrated by color Doppler in transverse fetal head position. In normal pregnancy, at 28–30 weeks, MCA is characterized by high systolic velocities and minimal diastolic velocities, resulting in high PI values > 1.45 **(Figs. 15.12A and B)**. In IUGR, deficiency of oxygen causes the redistribution of blood flow, resulting in increased blood flow to the brain causing a drop in the cerebral resistance. These changes can be attributed to the "brain sparing effect," in which there is preferential perfusion of the brain, heart, and adrenals at the expense of the integument and viscera, gut, and kidneys in the hypoxic fetuses. This leads to a decrease in the S/D ratio as well as the PI and resistance index (RI) in the MCA **(Fig. 15.13)**. At the same time, there is reduced flow to the peripheral and placental circulations, resulting in decreased end diastolic velocity in umbilical vessels and thereby increase in the S/D ratio, PI, and RI. With the worsening of the fetal condition, as the blood flow to the brain also reduces, MCA blood flow velocity may return to normal. Changes in the cerebral flow parameters, however, have not been observed to correlate with the degree of asphyxic compromise. Therefore, these parameters are not helpful in choosing timing for delivery.

Umbilical Artery Doppler

In normal pregnancy, the placental vascular bed is a low-resistance bed, where impedance decreases with the advancing gestational age. The assessment of umbilical blood flow provides information regarding blood perfusion of the fetoplacental unit. In normal pregnancy, the fetal umbilical circulation is characterized by continuous forward flow **(Fig. 15.14)**. Characteristic umbilical blood flow has sawtooth appearance of arterial flow in one direction and continuous umbilical venous blood flow in the other **(Fig. 15.15A)**. The S/D ratio serves as an index of measurement, which compares the systolic with diastolic

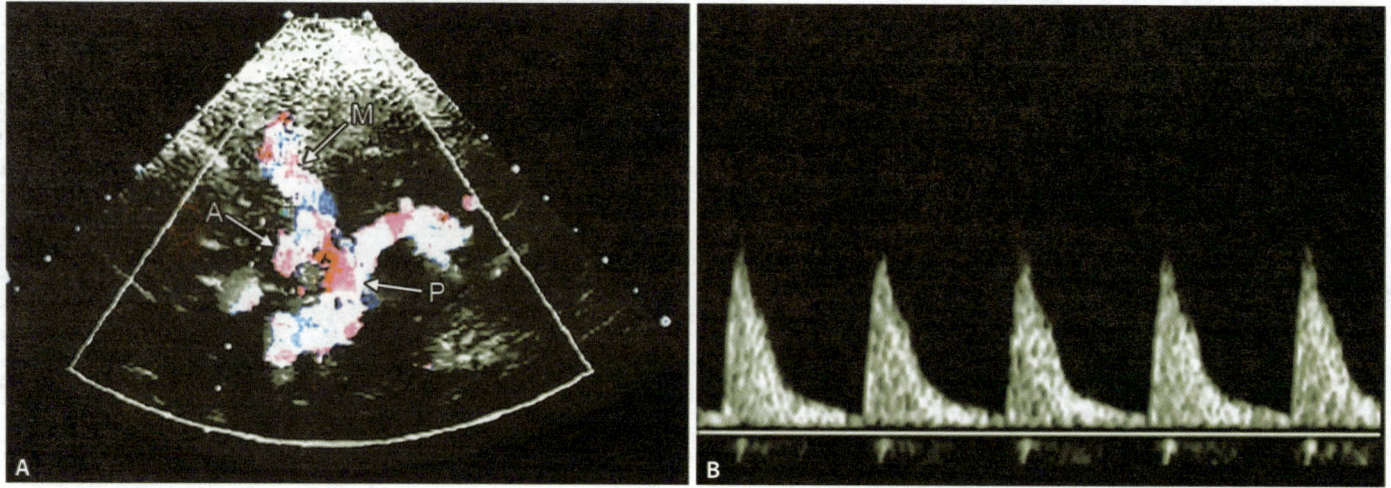

Figs. 15.12A and B: (A) Color Doppler evaluation of middle cerebral artery (MCA) showing circle of Willis; (B) Normal Doppler velocity waveforms in MCA showing high systolic velocities and minimal diastolic velocities. (A: anterior cerebral artery; M: middle cerebral artery; P: posterior cerebral artery)

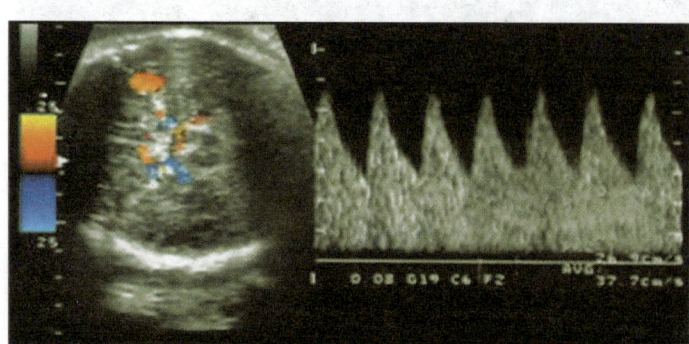

Fig. 15.13: Increased diastolic flow in the middle cerebral artery during the initial stages of IUGR due to the brain sparing effect.

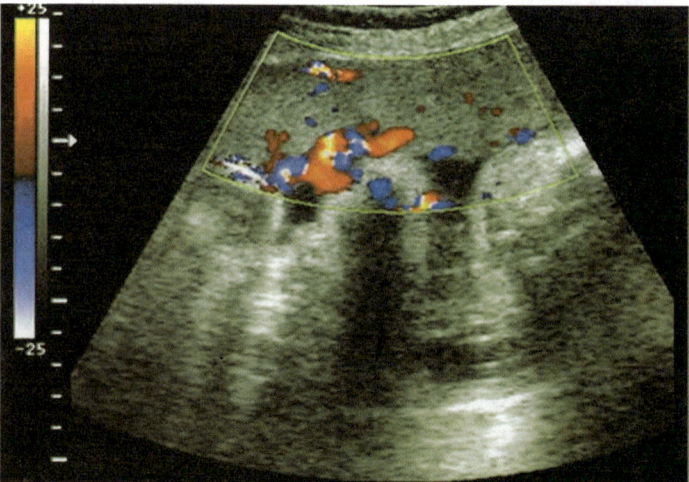

Fig. 15.14: Umbilical artery circulation on color Doppler ultrasonography.

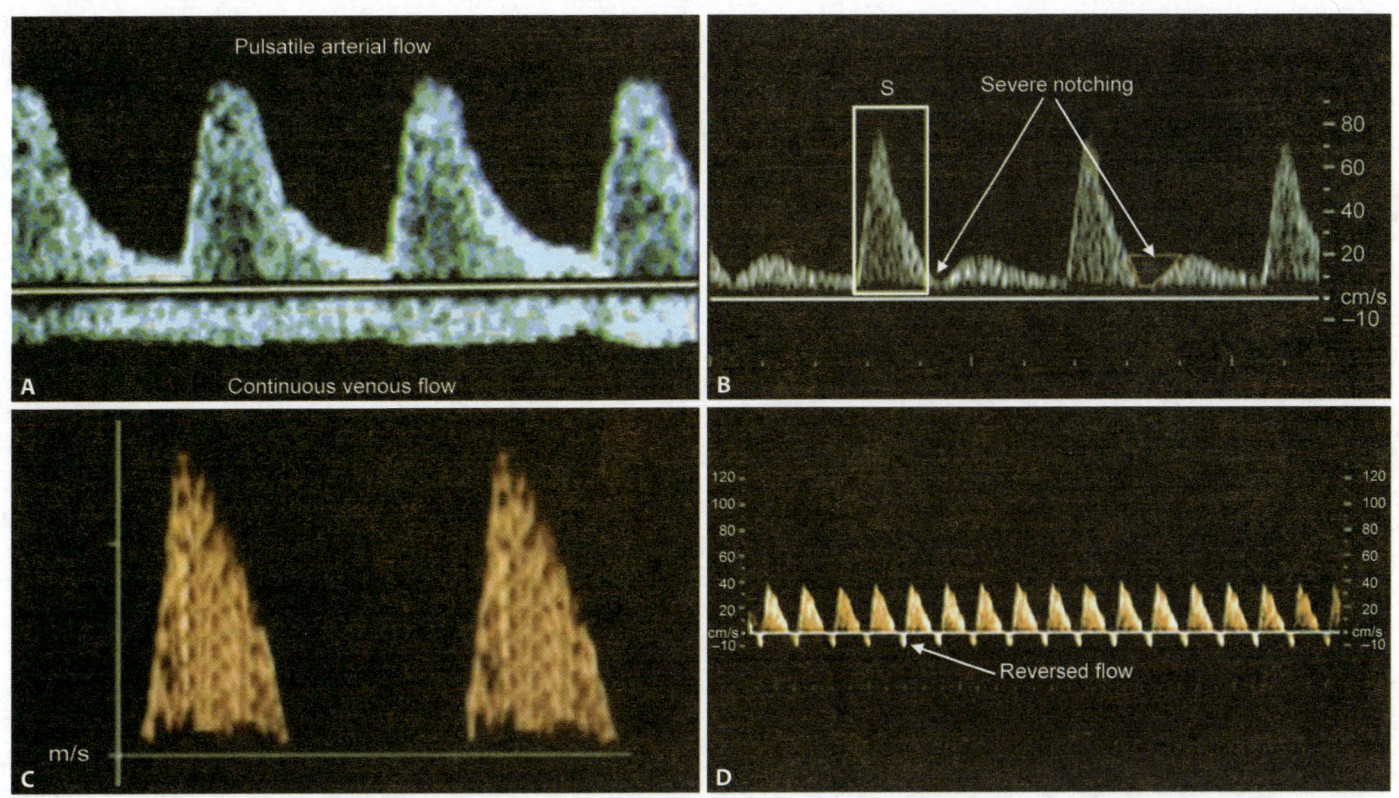

Figs. 15.15A to D: Umbilical artery blood flow patterns. (A) Normal umbilical artery Doppler ultrasound waveforms; (B) Early diastolic notching; (C) Absent end-diastolic flow; (D) Reversed end-diastolic flow.

TABLE 15.12: Types of Doppler indices.	
Doppler index	**Calculation of Doppler index**
S/D ratio (Stuart, 1980)	Peak systolic blood flow/end diastolic velocity
PI (Pourcelot, 1974)	(Peak systolic velocity—end-diastolic velocity)/mean systolic velocity
RI (Gosling and King, 1977)	(Peak systolic velocity—end-diastolic velocity)/peak systolic velocity

(PI: pulsatility index; RI: resistance index; S/D: systolic/diastolic)

flow in the umbilical arteries and identifies the amount of resistance in the placental vasculature. The end diastolic blood flow in umbilical artery increases with advancing gestation in normal pregnancies. As a result, there is a decline in both PI and S/D ratio with increasing gestation. As resistance decreases, RI values approach zero. On the other hand, when the resistance increases, end diastolic flow approaches zero; therefore, RI approaches one. If the end diastolic flow is absent, according to the equations mentioned in **Table 15.12**, S/D ratio would be equal to infinity and RI would be equal to one. Therefore in these cases, the blood flow is assessed with the help of PI.

In cases of IUGR (especially due to placental insufficiency) if the resistance to blood flow does not decrease sufficiently, the umbilical circulation is characterized by the presence of abnormal S/D ratio, PI, or RI. The umbilical artery indices are considered as abnormal if they become >95th percentile for the gestational age or there may be early diastolic notching (**Fig. 15.15B**) or the end-diastolic flow may be either absent or reversed (**Figs. 15.15C and D**). Generally, an S/D ratio of ≤3.0 is considered as normal. A rising S/D ratio indicates a worsening fetal prognosis and warrants a closer, more frequent monitoring. Absent end-diastolic waveforms in umbilical arteries imply that nearly 75% of the vascular bed has been obliterated. There are 85% chances that the fetus would be hypoxemic. Reverse end diastolic frequencies, on the other hand, are associated with a ten-fold increase in perinatal mortality. Abnormal waveforms on umbilical artery Doppler ultrasound should be followed-up with methods for enhanced fetal surveillance or delivery. Various changes in Doppler waveform analysis with increased resistance in umbilical vessels are summarized in **Box 15.2**.

Ductus Venosus Doppler

The DV (**Fig. 15.16**) is a very important part of fetal venous circulation. This vessel acts as a shunt and helps in directly connecting the umbilical vein to the inferior vena cava (IVC). The fetus receives oxygenated blood from the mother through placenta in the form of umbilical veins. As this oxygenated blood bypasses DV, some of the oxygenated blood goes to the liver, but most of it bypasses the liver and empties directly into the IVC, which enters the right atrium. This highly oxygenated and nutrient-rich umbilical venous blood is eventually supplied to the fetal brain and myocardium instead of the fetal liver. It has been estimated that during the periods of fetal hypoxia, a compensatory mechanism occurs. This results in transient dilatation of the ductus, which is supposed to increase oxygenated blood flowing through it during these periods of hypoxia or reduced umbilical flow. In order to increase the cerebral blood flow at the time of hypoxia, the blood flow shunted through the DV increases and could amount to as much as 70% of the umbilical blood flow.

However, in normal pregnancies with increasing gestation there is significant reduction in the umbilical blood flow shunted through the DV from 40% at 20 weeks of gestation to 15% at 38 weeks of gestation. This is so, as late in normal pregnancy DV plays a less important role in shunting well-oxygenated blood to the brain and myocardium in comparison to that in the early gestation. The typical waveform for the blood flow in the venous vessels consists of three phases related to cardiac cycle **(Figs. 15.17A and B)**. Peak S wave corresponds to ventricular systole, peak D wave to early diastole, and peak A wave to atrial contraction **(Fig. 15.17B)**. In normal fetuses, the blood flow in DV is always in the forward direction throughout the cardiac cycle **(Fig. 15.17A)**. Forward blood flow in the venous system is a function of cardiac compliance, contractibility, and afterload. A decline in forward velocities in venous system results in increased Doppler indices and suggests impaired circulation. An absence or even reversal of the A waves in the DV is the hallmark of the advancing circulatory deterioration since this documents the inability of the heart to accommodate venous return **(Fig. 15.18)**.

Since the DV shunt would increase during fetal hypoxia, examination of dilated DV would help in the identification of patients with IUGR, preeclampsia, etc., who are at a high risk for fetal distress. The presence or absence of fetal cardiac failure secondary to hypoxia and acidosis is indicated by Doppler studies of DV.

Sequence of Changes Occurring in Various Doppler Velocity Waveforms in IUGR Fetuses

Doppler velocimetry is one of the best methods of fetal surveillance during IUGR and helps in diagnosing the

> **BOX 15.2:** Changes in umbilical blood flow with increasing vascular resistance.
> - Elevated pulsatility index and resistance index
> - Early diastolic notch **(Fig. 15.15B)**
> - Absent end-diastolic blood flow **(Fig. 15.15C)**
> - Reversed end-diastolic blood flow **(Fig. 15.15D)**

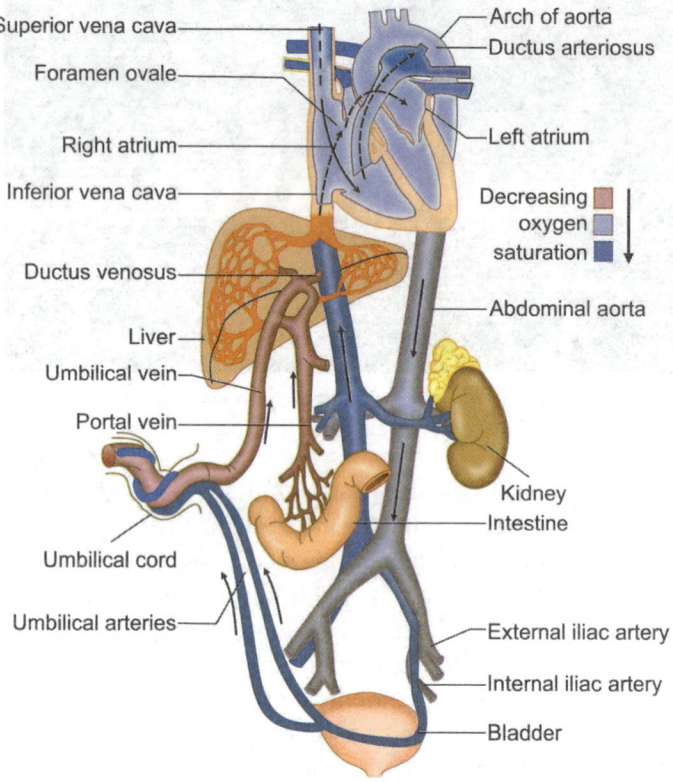

Fig. 15.16: Fetal circulation just before birth showing ductus venosus.

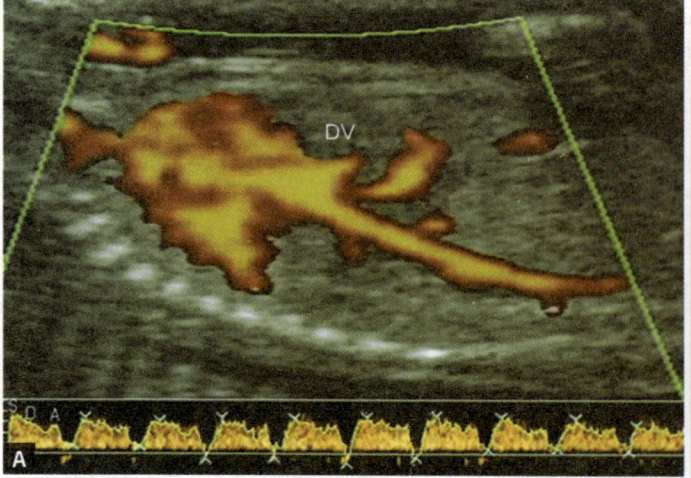
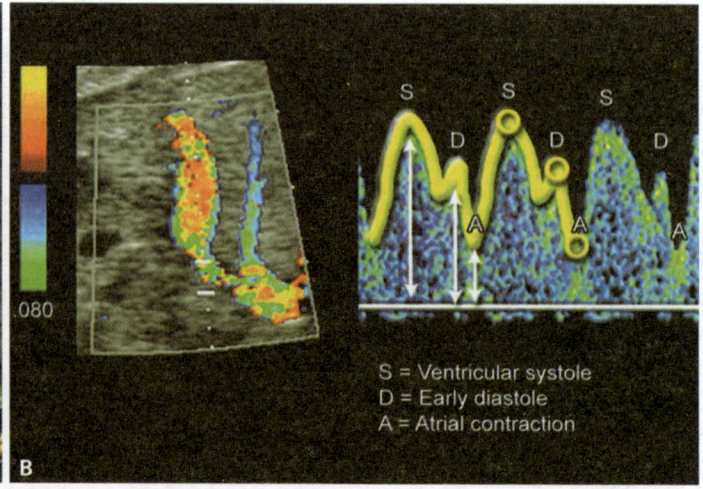

Figs. 15.17A and B: Blood flow in ductus venosus (DV). (A) Normal blood flow in the DV; (B) Normal DV waveform at 25 weeks of gestation showing S, D, and A wave with positive flow during atrial contraction.

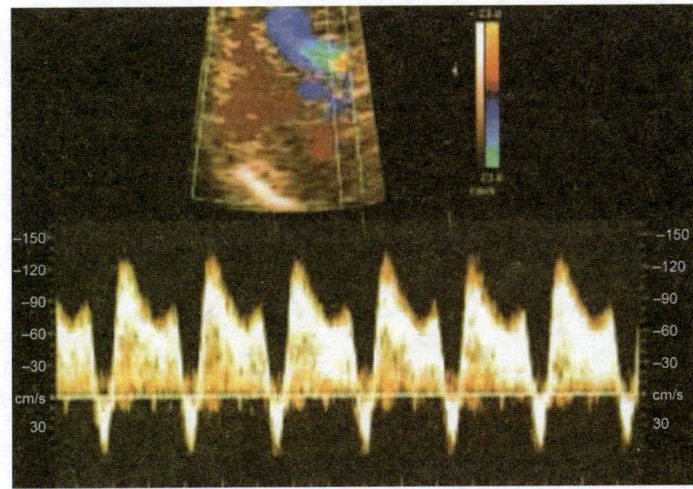

Fig. 15.18: Reversed blood flow during atrial contraction in the ductus venosus.

TABLE 15.13: Volume of amniotic fluid inside the amniotic cavity (based on ultrasound findings).

Amount of amniotic fluid	Total amount of amniotic fluid	Maximum vertical pool of liquor	AFI
Normal	700 mL to 1L at full term	Adequate fluid, seen everywhere	5–25 cm
Oligohydramnios	<200 mL of amniotic fluid	Maximum vertical pool of liquor < 2 cm	<5 cm
Polyhydramnios	Amniotic fluid volume of 2,000 mL or greater at term	Presence of maximum vertical fluid pocket seen >8 cm in diameter	>25 cm

associated fetal acidosis and hypoxia. The sequences of changes occurring in fetal vessels occur in parallel to the extent of the fetal compromise. Initially, there is appearance of changes on fetal artery Doppler analysis, followed by changes on fetal venous Doppler analysis. This is followed by changes on BPP and CTG. The usual order of the findings on CTG trace indicating fetal hypoxia include the initial loss of accelerations, followed by decreasing variability and the presence of late decelerations. The arterial changes on Doppler analysis are indicative of brain damage, whereas venous changes point toward fetal heart failure. The normal placental sufficiency is indicated by normal Doppler waveforms in the uterine, umbilical, and fetal MCAs. Increased S/D ratio in the uterine artery suggests increased resistance at the maternal end, whereas increased S/D ratio in the umbilical artery suggests increased resistance at the fetal end.

CEREBROPLACENTAL RATIO

Cerebroplacental ratio (CPR) can be defined as the ratio of PI of MCA and umbilical artery. It reflects provision of oxygenated blood to the brain. CPR values of <5th centile indicate redistribution of blood flow or centralization of flow. Therefore, CPR values of <5th centile are associated with a higher risk of cesarean delivery for fetal distress, low Apgar scores, and higher rates of admission to the NICU.

AMNIOTIC FLUID VOLUME

Measurement of amniotic fluid volume is an important method of fetal surveillance. Estimation of amniotic fluid can be done in two ways: maximal vertical pocket depth of amniotic fluid and AFI. The classification of amniotic fluid volume based on these two parameters is shown in **Table 15.13**. Determination of maximal vertical pool of liquor involves the measurement of maximum vertical diameter of the deepest pocket of amniotic fluid identified upon ultrasound examination. AFI is obtained by measuring the vertical depth of the largest fluid pockets in each of the four uterine quadrants. These four measurements are added in order to obtain a total AFI. The AFI uses the 5th and 95th percentiles for gestational age to signify oligohydramnios and polyhydramnios, respectively. If the AFI measures <5 cm (5th centile), the pregnant woman is supposed to have oligohydramnios.

If amniotic fluid levels add up to >25 cm (95th centile), she is supposed to have polyhydramnios. The use of amniotic fluid volume evaluation has become important in the assessment of pregnancy at risk for an adverse pregnancy outcome as it forms basis of two important tests of fetal well-being used commonly, namely the BPP and the modified BPP, both of which include ultrasound estimation of amniotic fluid volume. If the amount of amniotic fluid is reduced, the frequency of NST must be increased.

NONSTRESS TEST

The fetal NST is a simple, noninvasive test performed in pregnancies over 28 weeks of gestation. The test is named "nonstress" because no stress is placed on the fetus during the test. Antepartum NST performed on weekly basis may be considered as a method of fetal surveillance in IUGR fetuses.

Procedure

1. The test involves attaching one belt to the mother's abdomen to measure FHR and another belt to measure uterine contractions **(Fig. 15.19A)**. Fetal movement, heart rate, and "reactivity" of fetal heart (acceleration of FHR) are measured for 20–30 minutes. If the baby does not move, it does not necessarily indicate that there is a problem; the baby could just be asleep.
2. The mother is handed a probe, which she is asked to press whenever she feels a fetal movement. The fetal heart tracing is observed for FHR accelerations that peak

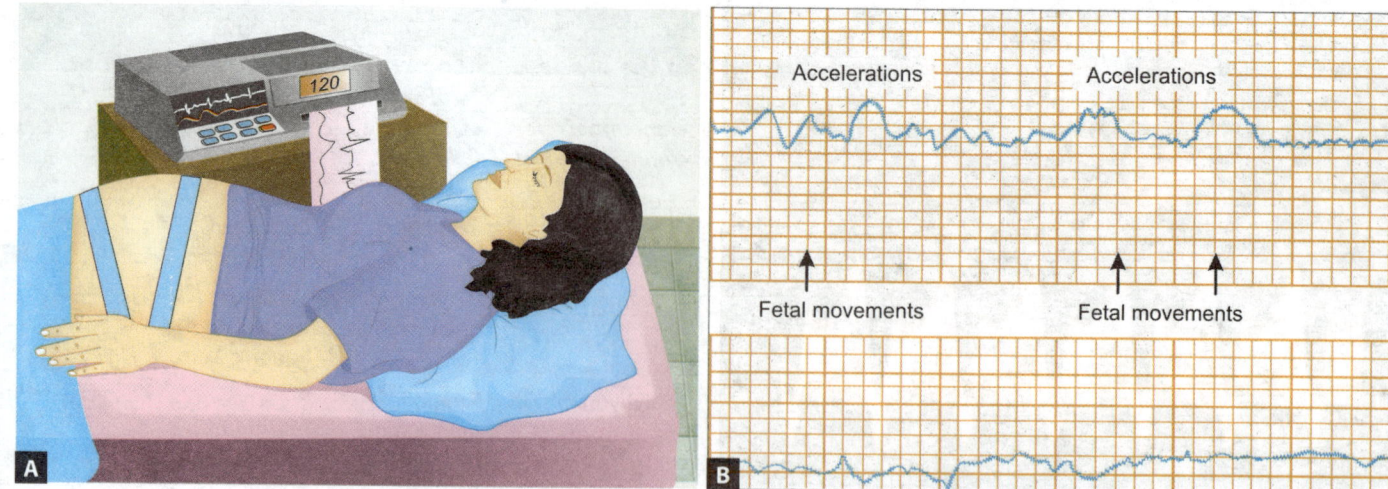

Figs. 15.19A and B: NST. (A) Procedure of performing an NST; (B) Reactive NST.

(but do not necessarily remain) at least 15 beats/min above the baseline and last for 15 seconds from baseline to baseline. NST is defined as reactive if there is a presence of two or more accelerations that peak 15 beats/min above the baseline, each lasting for 15 seconds or more and all occurring within a 20-minute period from beginning the test **(Fig. 15.19B)**. Fetal movement may or may not be recognized by the patient. The test is defined as nonreactive if there are no FHR accelerations over a 40-minute period **(Table 15.14)**.

3. It may be necessary to continue the tracing for 40 minutes or longer to take into account the average period of nonrapid eye movement (NREM) sleep when fetal movement and subsequently heart rate variability are reduced.
4. When the fetal heart tracing is continued for 40 minutes, it is termed as an "extended NST."

Implications of a Reactive (Normal) Nonstress Test

A reactive nonstress result indicates fetal well-being, i.e., the fetus is receiving an adequate supply of blood and oxygen. In most cases, a normal NST is predictive of good perinatal outcome for 1 week (provided that the fetomaternal condition remains stable), except in women with IUGR, in which case, NSTs are recommended at least twice weekly.

Implications of a Nonreactive (Abnormal) Nonstress Test

A nonreactive test could be due to fetal hypoxia or fetal inactivity (i.e., fetal sleep patterns, certain maternal drugs). A nonreactive NST does not indicate definite fetal compromise. It just requires additional testing to determine whether the result is truly due to poor oxygenation, or whether there are other reasons for fetal nonreactivity. The additional testing can be in the form of prolonged NST, a contraction stress test, or a BPP.

TABLE 15.14: Classification of NST as either reactive or nonreactive.

Test result	Interpretation
Reactive nonstress	If there are accelerations of the FHR of at least 15 beats/min over the baseline, lasting for at least 15 seconds, occurring within a 20-minute time block
Nonreactive nonstress	If these accelerations do not occur, the test is said to be nonreactive. Additional testing may be required to determine whether the result is truly due to poor oxygenation

BIOPHYSICAL PROFILE

When the primary surveillance with umbilical artery Doppler is abnormal, BPP is likely to be a useful surveillance tool as it has good negative predictive value in high-risk populations. The BPP was first described by Manning in 1980. It utilizes multiple ultrasound parameters of fetal well-being and NST. It is more accurate than a single test as it correlates five measurements to give a score. As a result, it is associated with much lower rates of false positives and false negatives. The ultrasound parameters of the test are fetal tone, fetal movement, fetal breathing, and amniotic fluid volume. **Table 15.15** and **Figure 15.20** show the parameters of each observation. An NST, which is not an ultrasonic measurement, is also performed. Two points are given if the observation is present, and zero points are given if it is absent. A BPP test score of at least 8 out of 10 is considered as reassuring. A score of 6 or 7 out of 10 is equivocal and must be repeated within 24 hours. A score of 4 or less out of 10 is a positive test and strongly indicates fetal compromise. If the BPP falls below 4, the patient should be urgently prepared for delivery. Initially, the performance of a BPP score included analysis of all five components in every pregnancy. Of the various parameters recorded by BPP, the first one to get affected is NST, followed by fetal breathing, fetal movements, and lastly the fetal tone. First sign of acidosis (cord arterial pH < 7.2) was thought to result in an abnormal NST and absent fetal breathing. Advanced or chronic acidosis was thought

Intrauterine Growth Restriction

TABLE 15.15: BPP criteria.

Component	Score of 2	Score of 0
Amniotic fluid volume	Single vertical pocket of amniotic fluid > 2 cm in two perpendicular planes	Largest vertical pocket of amniotic fluid is 2 cm or less
Fetal breathing movements	One or more episodes of rhythmic fetal breathing movements of 30 seconds or more within 30 minutes	Abnormal, absent, or insufficient breathing movements
Fetal movement	Three or more discrete body or limb movements within 30 minutes	Abnormal, absent, or insufficient movements
Fetal tone	At least one episode of flexion extension of fetal extremity with return to flexion, or opening or closing of hand within 30 minutes	Abnormal, absent, or insufficient fetal tone
NST	Reactive (normal)	Nonreactive (abnormal)

(BPP: biophysical profile; NST: nonstress test)

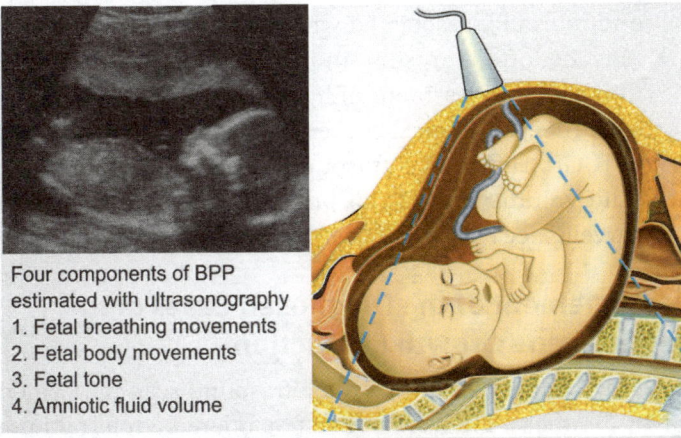

Four components of BPP estimated with ultrasonography
1. Fetal breathing movements
2. Fetal body movements
3. Fetal tone
4. Amniotic fluid volume

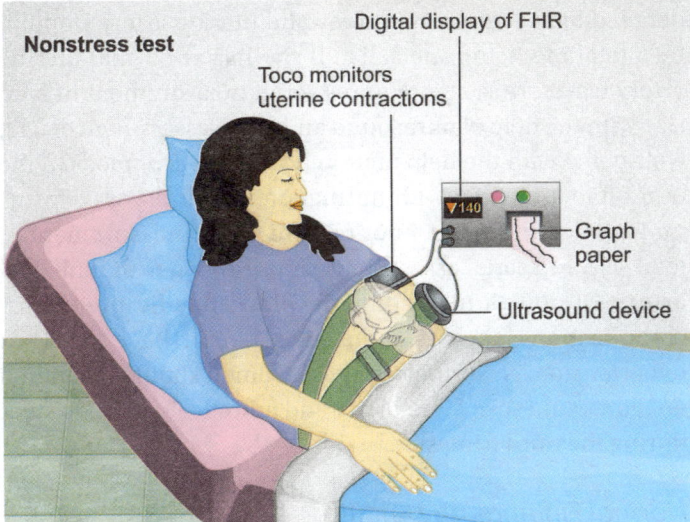

Fig. 15.20: Components of BPP.

to compromise fetal tone and movement. Assessment of amniotic fluid volume helps in quick evaluation of long-term uteroplacental function as in the late second and all through the third trimester, amniotic fluid is essentially fetal urine. With uteroplacental dysfunction, redistribution of blood flow takes place. This leads to decreased renal perfusion and thus oligohydramnios. Manning described the modified BPP in 1990, combining an NST, amniotic fluid volume, and fetal breathing. It was less cumbersome than the original BPP, and its results were just as predictive.

However, the recent approach is to carry out only the ultrasound components of the test in the beginning. If there appears to be an abnormality in either of the ultrasound components, NST is performed. If all the ultrasound components are within normal limits, there is no need to perform an NST. This approach is based on the fact that the ultrasound fluid index is the indicator of long-term uteroplacental function, while the NST is the short-term indicator of fetal acid–base status. Weekly BPP is recommended for evaluation of fetal well-being in the pregnancies complicated with IUGR.

Modified Biophysical Profile

In the late second or third trimester fetus, amniotic fluid volume reflects fetal urine production. Placental dysfunction may result in diminished fetal renal perfusion, leading to oligohydramnios. Amniotic fluid volume assessment can therefore be used to evaluate long-term uteroplacental function.

This observation encouraged the development of "modified BPP" as a primary method for antepartum fetal surveillance. The modified BPP combines NST (with the option of acoustic stimulation in case of nonreactive NST after 20 minutes) with the AFI. While NST is a short-term indicator of fetal acid–base status, the AFI serves as an indicator of long-term placental function. An AFI > 5 cm is generally considered to represent an adequate volume of amniotic fluid. Thus, the modified BPP is considered normal if the NST is reactive and the AFI is >5 and abnormal if either the NST is nonreactive or the AFI is 5 or less. If the results of a modified BPP indicate a possible abnormality, then the full BPP is performed.

PRENATAL SCREENING

The Society of Obstetricians and Gynecologists of Canada (2014) in a joint guideline with the Canadian College of Medical Geneticists (CCMG) has recommended that screening early in pregnancy may help identify those pregnancies at risk for chromosomal anomalies, which may be associated with SGA, IUGR, and stillbirths. Noninvasive screening (serum alpha fetoprotein levels and/or ultrasound examination) for trisomy 13, 18, and 21 may be done through first-trimester or second-trimester screening.

TREATMENT/OBSTETRIC MANAGEMENT

PREVENTION

Interventions to be considered in the prevention of SGA fetuses are as follows:

- *Lifestyle and dietary modifications:* Presently, there is no reliable evidence that dietary modification, or the use of agents such as progesterone or calcium, may help in preventing birth of an SGA infant and therefore must not be used in these cases. However, the use of interventions, which help in cessation of smoking, may prevent delivery of an SGA infant. Therefore, these interventions should be offered to all pregnant women who smoke.
- *Antiplatelet agents:* They may be effective in preventing SGA birth in women who are at a high risk of preeclampsia. Therefore, in women at a high risk of preeclampsia, antiplatelet agents should be started at 16 weeks of pregnancy.
- *Antithrombotic therapy:* Though presently there is insufficient evidence regarding the use of antithrombotic therapy in cases of SGA infants, it might have some role in preventing delivery of SGA babies in high-risk pregnancy. However, its use may be associated with serious adverse effects. Therefore, its use is usually not recommended.

ANTENATAL PERIOD

The first step in the management of these patients is identifying the underlying risk factors for IUGR.

Identification of Major Risk Factors

Women who have a major risk factor (OR > 2.0) as described in **Table 15.8** should be referred for serial ultrasound examination involving the measurement of fetal size as well as assessment of well-being with umbilical artery Doppler from 26 to 28 weeks of gestation.

Identification of a Minor Risk Factor

Women who have three or more minor risk factors **(Table 15.8)** should be referred for uterine artery Doppler at 20–24 weeks of gestation. Subsequent normalization of flow velocity indices in women with an abnormal uterine artery Doppler at 20–24 weeks of pregnancy is still associated with an increased risk of an IUGR fetus. Therefore, repeating uterine artery Doppler is associated with limited value. Serial ultrasound measurement of fetal size and assessment of well-being with umbilical artery Doppler starting at 26–28 weeks of pregnancy must be done in women who have an abnormal uterine artery Doppler at 20–24 weeks (defined as a PI > 95th percentile) and/or notching.

- Women must be advised to take rest in the left lateral position for a period of at least 10 hours every day.
- *Daily fetal movement count:* In case the woman perceives <6 fetal movements within 2 hours, she should be advised to immediately consult her doctor.
- *Fetal surveillance in IUGR fetuses:* Umbilical artery Doppler should be considered as the primary tool for surveillance in case of IUGR fetuses. Its use in high-risk population has been shown to reduce perinatal morbidity and mortality associated with IUGR. Oligohydramnios may be often present in IUGR fetuses. Therefore, ultrasound assessment of liquor volume, based on the single deepest vertical pocket, is often performed in cases of IUGR. However, ultrasound assessment of amniotic fluid volume should not be used as the only form of surveillance in SGA fetuses.

Management of the Diagnosed Cases of Intrauterine Growth Restriction

If IUGR is identified during the ultrasound scan performed at 18–20 weeks, the woman must be offered a referral for a detailed fetal anatomical survey and uterine artery Doppler by a fetal medicine specialist. If she has abnormal uterine artery waveforms, she requires serial measurement of fetal size with the help of ultrasound and serial assessment of fetal well-being with the help of umbilical artery Doppler. On the other hand, women with normal uterine artery waveforms on Doppler analysis do not require serial measurement of fetal size and serial assessment of well-being with umbilical artery Doppler unless they develop specific pregnancy complications, such as antepartum hemorrhage (APH) or hypertension. Nevertheless, these women should be offered an ultrasound scan for fetal size and umbilical artery Doppler during the third trimester.

Normal Findings on Umbilical Artery Waveform Analysis

- If findings on umbilical artery waveform analysis are within normal limits, ultrasound examination must be repeated every fortnightly for estimation of AC and expected fetal weight. Umbilical artery and MCA Doppler must be performed in the third trimester after 32 weeks.
- *Timing of delivery:* In these cases, delivery must be offered after 37 weeks with the involvement of a senior clinician. The patient should preferably be delivered by 37 weeks if MCA Doppler PI is <5th percentile. Delivery

may be considered after 34 weeks if the growth appears to be static over 3 weeks.

Abnormal Findings on Umbilical Artery Waveform Analysis

- If the findings on umbilical artery Doppler analysis are abnormal, i.e., PI or RI greater than 2.5 S/D, but EDV is present, then ultrasound (AC and expected fetal weight) must be repeated at every weekly interval. Umbilical artery Doppler analysis must be performed twice weekly. Delivery is recommended by 37 weeks. Steroids must be considered if the patient is being delivered by caesarean section. Delivery after 34 weeks must be considered if growth appears to be static over 3 weeks.
- If Doppler waveform analysis shows absent or reversed end diastolic volume (AREDV), ultrasound examination (for assessment of AC and EFW) must be repeated on weekly basis. Investigations such as umbilical artery Doppler, DV Doppler, and computerized cardiotocographic examination (cCTG) must be performed on daily basis. Delivery may be considered before 32 weeks after a course of corticosteroids in case of abnormal DV Doppler or cCTG results, provided that the period of gestation is ≥24 weeks and EFW is ≥500 g. Even if the results of DV Doppler examination are within normal limits, delivery must be considered between 30 and 32 weeks in these cases.

■ INTRAPARTUM PERIOD

- Early admission to the labor ward is recommended for women in spontaneous labor with an IUGR fetus in order to initiate continuous FHR monitoring in these patients.
- Presently, the RCOG (2013) recommends that the clinician needs to individualize each patient and decide the time for delivery by weighing the risk of fetal demise due to delayed intervention against the risk of long-term disabilities resulting from preterm delivery due to early intervention.
- Since the growth-restricted fetus is especially prone to develop asphyxia, continuous fetal monitoring using external or internal CTG needs to be done in the intrapartum period. However, CTG must not be used as the only form of surveillance in SGA fetuses. CTG tracing should preferably be interpreted based on short-term FHR variation from computerized analysis. If, at any time, the FHR appears to be nonreassuring, an emergency cesarean may be required. However, elective cesarean section is not justified for delivery of all IUGR fetuses.

Timing of Delivery

There is wide variation in practice in the timing of delivery of growth-restricted fetuses. The most important goal of

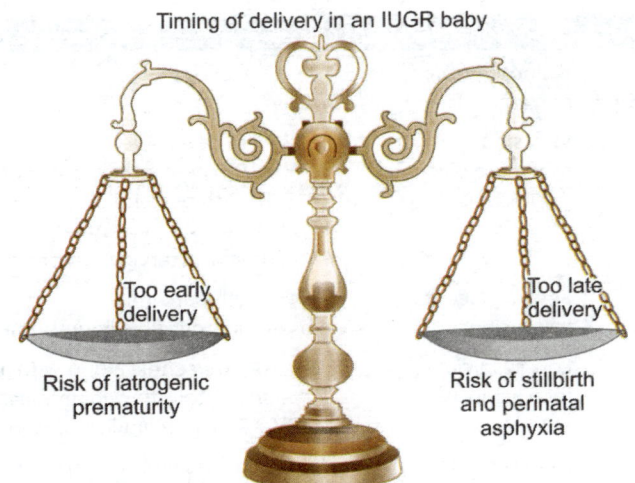

Fig. 15.21: Deciding the time of delivery in IUGR babies.

management is to deliver the most mature fetus in the least compromised position and at the same time cause minimum harm to the mother (**Fig. 15.21**). Preterm IUGR fetus with absent/reversed EDV in the umbilical artery, prior to 32 weeks of gestation, must be delivered when DV Doppler becomes abnormal or umbilical vein pulsations appear, provided the fetus has attained viability. The course of corticosteroids must be administered prior to delivery in these cases. Even when DV Doppler waveforms are normal, delivery is recommended by 32 weeks of gestation in these cases and should be considered between 30 and 32 weeks of gestation.

A senior obstetrician should preferably be involved in determining the timing and mode of delivery for IUGR fetuses having normal umbilical artery Doppler waveforms after 32 weeks of gestation. Delivery should be offered at 37 weeks of gestation in these cases. IUGR fetus with abnormal umbilical artery Doppler waveforms detected after 32 weeks of gestation should be delivered no later than 37 weeks of gestation.

In the term SGA fetus with normal umbilical artery Doppler, MCA Doppler waveforms should be used for deciding the timing for delivery. If MCA Doppler is abnormal (PI < 5th percentile), delivery should be recommended no later than 37 weeks of gestation. In the preterm SGA fetus, MCA Doppler has limited accuracy to predict acidemia and adverse outcome. Therefore, MCA Doppler should not be used to time delivery in case of preterm IUGR fetuses with abnormal umbilical artery Doppler waveform. In these cases, DV Doppler should be used for surveillance and for timing the delivery.

The PORTO (Prospective Observational Trial to Optimize Pediatric Health in IUGR) study (2013) evaluated multivessel Doppler changes in a large cohort of IUGR fetuses and has demonstrated multiple potential patterns of Doppler deterioration in this large prospective cohort of IUGR pregnancies, thereby asserting the usefulness of

TABLE 15.16: Eduard Gratacos criteria.

Stage	Pathophysiological correlations	Criteria	Monitoring	GA (in weeks)	Mode of delivery

I	Very small EFW or moderate placental insufficiency	• EFW < 3rd percentile
		• EFW < 10th percentile along with any of the criteria:
		  – CPR < 5th percentile*
		  – PI MCA < 5th percentile*
		  – PI uterine artery > 95th percentile
			Weekly	37	IOL

II	Severe placental insufficiency	• EFW < 10th percentile • Absent diastolic flow in umbilical artery†	Biweekly	34	CS
III	Low suspicion of fetal acidosis	EFW < 10th percentile along with any of the criteria: • Reverse diastolic flow in umbilical artery† • PI-DV > 95th percentile or absent diastolic flow in DV‡	1–2 days	30	CS
IV	High suspicion of fetal acidosis	EFW < 10th percentile along with any of the criteria: • Reverse diastolic flow in DV‡ • Pathological CTG	12 hours	26	CS

(CPR: cerebroplacental ratio; CS: cesarean section; CTG: cardiotocography; DV: ductus venosus; EFW: estimated fetal weight; GA: gestational age; IOL: induction of labor; MCA: middle cerebral artery; PI: pulsatility index)

Note:
*On two separate occasions > 12 hours.
†>50% of cycles, in free cord loop in both arteries on two separated occasions > 12 hours.
‡On two separated occasions > 6–12 hours.
Sources: Gomez MD, Llurbaa E, Gratacos E, Oros D, Garcia O, Rodriguez G. Defectos del crecimiento fetal. Documento de Consenso. Madrid: SEGO (Sociedad Española de Ginecologiay Obstetricia); 2015.
Figueras F, Gomez L, Eixarch E, Paules C, Mazarico E, Perez M, et al. (2019). Defectos del crecimiento fetal. [Online] Available from https://medicinafetalbarcelona.org/protocolos/es/patologia-fetal/defectos-del-crecimiento-fetal.html. [Last accessed December, 2022].

multivessel Doppler assessment for fetal surveillance and timing of delivery of IUGR fetuses. A general plan for delivery in IUGR fetuses based on the criteria by Eduard Gratacos is described in **Table 15.16**.

Delivery Decisions in Early-onset FGR

Fetal growth restriction prior to 32 weeks' gestation is a rare but serious complication of pregnancy due to its association with adverse perinatal outcome. Treatment of the underlying condition is impossible, and the challenge therefore lies in optimizing the timing of delivery. The risks associated with prematurity, namely neonatal complications and impaired neurodevelopment, have to be balanced against the risks associated with prolonged fetal exposure to hypoxemia and acidemia, which may result in stillbirth or brain damage. The optimal indication for timing of delivery still remains controversial.

A randomized controlled trial [Growth Restriction Intervention Trial (GRIT)] aimed at comparing the effect of early delivery to prevent terminal hypoxemia versus delaying the delivery for as long as possible to increase maturity in cases of early-onset FGR (fetal compromise between 24 and 36 weeks). The results of the trial showed no difference in overall mortality. Therefore, the study concluded that conversative management can be recommended in FGR fetuses with regular monitoring of Doppler parameters.

In the TRUFFLE (Trial of Randomized Umbilical and Fetal Flow in Europe) study on the outcome of early FGR, women were allocated to one of the three groups of indication for delivery according to the following monitoring strategies: (1) reduced FHR short-term variation (STV) on CTG, (2) early changes in fetal DV waveform (DV-p95), and (3) late changes in fetal DV waveform (DV-no-A). The results of this trial showed that the optimal timing of delivery of fetuses with early IUGR may therefore be best determined by monitoring them longitudinally, with both DV and cCTG monitoring.

Delivery Decisions in Late-onset FGR

As discussed previously, approximately 80% of IUGR infants are born at term. They are likely to be associated with an increased perinatal mortality and morbidity including behavioral problems, minor developmental delay, and spastic cerebral palsy. Management remains controversial, regarding the decision between induction of labor or awaiting spontaneous delivery with strict fetal and maternal surveillance. A multicenter randomized controlled trial comparing induction of labor versus expectant management in women with a suspected IUGR fetus at term between 36^{+0} and 41^{+0} weeks [DIGITAT (Disproportionate Intrauterine Growth Intervention Trial At Term) trial] showed no significant differences in adverse outcomes between the two groups. Patients who do not desire any intervention can safely choose expectant management with intensive maternal and fetal monitoring. However, sometimes it may be a practical option to choose induction of labor for preventing possible neonatal morbidity and stillbirth.

Presently, the RCOG (2002) recommends that the clinician needs to individualize each patient and decide the time for delivery by weighing the risk of fetal demise due to delayed intervention against the risk of long-term disabilities resulting from preterm delivery due to early intervention. The two main parameters for deciding the optimal time of delivery include results on various fetal surveillance techniques and gestational age. Also, the patient needs to be counseled regarding the potential risks associated with the two strategies.

Preterm delivery could be associated with future disabilities, intraventricular hemorrhage, sepsis, retinopathy of prematurity, etc. (the EPICURE Study Group, 2000). Delayed delivery, on the other hand, may be associated with ischemic brain injury, periventricular leukomalacia, intraventricular hemorrhage, and intrauterine death.

The management plan for patients with IUGR is presented in **Flowchart 15.4**. The various tests used for fetal surveillance vary from one center to the other. However, the main method of fetal surveillance which helps in determining the decision for delivery is Doppler analysis of umbilical blood vessels at most tertiary centers. The other methods used for fetal surveillance include NST and CTG. Doppler sonography in combination with other methods of antepartum surveillance such as antepartum CTG and BPP score should be used in everyday practice for fetal monitoring, especially in cases of high-risk pregnancy (IUGR, preeclampsia, etc.). Umbilical artery Doppler velocimetry is a highly sensitive and specific, noninvasive, simple, outpatient procedure for detection of chronic fetal hypoxia and acidosis in cases of IUGR. This technique allows fetal umbilical blood flow patterns to be observed from as early as 12 weeks of gestation.

When end diastolic flow is present on Doppler analysis of umbilical vessels, delivery must be delayed until at least 37 weeks, provided other surveillance findings are normal. Absent end diastolic blood flow in the umbilical artery is associated with increasing hindrance of flow toward the placenta along with decrease in the number of functioning

Flowchart 15.4: Management plan for IUGR fetuses.

(ANC: antenatal care; APH: antepartum hemorrhage; BMI: body mass index; MoM: multiples of the median; PAPP-A: pregnancy-associated plasma protein-A; SFH: symphysis-fundal height))

tertiary villi. This finding has been found to be associated with significant increase in the rate of fetal acidosis, fetal compromise, and perinatal mortality and morbidity.

If the umbilical artery end diastolic flow is reduced, absent, or reversed, this is taken as an indication for enhanced fetal surveillance or delivery. If preterm delivery is required, improved lung maturity should be achieved through maternal administration of glucocorticoids. Fetuses with reversed end diastolic umbilical flow should be provided intensive fetal surveillance until the time of delivery. In case abnormal findings on Doppler ultrasound are recognized along with abnormalities in other antenatal measures of fetal surveillance (CTG, BPP, contraction stress test, etc.), urgent delivery may be required. If gestation is over 34 weeks, even if other results are normal, delivery may be considered. The major dilemma for the clinician occurs when the fetal gestation is <34 weeks and the results of various antepartum surveillance tests are abnormal. In these cases the tests of fetal lung maturity (L:S ratio, presence of phosphatidylglycerol, etc.) must be done. If these tests indicate pulmonary maturity, the fetus can be delivered. Until the fetal lung maturity is achieved, IM corticosteroids must be administered to the mother. Also, while awaiting fetal lung maturity, fetal surveillance must be done using daily CTG, biweekly BPP, and weekly Doppler studies. The frequency of fetal testing can be changed depending on the severity of fetal compromise.

Mode of Delivery

Delivery via cesarean section is recommended in the case of IUGR fetus with reversed or absent umbilical artery velocity. Induction of labor can be offered to the IUGR fetuses having normal umbilical artery Doppler waveforms or those where there is abnormal umbilical artery PI or RI but end diastolic velocity is present. However, in these cases, the rates of emergency cesarean section are increased. Therefore, continuous FHR monitoring is recommended from the onset of uterine contractions. Women in spontaneous labor with an SGA fetus are advised early admission to the hospital so that continuous FHR monitoring can be initiated early in labor. Indications for emergency cesarean section in growth-restricted babies are described in **Box 15.3**.

Preterm Intrauterine Growth-restricted Fetus

Following steps may be required in preterm IUGR fetuses:
1. Administration of a single course of corticosteroids is required in case the delivery takes place between 24^{+0} and 35^{+6} weeks of gestation.
2. Surveillance with umbilical artery Doppler must be repeated after every 14 days in case the initial studies are normal. More frequent Doppler surveillance may be appropriate in a severely SGA fetus.

BOX 15.3: Indications for emergency cesarean section in growth-restricted babies.
- IUGR along with reduced fetal movements
- Presence of an obstetric complication (placenta previa, abruption placenta, etc.)
- Nonreassuring fetal heart sounds
- Meconium-stained liquor
- IUGR fetus with breech presentation
- Absent or reversed umbilical artery blood flow on Doppler examination
- BPP becomes less than four

3. In a preterm baby, when umbilical artery Doppler flow indices are abnormal, i.e., PI or RI are greater than two standard deviations above mean for gestational age and the delivery is not indicated, the following needs to be done:
   a. Surveillance to be repeated twice weekly in fetuses where end diastolic velocities are present.
   b. Surveillance to be done on a daily basis in fetuses where there is absent or reversed end diastolic velocities.
   c. DV Doppler should be used for surveillance in the preterm SGA fetus with abnormal umbilical artery Doppler and may also be used for deciding the time for delivery.

Therapeutic Interventions

There is a high risk of preterm birth and an overall grim fetal prognosis, especially in pregnancies complicated by early-onset extreme FGR. Presently, there is no form of therapy available which can reverse FGR. Presently, the most important intervention in these cases is to deliver the baby. Several therapeutic interventions have been tried, most effective of which includes aspirin, which acts by inactivating platelet cyclooxygenase and reducing the levels of thromboxane. The CLASP (Collaborative low-dose aspirin study in pregnancy) trial has shown that it may be appropriate to start prophylactic low-dose aspirin (dosage of 1–2 mg/kg body weight) early in the second trimester (typically at 16 weeks) in women who are at a risk of early-onset preeclampsia, which may be severe enough to result in growth-restricted fetuses, requiring very preterm delivery.

Several other therapeutic interventions have been tried, e.g., low-molecular-weight heparin (LMWH) and phosphodiesterase inhibitors (e.g., Sildenafil).

However, none of these agents have been shown to have a beneficial role for prevention of FGR. The STRIDER (Sildenafil Therapy In Dismal prognosis Early-onset intrauterine growth Restriction) trial has not shown any beneficial effect of sildenafil in prolonging pregnancy or improving pregnancy outcomes in severe early-onset FGR. As a result, sildenafil must not be prescribed for this indication outside of research studies, that too after taking appropriate consent from the participants. A 6-year European multicenter prospective cohort study, the EVERREST clinical trial, is a phase I/IIa trial for assessing the safety and efficacy of maternal vascular endothelial growth factor (VEGF) gene therapy in severe cases of early-onset FGR. The results of this trial are still awaited and if positive would support the development of a novel therapy in cases of severe early-onset FGR.

COMPLICATIONS

FETAL COMPLICATIONS

Antepartum Complications

Antepartum complications may include the following:
- Fetal hypoxia and acidosis
- Meconium aspiration/infection
- Stillbirth
- Oligohydramnios
- Iatrogenic prematurity

Intrapartum Complications

Neonatal asphyxia and acidosis are especially common in these fetuses. Some of the neonatal complications associated with this include the following:
- *Respiratory distress syndrome:* The pulmonary system of growth-restricted babies is often immature at birth, resulting in the development of respiratory distress syndrome.
- *Meconium aspiration syndrome:* Aspiration of meconium is a significant cause of mortality and morbidity in a FGR baby.
- *Persistent fetal circulation:* This condition is characterized by severe pulmonary vasoconstriction and persistent blood flow through the DV, even after birth. This is responsible for producing hypoxia, hypercarbia, and signs of right-to-left shunting.
- *Intraventricular bleeding:* This condition is produced as a result of bleeding inside or around the cerebral ventricles in a growth-restricted baby.
- *Neonatal encephalopathy:* This condition can occur as a consequence of severe birth asphyxia and can produce a constellation of neurological signs and symptoms (seizures, twitching, irritability, apnea, etc.).

NEONATAL COMPLICATIONS

The newborn child typically shows an old man-like appearance. There are signs of soft-tissue wasting including reduced amount of subcutaneous fat and loosened, thin skin. The muscle mass of arms, buttocks, and thighs is greatly reduced. The abdomen is scaphoid, and the ribs are protuberant. The HC may appear to be obviously larger than the AC. Some of the metabolic complications which can be frequently encountered in these babies include the following:

- *Hypoglycemia:* Neonatal hypoglycemia can be defined as blood glucose levels of <30 mg/dL. It can be associated with symptoms such as jitteriness, twitching, and apnea. It can occur due to reduced glycogen stores/glycogenolysis/gluconeogenesis, increased metabolic rate, and deficient release of catecholamines in an IUGR baby. Early feeding of the newborn baby can help prevent hypoglycemia.
- Hypoinsulinemia
- Hypertriglyceridemia
- *Hypocalcemia:* It may be common in the first few days of life due to relative hypoparathyroidism. Hypocalcemia is often associated with perinatal stress, asphyxia, and prematurity in the newborn baby.
- Polycythemia
- Meconium aspiration
- Hyperphosphatemia
- Birth asphyxia
- *Hypothermia:* The growth-restricted fetus has a poor temperature control due to which there is an increased tendency to develop hypothermia. Other factors responsible for producing hypothermia include reduced amount of subcutaneous fat, increased surface–volume ratio, decreased heat production, etc.
- Hyperbilirubinemia
- Sepsis
- Thrombocytopenia
- Respiratory distress
- Necrotizing enterocolitis
- *Hyperviscosity syndrome:* It is mainly associated with polycythemia and increased hematocrit levels above 65%.

Long-term Sequel of Intrauterine Growth Restriction

Postnatal growth: In some cases, catchup growth may occur in the first 6 months of life.

Cerebral palsy

Adult disease: These children are supposed to be at an increased risk of developing disorders such as obesity, diabetes mellitus, hypertension, cardiovascular disease, and ischemic heart disease later in life.

EVIDENCE-BASED CLINICAL TRIALS

List of references can be scanned through QR code to enable the readers gain deeper insight of the subject by referring to the entire article or its abstract.

CHAPTER 16

Preterm Labor

CASE STUDY

A 28-year-old G2P1A0L1 unbooked patient presents at 32 weeks of gestation with complaints of experiencing abdominal cramps at every 5-minute interval since morning (last 2–3 hours). Initially, the pain was coming at the intervals of 15–20 minutes. However, it has progressively increased in intensity and frequency since morning. There is no history of leakage of any fluid or passage of any kind of vaginal discharge or bleeding. Previous baby was born at 34 weeks of gestation. He is presently healthy and 3 years old.

INTRODUCTION

Q. Write a short essay describing preterm labor.

Preterm labor can be defined as onset of labor prior to the completion of 37 weeks of gestation, once the period of viability (20 weeks) has been attained. The degree of severity of preterm birth is described in **Table 16.1**. The gestational age included in the extreme preterm birth category varies but also includes birth between 20 and 28 weeks of gestation. Resuscitation of extremely preterm infants may present with an ethical, moral, and financial dilemma. The mortality rates amongst these infants are high, and the surviving infants may have a high rate of complications such as bronchopulmonary dysplasia, necrotizing enterocolitis, intraventricular hemorrhage (IVH), and sepsis. Neonatologists attempt resuscitation for infants born at <24 weeks of gestation only in very few countries worldwide due to reduced chances of survival below this gestational age. Nearly 50–60% of preterm births can occur as a result of preterm labor. Preterm birth can be associated with low-birth-weight babies and an increased rate of neonatal death and morbidity, resulting in lifetime disabilities such as learning disabilities, visual and hearing problems. Presently, prematurity is the second leading cause of death after pneumonia in children under the age of 5 years. India presently shows the highest burden of preterm births. As per the Times of India (2012), nearly 24% or one in every four children born prematurely across the globe were from India.

Diagnosis of preterm labor is established in case of the presence of the following:
- Uterine contractions of at least four in 20 minutes or eight in 60 minutes
- Cervical changes having effacement of 80% or more (corresponding to the cervical length of <20 mm) and cervical dilatation of >3 cm.

Babies born before 37 weeks of pregnancy are called premature babies. Even babies born between 37 and 39 weeks are likely to be associated with suboptimal outcome. Hence, induction of labor or cesarean delivery should not be preferably planned prior to 39 weeks of gestation.

Premature delivery may be preceded either by contractions or premature rupture of membranes (PROM). When the bag of membranes ruptures before the commencement of labor, this is known as premature/prelabor ROM. When the rupture of membranes occurs prior to 37 weeks of gestation, it is known as preterm PROM (PPROM).

TABLE 16.1: Classification of preterm birth.

WHO criteria	
Severity of preterm birth	**Period of gestation**
Extreme preterm birth	<28 weeks
Very preterm birth	28–31 weeks
Early preterm	32–34 weeks
Moderate/late preterm birth	34–37 weeks
Birth weight criteria	
Severity of low birth weight	**Birth weight**
Low birth weight	1,500–2,500 g
Very low birth weight	1,000–1,500 g
Extremely low birth weight	500–1,000 g

PATHOGENESIS

Q. Discuss the ethology and prediction of preterm labor with the help of a short essay.

Q. Write a short essay on etiopathogenesis of preterm labor.

The four most important pathogenic processes, which are likely to be implicated in the pathogenesis of preterm labor, are described in **Box 16.1**. Cytokines play a major role in the initiation of preterm labor **(Table 16.2)**. Pathogenesis of preterm labor has been described in **Flowchart 16.1**.

HISTORY AND CLINICAL PRESENTATION

RISK FACTORS

Although the actual cause remains unknown, some risk factors for preterm labor **(Fig. 16.1)** are described next. An attempt must be made to identify the possible risk factor at the time of taking history.

- *Multiple births:* An increased incidence of multiple births is associated with the increasing use of fertility drugs and assisted reproductive techniques. Various methods, such as cervical cerclage, prophylactic bed rest, and empiric use of tocolytics and progestogens, have been tried for prevention of preterm births in case of multifetal gestation. However, none of them have proved to be really successful.
- *Extremes of maternal age:* Maternal age < 18 years or >35 years can be considered as a risk factor for preterm labor.
- *Infection:* Infection is an important etiological factor in the pathogenesis of preterm labor and can include various causes such as asymptomatic bacterial vaginosis (BV), *Trichomonas vaginalis*, and infection by *Chlamydia trachomatis, Ureaplasma urealyticum, Mycoplasma hominis*, etc. Infections such as asymptomatic bacteriuria, pyelonephritis, pneumonia, and acute appendicitis may also be responsible for producing intra-amniotic inflammatory response, which may trigger uterine contractions. The role of group B *Streptococcus* (GBS) is not clear but is also found to be associated with

BOX 16.1: Pathogenesis of preterm labor.

- Premature activation of maternal or fetal hypothalamopituitary axis
- *Exaggerated inflammatory response:* TNF-α, IL-1, IL-6, etc./infection and altered genital tract microbiome, resulting in fetal rejection
- *Abruption (decidual hemorrhage):* Causes extravasation of the clotting factors, which activates factor VIIIa, resulting in the activation of thrombin. This acts on the myometrium to cause contractions. This also causes cervical changes and ROM
- *Pathogenic uterine distension (due to multiple gestation, hydramnios, etc.):* This causes release of IL-6 and IL-8, resulting in uterine contractions

(IL: interleukin; TNF: tumor necrosis factor)

TABLE 16.2: Role of cytokines in the pathogenesis of preterm labor.

Cytokines	Action	Effect
IL-6, IL-8, IL-1, TNF-α	Degradation of collagen fibers	Cervical ripening
IL-1, TNF-α	Induction of matrix metalloproteinases	Membrane rupture
IL-1, IL-2, IL-6, TNF-α	Increase in PGE2, PGF2α	Uterine contractions

(IL: interleukin; PGE2: prostaglandin E2; PGF2α: prostaglandin F2 alpha; TNF: tumor necrosis factor)

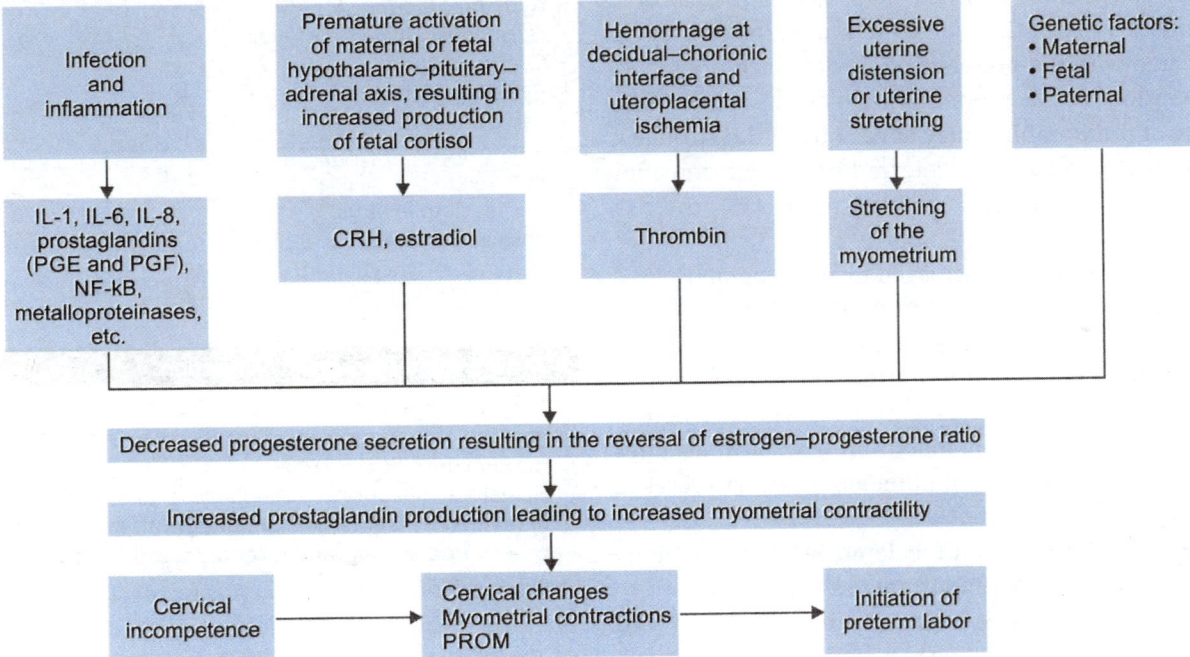

Flowchart 16.1: Pathogenesis of preterm labor.

(CRH: cortiotropin-releasing hormone; IL: interleukin; NF-kB: nuclear factor kappa B cells; PGE: prostaglandin E; PROM: premature rupture of membranes)

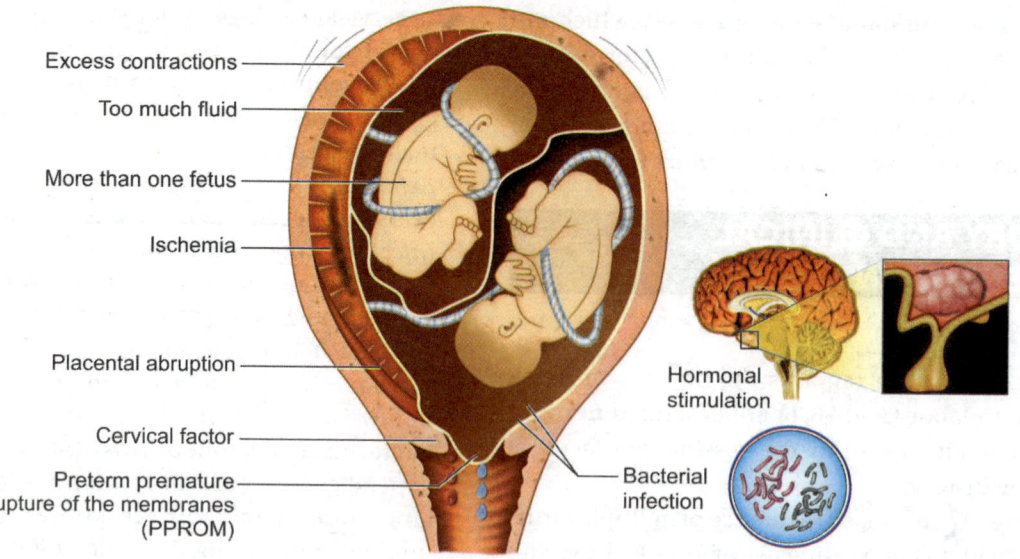

Fig. 16.1: Risk factors for preterm labor.

preterm labor. Infections may lead to preterm labor and PROM by causing the following three mechanisms: (1) maternal inflammatory response, (2) fetal infection, and (3) fetal inflammatory response. Microorganisms responsible for causing intrauterine infection, which may eventually result in preterm labor and PROM, are listed in **Box 16.2**. Various routes for spread of infection are given in **Box 16.3**.

- *PPROM:* Nearly 30% of preterm births could be due to PPROM. It usually results from intra-amniotic infections (especially BV, *U. urealyticum*, and *M. hominis*).
- *Previous obstetric history:* Taking the woman's past obstetric history is important because previous history of preterm births or second-trimester pregnancy loss may be associated with 17–20% risk of recurrence. Previous history of three or more miscarriages may be associated with the presence of cervical incompetence. Of the various risk factors for preterm birth, past obstetric history of preterm birth may act as one of the strongest predictors for recurrent preterm birth. If we consider the baseline risk for preterm birth as 10–12%, the risk of recurrent preterm births after 1, 2, and 3 consecutive preterm births may be increased to approximately 15%, 30%, and 75%, respectively **(Table 16.3)**. Cervical length of ≤25 mm has a likelihood ratio for preterm birth of 2.9 in women with history of previous preterm births. Therefore, the clinician must get alert if cervical length is ≤25 mm. The risk of spontaneous preterm birth declines by 6% for every additional millimeter increase in cervical length.
- *Preeclampsia:* History of preeclampsia in the previous pregnancy serves as an important risk factor.
- *Antepartum hemorrhage* (especially that associated with placental abruption resulting in hemorrhage at decidual–chorionic interface)

BOX 16.2: Microorganisms causing intrauterine infections.

Bacteria:
- *Ureaplasma urealyticum* (the most commonly isolated organism from amniotic fluid in women with preterm birth)
- *Mycoplasma hominis* (common)
- *Bacteroides, Fusobacterium* species (common)
- *Gardnerella vaginalis*
- *Staphylococcus aureus*
- *Streptococcus viridans*
- *Peptostreptococcus* species
- Group B *Streptococcus*
- *Lactobacillus* species
- *Escherichia coli*
- *Proteus*
- *Pseudomonas*
- *Enterococcus*
- *Neisseria gonorrhoeae*
- *Haemophilus influenzae* (rarely)

Viruses:
- Cytomegalovirus
- Parvovirus B19
- Adenovirus
- Enterovirus
- Herpes simplex virus
- Epstein–Barr virus
- Respiratory syncytial virus

BOX 16.3: Routes for spread of infection.

- Ascending infection from the cervix and vagina
- Invasion of the uterus by migration from the abdominal cavity through the fallopian tubes
- Hematogenous spread through placenta
- Inadvertent needle contamination at the time of invasive procedures, such as amniocentesis, chorionic villus sampling, and cordocentesis.

- Second-trimester bleeding not associated with placental causes

TABLE 16.3: Previous pregnancies and risk of preterm delivery.

No of prior preterm births	Subsequent preterm deliveries
1	14–23%
2	28–42%
3	75%

- *Idiopathic preterm labor:* Spontaneous unexplained preterm labor can occur with either intact or ruptured membranes.
- *Iatrogenic causes for inducing preterm labor:* Iatrogenic causes where labor is induced or infant is delivered by a prelabor cesarean section can include preeclampsia, fetal distress, intrauterine growth restriction, abruption, intrauterine death, etc.
- *Race and ethnicity:* Black women are twice at risk in comparison to white women.
- *Body mass index:* Women with low body mass index and poor maternal weight gain during pregnancy are at an increased risk.
- *Past medical history:* Past history of medical and surgical illnesses such as chronic hypertension, acute pyelonephritis, diabetes, renal diseases, and acute appendicitis
- *Stressful life event:* Stressful life events such as anxiety, depression, and negative life events could be responsible for triggering preterm labor. Maternal or fetal stress can precipitate preterm labor by increasing the secretion of corticotropin-releasing hormone.
- Uterine/cervical malformations/abnormalities
- *Cervical trauma:* Cervical trauma and injury resulting in cervical incompetence may act as another risk factor for preterm labor. The most common causes for cervical injury may include procedures for elective abortion (especially where the cervix is forcefully dilated to more than 10 mm), surgeries to treat cervical dysplasia, and cervical injury occurring at the time of normal delivery. Patients with a history of multiple first-trimester elective terminations or one or more second-trimester elective abortions may be at an increased risk for preterm delivery. Cervical dilatation with Laminaria tents or cervical ripening agents, such as misoprostol, appears to be less traumatizing to the cervix than mechanical dilation. Surgeries for treating cervical dysplasia, e.g., cold knife cone, cryoconization, laser cone, and loop electrical excision procedure (LEEP), may increase the risk of subsequent preterm deliveries. Chances of preterm labor are also increased if procedure to pregnancy interval is <6 months. Since obstetric trauma is an important risk factor for midtrimester loss or preterm birth, the cervix must be visually inspected to assess the degrees of injury and risk. Defects that involve >50% of the cervical length may be associated with a higher risk for midtrimester loss.
- Pregnancy with an intrauterine contraceptive device in situ
- Drug abuse, smoking, alcohol consumption
- Genetic and hereditary predisposition
- Poor socioeconomic status
- Undernutrition and poor weight gain during pregnancy
- *Recurrent midtrimester loss:* It may be associated with many causes such as infection (e.g., syphilis), antiphospholipid syndrome, diabetes, substance abuse, genetic disorders, congenital Müllerian abnormalities, cervical trauma, and cervical incompetence. Unfortunately, many midtrimester losses remain unexplained. A complete workup in cases of recurrent miscarriage may be required. Kindly refer to Chapter 13 for details. If antiphospholipid syndrome is suspected, its workup should include assessment of anticardiolipin and lupus anticoagulant antibodies.
- *Assisted reproductive technologies:* They are associated with an increased risk of preterm labor due to a high rate of multiple pregnancies. Reduction of multifetal pregnancy reduces the incidence of preterm birth.

CLINICAL PRESENTATION

The patient may give history of experiencing symptoms such as menstrual cramps, pelvic pressure, backache, and/or vaginal discharge or bleeding. A typical clinical presentation of preterm labor includes the following:

- Regular uterine contractions (with the frequency of one in every 10 minutes or six contractions per hour) along with cervical changes between 20 and 37 weeks of gestation
- Associated cervical changes include:
  - Cervical length < 1 cm
  - Cervical dilatation > 2 cm
  - Vaginal bleeding or ROM
- Patient may give a history of breaking her membranes, followed by a sudden gush of watery fluid.
- ROM may be associated with a history suggestive of chorioamnionitis. These may include fever (temperature > 100.4°F or 37.8°C), tachycardia (>120 bpm), foul-smelling vaginal discharge, uterine tenderness, and maternal leukocytosis (total leukocyte blood count > 15,000–18,000 cells/mL).

GENERAL PHYSICAL EXAMINATION

There is no clinical sign specific to preterm labor, which may be present in these patients. Tachycardia/fever may be present in cases of chorioamnionitis.

SPECIFIC SYSTEMIC EXAMINATION

PER SPECULUM EXAMINATION

- Integrity of the cervix and the extent of any prior injury to the cervix may be assessed by speculum and digital examinations.

- On sterile speculum examination, there is copious pooling of fluid in the vagina or leakage of fluid from the cervical os. Vaginal fluid sample must be collected for pH determination.
- Sterile speculum examination helps in detecting ruptured membranes.
- Endocervical samples can be collected for detection of gonorrhea and Chlamydia infections. Wet smear examination helps in the diagnosis of BV and trichomonal infection.

VAGINAL EXAMINATION

The following are clinical presentations suggestive of preterm labor on digital examination:
- Cervical dilatation of ≥1 cm and effacement of 80% or more
- Bishop's score may be 4 or greater. Lower uterine segment may be thinned out, and the presenting part may be deep in the pelvis.
- Cervical length on transvaginal sonography may be ≤2.5 cm and there may be funneling of internal os. Based on the findings of clinical examination, preterm labor can be of two types:
  1. *Early preterm labor:* In cases of early preterm labor, cervical effacement is ≥80% and cervical dilatation is ≥1 cm, but <3 cm.
  2. *Advanced preterm labor:* In cases of advanced preterm labor, cervical dilatation is ≥3 cm.

ABDOMINAL EXAMINATION

Uterine contractions of greater than or equal to four per 20 minutes or greater than or equal to eight per hour, lasting for >40 seconds, may be felt on abdominal examination.

In case preterm labor is related to the presence of multifetal gestation, the finding relevant to the presence of multifetal gestation may be observed on abdominal examination (see Chapter 9).

DIFFERENTIAL DIAGNOSIS

Threatened preterm labor: This is characterized by the presence of uterine contractions in the absence of cervical changes. Options for management in these cases include continued observation or therapeutic sleep (e.g., morphine sulfate 10–15 mg through subcutaneous route).

MANAGEMENT

Management strategies to be adopted in cases of preterm labor are mentioned in **Box 16.4**. The algorithm for management of patients with preterm labor is described in **Flowchart 16.2**. Management comprising investigations and definitive obstetric management is discussed next.

> **BOX 16.4:** Management strategies in case of preterm labor.
> - Treatment with corticosteroids to promote lung maturity
> - Tocolysis
> - Antibiotics in cases of preterm PROM
> - Judicious use of magnesium sulfate for neuroprotection of the newborn
>
> (PROM: premature rupture of membranes)

> Q. With the help of a long essay, discuss the etiology and management of a primigravida with preterm pregnancy.
>
> Q. Write a long essay discussing the current concepts in the management of PROM.
>
> Q. Discuss in detail the management of a 25-year-old G2P1A0L1 woman with a history of preterm labor at 30 weeks in the previous pregnancy. She has presented now at 28 weeks of gestation having strong uterine contractions.
>
> Q. What is the next step of management in the case study mentioned in the beginning of the chapter?

INVESTIGATIONS

CLINICAL EXAMINATION

Diagnosis of preterm labor is usually made at the time of clinical examination. Uterine contractions of sufficient frequency and intensity causing progressive effacement and dilation of the cervix prior to 37 weeks of gestation are indicative of active preterm labor. Following the suspicion of preterm labor on clinical examination, the diagnosis of preterm labor can be predicted with the help of the following tests:
- Fetal fibronectin (fFN) levels
- Ultrasound measurement of cervical length

If on history and abdominal examinations the diagnosis of preterm labor is suspected, but not confirmed, a vaginal fFN sample must be obtained before proceeding for pelvic cervical examination. If the diagnosis of preterm labor becomes obvious after the pelvic examination, the fFN specimen can be later discarded.

However, if the diagnosis still remains doubtful, the fFN specimen can be sent to the lab for analysis.

The EQUIPP study, 2015 (evaluation of a quantitative instrument for prediction of preterm labor) was the first prospective study to show the enhanced value of quantitative testing of fFN in asymptomatic women at high risk of preterm birth between 22 and 27 weeks of gestation.

Presently, ultrasonography to determine cervical length and estimation of fFN levels or a combination of both serve as the most useful tools for determining women at high risk for preterm labor. The clinical usefulness of both these tests rests primarily with their negative predictive value due to the lack of any definite treatment options for prevention of preterm birth.

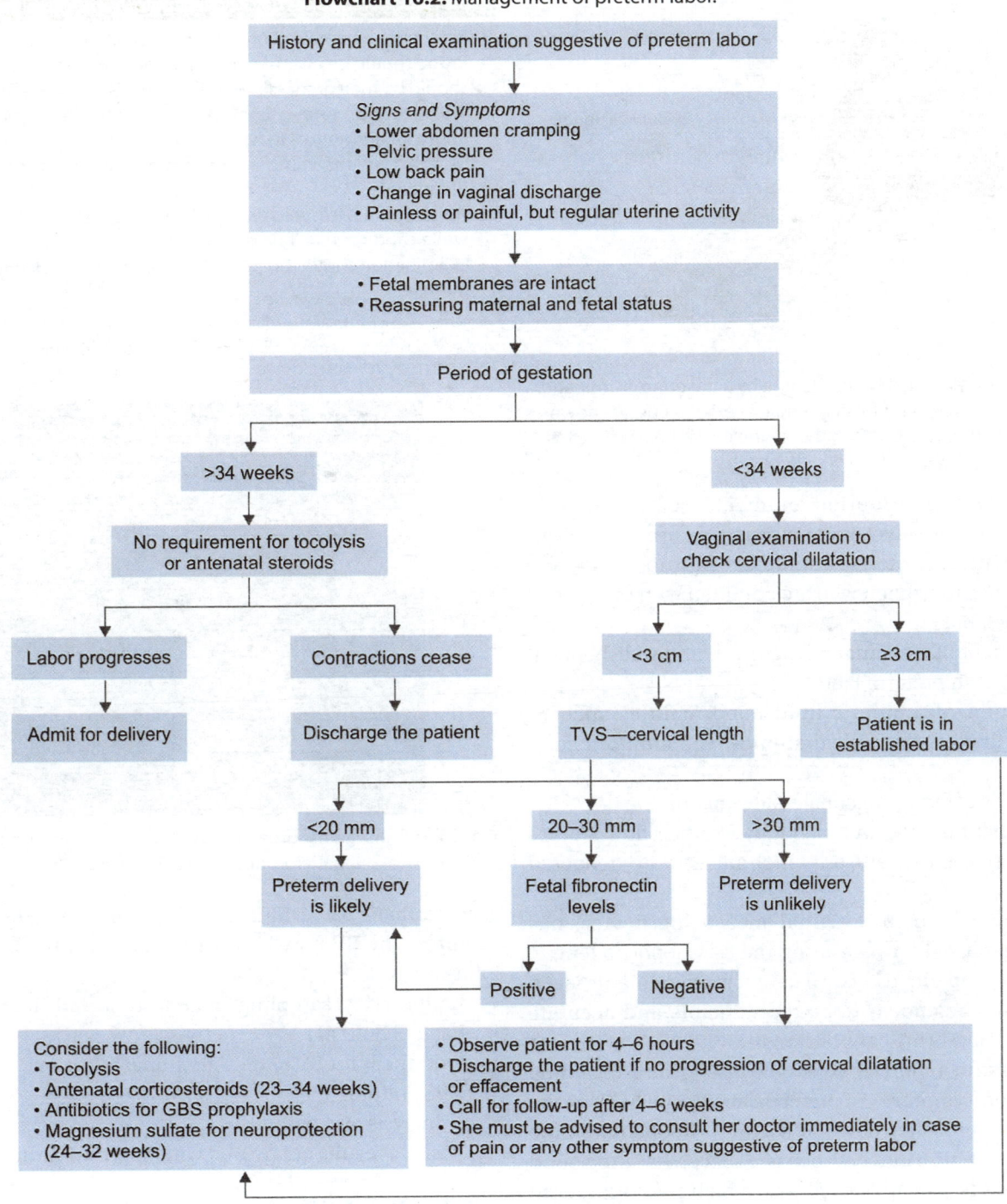

Flowchart 16.2: Management of preterm labor.

(GBS: group B *Streptococcus*; TVS: transvaginal sonography)

ULTRASOUND ASSESSMENT OF CERVICAL LENGTH

Presently, transvaginal screening of cervical length with an empty bladder during mid-gestation (16–24 weeks) is the gold standard test for predicting preterm labor, which must be offered to all pregnant women. Cervical length is measured between internal and external os **(Fig. 16.2)**. The parameters which are assessed include cervical dilatation, funneling of membranes, and cervical length. Cervical length of <2.5 cm and/or cervical score* of <0 in the second trimester is associated with high chances of having preterm birth at <35 weeks of gestation. In case of multiple pregnancy, the cervical length cutoff of 1.5–2 cm can be considered.

Besides identifying the women at an increased risk for preterm delivery, ultrasound assessment also helps in the following:

---

*[Cervical score = cervical length (cm) – cervical dilation (cm) at the internal os]

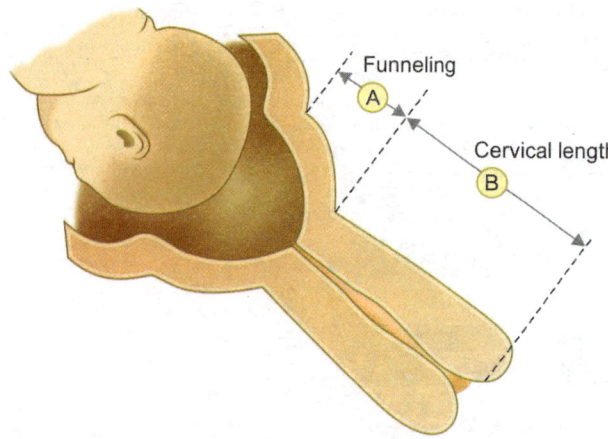

Fig. 16.2: Measurement of cervical length by ultrasound examination. The distance B, extending from internal to external os, is known as the cervical length. The length of the "funneled" cervix, denoted as A, should not be included in the cervical length.

- Detection of any uterine anomalies such as uterine malformations (bicornuate uterus, unicornuate uterus, septate uterus, etc.), submucous fibroids, and scar dehiscence in women who are admitted with threatened preterm labor
- Assessment of fetal anatomy, growth, and well-being in patients with preterm labor
- Evaluation of amniotic fluid abnormalities such as oligohydramnios, polyhydramnios, and amniotic fluid sludge
- Diagnosis of fetal congenital malformations
- Assessment of fetal well-being by Doppler flow studies will help identify fetuses, which need to be delivered preterm.

Cervilenz™, an intravaginal measuring device, has recently been used for measuring the cervicoportio length. The manually obtained cervical length measurements taken using CerviLenz appear to be reproducible and accurate method for measuring cervical length.

Patients with a short cervix should be educated regarding the signs and symptoms of preterm labor, especially as the pregnancy approaches potential viability. Reduction in the length of cervix of >6 mm between two successive ultrasound examinations is also associated with a high risk for preterm labor. Funneling or change in the diameter of internal os by ≥5 mm can also be considered as an independent risk factor for the development of preterm labor. Criteria to be taken into consideration before performing transvaginal sonography are listed in **Box 16.5**. **Figure 16.3** shows short cervical length as observed on transvaginal sonography observed in a woman with preterm labor at 30 weeks of gestation.

ASSESSMENT OF LOWER GENITAL TRACT INFECTION

Patients with preterm labor may be assessed for the presence or absence of lower genital tract infection. The presence of

> **BOX 16.5:** Prerequisites before performing transvaginal sonography.
> - Bladder to be emptied prior to the procedure
> - Probe should be inserted in such a way as to contact the cervix. It should be then gradually withdrawn until the image gets blurred
> - The anterior and posterior lips of the cervix should be approximately equal in width
> - Contrast agents can be used if the external os is not readily identifiable
> - Transfundal pressure is applied for a period of 15–30 seconds while capturing the image
> - Examination should be performed carefully and slowly over 3–5 minutes
>
> *Source:* Berghella V, Bega G, Tolosa JE, Berghella M. Ultrasound assessment of the cervix. Clin Obstet Gynecol. 2003;46:947-62.

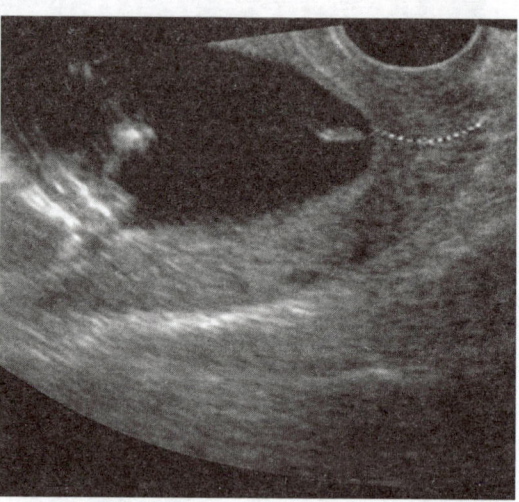

Fig. 16.3: Transvaginal ultrasound showing cervical length < 2 cm in a patient undergoing preterm labor.

asymptomatic bacteriuria, sexually transmitted disease, and symptomatic BV may be investigated with the help of the following tests:
- Endocervical sampling for gonorrhea and chlamydia
- Vaginal fluid pH
- Wet smear for BV and trichomonal infection
- GBS culture
- Urinalysis and culture
- Positive results are treated with appropriate antibiotics.

METHODS FOR PREDICTING PRETERM BIRTHS

> **Q.** Using a short note, discuss the etiology and prediction of preterm labor.

The ACOG, 2001 recommendations on assessment of risk factors for preterm birth include the following biological markers.

Home Uterine Activity Monitoring

Home uterine activity monitoring (HUAM) has been suggested as a method for predicting preterm birth in high-risk women. It combines telemetric recordings of uterine contractions using a tocodynamometer and daily telephone calls from a physician to offer support and advice. This method was based on the observation that some women who give birth early have an increase in uterine activity earlier in pregnancy than women who give birth at term, and that these uterine contractions may not be recognized by the patient.

Presently, there is uncertainty regarding the usefulness of HUAM. According to the US Preventive Services Task Force and the US Food and Drug Administration (FDA), the device has been deemed ineffective and its use is not recommended.

Screening for Bacterial Vaginosis

The presence of BV has been considered as an independent risk factor for prediction of preterm labor. BV is associated with the alteration of the normal vaginal flora. Therefore, screening and treatment for BV in pregnant women are likely to reduce the incidence of preterm births. However, presently there is insufficient data to support screening and treatment of women at high risk for the prevention of preterm labor.

Fetal Fibronectin Levels

Fibronectin is a glycoprotein, secreted by the chorionic tissue at the maternal-fetal interface, due to which it may be present in the amniotic fluid, placental tissues, and decidua basalis **(Fig. 16.4)**. It acts as a biological glue, which helps in binding blastocyst to endometrium. It is normally present in the cervicovaginal secretions up to 20–22 weeks of gestation. From around 22 weeks, the chorion fuses completely with the underlying decidua. Therefore, this prevents the leakage of fibronectin into the vaginal secretions until at the time of labor when the membranes rupture or the cervix dilates. Therefore, the presence of fibronectin in the vaginal secretions between 27 and 34 weeks serves as an important marker of preterm labor. Swabs can be taken from the ectocervix or posterior vaginal fornix for collection of cervicovaginal secretions. This will help in ruling out GBS infection. ELISA with FDC-6 monoclonal antibody is used for detecting fFN. A cutoff value of 50 ng/mL is considered positive. The presence of fibronectin is associated with sensitivity of 89% and specificity of 86%. On the other hand, the absence of fibronectin from the cervicovaginal secretions is associated with a low risk for preterm delivery. Although a negative test result appears to be useful in ruling out preterm delivery within 2 weeks, a positive fFN has limited value in predicting women who will deliver preterm. Nevertheless, fFN has a predictive value in identifying patients who will or will not deliver within the subsequent 1–2 weeks. The clinical implications of a positive result have not been evaluated fully because no intervention has been shown to decrease the risk of preterm delivery. The test has limited usefulness in low-risk women. For high-risk women, the following criteria should be met: intact amniotic membranes, minimal cervical dilatation, testing should be performed no earlier than 24 weeks, zero days of gestation, and no later than 34 weeks, 6 days of gestation, and results must be available in time to allow for decision-making, ideally within 24 hours.

INVESTIGATIONS FOR MIDTRIMESTER LOSS

Laboratory tests, which may be required in cases of midtrimester loss, include the following:

- Rapid plasma reagent test
- Gonorrheal and chlamydial screenings
- Vaginal pH/wet smear/whiff test
- Anticardiolipin antibody, lupus anticoagulant antibody
- Activated partial thromboplastin time
- 1-hour glucose challenge test
- TORCH, immunoglobulin G, and immunoglobulin M screening whenever historical or clinical suspicion is present

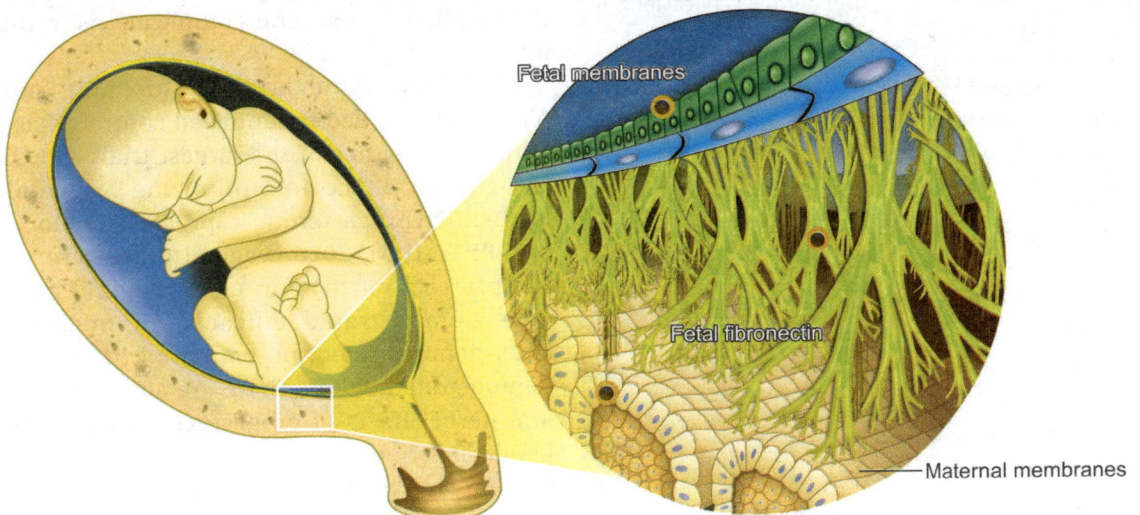

Fig. 16.4: Fetal fibronectin at maternal-fetal interface.

- *Tests for cervical incompetence:* A preconceptual hysterosalpingogram may be of benefit in patients with a history of two or more midtrimester losses. One can also attempt to pass a No. 8 Hegar's dilator into the nonpregnant cervix; easy passage may be a sign of cervical incompetence. Baseline transvaginal ultrasonography scan must be performed to assess cervical length, especially at 13–17 weeks' gestation; abnormal findings include a length < 2.5 cm, funneling > 5 mm, or dynamic changes.

TREATMENT/OBSTETRIC MANAGEMENT

PREVENTION

Some interventions with proven benefits for the prevention of preterm labor and those with no proven effect for the prevention of preterm labor are described in **Box. 16.6**.

Antibiotics: Antibiotic therapy at 24 weeks and then repeated during labor is likely to reduce the incidence of BV and trichomoniasis but is unlikely to have a significant effect in the prevention of preterm labor. The use of prophylactic antibiotics in patients with intact membranes is not likely to show any definite benefit on neonatal outcomes (ORACLE II trial). However, if the ROM has occurred preterm prior to the onset of labor, administration of antibiotics is helpful in prolongation of pregnancy and in the improvement of neonatal outcomes along with a decrease in perinatal complications (ORACLE I trial). However, caution must be observed prior to the prescription of Augmentin, (amoxicillin and clavulanate potassium) because its use may be associated with necrotizing enterocolitis. The antibiotic of choice is presently erythromycin.

Use of progesterone therapy to reduce preterm birth: Progesterone therapy must not be routinely used in all women with preterm birth. The ACOG (2016) recommends the use of progesterone supplementation to reduce preterm birth in patients at high risk for recurrent preterm delivery (i.e., prior preterm birth < 37 weeks' gestation, very short cervical length ≤ 25 mm). It is recommended that administration of progesterone therapy must be initiated from 16 to 24 weeks of gestation. The following preparations of progesterone can be used: natural micronized progesterone (route of administration: oral or vaginal in the form of gel or tablets) or a synthetic analog of its metabolite, 17-hydroxyprogesterone caproate (17-OHPC), administered through intramuscular route. Bioavailability of vaginal formulations is 90%, whereas that of oral formulations is 10%. Dydrogesterone is an orally available progesterone administered in the dosage of 10 mg BD. If indicated, vaginal progesterone should be administered in the dosage of 200–400 mg daily or 17-hydroxyprogesterone in the dosage of 250 mg via intramuscular route administered in the hip every week until 34–36 weeks of gestation or ROM or birth, whichever occurs earlier. Formulations of 17-OHPC available in India include Proluton and uniprogestin. Formulation of micronized progesterone available in India is endogest.

The results of the PREGNANT trial (2011) showed that treatment using 100 mg of progestogen gel intravaginally resulted in a 45% reduction in the rate of earlier preterm birth, at <33 weeks, along with an improved neonatal outcome. Weekly injections of 17-alpha-hydroxyprogesterone caproate are thought to cause a substantial reduction in the rate of recurrent preterm delivery amongst women who are at a high risk for preterm delivery. This is also likely to reduce the likelihood of several complications in the premature infants.

Although some large multicenter, multinational, placebo-controlled randomized control trials support this approach, neither of the largest trials—PROLONG, 2018 (Progestin's ROLe in Optimizing Neonatal Gestation) for hydroxyprogesterone caproate injection, 250 mg/mL or OPPTIMUM, 2016 (Vaginal progesterone prophylaxis for preterm birth) for using vaginal progesterone—have demonstrated efficacy. Although no harm has been demonstrated, no benefit of this therapy has been demonstrated either. There are almost no data regarding long-term effects of progestogens or benefit beyond the neonatal period.

- *GBS prophylaxis:* All patients in preterm labor should be considered at high risk for neonatal GBS sepsis. Patients in preterm labor with the potential to deliver should

BOX 16.6: Interventions for prevention of preterm labor.

Interventions with proven benefits	Interventions without any proven benefits
• Diagnosis and treatment of asymptomatic bacteriuria and bacterial vaginosis • Cervical cerclage with prior preterm birth (<34 weeks), singleton pregnancy, CL < 25 mm, and period of gestation < 24 weeks • Progesterone therapy in cases of prior preterm labor and cervical length < 25 mm [as per the recommendations by SMFM (2018), all women with a prior spontaneous preterm birth of a singleton pregnancy should be offered (17OHP-C) therapy in a subsequent pregnancy with a singleton gestation] • Smoking cessation • Increasing interpregnancy interval • Improving prepregnancy health • Treatment of malaria	• Bed rest • Empirical use of antibiotics • Cervical cerclage in women with previous history of preterm birth but normal cervical length

(17OHP-C: 17-alpha hydroxyprogesterone caproate; CL: cervical length; SMFM: Society for Maternal Fetal Medicine)

receive prophylactic antibiotics against GBS, unless GBS culture is negative. Prophylactic antibiotics should be administered when the diagnosis of preterm labor is made and should be continued until delivery or for a minimum of 72 hours. Patients should be retreated if preterm labor recurs or when the patient enters labor at term, depending upon culture results.

> **Q.** Write a short note on the role of cervical cerclage in case of preterm labor.

- *Use of cervical cerclage:* As per the Cochrane review (2017), cervical cerclage is associated with a reduced risk of preterm delivery in women who are at a high risk for preterm birth. If the cervical length is <25 mm along with a previous history of preterm labor, surgical intervention with cervical cerclage may help prevent preterm labor. Progesterone supplementation can be administered simultaneously. Cerclage is not recommended in cases of multiple pregnancy, uterine anomalies, previous cervical surgery, and women with short cervix (without a history of prior preterm birth). In case of multiple pregnancy, there is no evidence that the use of cerclage could help in preventing preterm births and reducing perinatal deaths or neonatal morbidity. The optimum time for insertion of cerclage is 13–23 weeks, and it must be routinely removed at around 37 weeks. The patient with cerclage must be advised to report in case they experience symptoms such as abdominal pain, ROM, foul-smelling vaginal discharge, and vaginal bleeding. In case the woman experiences premature uterine contractions which cannot be arrested with the help of a tocolytic agent, the cerclage may require removal.

Different types of cerclage procedures are enumerated in **Table 16.4**. The technique of application of stitches via transvaginal route, McDonald stitch (at the cervicovaginal junction), and Shirodkar stitch (at the level of internal os) has been described in Chapter 13. Transabdominal stitches applied either through laparotomy or via laparoscopic route are likely to be more effective. However, transabdominally placed stitches would require another laparotomy procedure for removal of the cerclage stitch. The indications for cervical cerclage could be as follows:

- *History-indicated cerclage:* Previous history of preterm deliveries or midtrimester miscarriages is an indication for early cerclage (around 13 weeks).
- *Ultrasound-indicated cerclage:* Short cervix on ultrasound
- *Physical examination-related cerclage:* This is indicated in the presence of bulging bag of membranes on per speculum examination. Also known as emergency or rescue cerclage, this is the only type of cerclage which can be performed at 28 weeks of gestation.
- *Silicone Arabin pessary:* The use of Arabin pessary was supposed to prevent premature dilatation of cervix and PPROM. The use of this pessary is likely to help in changing the angulation between uterus and cervix, thereby preventing the transmission of intrauterine force to cervix. The pessary is also likely to support the immunological barrier between the chorion and vaginal microbiological flora, thereby helping in preventing preterm labor. Presently, there is inadequate evidence regarding the efficacy of this pessary for prevention of preterm labor. Therefore, this therapy is presently being used in research settings and not in clinical settings.

Flowchart 16.3 shows the algorithm for prevention of preterm labor.

GOALS OF OBSTETRIC MANAGEMENT

Goals of obstetric patient management of preterm labor include the following:

- Early identification of risk factors associated with preterm birth
- Timely diagnosis of preterm labor
- Identifying the etiology of preterm labor
- Evaluating fetal well-being
- Provision of prophylactic pharmacologic therapy to prolong the period of gestation and reduce the incidence of complications such as respiratory distress syndrome and intra-amniotic infection
- Initiation of tocolytic therapy when indicated
- Establishing a plan of maternal and fetal surveillance in order to improve neonatal outcome
- Deciding the time of delivery

DECIDING THE TIME OF DELIVERY

For a majority of patients, prolonging pregnancy does not offer any benefit because in a majority of cases, preterm labor serves as a protective mechanism for fetuses threatened by problems such as infection or placental insufficiency. Preterm labor is often associated with PROM. The following considerations should be given regarding delivery in women with preterm labor.

TABLE 16.4: Classification of cervical cerclage.

Criterion	Classification
Time of insertion	Prophylactic or after evidence of cervical change
Route of insertion	Transvaginal, transabdominal, laparoscopic
Technique of insertion	Shirodkar, McDonald
Indication of cerclage	History-indicated, ultrasound-indicated, physical examination-indicated (emergency or rescue) cerclage

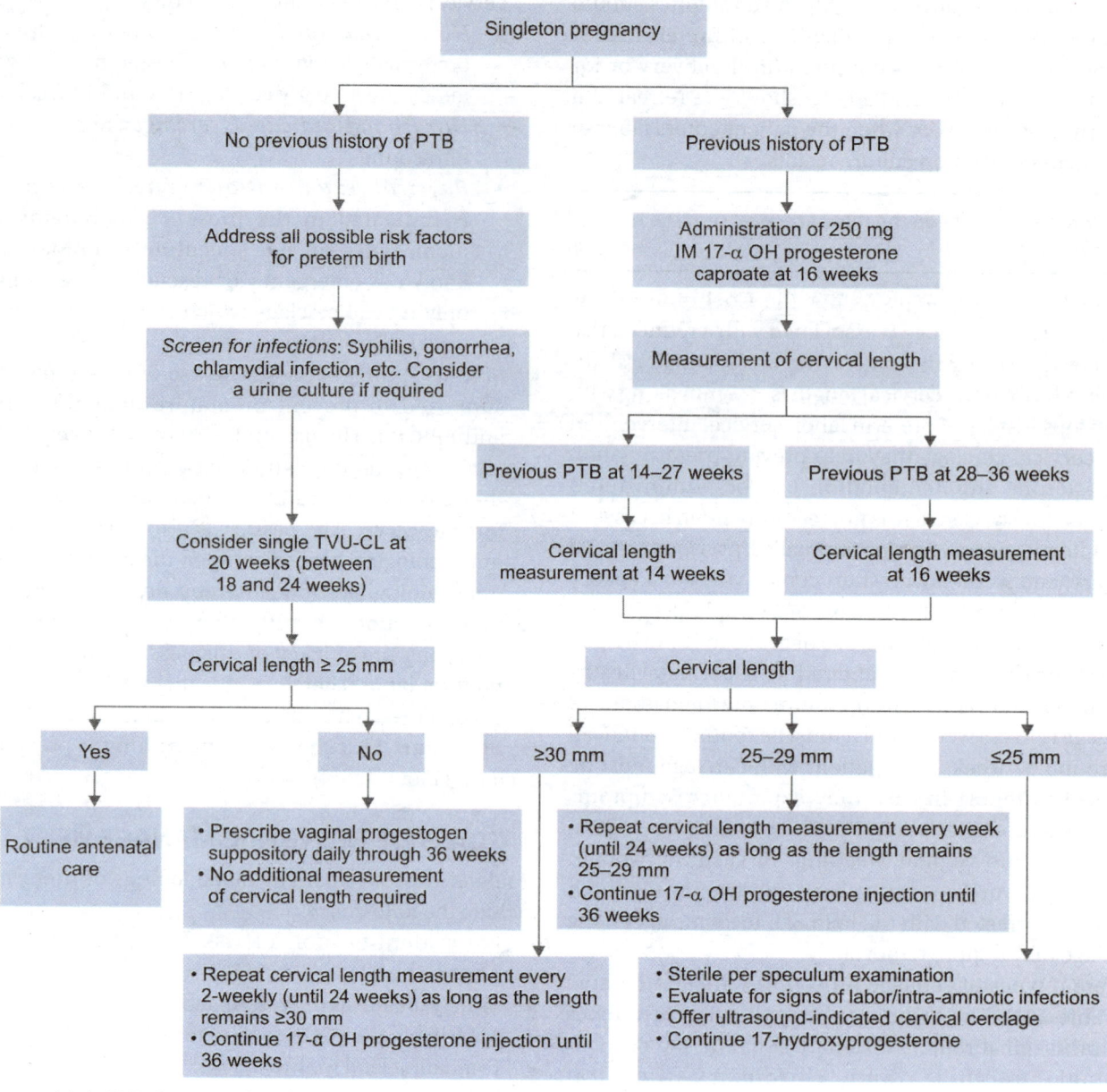

Flowchart 16.3: Algorithm for prevention of preterm labor.

(PTB: preterm birth; TVU-CL: transvaginal ultrasound cervical length)
Source: American College of Obstetricians and Gynecologists' Committee on Practice Bulletins—Obstetrics. Practice Bulletin No. 171: management of preterm labor. Obstet Gynecol. 2016 Oct;128(4):e155-64. doi: 10.1097/AOG.0000000000001711. PMID: 27661654.

Period of Gestation Less Than 34 Weeks

For pregnancies < 34 weeks of gestation in women with no maternal or fetal indication for delivery, expectant management comprising the following may be used:
- Close monitoring of uterine contractions
- Fetal surveillance
- Corticosteroids may be used for enhancing pulmonary maturity.
- Use of magnesium sulfate infusion for 12–24 hours helps in providing neuroprotection.
- Prophylactic therapy for group B streptococcal infection should be administered, especially in cases where the membranes have also ruptured.

- *Progesterone therapy:* This can be used to reduce the occurrence of preterm birth.
- *Tocolytic therapy:* This may be required to delay delivery for up to 48 hours, thereby buying time to allow the maximum benefit of corticosteroids in order to reduce the incidence of respiratory distress syndrome. This time delay may also be useful in transferring the patient to a tertiary care center. Once the episode of preterm labor has been controlled with tocolytic agents, women in early preterm labor should be managed on OPD basis, except those patients who have a positive fibronectin test. In these patients, the risk of preterm delivery is substantial, and they should be admitted to the hospital for bed rest.

- *Corticosteroid therapy:* The administration of corticosteroids is recommended in patients with preterm labor, whenever the gestational age is between 24 and 34 weeks.

Period of Gestation 34 Weeks or More

For pregnancies at 34 weeks or more, women with preterm labor must be monitored for labor progression and fetal well-being.

Inpatient Care of the Patient

Once the episode of preterm labor has been arrested, the patient must be encouraged to return to the level of limited activity before discharge from the hospital. The factors which may be taken into consideration before taking the decision for discharging these patients are as follows:
- Cervical dilation
- Fetal presentation
- Number of fetuses
- Gestational age
- Access to the hospital (availability of transportation facilities, telephone facilities)
- Social support at home
- Ability to maintain limited activity and pelvic rest
- Good patient compliance

The patient should be informed regarding the signs and symptoms of recurrent preterm labor. She should be asked to contact her doctor if she experiences any of the symptoms suggestive of preterm labor.

Outpatient Care of the Patient

Once the patient's symptoms of preterm labor are in control, she can be discharged home. She must not be advised complete bed rest because that is likely to result in thromboembolism. However, she must be asked to avoid strenuous activity, coitus, driving, going to office, etc. The healthcare provider should call the patient for frequent antenatal visits even after the patient has been discharged home. The patient should be instructed to immediately report symptoms of preterm labor or complications. The contact may be via a combination of telephone contacts and office visits. If genital tract infection had previously played a role in the pathogenesis of preterm labor (positive culture results), a repeat culture may be recommended 2–4 weeks after discharge.

A cerclage may be indicated after two or more midtrimester losses consistent with incompetent cervix or in whom the etiology is unknown and is usually performed electively at 13–17 weeks of gestation.

INTRAPARTUM MANAGEMENT

Intrapartum management in these cases comprises the following steps:

1. *Requirement of NICU facilities:* Delivery should preferably be undertaken in a tertiary care setting having good neonatal intensive care facilities. Also, the parents must be counselled regarding the likely fetal outcome as well as requirement for NICU facilities. Senior obstetrician must be involved if the period of gestation is between 23 and 25^{+6} weeks.
2. *Fetal surveillance and monitoring:* Since the preterm babies are susceptible to the development of fetal hypoxia and acidosis, these fetuses must be carefully monitored for signs of hypoxia during labor, preferably by continuous electronic fetal monitoring.
3. *Fetal scalp electrode:* It is usually not performed prior to 34 weeks except in the presence of the following: not possible to monitor externally, the issue has been discussed with senior obstetrician, benefits outweigh risk, and the patient does not accept the options for fetal alternative methods of monitoring or no monitoring.
4. *Antibiotic prophylaxis:* This may be particularly useful in cases of group B streptococcal infection. 2g ampicillin is given stat followed by 2 g 6-hourly for 48 hours.
5. *Tocolysis:* Magnesium sulfate is administered for neuroprotection of the premature neonate in some countries. However, it should not be combined with calcium channel blockers due to the possibility of severe maternal hypotension.
6. *Epidural analgesia:* It can be administered to the mother.
7. *Delivery:* This must be conducted in the presence of an expert neonatologist capable of dealing with the complications of prematurity. Ventouse application is contraindicated in preterm deliveries, especially prior to 34 weeks.
    a. *Cesarean delivery:* There are no known harms or benefits of cesarean delivery. However, it is indicated only in case of obstetric indications. It must be considered between 26 and 36 weeks of gestation with breech presentation. If the baby is very premature and/or hypoxic, cesarean delivery may be associated with better outcomes. Possibility of vertical incision in the upper segment must be taken into consideration.
    b. *Episiotomy:* At the time of delivery, an episiotomy may be given to facilitate the delivery of fetal head. However, there is no need for routine administration of an episiotomy or routine application of forceps.
    c. *Cord clamping:* Delayed clamping of the cord is to be considered in cases of preterm delivery. The cord must be kept at least 10 cm long in these cases. Umbilical cord must be clamped after milking the cord three times, if the baby has to be taken away. However, in case of stable mother and baby, clamping of the cord can be delayed by 30 seconds to 3 minutes (no longer). This strategy helps in transferring extra

80 mL blood or 50 mg iron to the baby. Also, the baby must be positioned below the level of placenta.

Precautions to be Taken at the Time of Delivery

- Bed rest, hydration, and pelvic rest do not appear to improve the rate of preterm birth and are not routinely recommended.
- Amniocentesis may be used in women with preterm labor to assess fetal lung maturity and intra-amniotic infection.
- Delaying cord clamping for 30–45 seconds after delivery of infants with very low birth weight (weighing <1,500 g) is associated with significant reductions in intraventricular hemorrhage (IVH) and late-onset sepsis. Infants where the cord clamping has been delayed also show improved hemodynamic parameters and reduced requirement for transfusion during their hospitalization.
- Prevention of hypothermia [skin-to-skin (kangaroo) care **(Fig. 16.5)**]
- Provision of adequate oxygenation
- Provision of intensive respiratory support starting right from the delivery room
- Provision of neonatal intensive care support
- Provision of optimal nutrition primarily with mother's own breast milk
- Early feeding of the newborn child must be initiated to prevent hypoglycemia.
- Magnesium sulfate provides neuroprotection for the neonate.
- The chances of sepsis can be minimized by observing adequate aseptic precautions.
- Prevention of long-term disability should be the goal.
- Initiation of surfactant therapy in the newborn baby may take care of its immature lungs.

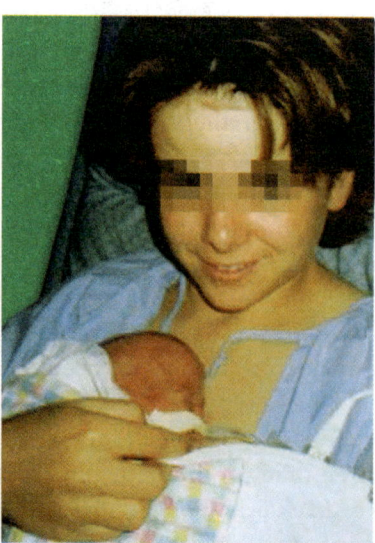

Fig. 16.5: Photograph of a mother giving kangaroo care to her newborn preterm child.

MEDICAL MANAGEMENT WITH TOCOLYSIS

> Q. Evaluate the role of tocolytic agents in case of preterm labor with the help of a short note.

Tocolysis should be used with caution only when the fetus is salvageable (≥24 weeks of gestation) because the expected prolongation of the pregnancy is limited. The chances of fetal survival are minimal at <23 weeks. Moreover, the chances of survival are further reduced in the presence of significant medical complications, such as intra-amniotic infection. Contraindications for tocolytic therapy are described in **Box 16.7**.

Since the risk of neonatal mortality and morbidity is low after 34 completed weeks of gestation, aggressive tocolytic therapy is generally not recommended beyond 34 weeks, due to potential maternal complications. Between 24 and 33 weeks of gestation, tocolytic therapy must be initiated if the benefits associated with its use outweigh the risk of maternal and/or fetal complications. Even though aggressive tocolysis is not typically used beyond 34 weeks of gestation, clinicians are advised not to deliver patients at this gestation without indication because of a higher risk of neonatal morbidity in infants born at 34–36 weeks' gestation.

Tocolytic agents have not proven to be efficacious in preventing preterm birth or reducing neonatal mortality or morbidity. The goals of tocolytic therapy are enumerated in **Box 16.8**. The primary purpose of tocolytic therapy today is to delay delivery for 48 hours to allow the maximum benefit of glucocorticoids to decrease the incidence of respiratory distress syndrome. While tocolytics can be successful for 48 hours when membranes are intact, some clinical studies suggest that the effectiveness of tocolytics is only slightly

BOX 16.7: Contraindications for tocolytic therapy.

- Advanced labor
- Chorioamnionitis
- Severe preeclampsia
- Abruption placenta
- Fetal distress
- Fetal demise
- Fetal anomaly
- Hyper/hypothyroidism
- Severe anemia
- Patients with heart disease/diabetes

BOX 16.8: Goals of tocolytic treatment for women in preterm labor.

- Delay in delivery to optimize the place, time, and type of delivery
- Allow time for administration of antenatal corticosteroids to accelerate fetal lung maturity
- Antibiotic administration in labor to reduce neonatal infection, specifically group B *Streptococcus* infection
- Administration of magnesium sulfate before the anticipated delivery for fetal neuroprotection

better than bed rest and hydration, both of which have fewer adverse effects than tocolytic therapy. Criteria for considering tocolytic therapy are enumerated in **Box 16.9**.

Prerequisites for Initiation of Tocolytic Therapy

The parameters which must be assessed before initiating the tocolytic therapy are mentioned in **Box 16.10**. One should always attempt to determine the gestational age by first identifying the first day of LMP and confirming it by one or more of the following:

- Positive pregnancy test (home or clinic) prior to the expected date of second missed period
- Estimation of uterine size determined by bimanual examination prior to 12 weeks' gestation
- Doppler fetal heart tones noted prior to 12 weeks' gestation
- Ultrasonographic estimation of gestational age (preferably in the first trimester). When the LMP is not reliable, the gestational age is determined by the first ultrasonography.

Specific tocolytic agents should not be used whenever known allergies exist. Indomethacin is contraindicated in the presence of aspirin-induced asthma, coagulopathy, or significant liver disease. Magnesium sulfate should not be used in combination with certain medications, such as calcium channel blockers, or when myasthenia gravis or neuromuscular disorders exist. Betamimetics (e.g., terbutaline) may be contraindicated in the presence of cardiac arrhythmia, valvular disease, ischemic heart disease, etc. It may also alter glucose homeostasis in patients with diabetes and abnormal glucose tolerance test results.

> **BOX 16.9:** Criteria for considering tocolytic therapy.
>
> - Presence of more than six contractions per hour, resulting in a demonstrated cervical change
>   or
> - Presumed prior cervical change (transvaginal cervical length < 2.5 cm, >50% cervical effacement, or cervical dilation ≥ 2 cm)

> **BOX 16.10:** Criteria to be assessed before initiating tocolytic therapy.
>
> - Accurate determination of the gestational age
> - No evidence of chorioamnionitis
> - Absence of any congenital anomaly incompatible with life
> - Reactive nonstress test results or negative contraction stress test results
> - Absence of any decelerations on cardiotocographic examination
> - Normal diastolic flow upon Doppler examination of umbilical blood flow
> - Absence of significant vaginal bleeding (indicative of abruption)
> - Absence of any underlying medical condition, particularly cardiac disease
> - No known allergy/contraindication to the particular tocolytic agent being used

Tocolytic Agents

The most common tocolytic agents used for the treatment of preterm labor are indomethacin and nifedipine. In the past, betamimetic agents, such as terbutaline or ritodrine, were the agents of choice, but in recent years their use has been significantly curtailed due to maternal and fetal side effects, such as maternal tachycardia, hyperglycemia, arrhythmia, myocardial ischemia, palpitations, arrhythmia, bronchospasm, pulmonary edema, and abnormal glucose tolerance tests. The FDA (2011) concluded that the risk of serious adverse events caused by the betamimetic agents outweighs any potential benefit to pregnant women receiving prolonged treatment with these agents. The various tocolytic agents which can be used to treat preterm labor are summarized in **Table 16.5**. The first-line tocolytic agent of choice is nifedipine. The second tocolytic agent of choice is indomethacin.

Nifedipine

Calcium channel blockers, such as nifedipine, act as uterine relaxants by reducing the influx of Ca^{2+} into the cell membranes, thereby reducing the tone of smooth muscles. As a result, nifedipine has emerged as an effective and safe alternative tocolytic agent for the management of preterm labor. Several randomized studies have shown that the use of nifedipine in comparison with other tocolytics is associated with a more frequent and successful prolongation of pregnancy, resulting in significantly fewer maternal side effects and neonatal complications.

It is administered in the dosage of 20–30 mg stat followed by 10–20 mg 6-hourly for 48–72 hours. Nifedipine can be considered in case of preterm labor between 24 and 25^{+6} weeks of gestation and must be definitely offered between 26 and 33^{+6} weeks of gestation.

Contraindications of nifedipine therapy include allergy to nifedipine, hypotension, hepatic dysfunction, concurrent use of betamimetics or $MgSO_4$, transdermal nitrates, or other antihypertensive medication. Some commonly reported side effects associated with nifedipine therapy include hypotension, palpitations, flushing, nausea, dizziness, headaches, feeling of nervousness, etc.

Serious side effects, which can rarely occur, include myocardial infarction, gastrointestinal obstruction, and very rarely, aplastic anemia. There are no known fetal side effects related with the use of nifedipine.

If nifedipine is contraindicated, oxytocin receptor antagonists can be offered. However, betamimetics must not be offered for tocolysis.

Prostaglandin Synthetase Inhibitors

Prostaglandin synthetase inhibitors include drugs such as indomethacin, aspirin, ibuprofen, and sulindac. Of these

TABLE 16.5: Various tocolytic agents used in cases of preterm labor.

Tocolytic agent	Dosage and administration	Maternal side effects	Fetal and neonatal side effects
Betamimetics	• Terbutaline, 0.25 mg subcutaneously every 20 minutes to 3 hours (withhold administration for pulse rate > 120 bpm) • Ritodrine initial dose of 50–100 µg/min, IV, increase by 50 µg/min every 10 minutes until contractions cease or side effects develop. Maximum dose is 350 µg/min	• Cardiac or pulmonary arrhythmias, pulmonary edema, myocardial ischemia, hypotension, tachycardia, shortness of breath, etc. • Metabolic hyperglycemia, hyperinsulinemia, antidiuresis, altered thyroid function, hypokalemia, tremor, nervousness, nausea or vomiting, etc.	Tachycardia, hyperinsulinemia, fetal hyperglycemia, neonatal hypoglycemia, hypocalcemia, hypotension, myocardial and septal hypertrophy, myocardial ischemia, etc.
Magnesium sulfate	4–6 g bolus for 20 minutes, then 2–3 g/h	Flushing, lethargy, muscle weakness, diplopia, dry mouth, pulmonary edema, cardiac arrest	Lethargy, hypotonia, respiratory depression, demineralization
Calcium channel blockers: Nifedipine	30 mg loading dose, then 10–20 mg every 4–6 hours for 48–72 hours (Maximum dose is 180 mg in 24 hours)	Flushing, hypotension, headache, dizziness, nausea, facial flushing, hypotension, transient tachycardia, palpitations	Sudden fetal death, fetal distress
Prostaglandin synthetase inhibitors: Indomethacin	*Indomethacin:* Loading dose of 50 mg rectally or 50–100 mg orally, then 25–50 mg orally every 6-hourly for 48 hours	Nausea, heartburn, gastritis, proctitis with hematochezia, impairment of renal function, increased postpartum hemorrhage, heartburn, headache, dizziness, depression	Constriction of ductus arteriosus, pulmonary hypertension, reversible decrease in renal function with oligohydramnios, intraventricular hemorrhage, hyperbilirubinemia, necrotizing enterocolitis
Nitric oxide donors	Glyceryl trinitrate 10 mg patch for every 12 hours, continuing until contractions cease, up to 48 hours	Headache, neonatal hypotension	Neonatal hypotension
Oxytocin antagonists	Atosiban initial bolus dose: 6.75 mg over 1 minute, followed by an infusion of 18 mg/h for 3 hours and then 6 mg/h for up to 45 hours	Nausea (short duration), allergic reaction, headache (short duration)	None noted as yet

Source: Hearne AE, Nagey DA. Therapeutic agents in preterm labor: tocolytic agents. Clin Obstet Gynecol. 2000;43:787-801.

various agents, indomethacin is most commonly used and acts as an appropriate tocolytic agent for the pregnant patient in early preterm labor or preterm labor associated with polyhydramnios. Indomethacin also decreases the synthesis of prostaglandins from decidual macrophages. The fetal renal effects of indomethacin may be helpful in reducing the amount of amniotic fluid. Therefore, besides treating polyhydramnios, the use of indomethacin can be associated with complications such as oligohydramnios, premature closure of ductus, neonatal pulmonary hypertension, and necrotizing enterocolitis. Since premature closure of the ductus is common after 32 weeks of gestation, the use of indomethacin at a gestational age of ≥32 weeks is not recommended.

Prostaglandin synthetase inhibitors, such as indomethacin, have been shown to have efficacy similar to that of terbutaline but are associated with infrequent maternal side effects. Baseline laboratory investigations, including CBC and liver function tests, should be ordered prior to the initiation of therapy.

- During treatment, parameters such as urine output, maternal temperature, and amniotic fluid index should be evaluated periodically.
- The loading dose of indomethacin is 60 mg stat by oral route followed by 25 mg every 4 hours for 48–72 hours. It must not be administered beyond 72 hours. It is also likely to cause oligohydramnios, so the clinician needs to be careful about that.
- Maternal side effects which can occur with indomethacin include dizziness, headaches, vertigo, and tinnitus. Serious side effects include gastrointestinal bleeding and perforation, aplastic anemia, hepatic necrosis, renal failure, and reduced platelet count. Therefore, administration of indomethacin must be avoided in patients with hepatic, renal, and ulcerative disorders, as well as asthmatic patients.

Oxytocin Antagonists

Oxytocin antagonists, such as atosiban, are now licensed for use in the UK and are considered as the tocolytic agents of choice in cases of preterm labor. However, their high cost might prevent their frequent use in developing countries. Moreover, administration of atosiban requires the patient to be admitted for monitoring in the hospital for 48 hours. Nevertheless, this drug is increasingly being used at several centers across India. Atosiban is administered in an initial bolus dose of 6.75 mg over 1 minute, followed by an infusion of 37.5 mg in 3 hours (high-dose infusion), then 37.5 mg for up to 45 hours.

Nitric Oxide Donors

Nitric oxide donors, such as nitroglycerine, have been sometimes used for causing smooth muscle relaxation.

Beta Agonists

Beta 2 agonists: These comprise agents such as Isoxsuprine, ritodrine, terbutaline, and salbutamol. These agents can cause vasodilatation, bronchodilation, and uterine muscle relaxation. In lieu of several safer tocolytic agents available, beta agonists are nowadays rarely used as tocolytic agents. If these drugs are ever used as tocolytic agents, the clinician must be careful to closely monitor the pulse rate and not to let it go beyond 120 bpm.

Neuroprotection

Magnesium Sulfate

Though previously magnesium sulfate was commonly used as a tocolytic agent in the USA, it is now commonly being used worldwide for neuroprotection. However, the tocolytic activity of magnesium sulfate is quite weak. It has been demonstrated to provide neuroprotection by reducing the risk of cerebral palsy and gross motor dysfunction. In case it is being used for providing neuroprotection, it should not be used concomitantly with nifedipine (as a tocolytic agent) in order to prevent maternal complications. The ACTOMgSO$_4$ (Australian Collaborative Trial of Magnesium Sulfate) trial (2003) has shown that administration of magnesium to women immediately before very preterm birth may improve important pediatric outcomes. No serious harmful effects were seen. In this study, a loading dose of 4 g was given followed by 1 g/h for maximum of 24 hours. A randomized controlled BEAM (Beneficial Effects of Antenatal Magnesium Sulfate) trial, 2008 has shown that although fetal exposure to magnesium sulfate before anticipated early preterm delivery is not likely to reduce the combined risk of cerebral palsy or death, the rate of cerebral palsy is likely to be significantly reduced amongst the survivors in the group that received magnesium sulfate. In this study, a loading dose of 6 g was given followed by a maintenance dose of 2 g/h for a maximum of 12 hours. The PREMAG (PREterm brain protection by MAGnesium sulfate) trial (2007) has shown that the rate of combined death or gross motor dysfunction at 2 years was lower in the magnesium sulfate group. In this study, a loading dose of 4 g was only administered and no maintenance dose was given.

- The loading dose of magnesium sulfate used for neuroprotection is 4–6 g in 15 minutes followed by 1–2 g/h for 12–24 hours. If the preterm pain has subsided, the use of magnesium sulfate must be discontinued because its use over a period of 1 week may result in the development of fetal osteopenia.
- Between 23 and 23^{+6} weeks of gestation, administration of magnesium sulfate must be discussed with the woman and her family in context of individual circumstances. Magnesium sulfate must be offered to the women between 24 and 29^{+6} weeks of gestation if established labor and birth appears likely within 24 hours. It should be preferably used prior to 32 weeks.
- Common maternal side effects associated with the use of magnesium sulfate include flushing, nausea, headache, drowsiness, and blurred vision. The mother should be monitored for toxic effects such as respiratory depression or even cardiac arrest that can occur at supratherapeutic levels. In addition, magnesium sulfate readily crosses the placenta and may lead to respiratory and motor depression of the neonate.
- Before starting magnesium sulfate, the following baseline investigations must be performed, including, CBC, serum creatinine level, and urine output (normal value is >30 mL/h). A baseline maternal neurological examination must also be performed to assess maternal mentation.
- Serum magnesium levels may be obtained 1 hour after the loading dose and then every 6 hours, and the maintenance dosage should be titrated to maintain a serum level of 4–8 mg/dL.
- If the toxicity symptoms are life-threatening, administration of 1 g of calcium gluconate by slow IV push may prove to be helpful.
- Contraindications for the use of magnesium sulfate are enumerated in **Box 16.11**.

Corticosteroid Therapy

Corticosteroid therapy helps in reducing the incidence of complications such as respiratory distress syndrome, IVH, and neonatal mortality. This therapy is recommended in the absence of clinical infection whenever the gestational age is between 23 and 33^{+6} weeks of gestation. Corticosteroids must be recommended if there is a high likelihood of spontaneous or indicated preterm delivery. An attempt should be made to delay delivery for a minimum of 12 hours to obtain maximum benefits of antenatal steroids. The recommended dosage of corticosteroids includes the following:

- Two 12 mg doses of betamethasone 24 hours apart (to be administered intramuscularly)

BOX 16.11: Contraindications for the use of magnesium sulfate.

- Active labor
- Major congenital anomalies
- Pulmonary hypertension
- Myasthenia gravis
- Class II–IV cardiac disease
- Severe acute pulmonary disease
- Renal insufficiency

- Four doses of 6 mg of dexamethasone should be administered at 6-hour intervals (to be administered intramuscularly).
- For period of gestation between 23 and 23^{+6} weeks of gestation, the option of prescribing steroids must be discussed with the woman and her family after explaining to them the poor fetal prognosis. Corticosteroids must be offered between 24 and 33^{+6} weeks of gestation. They can be considered between 34 and 35^{+6} weeks of gestation after discussing the potential risks and benefits with the woman. Whenever the following clinical conditions exist, the glucocorticoid regimen may require modification:
    - In the presence of insulin-dependent or gestational diabetes, the provider should be prepared for control of blood sugars.
    - In case of severe fetal hypoxia, the use of prophylactic steroids should not delay the delivery of an acutely distressed fetus.
- The use of repeated doses of glucocorticoids in women at risk of preterm delivery remains controversial. Most clinicians consider the use of a single repeated dose of corticosteroids if the woman has crossed 2 weeks of prior corticosteroid injection and the patient remains at a significant risk for preterm delivery within the next 7 days, at a gestational age of <34 weeks. Corticosteroids can also be administered even between 34 and 36 weeks of gestation, if not given previously (<34 weeks) because steroids are likely to protect the newborn baby against respiratory distress syndrome, IVH, and necrotizing enterocolitis.

SURGICAL MANAGEMENT

Correction of Uterine Anomalies

Cervical screening and routine prophylactic cerclage can be considered in cases of preterm labor with underlying uterine anomalies. Hysteroscopic metroplasty is useful in patients with septate and subseptate uteri and helps in improving the pregnancy outcome. Hysteroscopic myomectomy can be used for removing the submucosal myomas. If pregnancy occurs with an intrauterine device (IUD) in situ, the device needs to be removed at the earliest opportunity in order to reduce the risk of preterm labor.

Therapeutic Interventions for Premature Cervical Shortening

Use of cervical cerclage in cases of preterm labor has been previously described in the text.

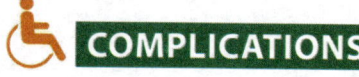

Maternal and fetal complications related to preterm labor are tabulated in **Table 16.6**.

TABLE 16.6: Complications related to preterm labor.

Maternal complications	Neonatal complications
• Preterm ROM and/or preterm delivery • Chorioamnionitis • Placental abruption • Retained placenta • Postpartum hemorrhage • Endometritis	• Prematurity • Pneumonia and early neonatal sepsis • Pulmonary hypoplasia • Fetal death

MATERNAL COMPLICATIONS

Premature Rupture of Membranes

 Q. Discuss the prelabor ROM with the help of a long essay.

Introduction

Premature rupture of membranes (PROM) can be defined as spontaneous rupture of membranes, beyond 28 weeks of pregnancy, but before the onset of labor. ROM occurring beyond 37 weeks of gestation, but before the onset of labor, is known as "term PROM". On the other hand, ROM occurring before 37 completed weeks of gestation but before the onset of labor is called Preterm premature rupture of membranes (PPROM). If ROM is present for >24 hours before delivery, it is known as prolonged ROM. PROM is not actually a complication, rather a cause for preterm labor because this condition may be followed by a preterm delivery (if PROM occurs at <37 weeks of gestation).

Etiology

- Increased friability and reduced tensile strength of the membranes
- Polyhydramnios
- Cervical incompetence
- Multiple pregnancy
- Intrauterine infection such as chorioamnionitis, urinary tract or lower genital tract infection

Diagnosis

Clinical presentation: There may be escape of watery discharge per vaginum in the form of either gush of fluid or slow leakage. The diagnosis of PROM can be confirmed by performing the following tests:

- *Sterile per speculum examination:* Per speculum examination must be conducted after observing all aseptic precautions as the risk for chorioamnionitis is high in these cases. Clear fluid coming out of cervical os or a speculum pool of amniotic fluid is indicative of PROM. A high vaginal swab can be taken at the time of this examination. Also, clinicians must be careful not to perform a digital examination unless they have decided to terminate the pregnancy. If no amniotic fluid is observed, perform a phosphorylated insulin-like growth factor binding protein (PIGFBP) test or placental alpha macroglobulin-1 (PAMG-1) test of vaginal fluid. Both these tests have a high negative predictive value, but poor positive predictive value, thereby supporting their role as useful "rule-out tests." If PlGFBP or PAMG-1 tests are positive, the clinician must consider the patient's clinical condition, medical history, obstetric history, and gestational age. In case these tests are negative, PPROM is unlikely, and she must be asked to return in case any further symptoms occur.

- *Nitrazine paper test:* A per speculum examination must be performed to collect the fluid from posterior fornix (vaginal pool). The pH of the fluid collected from the vaginal fornix must be detected using litmus or nitrazine paper. Since the liquor is normally alkaline in nature (pH 7–7.5), the normally acidic vaginal pH (4.5–5.5) turns alkaline in the presence of PROM, causing the color of the nitrazine paper to change from yellow to blue.
- *Ferning:* The liquor-smeared slide when examined under the microscope shows appearance of a characteristic ferning pattern.
- *Staining of the centrifuged cells with 0.1% Nile blue sulfate:* There may be orange–blue discoloration of the cells due to the presence of exfoliated fat-containing cells from sebaceous glands of the fetus.
- *Intra-amniotic dye injection:* Presence of blue discoloration of the fluid emanating from cervical os following the injection of 2–3 mL of sterile solution of the dye indigo carmine into the amniotic cavity is indicative of PROM.
- *Alpha-fetoproteins:* Presence of alpha-fetoproteins in the vaginal secretions is indicative of PROM.
- *AmniSure test:* This is an immunochromatographic method, which detects the presence of placental alpha microglobulin-1 (PAMG-1).
- *Ultrasound examination:* There may be the presence of oligohydramnios on ultrasound examination.

No diagnostic test is required if the woman is in established labor.

Investigations

- Full blood count
- White cell count
- Differential count
- Determination of levels of C-reactive protein
- Urine routine microscopy and culture
- *Speculum examination:* This helps in confirming the diagnosis of PPROM, obtaining fluid for determining pulmonary maturity, and obtaining endocervical samples for *Chlamydia* and *Neisseria gonorrhoeae*.
- Ultrasound for biophysical profile, estimation of gestational age and weight, measurement of cervical length and amniotic fluid volume
- Nonstress test

Management

> Q. With the help of a long essay, discuss the management of a 34-year-old para 3 woman with no live child admitted with PPROM at 32 weeks of gestation.
>
> Q. If the case study mentioned in the beginning of the chapter had been accompanied by ROM, in what way would the management change?
>
> Q. With the help of a short essay, discuss the management of preterm PROM.

Further management after confirmation of the diagnosis of PROM is described in **Flowchart 16.4**.

Deciding the time of delivery: Management of PROM basically depends on gestational age and fetal status. The main aim of management in case of PROM is to avoid delivery prior to 34 weeks of gestation. Delivery should be preferably considered at 34 weeks of gestation. The clinician should avoid going beyond 34 weeks.

In women with PROM at term, labor should be induced immediately, generally with oxytocin infusion, to reduce the risk of chorioamnionitis.

Women who need to be delivered irrespective of the period of gestation include the following:

- Those with acute chorioamnionitis/subclinical infection/inflammation or those at a high risk of infection
- Patients with placental abruption, or evidence of fetal compromise
- Those with mature lungs or with period of gestation > 36 weeks
- Nonreassuring fetal heart sounds
- Fetuses with lethal congenital anomalies
- Women in advanced labor, with cervical effacement of 80% or more and cervical dilatation of 5 cm or more

Expectant management: It may be considered if the period of gestation is <34 weeks or the pulmonary maturity has not been attained. It comprises the following steps:

1. Women should be observed for signs of clinical chorioamnionitis at least every 12-hourly.
2. A weekly high vaginal or rectal swab and at least a weekly maternal full blood count should be considered. Although weekly culture of swabs from the vagina is often performed as part of the clinical management of women with PPROM, there is little evidence regarding the efficacy of this practice. Antibiotics may be commenced based on the results of culture.
3. Antibiotics should be administered for 7 days. Ampicillin is the antibiotic of choice administered in the dose 2 g stat followed by 2 g every 6 hours for 48 hours. Erythromycin can be added in the dosage of 250 mg 6-hourly for 48 hours in order to provide neonatal benefits. Instead of erythromycin, azithromycin can be administered as 1 g stat dose. Following this, oral amoxycillin can be administered in the dosage of 500 mg TDS for next 5 days.

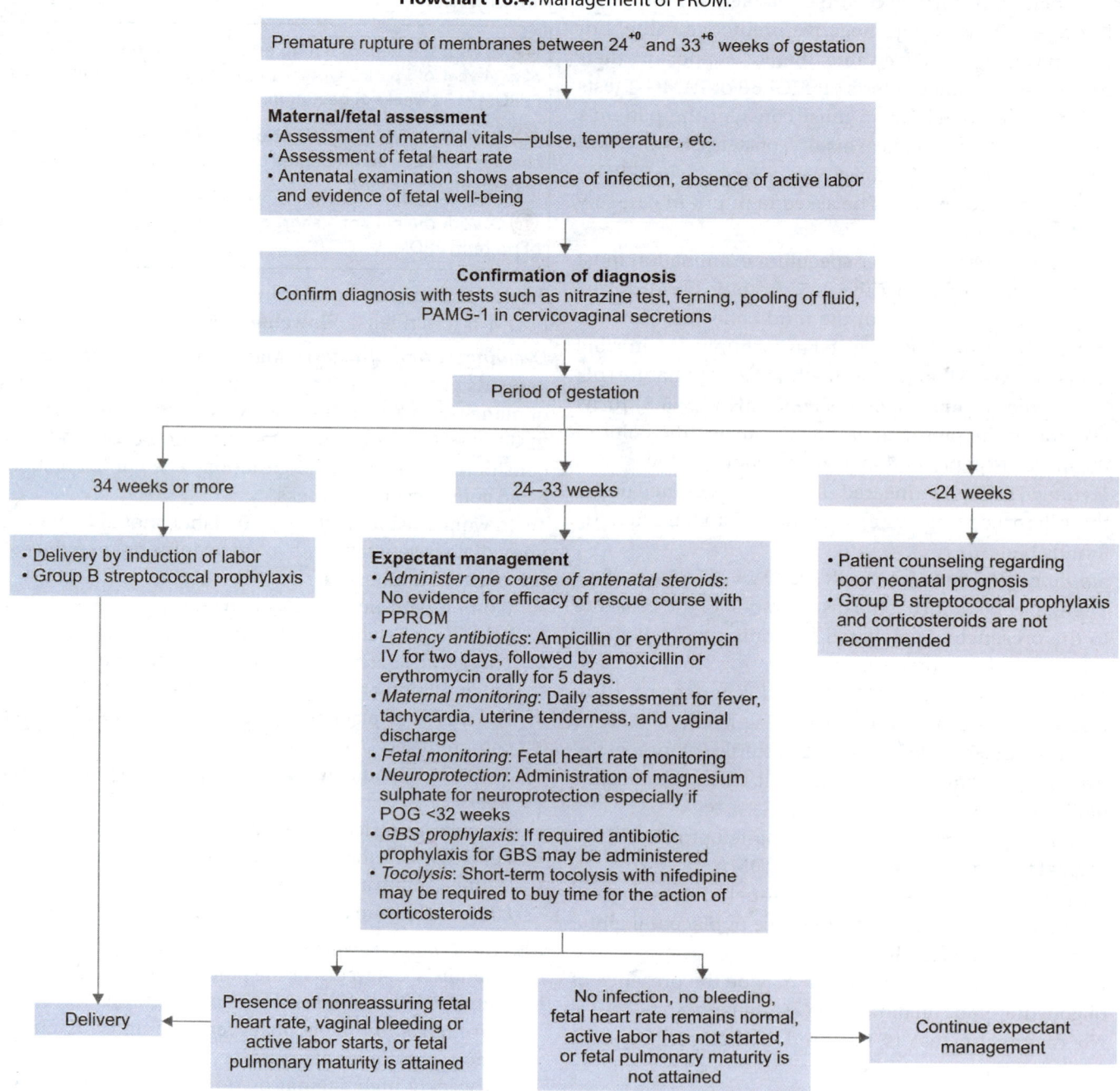

Flowchart 16.4: Management of PROM.

(GBS: group B streptococcus; PAMG-1: placental alpha macroglobulin-1; POG: period of gestation)

4. Fetal monitoring using cardiotocography should be considered where regular fetal surveillance is required.
5. Biophysical profile scoring or Doppler velocimetry should not be considered as first-line surveillance tests.
6. Prophylactic tocolysis in women with PPROM without uterine activity is not recommended. Women with PPROM and uterine activity who require antenatal corticosteroids should be considered for tocolysis. The tocolytic agent of choice for women with PPROM is nifedipine. It is given in the initial dosage of 20–30 mg followed by 10–20 mg at every 6 hours' interval.
7. Digital cervical examination should be avoided in patients with PROM unless they are in active labor or imminent delivery is anticipated.
8. Cesarean section is not routinely required, but may be required in the presence of an obstetric indication.
9. A single course of antenatal corticosteroids should be given to women with PROM at 24–31 weeks' gestation to reduce the risk of perinatal mortality, respiratory distress syndrome, and other morbidities.
10. Routine amniocentesis is not recommended for women with PPROM.
11. All women with PROM and a viable fetus, including those who are known carriers of GBS or who deliver before their GBS status can be determined, should receive intrapartum chemoprophylaxis to prevent vertical transmission of GBS. Recommended

prophylaxis for group B streptococcal infection is described in **Box 16.12**.
12. Transvaginal/transabdominal amnioinfusion in labor is not recommended for women with PROM.
13. A few studies have described transvaginal or transabdominal injection of fibrin into the amniotic fluid of patients with second-trimester PROM with the aim of sealing the membranes. Presently, fibrin sealants are not recommended as routine treatment for second-trimester oligohydramnios.

Complications

Maternal complications: These are as follows:
- *Infection*: It could be related to acute or chronic chorioamnionitis. There are high chances of ascending infection if ROM is present for >24 hours.
- *Preterm labor*: PROM is an important cause for preterm labor. In about 80–90% of the cases, labor starts within 24 hours.
- *Cord prolapse*: Sudden gush of amniotic fluid may be associated with an increased incidence of cord prolapse, premature placental separation (placental abruption), and/or oligohydramnios.

Fetal/neonatal complications: These are as follows:
- *Respiratory distress syndrome/hyaline membrane disease*: The newborn infant may suffer from severe respiratory distress, thereby requiring ventilator support after birth.
- *Nonreassuring fetal heart rate pattern*: Most common abnormality is variable decelerations associated with umbilical cord compression as a result of oligohydramnios. Moderate or severe variable/late decelerations may be present as a result of placental insufficiency and are indicative of intrapartum fetal distress.
- *Pulmonary hypoplasia*: This condition may be characterized by the presence of multiple pneumothoraxes and interstitial emphysema.
- *Cerebral palsy*: This may be the result of intraventricular bleeding, intrapartum fetal acidosis, and hypoxia.
- *Fetal deformities*: These may especially include facial and skeletal deformities.
- *Fetal trauma*: This could be related to fetal macrosomia, which may be responsible for producing injury to the brachial plexus, fracture of humerus or clavicle, cephalic hematomas, skull fracture, etc.

BOX 16.12: Recommended prophylaxis for group B streptococcal infection.

- *Penicillin G:* 5 million units IV initial dose, then 2.5 million units IV at every 4-hour-interval until delivery

  or

- *Ampicillin:* 2 g IV initial dose, then 1 g IV at every 4 hours or 2 g at every 6 hours until delivery

  or

- *Cefazolin:* 2 g IV initial dose, then 1 g IV at every 8-hour-interval until delivery

- *Postmaturity syndrome:* This is characterized by the presence of wrinkled skin due to reduced amount of subcutaneous fat. These fetuses are small, tolerate labor poorly, and may be acidotic at birth.

 Q. Write a short note on chorioamnionitis.

Chorioamnionitis

Diagnosis of chorioamnionitis is made in case of temperature > 38.0°C (100.0°F) and the presence of two out of the following five signs:
1. WBC count > 15,000 cells/mm^3
2. Maternal tachycardia > 100 bpm
3. Fetal tachycardia > 160 bpm
4. Tender uterus
5. Foul-smelling discharge

In situations in which the diagnosis remains unclear, an amniocentesis for fluid culture (aerobic/anaerobic bacteria), Gram stain (gram-positive bacteria present if Gram stain is positive or if WBC count is >50 cells/mm^3), glucose level (positive if <15 mg/dL), or leukocyte esterase evaluation may be considered.

FETAL COMPLICATIONS

Figure 16.6 shows the photograph of a preterm baby born at 30 weeks of gestation, weighing about 1,000 g. The preterm baby is usually deficient in subcutaneous fat. As a result, the baby's skin appears pink in color, feels very thin, and can easily wrinkle. The preterm baby's head circumference may exceed the waist circumference. Birth weight of a normal-term infant varies from 2,500 to 3,999 g. Most preterm babies may be of low weight. Low birth weight can be defined as weight < 2,500 g. Length of a preterm baby may be <47 cm. Dubowitz (Ballard) examination is used for assessing fetal maturity based on the physical characteristics as well as the maturity of neuromuscular system **(Fig. 16.7)**. Care of a premature baby should comprise the following steps:

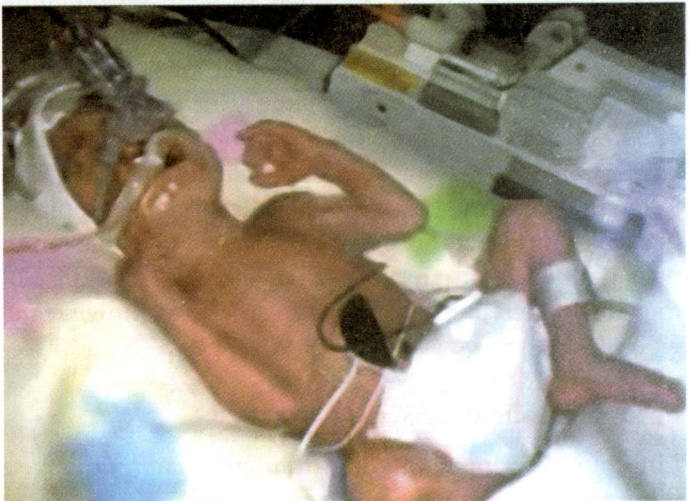

Fig. 16.6: Photograph of a preterm baby born at 30 weeks of gestation.

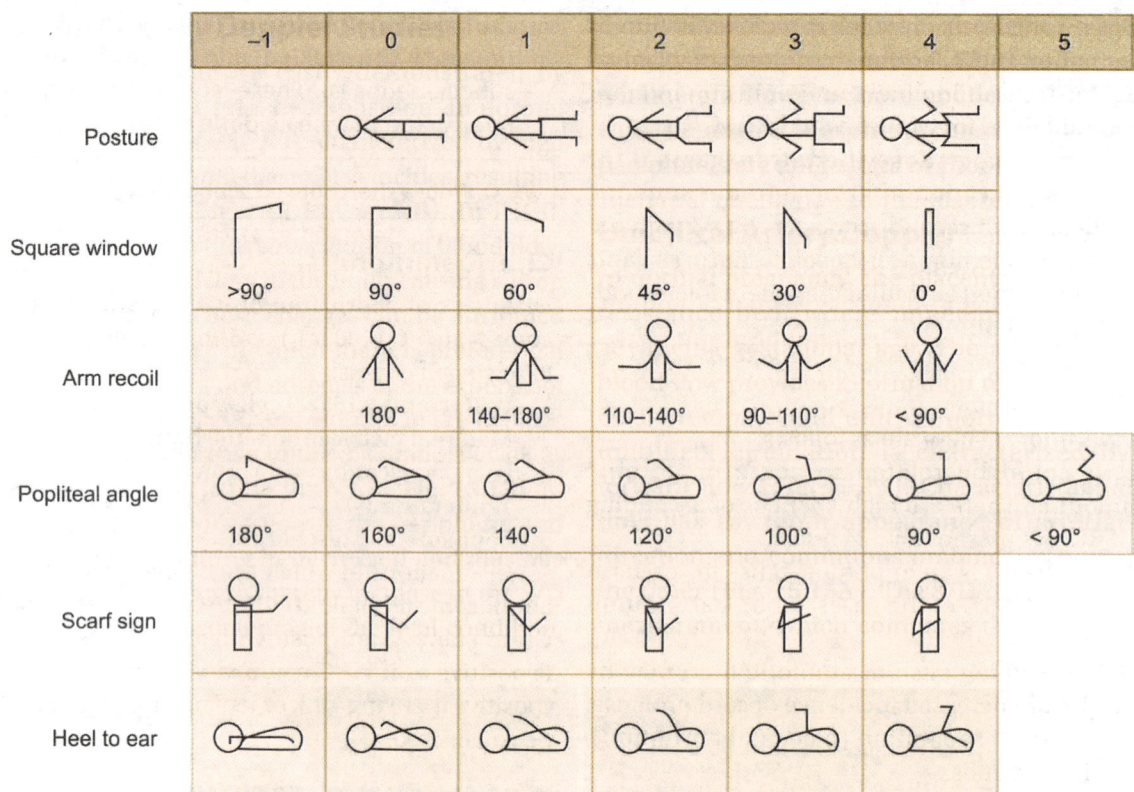

Fig. 16.7: Dubowitz (Ballard) examination for a newborn.

1. Comprehensive neonatal care, chlorhexidine cord care, control of respiratory distress syndrome, infection, etc.
2. Kangaroo mother care wherever possible

As per the WHO (2018), the goal of care is to reduce neonatal morbidity by 50% where presently it is ≥5/1,000 or to eliminate it completely in countries where it is less (by 2025).

Dubowitz (Ballard) examination for newborn: Points are given for each parameter, which is assessed. Low scores (–1 or 0) are given in case of extreme prematurity. High scores (4, 5) are given in case of postmaturity.

Physical characteristics, which are assessed, include parameters such as skin texture, lanugo hair, plantar creases, breasts, eyes and ear, and appearance of the genitalia. Assessment of neuromuscular maturity includes evaluation of parameters such as posture, square window (flexion of baby's hand toward the wrist), arm recoil (angle of recoil following very brief extension of the upper extremity), heel-to-ear movement (passive resistance to extension of posterior hip flexor muscles), popliteal angle (resistance of the baby's knee to extension), and scarf sign (how far the elbow can be moved across the baby's chest).

Fetal Complications

Children of women suffering from chorioamnionitis are more likely to experience complications such as sepsis, respiratory distress syndrome, early onset seizures, IVH and periventricular leukomalacia, necrotizing enterocolitis, bronchopulmonary dysplasia, myocardial dysfunction, and neonatal sepsis. Some of the complications which can occur in preterm infants include:

- *Pulmonary complications:* Respiratory distress, bronchopulmonary dysplasia, etc.
- *Gastrointestinal complications:* Hyperbilirubinemia, necrotizing enterocolitis, failure to thrive, etc.
- *Central nervous system complications:* IVH, hydrocephalus, cerebral palsy, neurodevelopmental delay, and hearing loss
- *Ophthalmological complications:* Retinopathy of prematurity, retinal detachment, etc.
- *Cardiovascular complications:* Hypotension, patent ductus arteriosus, pulmonary hypertension, etc.
- *Renal complications:* Water and electrolyte imbalance, acid–base disturbances, etc.
- *Hematological complications:* Iatrogenic anemia, requirement for frequent blood transfusions, anemia of prematurity, etc.
- *Endocrinological complications:* Hypoglycemia, transiently low thyroxine levels, cortisol deficiency, and increased insulin resistance in adulthood

 EVIDENCE-BASED CLINICAL TRIALS

 List of references can be scanned through QR code to enable the readers gain deeper insight of the subject by referring to the entire article or its abstract.

CHAPTER 17

Postdated Pregnancy and Intrauterine Death

PART 1: POSTDATED PREGNANCY

CASE STUDY

A 28-year-old primiparous patient presented to the obstetrics and gynecology clinic with the pregnancy, which was postdated by 2 weeks both according to dates and according to an ultrasound examination done during the first trimester. She has yet not started feeling any labor pains. She is however experiencing normal fetal movements.

INTRODUCTION

Post-term or postmature pregnancy can be defined as any pregnancy continuing beyond 2 weeks of the expected date of delivery (EDD) (>294 days or >42 weeks). The normal duration of pregnancy is 37–42 weeks, which is referred to as "term". The estimated delivery date is calculated by adding 40 weeks or 280 days to the first day of the last menstrual period (LMP). Post-term pregnancy is associated with increased perinatal mortality and morbidity.

Definitions of various terminologies used to define term and post-term pregnancies as devised by the ACOG (2013) have been described in **Table 17.1**. Nearly 10% of pregnancies are likely to go beyond 41 weeks, whereas 1–2% of pregnancies are expected to go beyond 42 weeks. As per the WHO longitudinal study, median gestational age of Indian women at birth was 38 weeks plus 4 days.

Physiological changes associated with post-term gestation are described in **Table 17.2**. Placental aging/senescence causes critical reduction in the supply of nutrients and oxygen to the fetus, resulting in fetal compromise. Moreover, oligohydramnios in post-term babies is associated with an increased morbidity related to disorders such as hypertension/ preeclampsia, diabetes mellitus, placental abruption, IUGR, and multiple gestation.

TABLE 17.1: Definition of various terminologies used to define pregnancy where period of gestation has exceeded the expected date of delivery.

Terminology used	Period of gestation (in weeks)
Early term	37–38^{+6}
Full term	39–40^{+6}
Late term	41–41^{+6}
Post term	42 weeks or beyond

TABLE 17.2: Physiological changes associated with post-term gestation.

Organ affected	Physiological changes
Placental changes	• Senescence/aging (increased placental grading on ultrasound examination) • Placental infarcts • Calcification
Amniotic fluid changes	• Oligohydramnios (diminished fetal urination) • Cloudiness of amniotic fluid (flakes of vernix) • L:S ratio = 4:1 • Presence of meconium in the amniotic fluid, resulting in MAS and inflammation of the lungs
Fetal changes	• Macrosomia (45%) • Intrauterine malnutrition

(L:S ratio: lecithin/sphingomyelin ratio, MAS: meconium aspiration syndrome)

HISTORY AND CLINICAL PRESENTATION

Q. With the help of a long essay, discuss the etiology and management of post-term labor.

RISK FACTORS

The exact cause of postdated pregnancy remains unknown, and majority of post-term pregnancies have no known causes. The process of initiation of labor is described in **Flowchart 17.1**. Interruption of the process at any stage is

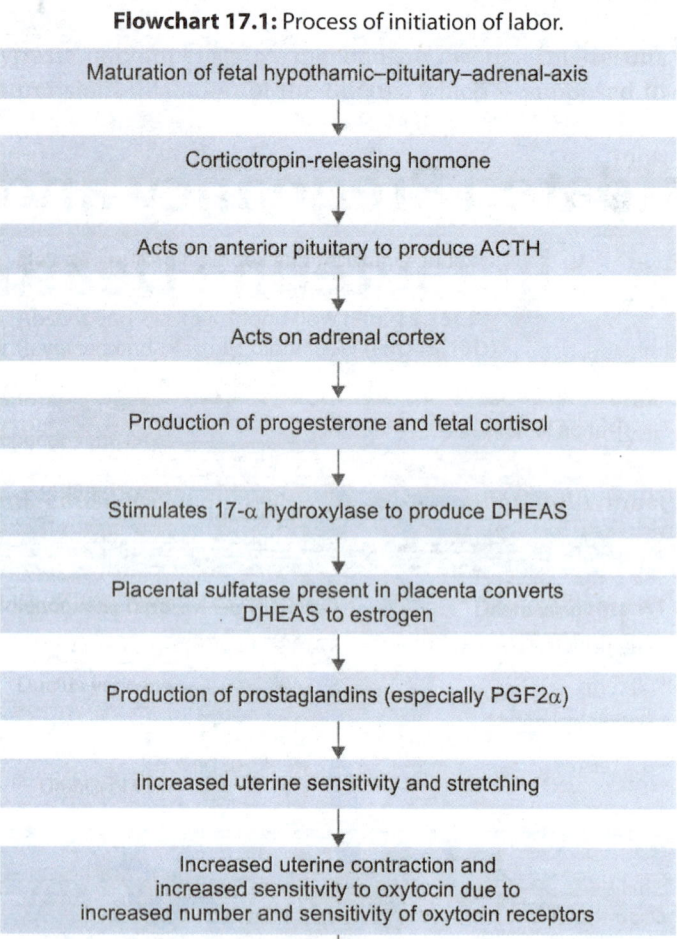

Flowchart 17.1: Process of initiation of labor.

(ACTH: adrenocorticotropic hormone; DHEAS: dehydroepiandrosterone sulfate; PGF2α: prostaglandin F2α)

likely to result in postdated pregnancy. Some of the likely causes for postdated pregnancy are as follows:

- *Wrong dates:* This can be considered as the most common cause of postmaturity. In these cases, the use of ultrasonography helps in determining the accurate estimation of gestational age.
- *Previous history of post-term pregnancy:* This can be considered as the most important risk factor for post-term pregnancy. One previous post-term pregnancy is associated with a two-to-three-fold increase in the risk of post-term pregnancy, whereas two previous post-term pregnancies are associated with nearly four-fold increased risk.
- *Maternal factors:* These include factors such as primiparity, previous history of prolonged pregnancy, sedentary habits, genetic predisposition, and elderly multipara. However, there is not much evidence available regarding each of these risk factors.
- *Fetal factors:* Fetal disorders such as anencephaly may be implicated in the causation of postmaturity. Anencephaly is likely to result in post-term pregnancy by causing the disruption of fetal pituitary–adrenal axis. Fetal male sex has also been implicated as a cause of postmaturity.
- *Placental factors:* Placental factors such as sulfatase deficiency (X-linked recessive disorder) may be also involved. As the pregnancy passes from week 40 to 42, there is placental insufficiency.
- *Genetic factors:* Genetic disorders such as congenital adrenal hyperplasia may be associated with post-term pregnancy due to the likely adrenal hypofunction.

CLINICAL PRESENTATION

At the time of taking history in case of post-term pregnancy, it is important to accurately calculate the gestational age. LMP tends to be reliable in calculation of period of gestation if the patient definitely remembers her LMP, she had been experiencing normal and regular menstrual cycles, there is no history of intake of oral contraceptives during the past 3 months, and the pregnancy was planned. Note that the length of gestation increases approximately by 1 day for each day the menstrual cycle is >28 days. In case of any discrepancy between the period of gestation calculated by applying Naegele's rule and that estimated using clinical examination in the first trimester, the following pointers can be used:

- *Time at which the mother can perceive quickening:* Maternal perception of fetal movements normally occurs at about 16–20 weeks.
- *Ultrasound examination:* Fetal heart sounds can be heard by 11 weeks of gestation. Crown-rump length (CRL) is most accurate in first trimester to within ±5 days. At the period of gestation ≥ 12 weeks, fetus begins to curve, and therefore this measurement becomes less accurate. Biparietal diameter (BPD) from 12–18 weeks of gestation is most accurate to ±7 days. Ultrasound examinations performed in the last half of pregnancy are less reliable for estimating the due date than those performed early in gestation.

GENERAL PHYSICAL EXAMINATION

The following findings can be observed on general physical examination (GPE):

- *Maternal weight record:* This may demonstrate a stationary or falling maternal weight.
- *False labor pains:* There may be appearance of labor pains which quickly subside.

SPECIFIC SYSTEMIC EXAMINATION

ABDOMINAL EXAMINATION

The following findings can be observed on abdominal examination:

- *Abdominal girth:* There may be gradually diminishing abdominal girth due to the progressively reducing liquor volume.

- *Abdominal palpation:* The uterus may feel "full of fetus" due to the diminishing volume of the liquor.

VAGINAL EXAMINATION

Hard skull bones may be felt through the cervix or vaginal fornix, thereby suggesting fetal maturity. Per vaginal examination also helps in assessing cervical inducibility by calculation of the Bishop's score.

MANAGEMENT

Management comprising investigations and definitive obstetric management is discussed next.

> Q. Write a short essay on post-term pregnancy. How will you manage such a patient?
>
> Q. Write a short essay on management of postdated pregnancy.
>
> Q. Write a long essay on effects and management of post-term pregnancy.
>
> Q. With the help of a long essay, discuss the management of a primi patient at 41 weeks' gestation with cephalic presentation and regular cycles.
>
> Q. What is the likely diagnosis in the case study mentioned in the beginning of the chapter?
>
> **Ans.** In the case study mentioned in the beginning of this chapter, a diagnosis of post-term pregnancy appeared to be likely based on the history and correlation of the period of gestation as calculated by LMP and that based on the CRL measurement (as calculated by the first-trimester ultrasound examination).
> After taking the complete history, a GPE, per abdominal examination, and per vaginal examination were performed. No significant finding was observed on GPE. Per abdominal examination revealed a fundal height corresponding to 40 weeks of gestation. The baby appeared to be of average size, and liquor appeared to be adequate on per abdominal examination. On per vaginal examination, the cervix appeared long, posterior, and firm, and internal cervical os was closed. An ultrasound examination and NST were performed. Amniotic fluid was found to be reduced on ultrasound examination.
> The patient was admitted and posted for immediate delivery in view of reduced amniotic fluid on ultrasound examination. Since the cervix was extremely unfavorable and the patient was not willing for the use of cervical ripening agents, she was posted for a cesarean delivery.

PREVENTION

Sweeping/stripping of membranes at term may help in prevention of post-term pregnancy in case of the absence of any vaginitis, malpresentation, or placenta previa. Present evidence does not show any significant effect associated with sweeping/stripping of fetal membranes in prevention of post-term pregnancy. Moreover, there is no evidence to show that stimulation of the breasts and nipples during the antenatal period may help reduce the incidence of post-term pregnancy.

INVESTIGATIONS

- *Ultrasonography:* Ultrasound parameters, such as CRL, BPD, and femur length (FL), help in the assessment of gestational age. Ultrasound scans performed early in gestation are more helpful in the accurate assessment of gestational age. Amniotic fluid pocket of <2 cm and AFI ≤ 5 cm on ultrasound examination are an indication for induction of labor or delivery. Absent end-diastolic flow on umbilical artery Doppler is another indicator of fetal jeopardy.
- *Tests for fetal well-being:* These include tests, such as NST, BPP, and ultrasound assessment of the amniotic fluid volume, which may be performed on a biweekly basis in case of a post-term pregnancy.

TREATMENT/OBSTETRIC MANAGEMENT

The obstetric management is based on two principles, the first being determination of accurate gestational age and the second being increased fetal surveillance. According to the ACOG, two strategies which may reduce the risk of an adverse fetal outcome related to post-term pregnancies include antenatal surveillance and induction of labor. Management of post-term pregnancy has been described in the **Flowchart 17.2** and comprises of the following.

ESTIMATION OF ACCURATE GESTATIONAL AGE

Obtaining an accurate estimate of gestational age at the time of taking history and using results of ultrasound examination performed early in the pregnancy can help reduce the incidence of pregnancies wrongly diagnosed as post-term, thereby minimizing unnecessary interventions. However, routine early ultrasonography has not been recommended as standard modality for care in the United States.

ANTEPARTUM FETAL SURVEILLANCE

Although the current evidence does not suggest that antenatal fetal surveillance for post-term pregnancies reduces perinatal mortality and improves perinatal outcome, this has become a common, universally accepted practice, which is often performed between 40 and 42 weeks of gestation. Antepartum fetal surveillance is particularly important in cases of post-term pregnancies because perinatal morbidity and mortality increase with advancing gestational age.

342 Complications of Pregnancy

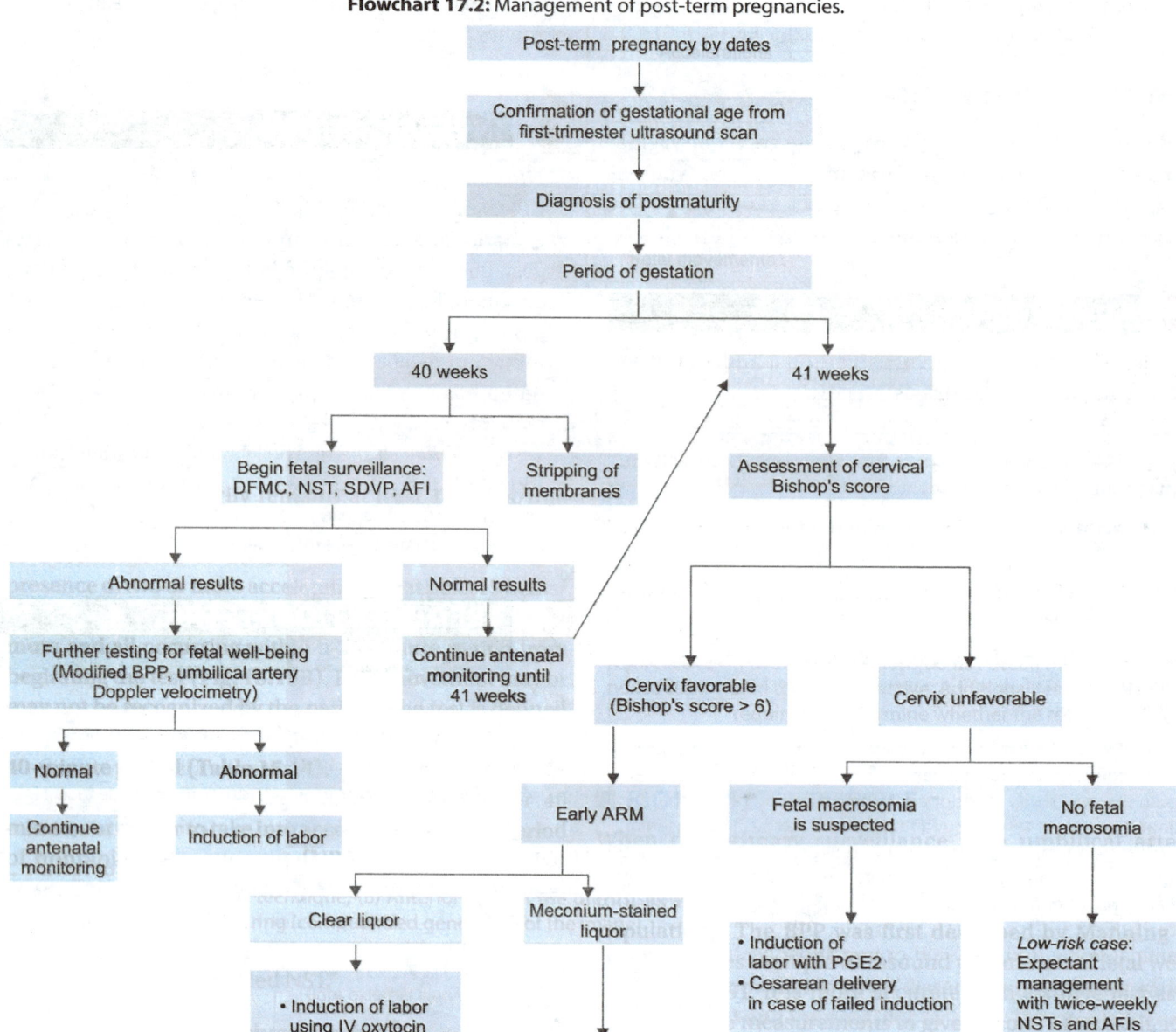

Flowchart 17.2: Management of post-term pregnancies.

(AFI: amniotic fluid index; ARM: artificial rupture of membranes; BPP: biophysical profile; DFMC: daily fetal movement count; NST: nonstress test; PGE: prostaglandin; SDVP: single deepest vertical pocket)

Various options for evaluating fetal well-being which are used include DFMC, NST, BPP or modified BPP (NST plus amniotic fluid volume estimation), and a combination of these modalities **(Table 17.3)**. Twice-weekly modified BPP is usually sufficient instead of a complete BPP, which can be performed in case of nonreactive or equivocal NST results. Amniotic fluid volume should be assessed using single deepest vertical pocket (SDVP), not containing umbilical cord or fetal extremities. A diagnosis of oligohydramnios is made when the pocket is 2 cm or less. SDVP is usually preferable to AFI, which has been shown to overdiagnose oligohydramnios, thereby resulting in unnecessary interventions. Delivery is recommended if there is evidence of fetal compromise or oligohydramnios.

However, none of these methods have been shown to be superior to the other. While presently there is no recommendation regarding the frequency of antenatal surveillance, most practitioners follow twice-weekly testing regime.

INDUCTION VERSUS SURVEILLANCE

The debate still continues between the use of routine induction and surveillance for care of post-term pregnancies. The risk of uteroplacental insufficiency and stillbirth gradually increases at term. Therefore, termination of pregnancy appears to be the best option for preventing adverse outcomes. The most appropriate gestation at which labor must be induced is chosen by maintaining a balance between reduction in the risk of stillbirth brought about by

Postdated Pregnancy and Intrauterine Death

TABLE 17.3: Tests of fetal surveillance.

Test of fetal surveillance	Characteristics
DFMC	Noninvasive and extremely simple method
NST	• Noninvasive test of fetal activity that correlates with fetal well-being • NST is not adequate to preclude an acute asphyxial event because fetal death has been reported to occur within 7 days of normal NSTs due to meconium aspiration • External monitor is used to record fetal heart rate, and mother participates in the test by indicating fetal movement • Further testing may be needed if these increases are not observed after monitoring for 40 minutes • NST can be reactive or nonreactive
BPP	• It comprises a combination of tests designed to identify a compromised fetus during antepartum period • It consists of five components, NST, and ultrasound measurement of four fetal parameters: fetal body movements, breathing movements, fetal tone (flexion and extension of an arm, leg, or the spine), and amniotic fluid volume • Each component is scored individually, 2 points if normal and 0 points if not normal • The maximum possible score in BPP is 10
Ultrasound examination	*Assessment of amniotic fluid volume:* Low amniotic fluid volume in post-term pregnancy can be defined as the largest vertical pocket of amniotic fluid depth of <2–3 cm, AFI < 5 cm, product of length × width × depth of the largest pocket < 60 • Macrosomia • Placental grading

(BPP: biophysical profile; DFMC: daily fetal movement count; NST: nonstress test)

delivering the baby and the potential iatrogenic risk related to induction of labor because induction of labor is likely to increase the risk of maternal and neonatal morbidity and operative delivery.

SWEPIS (SWEdish Post-term Induction Study) was multicentric, open label, randomized, superiority trial conducted in Sweden between May 2016 and October 2018. A total of 2,760 women with low-risk, uncomplicated, singleton pregnancy were randomized to either induction of labor at 41 weeks or expectant management and induction of labor at 42 weeks. The study was stopped due to a significantly higher rate of perinatal mortality in the expectant management group. While no perinatal death occurred in the induction group, six deaths occurred in the expectant management group.

The WHO (2018) guidelines also recommend routine induction of labor at 41 completed weeks in uncomplicated pregnancies.

Multicentric randomized controlled trial by Grobman et al. (2018) has shown that induction of labor at 39 weeks in low-risk nulliparous women was not associated with significantly reduced frequency of adverse perinatal outcomes. However, it did result in a significantly reduced frequency of cesarean delivery. As per the Cochrane review by Middleton et al. (2020), induction of labor at or beyond term in comparison with expectant management is likely to be associated with fewer perinatal deaths and cesarean sections. The rate of admission to the NICU were lower, and low APGAR scores were also encountered in fewer babies in the group who underwent induction. However, the rate of operative vaginal births was higher.

Therefore, it can be concluded that induction of labor at 41 weeks in comparison with the expectant management is likely to be associated with a better maternal and perinatal outcome.

- *Estimation of the accurate gestational age:* Prior to any decision, it is important to establish the patient's accurate gestational age. Dating scan should be preferably performed between 11^{+0} and 13^{+6} weeks of gestation when CRL measurement is between 45 and 84 mm.
- *Role of prostaglandin preparations in managing a post-term pregnancy:* Prostaglandin is a valuable tool for improving cervical ripeness and inducing labor; however, no standardized dose or dosing interval has been established. Lower doses of prostaglandins are preferred, because higher doses have been associated with an increased risk of uterine hyperstimulation leading to nonreassuring fetal testing results. Therefore, when prostaglandins are used, routine fetal heart monitoring should be performed due to the risk of uterine hyperstimulation.
- *Membrane sweeping or stripping:* This must be offered to nulliparous women from 39 to 40 weeks and to multiparous women at around 40 weeks. Stripping of membranes is likely to provoke the release of prostaglandins.
- *Fetal surveillance:* Expectant management includes antepartum fetal surveillance in late term and post-term with DFMC, twice-weekly NST, BPP, SDVP of amniotic fluid, etc.
- *Role of cesarean delivery:* Cesarean delivery may be required in the presence of circumstances mentioned in **Box 17.1**.
- *Role for vaginal birth after cesarean delivery in the management of post-term pregnancy:* Due to the presence of limited evidence regarding the safety or efficacy of VBAC in post-term pregnancies, presently there is no recommendation regarding the use of VBAC as an alternative to elective repeat cesarean deliveries for some women with post-term pregnancy.

344 Complications of Pregnancy

TIMING OF DELIVERY

- Delivery is recommended when the risks to the fetus due to continuation of pregnancy are greater than those faced by the neonate after birth. High-risk pregnancies must be particularly not allowed to become post-term. In these cases, delivery is preferred around 38–39 weeks of gestation.
- Management of low-risk patients is more controversial and depends upon the following factors:
  - Results of antepartum fetal assessment
  - Cervical favorability
  - Gestational age
  - Maternal preference following the discussion of risks versus benefits of both induction and expectant management

INTRAPARTUM MANAGEMENT

The following precautions must be taken during the antepartum period:

- Patient must be made to lie in the left lateral position.
- Continuous electronic fetal monitoring must be done in anticipation of intrapartum asphyxia.
- Initiating artificial rupture of membranes in the early active phase helps in hastening progress and also helps in an early detection of meconium.

  Other precautions which must be taken at the time of delivery in case of meconium-stained liquor are listed in **Box 17.2**. As per the new recommendation of the American Academy of Pediatrics and the American Heart Association (adapted by the ACOG, 2017), routine intrapartum suctioning is no longer required for infants with meconium-stained amniotic fluid, regardless of whether they are vigorous or not.
- Pediatrician must be present at the time of delivery.
- When fetal macrosomia is suspected, ultrasound should be performed to estimate fetal weight. In case of vaginal delivery, clinician should always be prepared to deal with a potential shoulder dystocia. Most clinicians favor cesarean delivery for infants in whom expected fetal weight is >4.5 kg.

COMPLICATIONS

 Q. Write a long essay on problems of postmaturity.

Various complications which can occur in the mother and fetus as a result of prolonged pregnancy are tabulated in **Table 17.4**.

FETAL COMPLICATIONS

Perinatal Mortality

There is nearly 30% greater risk of mortality compared with a term neonate due to placental aging, continued placental function, and fetal macrosomia.

Fetal Distress

Consequences of post-term pregnancy on placental function are described in **Flowchart 17.3**. In case of postdated pregnancy if the placental function remains maintained, it results in a macrosomic baby (described next in the text). In case there is deterioration of placental function with increasing period of gestation, it is likely to result in fetal distress and/or acidosis. Fetal distress indicates intrauterine fetal compromise, implying that the fetus is at risk. Fetal distress during labor is assessed mainly on the basis of two parameters: fetal heart rate pattern and the presence or absence of meconium. Babies with fetal distress are generally delivered in good health, but in some cases fetal distress can lead to problems such as learning disabilities, cerebral palsy, mental retardation, hypoxic ischemic encephalopathy, and

---

BOX 17.1: Indications for cesarean delivery.

- Macrosomic fetus (weight ≥ 4,500 g)
- A history of previous cesarean delivery
- Presence of fetal compromise on tests of fetal surveillance
- Patient's personal preference
- Failure of induction of labor

BOX 17.2: Precautions to be taken at the time of delivery in case of meconium staining of liquor.

- No requirement for intrapartum suctioning
- Availability of a team, well versed with complete resuscitation skills, including endotracheal intubation at the time of delivery
- Similar resuscitation principles must be followed for infants with meconium-stained fluid as for those with clear fluid
- If required, gentle clearing of meconium from the mouth and nose with a bulb syringe may be done
- Initiate appropriate intervention to support ventilation and oxygenation for each infant. In case of airway obstruction, intubation and suction may be required

---

TABLE 17.4: Complications related to prolonged pregnancy.

Fetal	Maternal
Increased perinatal morbidity and mortality	Increased maternal anxiety and stress
Low umbilical artery pH levels at delivery	Increase in labor dystocia
Low 5-minute APGAR scores	Increase in severe perineal injury related to macrosomia
Dysmaturity syndrome	Doubling in the rate of cesarean delivery
Increased risk of death within the first year of life	Increased anxiety for the pregnant woman
Fetal distress	Traumatic vaginal delivery (severe perineal lacerations)—shoulder dystocia
Neonatal seizures	
Fetal macrosomia	
MAS	
Fetal trauma	Increased requirement for instrumental delivery
Brachial plexus injuries, clavicle fracture	Increased risk for developing postpartum hemorrhage
Increased perinatal mortality	

(MAS: meconium aspiration syndrome)

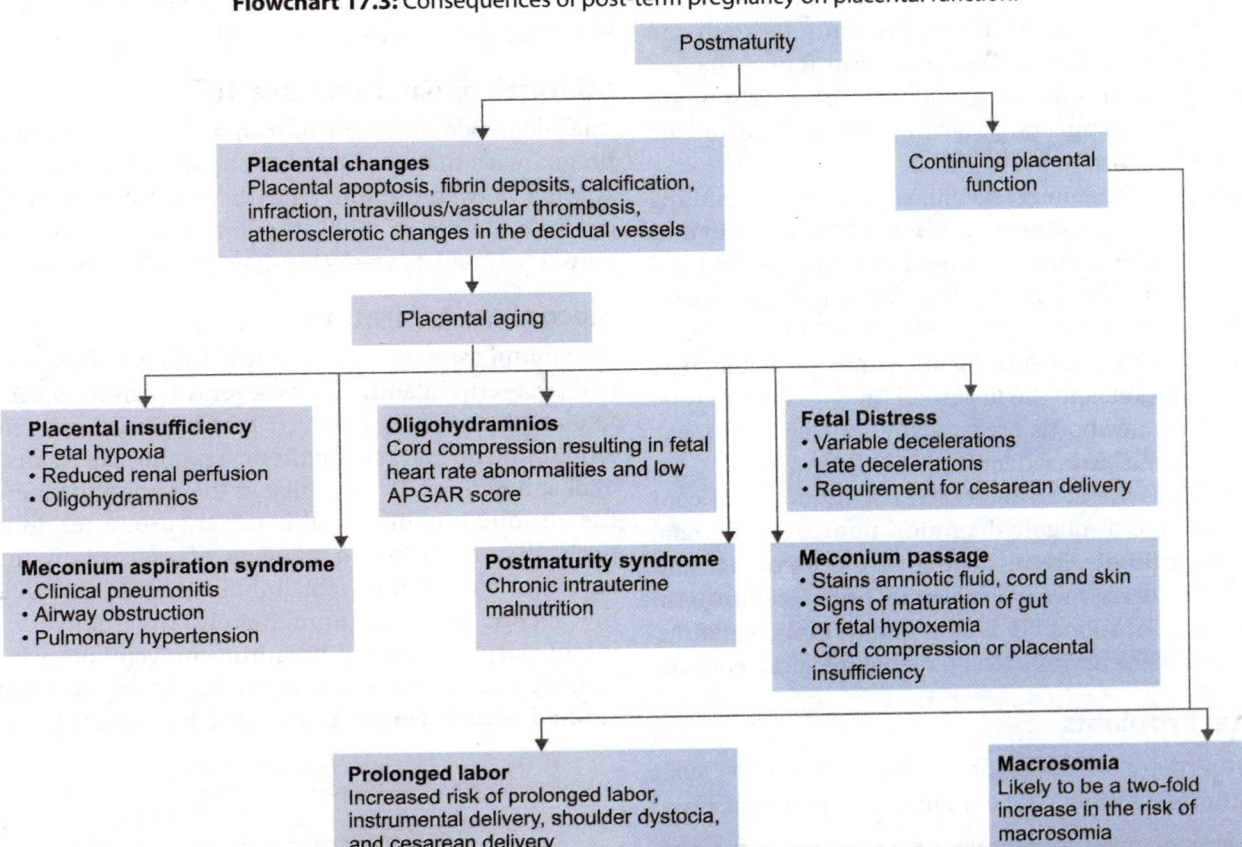

Flowchart 17.3: Consequences of post-term pregnancy on placental function.

Macrosomia

Macrosomia can be defined as expected fetal weight between 90 and 95 percentiles of gestational age. Birth weight is usually >4,000–4,500 g or greater (Fig. 17.1). Besides postdated pregnancy, other risk factors for development of macrosomia include gestational diabetes mellitus, prolonged gestation, maternal obesity, excessive pregnancy weight gain, etc. This is associated with an increased incidence of cephalopelvic disproportion, prolonged labor, shoulder dystocia, and operative delivery. Shoulder dystocia may be associated with resultant orthopedic risks (e.g., clavicular fractures) or neurologic injury (e.g., brachial plexus palsy). Presently, there is no method for predicting macrosomia. The woman must be posted for an elective cesarean delivery in case the expected fetal weight is >4,500 g in a diabetic mother and >5,000 g in a nondiabetic mother. Early induction has been tried in some cases. However, it is associated with an increased rate of failed induction.

Birth Trauma

There is an increased incidence of traumatic birth deliveries due to large size of the baby and nonmolding of fetal head due to hardening of skull bones.

seizures. Detection of fetal compromise at an early stage allows the obstetrician to undertake appropriate and timely interventions to expedite the baby's delivery.

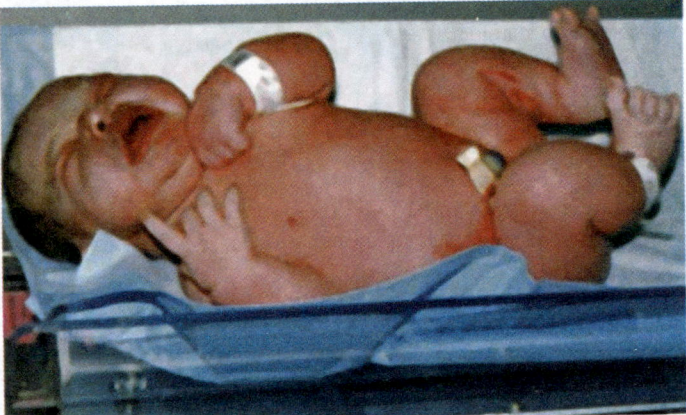

Fig. 17.1: Macrosomic baby.

Intrauterine Growth Restriction

Post-term fetuses, where there is deterioration of placental function, may suffer from IUGR. Such fetuses are at increased risk of complications such as umbilical cord compression from oligohydramnios, nonreassuring results on fetal antepartum or intrapartum assessment, and an increased rate of cesarean delivery.

Dysmaturity Syndrome

Dysmaturity syndrome refers to a fetus whose growth in the uterus after the due date has been restricted, resulting in chronic IUGR. This is usually related to a problem due to uteroplacental insufficiency, resulting in an inadequate supply of blood and nutrients to the fetus through the placenta. Approximately 20% of post-term fetuses have a syndrome of fetal dysmaturity, where the post-term infant shows a distinctive appearance having unique characteristic features **(Box 17.3)**.

The baby may have long and thin arms and legs, resulting in a long, thin, wasted appearance **(Fig. 17.2)**. The skin may appear dry, wrinkled, and parchment-like, with peeling and sometimes meconium staining. The skin may appear loose, especially over the thighs and buttocks. Wrinkling of the skin is typically prominent on the soles and palms. Scalp hair may be longer or thicker, and the fingernails and toenails may be long. Post-term newborns are typically very alert, and may have a "wide-eyed", worried look.

These babies are at an increased risk of umbilical cord compression due to oligohydramnios, nonreassuring fetal heart rate cardiotocograph tracing in the antenatal and intrapartum periods, meconium aspiration, and short-term neonatal complications such as hypoglycemia, seizures, respiratory insufficiency, and long-term neurological sequelae.

Neonatal Problems

After birth, many neonatal complications can arise, such as hypothermia, poor subcutaneous fat, hypoglycemia, hypocalcemia, and increased incidence of injuries such as brachial plexus injuries.

Stillbirth or Neonatal Death

The incidence of stillbirth or infant death is increased in pregnancies that continue beyond 42 weeks, with the risk varying between 4 and 7 deaths per 1,000 deliveries. In contrast, the risk of stillbirth or infant death in pregnancies between 37 and 42 weeks is 2–3 per 1,000 deliveries.

Meconium Aspiration

Meconium aspiration syndrome (MAS) is a disease of term and post-term infants, and its severity is linked to coexisting fetal asphyxia. It is believed that hypoxia and acidemia stimulate the parasympathetic system. This causes the anal sphincter to relax, whilst at the same time increasing the production of motilin, which promotes intestinal peristalsis resulting in passage of meconium into the amniotic cavity. Postnatal inhalation can occur late in the second stage or immediately after delivery if the infant gasps or makes breathing movements while the oropharynx, nasopharynx, or trachea contains meconium-stained liquor **(Figs. 17.3A and B)**. Meconium has a

> **BOX 17.3:** Characteristic features of fetal dysmaturity syndrome.
> - Long, thin, malnourished infant
> - Meconium staining
> - Wrinkled, peeling skin
> - Loss of subcutaneous fat
> - Dry, cracked skin
> - Long nails
> - Unusual degree of alertness
> - Poor glycogen stores
> - Increased risk of fetal hypoxia and MAS
>
> (MAS: Meconium aspiration syndrome)

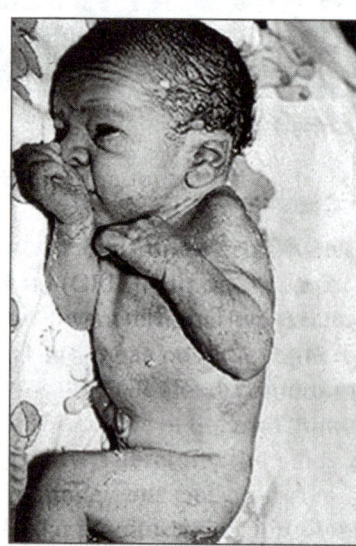

Fig. 17.2: Photograph of a post-term baby born at 42 weeks of gestation.

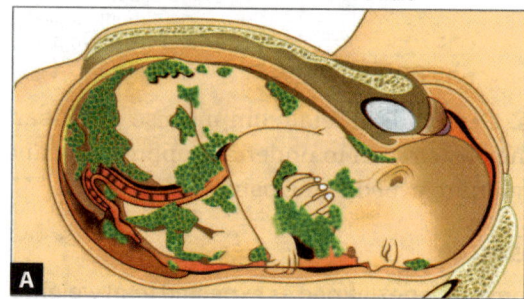
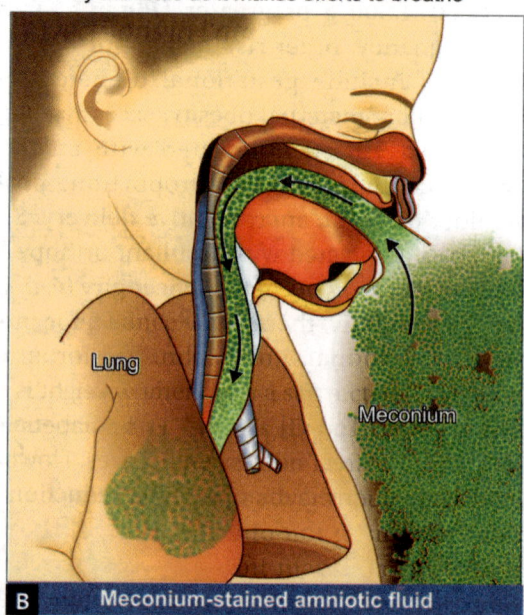

Figs. 17.3A and B: Aspiration of meconium by the newborn baby as it makes efforts to breathe.

number of adverse effects on the neonatal lung, which may ultimately result in the development of MAS that can lead to respiratory failure and hypoxemia. The ways through which the presence of meconium inside the fetal lungs can result in adverse effects are shown in **Figures 17.4A and B**. Aspiration of meconium can result in mechanical blockage of airways, chemical irritation, and secondary bacterial infection. Chemical irritation may produce an inflammatory reaction resulting in pneumonitis, alveolar collapse, and cell necrosis. This can eventually result in respiratory failure and hypoxemia. **Figure 17.5** shows the classic radiographic findings of MAS, namely atelectasis, pneumothorax, and hyperexpanded areas of the lung.

Respiratory Distress

Respiratory distress can occur due to chemical pneumonitis, atelectasis, and pulmonary hypertension. This may occur following meconium aspiration and eventually result in hypoxia and respiratory failure.

Increased Perinatal Mortality and Morbidity

All the previously mentioned fetal complications result in an overall increased rate of perinatal morbidity and mortality. **Figure 17.6** illustrates the effect of post-term pregnancy on maternal and fetal outcomes. With an increase or decrease in the duration of pregnancy on weekly basis, the perinatal mortality increases exponentially. At 42 weeks of gestation, the risk of perinatal mortality is double of that at 40 weeks. Lowest perinatal mortality is between 39 and 41 weeks. In cases of both preterm and post-term pregnancies, the rate of perinatal mortality and morbidity increases exponentially.

Long-term Outcomes

Though there are only a few studies for assessing long-term outcomes (e.g., growth and development patterns, and intelligence) of post-term infants, in general, the long-term outcome amongst post-term infants does not appear to be significantly different from that of term infants.

■ MATERNAL COMPLICATIONS

Various complications which can occur in the mother due to prolonged pregnancy include labor dystocia, increased rate of severe perineal injuries due to macrosomia, doubling of rate of cesarean delivery, etc.

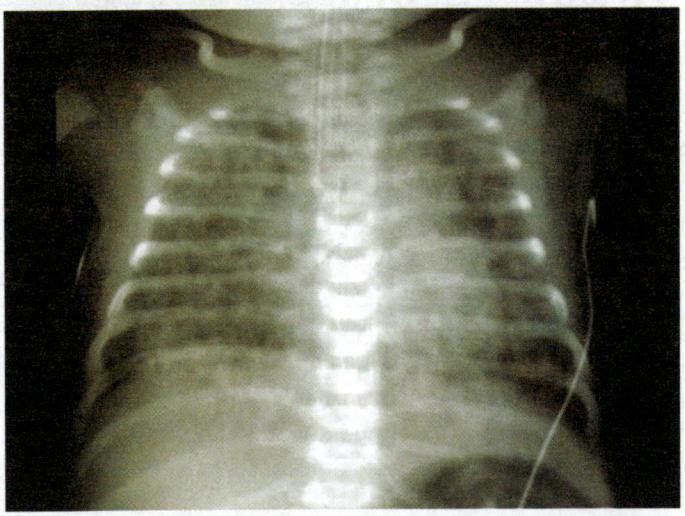

Fig. 17.5: Chest X-ray of a 2-day-old infant showing signs of MAS. There are classical radiographic findings of MAS, namely atelectasis, pneumothorax, and hyperexpanded areas of the lung.

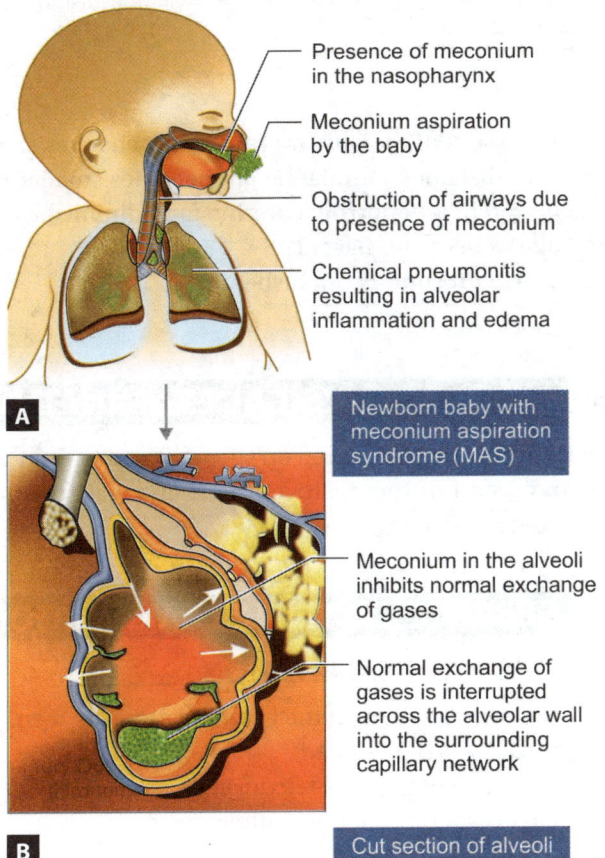

Figs. 17.4A and B: Consequences of meconium aspiration.

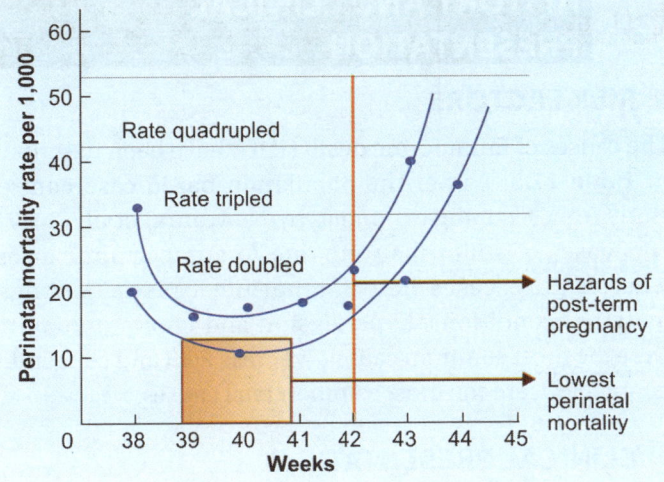

Fig. 17.6: Consequences of post-term pregnancy on perinatal outcome.

PART 2: INTRAUTERINE DEATH

 Q. Write a short essay on intrauterine death (IUD).

CASE STUDY

A 35-year-old G3P2A0L2 patient presented to the accident and emergency (A&E) department with a history of fall over her abdomen a few hours back. She has been experiencing pain in the abdomen and has not felt any fetal movements since that time. There is a history of slight vaginal bleeding. Period of gestation according to her LMP was calculated to be 33 weeks. Her antenatal period had been otherwise normal, and the clinical findings during her previous antenatal visits were within the normal limits.

INTRODUCTION

As per the definition by the International Classification of Disease (ICD) (10th revision), fetal death can be defined as follows: *"death prior to the complete expulsion or extraction from its mother of a product of conception, irrespective of the duration of pregnancy."*

The WHO/ICD defines stillbirths as the death of a fetus that has reached a birth weight of 500 g, or if birth weight is unavailable, gestational age of 22 weeks or crown-to-heel length of 25 cm. Within this category, late fetal deaths are defined as fetal weight of 1,000 g or more, or 28 weeks of gestation or more, or crown-to-heel length of 35 cm or more. Early fetal deaths are defined as fetal weight between 500 and 1,000 g or period of gestation of 22–28 weeks or crown-to-heel length of 25 cm.

On the other hand, miscarriage is defined as pregnancy loss prior to 22 completed weeks of gestation.

HISTORY AND CLINICAL PRESENTATION

RISK FACTORS

The causes of intrauterine death (IUD) have been described in **Table 17.5**. As per the population-based case control study from Chandigarh, India, by Newtonraj et al. (2017), 68% cases of stillbirths were due to antepartum causes, whereas 32% cases had intrapartum causes. Amongst maternal conditions, hypertension and chorioamnionitis were the most common causes, whereas FGR and congenital anomalies were the most common fetal causes.

CLINICAL PRESENTATION

- There is absence of fetal movement interpretation by the mother for more than a few hours.

TABLE 17.5: Causes of intrauterine death.

Maternal causes	Fetal causes
• Advanced maternal age > 35 years • Obesity (>30 kg/m^2) • Hypertensive disorders • Chromosomal anomalies • *Antepartum hemorrhage*: Placenta previa, abruptio placentae, etc. • Preexisting medical disease such as chronic hypertension, chronic nephritis, diabetes, severe anemia, hyperpyrexia, syphilis, hepatitis, systemic lupus erythematosus, thrombophilia, and cholestasis of pregnancy • Rh incompatibility • Gestational diabetes • Severe anemia • Hyperpyrexia • Previous history of stillbirth • Post-term pregnancy • Maternal infection (chorioamnionitis) • Antiphospholipid syndrome • Smoking, alcohol, drugs, etc.	• Congenital malformations • Chromosomal anomalies • Fetal infections [Parvovirus B19, cytomegalovirus (CMV), rubella, toxoplasmosis, malaria, etc.] • Rh incompatibility • Multiple gestation • Fetal growth restriction • Prematurity • Iatrogenic causes such as external version
Placental causes	
Placental insufficiency, antepartum hemorrhage, cord accidents (cord prolapse, knotted cord, etc.), twin-to-twin transfusion syndrome, etc.	

- Retrogression of the positive pregnancy changes (breast changes disappear, fundal height becomes smaller than the period of amenorrhea, uterine tone diminishes, and the uterus becomes flaccid).
- No fetal heart sounds can be heard.

GENERAL PHYSICAL EXAMINATION

No specific finding is observed on GPE except that there may be retrogression of the positive breast changes (normally seen during pregnancy).

SPECIFIC SYSTEMIC EXAMINATION

ABDOMINAL EXAMINATION

- Gradual retrogression of the height of uterus is seen.
- Uterine tone is diminished.
- Fetal movements are not felt during palpation.
- Fetal heart sounds are not audible.
- Fetal head shows eggshell cracking feeling upon palpation (late sign).

MANAGEMENT

Management comprising investigations and definitive obstetric management is discussed next.

> **Q. What is the next step of immediate management in the case study mentioned in the beginning of this topic?**
> **Ans.** In the case study described in the beginning of the chapter, the patient was immediately admitted in the emergency ward. On GPE, her vitals were stable. An IV line was secured, and blood samples were collected for blood grouping and crossmatching, and a coagulation profile.
> On per abdominal examination, fundal height corresponded to 34 weeks of gestation and there was extreme abdominal tenderness. Fetal heart sounds were not heard on fetal Doppler examination. On vaginal examination, slight vaginal bleeding was present, the cervical os was dilated by 2–3 cm and was about 50% effaced, and fetal membranes were present. An ultrasound examination was performed immediately. Fetal heart rate was found to be absent. The placenta was fundal, but a retroplacental clot was detected. A provisional diagnosis of abruptio placentae and IUD due to abdominal trauma was made. Since the cervix was favorable, vaginal mode of delivery was chosen. An ARM was performed. In the absence of good uterine contractions, an oxytocin infusion was started.

PREVENTION

Intrauterine death can be prevented by observing the following precautions:

- Regular antenatal care
- Screening out the high-risk patients to carefully monitor the fetal well-being and to terminate the pregnancy at the earliest evidences of fetal compromise. Regular antepartum surveillance is required in these cases in order to prevent fetal death.

INVESTIGATIONS

Various tests, which need to be done in cases of IUD, aim at the identification of underlying etiology and are listed in **Table 17.6**. The tests performed in an individual patient are based on the clinical presentation. Some of those which are commonly performed are:

- Blood grouping (ABO and Rh) and crossmatching
- *Tests for detecting the underlying cause:* Blood sugar, thyroid function tests, TORCH screening, VDRL, thrombophilia studies, lupus anticoagulant and anticardiolipin antibodies, urine routine microscopy for pus cells and casts
- *Absent fetal heart:* Inability to detect a fetal heartbeat via Doppler
- *Sonography:* Definitive diagnosis is made by observing the lack of fetal cardiac motion during a 10-minute period of careful examination with real-time ultrasound.

TABLE 17.6: Tests for evaluation of intrauterine fetal death.

Parameters	Investigations
Maternal/family history	History related to risk factors mentioned in **Table 17.5**
Maternal investigations	• Indirect Coombs test • Serologic test for syphilis • Testing for fetal–maternal hemorrhage (Kleihauer–Betke or other) • Parvovirus serology • Lupus anticoagulant, anticardiolipin anticoagulant, for antiphospholipid testing • Anti-β-2-glycoprotein 1 IgG or IgM antibodies • Diabetes testing using hemoglobin A1c and a fasting blood glucose • Syphilis screening using the VDRL or rapid plasma reagin test • Thyroid function testing (i.e., TSH, FT4) • Urine toxicology screening • Factor V Leiden • Prothrombin mutation • TORCH titers • Protein C, protein S, and antithrombin III deficiency (useful in some circumstances)
Cytogenic evaluation	• Amniocentesis* for cytogenic evaluation/karyotyping (10–25 mL of amniotic fluid is aspirated) • Cord • Cardiac tissues • Placental tissues
Examination of stillbirth	• External/physical examination • Fetal autopsy • Clinical examination • Postmortem ultrasound scan or MRI, especially if permission for autopsy has not been given
Cord examination and cord blood or infant cardiac blood investigations	• Gross/macroscopic/clinical examination • Histopathology • Culture • Cytogenetic studies • Syphilis serology • IgG and IgM antibodies for parvovirus, CMV, rubella, toxoplasmosis, herpes, etc.

Examination of placenta and placental tissues	• Gross/macroscopic/clinical examination:
	  – Placental size/morphology/cord insertion
	  – Presence of hematomas, edema, infracts, etc.
	• Histopathology
	• Culture
	• Cytogenetic studies

Note: *Amniocentesis for karyotyping is associated with the highest yield because cardiac failure is likely to have occurred in the macerated tissues. (CMV: cytomegalovirus; FT4: free thyroxine index)

Late signs are oligohydramnios and collapse of cranial bones.

- *X-ray abdomen:* Abdominal X-ray may show the presence of Spalding sign (irregular overlapping of the cranial bones), which usually occurs approximately

within 7 days after death; hyperflexion of the spine; and crowding of ribs and appearance of gas shadows in the heart and great vessels (Robert's sign), which usually appears by 12 hours after birth. Spalding sign can be also observed on ultrasound examination (**Fig. 17.7**).
- *Clotting profile:* Tests, such as blood fibrinogen levels and partial thromboplastin time, may especially be required, if the fetus has been retained for >2 weeks.

℞ TREATMENT/OBSTETRIC MANAGEMENT

- *Counseling:* Since the news is likely to be extremely traumatic for the patient and her family, proper counseling and reassurance must be provided to the bereaving parents. This must include explanation about the possible cause of death, requirement for various investigations, and autopsy of the dead infant. This information must be conveyed to the mother in an unhurried/sympathetic manner. She should be given adequate time to decide the further course of management (immediate termination or expectant management).
- Diagnosis and treatment of abnormality, if possible. In most of the cases, spontaneous expulsion occurs within 2 weeks of birth. In cases where spontaneous expulsion does not occur, induction by oxytocin infusion or prostaglandins (PGE2 gel or 25–50 µg of misoprostol) may be required.
- Fibrinogen levels to be estimated on a weekly basis. Falling fibrinogen levels should be arrested by controlled infusion of heparin.
- *Postmortem examination:* Examination of the dead baby and placenta (placental cultures for suspected infection) needs to be done in order to detect the cause of death.

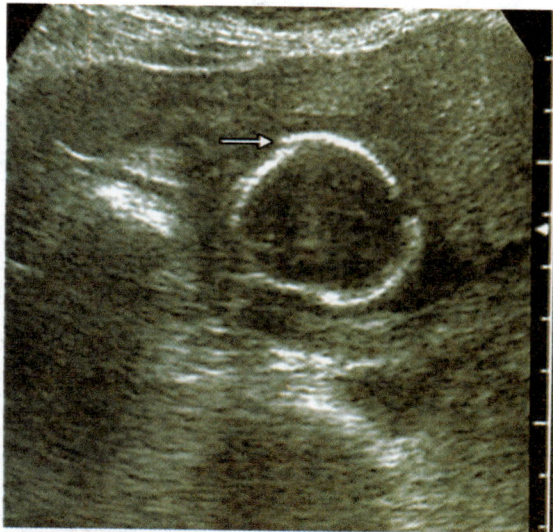

Fig. 17.7: *Spalding sign:* Showing overlapping of the fetal skull bones (indicated by arrow).

Autopsy and chromosomal analysis for detection of fetal anomalies and dysmorphic features need to be done.

■ MODE OF DELIVERY OF THE DEAD FETUS

Once the fetal death has been diagnosed, the options of expectant or active management must be discussed with the patient.

Expectant Management

The following need to be done in case expectant management is planned:
- The obstetrician must await spontaneous onset of labor during the coming 4 weeks.
- The woman must be assured that in 90% of cases the fetus would be expelled spontaneously during the waiting period with no complications.
- In those women who do not go into labor, there is a rare risk for hypofibrinogenemia and consumptive coagulopathy. This usually does not occur prior to 3–4 weeks of retention of dead fetus. This risk further increases in case of maternal sepsis, placental abruption, and preeclampsia. Moreover, there is a risk of infection, in case the fetal membranes have ruptured.
- If platelet levels are found to be decreasing on serial examinations or 4 weeks have passed without onset of spontaneous labor or fibrinogen levels are found to be low or the woman requests active management, the obstetrician must consider induction of labor.

Induction of Labor

- Prior to induction, the patient must be counseled regarding different methods for induction of labor. She should also be counseled regarding the induction-to-delivery interval.
- In case induction of labor is planned, cervix must be firstly assessed.
- If the cervix is favorable, labor can be induced with oxytocin. If cervix is unfavorable, it must be ripened using vaginal PGE2 or synthetic PGE1 analog (misoprostol). Mifepristone (RU-486), an antiprogestogen, can be used for induction of labor in women with fetal death. Combination of mifepristone with misoprostol helps in increasing the efficacy and reducing the induction-to-delivery interval. As per the NICE guidelines (2021), oral mifepristone followed by vaginal PGE2 or vaginal misoprostol should be used for induction of labor.
- Infusion of oxytocin may be required if the woman is not experiencing uterine contractions of sufficient intensity.
- Dosage of misoprostol as recommended by the FIGO (2017) is described in **Table 17.7**.
- Misoprostol must preferably not be used in a woman with previous uterine scar due to the risk of uterine rupture. The membranes must be preferably not ruptured.

TABLE 17.7: Dosage of misoprostol as recommended by the FIGO.	
Period of gestation	**Dosage of misoprostol**
13–26 weeks	200 µg PV/SL/buccal every 4–6 hours
27–28 weeks	100 µg PV/SL/buccal every 4 hours
>28 weeks	25 µg PV every 6 hours or 25 µg PO every 2 hours

(PV: vaginal; SL: sublingual)

COMPLICATIONS

- Psychological upset/trauma
- Infection (typically with anaerobic infections such as *Clostridium welchii*)
- Blood coagulation disorder (disseminated intravascular coagulation)
- *During labor:* Uterine inertia, retained placenta, and postpartum hemorrhage.

EVIDENCE-BASED CLINICAL TRIALS

List of references can be scanned through QR code to enable the readers gain deeper insight of the subject by referring to the entire article or its abstract.

SECTION 3

Medical Disorders Related to Pregnancy

18. Preeclampsia
19. Gestational Diabetes
20. Anemia in Pregnancy
21. Heart Disease During Pregnancy

CHAPTER 18

Preeclampsia

CASE STUDY

A 34-year-old primigravida patient with 39 completed weeks of gestation presented with complaints of headache since last 10 days. Her BP was 144/95 mm Hg, and dipstick examination revealed a 1+ proteinuria. She had never been diagnosed to be suffering from hypertension prior to the present pregnancy.

INTRODUCTION

> **Q. Enumerate the classification of hypertension in pregnancy. Write a long note on management of a primigravida with severe hypertension at 32 weeks of gestation.**

Increased BP is a problem commonly encountered amongst pregnant women. Management of high BP is of utmost importance during pregnancy because it is a major cause of preterm birth amongst fetuses and an early marker for future cardiovascular and metabolic diseases in children, as well as a cause of maternal morbidity and mortality.

High BP could occur as a syndrome specific to pregnancy (preeclampsia/gestational hypertension) or as a manifestation of chronic hypertension present before pregnancy. BP normally falls in the first and second trimesters of pregnancy; therefore, women with high BP before the 20th week of gestation are assumed to have preexisting hypertension. According to the revised classification system proposed by the International Society for the Study of Hypertension in Pregnancy (ISSHP, 2021) and United States Prevention Services Task Force (USPSTF, 2021), hypertensive disorders in pregnancy can be classified as gestational hypertension, preeclampsia–eclampsia, chronic hypertension in pregnancy, and preeclampsia superimposed on chronic hypertension **(Table 18.1 and Flowchart 18.1)**. Both preeclampsia and eclampsia develop during pregnancy, but 25% cases of eclampsia also develop postpartum, most often in the first 4 days. Patients should be evaluated every 1–2 week postpartum with periodic BP measurement. If BP remains high even after 8 weeks postpartum, chronic hypertension should be considered.

PREECLAMPSIA

Preeclampsia can be defined as a pregnancy-specific, multifactorial disease, which presents as a syndrome of specific signs and symptoms. This condition is characterized by placental dysfunction and a maternal response highlighting systemic inflammation with activation of the endothelium and coagulation. The condition is associated with characteristic hematological and biochemical abnormalities.

Preeclampsia can be considered as a potentially serious disorder, which is characterized by high BP and either proteinuria or other findings suggestive of maternal end-organ dysfunction. It usually develops after the 20th week of pregnancy and goes away after the delivery. Proteinuria is defined by excretion of protein ≥ 300 mg/24 hours, a urine protein/creatinine ratio of ≥0.3, or a reading of ≥ 1 on urine dipstick test. As per the revised criteria by the ISSHP and USPSTF (2021), proteinuria is no longer an essential criterion for diagnosis of preeclampsia. In the absence of proteinuria, symptoms suggestive of maternal end-organ damage or symptoms suggestive of uteroplacental dysfunction are also considered diagnostic of preeclampsia. It is also recommended that women with gestational hypertension having severe range of BP (systolic ≥ 160 mm Hg or diastolic ≥ 110 mm Hg) should be diagnosed as preeclampsia with severe features. Gestational hypertension and preeclampsia are now being considered as two separate disease processes having different mechanisms. **Table 18.2** lists the differences between these two entities.

Characteristic clinical features of preeclampsia are illustrated in **Figure 18.1**. Classification of hypertension by the NICE, 2010 based on its severity has been described in **Table 18.3**. According to the ACOG, acute-onset, persistently high BP (lasting 15 minutes or more), where systolic BP (≥160 mm Hg) or diastolic BP (≥110 mm Hg) or a combination of both in pregnant or postpartum women with preeclampsia or eclampsia is considered as a hypertensive emergency.

TABLE 18.1: Classification of hypertensive disorders in pregnancy.

Type of disorder	Characteristics
Gestational hypertension	• Appearance of high BP (>140/90 mm Hg) for the first time during pregnancy after 20 weeks of gestation • No proteinuria • BP returns to normal within 12 weeks of postpartum period

Preeclampsia/ eclampsia	• Appearance of high BP (>140/90 mm Hg) for the first time during pregnancy after 20 weeks of gestation
	• Presence of proteinuria ≥ 300 mg/24 hours or >1+ on the dipstick or urine protein to creatine ratio of ≥0.3)
	or
	• In the absence of proteinuria, other symptoms suggestive of maternal end-organ dysfunction:
	  – Neurological complications (e.g., eclampsia, altered mental status, blindness, stroke, clonus, severe headaches, or persistent visual scotomata)
	  – Pulmonary edema
	  – *Hematological complications*: Such as thrombocytopenia or platelet count < 100,000 × 10^9/L, DIC, and hemolysis
	  – *Renal insufficiency*: AKI, creatinine ≥ 90 μmol/L, or ≥ 1 mg/dL
	  – *Impaired liver function*: Liver involvement evident in the form of elevated transaminases such as ALT or AST > 40 IU/L (with or without right upper quadrant or epigastric/abdominal pain)
	or
	• Uteroplacental dysfunction (e.g., placental abruption, angiogenic imbalance, fetal growth restriction, abnormal umbilical artery Doppler waveform analysis, or intrauterine fetal death)
	• BP returns to normal within 12 weeks of postpartum period
	• Eclampsia is the occurrence of seizures in a pregnant woman with preeclampsia

Chronic hypertension	• Appearance of high BP (>140/90 mm Hg) before 20 weeks of gestation or even before pregnancy • No proteinuria • BP does not return to normal within 12 weeks of postpartum period
Preeclampsia superimposed on chronic hypertension	• New-onset proteinuria in women with the presence of hypertension and no proteinuria early in pregnancy (<20 weeks) • A sudden increase in BP in a woman whose hypertension has previously been well controlled • Thrombocytopenia (platelet count < 100,000 cells/mm³) • An increase in ALT or AST to abnormal levels

(AKI: acute kidney injury; ALT: alanine transaminase)
Source: Magee LA, Brown MA, Hall DR, Gupte S, Hennessy A, Karumanchi SA, et al. The 2021 International Society for the Study of Hypertension in Pregnancy classification, diagnosis and management recommendations for international practice. Pregnancy Hypertens. 2022;27:148-69.

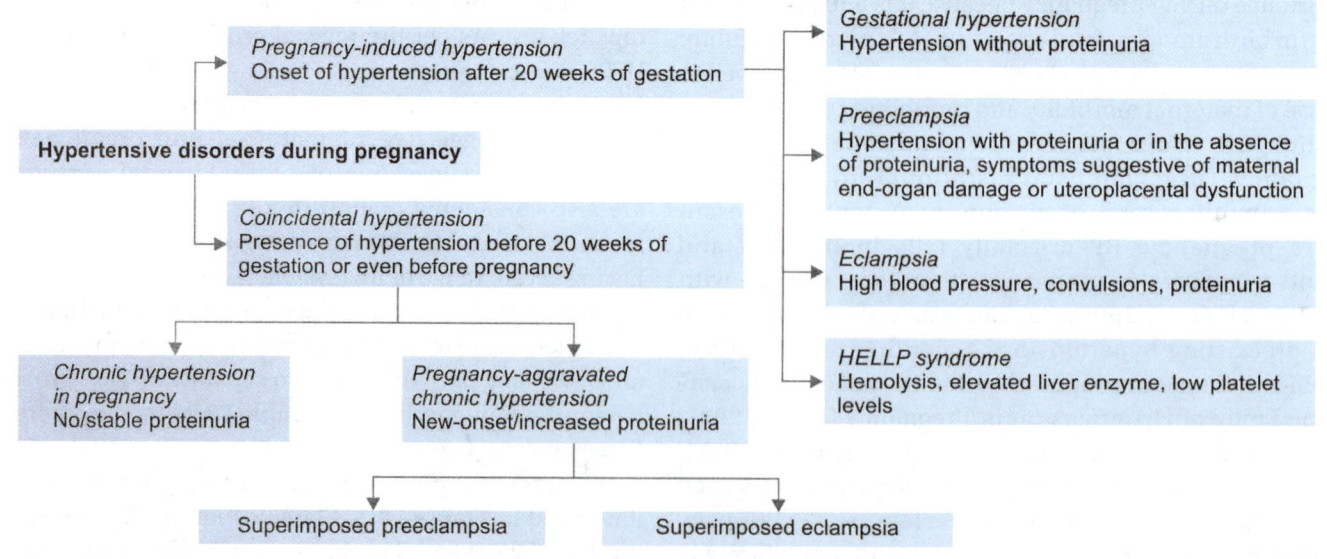

Flowchart 18.1: Classification of hypertensive disorders in pregnancy.

(HELLP: hemolysis, elevated liver enzymes, and low platelets)

Clinical classification of preeclampsia based on its time of onset (prior to 34 weeks or after 34 weeks) has been described in **Table 18.4**.

Atypical preeclampsia: Occurrence of hypertension and proteinuria before 20 weeks of gestation (e.g., in gestational trophoblastic disease) can be designated as atypical

Preeclampsia

TABLE 18.2: Differences between gestational hypertension and preeclampsia.

Parameter under consideration	Gestational hypertension	Preeclampsia
Nulliparity	Not a strong risk factor	Strong risk factor
Histological changes in placenta and kidneys	Not seen	Seen
Increase in angiogenic peptides	Not seen	Seen
Total circulatory blood volume	Normal	Lower

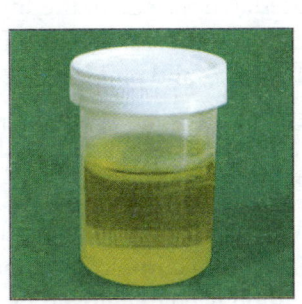
Proteinuria

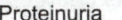
Proteinuria

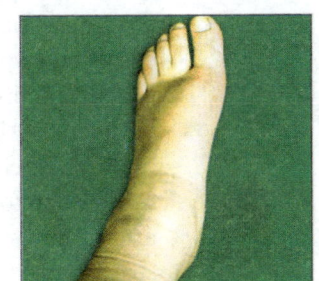
Pedal edema

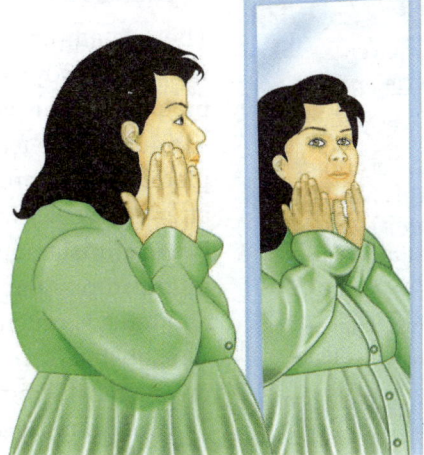
Swollen hands or face

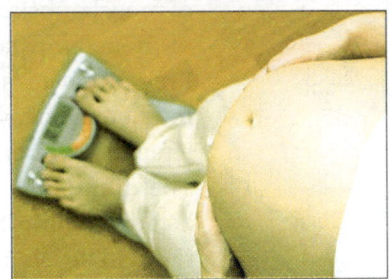
Weight gain during pregnancy

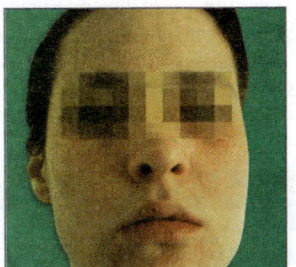
Facial puffiness

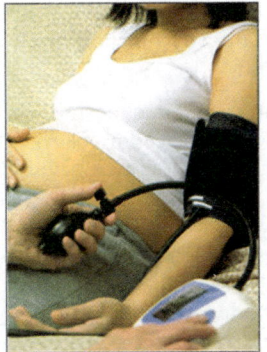
Increased blood pressure during pregnancy

Fig. 18.1: Clinical features of preeclampsia.

preeclampsia. Preeclampsia arising for the first time after 48 hours of delivery can also be included in this definition.

GESTATIONAL HYPERTENSION

This form of high BP develops after the 20th week of pregnancy and goes away after delivery. Affected women do not have proteinuria. However, some women with gestational hypertension may develop preeclampsia later during pregnancy. Gestational hypertension is often also known as transient hypertension. Sometimes, women with gestational hypertension, besides showing the absence of proteinuria, may develop other signs of preeclampsia including symptoms such as headache and epigastric pain. Worsening hypertension even in the absence of proteinuria may present significant risk to both the mother and the fetus, especially in the second half of the pregnancy.

TABLE 18.3: Classification of hypertension based on the degree of severity.

Degree of hypertension	Systolic BP (mm Hg)	Diastolic BP (mm Hg)
Mild	140–149	90–99
Moderate	150–159	100–109
Severe	≥160	≥110
Hypertensive emergency (crisis)	≥180	≥120 (evidence of impending or progressive target organ dysfunction)
Hypertensive urgency	≥180	≥120 (no progressive target organ dysfunction)

Source: National Institute for Health and Clinical Excellence. (2010). The management of hypertensive disorders during pregnancy. [online] Available from www.nice.org.uk/nicemedia/live/13098/50418/50418.pdf. [Last accessed November, 2022].

TABLE 18.4: Clinical classification of preeclampsia.

Characteristics	Early onset preeclampsia	Late-onset preeclampsia
Time of onset	<34 weeks	>34 weeks
Underlying etiology	Fetal disorder which is associated with placental dysfunction	Maternal disorder due to underlying maternal constitutional factors
Placental volume	Reduction in placental volume	Normal or larger placental volume
Fetal growth	Fetal growth restriction	Normal fetal growth
Uterine and umbilical artery Doppler evaluation	Abnormal	Normal
Baby's birth weight	Low	Normal
Maternal and neonatal outcomes	Usually adverse/less favorable	More favorable
Maternal and fetal morbidity	More	Less

Gestational hypertension was previously termed as PIH and considered as a benign condition. The old terminology is no longer used because it denoted all forms of hypertension during pregnancy. Also, the condition is no longer considered benign because nearly half of the women with gestational hypertension would eventually progress to develop proteinuria or other forms of end-organ dysfunction, consistent with the diagnosis of preeclampsia, especially when the condition develops prior to 32 weeks. As mentioned previously, women with gestational hypertension having severe range BP are now termed as severe preeclampsia and are managed with the same approach.

CHRONIC HYPERTENSION

Chronic hypertension can be defined as high BP that is diagnosed before pregnancy or before the 20th week of pregnancy in the absence of gestational trophoblastic disease. Hypertension should be documented on at least two occasions 4 hours apart. The condition does not return to normal following delivery. BP elevation that persists >12 weeks postpartum is also retrospectively considered as chronic hypertension. Most women in this category have essential hypertension, i.e., there is no underlying cause for chronic hypertension. This hypertension is mostly mild (≤105 mm Hg diastolic) in intensity. Pregnancy usually remains uncomplicated. On occasion, the high BP may be secondary to disorders such as endocrine tumors, renal artery stenosis, renal disease, and pheochromocytoma.

PREECLAMPSIA SUPERIMPOSED UPON CHRONIC HYPERTENSION

There is ample evidence that preeclampsia may occur in women already suffering from chronic hypertension prior to pregnancy. This condition is characterized by development of one or more features of preeclampsia (e.g., low enzymes, platelets, and proteinuria) for the first time in pregnancy after 20 weeks in a woman with chronic hypertension. Preeclampsia superimposed upon chronic hypertension holds importance because prognosis for both mother and fetus is much worse than with either condition alone. The obstetrician's task is to distinguish superimposed preeclampsia from worsening chronic hypertension.

Preeclampsia–eclampsia can be considered as a serious multisystemic disorder having a broad clinical spectrum with preeclampsia at one end and the most severe manifestation of preeclampsia, i.e., eclampsia at the other. Clinical course of preeclampsia can vary from one patient to the other. Preeclampsia always presents potential danger to the mother and baby. Sometimes, mild preeclampsia (especially if remains untreated) can progress into severe preeclampsia. The difference between mild and severe preeclampsia is listed in **Table 18.5**. Severe preeclampsia may ultimately result in development of eclampsia, which can be defined as the occurrence of seizures that cannot be attributed to other causes, in a woman with preeclampsia. Some indicators of severe preeclampsia during pregnancy are listed in **Box 18.1**.

PATHOPHYSIOLOGY OF PREECLAMPSIA

> Q. With the help of a long essay, discuss the pathophysiology of preeclampsia.
>
> Q. Discuss in brief about angiogenesis and its role in uteroplacental dysfunction.
>
> Q. Discuss in brief the etiopathogenesis of preeclampsia.

TABLE 18.5: Difference between mild and severe preeclampsia.

Characteristics	Mild preeclampsia	Severe preeclampsia
Time of presentation	Presents at gestational age ≥ 34 weeks	Presents at gestational age < 34 weeks
Diastolic BP	<100 mm Hg	>110 mm Hg
Symptoms showing neurological involvement such as headache, visual disturbances, and hyperreflexia, and abdominal pain	Absent	May be present
Presence of ominous features such as convulsions (eclampsia), congestive heart failure, or pulmonary edema	Absent	May be present
Oliguria	Absent	Present
Elevated liver enzymes [lactate dehydrogenase (LDH), AST]	Absent	Present
Thrombocytopenia (platelet count < 100,000/μL)	Absent	May be present
Serum creatinine levels	Normal	Elevated
Proteinuria	Mild to moderate	Severe (in nephrotic range) > 3 g/24 hours (especially in association with ominous features)
Nonreassuring FHR with or without fetal growth restriction	Absent	Present

(AST: aspartate aminotransferase)

BOX 18.1: Indicators of severe preeclampsia during pregnancy.
- Diastolic BP ≥ 110 mm Hg and/or systolic BP ≥ 160 mm Hg
- Proteinuria 2+ or more on the dipstick
- Presence of symptoms such as headache, visual disturbances, oliguria (urine volume ≤ 500 mL/ 24 hours), and convulsions
- Investigations show the presence of thrombocytopenia (platelet count < 100,000 cells/mm^3), elevated serum creatinine levels (>1.2 mg/dL, unless known to be previously elevated), serum uric acid of >4.5 mg%, elevated liver enzymes (ALT or AST), evidence of microangiopathic hemolytic anemia, fetal IUGR, etc.

(AST: aspartate aminotransferase; ALT: alanine aminotransferase)

The exact pathophysiology of preeclampsia is not yet understood. The most likely causes for preeclampsia and their underlying mechanisms are tabulated in **Table 18.6** and described in **Flowchart 18.2**. Preeclampsia can occur in two stages, which are described next:

TABLE 18.6: Pathophysiology of preeclampsia.

Likely cause for preeclampsia	Underlying mechanism
Inadequate trophoblastic invasion	Insufficient blood flow to the uterus
Prostacyclin/thromboxane imbalance	Disruption of the balance of the hormones that maintain the diameter of the blood vessels
Endothelial activation and dysfunction	Damage to the endothelial lining of the blood vessels that regulates the diameter of the blood vessels, keeping fluid inside and preventing leakage of proteins
Calcium deficiency or insufficient magnesium oxide	Calcium helps maintain vasodilation, so a deficiency would impair the function of vasodilation; magnesium stabilizes vascular smooth muscles and helps regulate vascular tone
Hemodynamic vascular injury	Injury to the blood vessels due to too much blood flow
Dysfunctional immunological tolerance	There is abnormal immunological tolerance between maternal, paternal (placental), and fetal tissues
Nutritional problems/poor diet	Insufficient protein, excessive protein, not enough fresh fruits and vegetables (antioxidants)
Genetic factors	Includes predisposing genes and epigenetic influences. However, the exact genes have yet not been identified
Maternal maladaptation	Inability of the mother to adapt to cardiovascular or inflammatory changes of normal pregnancy

Stage 1: Placental Syndrome (Inadequate Trophoblastic Invasion)

Preeclampsia occurs only in the presence of a placenta. Some cases of preeclampsia are associated with a failure of the normal invasion of trophoblast cells, resulting in the maladaptation of maternal spiral arterioles **(Figs. 18.2A and B)**. The maternal arterioles are the source of blood supply to the fetus, and inadequate trophoblastic invasion of these spiral vessels, which causes placental insufficiency, can interfere with normal villous development. In most cases, poor villous development results in placental insufficiency. Secondary damage, such as fibrin deposition and thrombosis, can then occur within the placenta. These features result in placental insufficiency, which is characteristically present in preeclampsia. These pathological changes may be aggravated due to disorders such as diabetes, hydatidiform mole, and multiple pregnancy. **Figure 18.3** shows the histopathological picture in case of preeclampsia demonstrating hypertrophic decidual vasculopathy. There is thickening of the walls of maternal blood vessels and narrowing of their lumen due to lipid deposition.

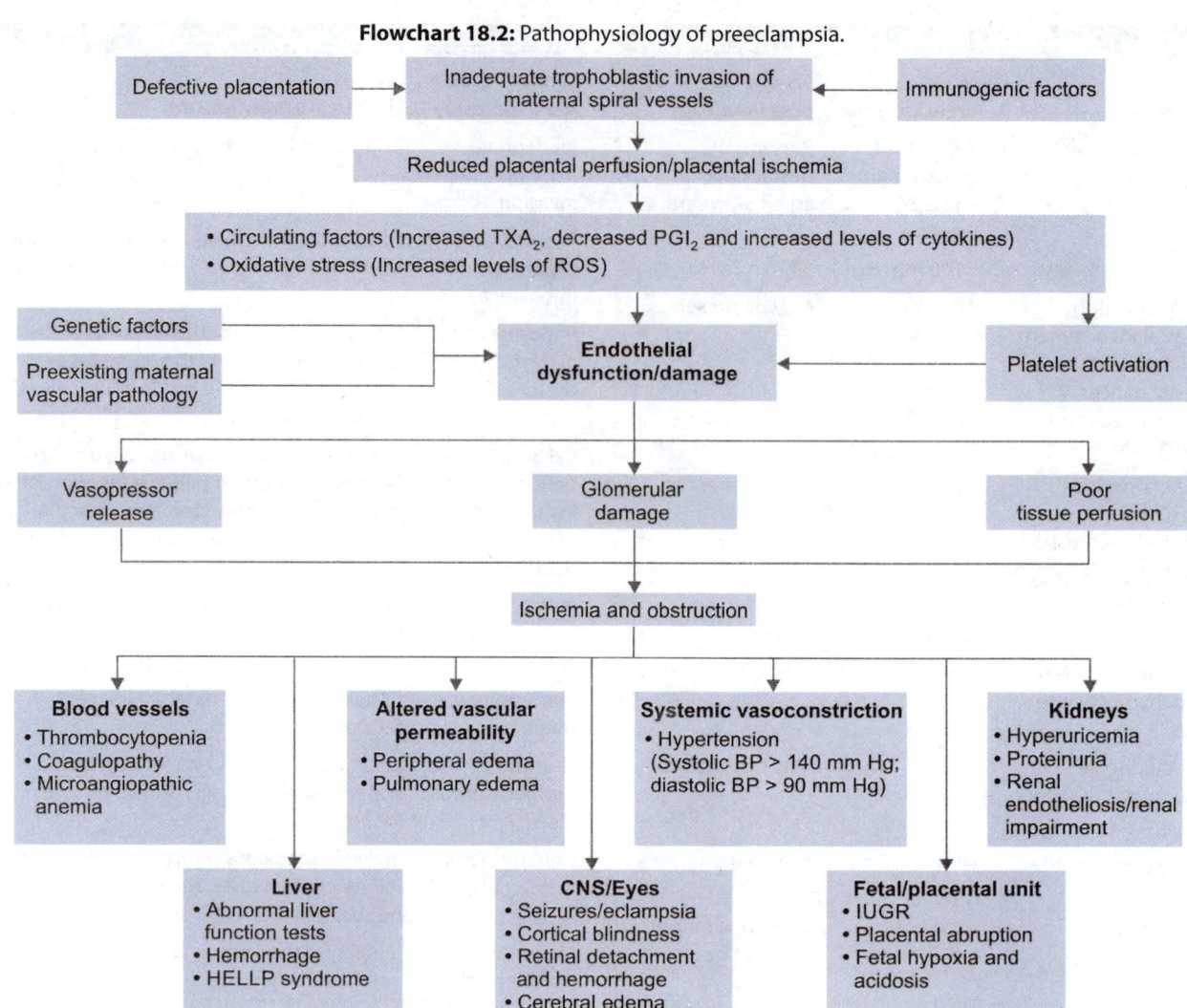

Flowchart 18.2: Pathophysiology of preeclampsia.

(CNS: central nervous system; HELLP: hemolysis, elevated liver enzymes, and low platelets; IUGR: intrauterine growth restriction; PGI_2: prostaglandin I_2; TXA_2: tranexamic acid; ROS: reactive oxygen species)

Stage 2: Maternal Syndrome (Maternal Inflammatory Response)

Although preeclampsia is a multisystem disorder, the chief pathology underlying preeclampsia is a vascular endothelial dysfunction. Inflammatory changes are considered to be a continuation of the placental syndrome. This could be related to strong maternal inflammatory response. Antiangiogenic markers, metabolic factors, other inflammatory leukocyte mediators, and cytokines such as tumor necrosis factor (TNF-α) and interleukins are responsible for producing inflammatory damage.

Some of the causes for preeclampsia are as follows:

Hereditary Factors

Preeclampsia has been considered to be a multifactorial polygenic disease. However, the exact genetic defects or preeclampsia genes have not yet been identified. A single preeclampsia gene is unlikely; there are probably several modifier genes along with environmental factors. The various genes which have been thought to be the likely candidates include the genes which encode angiotensinogen, superoxide dismutase, TNF-α, methylene-tetrahydrofolate reductase, factor V Leiden, and endothelial nitric oxide synthase.

Immunological Factors

The risk of development of preeclampsia is especially increased when there is impairment in the production of blocking antibodies to various placental antigenic sites. These antigens are responsible for producing damage similar to that occurring in case of acute graft reflection.

Endothelial Dysfunction and Vasospasm

In normal pregnancy, the vascular system is refractory to the effect of a potent vasoconstrictor, angiotensin II, due to the increased production of an enzyme, angiotensinase. This enzyme is produced by the placenta and destroys angiotensin II. In preeclampsia, there is increased vasoconstriction due to reduced refractoriness to the action of angiotensin II and due to the imbalance in production of various prostaglandins. There is increased production

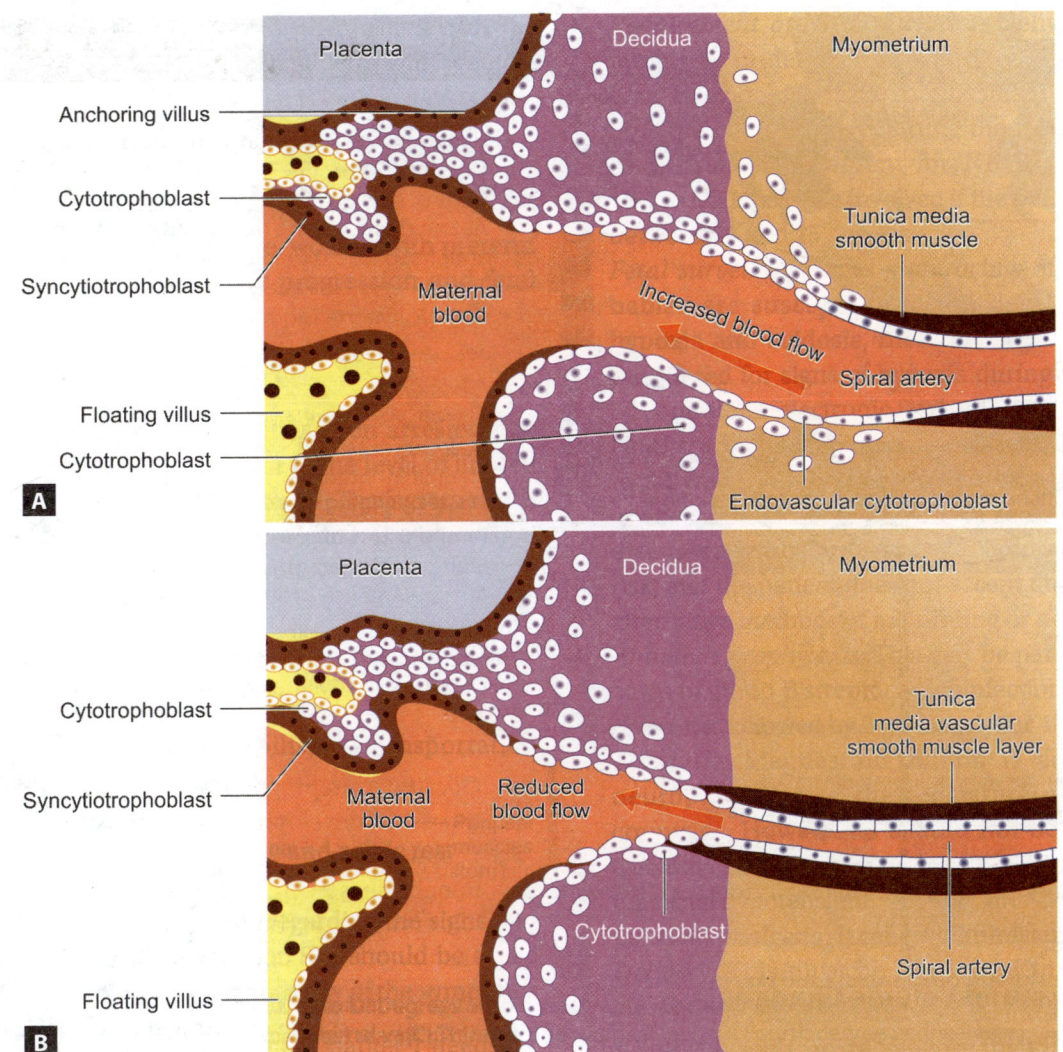

Figs. 18.2A and B: Inadequate trophoblastic invasion. (A) Trophoblastic invasion of spiral arterioles in normal pregnancy; (B) Reduced trophoblastic invasion of spiral vessels in preeclampsia.

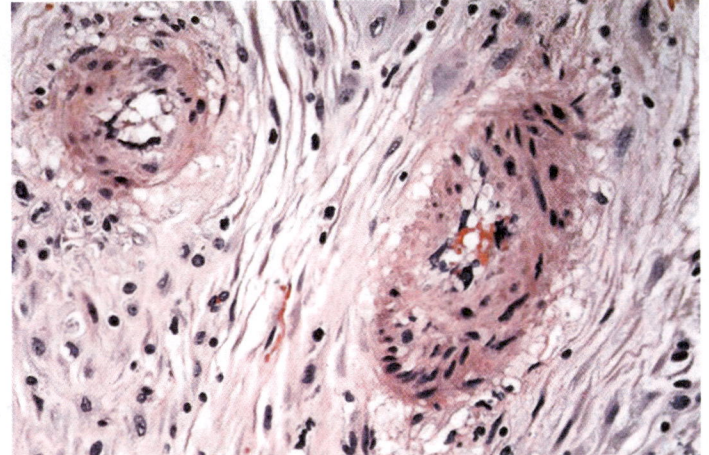

Fig. 18.3: Histopathological appearance in case of preeclampsia showing hypertrophic decidual vasculopathy.

of vasoconstrictors such as thromboxane A_2 and reduced production of vasodilatory prostaglandins such as prostacyclins.

Nitric oxide is a potent vasodilator synthesized from L-arginine in endothelial cells with the help of an enzyme, nitric oxide synthase. Inhibition of nitric oxide synthesis is likely to result in the following:

- Rise of mean arterial pressure
- Lowering of heart rate
- Reversal of pregnancy-induced refractoriness to vasopressors

Therefore, reduced expression of endothelial nitric oxide synthase and lower activity of nitric oxide are likely to be associated with preeclampsia.

Difference between Preeclampsia, Toxemia, Preeclamptic Toxemia, and Pregnancy-induced Hypertension

Toxemia is an older term based on a belief that the condition was the result of toxins (poisons) in the blood. Preeclamptic toxemia (PET) is a term used by older physicians in the UK and elsewhere in Europe. PIH, a newer term, stands for pregnancy-induced hypertension. The Preeclampsia Foundation uses the term "preeclampsia" as an umbrella

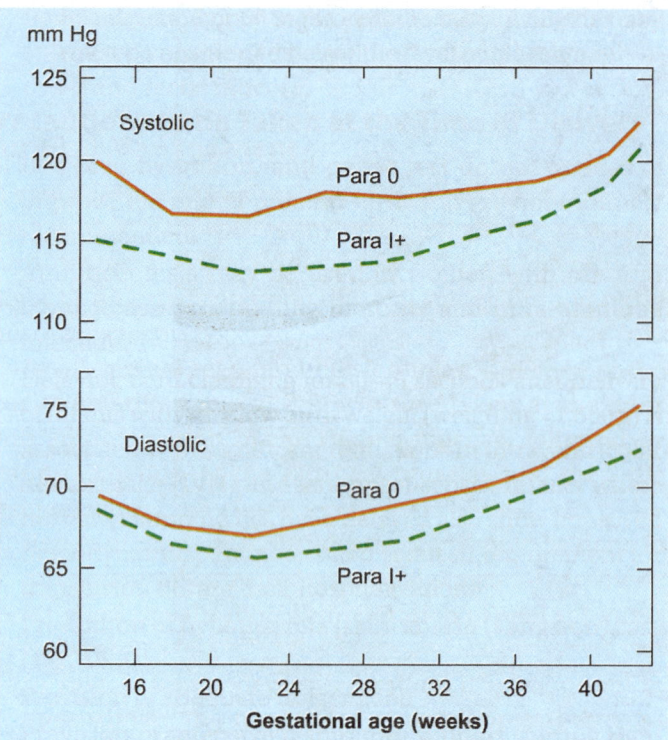

Fig. 18.4: Changes in systolic and diastolic BPs in relation to gestational age during normal pregnancy.

> **BOX 18.2:** Risk factors to identify women at an increased risk of preeclampsia.
>
> *High-risk factors*
> - Hypertensive diseases in a previous pregnancy
> - Obesity
> - Chronic kidney disease
> - Autoimmune disease (e.g., lupus erythematosus or antiphospholipid syndrome)
> - Type 1 or type 2 diabetes
> - Chronic hypertension
>
> *Moderate-risk factors*
> - Primiparity
> - Age 40 years or older
> - New paternity
> - Pregnancy interval of 10 years or more
> - Elevated BMI; >35 kg/m² at first visit
> - Family history of preeclampsia
> - Multiple pregnancy
> - African–American ethnicity
>
> (BMI: body mass index)
> *Source:* Waugh JJ, Smith MC. In: Edmonds DK (Ed). Dewhurst's Textbook of Obstetrics and Gynecology. Oxford: John Wiley & Sons Ltd; 2012. pp. 101-10.

term to cover all variants of various hypertensive disorders occurring during pregnancy.

Cardiovascular and Volume Changes in Normal Pregnancy

There is a fall in the systemic vascular resistance during normal pregnancy. Also, due to an increase in plasma volume, accompanied by marked increases in intravascular and extracellular volumes, there is an increase in cardiac output during normal pregnancy. Despite an increase in the cardiac output, there is a fall in BP due to a reduction in systemic vascular resistance. As a result, there is an overall fall in the diastolic pressure and mean arterial pressure during pregnancy, with decrease starting in early gestation and reaching a nadir near midpregnancy **(Fig. 18.4)**. Clinical relevance of these changes is that undiagnosed chronic hypertension may be masked in early pregnancy because of the initial decrease in pressure.

HISTORY AND CLINICAL PRESENTATION

RISK FACTORS

The various factors which are associated with increased risk of preeclampsia are listed in **Box 18.2** and need to be elicited while taking history. The various risk factors include the following:

- *Obesity:* A prepregnancy BMI of ≥35 almost quadruples the risk of developing preeclampsia.
- Diabetes
- Renal disease
- Extremes of age (under 18 or over 40 years)
- History of having preeclampsia in a previous pregnancy, particularly if its onset was before the third trimester. Women with severe preeclampsia in their previous pregnancies are at an increased risk of recurrence during their next pregnancies. However, the disorder is generally less severe and manifests 2–3 weeks later than in the first pregnancy.
- Certain autoimmune conditions, including antiphospholipid antibody syndrome, are associated with an increased risk for preeclampsia (Chapter 13).
- Previous history of chronic hypertension
- African–American or Hispanic ethnicity
- *Family history of preeclampsia:* Having a sister, mother, or daughter who has had preeclampsia or high BP in pregnancy increases the chances of the woman to develop preeclampsia during her present pregnancy.
- *A change of male partner:* Having a male partner whose previous partner had preeclampsia may increase the woman's risk of developing preeclampsia during her future pregnancies. This suggests that the father's genetic material, passed onto the fetus and its placenta, may play a role, thereby suggesting the role of genetic factors in the etiopathogenesis of preeclampsia.
- Nulliparity
- Multifetal gestation
- *History of smoking:* Although smoking is associated with an increased risk of various adverse pregnancy-related

outcomes, ironically it is associated with a reduced risk of hypertension during pregnancy.
- Family history of preeclampsia
- A time duration of ≥10 years since the last pregnancy
- Raised BP at the time of booking

CLINICAL PRESENTATION

Presenting symptoms of preeclampsia which need to be elicited while taking the history include the following:
- *Edema of the hands and face:* Since edema is a universal finding in pregnancy, it is not considered as a criterion for diagnosing preeclampsia. The best way to ask the patient about development of edema is to inquire if she has been experiencing tightening of rings on the fingers of her hands or facial puffiness and swelling of feet on getting up from the bed. Some swelling of the feet and ankles is considered normal with pregnancy. Nondependent edema such as facial or hand swelling (the patient's ring may no longer fit her finger) is more specific than dependent edema. Vulvar edema or the presence of edema over ankles in the morning on getting up from the bed is also pathological.

  Virtually, any organ system in the body may be affected due to severe preeclampsia. Some of the symptoms which may be sometimes observed, especially in association with severe disease may include the following:
- *Headache:* Dull, throbbing headache, often described as migraine-like, which would just not go away
- *Visual problems:* Vision changes include temporary loss of vision, sensations of flashing lights, sensitivity to light auras, and blurry vision or spots. The problems related to vision are usually related to the spasm of retinal vessels.
- *Epigastric or right upper quadrant abdominal pain:* It is usually indicative of hepatocellular necrosis, ischemia, edema, etc. all of which are responsible for stretching the Glisson's capsule of the liver. This pain is usually associated with elevation in liver enzymes such as AST (aspartate aminotransferase) and ALT (alanine aminotransferase) (reflecting hepatic ischemia or derangement). There may be associated nausea and vomiting as well. The liver may swell as a result of local edema secondary to the presence of inflammatory infiltrates and obstruction to the blood flow in the sinusoids. Hemorrhage can occur beneath the liver capsule and may be so extensive as to cause rupture of the capsule into the peritoneal cavity. If a hematoma or hemorrhage is suspected, the liver should be examined by ultrasonography. Liver involvement could be a part of HELLP (hemolysis, elevated liver enzymes, and low platelets) syndrome, which would be discussed later.
- Substantial hepatic dysfunction can also result in the development of coagulation abnormalities.
- *Shortness of breath or dyspnea:* This could be reflective of pulmonary edema or acute respiratory distress syndrome.
- *Oliguria:* Reduced urinary output of <300–400 mL in 24 hours could be indicative of reduced plasma volume or ischemic acute tubular necrosis.
- *Reduced fetal movements:* The patient may give a history of experiencing reduced fetal movements especially in association with IUGR and oligohydramnios.

GENERAL PHYSICAL EXAMINATION

Since the diagnostic features of preeclampsia include high BP and proteinuria, both of these would be described first.

INCREASED BLOOD PRESSURE

The presence of increased BP (>140/90 mm Hg) for the first time during pregnancy, after 20 weeks of gestation, can be considered as one of the diagnostic features of preeclampsia.

Method of Taking Blood Pressure

According to the current consensus, BP during pregnancy must be measured with the woman sitting quietly for several minutes, the arm cuff at heart level. The right upper arm must be used, and the arm must be taken out of the sleeve. The BP should be taken after 5 minutes of rest. The BP cuff should be of the appropriate size (12 cm wide and 35 cm in length) and should be placed at the level of the heart. If the arm is very fat, a wider cuff must be used to obtain correct reading **(Fig. 18.5)**. A BP cuff that encompasses about 80% of arm length and 40% of the width of arm circumference must be used. The cuff must be applied firmly around the arm, not allowing more than one finger between the cuff and the patient's arm. The woman should not use tobacco or caffeine within 30 minutes of the measurement. The RCOG recommends that mercury sphygmomanometers should be

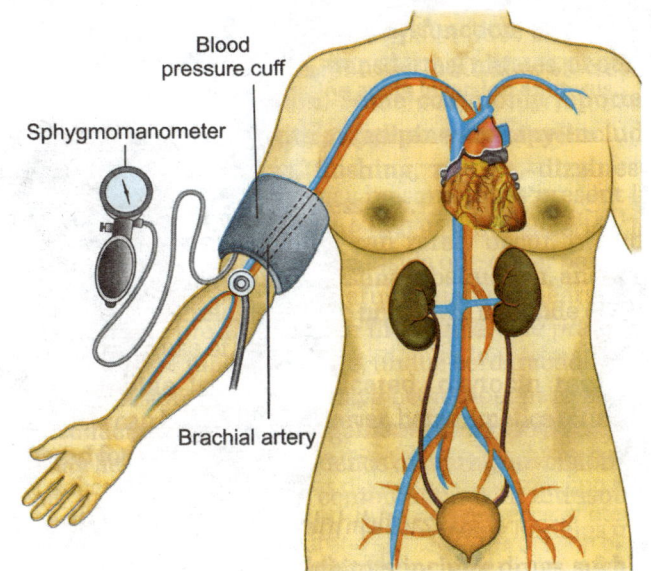

Fig. 18.5: Method of accurately recording the BP.

used at least to establish baseline BP as a reference, since this reading is supposed to be most accurate. Automated systems for BP measurement are not reliable in cases of severe preeclampsia and are likely to under-record these values, particularly the systolic BP.

Measurement of Blood Pressure Reading

Korotkoff phase 5 (disappearance of heart sounds and not simply muffling of sounds) is considered as the appropriate measurement of diastolic BP. In cases where K5 is absent, fourth Korotkoff sound should be accepted. On the other hand, the systolic BP is taken at Korotkoff phase 1 (the first sound heard after the cuff pressure is released). It is also recommended that elevation of gestational BP must be defined based on at least two readings of high BP obtained at least 6 hours apart within a span of 1 week.

MEASUREMENT OF PROTEINURIA

The usual screening test for proteinuria is visual assessment of dipstick or a regent strip **(Figs. 18.6A and B)**. Dipstick is a device in which a strip of paper impregnated with a reagent (used for testing proteins) is dipped into urine to measure the quantity of proteins present in the urine. The reagent strips for measuring proteins in the urine have the markings for "trace", 1+, 2+, etc. A reading of trace protein is relatively common and is usually not a cause for concern. A 2+ dipstick measurement can be taken as evidence of proteinuria. However, this must be confirmed by a 24-hour urine collection for protein estimation.

Though visual dipstick assessment is associated with both false-positive and false-negative test results, this test is most used for estimation of proteinuria. Despite this, it remains an important screening test due to easy availability, convenience, and low cost. The approximate equivalence of the dipstick result and amount of protein in the urine are shown in **Table 18.7**, with the results of 1+ = 0.3 g/L, 2+ = 1 g/L, 3+ = 3 g/L, and 4+ = 10g/L. Proteinuria is defined as significant if the excretion of proteins exceeds 300 mg/24 hours or urine protein/creatinine ratio ≥ 30 mg/mmol. This correlates with a persistent presence of the protein (30 mg/dL or 1+ dipstick) in two random urine samples collected 4–6 hours apart in the absence of any evidence of urinary tract infection. In view of the high false-positive rates with visual dipsticks assessment, a 24-hour urine collection for protein estimation or a timed collection corrected for creatinine excretion is sometimes recommended by the obstetrician to confirm significant proteinuria. According to the NICE guidelines (2010), repeated measurements are not necessary once proteinuria is detected, and clinical interventions must be immediately started.

Proteinuria is generally associated with the classic pathological finding of glomeruloendotheliosis, which is not permanent but recovers after delivery. Increased urinary excretion of proteins and an increase in capillary endothelial permeability lead to an increase in extracellular volume and a reduction in intravascular volume. These changes may be responsible for the development of tissue edema in cases of preeclampsia.

Procedure for Determining Proteinuria

1. Fresh specimen of urine must be collected. Reagent strips may give false-positive result if a very concentrated specimen of urine is used. The first urine specimen passed in the morning may be concentrated and may give a falsely high reading. Therefore, the first morning specimen must preferably not be used.
2. Following the removal of reagent strip from the bottle, the cap must be replaced.
3. The reagent strip must be dipped into the urine in such a way that the entire test area is completely covered,

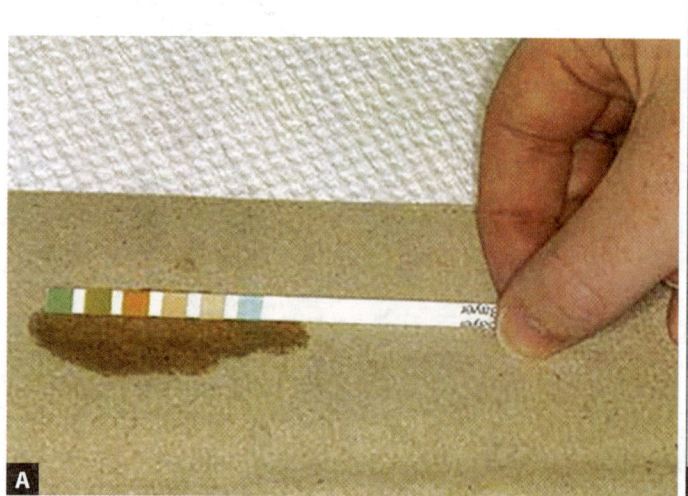
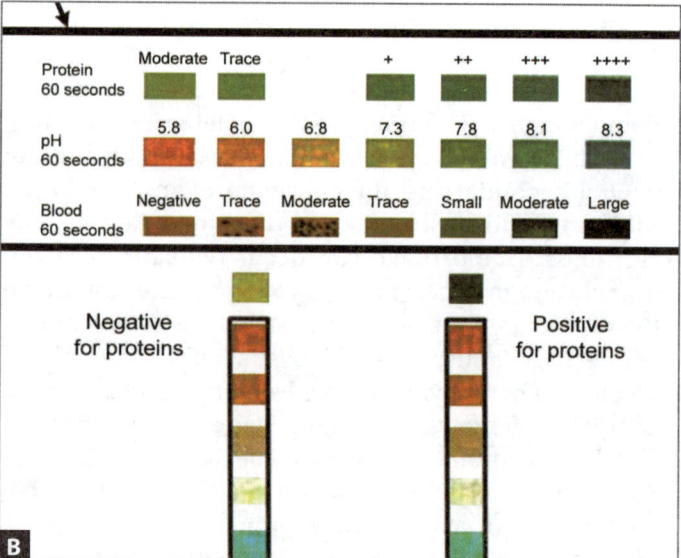

Figs. 18.6A and B: (A) Method of measuring proteinuria using dipstick; (B) Measurement of proteinuria through visual assessment of dipstick.

TABLE 18.7: Grading of proteinuria in the urine.	
Dipstick result	**Amount of protein in the urine**
Trace	0.15–0.3 g/L
1+	0.3 g/L
2+	1 g/L
3+	3 g/L
4+	10 g/L

following which the strip should be immediately removed from the urine sample.
4. For the accurate color changes to take place, the clinician must wait for at least 60 seconds and let the tested area get air-dried.
5. The reagent strip must be held horizontally, and the color must be compared with that of the color blocks on the side of the bottle. The darker the color of the reagent strip, the greater is the amount of proteinuria.

Likely Cause for the Occurrence of Proteinuria

Proteinuria is primarily due to the vasospasm and endothelial dysfunction of the endothelial cells lining the afferent glomerular arterioles. This results in an increased permeability of the vessels causing the development of proteinuria. Albumin forms the major component of this proteinuria. However, it is not admissible to use the term albuminuria as small amounts of globulins are also present.

OTHER FEATURES ON GENERAL PHYSICAL EXAMINATION SUGGESTIVE OF PREECLAMPSIA

The other features on general physical examinations which are suggestive of severe preeclampsia are described below:
- *Edema of the hands and face:* As previously mentioned, pedal edema is no longer considered as the diagnostic criteria of preeclampsia as it can be present in the normal pregnancy as well. Nondependent edema such as facial edema or hand swelling (edema in the fingers) is more specific than dependent edema. The obstetrician must specifically look for vulvar edema, facial edema, and edema over the fingers.
- *Weight gain:* The weight of a patient with suspected or diagnosed preeclampsia must be taken at each antenatal visit because preeclampsia is associated with a significant weight gain. Weight gain of >2 pounds per week or 6 pounds in a month or a sudden weight gain over 1–2 days can be considered as significant.
- *Petechiae:* Presence of petechiae may reflect a bleeding tendency, which may serve as an indicator of HELLP syndrome. Platelet count may fall below $100 \times 10^6/L$.
- *Ankle clonus:* Presence of ankle clonus is indicative of excessive neuromuscular irritability, which can progress to seizures (eclampsia).
- *Knee jerks:* Evaluation of knee jerks is especially important in patients receiving magnesium sulfate as reduced or absent knee jerks in a patient on magnesium sulfate therapy are usually indicative of magnesium toxicity.
- *Papilledema:* This can be described as the swelling of optic disk diagnosed on ophthalmoscopy or slit-lamp examination in very severe cases of hypertension. Papilledema occurs due to increased intracranial pressure, usually in association with malignant hypertension.

SPECIFIC SYSTEMIC EXAMINATION

ABDOMINAL EXAMINATION

On abdominal examination, there may be evidence of placental insufficiency in the form of oligohydramnios or/and IUGR. Oligohydramnios can be defined as the presence of <200 mL of amniotic fluid at term or an AFI of <5 cm or the presence of the largest pocket of fluid, which does not measure >2 cm at its largest diameter. For specific abdominal findings in relation to IUGR, refer to Chapter 15. Findings on abdominal examination suggestive of oligohydramnios are as follows:
- The fundal height is less than that estimated on the basis of last menstrual period (LMP).
- Uterus may appear full of fetus, and/or evidence of IUGR may be present.

DIFFERENTIAL DIAGNOSIS

It is important for the obstetrician to differentiate between preeclampsia, gestational hypertension, and chronic hypertension. The differentiating features of all these have been described in the introduction previously.

In case of seizures (eclampsia), the differential diagnosis may include abnormalities such as epilepsy, intracranial hemorrhage and thrombosis, rupture of cerebral aneurysm, meningitis, encephalitis, cerebral tumors, and cerebral malaria. Despite these possible differential diagnoses, the rule of thumb is that "any convulsion in the later part of pregnancy should be considered as eclampsia unless proved otherwise."

MANAGEMENT

> **Q. Describe the management of the patient described in the case study described at the beginning of the chapter.**

Management comprising investigations and definitive obstetric management is discussed next.

INVESTIGATIONS

LABORATORY TESTS

Laboratory tests which must be performed in these patients include the following:
- CBC, platelet count

- LFTs
- Measurement of serum electrolytes, blood urea nitrogen (BUN)
- Kidney function tests (KFTs) (creatinine, creatinine clearance, and 24-hour urine protein)
- Urinalysis
- Ophthalmoscopic examination

Hematocrit

The decrease in blood volume in preeclampsia can lead to an increase in maternal hemoglobin concentration, resulting in increased hematocrit.

Platelet Count

In normal pregnancy, the platelet count can fall below 200×10^9/L due to the normal maternal blood volume expansion.

In preeclampsia, the platelet count falls further and is associated with progressive disease. This fall is probably a result of both increased platelet consumption and intravascular destruction related to preeclampsia. Coagulation abnormalities are unlikely to occur if the platelet count remains above 100×10^9/L. Normal platelet count varies between 150×10^9/L and 400×10^9/L. A low platelet count could also be indicative of the HELLP syndrome, which would be discussed later in the chapter.

Kidney Function Tests

Renal function is generally maintained in preeclampsia until the late stage, unless the HELLP syndrome develops.

Serum Creatinine Levels

In normal pregnancy, there is an increase in creatinine clearance with a concomitant decrease in serum creatinine and urea concentrations. If creatinine is found to be elevated early in pregnancy, underlying renal disease should be suspected. In severe preeclampsia, serum creatinine can be seen to rise and is associated with a worsening outcome. However, with increase in the use of antihypertensive drugs and magnesium sulfate in patients with preeclampsia, the incidence of renal failure is progressively decreasing. When renal failure does occur, it is usually associated with hemorrhage, HELLP syndrome, or sepsis.

Serum Uric Acid Levels

Serum concentrations of uric acid fall in normal pregnancy because renal excretion increases.

In preeclampsia, there can be a rise in uric acid concentrations mostly due to decrease in renal excretion but could also be related to increased production secondary to tissue ischemia and oxidative stress. Increased serum uric acid levels are usually related to poorer outcomes for both the mother and the baby.

Liver Function Test

- LFTs including the measurement of ALT and AST, and lactate dehydrogenase (LDH) activities must be performed.
- An AST level of above 75 IU/L is seen as significant, and a level above 150 IU/L is associated with increased morbidity to the mother.

Ophthalmoscopic Examination

The following findings may be observed on the ophthalmoscopic examination:
- Presence of retinal edema
- *Constrictions of the retinal arterioles:* Narrowing of the retinal arterioles is related to the severity of hypertension.
- *Alteration of normal ratio of vein:arteriolar diameter:* Due to the arteriolar narrowing, the vein:arteriolar diameter is altered from 3:2 to about 3:1.
- There is nicking of the veins where they are crossed by the arterioles.

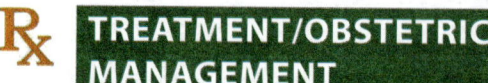

TREATMENT/OBSTETRIC MANAGEMENT

PREVENTION

Although there is no known way to prevent preeclampsia, it is important for all pregnant women to start prenatal care early and continue it throughout the pregnancy. This allows the healthcare provider to find and treat conditions such as preeclampsia early. Some methods for preventing preeclampsia, which have been evaluated in the randomized trials, include the following:

- *Dietary manipulation:* Low salt diet, calcium, or fish oil supplementation
- *Exercise:* Physical activity, stretching, etc.
- *Cardiovascular drugs:* Antihypertensives and diuretics
- *Antioxidants:* Vitamin C (ascorbic acid), vitamin E (α tocopherol), and vitamin D
- *Antithrombotic drugs:* Low-dose aspirin, dipyridamole, combination of aspirin and heparin, or combination of aspirin and ketanserin
- *Salt-restricted diet:* Randomized controlled trial by Knuist et al. (1998) has shown that salt-restricted diet is insufficient in preventing preeclampsia.
- *Exercise during pregnancy:* Regular exercise during pregnancy is linked to a lower risk of developing preeclampsia. A systemic review by Kasawara et al. (2012) has shown a probable protective effect of physical activity in the prevention of preeclampsia.
- *Bed rest during pregnancy:* Study by Abenhaim (2008) has shown that bed rest is associated with a significantly reduced risk of developing preeclampsia. Meher (2006) has also shown that 4–6 hours of bed rest daily at home

was successful in lowering the incidence of preeclampsia in women with normal BP.
- *Supplementation with calcium:* Cochrane reviews by Palacios et al. (2019) and Hofmeyr (2018) have shown that supplementation with vitamin D and calcium usually offers no benefits in prevention of preeclampsia unless the women are calcium deficient.
- *Supplementation with antioxidants:* The combined antioxidant and preeclampsia prediction study (CAPPS) by Maternal–Fetal Medicine Unit (MFMU) network has not shown reduced rate of preeclampsia in women supplemented with vitamins C and E.
- *Supplementation with heparin:* Rodger et al. (2016) have shown that the risk of recurrent preeclampsia, abruption, or fetal growth restriction (FGR) in women receiving low-molecular-weight heparin was similar to those receiving placebo.
- *Supplementation with aspirin:* At present, the use of aspirin appears to be the only method having a significant role in prevention of preeclampsia amongst high-risk women. According to a multicentric, double blind placebo control trial by Rolnik et al. (2017), the use of low-dose aspirin prophylaxis in women at high risk for preterm preeclampsia was associated with a 1.6% risk of preeclampsia in comparison with a risk of 4.3% in the placebo group. Roberge et al. (2017) found that aspirin prophylaxis initiated at <16 weeks was associated with 60% risk reduction for both preeclampsia and IUGR. However, low-dose aspirin initiated at ≥16 weeks was associated with an insignificant impact on the risk of preeclampsia. A systemic review and meta-analysis by Roberge et al. (2018) has shown that aspirin prophylaxis at ≤16 weeks of gestation in a dosage ≥ 100 mg is likely to reduce the risk of preterm, but not term, preeclampsia. Turner et al. (2020) have reported that the use of aspirin commenced at ≤16 weeks in the dosage ≥ 100 mg also improves perinatal outcomes independent of the concomitant beneficial effects on reducing the risk of preeclampsia. Review by Chaemsaithong (2020) found no benefits in reducing the risk of preeclampsia when low-dose aspirin was given prior to 11 weeks of gestation in high-risk women.

The USPSTF, 2021 recommends low-dose aspirin prophylaxis (81 mg/day) for women at high risk for preeclampsia. The ACOG (2020) has recommended low-dose aspirin to be administered between 12 and 28 weeks of gestation for preventing preeclampsia in high-risk women. Candidates for aspirin prophylaxis include those with more than or equal to one of the following features:
- Prior preeclampsia
- Chronic hypertension
- Overt diabetes
- Renal disease
- Autoimmune disorders
- Multiple gestation

Supplementation must also be considered for those with more than one of the following:
- Nulliparous women
- >35 years of age
- Obese
- Family history of preeclampsia
- Vulnerable sociodemographics
- Prior history of low-birth-weight babies

Ayala (2019) has raised a question asking if all pregnant women should be given low-dose aspirin and there should be a transition toward universal aspirin prophylaxis. Presently, there is no answer to this question.

Predictive Tests for Preeclampsia

> Q. Write a short essay on the predictors of preeclampsia.
>
> Q. Discuss in brief the predictors of PIH.
>
> Q. With the help of a short note, discuss screening of preeclampsia.

Early prediction for development of preeclampsia is important as it could lead to early and appropriate surveillance of women in high-risk category, at the same time avoiding unnecessary intervention in those at low risk. Most obstetric units presently rely on clinical history, BP examination, and urinary protein testing for prediction of preeclampsia. Presently, there is no screening test for preeclampsia which can be considered reliable, valid, and economical. Some tests which are occasionally employed in the clinical practice include the following.

Testing the Vascular Resistance and Placental Perfusion

There are three tests based on this concept, which help in assessing the BP rise in response to a stimulus:

1. *Roll-over test:* The woman at 28–32 weeks of gestation is made to lie in the left lateral position and then roll over to lie in the supine position. Rise in BP in response to this maneuver indicates a positive test.
2. *Isometric exercise test:* BP is taken at rest and while doing isometric exercises such as squeezing a handball.
3. *Angiotensin II infusion test:* BP is measure before and after the infusion of angiotensin II.

All these tests are associated with sensitivity ranging between 55% and 70% and specificity ranging between 80% and 85%.

Uterine artery Doppler velocimetry previously was considered as a good predictor of preeclampsia by demonstrating faulty trophoblastic invasion of the spiral arterioles. However, this is no longer being used in view of its poor predictive value.

Endothelial Dysfunction and Oxidative Stress

Since endothelial activation and inflammation can be considered as the main parameters responsible behind the pathophysiology of preeclampsia, levels of some compounds which are elevated in these cases have been assessed for predicting the occurrence of preeclampsia. Markers of oxidative stress such as high levels of lipid peroxides along with decreased antioxidant activity have been observed in cases of preeclampsia. Other markers of oxidative stress such as ferritin, resistin, iron, transferrin, and antioxidants such as ascorbic acid and vitamin E have been assessed. However, none is associated with a sufficient predictive value.

Imbalance between Angiogenic and Antiangiogenic Factors

Imbalance between angiogenic and antiangiogenic factors has been implicated in the pathogenesis of preeclampsia. Usually there is a decline in the levels of angiogenic factors such as vascular endothelial growth factor (VEGF) and placental growth factor (PlGF) before the development of clinical features of preeclampsia. Also, the levels of some antiangiogenic factors such as placental soluble fms-like tyrosine kinase 1 (sFlt-1) and soluble endoglin (sEng) begin to rise. Blood levels of these factors are associated with a good predictive value in cases of early onset preeclampsia. These markers are likely to have a significant role in the first-trimester preeclampsia screening.

Other Markers

Circulating cell-free fetal deoxyribonucleic acid (cffDNA) of placental origin is detected in maternal plasma. cffDNA is believed to be released in preeclampsia due to an accelerated apoptosis of cytotrophoblasts. However, there is presently no evidence regarding its role in predicting the occurrence of preeclampsia.

Many other markers have been identified, including the glycosylated hemoglobin, serum cystatin-C, and first-trimester estimated placental volume. Some preliminary studies have indicated their role as predictor molecules. However, long-term studies are still awaited.

MANAGEMENT OF CASES OF GESTATIONAL HYPERTENSION

> **Q.** With the help of a long essay, discuss the management of a 30-year-old primi patient with gestational hypertension at 32 weeks of gestation.

Gestational hypertension may be associated with an increased risk of maternal and perinatal morbidity and mortality. Also, mild gestational hypertension may be associated with an increased incidence of obstetric interventions such as induction of labor or cesarean section, while severe gestational hypertension may be associated with an increased incidence of preterm births or small for gestational age (SGA) babies. The most important complication of gestational hypertension is progression to preeclampsia, which is commonly evidenced by the development of proteinuria. The risk of progression to preeclampsia depends on the severity of hypertension (directly proportional) and gestational age at the time of diagnosis (indirectly proportional). The most important risk factor to be considered while managing such patients is the degree of BP elevation. If the BP is severe (≥160 systolic or ≥110 diastolic), the patient should be managed as a case of severe preeclampsia. Another major risk factor to be taken into consideration is gestational age at the onset of disease. Earlier presentation is associated with an increased likelihood of complications and poor outcomes.

Gestational Hypertension without the Risk Factors

In case of gestational hypertension without the presence of risk factors, these women can be managed as outpatients. The aim of management in these cases is early detection of preeclampsia and prevention of the progression of the condition to a severe form. Such women are instructed to do the following and bring that information with them at the time of visit to the clinic:

- Self-assessment of symptoms suggestive of end-organ damage, e.g., blurred vision, headache, and epigastric pain. In case she experiences either of these symptoms, she must immediately report to the clinic.
- Daily recording of the BP at home. They must be advised to visit the clinic/hospital in case the BP is above the threshold (systolic ≥ 150 mm Hg and diastolic ≥ 100 mm Hg).
- Perform qualitative examination of their first-voided urine sample for proteins using dipstick at least twice weekly and visit the clinic if the result is ≥1+.
- She must perform daily fetal movement count. She needs to report to the clinic in case she experiences reduced fetal movements.
- Absolute bed rest as recommended in the past is not required. However, the women must be asked to avoid strenuous physical activity or activity involving standing for a prolonged period of time.
- There is no requirement for dietary restrictions, and normal activities are allowed.
- Well-balanced diet, rich in proteins and calories, is prescribed.
- They must visit the clinic/hospital on a weekly basis.
- In order to ensure fetal well-being, a baseline ultrasound for fetal growth, assessment of amniotic fluid volume, and umbilical artery Doppler are required at the time of diagnosis in the clinic. As per the recommendations by the ACOG (2020), ultrasound for fetal growth must

be repeated every 3–4 weeks and amniotic fluid volume assessment must be done on a weekly basis. Additionally, an antenatal test for fetal well-being (e.g., NST) must be done once or twice weekly in patients with gestational hypertension, even in the absence of severe features.

- Patients with no positive findings in their weekly assessment may be allowed to continue pregnancy until 38–39 weeks. The pregnancy should not be allowed to continue beyond the estimated due date. Ripening agents may be used in case the cervix is not ripe.
- Admission to the hospital for further evaluation is required in the presence of the conditions listed in **Box 18.3**.

Gestational Hypertension with Risk Factors

Women having gestational hypertension in the presence of risk factors (**Box 18.4**) require to be admitted in the hospital. The aim of management in these cases is control of BP and early detection of preeclampsia, end-organ damage, and fetal decompensation. The following are required in these cases:

- *Blood investigations:* These need to be repeated at weekly or twice-weekly intervals and include the following:
  - CBC with platelet count
  - LFTs including LDH and liver enzymes
  - Urea and electrolytes
- *BP:* This needs to be measured at intervals of 6 hours.
- *Fetal surveillance:* This is extremely important in these cases and includes the following:
  - Ultrasound examination for fetal growth and amniotic fluid volume to be done after every 2 weeks.
  - Umbilical artery and cerebral vessel Doppler examinations to be done after every 2 weeks.
  - CTG for assessment of fetal well-being to be done on weekly basis.
- *Bed rest:* There are no definite studies indicating that bed rest is likely to be useful. There are a few studies showing the beneficial effect of bed rest in cases of preeclampsia. Complete bed rest, however, must not be recommended due to a risk of venous stasis, thromboembolism, bone demineralization, and muscle atrophy.
- *Antihypertensive therapy:* As per the ACOG (2020) recommendations, treatment with antihypertensive agents is required in case of systolic BP ≥ 160 mm Hg and diastolic BP ≥ 110 mm Hg. The aim of treatment is to prevent the potential complications associated with uncontrolled hypertension, e.g., ischemic or hemorrhagic stroke, congestive heart failure, myocardial infraction, renal injury, and pulmonary edema. However, as per the NICE guidelines (2019), pharmacological therapy must be initiated if BP remains above 140/90 mm Hg and aim of the therapy is to achieve a BP of 135/85 mm Hg. The NICE also suggests using labetalol as the first-line therapy for gestational hypertension followed by nifedipine in women for whom labetalol may not be suitable. Methyldopa may be used if both labetalol and nifedipine are not found to be suitable. The choice of antihypertensive is based on the side effect profile as well as the woman's tolerance and preference.
- *Delivery:* Women with gestational hypertension who have risk factors or progress to develop preeclampsia must be managed as those with severe preeclampsia. Women with gestational hypertension whose BP is <160/110 mm Hg with or without antihypertensive treatment should not be offered planned early delivery prior to 37 weeks unless there are other medical indications. Indications for termination of pregnancy include the following:
  - When hypertension is uncontrollable
  - There is an evidence of end-organ damage.
  - Bleeding suggestive of abruption placenta
  - Arrest of fetal growth
  - Worsening of Doppler evaluation with absent or reserved umbilical artery diastolic flow or development of severe abnormality in the FHR

Route of delivery in women with severe gestational hypertension who require delivery depends on the result of digital pelvic examination and cervical length. Cervix is considered unripe in case cervical length is ≥2.5 cm. In case the cervix is ripe, vaginal delivery is appropriate.

MANAGEMENT OF PREECLAMPSIA

Immediate hospitalization is recommended even in cases where there is suspicion of preeclampsia because of the disease's potential to accelerate rapidly. Immediate delivery is indicated irrespective of the period of gestation if severe hypertension remains uncontrolled for 24–48 hours or whenever there is appearance of certain "ominous" signs such as coagulation abnormalities, signs of worsening renal/hepatic function, signs of impending eclampsia (headache,

---

BOX 18.3: Circumstances under which the woman must be admitted to the hospital for further evaluation.

- Development of proteinuria
- Elevation of BP above the threshold
- Reduced fetal movements
- Poor fetal growth
- Development of other signs of preeclampsia

BOX 18.4: Criteria to identify high-risk women with gestational hypertension.

- BP ≥ 150/100 mm Hg
- Gestational age < 32 weeks
- Evidence of end-organ damage
- Oligohydramnios
- Fetal growth restriction
- Abnormal uterine and/or umbilical Doppler velocimetry

epigastric pain, and hyperreflexia), or the presence of severe growth restriction or nonreassuring fetal testing. Immediate delivery of the baby remains the only known "cure." Preeclampsia remote from term is a special situation in which the patients should be hospitalized and closely monitored in tertiary obstetric care centers (preferably those with prenatal close observation units). Pregnancy may be allowed to continue as long as BP remains controlled, no ominous signs of life-threatening maternal complications occur, and there are no signs of imminent danger to the fetus (e.g., nonreassuring FHR). Eclamptic convulsions must be managed using parenteral magnesium sulfate, which has been shown to be superior to either diazepam or phenytoin for both prevention and treatment. IV magnesium is not without risk, and its use must be largely reserved for women with severe disease.

Antihypertensive agents are mainly used to treat severe hypertension to delay delivery for as long as it is safely possible in order to maximize the gestational age and prevent neonatal complications of extreme prematurity such as cerebral hemorrhage. The goal of antihypertensive therapy is to maintain BP at a level so as to prevent cardiovascular and central nervous system consequences related to severe hypertension in the mother without compromising uteroplacental blood flow and fetal perfusion. Eventually, this protects the mother and fetus from the dangers of severe hypertension and related morbidity, thereby allowing the pregnancy to continue and the fetus to grow and mature. However, antihypertensive medicines do not prevent preeclampsia, nor do they reverse the primary pathogenic process of placental underperfusion and severe preeclampsia.

Management of cases with preeclampsia is described in **Flowchart 18.3**. Management of preeclampsia would be discussed under two headings: management in cases of mild preeclampsia and management in cases of severe preeclampsia.

Management of Mild Cases

Maternal Management

When the mother is diagnosed with mild type of preeclampsia in the antenatal period, she should be admitted in the hospital in order to assess the severity of condition and decide further management. Domiciliary treatment has no role in an established case of preeclampsia, and the patient must be hospitalized. In an under-resourced setting where it might not be possible to admit every patient with mild preeclampsia, the patient must be at least referred to an antenatal day unit for further investigations. The following assessments need to be carried out in patients who are admitted:

- Daily detailed examination for symptoms indicative of severe preeclampsia, including history of headache, visual disturbances, epigastric pain, edema, etc.
- Regular weight measurement at weekly intervals to assess if the woman is gaining weight at a rapid rate
- Daily examination of the first-voided urine sample for the presence of proteins by dipstick. If proteinuria of 2+ or more on dipstick is present, 24-hour protein estimation may be required.
- BP measurement to be done every 4-hourly (at least four times a day).
- The following investigations to be done on weekly basis: hematocrit with platelet count, KFT (blood urea, serum uric acid, and serum creatinine), LFT (AST, ALT, and LDH), and ophthalmoscopic examination. The frequency of investigations can be changed depending upon the severity of symptoms and the results of investigations.
- Absolute bed rest, as recommended in the past, is not required. However, reduced physical activity throughout the day is likely to be beneficial.
- In case the woman is hospitalized, to avoid the risk of DVT secondary to prolonged bed rest compression stockings or external pneumatic compression cuffs may be used.
- Prescription of sedatives or tranquilizers is not required.
- Well-balanced diet, rich in proteins and calories, is prescribed. No salt or fluid restriction is required.
- No medications are required other than iron and vitamin supplements.

Fetal Evaluation

Most cases of gestational hypertension and mild preeclampsia respond to conservative management. However, fetal surveillance is required until the baby has attained maturity because the underlying pathophysiology behind preeclampsia would be corrected only following delivery of the baby. Until fetal maturity is attained, fetal surveillance comprises the following tests:

- Daily fetal movement count
- Weekly measurement of fundal height and abdominal girth in order to detect IUGR
- NST weekly
- Ultrasound examination for evaluating fetal growth at every 1–2 weekly intervals
- Assessment of liquor by measurement of AFI on weekly basis
- Doppler ultrasound at every 1–2 weekly intervals, especially in case of suspected FGR

Mode of Delivery

There is no advantage of performing a cesarean over normal delivery. There is no need to hasten the delivery in cases of mild preeclampsia.

- *Gestational age ≥ 37 weeks:* Delivery should be undertaken in pregnant women with mild preeclampsia at 37 weeks or more because gestational hypertension and mild preeclampsia are both known risk factors for fetal death. In women with gestational hypertension

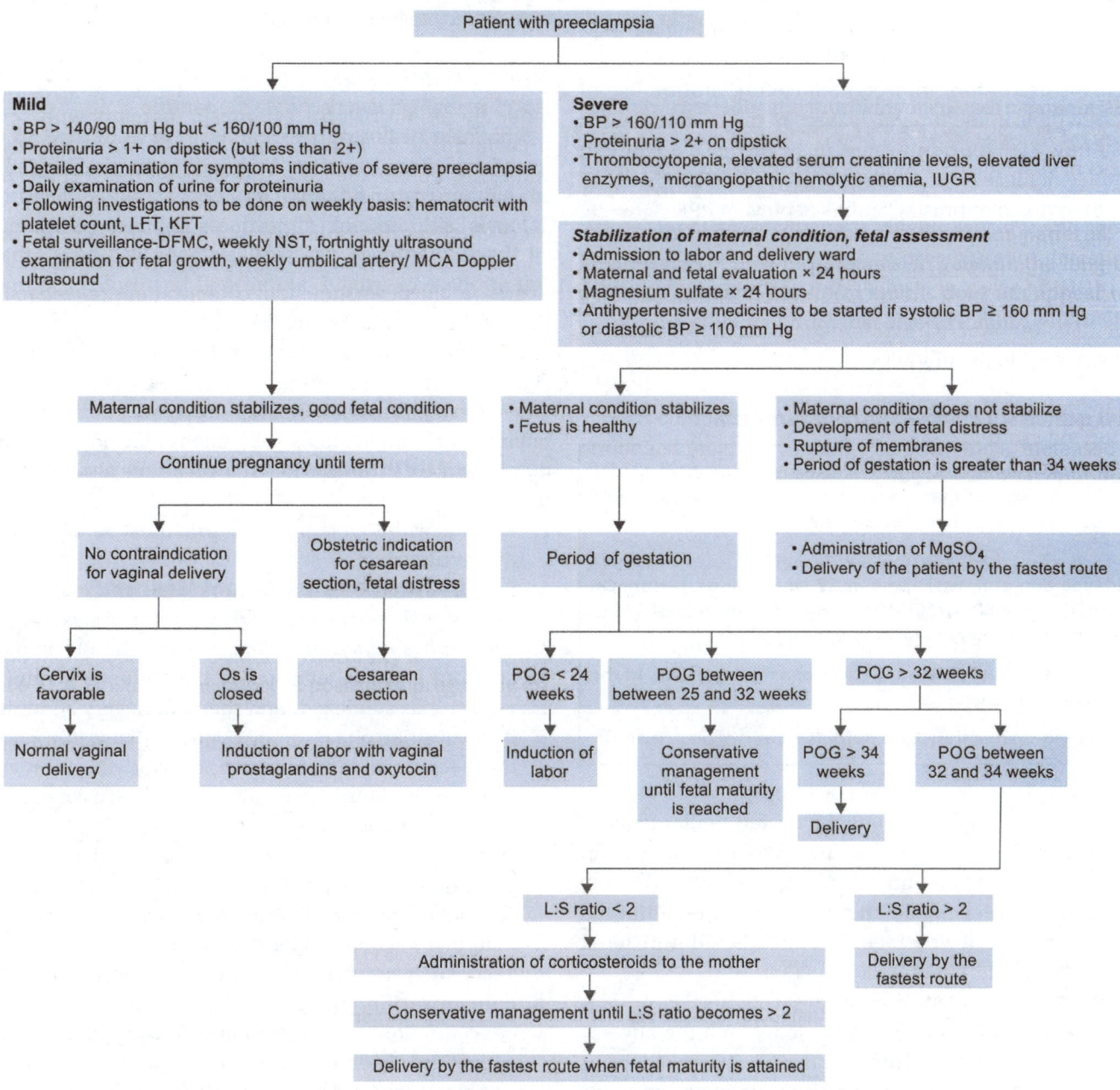

Flowchart 18.3: Management of cases with preeclampsia.

(DFMC: daily fetal movement count; IUGR: intrauterine growth restriction; LFT: liver function test; L:S ratio: lecithin: sphingomyelin ratio; MCA: middle cerebral artery; NST: nonstress test; POG: period of gestation)

or preeclampsia without severe features at or beyond 37 weeks of gestation, it is recommended that the patient be delivered rather than resorting to conservative management. HYPITAT (2009) (hypertension and preeclampsia intervention trial) has shown that women with gestational hypertension and preeclampsia are likely to have better maternal and neonatal outcomes with induction of labor at ≥37 weeks in comparison with expectant management.

- *24–36 weeks:* Between 24 and 36 weeks of gestation, management of patients with preeclampsia is dependent on maternal and fetal status at the time of initial clinical and laboratory evaluations. In case of preterm fetuses < 32 weeks' gestation, two doses of betamethasone, 12 mg IM 24 hours apart, are recommended. This may also be considered in fetuses between 35 and 36 weeks' gestation.

Intrapartum Period

- Such women require continuous monitoring of BP and symptoms suggestive of end-organ damage during labor to detect progression to severe disease.
- Antihypertensive therapy must be considered to maintain systolic BP < 160 mm Hg and diastolic < 100 mm Hg at the time of labor.
- Continuous fetal monitoring is indicated, especially in cases of FGR.

Postpartum Period

- The obstetrician must remain vigilant regarding the high chances of the occurrence of PPH.
  This is even more important since the routine use of methergine at the time of delivery of the baby's anterior shoulder is contraindicated in hypertensive women. Active management of third stage of labor can be done with oxytocin or prostaglandins to prevent PPH.
- Following delivery, the angiotensin-converting enzyme (ACE) inhibitors can be restarted.
- Use of methyldopa is to be stopped due to the risk of development of psychological changes, such as depression in the mother.

Management of Severe Preeclampsia

> Q. On examining a nulliparous patient having BP of 140/90 mm Hg, you observe that she has brisk knee jerks. How should this observation alter her management?
>
> Q. A 28-year-old primigravida patient presents with headache and epigastric pain at 32 weeks of gestation. On examination, her BP is 160/110 mm Hg. With the help of a long essay, discuss the management in this case.
>
> Q. Write a short note on the role of anticonvulsants in the treatment of preeclampsia.
>
> Q. Briefly discuss the role of steroids in cases of preeclampsia.

Increased tendon reflexes are a sign of imminent eclampsia. These patients should be treated similar to those with severe preeclampsia, irrespective of the degree of hypertension or the amount of proteinuria. To prevent the development of eclampsia, the patient must be admitted to the hospital and observed. She may be administered magnesium sulfate, if required.

The aim of treatment in cases of severe preeclampsia is to protect both the mother and the fetus from the adverse effects of high BP and to prolong the pregnancy as far as possible in order to prevent the risk of fetal prematurity. Maternal complications of high BP may include pulmonary edema, myocardial infraction, stroke, acute respiratory distress syndrome, retinal injury, coagulopathy, renal failure, etc. Management of severe preeclampsia must be preferably done in tertiary unit, following a multidisciplinary team approach involving the obstetrician, physician, pediatrician, and anesthetist. Management of cases with preeclampsia is all the more important because there is danger of progression to eclampsia (a stage in which the patient experiences fits), if the BP remains uncontrollably high. The management of severe preeclampsia is to be based on careful fetal assessment, maternal stabilization, continued monitoring, and delivery at the optimal time for the mother and her baby. The only cure for preeclampsia is the delivery of the baby. Therefore, while deciding the time for delivery, a fine balance between fetal maturity and maternal well-being needs to be maintained.

Maternal Stabilization

Since there is a risk for eclampsia, patients with severe preeclampsia or imminent eclampsia must always be stabilized before they are transferred to a tertiary unit, or before delivery is planned. One way of doing this is by prescribing antihypertensive medicines to keep BP under control. Prescriptions of antihypertensive medicines help to prevent the development of complications related to high BP (e.g., intracranial hemorrhage).

Another strategy, which is commonly employed, is starting magnesium sulfate (would be described later). These strategies usually help in preventing eclampsia and buying time until the fetus has gained sufficient maturity so that it can be delivered. The following steps also need to be taken:

1. Patients with severe preeclampsia must be hospitalized in a tertiary unit.
2. Senior obstetric and anesthetic staff and experienced midwives should be involved in the care of such patients.
3. *Continuous maternal BP monitoring:* The BP should be checked every 15 minutes in the beginning, until the woman has stabilized, and then after every 30 minutes in the initial phase of assessment. Once the patient has become stable and asymptomatic, the BP may be checked at 4-hourly intervals, especially if a conservative management plan is in place.
4. Urine should be carefully monitored for proteinuria twice daily. In the presence of significant proteinuria, a 24-hour estimation of urine proteins may be done.
5. Maternal weight must be measured every day.
6. Tests such as platelet count, KFTs (serum uric acid concentration, blood urea, and serum creatinine concentration), and tests of liver function must be done at the time of admission and then twice weekly.
7. Antihypertensive drugs must be used to keep the diastolic BP below 110 mm Hg.
8. Prophylactic use of magnesium sulfate prevents eclampsia.

Fetal Management

Rationale for fetal assessment: In cases of preeclampsia the fetuses are at risk, particularly due to prematurity as premature delivery may be required to save the mother's life. On the other hand, if the pregnancy is allowed to continue, placental insufficiency resulting from preeclampsia may cause IUGR. IUGR occurs in approximately 30% of pregnancies with preeclampsia. Thus, fetal monitoring forms an important aspect of management of patients with preeclampsia. The chronic hypoxia caused by preeclampsia results in poor fetal reserves. There are high chances of abnormal FHR pattern, meconium-stained amniotic fluid, and overall poor fetal outcomes in labor, which may at times be related to severe complications such as placental abruption and fetal death. The rationale behind fetal assessment is that if there occurs even a slight evidence of poor perinatal outcome, obstetric intervention must be undertaken immediately before irreversible damage occurs. The obstetric intervention in such situations is usually delivery. An earlier period of gestation may be associated with prematurity-related complications such as respiratory distress, intraventricular hemorrhage, necrotizing enterocolitis, metabolic disturbances, and sepsis. A balance has to be maintained between intervention and conservation following fetal assessment. In cases of hypertensive disorders in pregnancy, it is important to identify fetuses which may be at risk of growth restriction. Surveillance and monitoring of these fetuses should then be undertaken by umbilical artery Doppler.

Expectant Management

Before resorting to the expectant management, the obstetrician needs to adhere to the principles of shared decision-making and appropriately discuss the maternal and fetal risks and benefits with the mother and her partner. In case of deterioration of maternal or fetal condition at any time or in the presence of conditions listed in **Box 18.5**, the expectant management needs to be abandoned, and delivery must be recommended. If conservative management is planned, until fetal maturity is attained, the following investigations need to be done:

- *Daily fetal movement count:* The fetus responds to chronic hypoxia by conservation of energy and subsequent reduction of fetal movements.
- Weekly measurement of fundal height and abdominal girth in order to detect IUGR

BOX 18.5: Indications for termination of expectant management.

Maternal:
- Uncontrollable BP in severe range (systolic ≥ 160 mm Hg)
- Refractory persistent headaches
- Epigastric pain or right upper quadrant pain
- Visual disturbances
- Motor deficit or altered sensorium
- Stroke
- Myocardial infraction
- HELLP syndrome
- New or worsening renal dysfunction
- Pulmonary edema
- Eclampsia
- Acute placental abruption

Fetal:
- Abnormal FHR
- Fetal death
- Extreme fetal prematurity (no expectation of fetal survival)
- Persistent reversed end diastolic flow in the umbilical artery

(FHR: fetal heart rate; HELLP syndrome: hemolysis, elevated liver enzymes, low platelet count)

- Ultrasound measurement of fetal growth after every 2 weeks
- *Umbilical/cerebral artery Doppler analysis:* Serial assessment of umbilical blood flow or middle cerebral artery velocity by Doppler ultrasonographic assessment must be done twice every week.
- *Electronic FHR monitoring (EFHRM):* At present, most authorities recommend a weekly NST for women with mild hypertensive diseases of pregnancy and twice weekly for women with severe disease or evidence of fetal compromise (growth restriction or oligohydramnios). Based on the fetal condition, sometimes NST may be required on a daily basis.
- *Amniotic fluid index:* Reduced liquor volume is also associated with placental insufficiency and FGR. Serial estimations of liquor volume twice weekly can help to detect fetal compromise.

The frequency of various tests for fetal and maternal surveillance is not fixed. It can vary from patient to patient based on the clinical situation.

Delivery is Planned

In case the delivery is planned and a preterm fetus needs to be delivered, the following steps need to be undertaken:
1. Administration of corticosteroids
2. Measurement of L:S ratio in the amniotic fluid; L:S ratio > 2 is indicative of fetal maturity.
3. Fetus should be closely monitored at the time of labor, preferably with continuous electronic fetal monitoring.
4. Delivery must be conducted in an obstetric unit, which can offer a reasonable chance of survival to the neonate in terms of outcomes of prematurity.

Timing of Delivery

The only way to cure preeclampsia is to deliver the baby. Therefore, termination of pregnancy is the treatment of choice in all patients with severe preeclampsia where the fetus has attained maturity. The timing of delivery needs to be decided based on various parameters enumerated in **Box 18.6**. The timing of delivery based on the period of gestation in cases with severe preeclampsia is described below.

- *More than 34 weeks of gestation:* In cases of severe preeclampsia, when the pregnancy is >34 weeks of gestation, delivery is the treatment of choice.
- *Before 24 weeks of gestation:* In women with severe preeclampsia before 24 weeks of gestation, prolonging

BOX 18.6: Parameters for deciding the timing of delivery in cases with severe preeclampsia.

- Fetal maturity
- Fetal condition
- Maternal condition
- Bishop's score
- Period of gestation

the pregnancy at this gestational age may result in severe maternal and neonatal morbidity and mortality. Therefore, labor must be induced for pregnancies < 24 weeks, although it is quite unlikely that the fetus would survive at this time.

- *Between 25 and 33 weeks of gestation:* Pregnancies between 25 and 33 weeks represent a "gray zone." In case the period of gestation is <32 weeks, prophylactic steroids should be given to induce fetal lung maturity. A policy of administering corticosteroids, 12 mg betamethasone IM every 24 hours for two doses or 6 mg dexamethasone IM every 12 hours for four doses to women who are likely to have a preterm delivery can be expected to achieve substantial reduction in neonatal morbidity and mortality.

The obstetrician needs to balance the risk of prolonging the pregnancy, thereby increasing the maternal risk of developing complications related to severe preeclampsia against the risk of delivering a premature fetus, which may not even survive.

If the obstetrician decides to continue pregnancy, close maternal and fetal monitoring require to be done, because simply lowering the BP under conservative management will not slow down the disease process. The risk for preeclampsia-related complications, such as abruption, still remains. Expectant management must be adopted in women who are not showing any symptoms suggestive of end-organ damage, and only the BP criteria is elevated. Also, prior to initiating expectant treatment, maternal and fetal conditions must be stabilized. Expectant management must be practiced in tertiary healthcare centers having adequate facilities for maternal and neonatal intensive care. The woman should be counseled about the maternal and fetal risks (placental abruption, pulmonary edema, eclampsia, HELLP syndrome, cerebrovascular hemorrhage, acute renal failure, maternal death, fetal hypoxemia, perinatal death, etc.). The decision to continue such management should be made on a day-to-day basis.

In case of a woman with severe hypertension and premature fetus, if conservative management is desired, treatment with magnesium sulfate is not advisable until the decision to deliver the baby has been made.

Mode of Delivery

> **Q. By what method should the woman in the case study described at the beginning of chapter be delivered?**

Severe preeclampsia per se is not an indication for cesarean section. In the presence of an obstetric indication (fetal malpresentation, placenta previa, etc.) or a fetal indication (fetal distress), a cesarean section should be performed. Otherwise, there is no requirement for a cesarean delivery, and vaginal route should be the delivery modality of choice. A surgical induction of labor (artificial rupture of membranes) should be performed if the cervix is favorable. If the cervix is not favorable, medical induction of labor using cervical priming with prostaglandin E2 gel followed by induction with oxytocin may be done.

Labor may be induced if any of the conditions mentioned in **Box 18.7** occur. In case of presence of unfavorable cervix or other complications (e.g., breech presentation and fetal distress), a cesarean section needs to be done. If delivery has been decided upon before 32 weeks of gestation, the practice in the UK and US is to deliver by elective cesarean section; after 32 weeks of gestation, a vaginal delivery is more likely. This is so as labor can aggravate fluid overload and BP control, and therefore vaginal delivery may not be successful in >50% of cases. However, most other healthcare centers with limited neonatal resuscitation facilities throughout the world prefer attempting a vaginal delivery with varied results.

Maternal Management during Labor

Two main goals for management of women with severe preeclampsia during labor and delivery are prevention of seizures and control of hypertension. The parameters which need to be taken care of at the time of labor in a patient with severe preeclampsia are enumerated in **Box 18.8** and would be described below in detail.

Monitoring of Maternal Vitals

Monitoring of maternal vitals involves monitoring of vitals, especially maternal pulse and BP, at hourly intervals. Urine protein levels using a dipstick must be monitored at every 6-hourly interval.

BOX 18.7: Indications for induction of labor in patients with severe preeclampsia.

- Signs of impending eclampsia including abdominal pain, blurring of vision, severe persistent headache, etc.
- Abnormal biophysical profile, nonreassuring results on electronic fetal monitoring
- Diastolic BP over 110 mm Hg
- Abnormal LFTs (lactate dehydrogenase > 1,000 IU/L)
- Eclampsia
- IUGR
- HELLP syndrome
- Rising serum creatinine levels
- Fetal death
- Placental abruption
- Urine output < 500 mL/24 hours

(HELLP: hemolysis, elevated liver enzymes, and low platelet count; IUGR: intrauterine growth restriction)

BOX 18.8: Parameters which need to be taken care of at the time of labor in a patient with severe preeclampsia.

- Monitoring of maternal vitals
- Use of IV fluids
- Use of antihypertensive medication
- Use of magnesium sulfate
- Choice of anesthesia in case of cesarean delivery

Choice of Anesthesia

The choice of anesthetic in cesarean section is important, because tracheal intubation can cause a rise in both systolic and diastolic BP. With an epidural or spinal block, care should be taken to keep the fluid load to a minimum level. However, these methods can be safely used with appropriate supervision. If required and in the absence of coagulopathy, regional or neuraxial analgesia/anesthesia is preferred.

Antihypertensive therapy should be continued throughout labor. An epidural analgesia, by allowing adequate pain relief, can reduce the rise in BP commonly associated with labor. It also allows a planned delivery and easy transition to cesarean section, if necessary.

Antihypertensive agents are used to control persistent increase in BP, especially when diastolic BP is above 110 mm Hg.

Magnesium sulfate may act synergistically with the muscle relaxants used at the time of general anesthesia. Obstetric anesthesiologists must prescribe a smaller dose of such medications at the time of administering general anesthesia to the patients on magnesium sulfate.

Use of IV Fluid in Women with Severe Preeclampsia or Eclampsia

While in normal pregnancy there is an increase in plasma volume, in preeclampsia there is contracted plasma volume and hemoconcentration. These patients usually have intravascular volume depletion, with high peripheral vascular resistance. Therefore, administration of IV fluids in women with severe preeclampsia and eclampsia must be monitored carefully. Infusion of excessive fluid may result in the development of pulmonary edema and adult respiratory distress syndrome.

Invasive hemodynamic monitoring (e.g., pulmonary artery catheter) may be useful in women with preeclampsia who have severe cardiac or renal disease, pulmonary edema, treatment-refractory hypertension, or unexplained oliguria. Central venous pressure (CVP) or pulmonary artery pressure monitoring may be done in critical cases. CVP of 4 mm Hg in women with no heart disease indicates sufficient intravascular volume, and in these cases the use of maintenance fluids alone is sufficient. Total fluids should generally be limited to 80 mL/h or 1 mL/kg/h.

On the other hand, if CVP is between 4 and 8 mm Hg, it could be indicative of volume overload. In these cases, the obstetrician must look for the clinical signs of pulmonary edema, such as crepitations in the base of lungs. If crepitations are present, 20 mg of furosemide must be administered via IV route. If no response is seen to furosemide, dopamine infusion (1 up to 5 µg/kg/min) must be given to enhance renal perfusion. One of the complications of pulmonary edema is poor oxygen saturation, so one of the best methods for monitoring fluid status is continuous measurement of oxygen saturation with a pulse oximeter.

> **Q. Discuss in detail the use of antihypertensive drugs in preeclampsia.**

Use of Antihypertensive Medication

Uncontrollable hypertension can result in several complications such as cerebrovascular hemorrhage, hypertensive crisis, congestive heart failure, eclamptic seizures, and abruption. The aim of treatment with antihypertensives is to prevent intracranial bleeding and left ventricular failure. Treatment with antihypertensives is also likely to be useful for preventing eclamptic seizures by lowering the perfusion pressure and preventing vasogenic edema by reducing cerebral arterial vasospasm. Vasospasm is likely to result in tissue ischemia and per capillary bleeding.

Presently, there is little evidence regarding the antihypertensive drug of choice to be used for lowering BP in case of women with severe preeclampsia or the threshold of BP at which therapy with antihypertensive drugs must be initiated.

If BP is above 160/110 mm Hg, the antihypertensive drugs must be definitely used for controlling the raised BP. The aim of treatment must be to maintain diastolic BP between 95 and 105 mm Hg. Treatment with antihypertensive agents must be initiated within 30–60 minutes. In mild-to-moderate cases of preeclampsia, the role of antihypertensive therapy is less clear. If the BP is below 160/100 mm Hg, there is no immediate requirement for antihypertensive therapy as per the ACOG. However, as per the NICE (2019) guidelines, treatment with antihypertensives must be initiated in cases of moderate hypertension (BP of greater than 140/90 mm Hg), and the aim is to maintain the BP < 135/85 mm Hg. Below the BP of 140/90 mm Hg, there is no immediate requirement for antihypertensives unless there are markers of potential severe disease or signs of end-organ dysfunction or the presence of underlying comorbid conditions (e.g., diabetes, chronic hypertension, and renal disease) When the BP remains uncontrollable despite the use of antihypertensive medications, delivery is the only option.

The most commonly used drugs include labetalol, nifedipine, hydralazine, and α-methyldopa. While these medications to lower BP are safe during pregnancy, others, including drugs such as ACE inhibitors, beta blockers (atenolol), angiotensin-receptor blockers (ARBs), and diuretics, can harm the fetus. The use of atenolol and diuretics has been found to be associated with fetuses having lower birth weights and/or IUGR by decreasing the uteroplacental blood flow. ACE inhibitors and ARBs, when administered in the second and third trimesters, have been found to be associated with a characteristic fetopathy, oligohydramnios, neonatal renal failure, and death.

Thus, the use of these drugs should be avoided during pregnancy. The use of diuretics should be limited to the cases described in **Box 18.9**.

Labetalol and nifedipine are the most commonly used drugs, followed by α-methyldopa as the second-line agent in developing countries, including India. No single therapy can be successful in all patients and increasing doses and combinations of drugs are generally required. IV labetalol or oral nifedipine is as effective as IV hydralazine, with fewer adverse effects. Other rapidly acting agents, such as nitroglycerin, diazoxide, and sodium nitroprusside, are usually preserved for use in an ICU setting or in the OT. In treating severe hypertension, it is important to avoid hypotension, because aggressive lowering of maternal BP may result in fetal distress. In women with preeclampsia, treatment of acute severe hypertension must be started at lower doses, because these patients may be having depleted intravascular volume and thereby may be at an increased risk for hypotension. Drugs used for emergency control of severe hypertension in pregnancy are listed in **Table 18.8**. The most commonly used drugs are labetalol, hydralazine, and nifedipine. Nitroprusside, previously recommended for emergency control of high BP during pregnancy, has now largely been discontinued due to the risk of possible cyanide toxicity. Drugs used for control of chronic hypertension in pregnancy are listed in **Table 18.9**.

Labetalol

Presently, labetalol is considered as the medication of choice for treatment of acute severe hypertension in pregnancy and for the maintenance treatment of hypertensive disorders during pregnancy. The features which make labetalol the drug of choice include high efficacy, low incidence of side effects, and availability of oral as well as parenteral preparations.

> **BOX 18.9:** Indications for the use of diuretics.
> - Severe pulmonary edema
> - Massive edema, not relieved by rest
> - Cardiac failure

Labetalol is a nonselective β-blocker, which also has vascular α-1 receptor blocking capabilities. It has gained wide acceptance in pregnancy because it helps in lowering BP smoothly but rapidly, without causing tachycardia.

Dose: Labetalol can be administered via intermittent or continuous infusion. For intermittent infusion, it is given as a 20 mg IV bolus, followed by 40 mg after 10 minutes. If the first dose is not effective, then 80 mg is administered every 10 minutes. A maximum total dose of 220 mg can be administered. It can also be administered in the form of a continuous infusion—250 mg of labetalol in 250 mL of normal saline, administered at the rate of 20 mg/h (20 mL/min). Orally, labetalol is administered in the dose of 100 mg 8-hourly, which may be increased to 800 mg/day. The onset of action of IV dosage is within 5–10 minutes.

Side effects: This drug can produce side effects such as flushing, headache, nausea, and vomiting. It is contraindicated in women with asthma and first-degree heart block. Therefore, its use must be avoided in women with asthma or congestive heart failure. Due to a lower incidence of side effects such as maternal hypotension, the use of labetalol now supplants that of hydralazine. When administered orally to women with chronic hypertension, it seems to be as safe and effective as methyldopa, although neonatal hypoglycemia can occur with higher doses.

Nifedipine

Nifedipine is a calcium channel blocker, which should be given orally and not sublingually for control of high BP. Recently, it has gained popularity for its efficacy in controlling acute hypertension related to pregnancy. This medication is also an excellent peripheral vasodilator and a good tocolytic agent.

Dosage: Nifedipine should be given in the dose of 5–10 mg orally, which can be repeated after 30 minutes, if necessary, followed by 10–20 mg every 3–6 hours. The slow-release preparation is given in the dosage of 30–120 mg/day. Nifedipine can also be administered via intragastric route using a Ryles tube. The dose should not exceed 10 mg

TABLE 18.8: Drugs used for urgent control of severe hypertension in pregnancy.		
Drug	**Dose and rate**	**Comments**
Labetalol	20 mg IV, then 20–80 mg every 20–30 minutes, up to a maximum of 300 mg; or constant infusion of 1–2 mg/min	Less risk for tachycardia and arrhythmia in comparison to other vasodilators
Nifedipine	Tablets recommended only; 10–30 mg orally, repeat in 45 minutes if needed	Possible interference with labor
Hydralazine	5 mg, IV or IM, then 5–10 mg every 20–40 minutes, or constant infusion of 0.5–10 mg/h	Drug of choice for severe hypertension according to the National High Blood Pressure Education Program (NHBPEP) working group; long-term experience of safety and efficacy

Source: Alpern RJ, Hebert SC. Seldin and Giebisch's The Kidney: Physiology and Pathophysiology, 4th edition. San Diego, California: Academic Press, Elsevier; 2008. p. 2387.

TABLE 18.9: Drugs for chronic hypertension in pregnancy.

Drug	Dose	Comments
Methyldopa	0.5–3.0 g/day in two divided doses	Drug of choice according to the NHBPEP working group. The safety of this drug after the first trimester has been well documented
Labetalol	200–1,200 mg/day in two to three divided doses	The use of this drug during pregnancy is gaining popularity and becoming the drug of first choice for treatment of chronic hypertension during pregnancy because no real adverse effects have been demonstrated
Nifedipine	30–120 mg/day of a slow-release preparation	Nifedipine may inhibit labor and have synergistic interaction with magnesium sulfate, causing the possible risk of neuromuscular blockade and myocardial depression. There has been little experience with other calcium channel blockers
Hydralazine	It is used for urgent control of severe hypertension or as a third-line agent for multidrug control of refractory hypertension in the dosage of 50–300 mg/day in two to four divided doses	Though there are a few controlled trials, long-term experience with a low risk for adverse events has been documented. It is useful only in combination with sympatholytic agent. Its use may be associated with neonatal thrombocytopenia
β-receptor blockers	• Dosage varies with different agents. Propranolol is initiated at a dosage of 40–60 mg daily. The maximum dosage is 480–640 mg/day • Dosage of labetalol has been previously mentioned	Use of β-blockers in general may cause fetal bradycardia and reduced uteroplacental blood flow. None of them has been found to be associated with teratogenicity. However, there is a risk for fetal growth restriction with the use of atenolol in the first or second trimesters. Use of atenolol must be avoided during pregnancy
ACE inhibitors	To be avoided in all trimesters of pregnancy	Exposure during the first trimester has been found to be associated with the congenital malformations of the cardiovascular and central nervous systems. Exposure during the second and third trimesters can result in complications such as oligohydramnios, fetal growth restriction, bony malformations, hypocalvaria, limb contractures, persistent patent ductus arteriosus, and pulmonary hypoplasia
AT1-receptor antagonists	Classified as category X drug during second and third trimesters of pregnancy. Its use should be avoided in all trimesters of pregnancy	Its use may be associated with various fetal anomalies
Sodium nitroprusside	An excellent drug to gradually reduce the elevated BP. However, must be avoided due to the risk of fetal toxicity	Metabolic degradation of sodium nitroprusside may result in the formation of cyanides, which may be associated with significant fetal toxicity
Diazoxide	Though this drug can cause a dramatic, sudden hypotensive response, it must be preferably avoided during pregnancy	It must be avoided during pregnancy because it can cause fetal and maternal hyperglycemia, inhibition of uterine contractions and sodium and water retention
Reserpine	To be preferably avoided during pregnancy	It is likely to result in nasal stuffiness, which may be a problem because newborns show an obligatory nasal breathing pattern

(ACE: angiotensin-converting enzyme; AT1: angiotensin 1; NHBPEP: National High Blood Pressure Education Program)
Source: Alpern RJ, Hebert SC. Seldin and Giebisch's The Kidney: Physiology and Pathophysiology, 4th edition. San Diego, California: Academic Press, Elsevier; 2008. p. 2386.

at a time and should not be repeated more frequently than every 30 minutes. The oral drug starts producing its effect between 10 and 15 minutes, whereas the slow-release drug preparation starts producing its effect within 60 minutes.

Side effects: It can produce side effects such as flushing, headache, tachycardia, and nausea. Fetal safety of this drug has not yet been established. It has also been shown to inhibit labor and may have synergistic action with magnesium sulfate in lowering of BP. Therefore, a combination of magnesium sulfate and nifedipine is to be avoided as it can cause sudden hypotension.

Hydralazine

Hydralazine is a directly acting arterial vasodilator, which acts directly on the arteriolar smooth muscles. It helps in the rapid lowering of the BP in obstetrics. Meta-analysis by Magee et al. (2003) has shown that hydralazine should not be used as the first-line drug for treatment of severe hypertension in comparison with labetalol and nifedipine.

Positive ionotropic effect of hydralazine can result in the development of hyperdynamic circulation following its administration.

Dosage: For controlling hypertensive crisis during pregnancy, hydralazine is given in the dose of 5–10 mg intravenously, repeated every 20 minutes until the desired response is achieved. It can also be administered in the form of continuous infusion, given at the rate of 0.5–10 mg/h. Hydralazine can also be administered orally in the dose of 50–300 mg/day in two to four divided doses for control of gestational hypertension or chronic hypertension during pregnancy. The time for onset of action is 10 minutes via IV route and 10–30 minutes via IM route.

Side effects: The most frequent side effects of hydralazine are reduced uteroplacental perfusion and hyperdynamic circulation. While hyperdynamic circulation is manifested in the form of maternal tachycardia, flushing, etc., reduced uteroplacental circulation may manifest in the form of late decelerations in the CTG trace of women who previously had a normal trace. Therefore, monitoring of fetal heart trace is mandatory when hydralazine is used. Recovery from this abnormal pattern occurs once hydralazine is discontinued. Other side effects related with the use of hydralazine are nausea, vomiting, hypotension, headache, CNS depression, anxiety, restlessness, hyperreflexia, etc. Hydralazine is contraindicated in women with myocardial insufficiency and heart failure. It is associated with an increased maternal risk of complications such as tachycardia and palpitations, whereas labetalol may cause complications such as bradycardia and hypotension. However, efficacy of both the drugs is more or less the same.

Alpha-methyldopa

Methyldopa is α-methyl analog of dopa and results in the formation of methylnoradrenaline (a centrally acting α-2-adrenergic agonist), which helps in decreasing the efferent sympathetic activity. BP control occurs gradually over a period of 6–8 hours and lasts for about 12–24 hours. It is not thought to have any teratogenic effect in pregnancy. α-methyldopa is frequently used in pregnant women with chronic hypertension and in cases of gestational hypertension/mild preeclampsia. However, it is not used in cases of severe preeclampsia due to its delayed onset of action.

Dosage: The dose of α-methyldopa commonly in use is 0.5–3.0 g/day in two to four divided doses.

Side effects: α-methyldopa can commonly produce side effects such as sedation, lethargy, cognitive impairment, dryness of mouth, nasal stuffiness, headache, fluid retention, and weight gain.

Magnesium Sulfate

> **Q. Discuss the management of the case of imminent eclampsia at 34 weeks.**
>
> **Q. Discuss in detail the use of magnesium sulfate in obstetrics.**
>
> **Q. Write a short note on fulminant eclampsia.**

- *Use of magnesium sulfate in severe preeclampsia:* As per the ACOG recommendations, magnesium sulfate should be considered for prevention and treatment of seizures in women with severe preeclampsia, gestational hypertension with severe features, impending eclampsia, etc., especially in those women where there is a concern about the risk of eclampsia. In women with less severe disease, the decision is less clear and usually depends on individual case assessment. Magnesium sulfate is usually used in patients with severe preeclampsia, once the decision for delivery has been made. The Magpie study (2002) has demonstrated that administration of magnesium sulfate to women with preeclampsia reduces the risk of an eclamptic seizure. Magnesium sulfate must be administered while awaiting delivery and in the immediate postpartum period for up to 24 hours following delivery or 24 hours after the last seizure, whichever is the later, unless there is a clinical reason to continue. It is now also considered as an anticonvulsant of choice for treating eclampsia. This agent had commonly been used in the US, following the results of the Collaborative Eclampsia trial (1995). However, following the demonstration of its efficacy in Magpie trial (2002), it is commonly being used in the UK as well for prevention of eclampsia. In 1995, the Eclampsia Trial Collaborative Group did an impressive study in developing countries and showed unequivocally that magnesium sulfate given intramuscularly or intravenously was superior to either phenytoin or diazepam in reducing recurrent eclamptic seizures. This study showed that the women on magnesium sulfate had a significantly lower risk of recurrent seizures than those on diazepam or phenytoin. Also, the women who received magnesium sulfate were at a lower risk of maternal death in comparison to those on diazepam or phenytoin. However, these results were not statistically significant. Babies of mothers on magnesium were in better condition after delivery and less likely to require special care. Recent Cochrane reviews have, however, also indicated a significant reduction in maternal mortality with magnesium. The Magpie trial (2002), which had recruited over 10,000 women with preeclampsia, showed that there was more than a halving in the risk of eclampsia associated with the use of magnesium sulfate rather than placebo.
- *Mode of action of magnesium sulfate:* Magnesium sulfate is associated with cerebral vasodilatation and is a blocker

of N-methyl-D-aspartate (NMDA) receptors in the brain, the pathway for anoxic cell damage.
- Magnesium sulfate also reduces systemic vascular resistance and mean arterial pressure. Simultaneously, it also increases cardiac output without myocardial depression.
- *Dosage:* A total dose of 14 g is administered in the form of loading and maintenance doses.
- *Magnesium sulfate regimens:* The various regimens which can be administered are described in the **Table 18.10**.

Intramuscular injection must be given in the upper outer quadrant of each buttock using a 3 inch, 20-gauge needle. At the time of IM injection, the medication can be mixed with 1 mL xylocaine (2% solution) because the IM injection can be painful. In case of the Pritchard regimen, IM injection must be given immediately following the IV loading dose in a patient having convulsions. In a patient without convulsions, only IM loading dose needs to be given. For women who require cesarean delivery, infusion should be started prior to surgery, continued during the surgery as well as 24 hours after the surgery. For women who deliver vaginally, infusion should continue for 24 hours after the delivery. In case the woman has had an eclamptic fit after delivery, infusion should continue 24 hours after the last fit.

Recurrent seizures should be treated with either a further bolus of 2–4 g magnesium sulfate IV over 5 minutes or an increase in the infusion rate to 1.5 g/h or 2.0 g/h in case the previous infusion rate was 1 g/h.

Monitoring of dosage of magnesium sulfate: Magnesium sulfate must always be administered slowly because if it is given too quickly, it can result in the development of cardiac arrhythmia or arrest. An overdose of magnesium sulfate causes respiratory and cardiac depression. Thus, at the time of administration of magnesium sulfate, the parameters mentioned in **Box 18.10** must be regularly assessed. Reevaluation of the rate of administration is required in case of any change in any of the indices.

After magnesium sulfate has been administered, a Foley's catheter is inserted into the patient's bladder to monitor the urinary output. If available, serum levels of magnesium should be regularly monitored. With the dose regimen as described previously (5 g IM every 4 hourly), there is no need for magnesium concentrations to be checked regularly. However, in many parts of the world, infusions of 1–3 g/h (Zuspan's and Sibai's regimens) are used. Although checking of magnesium concentrations may be necessary when a higher infusion rate is used, toxic effects are unlikely when deep tendon reflexes are still present. The therapeutic levels of magnesium range from 4 to 7 mEq/L or 4–8 mg/dL. Further dose of magnesium is adjusted based on the patient's reflexes, BP, urinary output, and serum magnesium levels.

The aim should be to maintain magnesium concentration at 4 mEq/L. If the magnesium levels reach 7 mEq/L (9 mg/dL), the patellar reflex is lost, and at 10 mEq/L (12 mg/dL) respiratory depression sets in. Cardiac arrest is likely to occur at the magnesium concentration of 25 mEq/L (30 mg/dL).

Thus, if the IM regime is used, it is important to ensure the following parameters before the administration of a repeat dose:
- Urine output is >30 mL/h.
- Patellar reflexes are intact.
- Respiratory rate is above 16/min.

Pulse oximetry is an excellent marker of magnesium toxicity because oxygen saturation begins to drop before the onset of respiratory distress. However, the obstetrician needs to consider the fact that sometimes reduced oxygen saturation and respiratory distress in patients with severe preeclampsia may be the initial manifestations of pulmonary edema. In these cases, 20–40 mg of furosemide IV must be administered.

TABLE 18.10: Various regimens for magnesium sulfate.

Pritchard regimen	
Loading dose	**Maintenance dose**
4 g IV slowly over 3–5 minutes (20 mL of 20% MgSO$_4$ solution) followed by 5 g deep IM in each buttock (10 mL of 50% MgSO$_4$ solution)	5 g (10 mL of 50% MgSO$_4$) deep IM injection in alternate buttock every 4 hours
Zuspan regimen	
4 g IV (20 mL of 20% MgSO$_4$ solution) in 100 mL of normal saline over 15–20 minutes	1 g/h IV infusion (add two 10 mL ampoules of 50% MgSO$_4$ to 1,000 mL of normal saline and give IV at the rate of 100 mL/h or 1 g/h); to be maintained for 24 hours after delivery or the last seizure
Sibai regimen	
6 g IV (30 mL of 20% MgSO$_4$ solution) in 100 mL of normal saline over 15–20 minutes	2 g/h IV infusion (Add four 10 mL ampoules of 50% MgSO$_4$ to 1,000 mL of normal saline and give IV at the rate of 100 mL/h or 2 g/h); to be maintained for 24 hours after delivery or the last seizure

Note:
50% MgSO$_4$ ampoule: 5 g/10 mL or 1 g/2 mL
20% MgSO$_4$ ampoule: 200 mg/mL

BOX 18.10: Parameters for monitoring MgSO$_4$ regimen.
- Urine output (at least 30 mL/h or 100 mL in 4 hours)
- Maternal deep tendon reflexes should be present (patellar reflexes must be intact)
- Respiratory rate ≥ 14/min
- Pulse oximetry ≥ 96%

The patellar reflex acts as a convenient warning. If the reflex is present, the drug may safely be given, as there is no danger of magnesium toxicity. If the reflexes are absent or reduced, there is a danger of magnesium toxicity, and the drug must be discontinued until the reflex reappears. Toxicity to magnesium sulfate is a life-threatening emergency and the following steps must be taken immediately:

1. Intubation and bag and mask ventilation must be done.
2. External cardiac massage may also be required.
3. 10 mL of 10% calcium gluconate must be slowly administered intravenously. This serves as an antidote for magnesium sulfate poisoning. IV furosemide must also be simultaneously administered to speed up the rate of urinary excretion. Calcium ions by increasing the amount of acetylcholine liberated by the action potentials at the neuromuscular junction help in antagonizing the action of magnesium.

The fetus is also not immune to the potential effects of magnesium because it can readily cross the placenta. Hypermagnesemia in the neonate is associated with flaccidity, lethargy, hypotonia, hyporeflexia, and respiratory depression. Magnesium sulfate is also likely to cause a decrease in FHR variability. However, reduced or absent variability on FHR tracing in patients with preeclampsia on magnesium sulfate therapy should not be ascribed to treatment unless there are definitive signs of fetal well-being.

No response to first dose of magnesium sulfate: After giving the first dose of magnesium sulfate, the BP must be measured again. If the diastolic BP is still 110 mm Hg or higher, dihydralazine or oral nifedipine is given as follows:

- 6.25 mg dihydralazine by IM injection or 10 mg (one capsule) nifedipine should be administered orally.
- Patients who have received 10 mg nifedipine can be given a second dose of 10 mg nifedipine orally if the diastolic BP remains 110 mm Hg or more even after 30 minutes.
- If necessary, it can be repeated half-hourly up to a maximum dose of 50 mg.
- In case of nonavailability of MgSO4, drugs such as diazepam (valium) or phenytoin (Dilantin) must be used. Thiopentone is reserved for status eclampticus. However, only single dose of these drugs must be administered. Prolonged use of diazepam is associated with an increase in maternal death rate. If convulsions persist, intubation may be required to protect the airway and maintain oxygenation. Transfer to intensive care facilities with intermittent positive pressure ventilation may appear to be appropriate in these circumstances.

Phenytoin

Phenytoin acts by preventing the spread of abnormal activity from the seizure foci to the motor cortex. A large randomized controlled trial involving 2,000 subjects by Lucas (1995) has demonstrated the superiority of magnesium sulfate over phenytoin in prevention of eclamptic seizures.

Magnesium sulfate is more effective than phenytoin, diazepam, or nimodipine in reducing preeclampsia and should be considered as the drug of choice for preventing eclampsia in intrapartum and postpartum periods.

The use of phenytoin and benzodiazepines as an antiepileptic treatment is justified only in cases where magnesium sulfate is contraindicated or unavailable (e.g., myasthenia gravis, hypocalcemia, moderate-to-severe renal failure, and cardiac ischemia).

The loading dose of phenytoin is 15–25 mg/kg IV. In general, the loading dose is 1 g IV, diluted in 200 mL of normal saline given by slow infusion over 20 minutes. This must be followed by 100 mg 6 hourly. The first 750 mg is given at the rate of 25 mg/min and the remaining at the rate of 12.5 mg/min. Side effects include cardiac toxicity, nystagmus, hypertension, ataxia, and lethargy.

Diazepam (Lean Regimen)

A loading dose of 10 mg IV is administered over 2 minutes, followed by IV infusion of 40 mg in 500 mL normal saline for the next 24 hours. This drug is nowadays not preferred as it causes lethargy and apnea of the newborn.

The Lytic cocktail regimen or Krishna Menon regimen comprising chlorpromazine, Phenergan, and pethidine is no longer used.

Fluid Balance

Since pulmonary edema has been found to be a significant cause of maternal death, fluid restriction is advisable to reduce the risk of fluid overload in the intrapartum and postpartum periods. In usual circumstances, total fluids should be limited to 80 mL/h or 1 mL/kg/h.

The regime of fluid restriction should be maintained until there is a postpartum diuresis, as oliguria is common with severe preeclampsia. If there is an associated maternal hemorrhage, fluid balance is more difficult, and fluid restriction may be inappropriate in these cases.

Management of Postpartum Hypertension

Postpartum hypertension commonly occurs 3–6 days after delivery, with the maximum increase in BP occurring toward the end of the first postpartum week. The following steps need to be taken in the postpartum period:

1. An initial improvement in BP, followed by a relapse of high BP, is commonly observed within 24 hours of delivery. Therefore, continued close monitoring must be done following delivery.
2. Antihypertensive drugs should be given if the BP exceeds 150 mm Hg systolic or 100 mm Hg diastolic in the first 4 days of the puerperium. The medication may then be discontinued when BP normalizes. This may occur days to several weeks postpartum, and home BP monitoring by the patient may be helpful in this regard.
3. After delivery, ACE inhibitors can be started; methyldopa is to be stopped due to the risk of development of

psychological changes, particularly depression. Diuretics are usually avoided as they may reduce milk production.

4. In the postpartum period, previously normotensive women have been noted to have a rise in BP, which reaches a maximum on the fifth postpartum day, probably as a consequence of physiological volume expansion and fluid mobilization in the postpartum period.

Women with Eclampsia in the Postpartum Period

- Most postnatal convulsions occur within the first 24 hours after delivery, so anticonvulsant therapy is generally continued for at least 24 hours after delivery.
- Clinicians should be aware of the risk of late seizures and ensure that women have a careful review before discharge from hospital. Obstetricians must remember that nearly half the cases of eclampsia occur postpartum, especially at term, so women with signs or symptoms compatible with preeclampsia should be carefully observed postnatally.
- Most women with severe preeclampsia or eclampsia will need inpatient care for 4 days or more following delivery.
- Antihypertensive medication should be continued after delivery depending on the BP recordings. During this time, BP should not be allowed to exceed 160/110 mm Hg. In most cases, the antihypertensives are not required 12 weeks following delivery, although most women can have their treatment stopped much earlier than this. Currently, there is insufficient evidence to recommend any particular antihypertensive. The most commonly used drugs in the postpartum period include:
    - β-blockers (e.g., atenolol 50–100 mg OD), with addition of a calcium antagonist (e.g., slow-release nifedipine 10–20 mg OD) and/or an ACE inhibitor (e.g., enalapril 5–10 mg BD)
    - Drugs such as labetalol, nifedipine, enalapril, captopril, atenolol, and metoprolol have been known to be safe for breastfeeding women. There is insufficient evidence regarding the safety of other drugs such as amlodipine, ARB, and ACE inhibitors other than enalapril and captopril in breast-feeding women.
- A regular assessment of BP and proteinuria by the general practitioner at the 6th and 12th weeks following delivery is recommended. If hypertension or proteinuria persists, then further investigation to rule out chronic hypertension or chronic renal disease is recommended.

COMPLICATIONS

Q. Discuss in brief the complications of preeclampsia and eclampsia.

TABLE 18.11: Complications related to preeclampsia.

Maternal	Fetal
• HELLP (hemolysis, elevated liver enzymes, and low platelet count) syndrome • Abruption placenta • Cerebral hemorrhage • Sepsis/shock • Eclampsia • Risk of recurrence of preeclampsia in subsequent pregnancies • Impaired renal function • Impaired liver function • Pulmonary edema • Maternal death	• Oligohydramnios • Intrauterine death • Prematurity • IUGR • Intrauterine asphyxia and acidosis • Infant death

All forms of high BP increase the risk for development of pregnancy-related complications. However, the risk of complications is highest in women with chronic high BP accompanied by preeclampsia. Some of the maternal and fetal complications related to preeclampsia are enumerated in **Table 18.11**.

FETAL COMPLICATIONS

Prematurity

Premature delivery (before 37 completed weeks of pregnancy) may be required in women with severe preeclampsia in order to prevent severe complications to mother and baby.

These babies have been shown to be at an increased risk for health problems during the newborn period, such as learning disabilities and cerebral palsy.

Intrauterine Growth Restriction

Uteroplacental insufficiency in patients with preeclampsia restricts the placental blood flow, limiting the supply of essential nutrients and oxygen to the fetus. Blood flow in the baby may get restricted to the limbs, kidney, and abdomen in an effort to preserve the blood supply to vital areas such as the brain and heart, resulting in the development of growth-restricted fetuses. Details related to the management of a pregnancy complicated by IUGR are described in Chapter 15. IUGR in the long run can result in the development of fetal acidosis and hypoxia.

Hypertensive disorders of pregnancy and IUGR are leading causes of maternal and perinatal morbidity and mortality. Failure to diagnose IUGR in women at high risk has been identified as a significant preventable cause of serious fetal outcome. An observational study by Molvarec et al. (2013) compared the fetal flow using Doppler ultrasonography with a new test for PlGF to predict adverse fetal events. PlGF is a member of the VEGF family. It is produced mainly by the placenta and has potent proangiogenic effects. In normal uncomplicated pregnancy, PlGF levels rise until approximately 32 weeks of pregnancy and then fall until delivery. In pregnancies complicated by preeclampsia before the 37th week with or without IUGR, PlGF levels are significantly lower. PlGF is classified as normal (PlGF ≥ 100 pg/mL), low (12 < PlGF < 100 pg/mL), or very low (PlGF ≤ 12 pg/mL). Measurement of low serum PlGF levels before 35th week of gestation may help to identify fetuses at risk requiring urgent delivery in women with hypertensive disorders of pregnancy, where adverse fetal outcomes have not been identified by fetal flow Doppler ultrasonography.

MATERNAL COMPLICATIONS

Abruption Placenta

Abruption placenta refers to the premature separation of normally implanted placenta. Preeclampsia is an important cause for development of abruption placenta. Details regarding abruption placenta are described in Chapter 8.

Cerebral Hemorrhage

Untreated high BP serves as an important cause for the development of cerebral hemorrhage and stroke.

ECLAMPSIA

> **Q.** Write a short note on the management of eclampsia.
>
> **Q.** Briefly discuss how to go about controlling convulsions in a case of eclampsia.
>
> **Q.** Briefly discuss the role of cesarean delivery in cases of eclampsia.
>
> **Q.** With the help of a short note, discuss the critical assessment in a case of eclampsia and its management.
>
> **Q.** Discuss the management of cases of eclampsia in detail.

Eclampsia is one of the most serious complications of preeclampsia. This can be defined as the onset of tonic and clonic convulsions in a pregnant patient with preeclampsia, usually occurring in the third trimester of pregnancy, intrapartum period, or >48 hours postpartum.

Eclampsia is thought to be related to cerebral vasospasm, which can cause ischemia, disruption of the blood–brain barrier, and cerebral edema. Once the seizures and severe hypertension have been controlled, delivery is required for the treatment of eclampsia.

Prevention of Eclampsia

- In order to prevent the occurrence of eclampsia, the obstetrician needs to remain vigilant regarding the appearance of signs of imminent eclampsia in patients with severe preeclampsia.
- The decision for delivery must be made as soon as possible in patients with severe preeclampsia.
- Women with severe preeclampsia (BP > 160/100 mm Hg along with proteinuria) should be given magnesium sulfate as a prophylactic measure. Magnesium sulfate should be continued for 24 hours after delivery or 24 hours after the last convulsion, whichever is later.

Management of Eclampsia

Every maternity unit must be equipped to deal with this obstetric emergency and must institute emergency management effectively. There should preferably be a separate eclampsia room in each obstetric ward. This room should be especially reserved for patients with severe preeclampsia or eclampsia and should be free from noise. It should have a railed bed and equipment such as suction machine, equipment for resuscitation, syringes, tongue blade, and drug tray with drugs such as magnesium sulfate, nifedipine, and diazepam.

Early involvement of consultant obstetrician, anesthetic staff, and other specialists including a hematologist, ophthalmologist, neonatologist, etc. may be required. Care of patients with eclampsia requires the following steps:

1. Immediate care involves maintenance of airway, oxygenation, and prevention of trauma or injury to the patient. Injury to the patient can be prevented by placing her on a railed bed. A tongue blade can be used to prevent her from biting her tongue.
2. Patient should be placed in the left lateral position, and the airway must be secured. Oxygen should be administered through a face mask.
3. Monitoring of vitals including pulse, BP, respiratory rate, and oxygen saturation needs to be done every 15 minutes. Knee jerks and urine output need to be monitored every half hourly.
4. IV line must be secured, and the patient must be given IV Ringer's lactate or 0.9% normal saline solution. Fluids should be restricted to 80 mL/h or 1 mg/kg body weight.
5. RCOG recommends fluid restriction so as to avoid fluid overload and pulmonary edema. Close monitoring of fluid intake and urine output at every half-hourly interval is mandatory.
6. Treatment of choice to treat convulsions is the administration of magnesium sulfate. Magnesium sulfate is supposed to act by relieving cerebral vasospasm.
7. Once the patient has stabilized, an obstetric examination must be performed, and fetal status must be evaluated. An obstetric evaluation and plan to deliver the patient is required.
8. Continued fetal monitoring, preferably through continuous electronic monitoring, is required until the baby is delivered.

Though definitive treatment of eclampsia is delivery, the maternal well-being gets priority over fetal condition. Once the mother has stabilized, she should be delivered as soon as possible. However, it is inappropriate to deliver an unstable mother even if there is fetal distress. Once seizures and severe hypertension have been treated and hypoxia has been corrected, delivery can be expedited. The mode of delivery, either by vaginal or abdominal route, depends on obstetric evaluation of the individual patient. If the cervix appears unfavorable, vaginal prostaglandins can be used for induction of labor. Strict BP monitoring must be continued throughout labor. If the maternal condition stabilizes, convulsions are absent, and the fetus is preterm, the delivery can be delayed. During this time, corticosteroids should be administered to attain fetal maturity, and continuous fetal surveillance needs to be done. During this time, patient can be shifted to a tertiary care center having adequate neonatal resuscitation facilities.

Management in patients with eclampsia is shown in **Flowchart 18.4**. Parameters used for planning the delivery include gestational age, severity of disease, seizures/hypertension, and immediate danger to the mother/fetus. If the period of gestation is <26 weeks, both the maternal and the fetal prognoses would be bad if the pregnancy is allowed to continue in order to attain fetal maturity. In these cases, pregnancy must be terminated following maternal stabilization.

In case the period of gestation is between 26 and 34 weeks, expectant management plan can be followed, provided that the maternal condition remains stabilized. The mother must be administered IM corticosteroids, and the fetus must be adequately monitored. The fetus must be delivered when the amniotic fluid L:S ratio becomes >2, i.e., the fetal lung maturity has been attained. In case fetal maturity has not been attained, but either the maternal (high BP) or the fetal condition (fetal distress) deteriorates, the fetus needs to be delivered by the fastest route. In case the period of gestation is >34 weeks, there is no need to continue the pregnancy, and the baby may be delivered by the fastest route. The obstetrician may also be required to expedite the delivery in case there is a presence of any of the ominous features of eclampsia as described in **Box 18.11**.

If the delivery can be delayed for at least 24 hours and the fetus is premature, steroids for attaining lung maturity can be given (2 doses of 12 mg of betamethasone, 24 hours apart).

However, in patients with eclampsia, due to a requirement for urgent delivery, there may be unavailability of so much time. Therefore, a woman with severe preeclampsia may be administered the dose of corticosteroids in the antenatal

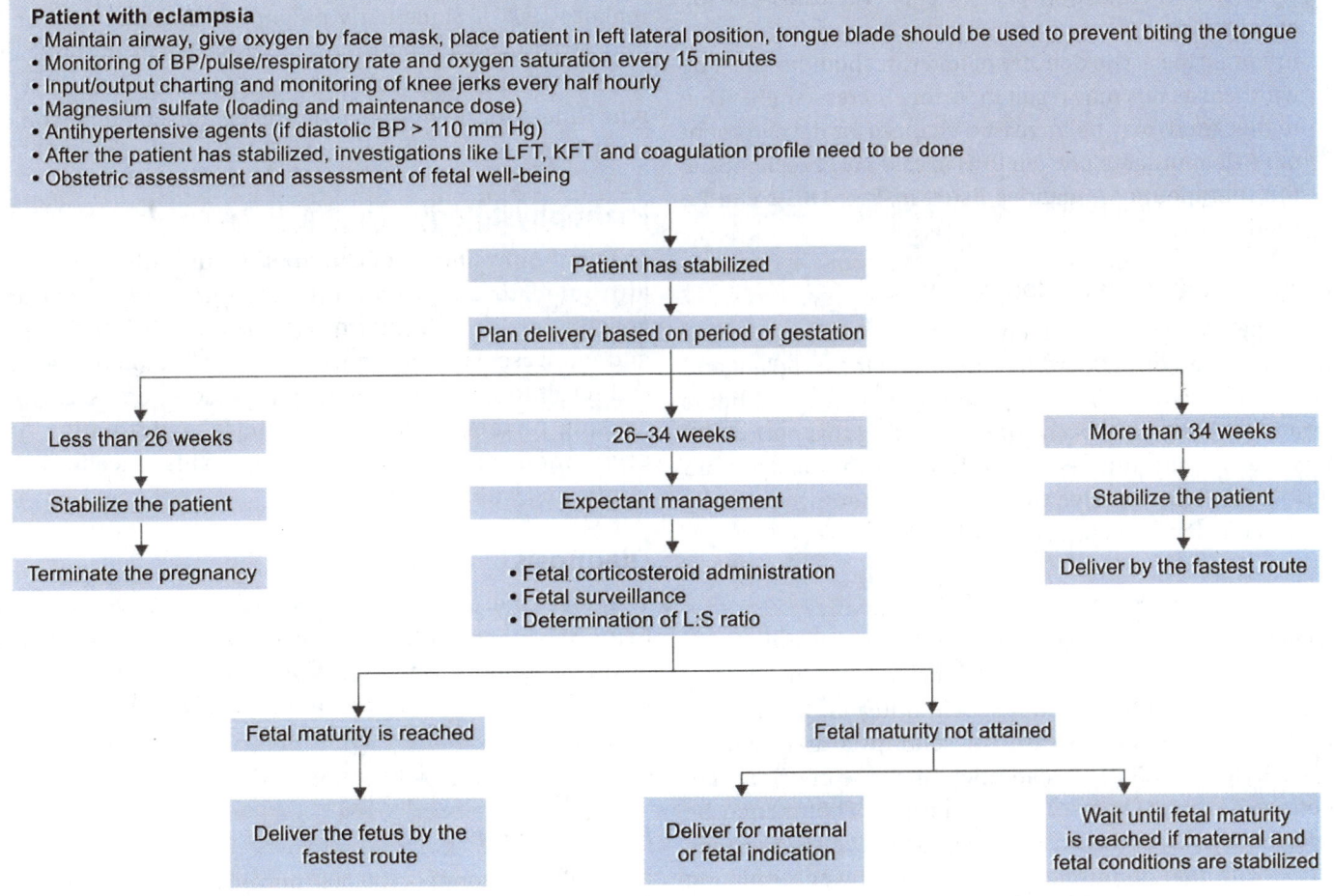

Flowchart 18.4: Management of patients with eclampsia.

(KFT: kidney function test; LFT: liver function test, L:S ratio: lecithin:sphingomyelin ratio)

> **BOX 18.11:** Ominous features of eclampsia.
>
> - Long interval between onset of fits and commencement of treatment
> - Antepartum eclampsia early in pregnancy
> - Number of seizures more than 10
> - Systolic BP > 200 mm Hg
> - Temperature > 102°F
> - Oliguria
> - Nonresponse to treatment
> - Jaundice

> **BOX 18.12:** Drugs for controlling PPH in cases with severe preeclampsia.
>
> - Oxytocin (10 units IV or IM)
> - Prostaglandin (PGF2α) 125 µg or 250 µg IM
> - Misoprostol 600–1,000 µg (rectal, vaginal, oral)

> **BOX 18.13:** Indications for cesarean section in cases with eclampsia.
>
> - Any obstetric indication (cephalopelvic disproportion, placenta previa, etc.)
> - Fetal distress
> - Vaginal delivery is unlikely to occur within a reasonable time frame after the first eclamptic fit

period in anticipation of an emergency preterm delivery. In case an urgent preterm delivery is required, the obstetrician must try to administer at least one dose of corticosteroids 1 hour prior to delivery. Patients with severe eclampsia or preeclampsia, who had received even a single dose of IV steroids 1 hour prior to delivery, have been observed to be associated with a reduced incidence of intraventricular hemorrhage and necrotizing encephalopathy amongst the preterm infants.

Intrapartum Management

The following steps should be taken during the intrapartum period amongst women with severe eclampsia undergoing normal vaginal delivery:

1. Second stage of labor should be cut short and assisted operative vaginal delivery (forceps/vacuum) can be considered.
2. Ergometrine at the delivery of anterior shoulder must be withheld as this may result in further increase in BP. Due to this, there may be increased chances for development of PPH. In order to prevent PPH in cases of preeclampsia, the therapeutic modalities listed in **Box 18.12** can be tried.

Management in the Postpartum Period

Following delivery, close monitoring should be continued for a minimum of 24 hours. It is important to be vigilant and continue anticonvulsive treatment for the first 24–48 hours because eclampsia is likely to occur during this period. BP needs to be continuously monitored in the postpartum period. Antihypertensive treatment can then be gradually tapered off, depending upon the BP levels.

Mode of Delivery

Eclampsia per se is not an indication for cesarean delivery. In case the cervix is not favorable, labor can be induced using vaginal prostaglandins and oxytocin infusion. Indications for cesarean section in cases of eclampsia are listed in **Box 18.13**. If LSCS is decided upon in a case of eclampsia, then the next $MgSO_4$ dose (to be given after 4 hours) may be deferred. This is so because $MgSO_4$ may have a synergistic action with that of muscle relaxants, thereby accentuating the action of muscle relaxants, resulting in uterine atony.

HELLP SYNDROME

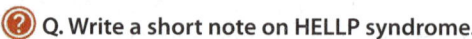

Q. What is HELLP syndrome? How will you diagnose and manage such a case?

Q. Write a short note on HELLP syndrome.

About 20% of women with severe preeclampsia may develop a complication called HELLP syndrome.

Symptoms

Symptoms may include nausea and vomiting (65%), headache (31%), upper abdominal pain (30%), and general malaise (90%). Since early diagnosis of this syndrome is critical, HELLP syndrome must be suspected in any pregnant woman who presents with malaise, epigastric pain, or a viral-type illness in the presence of preeclampsia. Such women must be evaluated with a complete blood cell count and LFTs.

Pathophysiology

The pathophysiology of this multisystem disease can be attributed to abnormal vascular tone, vasospasm and coagulation defects, microvascular endothelial damage, and intravascular platelet activation. Activation of platelets can result in the release of thromboxane A_2 and serotonin, causing further vasospasm, platelet agglutination and aggregation, and endothelial damage. This cascade is only terminated with delivery.

Diagnosis

The three chief abnormalities found in HELLP syndrome are hemolysis, elevated liver enzyme levels, and a low platelet count. Laboratory tests such as proteinuria and an increased uric acid concentration, which are usually elevated in cases with preeclampsia, may not be altered in cases with HELLP syndrome.

Platelet Count

A low platelet count (<100,000/mm^3) is the best indicator of HELLP syndrome. Thrombocytopenia has been attributed to increased consumption and/or destruction of platelets. Platelet counts can drop to as low as 6,000/mm³ (6 × 10⁹/L), but any platelet count < 150,000/mm³ (150 × 10⁹/L) warrants attention. Reduction in the values of various clotting parameters, such as prothrombin time, partial thromboplastin time, and fibrinogen level (<300 mg/dL), is usually not present in patients with HELLP syndrome, unless there is an associated DIC. Besides the reduction in above-mentioned clotting parameters, increase in the levels of D-dimer is a more sensitive indicator of subclinical coagulopathy and may be positive before other coagulation studies become abnormal.

Peripheral Smear

Hemolysis in HELLP syndrome results in microangiopathic hemolytic anemia. Red blood cells become fragmented as they pass through small blood vessels with endothelial damage and fibrin deposits. The peripheral smear may reveal evidence of hemolysis in the form of spherocytes, schistocytes, triangular cells, and burr cells. Excessive hemolysis may result in an increase in serum bilirubin levels ≥ 1.2 mg/dL.

Liver Function Tests

Obstruction of hepatic blood flow by fibrin deposits in the sinusoids is thought to result in periportal necrosis and in severe cases, intrahepatic hemorrhage, subcapsular hematoma formation, or hepatic rupture. This liver damage manifests in the form of elevated liver enzyme levels (AST and ALT ≥ 72 IU/L and LDH > 600 IU/L). Hepatic imaging regardless of the severity of the laboratory abnormalities is useful for assessment of subcapsular hematoma or rupture.

Physical Examination

Physical examination may be normal in patients with HELLP syndrome. However, right upper quadrant tenderness is present in as many as 90% of affected women. Hypertension and proteinuria may be absent or mild.

Differential Diagnosis

Differential diagnosis of HELLP syndrome includes acute fatty liver of pregnancy, thrombotic thrombocytopenic purpura, hemolytic uremic syndrome, viral hepatitis, gall bladder disease, gastroenteritis, kidney stones, pyelonephritis, encephalopathy, and hyperemesis gravidarum.

Classification

HELLP syndrome can be classified based on the number of abnormalities, namely hemolysis, thrombocytopenia, and elevated liver enzymes. According to this classification system, also known as the Tennessee classification, patients with one or two abnormalities are categorized as having partial HELLP syndrome, whereas those with all the three abnormalities are categorized as having full HELLP syndrome. Women with full HELLP syndrome are at higher risk for complications, including DIC, in comparison to women with the partial syndrome. Therefore, patients with the full syndrome should be considered for delivery within 48 hours. The second classification system, also known as the Mississippi or Martin classification of HELLP syndrome, is based on the platelet count and is described in **Table 18.12**. Patients with class I HELLP syndrome are at a higher risk for maternal morbidity and mortality than patients with class II or III HELLP syndrome.

Treatment

Management of HELLP syndrome is described in **Flowchart 18.5**. The mainstay of therapy is supportive management, including seizure prophylaxis and BP control in patients with hypertension. Women remote from term should be considered for conservative management, whereas those with period of gestation > 34 weeks must be delivered. Some patients may require transfusion of blood products or platelets. Rarely, patients with refractory HELLP syndrome require plasmapheresis.

Previously, when patients were diagnosed with HELLP syndrome, prompt delivery was recommended.

However, recent research suggests that morbidity and mortality does not increase when patients with HELLP syndrome are treated conservatively. The patient management should be decided on the basis of gestational age and the condition of the mother and fetus. In the past, delivery in patients with HELLP syndrome was routinely accomplished by cesarean section.

Patients with severe HELLP syndrome, superimposed DIC, or a gestation of <32 weeks should be delivered by cesarean section. A trial of labor is appropriate in patients with mild-to-moderate HELLP syndrome, who remain stable, have a favorable cervix, and have a period of gestation of 32 weeks or greater. Corticosteroids to achieve pulmonary lung maturity may be administered to women in whom delivery may be required before 32 completed weeks of gestation.

The laboratory abnormalities in HELLP syndrome typically worsen after delivery and then begin to resolve by 3–4 days postpartum.

The various other therapeutic options used in patients with HELLP syndrome are described next.

TABLE 18.12: Mississippi or Martin classification of HELLP syndrome.

Class of HELLP syndrome	Platelet count
Class I	<50,000/mm³ (50 ×10⁹/L)
Class II	50,000 to <100,000/mm³ (50–100 × 10⁹/L)
Class III	100,000–150,000/mm³ (100–150 × 10⁹/L)

Flowchart 18.5: Management of cases with HELLP (hemolysis, elevated liver enzymes, and low platelets) syndrome.

```
Patient diagnosed with HELLP syndrome
• Maternal stabilization
• Antihypertensive therapy to keep the blood pressure under control
• Magnesium sulfate to prevent eclampsia
• High-dose corticosteroids to improve laboratory abnormalities
  associated with HELLP syndrome
            │
            ▼
Plan delivery based on period of gestation
   │                    │                       │
   ▼                    ▼                       ▼
POG < 32 weeks     POG 32–34 weeks         POG > 34 weeks
   │                    │                       │
   ▼                    ▼                       ▼
Administration of   Administration of      Deliver the patient
corticosteroids     corticosteroids
to the mother       to the mother
   │                    │
   ▼                    ▼
Determination of    • Determination of L:S ratio
L:S ratio           • To determine patient's
   │                  eligibility for conservative
   │                  management
   ├──────┐                │
   ▼      ▼                │
L:S<2   L:S>2              │
   │      │                │
   ▼      ▼         ┌──────┴──────┐
Conservative  Deliver    ▼             ▼
management    patient   •L:S>2        •L:S<2
              by fastest •Not eligible •Eligible for
              route     for           conservative
   │                    conservative  management
   │                    management
   ▼                       │             │
Patient's  Patient's       ▼             ▼
condition  condition   Delivery by   Conservative
worsens    stabilizes  fastest route management
   │         │                           │
   ▼         │                           ▼
Delivery     │                       Transfer to
by fastest   │                       tertiary
route        │                       care unit
        ┌────┴────┐
        ▼         ▼
   Fetal       Fetal
   maturity    maturity
   is reached  not reached
        │         │
        ▼         ▼
   Delivery by  Continue conservative
   fastest      management until fetal
   route        maturity is reached
```

Corticosteroids

Patients with HELLP syndrome should be routinely treated with high-dose corticosteroids. The antenatal administration of dexamethasone (Decadron) in a high dosage of 10 mg intravenously every 12 hours has been shown to markedly improve laboratory abnormalities associated with HELLP syndrome. Corticosteroid therapy should be instituted in patients with HELLP syndrome who have a platelet count of <100,000/mm^3 (100 × 10^9/L) and should be continued until liver function abnormalities have started resolving and the platelet count becomes >100,000/mm^3 (100 × 10^9/L).

Magnesium Sulfate

Patients with HELLP syndrome should be treated prophylactically with magnesium sulfate to prevent seizures, whether hypertension is present or not.

Antihypertensive Therapy

Antihypertensive therapy should be initiated if BP remains consistently above 160/110 mm Hg despite the use of magnesium sulfate. This reduces the risk of maternal cerebral hemorrhage, placental abruption, and seizure. The goal is to maintain diastolic BP between 90 and 100 mm Hg.

Blood Transfusion

Nearly half of the patients with HELLP syndrome require transfusion with some form of blood product. Patients with a platelet count > 40,000/mm^3 (40 × 10^9/L) are unlikely to bleed. These patients do not require transfusion unless the platelet count drops to <20,000/mm^3 (20 × 10^9/L). Patients who undergo cesarean section should be transfused if their platelet count is <50,000/mm^3 (50 × 10^9/L). Prophylactic transfusion of platelets at delivery does not reduce the incidence of PPH or hasten normalization of the platelet count. Patients with DIC should be given fresh frozen plasma and packed red blood cells.

Plasmapheresis

Plasmapheresis has been successful in patients with severe laboratory abnormalities, i.e., a platelet count of <30,000/mm³ (30 × 10⁹/L) and continued elevation of liver function values and those who have required repeat transfusions to maintain their hematocrit at 72 hours postpartum. In these patients, plasmapheresis has resulted in an increase in the platelet count and a decrease in the LDH levels.

Complications

HELLP syndrome is associated with high rate of mortality and can cause numerous complications such as DIC, placental abruption, adult respiratory distress syndrome, hepatorenal failure, pulmonary edema, subcapsular hematoma, and hepatic rupture. Patients with HELLP syndrome are at an increased risk of developing recurrence in subsequent pregnancies.

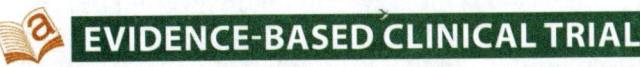

EVIDENCE-BASED CLINICAL TRIALS

List of references can be scanned through QR code to enable the readers gain deeper insight of the subject by referring to the entire article or its abstract.

CHAPTER 19

Gestational Diabetes

CASE STUDY

A 30-year-old G2P1L1 with previous history of giving birth to a baby with birth weight of 4.8 kg presented for routine ANC checkup at 20 weeks. The first baby was born by normal vaginal delivery. The diagnosis of gestational diabetes was confirmed in the previous pregnancy. However, the oral glucose tolerance test (OGTT) performed at 6 weeks postpartum at the time of previous pregnancy was found to be within normal limits.

INTRODUCTION

DIABETES MELLITUS

> Q. Write a short essay describing carbohydrate metabolism in pregnancy.
>
> Q. With the help of a long essay, discuss in detail carbohydrate metabolism in pregnancy and screening tests for gestational diabetes mellitus (GDM).

Diabetes mellitus is an endocrine disorder of carbohydrate metabolism resulting from the lack of action of hormone insulin, produced by the pancreatic β cells in the body. Due to insulin deficiency, the body is unable to utilize glucose efficiently and is associated with the development of symptoms such as polyphagia, polyuria, polydipsia, nocturia, weight loss, exhaustion, and electrolyte imbalance. Diabetes can be associated with development of numerous complications related to the disease process and treatment. This includes complications such as diabetic ketoacidosis (DKA), hyperosmolar nonketotic diabetic coma, lactic acidosis, and hypoglycemia. Longstanding diabetes can result in development of numerous macrovascular and microvascular complications. Macrovascular complications include complications such as myocardial infarction, peripheral vascular disease (ischemia, intermittent claudication, etc.), and stroke. Microvascular complications can include complications such as neuropathy, retinopathy, nephropathy, and erectile dysfunction. According to the classification system devised by the WHO and American Diabetes Association (ADA), diabetes mellitus has now been classified into two types: Type 1 and Type 2 diabetes. The previously used terms noninsulin-dependent diabetes mellitus (NIDDM) and insulin-dependent diabetes mellitus (IDDM) are no longer used. Metabolic changes taking place in diabetes mellitus are shown in **Flowcharts 19.1A and B**, whereas different types of diabetes are shown in **Table 19.1**.

TABLE 19.1: Etiological classification of disorders of diabetes mellitus.

Classification	Criteria
Type 1	Type 1A: Due to islet cell autoantibodies Type 1B: Idiopathic
Type 2	Predominantly due to insulin resistance with relative insulin deficiency
Other specific types	Genetic defects of β-cell function, genetic defect of insulin action, diseases of exocrine pancreas, endocrinopathies, drug- or chemical-induced diabetes, diabetes associated with genetic syndromes, immune-mediated diabetes, etc.
Gestational diabetes	Diabetes associated with pregnancy

CLASSIFICATION OF DIABETES IN PREGNANCY

About 2–5% of total pregnancies may be affected by diabetes. Among pregnancies complicated by diabetes, about 65% cases involve gestational diabetes, whereas 35% cases are associated with preexisting diabetes, of which 25% of cases may be associated with preexisting type 1 diabetes and 10% may involve preexisting type 2 diabetes. The WHO and National Diabetes Data Group (NDDG) have classified diabetic pregnancies as follows:
- *Preexisting diabetes:* Diabetes that antedates pregnancy
  - *Type I:* No endogenous insulin, ketosis prone
  - *Type II:* Late-onset diabetes, associated with obesity, insulin resistant

Gestational Diabetes

Flowchart 19.1A: Immediate metabolic consequences of diabetes mellitus.

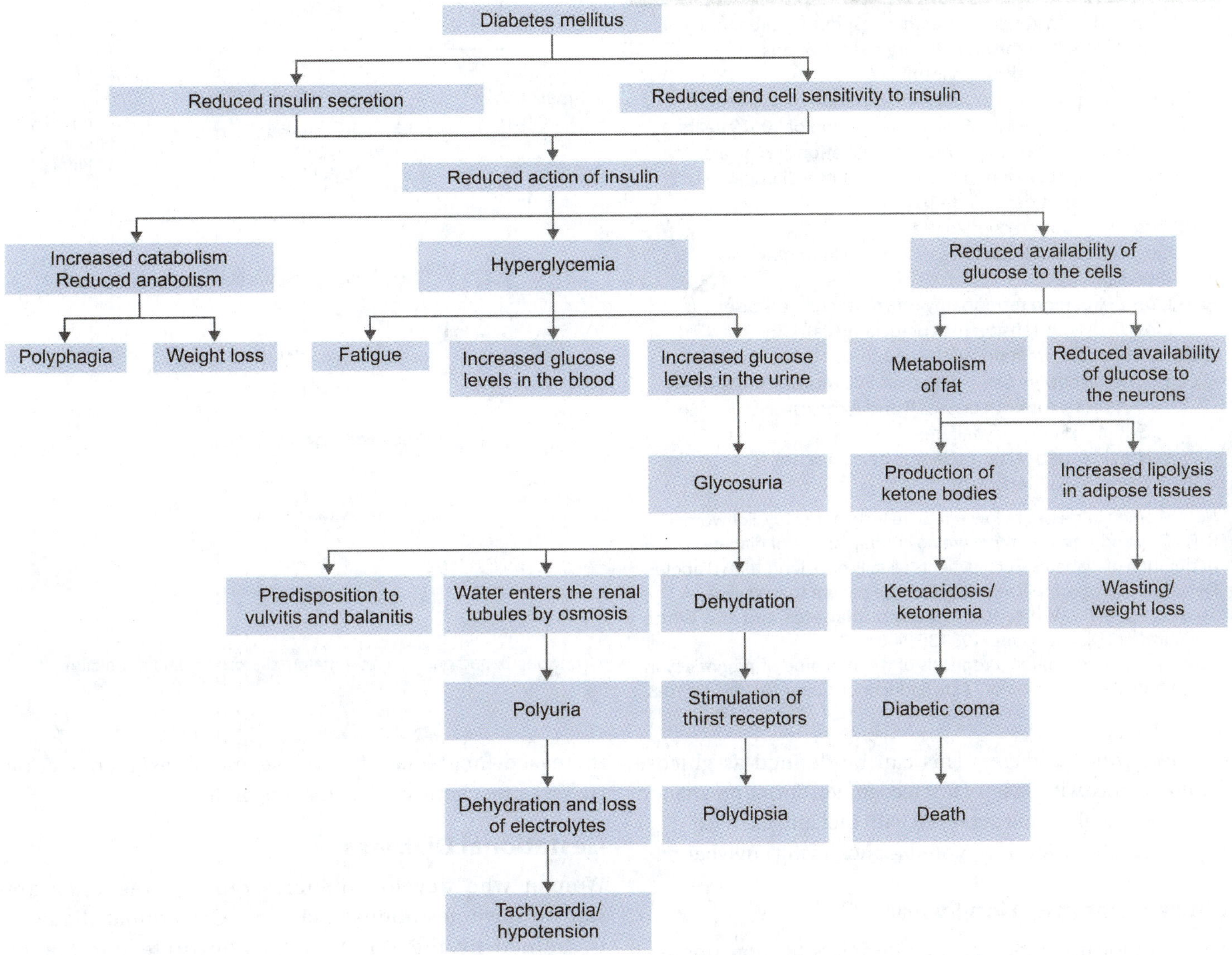

Flowchart 19.1B: Delayed complications of diabetes mellitus.

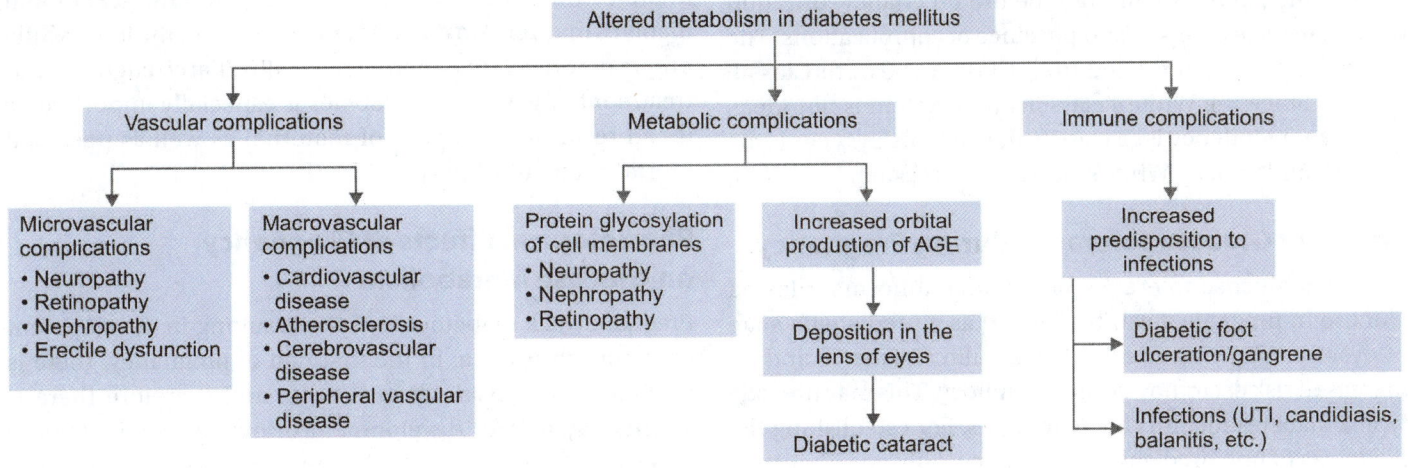

(AGE: advanced glycation end product; UTI: urinary tract infection)

> **BOX 19.1:** White's classification of diabetes (modified by Pedersen).
>
> - *Class A:* Abnormal glucose tolerance test during pregnancy
>   - *Class A1:* Treated through dietary modifications
>   - *Class A2:* Treated through insulin
> - *Class B:* Onset at age ≥ 20 years and duration of <10 years
> - *Class C:* Onset at age 10–19 years or duration of 10–19 years
> - *Class D:* Onset before 10 years of age, duration ≥ 20 years, benign retinopathy, or hypertension (not preeclampsia)
>   - *Class D1:* Onset before age 10 years
>   - *Class D2:* Duration over 20 years
>   - *Class D3:* Calcification of vessels of the leg (macrovascular disease)
>   - *Class D4:* Benign retinopathy (microvascular disease)
>   - *Class D4:* Hypertension (not preeclampsia)
> - *Class R:* Proliferative retinopathy or vitreous hemorrhage
> - *Class F:* Renal nephropathy with over 500 mg/day proteinuria
> - *Class RF:* Criteria for both classes R and F coexist
> - *Class G:* Many pregnancy failures
> - *Class H:* Evidence of arteriosclerotic heart disease
> - *Class T:* Prior renal transplant
>
> *Note:* Women in classes below A require insulin therapy. For women in R, F, RF, H, and T classes, there are no criteria for age of diabetes onset or duration of diabetes. Such patients usually have long-term diabetes. Development of complications moves the patient to next class.
> *Source:* Hare JW, White P. Gestational diabetes and the White classification. Diabetes Care. 1980;3:394-6.
> Pedersen J, Pedersen LM. Prognosis of the outcome of pregnancy in diabetes. A new classification. Acta Endocrinol (Copenh). 1965;50:70-8.

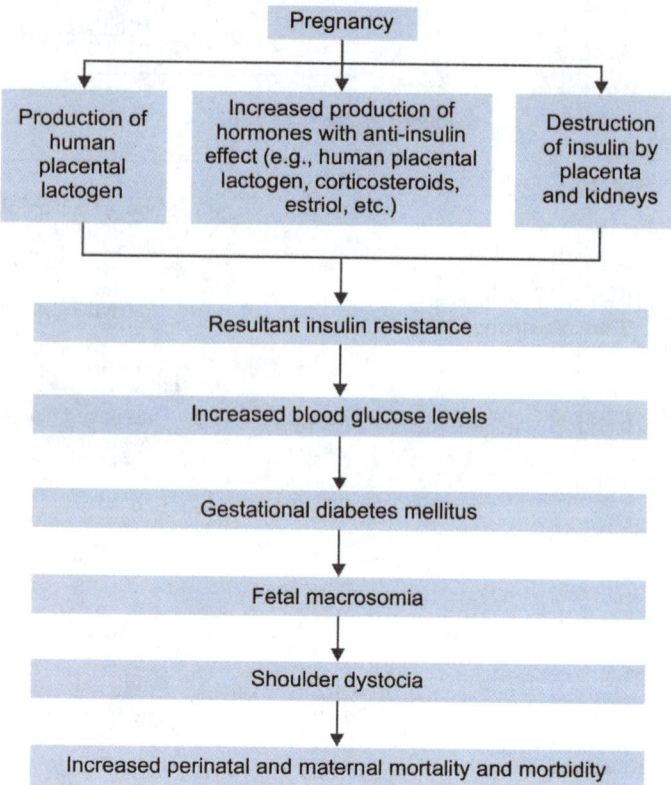

Flowchart 19.2: Pathogenesis of gestational diabetes.

- *Gestational diabetes:* This can be defined as glucose intolerance with onset or first recognition during pregnancy.
  - *A1:* Euglycemia achieved with diet and exercise
  - *A2:* Medications required for achieving euglycemia

White's Classification System

Many European centers apply White's classification modified by Pedersen **(Box 19.1)**. This classification system by Priscilla White helps in predicting the outcome of pregnancy based on various metabolic, obstetric, and other risk factors such as the patient's condition before pregnancy, duration of diabetes, age of onset, and presence of complications. The prognosis has been graded from Class A (best) to Class F (worst). Since the White's classification system is not ideal, the current tendency is to classify the patients by types (type I and II) and then by White's classification system.

Impaired Glucose Tolerance during Pregnancy

Impaired glucose tolerance or isolated abnormal plasma glucose in pregnancy can be defined as a prediabetic state of dysglycemia, characterized by insulin resistance and an increased risk of cardiovascular pathology. This may precede type 2 diabetes mellitus by many years. For establishing the diagnosis of impaired glucose tolerance, only one abnormal glucose value is required in 100-g glucose tolerance test. Impaired glucose tolerance is associated with an increased maternal and fetal morbidity. It is also associated with an increased incidence of lower segment cesarean section (LSCS), preeclampsia, and macrosomia.

Gestational Diabetes

Women who develop diabetes during pregnancy are said to have gestational diabetes. Gestational diabetes is defined by the WHO as "carbohydrate intolerance resulting in hyperglycemia of variable severity with onset or first recognition during pregnancy." It now includes both gestational impaired glucose tolerance and gestational diabetes mellitus (GDM). Some women with gestational diabetes may remain diabetic after delivery of the fetus, while others may revert to apparent normality. Early diagnosis and treatment of gestational diabetes is especially important as it can result in high rates of maternal as well as perinatal mortality and morbidity.

Physiological Effects of Pregnancy on Glucose Metabolism

Pregnancy is a diabetogenic state resulting in development of insulin resistance. In the first half of pregnancy, there is an increased sensitivity to insulin, and therefore there is a tendency toward development of hypoglycemia. On the other hand, the second half of pregnancy (especially after 24 weeks of gestation) is related with development of insulin resistance. This insulin resistance is thought to be the cause for pathogenesis of gestational diabetes **(Flowchart 19.2)**. As a result, insulin requirements decrease during the first trimester and increase progressively from the second trimester until the last month of gestation. Some of the physiological changes taking place during pregnancy are as follows:

- Human placental lactogen, which has anti-insulin and lipolytic effects, is produced late in pregnancy. As a result, the glucose levels in maternal plasma are increased.
- Steroid hormones (especially corticosteroids, estriol, and progesterone), which are produced late in pregnancy, show an anti-insulin effect.
- Some insulin may be destroyed by the placenta and kidneys.
- The diabetogenic effects of pregnancy are increased in the presence of maternal obesity and history of gestational diabetes in previous pregnancy.

The changes related to carbohydrate metabolism in early and late pregnancies are described in **Tables 19.2 and 19.3**, respectively. The net effect of the above-mentioned physiological changes is that of underutilization of exogenous fuel in the fed state (facilitated anabolism) and overproduction from endogenous source in the fasted state (hyperaccelerated starvation or starvation ketosis). Besides this, the changes in carbohydrate metabolism during pregnancy are also likely to result in fasting hypoglycemia, postprandial hyperglycemia, and glycosuria.

Pathogenesis of Gestational Diabetes Mellitus

Precise mechanisms related to the pathogenesis of GDM remain unknown. Hallmark of GDM is an increased insulin resistance. There is an inability to secrete sufficient insulin to compensate for the increased nutritional needs of gestation due to:

- Increased adiposity of pregnancy
- Increased levels of anti-insulin hormones such as human placental lactogen, prolactin, cortisol (potent), progesterone, and estrogen (weak)
- Increased production of enzymes with insulinase activity (oxytocinase, histaminase, and alkaline phosphatase)

- *Role of inflammatory mediators:* There is an increase in inflammatory mediators (tumor necrosis factor α, interleukin 6, etc.) and a decrease in anti-inflammatory mediators (e.g., adiponectin and interleukin 10).

The likely mechanism for pathogenesis of gestational diabetes is demonstrated in **Flowchart 19.2** and **Figure 19.1**.

HISTORY AND CLINICAL PRESENTATION

Q. Enumerate the risk factors which predispose a woman to develop gestational diabetes.

RISK FACTORS

The risk factors which predispose a woman to develop gestational diabetes and need to be elicited while taking the history are described in **Box 19.2**.

GENERAL PHYSICAL EXAMINATION

There are no specific findings related to gestational diabetes on general physical examination. However, signs suggestive of preeclampsia must be looked for as the women with GDM are especially prone to develop preeclampsia.

SPECIFIC SYSTEMIC EXAMINATION

ABDOMINAL EXAMINATION

Women with GDM are especially prone to develop polyhydramnios. Some signs suggestive of polyhydramnios on abdominal examination are as follows:

- Abdomen is markedly enlarged along with fullness of flanks. The skin of the abdominal wall appears to be tense, shiny, and may show appearance of large stria.
- Patients have a fundal height greater than the period of amenorrhea, and fetal parts may not be easily palpable.

TABLE 19.2: Carbohydrate metabolism in early pregnancy (up to 20 weeks).

Hormonal alteration	Effect	Metabolic change
Increased levels of estrogen and progesterone	Increased tissue glycogen storage	Net anabolic effect due to increased level of sex steroids
β-cell hyperplasia and increased insulin secretion	• Decreased hepatic glucose production • Increased peripheral glucose utilization • Decreased fasting plasma glucose	Hyperinsulinemia and reduced serum glucose levels help in protecting the developing embryo from elevated glucose levels

TABLE 19.3: Carbohydrate metabolism in late pregnancy (20–40 weeks).

Hormonal alterations	Effects	Metabolic changes
• Increased human chorionic somatomammotropin • Increased prolactin levels • Reduced levels of bound and free cortisol	• Increased insulin resistance • Decreased hepatic glycogen stores • Increased hepatic glucose production	• Facilitated anabolism during feeding • Accelerated starvation during fasting ensures supply of glucose and amino acids to the fetus

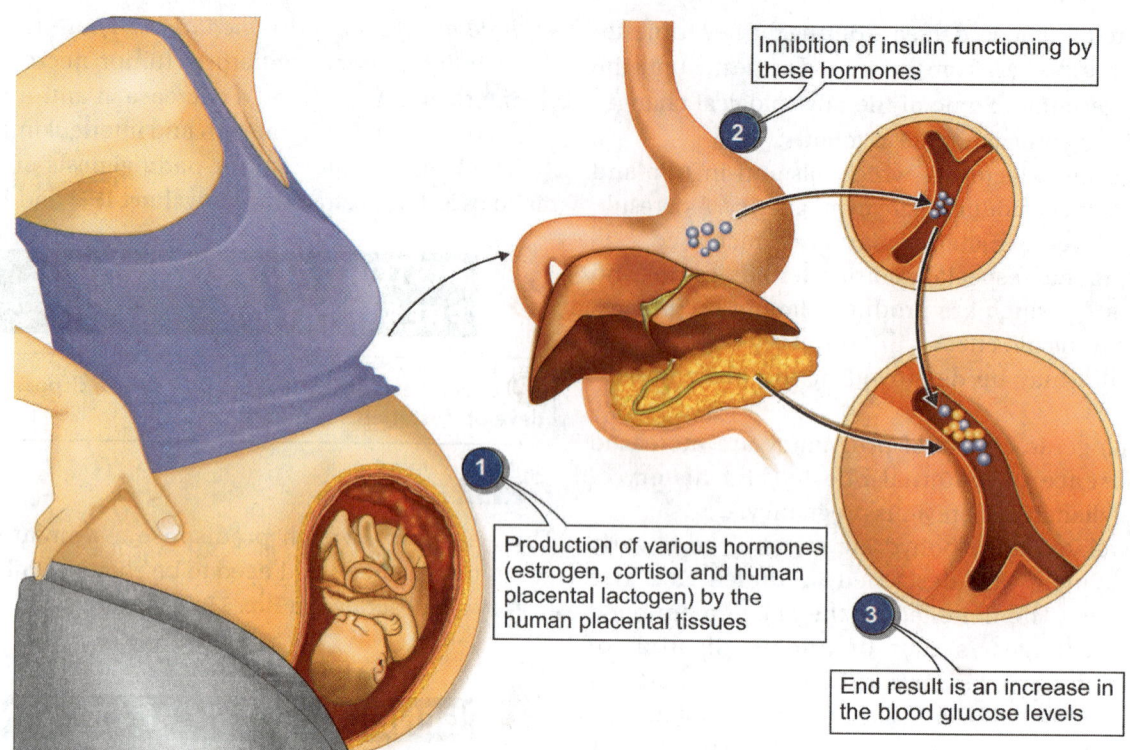

Fig. 19.1: Pathogenesis of gestational diabetes.

- Fetal heart sounds may appear muffled as if coming from a distance.
- A fluid thrill may be commonly present.
- It may be difficult to palpate the uterus or fetal presenting parts due to the presence of excessive fluid.

Since women with GDM are prone to develop macrosomic or IUGR fetuses, signs for both these features must be observed on clinical abdominal examination. Features suggestive of IUGR are described in Chapter 15. Macrosomic fetus is suggested in case expected fetal weight on Leopold's maneuver appears to be > 4.0 kg. However, estimation of fetal weight on Leopold's maneuver has been observed to be grossly inaccurate.

MANAGEMENT

Management comprising investigations and definitive obstetric management is discussed next.

INVESTIGATIONS

 Q. Discuss with the help of a short note how you would go about screening for gestational diabetes mellitus.

 Q. With the help of a long essay, describe the screening methods and current concepts in the management of gestational diabetes mellitus.

 Q. Write a detailed account regarding how the state of euglycemia is maintained during pregnancy.

 Q. Write a short essay on glucose challenge test.

Presently, there is no international consensus regarding timing and type of screening method and the optimal cutoff points for diagnosis and intervention of GDM.

SINGLE-STEP METHOD FOR SCREENING

The single-step method of screening is inclusive of screening as well as diagnostic tests.

Diabetes in Pregnancy Study Group of India Criteria

In the Indian scenario, as per the national guidelines, universal screening via the Diabetes in Pregnancy Study Group of India (DIPSI) is done using the single-step method (rather than a two-step method). This method is recommended during the first antenatal visit because a single-step method is more likely to correlate with the complications of diabetes. In this method, the pregnant lady is administered 75 g of glucose, mixed in 300 mL of water, irrespective of her fasting status or timing of her last meal. She is asked to drink this solution within 5 minutes. The interpretation of the DIPSI test is described in **Table 19.4**. If the patient's results are normal during this visit, it is repeated at 24–28 weeks. The importance of performing DIPSI in the first trimester is that it helps in differentiating between pregestational and gestational diabetes. However, since this criterion does not take fasting and 1 and 2 hours blood glucose values into consideration, it is likely to miss some women with GDM.

In case the woman vomits within half an hour of consuming glucose, the test is not considered valid and needs to be repeated after 3 days. However, if she vomits after half an hour, there is no need to repeat the test.

International Association of Diabetes in Pregnancy Study Group Criteria

As per the International Association of Diabetes in Pregnancy Study Group (IADPSG) consensus panel, a single-step approach for GDM is used. This is based on the results of the HAPO (Hyperglycemia and Adverse Pregnancy Outcomes) study (2008) and is being followed in most of the National Health Service (NHS) trusts across the UK. IADPSG **(Table 19.5)** also advocates first-trimester screening through following tests: fasting blood glucose (<92 mg/dL), glycated hemoglobin (HBA1c) < 6.5 g%, and a random blood glucose value < 200 mg/dL.

Selective screening rather than universal screening is followed in the UK, where the women with risk factors **(Box 19.2)** are offered testing for GDM.

According to these criteria, following a period of overnight fasting or fasting for 8–14 hours, a fasting glucose sample is taken, following which the woman is administered 75 g of glucose in 300 mL of water.

TABLE 19.4: Diabetes in Pregnancy Study Group of India (DIPSI) criteria of screening for gestational diabetes.

Plasma glucose value (mg/dL)	Interpretation
<120	Normal
120–139	Impaired glucose tolerance or gestational glucose intolerance
140–199	Gestational diabetes mellitus
>200	Overt diabetes

TABLE 19.5: International Association of Diabetes in Pregnancy Study Group (IADPSG) criteria for diagnosis of gestational diabetes.

Timing	Blood glucose values (mg/dL)
Fasting	<92
1 hour	<180
2 hours	<153

BOX 19.2: Risk factors for development of gestational diabetes.

- Age > 25 years
- Body mass index > 30 kg/m^2
- Previous history of macrosomic baby (>4.5 kg or above)
- Previous obstetric history of gestational diabetes/polyhydramnios/intrauterine death (IUD)/unexplained stillbirths
- Family history of diabetes (first-degree relatives with diabetes)
- Minority ethnic origin with a high prevalence of diabetes (e.g., South Asian and Middle Eastern)

As per the NICE guidelines (2015), women who have had GDM in a previous pregnancy must be offered early self-monitoring of blood glucose or a 75-g 2-hour OGTT as soon as possible after booking (first or second trimester) and a further 75-g OGTT at 24–28 weeks' period if the results of the first OGTT are normal.

In comparison to the DIPSI criteria, the IADPSG criteria requires a period of overnight fasting, which makes it less favorite in the busy Indian clinical setup. However, since DIPSI does not consider the fasting values, it may miss the fasting hyperglycemia. Also, 1-hour values as considered by the IADPSG criteria are not taken into consideration by DIPSI. This value holds importance because after 1 hour the blood glucose levels tend to come down in lieu of interaction between insulin and other counter-regulatory hormones.

TWO-STEP SCREENING TEST

Two-step method of screening is followed in the United States as well as some setups in India.

It comprises a glucose challenge test (GCT) and 3-hour 100-g OGTT for patients with an abnormal result on GCT. GCT involves measurement of plasma blood glucose levels 1 hour after administration of 50-g glucose load to the woman. It is not necessary for her to follow a special diet before test or to be in the fasting stage. A value of 140 mg/dL or higher indicates high risk for development of gestational diabetes. Some people prefer to use 130 mg/dL as a cutoff threshold, but the number of false-positive screening results would be much higher with the 130 mg/dL threshold. An abnormal result on GCT must be followed by a 100-g OGTT.

An abnormal result on GCT should be followed by a 100-g 3-hour OGTT. This test involves measurement of blood glucose levels at fixed time intervals following the intake of prefixed quantities of glucose. While a 100-g 3-hour OGTT is a standard in the United States, in the United Kingdom a 75-g 2-hour OGTT is preferred. If the 100-g 3-hour OGTT is used, the diagnosis can be made using either the Carpenter and Coustan criteria **(Table 19.6 and Fig. 19.2)** or the criteria defined by the NDDG **(Table 19.7)**. On the other hand, if the 2-hour 75-g OGTT is used, the diagnosis can be made using

TABLE 19.6: 100-g glucose load by O'Sullivan and Mahan: Criteria modified by Carpenter and Coustan.

Status	Plasma/serum glucose (mmol/L)	Plasma/serum glucose levels (mg/dL)
Fasting	≥5.3	95
1 hour	≥10.0	180
2 hours	≥8.6	155
3 hours	≥7.8	140

Source: Carpenter MW, Coustan DR. Criteria for screening tests for gestational diabetes. Am J Obstet Gynecol. 1982;144:768-73. doi: 10.1016/0002-9378(82)90349-0

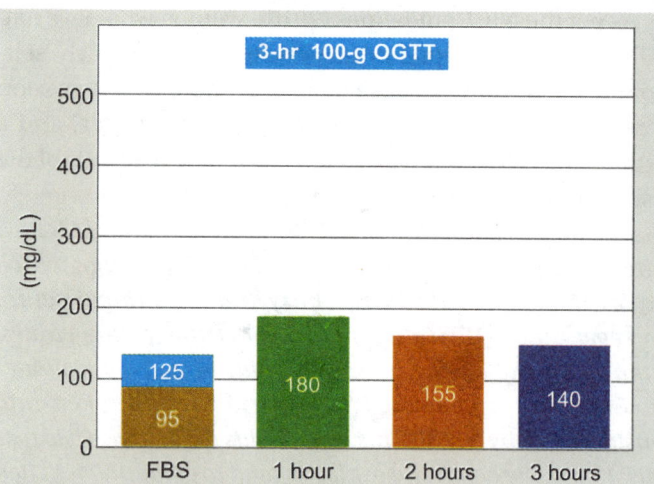

Fig. 19.2: 3-hour 100-g oral glucose tolerance test (OGTT) by O'Sullivan and Mahan: Criteria modified by Carpenter and Coustan. (FBS: fasting blood sugar)
Source: Carpenter MW, Coustan DR. Criteria for screening tests for gestational diabetes. Am J Obstet Gynecol. 1982;144:768-73.

TABLE 19.7: National Diabetes Data Group criteria for 100-g oral glucose tolerance test.

Status	Plasma/serum glucose levels (mmol/L)	Plasma/serum glucose levels (mg/dL)
Fasting	≥5.8	105
1 hour	≥10.6	190
2 hours	≥9.2	165
3 hours	≥8.0	145

Source: National Diabetes Data Group. Classification and diagnosis of diabetes mellitus and other categories of glucose intolerance. Diabetes. 1979;28:1039-57.

TABLE 19.8: WHO criteria for 75-g oral glucose tolerance test.

Status	Whole blood venous	Whole blood capillary	Plasma venous	Plasma capillary
Fasting	≥6.1 mmol/L	≥6.1 mmol/L	≥7.0 mmol/L (126 mg/dL)	≥7.0 mmol/L
2 hours	≥6.7 mmol/L	≥6.7 mmol/L	≥7.8 mmol/L (140 mg/dL)	≥8.9 mmol/L

Source: World Health Organization. (1999). Definition, diagnosis, and classification of diabetes mellitus and its complications: report of a WHO consultation. Part 1: diagnosis and classification of diabetes mellitus. [Online] Available from https://apps.who.int/iris/bitstream/handle/10665/66040/WHO_NCD_NCS_99.2.pdf?sequence=1&isAllowed=y. [Last accessed November, 2022].

TABLE 19.9: American Diabetes Association criteria for 75-g oral glucose tolerance test.

Status	Plasma glucose levels (mg/dL)	Plasma glucose levels (mmol/L)
Fasting	≥92	5.1
1 hour	≥180	10.00
2 hours	≥153	8.50

Source: American Diabetes Association. Standards of medical care in diabetes—2013. Diabetes Care. 2013;36(Suppl 1):S11-66. [Online] Available from https://doi.org/10.2337/dc13-S011.

the criteria defined by the WHO **(Table 19.8)** or the criteria by the ADA **(Table 19.9)**.

The patient cannot be diagnosed as gestational diabetic if only one value is abnormal in case of 100-g OGTT (criteria by Carpenter and Coustan) or in case of 75-g OGTT (criteria by the ADA). In these cases, two or more values must be abnormal to establish the diagnosis of gestational diabetes. However, with one abnormal value, the woman is at an increased risk for developing complications, such as macrosomia (18%) and preeclampsia–eclampsia (7.9%). Even patients who show no abnormal values in their 3-hour OGTT have risks of 6.6% and 3.3% for development of macrosomia and preeclampsia–eclampsia, respectively. This shows that even small alteration in maternal carbohydrate metabolism may have a significant impact on the fetus. Thus, the obstetrician needs to maintain strict glycemic control in order to decrease the frequency of abnormal outcomes to both the mother and the fetus at the time of pregnancy.

℞ TREATMENT/OBSTETRIC MANAGEMENT

Q. What is the likely diagnosis and management in the case described in the beginning of this chapter?

Q. Write a long essay on diagnosis and management of gestational diabetes mellitus (GDM).

Q. Write a long essay discussing the management of a gravida 2 woman, diagnosed to have GDM at 30 weeks of gestation.

Q. Discuss the medical and obstetric management of GDM.

Diagnosis and treatment of gestational diabetes are of extreme importance. If gestational diabetes is not detected and controlled on time, it can result in high rates of perinatal morbidity and mortality, primarily related to the development of complications such as macrosomia and shoulder dystocia. These complications may be associated with an increased risk of birth trauma, induction of labor, and cesarean section.

Gestational diabetes also increases the risk of the baby developing obesity and/or diabetes in later life. Controlling the patient's blood sugar level is the best way for preventing various diabetes-related complications, including the risk of miscarriage, stillbirth, and congenital malformations, particularly those affecting the brain, spine, heart, etc. The definitive management of the pregnant diabetic patient is best undertaken using a multidisciplinary team approach involving an obstetrician, midwife, physician,

endocrinologist, diabetologist, neonatologist, etc. The two main aims for management of diabetic patient during pregnancy are as follows:
1. Maintenance of blood glucose levels
2. Regular fetal monitoring

MONITORING IN THE PRECONCEPTIONAL PERIOD

> Q. Write a short essay discussing the care which needs to be given to the prepregnant woman who is a known case of diabetes.
>
> Q. What is diabetic retinopathy? How does the grading affect fetal outcome?

According to the ADA guidelines (2013) in women with overt pregestational diabetes, the cutoffs for diagnoses at the time of first prenatal visit are as follows:
- Fasting plasma glucose levels (126 mg/dL or 7.0 mmol/L)
- HbA1c values of ≥6.5%
- Random blood glucose values of ≥200 mg/dL (11.1 mmol/L)For women with pregestational diabetes, the blood glucose levels need to be controlled right since the preconceptional period. Nutritional and metabolic interventions must be initiated well before pregnancy begins, because birth defects occur during the critical 3–6 weeks after conception. The following steps need to be taken to monitor the women during the preconceptional period:
- *Measurement of HbA1c levels:* Monthly measurements of HbA1c levels give an idea about the patient's blood glucose levels over past few months. The clinician's aim must be to maintain the levels of HbA1c below 6.5%. Increased level of HbA1c is associated with higher rates of congenital malformations in the baby. If HbA1c is below 6.5% prior to conception, the incidence of congenital malformations is same as that of general population. However, this risk rises to 8% if HbA1c levels are >10%. Thus, the women whose HbA1c is above 10% should be strongly advised to avoid pregnancy and use contraception until their HbA1c levels come within the normal limits.
- *Self-monitoring of blood glucose levels:* Self-monitoring of blood glucose levels using a glucose meter and finger-prick method must be offered to all diabetic women planning for pregnancy **(Fig. 19.3)**. These women need to be educated regarding the importance of maintaining adequate levels of glucose in their body. They should be advised to test their blood glucose levels at least four times a day, including fasting blood glucose levels and blood glucose levels 1 hour after every meal.
- *Blood and urine investigations:* These include collection of 24-hour urine sample for proteins and creatinine clearance. Blood urea, serum creatinine, thyroid-stimulating hormone, and free thyroxine levels also

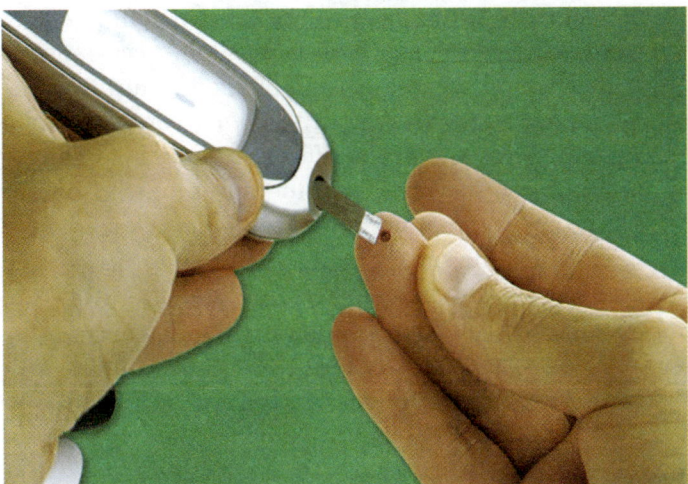

Fig. 19.3: Finger-prick method for blood glucose assessment.

need to be determined. Women with type 1 diabetes who are planning pregnancy should be advised to use ketone testing strips and test for ketonuria in their urine samples, especially if their blood glucose levels show hyperglycemia.
- *Discontinuation of various drugs during pregnancy:* Lipid-lowering drugs including statins (atorvastatin, Fluvastatin, pravastatin, rosuvastatin, simvastatin, etc.) should be discontinued before pregnancy or as soon as the pregnancy is confirmed.

If the woman has been using antihypertensive agents such as angiotensin-converting enzyme inhibitors and angiotensin II receptor antagonists, they should be discontinued before conception or as soon as pregnancy is confirmed because of the possible risk of congenital malformations (skull defects and oligohydramnios). She should be prescribed safer alternative antihypertensive drugs suitable for use during pregnancy.

Calcium channel blockers should be avoided throughout pregnancy because of the risk of disruption to labor and fetal hypoxia. However, in case the clinicians feel that the risk of uncontrolled maternal hypertension is greater than the fetal risk, nifedipine may be continued.

Whereas all the oral hypoglycemic drugs need to be discontinued before pregnancy, women with diabetes may be advised to use metformin as an adjunct or alternative to insulin in the preconception period and during pregnancy. There is strong evidence for the effectiveness and safety of metformin.
- *Retinal assessment in the preconception period:* Women with pregestational diabetes planning pregnancy must be offered retinal assessment at the time of their first preconception appointment. This may not be required if an annual retinal assessment has taken place within the last 6 months. If no changes related to diabetic retinopathy are found at the time of initial examination, annual retinal assessment is required. In case of presence

of proliferative retinopathy, she must be offered laser therapy before she conceives to avoid the occurrence of retinal hemorrhages (a cause of blindness) during labor.
- *Renal assessment in the preconception period:* Women with diabetes should be offered a renal assessment, including a measure of microalbuminuria, before planning pregnancy. She should be referred to a nephrologist if serum creatinine is abnormal (≥ 120 µmol/L) or the estimated glomerular filtration rate (eGFR) is < 45 mL/min/1.73 m².
- *Maintenance of adequate body weight:* Women with diabetes who are planning to become pregnant and who have a BMI above 27 kg/m² should be offered advice on how to lose weight.
- *Regular intake of folic acid:* Women with diabetes who are planning to become pregnant should be advised to take folic acid in the dose of 5 mg/day, starting right from the periconceptional period and throughout the period of gestation. This would help in reducing the risk of having a baby with neural tube defects.

MANAGEMENT DURING THE ANTENATAL PERIOD

> Q. Write a short essay discussing the nutritional requirements in a patient with gestational diabetes mellitus.

The following advice need to be given to the woman with GDM during antenatal period:
- Antenatal care in patients with GDM should preferably be hospital-based, involving a multidisciplinary team approach comprising an endocrinologist, obstetrician, and pediatrician. The blood glucose levels need to be assessed every 1–2 weeks throughout pregnancy.
- *Diet/medical nutrition therapy (MNT):* First line of management is MNT. This mainly involves lifestyle modification in the form of diet and exercise.
- *Glycemic targets to be achieved during pregnancy:* **Table 19.10** describes the glycemic targets, which need to be observed during pregnancy. In case the woman's fasting blood levels are <90 mg/dL and 2-hour postprandial levels are <120 mg/dL, MNT and physical exercise regimen may be continued. In these cases, fasting blood glucose and 2-hour postprandial values must be monitored at least once on a monthly basis.

TABLE 19.10: Glycemic targets in pregnancy.

Criteria	Blood sugar fasting (mg/dL)	1 hour (mg/dL)	2 hours (mg/dL)
ADA	≤95	≤140	≤120
*DIPSI	≤90	–	≤120

(ADA: American Diabetes Association; DIPSI: Diabetes in Pregnancy Study Group of India)
Note: DIPSI guidelines utilize plasma glucose.

Plasma values of glucose are approximately 12% higher than the whole blood values. Blood samples obtained by a finger stick (yielding arterialized blood) produce higher values in comparison to the venous samples. This is because the arterialized blood has not yet traversed muscles, and hence glucose removal by these tissues has not occurred.
- *Requirement for hypoglycemic therapy:* In case the woman's fasting blood levels are ≥ 90 mg/dL and 2-hour postprandial levels are ≥ 120 mg/dL on MNT and physical exercise regimen, the clinician needs to start hypoglycemic therapy [either oral hypoglycemic agents (OHAs) or insulin] in order to maintain their blood glucose levels within the normal (nondiabetic) range. The aim should be to maintain her HbA1c levels below 6.5%. HbA1c should not be used routinely for assessing glycemic control in the second and third trimesters of pregnancy. Fasting blood glucose levels and 2-hour postprandial levels should be checked every 3 days or more frequently in case of insulin and biweekly in case of metformin. Dose adjustments of insulin or OHA may be required in between in order to maintain normal blood glucose levels. Once these values are within normal limits, monitoring needs to be continued on a weekly basis with insulin and once every 2 weeks in case of OHAs.
- *Retinal assessment during pregnancy:* Pregnant women with preexisting diabetes should be offered retinal assessment by digital imaging with mydriasis using tropicamide. This can be offered following their first antenatal clinic appointment and again at 28 weeks if the first assessment is normal. If any diabetic retinopathy is present, an additional retinal assessment should be performed at 16–20 weeks. Women, in whom preproliferative diabetic retinopathy has been diagnosed during pregnancy, should have ophthalmological follow-up for at least 6 months following the birth of the baby. Diabetic retinopathy should not be considered a contraindication to vaginal birth.
- *Renal assessment during pregnancy:* Diabetic nephropathy is a progressive disease that can be divided into the following stages:
  - *Microalbuminuria:* Microalbuminuria (incipient nephropathy), which can be defined as albumin:creatinine ratio of ≥3.5 mg/mmol or 30–300 mg of protein in 24-hour urine collection specimen
  - *Macroalbuminuria:* Macroalbuminuria or proteinuria (overt nephropathy), which is defined as albumin:creatinine ratio of ≥30 mg/mmol or albumin concentration of >300 mg/24 hours collection specimen as a result of widespread glomerular sclerosis. Such patients are destined to have end-stage renal disease.

- *End-stage renal disease:* It is associated with decreasing creatinine clearance, increasing serum creatinine levels, and uremia.
- Women with diabetic nephropathy are at increased risk of adverse pregnancy outcomes, in particular IUGR, chronic hypertension, preeclampsia and preterm birth. If renal assessment has not been undertaken in the preceding 12 months in women with preexisting diabetes, it should be arranged at the time of first contact in pregnancy. If serum creatinine is abnormal (≥120 µmol/L) or if total protein excretion exceeds 2 g/day, referral to a nephrologist should be considered.
- *Diabetes education and information:* The obstetrician needs to discuss information regarding the effect of diabetes on pregnancy; importance of blood glucose control at the time of pregnancy; changes in the hypoglycemic therapy during and after birth; complications related to use of insulin therapy (e.g., hypoglycemia); advice regarding timing, mode of delivery, and management of birth; management of the baby after birth; and advice related to early parenting (including breastfeeding and initial care of the baby), contraception, and follow-up.

TABLE 19.11: Calorie intake in diabetic women based on their BMI.

BMI	Interpretation	Calorie intake
BMI ≤ 18.5	Underweight	35–40 kcal/kg/day
BMI of 18.5–24.9	Normal	30 kcal/kg/day
BMI of 25.0–29.9	Overweight	25 kcal/kg/day
BMI of 30.0–39.9	Moderate obesity	20 kcal/kg/day
BMI of 40–49.9	Severe obesity	20 kcal/kg/day
BMI ≥ 50	Very severe obesity	12 kcal/kg/day

(BMI: body mass index)

Exercise and Diet Therapy in the Antenatal Period

- The first-line therapy for women with gestational diabetes is exercise and diet therapy. The ADA recommends minimum 30 minutes of moderate exercise daily for women with gestational diabetes.
- Proper nutritional advice is one of the most important components of the care of women with GDM. The objective of nutritional treatment (often referred to as MNT) is to provide a healthy diet, which contains the necessary calories and nutrients, to both mother and fetus without causing postprandial hyperglycemia. Since the carbohydrate content of food is likely to increase the blood glucose levels, women with gestational diabetes should be preferably advised to choose carbohydrates having low glycemic index. The amount of calorie consumption per day based on the woman's basal metabolic rate (BMR) and physical activity level (PAL) is as follows:

Calorie requirement = BMR × PAL + 350 (kcal) for pregnancy, where:
BMR (18–30 years) = 14 × prepregnancy weight (kg) + 471
BMR (30–60 years) = 8.3 × prepregnancy weight (kg) + 788
PAL values: Sedentary work = 1.53, moderate work = 1.8, heavy work = 2.3

Total calories, which are calculated through this formula, must be divided into nine portions, which must be distributed into three major meals and three snacks. Therefore, each meal would comprise two portions and each snack would comprise one portion. A simpler way of calculating the calorie requirement is described in **Table 19.11**.

This total calorie intake must be distributed in the form of multiple, small, evenly spaced meals and snacks throughout the day, e.g., three small meals in morning, afternoon, and night and three snacks in midmorning, midafternoon, and bedtime. The bedtime snack is particularly important as it helps in avoiding overnight hypoglycemia and ketosis. Of the total calorie intake, 40–50% must come from carbohydrates, 30–40% from fats (two-thirds of which should be unsaturated fats and remaining one-third should be saturated fats), and 15–20% must come from proteins. The woman must be advised to consume lean proteins including oily fish and avoid red meat (beef, pork, etc.) and also must increase her consumption of polyunsaturated fats in comparison to the monounsaturated or saturated fats. She must also be advised to restrict her intake of refined sugars and increase her daily consumption of fibers. Recommendations regarding optimal distribution of total calories per day are as follows:

- *Breakfast:* 10% of total caloric allotment (carbohydrate intake is limited at breakfast since insulin resistance is greatest in the morning.)
- *Lunch:* 30% of calories
- *Dinner:* 30% of calories
- *Snacks:* 30% of calories

Composition of Indian Lunch and Dinner Plate (Thali)

As shown in **Figures 19.4A to C**, half the portion of this plate for women with gestational diabetes must comprise vegetables, which can be cooked or consumed in the form of salad. One-fourth of the plate should comprise cereals such as millets, starch, and grains and the remaining one-fourth of the plate must comprise protein-rich foods. Along with this, she must be given one serving fruit and one serving dairy product.

Insulin Therapy

As per the ACOG (2018) and ADA (2017), insulin is the preferred first-line agent for persistent hyperglycemia and in women with GDM. Though studies have supported the

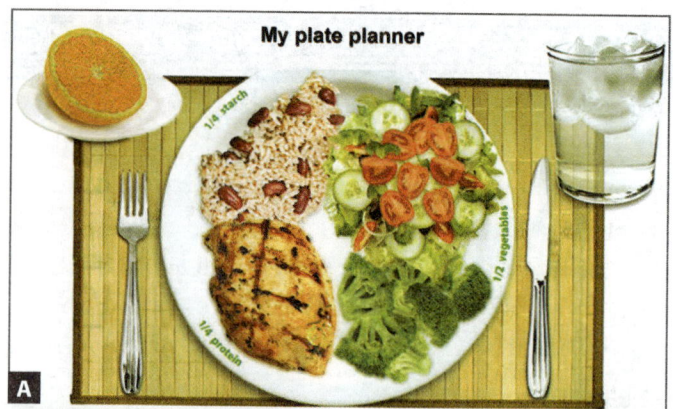
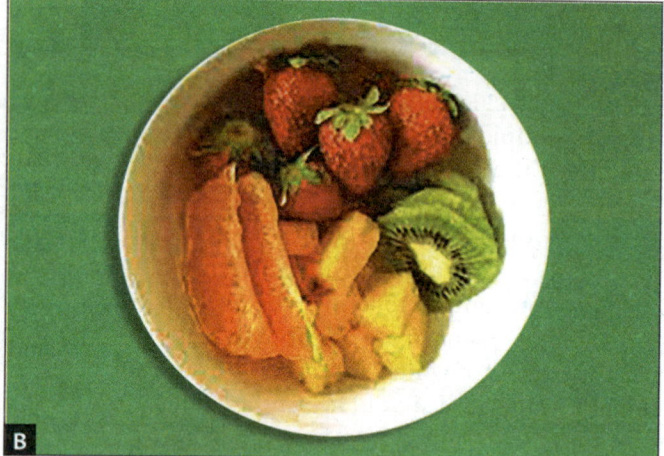
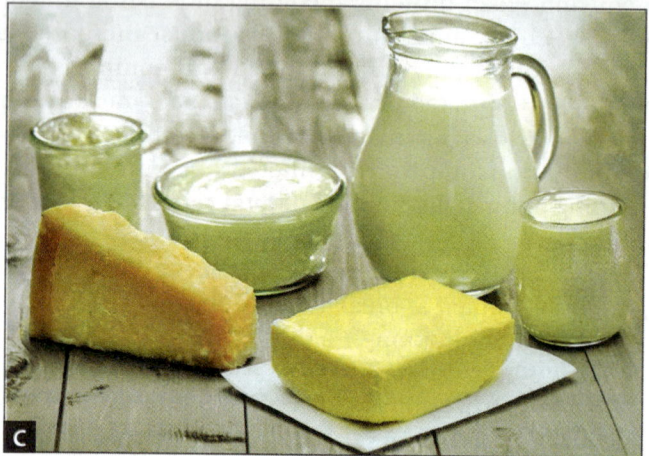

Figs. 19.4A to C: Components of a healthy diet for a patient with gestational diabetes. (A) 9-inch plate for adults. ½—vegetables, ¼—protein, ¼—starch; (B) One portion fruit to be added instead of orange; (C) One portion of dairy product to be added instead of glass.

TABLE 19.12: Different types of insulin preparations.		
Type of insulin preparation	Time for onset of action	Duration (hours)
Short acting		
Lispro	<15 minutes	2–4
Aspart	<15 minutes	2–4
Regular (subcutaneous)	30–60 minutes	3–6
Intermediate acting		
Neutral protamine Hagedorn (NPH)	1–4 hours	10–16
Long acting		
Detemir	1–4 hours	12–24
Glargine	1–4 hours	20–24

safety and efficacy of both metformin (Glucophage) and glyburide (also known as glibenclamide), the Food and Drug Administration (FDA) has not approved any of these drugs for treatment of GDM because both of them can cross placenta, and there are still some concerns regarding the data related to long-term safety for the offspring. The ACOG, however, recognizes both these drugs as a reasonable second-line therapy for glycemic control in women with gestational diabetes. On the other hand, as per the NICE guidelines (2015), metformin can be used as the first-line therapy in cases of gestational diabetes. In case metformin is contraindicated or unacceptable to the woman, insulin must be offered to her. Long-term safety data for this drug is still awaited. No teratogenic effects have been observed even though this drug crosses the placenta.

Various types of insulin preparations are tabulated in **Table 19.12**. In India, insulin preparations are available in two strengths: 40 (U 40) and 100 U/mL (U 100). These preparations should be carefully used because the use of a wrong syringe can result in serious dosage errors. Most used insulin regimens during pregnancy include intermediate-acting insulins such as isophane [neutral protamine Hagedorn (NPH)], short-acting insulins such as regular recombinant (Humulin R), and the rapid-acting insulin analogs such as aspart (Novolog) and lispro (Humalog). Short-acting insulin and intermediate-acting insulin are available in a combination called Mixtard. Mixtard comprises 30% short-acting insulin and 70% intermediate-acting insulin (NPH).

Presently, there is insufficient evidence regarding the use of long-acting insulin analogs (insulin glargine, protamine zinc insulin, detemir, etc.) during pregnancy. Clinicians must be aware that the rapid-acting insulin analogs (aspart and lispro) have advantages over soluble regular human insulin during pregnancy and therefore should be preferred over regular insulin. Insulin is usually started at a dosage of 0.3–1.0 units/kg/day (based on prepregnancy weight), administered in two divided doses. If the total dose of insulin is <10 units, it can be administered in the form of three doses of regular insulin prior to meals along with the administration of intermediate-acting insulin in the night. In case the total insulin requirement is >10 units, the most used dosage strategy involves administration of two-thirds of the total insulin dose in the morning before breakfast with the administration of remainder one-third in the evening before dinner. The morning dosage should comprise two-thirds NPH and one-third short-acting insulin, while the predinner dose should comprise equal parts of NPH and short-acting insulin.

Glucose monitoring in a patient with GDM on insulin must be done using 4-point sugars, which comprises fasting, 1 hour post-breakfast, 1 hour post-lunch, and 1 hour post-dinner blood glucose values. This method is considered favorable over the monitoring done using the 7-point sugars comprising fasting, 1 hour post-breakfast, 1 hour pre- and post-lunch, 1 hour pre- and post-dinner, and pre-bed blood glucose levels at 10 PM. If the patient on insulin therapy continues to experience fasting hyperglycemia in the morning, a 3:00-AM test may be required to differentiate between Dawn and Somogyi phenomena.

- *Somogyi phenomenon:* This phenomenon is associated with hypoglycemia at 3:00 AM and therefore requires a reduction in the insulin dosage. In these cases, posthypoglycemic hyperglycemia occurs due to the paradoxical tendency of the body to react to hypoglycemia by producing hyperglycemia. As per this phenomenon, drop in the blood glucose levels in the late evening/early morning (3:00 AM) causes activation of counter-regulatory hormones such as adrenaline, corticosteroids, and growth hormone, resulting in gluconeogenesis and resultant hyperglycemia in the morning, when the patient wakes up.
- *Dawn phenomenon:* This phenomenon is associated with hyperglycemia at 3:00 AM, thereby requiring an increase in the insulin dosage. Morning hyperglycemia in these cases is likely to be due to reduced levels of endogenous insulin secreted in the night.

Hypoglycemia and loss of hypoglycemic awareness are common during early pregnancy. Women with insulin-treated diabetes are especially at risk of developing hypoglycemia and hypoglycemia unawareness in pregnancy, particularly in the first trimester. The women must be educated about dealing with hypoglycemia. She must be advised to carry sugar candies or glucose tablets with her all the time. The woman, her partner, or other family members should be educated regarding the use of glucagon injections. The moment she experiences any symptoms related to hypoglycemia, she should eat the candies. In case of severe symptoms related to hypoglycemia, intramuscular glucagon injection may be required.

In case adequate blood glucose control is not achieved with insulin injections, the woman should be offered continuous subcutaneous insulin infusion (CSII). Presently, there are no randomized controlled trials which show advantage or disadvantage of using CSII pumps over intermittent insulin injections during pregnancy.

Oral Hypoglycemic Agents in the Antenatal Period

Q. Can oral hypoglycemic agents be used in diabetic women at the time of pregnancy?

Previously, the use of OHAs was not recommended during pregnancy due to safety concerns to the fetus and the risk of development of fetal hypoglycemia. This is so as most of the OHAs are capable of crossing placenta.

Metformin, a biguanide compound (glucophage), may be considered as an option for OHA in women with gestational diabetes. The MiG (Metformin in Gestational Diabetes) trial is the largest study so far regarding the use of metformin in pregnancy in which 751 women were randomized to receive either metformin or insulin. The results of the study demonstrated no significant difference in the composite fetal outcome between the two groups receiving either metformin or insulin, respectively, during pregnancy. It should also be noted that the group receiving metformin was associated with an increased incidence of preterm labor. Moreover, metformin crosses the placenta. Despite these concerns, metformin appears as a new alternative treatment for gestational diabetes. It is a biguanide, which acts by reducing hepatic gluconeogenesis, reducing intestinal absorption, and increasing peripheral uptake of glucose. It is administered in the dosage between 500 mg and 2 g (in divided doses) per day. A prospective randomized controlled trial by Picón-César (2021) has shown that treatment with metformin was likely to be associated with a better postprandial glycemic control, a lower risk of hypoglycemic episodes, reduced maternal weight gain, and a lower failure rate as a result of better compliance due to avoidance of injections in comparison to insulin in women with GDM.

Glibenclamide, also known as glyburide, is another oral hypoglycemic drug used for treating type 2 diabetes. Glyburide is a sulfonylurea, which acts by binding to the adenosine triphosphate (ATP)-linked potassium channel receptors in the pancreatic beta cells, thereby increasing insulin secretion and improving insulin sensitivity in the peripheral tissues. Several prospective and retrospective studies have demonstrated the effectiveness and probable safety of glyburide in the treatment of gestational diabetes. However, most of the studies on glyburide were of small size and therefore could not effectively prove the safety and efficacy of glyburide. Moreover, it is not yet clear as to whether glyburide crosses the placenta or not. A study by Langer et al. (2000), comprising 404 women with gestational diabetes, has shown that glyburide can be considered as a clinically effective alternative to insulin therapy in women with gestational diabetes. Therefore, treatment with glyburide can be considered as a practical alternative for women who are either unable to take insulin or are nonresponsive to it. This drug did not gain high popularity because it is associated with a higher incidence of neonatal and maternal hypoglycemia. Despite this, it is used at some centers. It can be administered in the dosage varying between 2.5 and 10 mg (in divided doses). In case either of the oral hypoglycemic drugs (metformin or glyburide) are unable to control the blood glucose levels in a woman with gestational diabetes, insulin can be added. Studies have shown that this requirement for insulin is more in case of glyburide in comparison to metformin.

Sites for Insulin Injections

The method of administration of insulin injection is shown in **Figures 19.5A to C**. Injections of insulin are commonly made into the subcutaneous tissues by lightly grasping a fold of skin and inserting the needle at an angle of 90°. The common sites in the body for injecting insulin include the following:

- Upper lateral area of the thighs
- Upper outer area of the back of the arms
- Buttocks
- Anterior abdominal wall (with the exception of a circle having a 2-inch radius around the navel)

Education Regarding Diabetes

Women with diabetes who are planning to become pregnant should be informed that establishing good glycemic control before conception and continuing this throughout pregnancy will help in reducing the risk of miscarriage, congenital malformation, stillbirth, and neonatal deaths. The importance of avoiding unplanned pregnancy should be an essential component of education for diabetic women, starting right from adolescence. The women must be advised to use contraception until pregnancy is planned. Women with diabetes who are planning to become pregnant and their families should be offered information regarding how diabetes affects pregnancy **(Box 19.3)** and how pregnancy affects diabetes **(Box 19.4)**. The information should cover:

- Role of diet, body weight, and exercise
- Risks of hypoglycemia and hypoglycemia unawareness during pregnancy
- How nausea and vomiting in pregnancy can affect glycemic control
- Increased risk of having a baby who is large for gestational age (LGA), which increases the likelihood of birth trauma, induction of labor, and cesarean section
- Need for assessment of diabetic retinopathy and nephropathy before and during pregnancy (especially in women with pregestational diabetes)

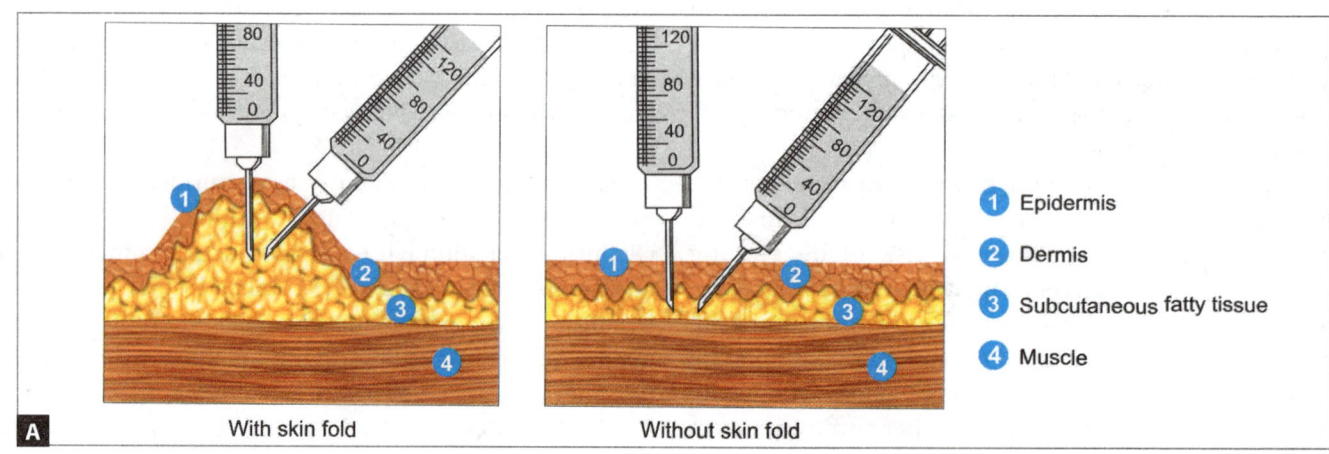

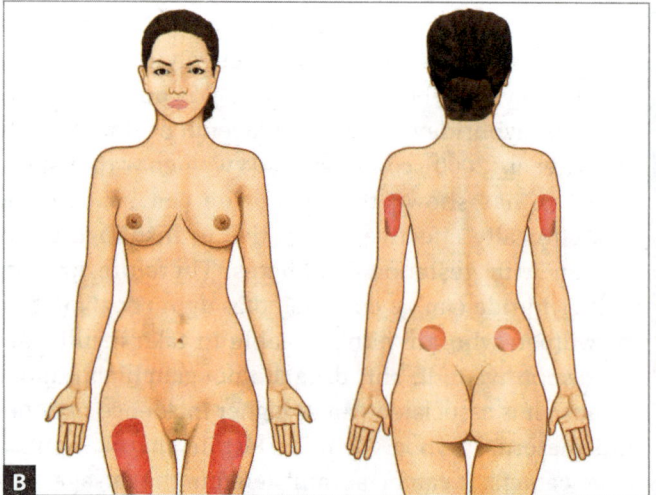

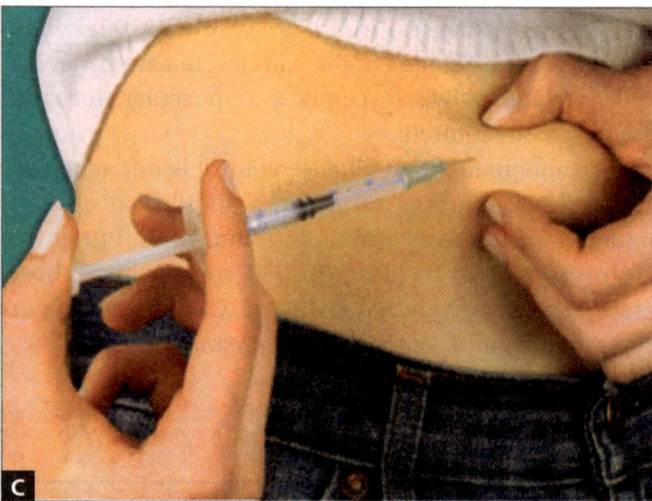

Figs. 19.5A to C: Injection of insulin. (A) Subcutaneous administration of insulin injection; (B) Sites of insulin injection; (C) Administration of insulin injection over the abdomen.

BOX 19.3: The effect of diabetes on pregnancy.

- Need for strict glycemic control during pregnancy
- Need for pregnancy planning
- Risk for increased fetal complications including the risk for congenital malformations, macrosomia, shoulder dystocia, birth injuries, etc.
- Increased risk for maternal complications including miscarriage, preeclampsia, hydramnios, preterm labor, increased rate of cesarean section, etc.
- Requirement for strict fetal surveillance
- General anesthesia in women with diabetes can increase the risk of hypoglycemia

BOX 19.4: The effect of pregnancy on diabetes.

- Changes in the eating pattern
- Decreased insulin requirement during the first half of pregnancy followed by increased insulin requirement during the second half of pregnancy
- Increased risk for hypoglycemia and decreased hypoglycemia awareness during pregnancy
- Deterioration of retinopathy and nephropathy in patients with pregestational diabetes
- Reduced renal threshold for glycosuria
- Disrupted blood glucose control due to nausea and vomiting during pregnancy
- Hyperemesis gravidarum in women with diabetes can lead to ketoacidosis

TABLE 19.13: Fetal surveillance during the antenatal period.

Test for fetal surveillance	Period of gestation	Parameter observed
• Third-trimester ultrasound scan • Daily fetal movement count	28, 32, 36 weeks	• Fetal growth assessment and amniotic fluid volume • <10 movements in 1 hour suggestive of fetal distress
Nonstress test	Twice weekly, starting from 28 weeks onward	Presence of two or more accelerations that peak 15 beats/minute above the baseline, each lasting for 15 seconds or more and all occurring within a 20-minute period from the beginning of test
Fetal BPP or at least amniotic fluid volume	To be done on weekly basis, starting from 28 weeks onward	• A BPP test score of at least 8 out of 10 is considered reassuring. A score of 6 or 7 out of 10 is equivocal and must be repeated within 24 hours • A score of 4 or less is a positive test and strongly suggests preparing the patient for delivery
Ultrasound	Monthly ultrasound examinations starting at 32–36 weeks	Estimation of fetal weight

(BPP: biophysical profile)

- Women should be explained about the importance of maternal glycemic control during labor and birth and early feeding of the baby to reduce the risk of neonatal hypoglycemia.
- The patient must be instructed to not skip doses of insulin. She should be advised to not smoke or drink alcohol or abuse illicit drugs.
- Monthly measurement of HbA1c levels in the preconceptional period and third trimester of pregnancy must be advised.

Fetal Monitoring during the Antenatal Period

Fetal surveillance involves screening for congenital anomalies, monitoring for fetal well-being, and ultrasound assessment for estimated fetal weight and macrosomia. The schedule of various tests for fetal surveillance during the antenatal period is described in **Table 19.13**.

Screening for Congenital Malformations

Since the fetuses of diabetic women are at a particularly high risk of congenital malformations, screening for these malformations must be started as soon as possible. The most common congenital anomaly includes congenital heart disease. The earliest anomaly related to pregestational diabetes is neural tube defects. Therefore, first-trimester ultrasound scan at 11–13 weeks must be done to look for nuchal translucency. Fetal echo scan needs to be done at 16 weeks to rule out any congenital heart anomaly. Second-trimester ultrasound scan for detailed scanning for fetal congenital anomalies must be done at 18–20 weeks. Fetal echo scan may again be repeated at 24 weeks if a cardiac lesion is suspected.

The methods of fetal surveillance for monitoring fetal well-being depend on whether the patients are at low or high risk, both of which are described below.

- *Low-risk patients:* Low-risk gestational diabetic patients who have achieved adequate glycemic control with diet and exercise and do not develop any of the complications related to gestational diabetes including macrosomia, polyhydramnios, or preeclampsia need not be admitted to the hospital. They must be seen in the clinic on biweekly basis from 36 weeks onward. In these cases, nonstress test must be done during each visit. Amniotic fluid determinations can be done on monthly basis.

- *High-risk patients:* High-risk gestational diabetics and patients on oral antihypoglycemic therapy and/or insulin should have antepartum fetal surveillance testing starting at 28–32 weeks of gestation. Biweekly nonstress tests are most commonly performed, starting from 28 weeks onward.

Ultrasound monitoring of fetal growth, estimated fetal weight, and amniotic fluid volume needs to be done on monthly basis, starting from 28 to 36 weeks. The BPP or at least the amniotic volume is performed on weekly basis from 28 weeks onward. Women with diabetes and a risk of IUGR (macrovascular disease and/or nephropathy) require an individualized approach for monitoring fetal growth and well-being. Umbilical artery Doppler ultrasound can be done at every 3–4 weeks in IUGR fetuses.

Mode of Birth

- *Low-risk patients:* There is no need to deliver low-risk gestational diabetic patients before term. These women may be allowed to develop spontaneous labor and deliver by 38–40 weeks of gestation. However, there is no need to wait beyond 40 completed weeks of gestation. Once the uncomplicated gestational diabetic patient reaches 40 weeks, labor should be induced. Cesarean delivery may be required if the estimated fetal weight is >4,000 g or some other obstetrical indication for cesarean delivery is present.
- *High-risk patients:* High-risk gestational diabetic patients should have their labor induced when they reach 38 weeks. Cesarean delivery may be required if the estimated fetal weight is >4,000 g (macrosomia) or some other obstetrical indication for cesarean delivery is present. If delivered vaginally, macrosomic babies are at an increased risk of shoulder dystocia.

Diabetes should not in itself be considered a contraindication for attempting vaginal birth after a previous cesarean section. Pregnant women with diabetes who have an ultrasound-diagnosed macrosomic fetus should be informed of the risks and benefits of vaginal birth, induction of labor, and cesarean section. The final decision regarding the mode of delivery depends on the patient's wishes and the obstetrician's judgment. The ACOG recommends an elective cesarean section in women with sonographically estimated fetal weight of 4.5 kg. The role of cesarean delivery in cases of expected fetal weight between 4 and 4.5 kg is controversial.

Timing of Delivery

Since an unexpected intrauterine death (IUD) may be associated with GDM and pregestational diabetes, the clinician must take steps for pregnancy extending beyond the EDD. **Table 19.14** likely describes the timing for delivery based on the patient's control of her blood glucose levels.

TABLE 19.14: Deciding the timing for induction of labor.

Indication	Timing of delivery (weeks)
Well-controlled glucose levels with the patient on medical nutrition therapy (MNT)	39–40
Patient on oral hypoglycemic agents	38–39
Patient on insulin	37–38

MANAGEMENT DURING THE INTRAPARTUM PERIOD

Q. Discuss management in labor of a patient with diabetes mellitus.

The two main goals of intrapartum management include avoidance of shoulder dystocia and maintenance of blood glucose levels. The following precautions should be taken during the intrapartum period:

- During the time of labor and birth, capillary blood glucose should be monitored on an hourly basis in women with diabetes and maintained at the levels between 80 and 120 mg/dL by using IV dextrose and insulin infusion.
- Consent must be taken in lieu of the anticipated instrumental delivery.
- Cross-matched blood samples must be available.
- Babies born with gestational diabetes are particularly at risk of developing neonatal hypoglycemia. Early feeding of the neonate is recommended for reducing the risk of neonatal hypoglycemia.
- Pediatrician must be present at the time of baby's delivery. The obstetrician must be well versed with the management of shoulder dystocia.
- Use of corticosteroids for pulmonary maturity in diabetic women, in whom preterm delivery may be required, is considered controversial as the administration of steroids in diabetic women may cause significant worsening of glycemic control requiring an increase in insulin dose.

However, diabetes should not be considered a contraindication for administration of antenatal steroids in order to achieve fetal pulmonary maturation. Insulin-treated diabetic individuals who are receiving steroids for fetal lung maturation should be closely monitored for their blood glucose levels for at least 5–7 days and can be given additional insulin according to a preagreed protocol.

- Anesthetic assessment must be offered to women with diabetes and comorbidities such as obesity or autonomic neuropathy during the third trimester of pregnancy. If general anesthesia is used at the time of cesarean section in women with diabetes, blood glucose levels should be monitored regularly, preferably at every half-hourly interval, starting right from the induction of general anesthesia until after the baby is born and the woman

becomes fully conscious. General anesthesia in women is associated with high risk of hypoglycemia. These women also have a high rate of Mendelson syndrome due to the higher resting gastric volume compared to women without diabetes.
- Betamimetic drugs should not be used for tocolysis in women with diabetes due to the tendency of betamimetics to cause hyperglycemia and ketoacidosis. Tocolytic agents of choice in these cases are nifedipine and magnesium sulfate.
- Delivery should be by the vaginal route unless there are obstetric contraindications. Some of the indications for cesarean delivery in these cases are described in **Box 19.5**.
- Since fetal distress is more common in diabetic women, continuous external or internal cardiotocographic monitoring is required at the time of labor. Fetal scalp blood may also be analyzed in case of nonreassuring fetal heart trace.
- Capillary blood glucose levels must be checked frequently using finger stick at every 1–2-hourly intervals and regular insulin must be administered accordingly **(Table 19.15)**. The target range for glucose concentration is 4.0–8.0 mmol/L or 80–120 mg/dL. Insulin requirement during labor may fall due to uterine contractions. Two separate IV lines must be started: one for IV infusion of short-acting insulin (50 units of Human Actrapid in 50 mL of normal saline to produce insulin concentration of 1 unit/mL) and second for dextrose with potassium (500 mL of 10% dextrose and 20 mmol/L of KCl at the rate of 100 mL/h). Potassium is added as insulin drives extracellular K^+ into the cells.
- Insulin requirements at the time of labor in diabetic women are shown in **Table 19.16**. It is important to reduce or omit the dose of long-acting insulin given on the day of delivery. Since the insulin requirements drop markedly after delivery, regular insulin must be used to meet most or all the insulin requirements of the mother.

BOX 19.5: Indications for cesarean delivery in women with gestational diabetes.
- Expected fetal weight > 4.5 kg (ACOG)
- Previous history of shoulder dystocia/stillbirths
- Presence of other obstetric indications for cesarean delivery

TABLE 19.15: Low-dose insulin infusion for diabetic women during the intrapartum period.

Blood glucose (g/dL)	Insulin dosage (U/h)	IV fluids (125 mL/h)
<120	0	D_5 lactated ringer
121–140	4	Normal saline
141–180	6	Normal saline
>180	8	Normal saline

In cases of vaginal delivery, prostaglandin gel should be used as early as possible in the morning.
- In case of elective cesarean delivery, the diabetic woman must be taken up as the first case in the morning. In these cases, the usual insulin dosage and meal must be given an evening before surgery. The woman must be put on fast from midnight onward.
- In case of women with type 1 diabetes mellitus or gestational diabetes already receiving insulin in the antenatal period, insulin requirements are described in **Tables 19.17 and 19.18**, respectively, depending on whether the insulin requirement is <40 or >40 units/day.

Neonatal Care

Q. Write a short essay discussing the management of a baby born to a diabetic mother.

- Women with diabetes should preferably be advised to give birth in hospitals where advanced neonatal resuscitation skills are available 24 hours a day.
- Routine admission of these babies to the neonatal unit is not required unless conditions mentioned in **Box 19.6** are present. Normal babies of women with diabetes should be kept with their mothers. Women should be encouraged to have skin-to-skin contact with their babies as soon as possible after birth. They should be advised to start breastfeeding as soon as possible after birth and ideally within an hour.
- Development of hypoglycemia (blood glucose <2.6 mmol/L or <40 mg/dL), i.e., in these babies is a major concern. The pathogenesis of fetal hypoglycemia is demonstrated in **Flowchart 19.3**. The obstetrician and

TABLE 19.16: Insulin requirements at the time of labor.

Day before induction	Day of induction
• Normal diet to be given • Normal insulin dose, an evening before induction • No overnight fasting	• Administration of half the morning dose of regular insulin before a light breakfast • IV infusion to be started once the labor establishes • Blood glucose levels need to be monitored so as to maintain levels between 80 to 120 mg/dL

TABLE 19.17: Low-dose insulin protocol for women with type 1 diabetes mellitus and gestational diabetes receiving <40 U/day of insulin antenatally.

Blood glucose (mmol/L)	Subcutaneous insulin injection
0–5	Nil
5.1–7.0	2 units
7.1–10.0	4 units
10.1–13.0	6 units
>13	8 units

TABLE 19.18: Low-dose insulin protocol for women with type 1 diabetes mellitus and gestational diabetes receiving >40 U/day of insulin antenatally.	
Blood glucose (mmol/L)	Subcutaneous insulin injection
0–5	Nil
5.1–7.0	4 units
7.1–10.0	6 units
10.1–13.0	8 units
>13	10 units

BOX 19.6: Indications for admission to the neonatal units.
- Hypoglycemia associated with abnormal clinical signs
- Respiratory distress
- Cardiac decompensation due to congenital heart disease or cardiomyopathy
- Signs of neonatal encephalopathy
- Signs of polycythemia
- Requirement for IV fluids and tube feeding
- Jaundice requiring intense phototherapy and frequent monitoring of bilirubinemia

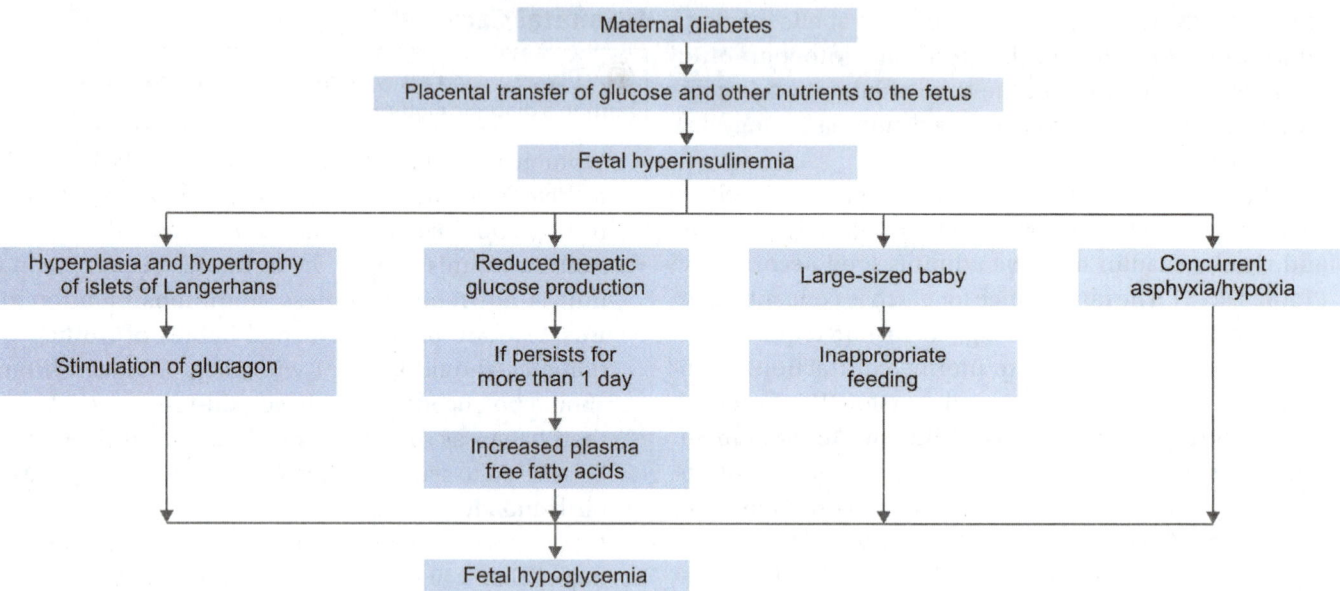

Flowchart 19.3: Pathogenesis of fetal hypoglycemia.

pediatrician must remain vigilant to anticipate and treat hypoglycemia. The following steps need to be taken:
1. Blood glucose testing should be carried out routinely at birth in babies of women with diabetes. This should be repeated at every 2–4-hour interval.
2. Early breastfeeding must be encouraged.
3. These babies should be fed as soon as possible after birth (within 30 minutes) and then at frequent intervals (every 2–3 hours) in order to maintain blood glucose concentration of at least 2.0 mmol/L.
4. If symptoms of hypoglycemia develop, a bolus dose of 2–4 mL/kg IV 10% dextrose may be administered.
5. In case the blood glucose values remain below 2.0 mmol/L on two consecutive occasions despite maximal maternal feeding, additional measures such as tube feeding or IV dextrose infusion (6–8 mg/kg/min) may be required.

- Blood tests for polycythemia, hyperbilirubinemia, hypocalcemia, and hypomagnesemia should be carried out in babies with clinical signs. Polycythemia, which is primarily responsible for hyperbilirubinemia, could be due to the fetal response to relative hypoxia.
- Newborns of women with pregestational and gestational diabetic pregnancies frequently have hypertrophic cardiomyopathy. Therefore, an echocardiogram may be performed if the baby shows clinical signs associated with congenital heart disease or cardiomyopathy.
- These babies should be discharged only when the healthcare professionals are satisfied that the babies are maintaining blood glucose levels and are feeding well.
- *Long-term follow-up:* It is required in these babies because they are at the risk of development of neurodevelopment defects such as autism spectrum disorders and developmental delay. Also, the disorder shows genetic tendency. If either of the parent is affected with type 1 diabetes, the risk of developing type 1 diabetes in the child varies between 3% and 5%. Type 2 diabetes is associated with an even stronger genetic component. If both the parents are diabetic, the offspring's risk of developing diabetes approaches 40%. Therefore, a long-term follow-up of these babies becomes important to detect the future development of diabetes.

Postnatal Care

> **Q. What is the risk for subsequent development of type 2 diabetes in women with gestational diabetes?**

- There is a significant risk that women who develop gestational diabetes will subsequently develop type 2 diabetes. It is now known that approximately 50% of women with gestational diabetes are likely to develop type 2 diabetes within the coming 5–10 years. These women are also likely to develop gestational diabetes in subsequent pregnancies at an earlier period of gestation. Thus, regular screening for type 2 diabetes in the form of an OGTT at 3-year intervals should be strongly encouraged. Also, these women must be advised to follow lifestyle recommendations in the form of regular exercising (of moderate intensity) and weight reduction.
- Immediately after birth, the insulin requirements may fall; therefore, insulin doses must be reduced immediately to prepregnancy levels, in order to avoid hypoglycemia. In case of patients with pregestational diabetes, the prepregnancy dose of insulin may be administered. In women with gestational diabetes, no insulin may be required post delivery. However, blood glucose monitoring needs to be continued for 2 hours post delivery and then postprandially for next 48 hours.
- In women with type 1 diabetes mellitus prior to pregnancy, insulin must be restarted in the dosage of 0.5–0.6 U/kg on day 2–5 post delivery.
- Women with preexisting type 2 diabetes who are breastfeeding can resume or continue to take metformin and glibenclamide immediately following birth, but other OHAs should be avoided while breastfeeding.
- These women are also at an increased risk of hypoglycemia in the postnatal period, especially when breastfeeding. Thus, they should be advised to have a meal or snack before or during each feed.

Women with diabetes who are breastfeeding should continue to avoid any drugs for the treatment of diabetes and its complications that were discontinued for safety reasons in the preconception period. The safety of OHAs, angiotensin-converting enzyme inhibitors, angiotensin II receptor blockers, statins, calcium channel blockers, and antiobesity drugs in women who are breastfeeding has not been established. However, according to the NICE guidelines (2008), women with preexisting type 2 diabetes who are breastfeeding can start taking metformin and glibenclamide immediately following birth.

Women who were diagnosed with gestational diabetes (including those with ongoing impaired glucose regulation) should be informed about the risks of gestational diabetes in future pregnancies. They should be offered screening with 75-g OGTT (as recommended by the WHO criteria) or fasting plasma glucose (as recommended by the NICE) for diabetes at 6-week postpartum checkup and annually thereafter and while planning future pregnancies.

The blood glucose values for postpartum evaluation of glucose intolerance in women with gestational diabetes are shown in **Table 19.19**. According to the NICE guidelines (2008), women who were diagnosed with gestational diabetes should also be offered lifestyle advice (including weight control, diet, and exercise) at the time of discharge. Women who are found to have diabetes even at 6-week follow-up should be managed accordingly.

These women should also be offered contraceptive advice and the need for preconception care when planning future pregnancies. Oral contraceptives (combination of low-dose estrogen and progestogens) can be used safely in low doses in uncomplicated diabetic patients. However, since oral contraceptives may increase blood pressure and enhance platelet aggregation, they are not recommended in cases of diabetes complicated by angiopathy or other risk factors such as smoking, hypertension, and age (over 35 years). Progestogen-only pills are usually not recommended due to the risk of development of type 2 gestational diabetes. The use of intrauterine contraceptive devices is also considered to be safe during pregnancy. For patients in whom pregnancy is contraindicated on the basis of medical grounds or who do not want to become pregnant anymore, permanent method of contraception can be offered.

TABLE 19.19: Postpartum evaluation for glucose intolerance in women with gestational diabetes.

Blood glucose levels	Normal (mg/dL)	Impaired glucose tolerance (mg/dL)	Diabetes mellitus (mg/dL)
Fasting	<110	110–125	≥126
2 hours postprandial	<140	140–199	≥200

Antenatal Banking of Colostrum

Babies of women with diabetes are at an increased risk of neonatal hypoglycemia and may require frequent early feeding for maintenance of normal blood glucose levels. Women with diabetes are encouraged to express and store colostrum before birth. Antenatal expression and storage of colostrum may be of benefit to babies of women with diabetes. This is especially so because increased risk of neonatal complications in babies born to diabetic women may require admission to intensive/special care units. This may prevent opportunities for early skin-to-skin contact and initiation of breastfeeding. Presently, there is no good evidence to support the effectiveness of antenatal banking of colostrum in women with diabetes. Future randomized controlled trials are required in order to determine the safety and cost-effectiveness of this practice. Until that time, it is better that the practice of antenatal colostrum banking is not strongly encouraged.

COMPLICATIONS

> **Q.** With the help of a long essay, discuss the maternal and fetal complications associated with gestational diabetes mellitus (GDM).
>
> **Q.** Discuss the complications in newborns to a diabetic mother.
>
> **Q.** A 26-year-old G2P1A0L1 woman is diagnosed with GDM at 24 weeks of gestation. Discuss in detail the maternal and fetal complications of GDM.

Diabetes in pregnancy is associated with numerous risks to the mother and the developing fetus as well as the newborn baby, which are enumerated in **Table 19.20**. Maternal hyperglycemia is likely to cause fetal hyperinsulinemia, which may result in the following:

- An overgrowth of insulin-sensitive tissues such as adipose tissues, especially around the chest, shoulders, and abdomen, which increases the risk of shoulder dystocia
- Increased risk for perinatal death, birth trauma, and rates of cesarean section
- Neonatal metabolic complications such as hypoglycemia
- Fetal hypoxia, which may increase the risk of intrauterine fetal death
- Fetal polycythemia, hyperbilirubinemia, and renal vein thrombosis
- Increased long-term risk of obesity and diabetes in the child

TABLE 19.20: Maternal and fetal complications related to gestational diabetes.

Maternal complications	Fetal complications
- Miscarriage - Preeclampsia - Preterm labor - Prolonged labor - Polyhydramnios (could be associated with fetal polyuria) - About 35–50% risk of developing type 2 diabetes later in life - Increased risk of traumatic damage during labor - Increased risk of shoulder dystocia - Diabetic retinopathy and nephropathy can worsen rapidly during pregnancy	- Fetal distress and birth asphyxia - Brachial plexus injuries - Cephalohematoma, resulting in more pronounced neonatal jaundice - Stillbirth, congenital malformations, macrosomia, birth injury, increased perinatal mortality - Hypoxia and sudden/unexplained intrauterine death after 36 weeks' gestation - Congenital malformations - Fetal hypoglycemia, polycythemia, hyperbilirubinemia, and renal vein thrombosis

MATERNAL COMPLICATIONS

Some of the maternal complications are described below in detail.

Polyhydramnios

Women diagnosed with pregestational diabetes or GDM having elevated HbA1c values are likely to develop hydramnios in the third trimester [amniotic fluid index (AFI) > 24 cm]. In case of polyhydramnios prior to 34 weeks of gestation, in the absence of preterm labor or PROM, indomethacin can be administered. In the presence of preterm labor, indomethacin is not administered due to the risk of premature closure of ductus arteriosus.

Preeclampsia

Gestational diabetes mellitus is commonly associated with the development of preeclampsia or hypertension during pregnancy. The ACOG recommends low-dose oral aspirin in the dosage of 81 mg/day between 12 and 28 weeks of gestation until delivery of the woman with type 1 or type 2 diabetes.

Preterm Labor/Preterm Rupture of Membranes

Women with gestational diabetes are at an increased risk of developing preterm labor or preterm premature rupture of membranes (PPROM). In these cases, the gestation age of the fetus becomes important because the lungs may not have attained sufficient maturity. Though administration of corticosteroids is likely to be associated with a rise in blood glucose levels, the benefit of administration of steroids to expedite fetal lung maturity outweighs its risk. Two doses of betamethasone (12 mg) must be administered 12 hours apart. These women are likely to be at an increased risk of infections, so antibiotics need to be administered. Tocolytics can also be used in these cases to inhibit premature uterine contractions. The tocolytic of choice in these cases is nifedipine. Beta adrenoceptor agonists such as isoxsuprine are to be largely avoided due to the problem of volume overload. Atosiban serves as a useful tocolytic drug. However, it is too expensive. Therefore, majority of centers in India may be unable to use it.

Infections

Such women are at an increased risk of developing infections, particularly candidiasis and urinary tract infections.

Unexplained Intrauterine Deaths/Stillbirths

Unexplained IUDs/stillbirths can be considered as the most dreaded complication of uncontrolled diabetes in pregnancy, with the risk of IUD with uncontrolled diabetes being about 30%. This risk is reduced to 3% if diabetes is well controlled. Some probable causes for stillbirths in pregnancy include, hypoxia, maternal ketoacidosis, electrolyte imbalance, abruption, etc.

Maternal Deaths

Maternal deaths, although rare, are mainly related to diabetic complications such as ketoacidosis, hypoglycemia, hypertension, and infection.

Complications Specific to Pregestational Diabetes

Diabetic Ketoacidosis

Diabetic ketoacidosis may develop in 1% pregnancies and is commonly encountered in women with type 1 diabetes. Therefore, it is commonly observed in cases of pregestational diabetes rather than GDM. DKA is a serious complication, which can cause fetal death at any stage. All diabetic women should also test their urine for ketones, especially if their blood glucose levels are high, if vomiting occurs or if they are unwell.

Risk factors for development of DKA are tabulated in **Box 19.7**. DKA occurs due to the deficiency of insulin in combination with an excess of counter-regulatory hormones, resulting in gluconeogenesis and formation of ketone bodies (especially hydroxybutyrate). The mainstay of management in these cases is rigorous rehydration with crystalloid solutions of normal saline or Ringer's lactate. Management of DKA is summarized in **Box 19.8**.

> **BOX 19.7:** Risk factors for development of diabetic ketoacidosis in pregnant women with pregestational diabetes.
>
> - Hyperemesis gravidarum
> - Infection
> - Insulin noncompliance
> - Insulin pump failure
> - Administration of beta-mimetic drugs for tocolysis or corticosteroids for lung maturation

> **BOX 19.8:** Management of diabetic ketoacidosis.
>
> - *Insulin:* Bolus dosage of 0.1–0.2 U/kg IV followed by infusion at the rate of 0.1 U/kg/h (rate is doubled if there is no fall in the blood glucose levels within 2 hours)
> - *IV fluids:* Initially, normal saline (NS) is infused at the rate of 1 L/h, reducing to 0.5 L/4 hours depending on the volume status. This must be changed to 0.45 NS (half-strength NS) once the BP and heart rate have stabilized and there is adequate renal perfusion. Switch to 5% glucose in 0.5 NS once blood glucose levels have reached 250 mg/dL
> - *Potassium:* Addition of 10–20 mEq/h KCl to the IV fluids after 2–3 hours
> - *Sodium bicarbonate:* If arterial pH is <7.0, 50 mEq of sodium bicarbonate is added to the IV fluids. Bicarbonate infusion is discontinued once blood pH > 7.1
> - *Phosphate:* Addition of 3–4 mol/h of potassium phosphate infusion is advocated if serum phosphate levels are within the low–normal range
> - *Antibiotics*

Diabetic Nephropathy

Diabetic nephropathy is the leading cause of end-stage renal disease. The first clinical feature of diabetic nephropathy is microalbuminuria. Macroalbuminuria may develop in patients destined to have end-stage renal disease. Such patients are often at a risk of developing hypertension and renal failure over a period of 5–10 years.

Diabetic Retinopathy

Retinal vasculopathy may occur with both type 1 and type 2 diabetes. The first lesion to appear in these cases is microaneurysm followed by blot hemorrhages, which occur due to the escape of erythrocytes from the aneurysms. Leakage of serous fluid results in the formation of hard exudates. This stage is known as nonproliferative or background retinopathy. With the progression of retinopathy, background vessels become occluded. There is formation of cotton wool exudates as a result of retinal ischemia and infraction. This stage is known as preproliferative retinopathy. Neovascularization soon sets in response to ischemia and begins to develop on the retinal surface and vitreous cavity, resulting in proliferative retinopathy. These vessels may bleed, resulting in obscuration of vision and blindness. Laser photocoagulation prior to hemorrhage is likely to reduce the progression of visual loss and blindness. Therefore, it is important for the woman with pregestational diabetes to get a fundus examination done in the preconception period. In case of proliferative retinopathy, she must get laser photocoagulation done before embarking upon pregnancy. Otherwise there remains a risk of retinal hemorrhages at the time of delivery, which can result in blindness.

Diabetic Neuropathy

Common manifestation of diabetic neuropathy in pregnancy is diabetic gastropathy. This may be associated with nutritional problems, nausea, vomiting, and difficult glucose control. This condition is likely to respond to treatment with metoclopramide, dopamine D2 receptor antagonists, and gastric neurostimulators.

■ FETAL COMPLICATIONS

Some of the fetal complications are mentioned in **Table 19.21** and are described below in detail.

Congenital Malformations

Infants of women with established IDDM have >10 times the risk in comparison to the general population for development of congenital malformations. While the risk of congenital malformation is increased, the risk of chromosomal malformations remains same as that of the general population. They also have five times the risk

TABLE 19.21: Fetal problems related to maternal hyperglycemia in the three trimesters of pregnancy.

First trimester	Second trimester	Third trimester
• Fetal congenital malformations • Growth retardation • Recurrent miscarriage	• Hypertrophic cardiomyopathy • Polyhydramnios • Placental insufficiency • Preeclampsia	• Hypoglycemia • Hypocalcemia • Hyperbilirubinemia • Respiratory distress syndrome • Macrosomia • Hypomagnesemia • Intrauterine death • Low intelligence quotient in the newborn

TABLE 19.22: Renshaw's (1978) classification of sacral agenesis.

Type	Characteristics
Type I	Unilateral sacral agenesis (partial or unilateral)
Type II	Bilateral, symmetrical, partial, sacral agenesis. The sacral vertebra may be normal or hypoplastic. There is stable articulation between the ilium and first sacral vertebra
Type III	There may be variable amount of sacral agenesis. The ilia may be articulating with the sides of the lowest vertebra present
Type IV	There may be variable amount of lumbar and total sacral agenesis with the caudal endplate of the lowest vertebra either articulating or fused with the ilia or iliac amphiarthrosis

BOX 19.9: Various types of congenital malformations associated with gestational diabetes.

- *Congenital heart disease:* Ventricular septal defect, transposition of great vessels, aortic stenosis, pulmonary atresia, dextrocardia, tetralogy of Fallot, truncus arteriosus, situs inversus, etc. (most common anomaly)
- *Neural tube defects:* Anencephaly, spina bifida, hydrocephaly, etc. (earliest anomaly to appear)
- Cystic fibrosis, in association with meconium ileus
- *Gastrointestinal abnormalities:* Ileal atresia, rectal/anal atresia, Hirschsprung's disease, etc.
- Congenital microcolon
- *Renal defects:* Agenesis, cystic kidney, duplex ureter, etc.
- Caudal regression sequence (most specific anomaly)

for stillbirth. If hyperglycemia is present during the first trimester of pregnancy when organogenesis is taking place, congenital malformations may occur. The risk of congenital malformations is also increased in cases of gestational diabetes, but this risk is less in comparison to the women with pregestational diabetes. Some of the congenital abnormalities commonly encountered in the babies of diabetic mothers are listed in **Box 19.9**.

Sacral Agenesis

Sacral agenesis, also known as caudal regression syndrome or sacral hypoplasia, is associated with abnormal development of the sacral bone. It is not the most common congenital anomaly encountered in cases of pregestational diabetes but is certainly the most specific one. It is likely to be 80 times more common in women with pregestational diabetes. Renshaw (1978) has classified sacral agenesis on the basis of amount of sacrum remaining and the characteristics of articulation between the spine and pelvis **(Table 19.22 and Figs. 19.6A and B)**.

Minor abnormalities may not cause any deformity and hence do not require any correction. Severe cases may present with spinal–pelvic instability and/or severe knee contractures with popliteal webbing of the knees. Reconstruction of limbs may be required in type IV defects, which may not be entirely successful. Bilateral subtrochanteric amputation may be done in some cases. Some surgeons have advocated spinal–pelvic fusion in order to protect the viscera from unphysiological compression and angulation. Knee flexion and foot deformities can be corrected at an early age using a combination of surgical release procedures, supracondylar femoral extension osteotomies, and serial casting.

Intrauterine Fetal Death

According to the ADA (1999), a fasting hyperglycemia of more than 105 mg/dL may be associated with an increased risk of fetal death during the last 4–8 weeks of gestation.

Macrosomia

The term macrosomia is often used to describe birth weight > 4,000 g or birth weight ≥ 90th percentile for gestational age. This is also referred to as LGA fetuses (ACOG, 2000). Fetal macrosomia occurs in 17–30% of pregnancies with gestational diabetes **(Figs. 19.7 and 19.8)** as compared with 10% in nondiabetic population. There are two types of macrosomia: symmetric and asymmetric. Symmetric macrosomia accounts for about 70% of cases. Asymmetric macrosomia is characterized by thoracic and abdominal circumference that is relatively larger than the head circumference. In symmetric macrosomia, the baby is symmetrically large on the whole. Symmetric macrosomia may also occur in women without diabetes. Some other causes of symmetric fetal macrosomia are listed in **Box 19.10**. The macrosomic baby is at an increased risk of shoulder dystocia, clavicular fracture, brachial palsy, and an overall increased rate of cesarean section. It has also been suggested that babies with asymmetric macrosomia may be at an increased risk of developing obesity, coronary heart disease, hypertension, and type 2 diabetes later in life. The pathogenesis of macrosomia is shown in **Flowchart 19.4**.

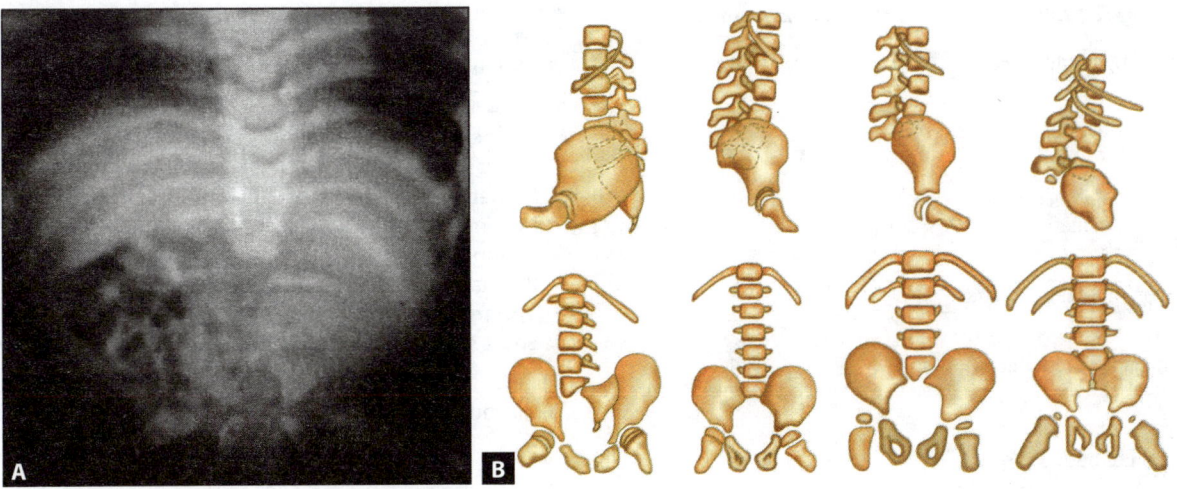

Figs. 19.6A and B: Sacral agenesis. (A) X-ray appearance: anterior–posterior view; (B) Renshaw's staging system for sacral agenesis.

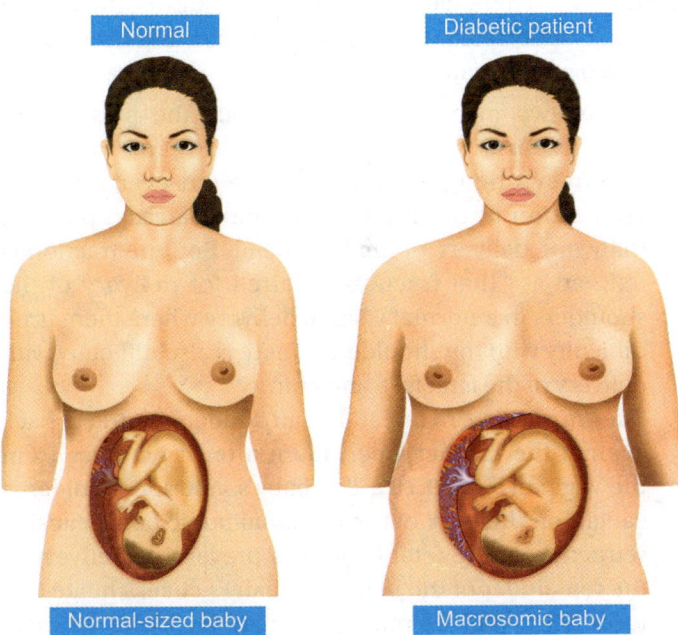

Fig. 19.7: Risk of development of macrosomia in diabetic patients.

Fig. 19.8: Macrosomic baby weighing 5.3 kg at birth.

BOX 19.10: Causes of macrosomia.
- Inaccurate dating of last menstrual period
- Familial, i.e., everyone in the family is large
- Chromosomal defects
- Hydrops fetalis
- Beckwith–Wiedemann syndrome

Management

The management of macrosomia is controversial. The ACOG (2020) concludes that presently the data is insufficient to determine if cesarean delivery must be performed in women with GDM having an ultrasonographically estimated weight ≥ 4.5 kg in order to avoid the risks associated with birth trauma. Nevertheless, the ACOG (2020) still acknowledges that prophylactic cesarean delivery may be considered in diabetic women with an estimated fetal weight ≥ 4.5 kg. The controversy arises when the expected fetal weight is between 4,000 and 4,500 g. Some investigators argue that a cesarean section must be routinely performed in these cases as the shoulder and trunk pads of these fetuses are relatively larger than the head, thereby favoring shoulder dystocia at the time of the birth. However, if trial of vaginal delivery is being performed, the clinician must remain extremely vigilant and must immediately perform a cesarean delivery with the development of any abnormality of labor such as delayed active phase, failure of descent, or secondary arrest of cervical dilatation. Assisted vaginal delivery in the form of vacuum or forceps application should not be used in these patients.

Gestational diabetes may reoccur in future pregnancies, and approximately 55% of the patients, usually those who are obese or with prior macrosomic infants, will show glucose intolerance in subsequent pregnancies. Gestational diabetics should be informed that they are at high risk for becoming type 2 diabetics later in their lives. Roughly, 40–60% will be overt diabetics when they are in their fifth decade.

Lifestyle changes such as weight loss, dietary control, and exercise will help in preventing overt diabetes later in life.

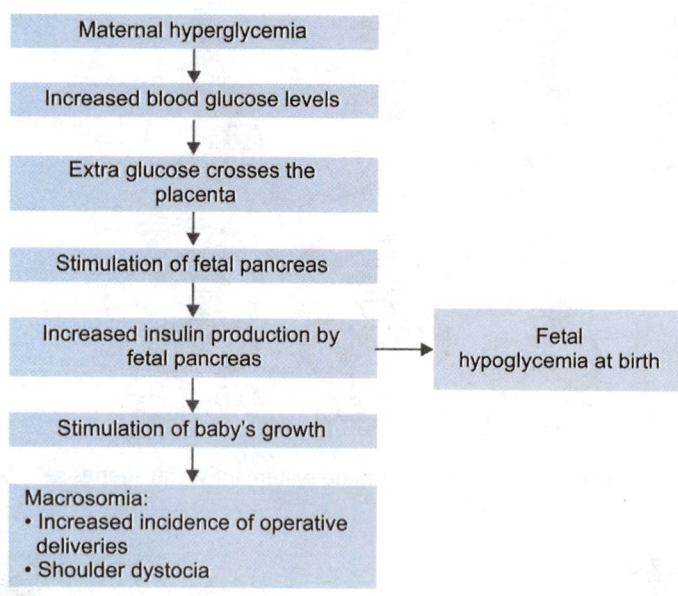

Flowchart 19.4: Pathogenesis of fetal macrosomia.

TABLE 19.23: Risk factors for development of shoulder dystocia.	
Prelabor factors	**Intrapartum factors**
• Previous history of shoulder dystocia • Macrosomia • Diabetes mellitus • Maternal BMI > 30 kg/m² • Multiparity • Postdated pregnancy • Abnormal pelvic anatomy • Short stature (<5 feet or 1.5 m)	• Prolonged first stage of labor • Secondary arrest • Prolonged second stage of labor • Oxytocin augmentation • Failure of descent of the head • Increased rate of assisted vaginal delivery
(BMI: body mass index)	

Intrauterine Growth Restriction

Women with diabetes are also at risk of having an IUGR baby, especially in the presence of accompanying preeclampsia. In these cases, fetal surveillance must be done using techniques such as umbilical artery Doppler ultrasound, fetal cardiotocography, and BPP.

Shoulder Dystocia

> **Q. What are the other risk factors besides gestational diabetes for development of shoulder dystocia? Describe various maneuvers used for managing a case of shoulder dystocia.**

Some of the risk factors for development of shoulder dystocia are described in **Table 19.23**.

Due to limitations in ultrasound-related predictive accuracy of macrosomia in uncomplicated cases, suspected macrosomia alone is not an indication for primary cesarean delivery. Despite the lack of evidence, most clinicians in the United States are of a view that cesarean delivery may be a reasonable management option in pregnancies with suspected fetal macrosomia when the estimated fetal weight is >5,000 g in a nondiabetic woman or >4,500 g in a woman with diabetes for the prevention of shoulder dystocia.

Shoulder dystocia can be defined as the inability to deliver the fetal shoulders after the delivery of the fetal head without the aid of specific maneuvers (other than the gentle downward traction on the head) **(Figs. 19.9A to C)**. It usually results when the diameter of the fetal shoulders (bisacromial diameter) is relatively larger than the biparietal diameter. Shoulder dystocia can be of two types: high shoulder dystocia and low shoulder dystocia. Low shoulder dystocia results due to the failure of engagement of the anterior shoulder and impaction of anterior shoulder over the maternal symphysis pubis. This type of shoulder dystocia is also known as unilateral shoulder dystocia. This is a more common type and is easily dealt with using standard techniques. There can be a high perinatal mortality and morbidity associated with the complication and needs to be managed appropriately.

There are two main signs that indicate the presence of shoulder dystocia:
1. The baby's body does not emerge out even after the application of routine traction and maternal pushing following delivery of the fetal head. Routine traction is defined as "that traction required for delivery of the shoulders in a normal vaginal delivery where there is no difficulty with the shoulders." There is also difficulty with delivery of the fetal face and chin.
2. *The "turtle sign"*: The fetal head suddenly retracts back against the mother's perineum after it emerges from the vagina **(Fig. 19.10)**. The baby's anterior shoulder is caught on the back of the maternal pubic bone, causing retraction of the fetal head and preventing delivery of the remainder of the baby. The baby's cheeks bulge out, resembling a turtle pulling its head back into its shell. There is failure of restitution of the fetal head and descent of shoulders.

Prediction of Shoulder Dystocia

Shoulder dystocia is a largely unpredictable and unpreventable event as a large majority of cases occur in the children of women with no risk factors. Clinicians should be aware of existing risk factors but must always be alert to the possibility of shoulder dystocia with any delivery. Shoulder dystocia has been observed to recur in about 1–16% cases.

Management

The immediate steps which need to be taken in case of an anticipated or a recognized case of shoulder dystocia include the following **(Flowchart 19.5)**:
1. Shoulder dystocia drill should form an important part of training for the junior doctor and nurses.

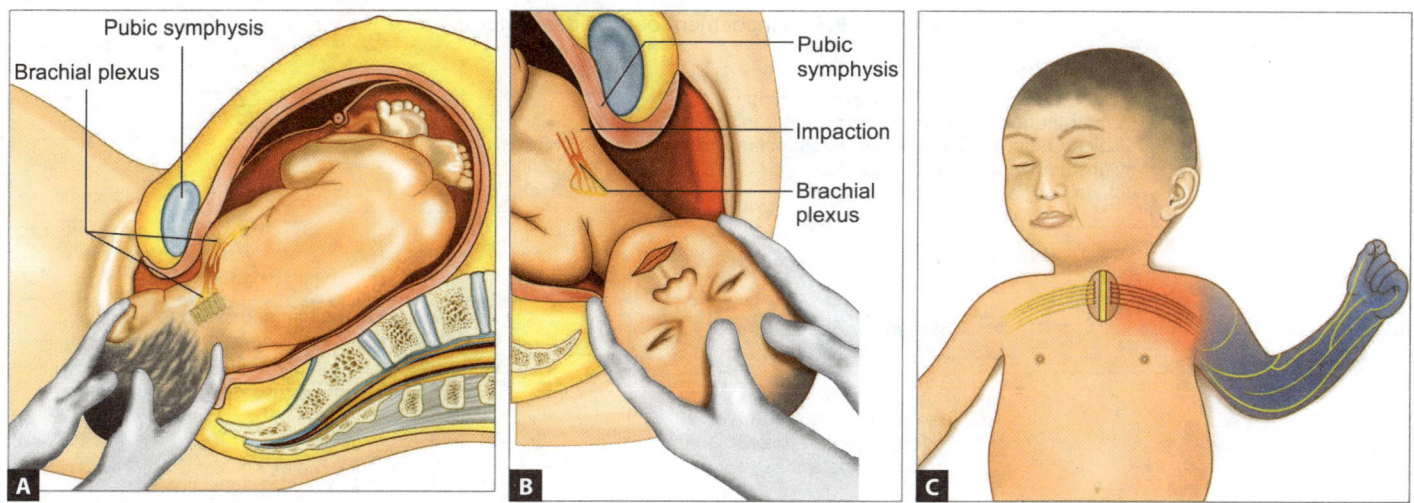

Figs. 19.9A to C: Shoulder dystocia. (A) Development of shoulder dystocia; (B) Injury to brachial plexus as a result of undue traction on fetal neck; (C) Effect on the baby's left arm due to the injury to left-sided brachial plexus.

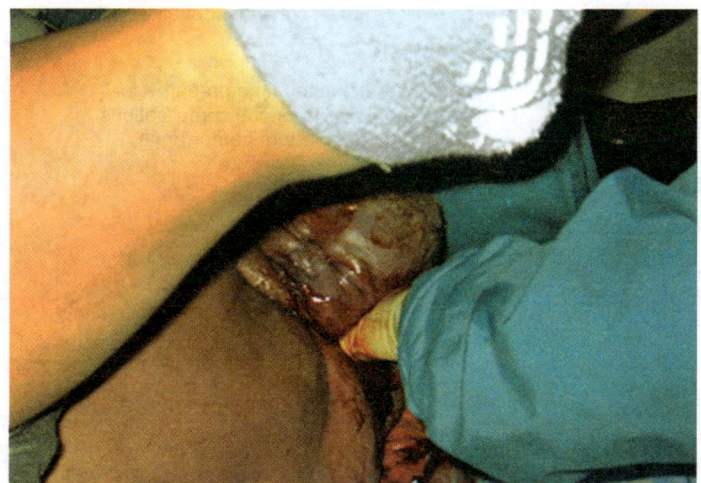

Fig. 19.10: Turtle sign. Neonatal face and head retracted up against the maternal perineum.

2. Immediately after recognition of shoulder dystocia, help should be summoned urgently. This should include further midwifery assistance, an obstetrician, a pediatric resuscitation team, and an anesthetist.
3. Maternal pushing and fetal pulling and pivoting should be discouraged as this may lead to further impaction of the shoulders.
4. The woman should be maneuvered to bring the buttocks to the edge of the bed.
5. Fundal pressure should not be employed. It is associated with a high rate of neonatal complications and may sometimes even result in uterine rupture.
6. Routine use of episiotomy is not necessary for all cases. Clinicians should apply their own discretion regarding whether an episiotomy needs to be given or not.
7. Management of shoulder dystocia needs to be done within 5–7 minutes of the delivery of the fetal head.
8. After delivery, the clinicians should be alert regarding the possibility of postpartum hemorrhage and third- and fourth-degree perineal tears.

McRoberts maneuver: If the above-mentioned steps do not prove to be useful, the McRoberts maneuver is the single most effective intervention, which is associated with success rates as high as 90% and should be performed first.

Prophylactic McRoberts position may also be recommended in cases where shoulder dystocia is anticipated. The McRoberts maneuver **(Figs. 19.11A and B)** involves sharp flexion and abduction of the maternal hips and positioning the maternal thighs on her abdomen. This maneuver helps in cephalad rotation of the symphysis pubis and the straightening of lumbosacral angle. This maneuver, by straightening the sacrum, tends to free the impacted anterior shoulder. In a large number of cases, this maneuver by itself helps to free the impacted anterior shoulder.

- *Suprapubic pressure:* Suprapubic pressure in conjunction with McRoberts maneuver is often all that is needed to resolve 50–60% cases of shoulder dystocia. It is the attempt to manually dislodge the anterior shoulder from behind the symphysis pubis during a shoulder dystocia. In this maneuver, the attendant makes a fist and places it just above the maternal pubic bone and pushes in a downward and lateral direction to push the posterior aspect of the anterior shoulder toward the fetal chest for a period of at least 30 seconds **(Fig. 19.12)**. Since shoulder dystocia is caused by an infant's shoulders entering the pelvis in a direct anterior–posterior orientation instead of the more physiologic oblique diameter, pushing the baby's anterior shoulder to one side or the other from above often helps in changing its position to the oblique, which would facilitate its delivery.

412 Medical Disorders Related to Pregnancy

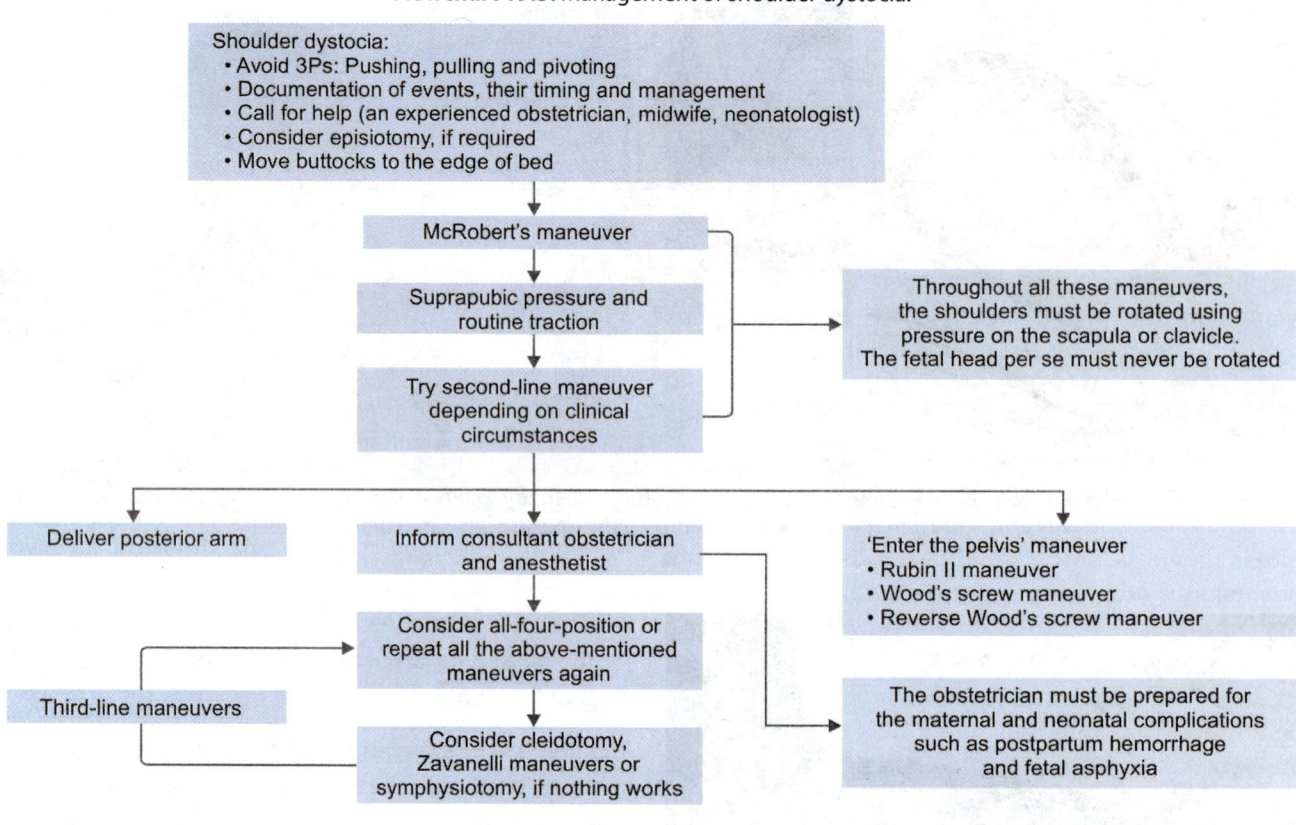

Flowchart 19.5: Management of shoulder dystocia.

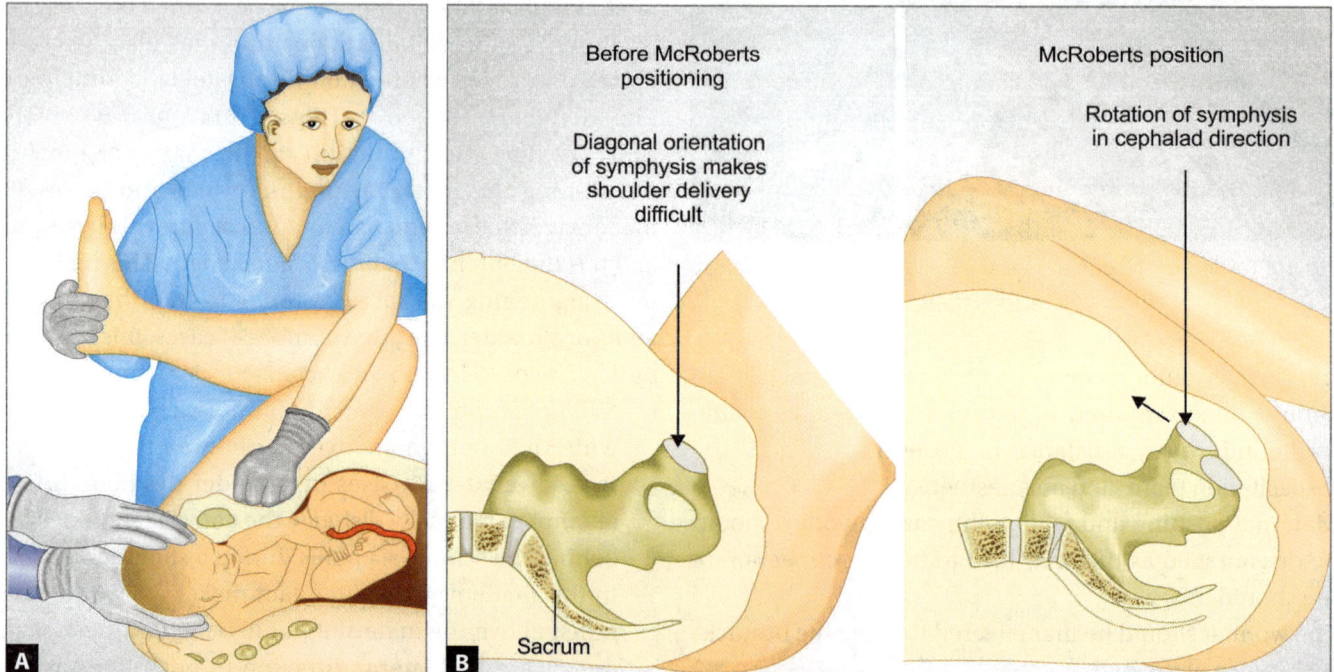

Figs. 19.11A and B: McRoberts maneuver. (A) Exaggerated hyperflexion of the thighs upon the maternal abdomen and application of suprapubic pressure; (B) McRoberts maneuver causes the rotation of pubic symphysis in cephalad direction and straightening of lumbosacral angle.

- Initial management in the cases of shoulder dystocia has also been summarized by the mnemonic HELPERR, which is elucidated in **Box 19.11**.
- If these simple measures (the McRoberts maneuver and suprapubic pressure) fail, then the obstetrician may have to resort to internal manipulation [enter the pelvis maneuvers **(Fig. 19.13)**].

The maneuvers for internal manipulation include Rubin II maneuver, Woods' screw maneuver, and reverse Woods' screw maneuver. At this juncture, it is to be noted that application of suprapubic pressure is known as Rubin I maneuver. Delivery of the posterior arm may be attempted in case of failure of "enter" maneuvers.

- *Enter maneuvers:* Firstly, Rubin II maneuver is attempted. If it fails, Woods' screw maneuver is attempted. Reverse Woods' screw maneuver is applied if even the Woods' screw maneuver fails.
  - *Rubin II maneuver:* In this maneuver, the obstetrician inserts the fingers of his/her right hand into the vagina and applies digital pressure onto the posterior aspect of the anterior shoulder, making an attempt to push it toward the fetal chest **(Fig. 19.14)**. This rotates the shoulders forward into the more favorable oblique diameter. The delivery is likely to be successful if attempted after the application of this maneuver.
  - *Woods' screw maneuver:* In this maneuver, the obstetrician's hand is placed behind the posterior shoulder of the fetus **(Fig. 19.15)**. The shoulder is rotated progressively by 180° in a corkscrew manner so that the impacted anterior shoulder is released. In addition to the corkscrew effect, pressure on the posterior shoulder has the advantage of flexing the fetal shoulders across the chest. This decreases the distance between the shoulders, thereby reducing the dimension that must come out through the pelvis.

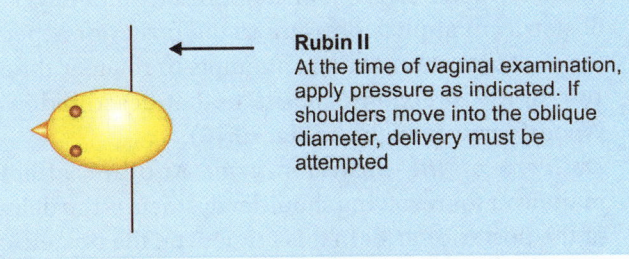

Rubin II
At the time of vaginal examination, apply pressure as indicated. If shoulders move into the oblique diameter, delivery must be attempted

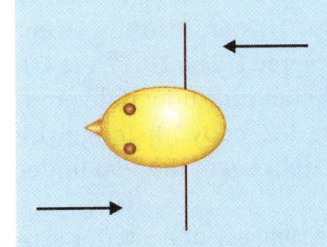

Rubin II + Woods' screw maneuver
If unsuccessful, add the Woods' screw maneuver and continue rotation in the same direction. Use both hands and apply pressure as indicated. If shoulders now move into the oblique diameter, delivery must be attempted. If this is unsuccessful, continue rotation by 180° and deliver

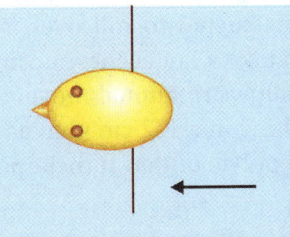

Reverse Woods' screw maneuver
If the last maneuver is unsuccessful, change to reverse Woods' screw maneuver. The obstetrician must slide fingers down to back of posterior shoulder and attempt 180° rotation in the opposite direction

Fig. 19.13: The "enter" maneuvers for shoulder dystocia, using the left occiput transverse position as an example.

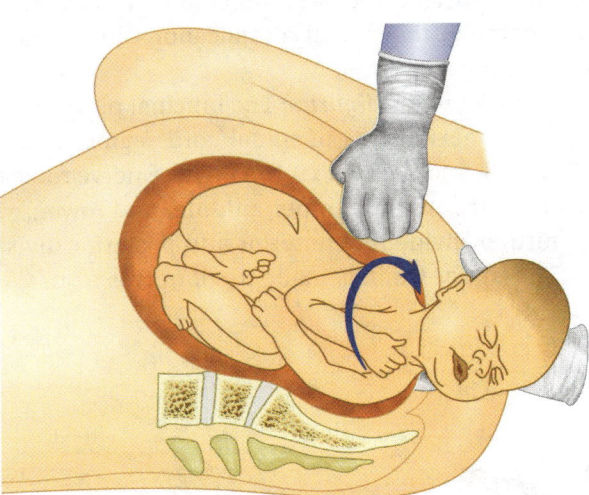

Fig. 19.12: Application of suprapubic pressure in the direction of fetal face.

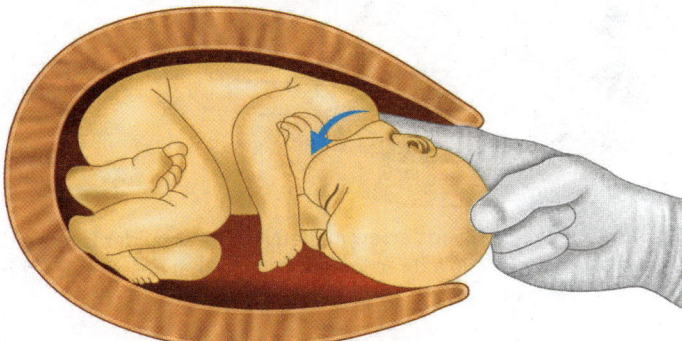

Fig. 19.14: Rubin II maneuver.

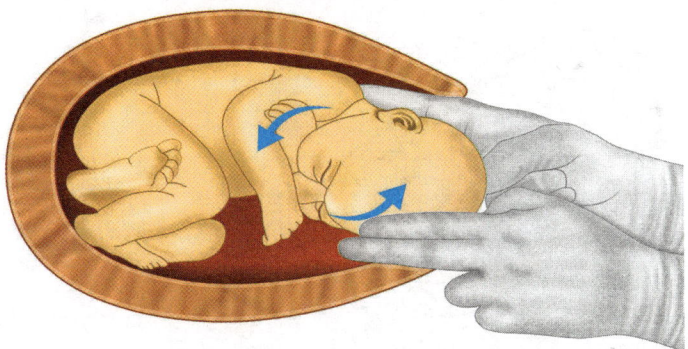

Fig. 19.15: Woods' screw maneuver. The hand is placed behind the posterior shoulder of the fetus. The shoulder is rotated progressively by 180° in a corkscrew manner so that the impacted anterior shoulder is released.

BOX 19.11: Mnemonic for describing initial management in the cases of shoulder dystocia.

H Call for help
E Evaluate for episiotomy
L Legs (the McRoberts maneuver)
P Suprapubic pressure
E Enter maneuvers (internal rotation)
R Remove the posterior arm
R Roll the patient

- *Reverse Woods' screw maneuver:* In this maneuver, the obstetrician applies pressure to the posterior aspect of the posterior shoulder and attempts to rotate it through 180° in the direction opposite to that described in the Woods' screw maneuver **(Fig. 19.16)**.
- *Delivery of the posterior arm:* Another effective maneuver for resolving shoulder dystocia is the delivery of the posterior arm. In this maneuver, the obstetrician places his or her hand behind the posterior shoulder of the fetus and locates the arm. This arm is then swept across the fetal chest and delivered **(Figs. 19.17A to C)**. With the posterior arm and shoulder now delivered, it is relatively easy to rotate the baby, dislodge the anterior shoulder, and allow delivery of the remainder of the baby.
- *All-four maneuver:* If even the delivery of posterior arm fails, an "all-four maneuver" must be employed. In this maneuver, the patient is instructed to roll over from her existing position and to take a knee–chest position on all her four limbs. This allows rotational movement of the sacroiliac joints, resulting in a 1–2 cm increase in the sagittal diameter of the pelvic outlet. It disimpacts the shoulders, allowing them to slide over the sacral promontory.

Third-Line Maneuvers (Last Resort Maneuvers)

Several third-line methods have been described for cases which are resistant to all simple measures. These are the last resort maneuvers in extremely resistant cases where nothing seems to work. Some of these maneuvers include cleidotomy (bending the clavicle with a finger or its surgical division), symphysiotomy (dividing the symphyseal ligament), the Zavanelli maneuver (cephalic replacement of the head followed by cesarean section), and administration of general anesthesia to cause uterine relaxation so as to facilitate delivery. These maneuvers are rarely employed in modern obstetric practice.

Zavanelli maneuver: It involves the rotation of fetal head back into its prerestitution position, i.e., occiput anterior **(Fig. 19.18A)**. Following this, the head is flexed and pushed back up into the vagina **(Fig. 19.18B)**. Once the fetal head gets back into the pelvis, an emergency cesarean section is performed to deliver a live baby.

Complications of Shoulder Dystocia

Following shoulder dystocia deliveries, 20% of babies will suffer some sort of injury, either temporary or permanent. The most common of these injuries are damage to the brachial plexus nerves, fracture of clavicles, fracture of humerus, contusions and lacerations, and birth asphyxia.
- *Fetal complications:* Fetal complications due to shoulder dystocia are as follows:
  - *Brachial plexus injuries:* The brachial plexus consists of the nerve roots of spinal cord segments C5, C6, C7, C8, and T1 **(Fig. 19.19A)**. These nerve roots form three trunks, i.e., upper, middle, and lower, which further divide into anterior and posterior divisions. The upper trunk is made up of nerves from C5 and

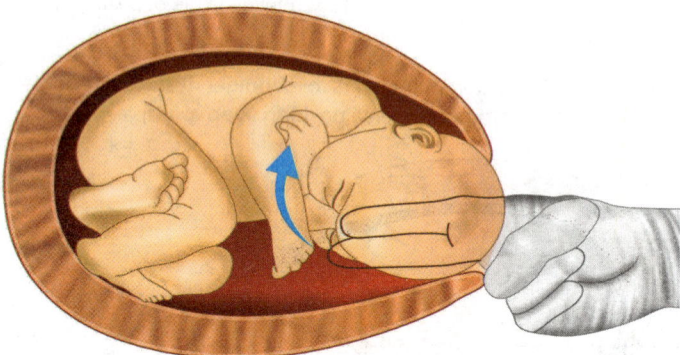

Fig. 19.16: Reverse Woods' screw maneuver. The shoulder is rotated progressively by 180° in a direction opposite to that described in the Woods' screw maneuver.

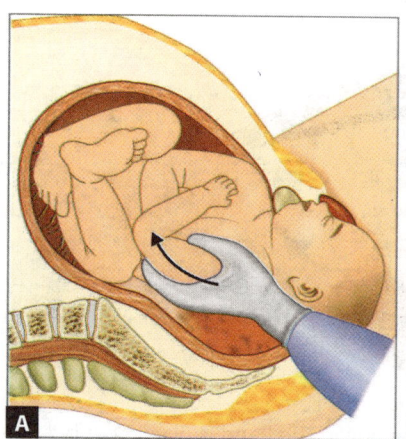 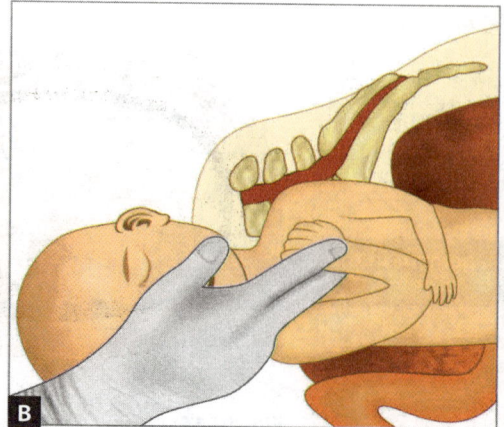 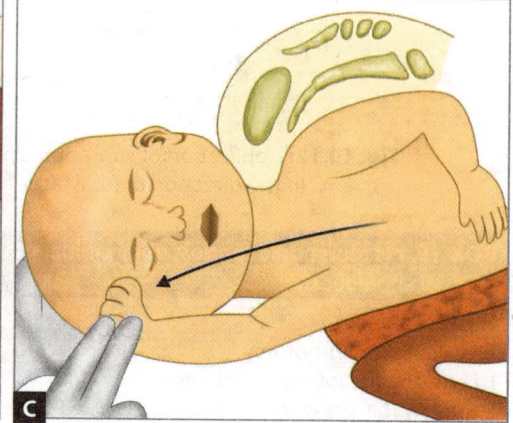

Figs. 19.17A to C: Delivery of posterior arm. (A) The clinician's hand is introduced into the vagina along the posterior shoulder. Keeping the arm flexed at the elbow, it is swept across the fetal chest; (B) The fetal hand is grasped and the arm is extended out along the side of the face; (C) The posterior arm and shoulder are delivered from the vagina.

C6, the middle trunk from undivided fibers of C7, and the lowermost trunk is made up of nerves from C8 and T1. Injury to the upper part of the brachial plexus is called Erb's palsy (C5–C7) while injury to the lower nerves of the plexus is called Klumpke's palsy (C8–T1) **(Fig. 19.19B)**. Both can cause significant, lifelong disability. Erb's palsy affects the muscles of the upper arm and shoulders, causing "winging" of scapula. This type of injury also causes adduction and internal rotation of humerus with the forearm extended. This has also been described as the "waiter's tip" position. Klumpke's palsy involves lower trunk lesions from nerve roots C7, C8, and T1. In this injury, the elbow becomes flexed and the forearm supinated (opened

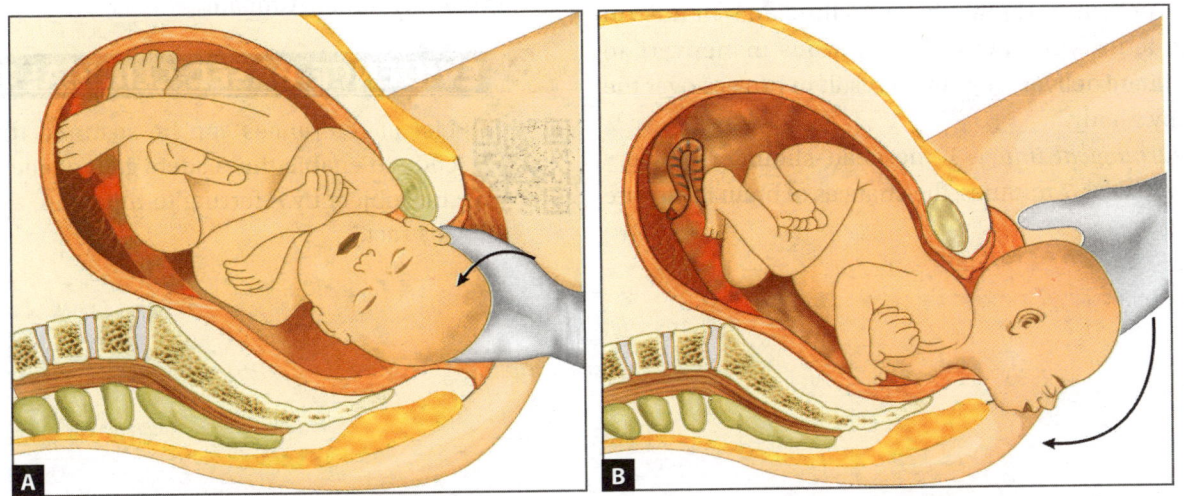

Figs. 19.18A and B: Zavanelli maneuver. (A) The head is manually rotated to occipitoanterior position; (B) Flexion of the fetal head and returning it into the vagina while applying constant pressure. This is followed by an immediate cesarean section.

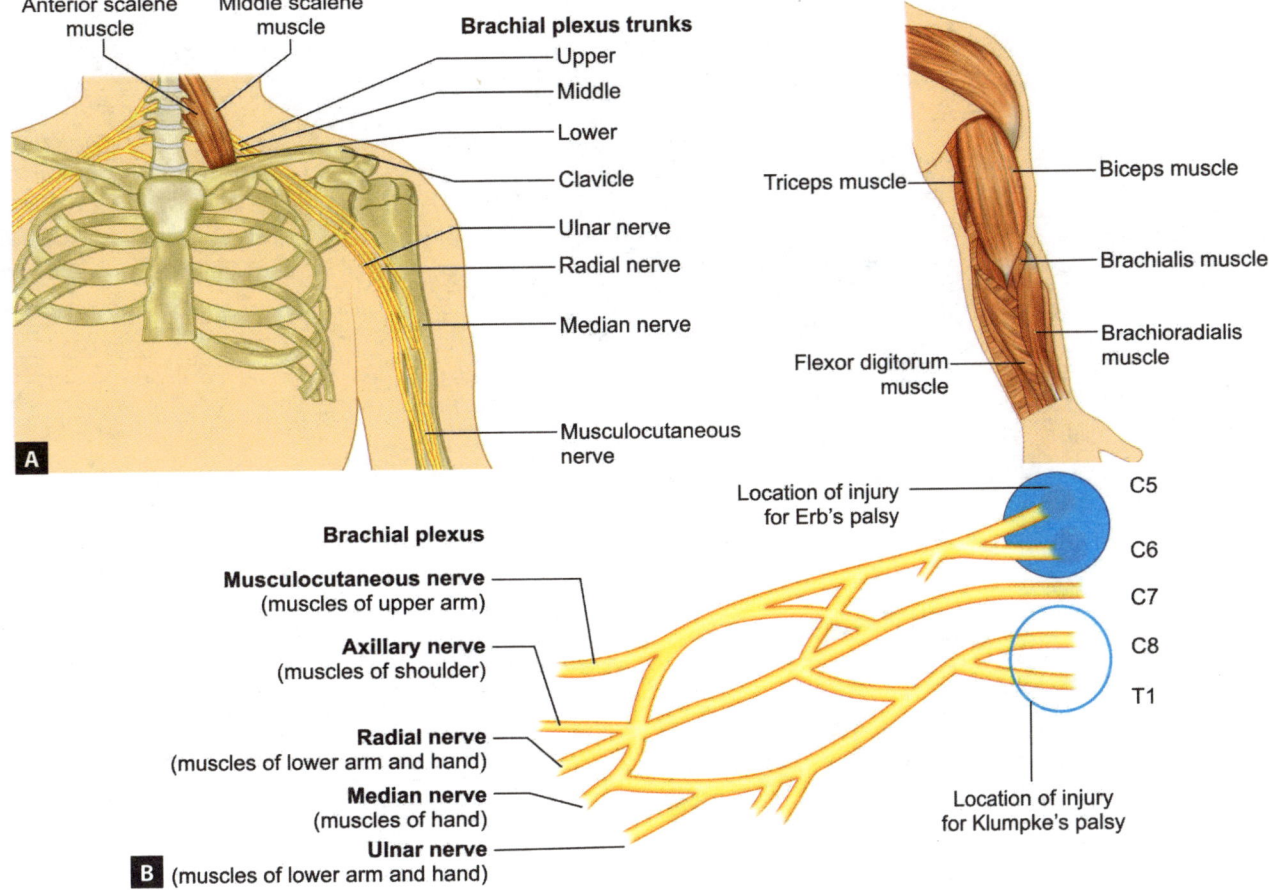

Figs. 19.19A and B: (A) Anatomy of brachial plexus; (B) Areas of brachial plexus injury due to shoulder dystocia.

up, palm upward) with a characteristic claw-like deformity of the hand.
- *Fractured clavicle:* The second most common type of injury suffered by infants following shoulder dystocia deliveries is a fracture of clavicle, having an incidence rate of nearly 10%.
- *Contusions:* The force with which the infant's shoulder is compressed against the maternal pubic bone and the pressure applied by the clinician's hands on the fetus while performing various maneuvers to facilitate delivery may often result in bruises over the baby's body.
- *Neurological injury:* If the head-shoulder delivery interval is >7 minutes, the chances of brain injury are high.
- *Maternal complications of shoulder dystocia:* Besides the fetal complications, shoulder dystocia can also produce some complications in the mother. The most common maternal complications include postpartum hemorrhage, second- and third-degree perineal tears, cervical lacerations, uterine rupture (in extreme cases), vaginal and vulvar lacerations, rectovaginal fistula, symphyseal separation, or diathesis with or without transient femoral neuropathy.

EVIDENCE-BASED CLINICAL TRIALS

List of references can be scanned through QR code to enable the readers gain deeper insight of the subject by referring to the entire article or its abstract.

CHAPTER 20

Anemia in Pregnancy

CASE STUDY

A 28-year-old G4P3L3 woman with 28-week period of gestation presents with complaints of easy fatigability and dyspnea since last 2 weeks. On general physical examination, pallor was observed on the lower palpebral conjunctiva, tongue, and palmar surface of hands. Pedal edema of pitting type was present. No other significant finding was observed on systemic examination. Abdominal examination revealed the presence of pregnancy corresponding to about 28-week period of gestation with cephalic presentation.

INTRODUCTION

DEFINITION

Anemia is one of the most common medical disorders present globally. It can be defined as reduction in circulating hemoglobin mass below the critical level. The WHO defines anemia as the presence of hemoglobin of <11 g/dL and hematocrit of <0.33 g/dL. The CDC (1990) has defined anemia as hemoglobin levels below 11 g/dL in a pregnant woman in first and third trimesters and <10.5 g/dL in second trimester. However, in India and most of the other developing countries, the lower limit is often accepted as 10 g%.

Hemoglobin is the iron-containing biomolecule present in the RBCs in the human blood vessels. It is responsible for transporting oxygen from the lungs to the various body organs and at the same time transporting carbon dioxide from various body tissues back to lungs **(Fig. 20.1)**. Each hemoglobin molecule is composed of heme group and four globin chains. The heme group consists of an iron ion held in the heterocyclic porphyrin ring. Iron is essential for carriage of oxygen by hemoglobin, oxidative metabolism, and normal growth.

GRADING OF ANEMIA

Depending on the levels of circulating hemoglobin in the body, the WHO has graded anemia as mild, moderate, and severe **(Table 20.1)**.

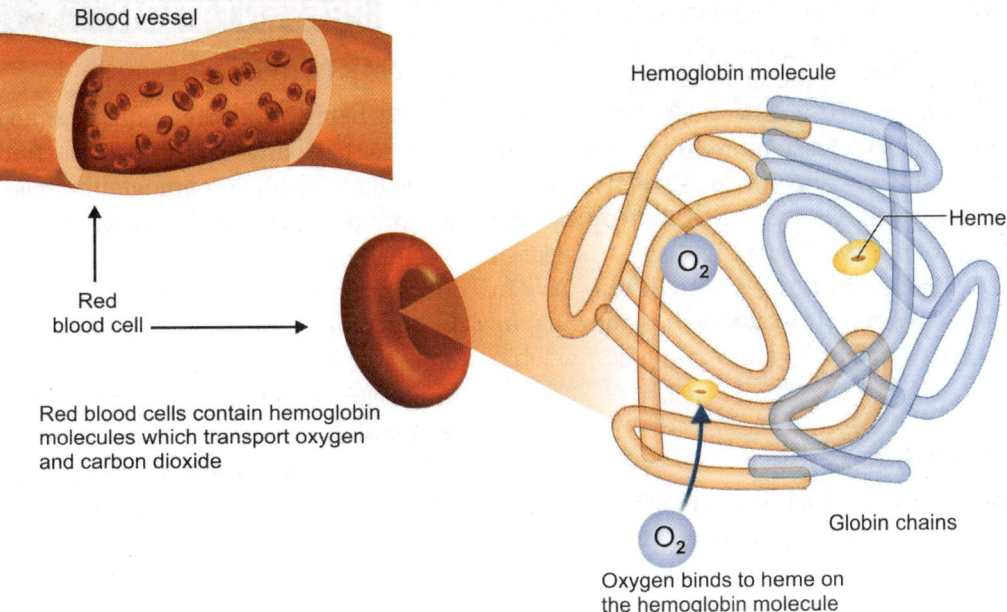

Fig. 20.1: Role of hemoglobin molecules in transportation of oxygen and carbon dioxide.

TABLE 20.1: Grading of anemia according to its severity.

Hemoglobin concentration (g/dL)	AIDS clinical trial group	WHO	National Cancer Institute	Indian Council of Medical Research
Normal	≥9.5	≥11	13.7–17.5 g/dL for men and 12–16 g/dL for women	≥11
Mild	8.0–9.4	10–10.9	10 to <lower normal limit	10.0–10.9
Moderate	7.0–7.9	8–9.9	8.0–9.9	7.0–9.9
Severe	6.5–6.9	7.9–7	6.5–7.9	<7.0
Very severe/life-threatening	<6.5	<7.0	<6.5	<4.0

Source: Brokering KL, Qaqish RB. Management of anemia of chronic disease in patients with the human immunodeficiency virus. Pharmacotherapy. 2003;23(11):1475-85.

TABLE 20.2: Cytometric classification of anemia.

Type	Laboratory value	Causes
Macrocytic, normochromic anemia	Increased MCV (>100 fL), normal MCHC (34%)	Vitamin B_{12} deficiency, folate deficiency
Microcytic, hypochromic anemia	Low MCHC (<30%), low MCV (<80 fL)	Thalassemia, iron deficiency anemia, anemia of chronic disease (rare cases)
Normocytic, normochromic anemia	Normal MCHC (34%), normal MCV (>80–99 fL)	Anemia due to chronic disease, anemia of acute hemorrhage, aplastic anemias, hemolytic anemias

(MCHC: mean corpuscular hemoglobin concentration; MCV: mean corpuscular volume)

Based on the findings of the peripheral smear and the results of various blood indices (explained later in the chapter), anemia can be classified into three types as shown in **Table 20.2**.

PHYSIOLOGICAL CHANGES TAKING PLACE IN ANEMIA

Decreased Hemoglobin Oxygen Affinity

In a normal person, when oxygen gets bound to hemoglobin, beta chains are pulled close together. On the other hand, when oxygen is released, beta chains move apart, permitting the entry of 2,3 diphosphoglycerate (2,3-DPG) molecules, resulting in lower affinity of hemoglobin for oxygen and improved delivery of oxygen to the tissues. These complex interactions are responsible for the sigmoid shape of oxygen dissociation curve. Increased levels of 2,3-DPG shift the curve to right and help to release more oxygen readily. In anemic individuals, there occurs an adaptive mechanism which increases the tissue levels of 2,3-DPG, thereby favoring increased availability of oxygen from red cells. Increased levels of 2,3-DPG also shift the hemoglobin–oxygen dissociation curve to the right **(Fig. 20.2)**, thus allowing the tissues to more easily extract oxygen from the hemoglobin molecules.

Redistribution of Blood Flow

In anemia, selective vasoconstriction of blood vessels helps in redistributing the blood from certain nonvital areas into critical areas. The blood flow is increased to areas such as brain, heart, and adrenals, and reduced to the skin and kidneys. Shunting of blood away from cutaneous sites is responsible for producing clinical finding of pallor, which can be considered as a cardinal sign of anemia.

Increased Cardiac Output

The heart tries to respond to tissue hypoxia by increasing the cardiac output. The increased output is associated with reduced peripheral vascular resistance and reduced blood viscosity, so that cardiac output can rise without an increase in blood pressure. Generally, anemia must be fairly severe (hemoglobin < 7 g/dL) before cardiac output rises.

HISTORY AND CLINICAL PRESENTATION

SYMPTOMS

In the beginning, pregnant women with mild anemia may not have any symptom as the body systems try to get adjusted to reduced hemoglobin mass. The symptoms are usually proportional to the severity of anemia. An acute hemorrhagic condition may produce symptoms with loss of as little as 20% of the total blood volume. On the other hand, anemia developing over long periods would allow compensatory mechanisms to operate, which would help in masking symptoms until the anemia becomes severe. In developing countries, it is not uncommon to see a patient with hemoglobin of 4 g/dL being reluctantly brought into a clinic by relatives with the complaint that she has been just looking a bit unwell.

With mild anemia, the woman may present with vague complaints of ill health, fatigue, loss of appetite, digestive upset, breathlessness, palpitation, dyspnea on exertion, easy

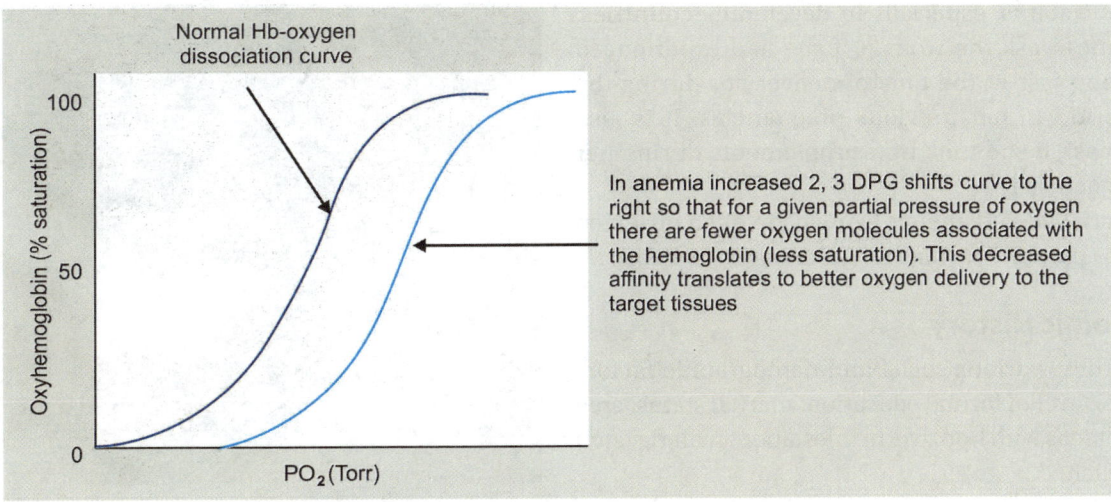

Fig. 20.2: Oxygen dissociation curve in anemic patients.

fatigability, fainting, lightheadedness, tinnitus, headache, etc. Fatigue is one of the most common complaints of anemic patients. In anemic patients, lack of circulating hemoglobin results in development of fatigue and diminished capability to perform hard labor. As a result, the woman may complain of reduced work performance, tiredness or reduced energy, severe fatigue, restlessness, tiredness or exhaustion, nocturnal leg cramps, etc. The woman may also experience headache, paresthesia and numbness in the extremities, oral and nasopharyngeal symptoms (e.g., burning of tongue), dysphagia (due to mucosal atrophy in the laryngopharynx), hair loss, etc. Pica, an unusual craving for nonnutritive substances, such as ice, dirt, starch, or paint in pregnant women, is a characteristic symptom of iron deficiency anemia (IDA).

The points in history which are important and should be elicited in these patients in order to know the etiology of anemia include the following.

Dietary History

- A detailed dietary history is important. Vegetarians are more likely to develop iron deficiency. In developing countries, due to poor socioeconomic conditions, patients may not be able to afford a good nutritious diet rich in iron and proteins.
- *History of pica:* Pica can be the etiology of iron deficiency amongst people who habitually eat either clay or laundry starch. One half of patients with moderate IDA may develop pagophagia, in which they develop strong craving to suck ice.

History of Hemorrhage

- Blood loss in any form from the body is an important cause of anemia. Two-thirds of body iron is present in circulating RBCs as hemoglobin. Each gram of hemoglobin contains 3.47 mg of iron; thus, each mL of blood lost from the body (hemoglobin 14 g/dL) results in a loss of approximately 0.5 mg of iron. The clinician needs to enquire about a history of bleeding from any of the orifices (hematuria, hematemesis, hemoptysis, melena, excessive menstrual loss, etc.). Since occult bleeding from the gastrointestinal tract often goes unrecognized, the patient needs to be specifically asked if she ever had ulcers in the gastrointestinal tract. History of chronic ingestion of aspirin or other NSAIDs needs to be elicited as this is commonly associated with occult gastric ulcerations.
- Malena usually points to upper gastrointestinal hemorrhage. History of melanotic stools can be elicited by asking the patient if she has ever passed black-colored stools (provided that she is not taking iron).

  Intake of iron tablets is also likely to cause black-colored staining of stools. The passage of black-colored stools can also be considered as the best way to find out if the patient is taking oral iron preparations or not. If she gives a history of passing normal-colored stools, she probably is not taking her iron tablets.
- The patient may not be able to give the correct estimate of menstrual blood loss, thus she should be specifically asked about the number of tampons or pads she needs to use in a day during the time of her periods and whether her menstrual flow is associated with passage of clots. Frequent pad changes and passage of clots signify greater blood loss.

Obstetric History

Obstetrical factors such as gravidity, parity and history of previous preterm or small for gestational age deliveries, and multifetal pregnancy are important. History of giving birth to babies at frequent intervals before the woman has a chance to replenish her depleted iron stores is an important reason for development of anemia in women with low socioeconomic status, especially in developing countries. It is important to ask the woman if she had experienced excessive blood loss at the time of delivery or during the antenatal period in her previous pregnancies. It is also important to ask if she took iron supplements during her previous pregnancies.

Undernourished and anemic women are often observed to give birth to preterm or small for gestational age babies.

Socioeconomic History

History regarding various social and demographic factors including age, level of formal education, marital status, area of residence (areas with hookworm infestation, malaria, etc.) needs to be elicited.

Behavioral History

Behavioral factors which must be taken into consideration include history related to smoking or tobacco usage, alcohol usage, utilization of prenatal care services, etc.

Medical History

Medical conditions (diabetes, renal or cardiorespiratory diseases, chronic hypertension, etc.) can further aggravate the development of anemia during pregnancy.

Menstrual History

It is important to take a detailed history of previous menstrual cycles including the amount of blood loss and the number of days the blood loss occurs. Small amount of menstrual blood loss occurring over a long period of time can also result in the development of anemia.

Treatment History

It is important to ask the woman if she has been taking iron supplements during this pregnancy. Due to continuous ingestion of iron tablets, the color of stools invariably turns black.

GENERAL PHYSICAL EXAMINATION

The following signs can be observed on general physical examination:
- *Pallor:* Reduced amount of oxygenated hemoglobin in anemic individuals results in development of nonspecific pallor of the mucous membranes. Paleness may be observed on the woman's face. Clinical examination may reveal pallor in lower palpebral conjunctiva (**Fig. 20.3**), pale tongue, pale nail bed, pale palmar surface of hands, lips, etc. (see Chapter 1). Mechanism of development of pallor is illustrated in **Flowchart 20.1**.
- *Epithelial changes:* The epithelial tissues of nails, tongue, mouth, hypopharynx, and stomach are affected, resulting

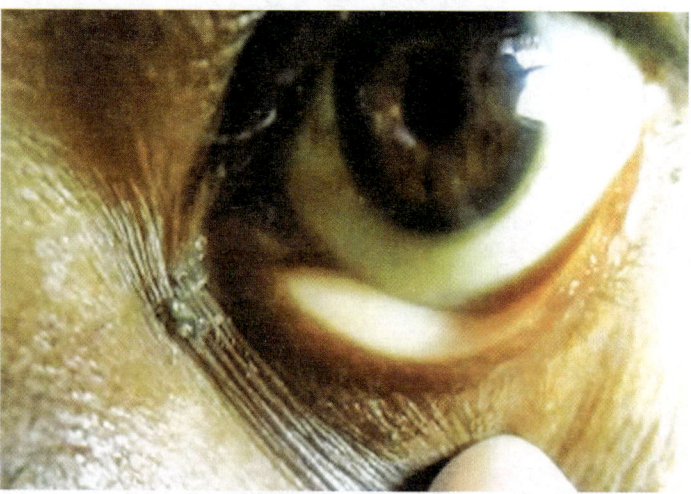

Fig. 20.3: Pallor in the lower palpebral conjunctiva.

Flowchart 20.1: Mechanism of development of pallor.

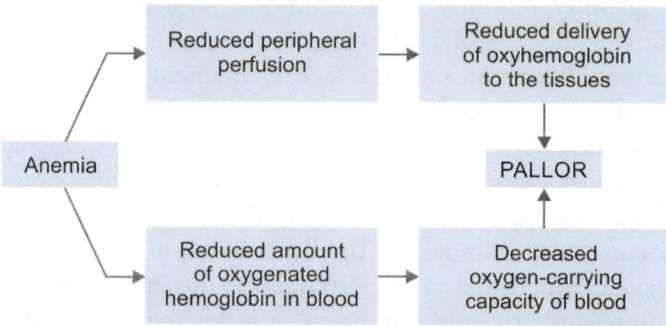

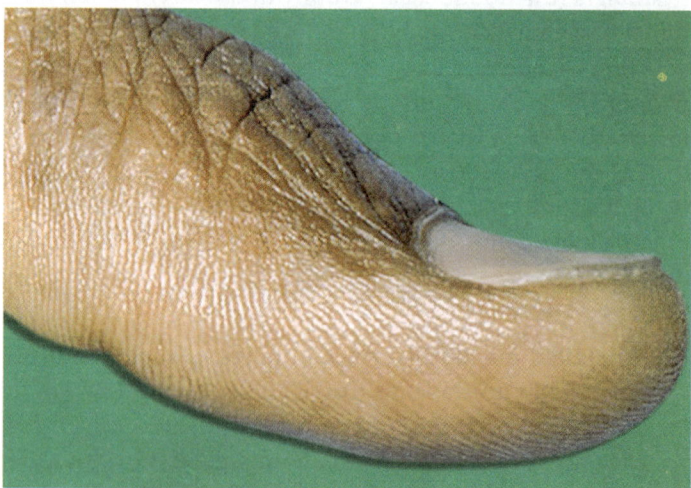

Fig. 20.4: Koilonychia.

in development of brittle, fragile, spoon-shaped nails, glossitis, angular stomatitis, atrophic gastritis, etc.
- *Nail changes:* Thinning, flattening, and finally development of concave "spoon-shaped nails," also known as koilonychias (**Fig. 20.4**), occurs.
- *Changes in the tongue or mouth:* There may be atrophy of lingual papilla accompanied by soreness or burning of the tongue. Glossitis and stomatitis can also develop. Angular stomatitis, characterized by development of

ulcerations or fissures at the corners of the mouth, is a less specific sign of anemia. It is commonly associated with deficiency of riboflavin or pyridoxine.

- *Pedal edema:* In severely anemic cases, there may be pedal edema **(Fig. 20.5)**.
- *Plummer-Vinson syndrome:* This syndrome is also known as Paterson-Kelly syndrome after the names of its discoverers. This is a rare condition characterized by the presence of IDA, nail abnormalities, and dysphagia. Some of the symptoms for Plummer-Vinson syndrome include pain in the throat during swallowing, burning sensation during swallowing, sensation of food being stuck in larynx, fatigue, pallor, difficulty in swallowing, development of mucosal webs in esophagus, etc.

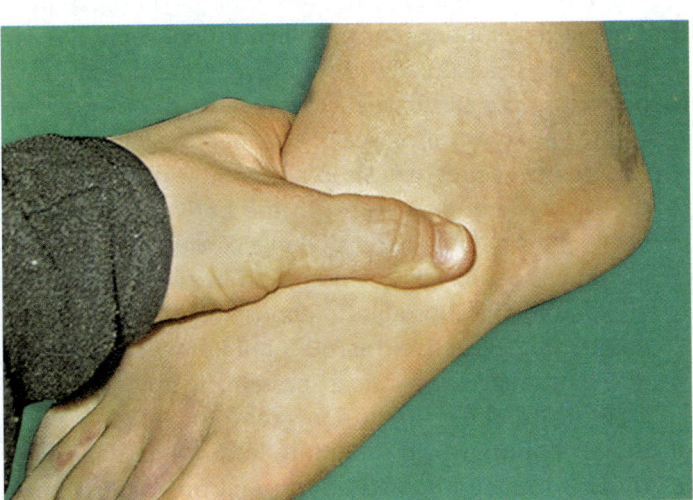

Fig. 20.5: Pedal edema.

SPECIFIC SYSTEMIC EXAMINATION

ABDOMINAL EXAMINATION

Splenomegaly may occur with severe, persistent, untreated IDA.

CARDIOVASCULAR SYSTEM

In cases of severe anemia increased blood flow to the heart results in the development of tachycardia and a systolic ejection murmur. In rapidly developing anemia (e.g., from hemorrhage), additional symptoms and signs may be noted, e.g., syncope on rising from bed, orthostatic hypotension (i.e., the blood pressure falls when the patient is raised from the supine to the sitting or standing positions), and orthostatic tachycardia.

DIFFERENTIAL DIAGNOSIS

NORMOCYTIC ANEMIA

The most important cause of normocytic anemia during pregnancy is physiological anemia due to hemodilution. Various other causes of anemia are listed in **Flowchart 20.2**.

> Q. Write a short essay discussing the hematological changes associated with normal pregnancy. Also discuss its obstetric implications.

Physiological Anemia due to Pregnancy

The two main reasons for development of physiological anemia due to pregnancy are:

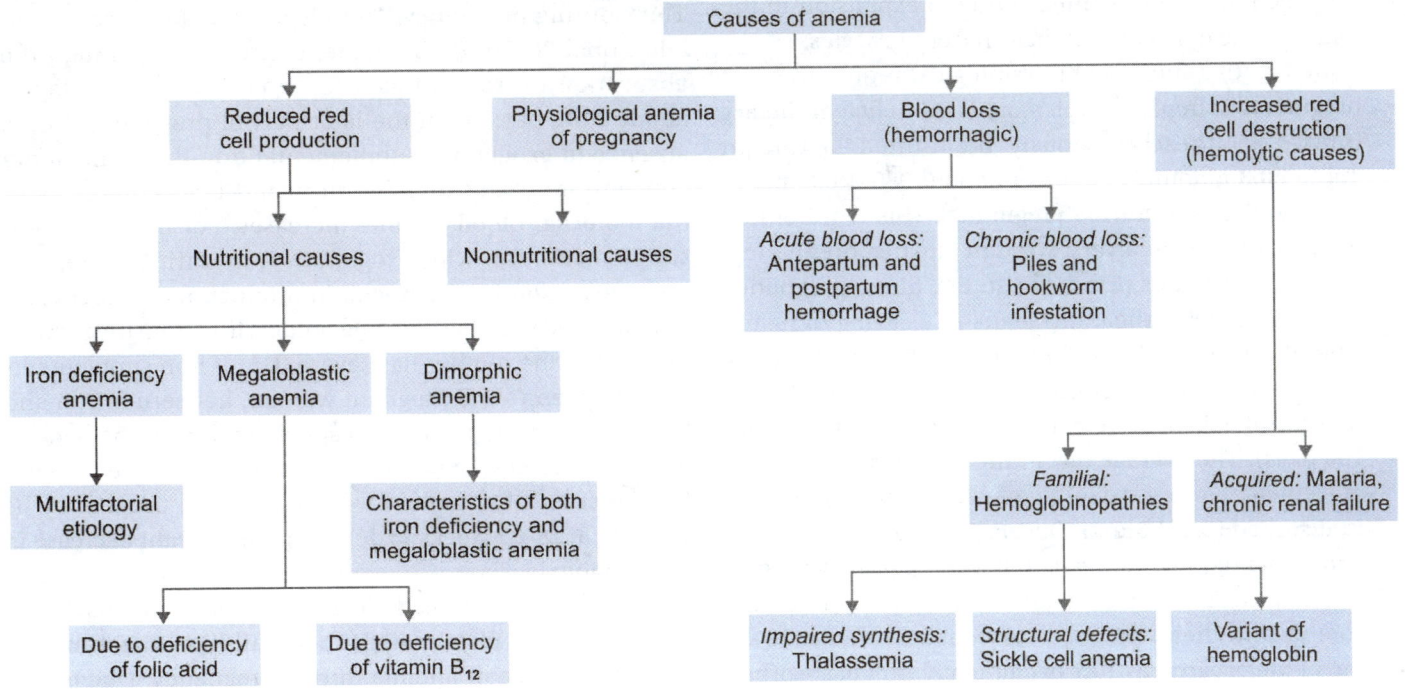

Flowchart 20.2: Various causes of anemia.

1. Physiological hemodilution resulting in disproportionate increase in plasma volume
2. Negative iron balance during pregnancy

Physiological hemodilution: Pregnancy causes a disproportionate increase in plasma volume, leading to an apparent reduction of RBC mass, hemoglobin, and hematocrit value. Normochromic normocytic anemia is produced as a result of this physiological dilution, which starts at 8–10 weeks of gestation and reaches a maximum during the second trimester of pregnancy. Maternal blood volume expands most rapidly during the second trimester, whereas in the third trimester the rate of rise considerably slows down, ultimately plateauing toward the last weeks of pregnancy. Blood volume expansion occurs, due to an increase in both plasma volume and erythrocyte volume. Initially, the increase in plasma volume is larger than the red cell volume. Thus, there is a drop in the hematocrit of approximately five units for a normal singleton pregnancy. Hemoglobin concentration at term averages to about 12.5 g% in normal women. Therefore, in most women hemoglobin concentration below 11 g/dL should be considered abnormal.

Negative iron balance during pregnancy: There is an increased iron requirement during pregnancy, amounting to about 1,000 mg **(Table 20.3)**. This increase is due to the following reasons:
- 270 mg of iron is actively transferred to the fetus. The fetus utilizes maternal iron for building up hemoglobin molecules.
- 170 mg is lost through various routes of excretion, primarily the gastrointestinal tract.
- Total amount of iron transferred to placenta and cord is 90 mg.
- 450–500 mg of iron is utilized due to expansion in the total volume of circulating maternal erythrocytes.
- Added to this increased physiological requirement of pregnancy is depleted iron stores and deficient dietary intake. All these previously mentioned factors in **Table 20.3** amount to a total of about 980–1,000 mg of iron requirement during pregnancy. This requirement of iron occurs in every woman during pregnancy, irrespective of her prior iron status. Since pregnancy results in amenorrhea, this leads to a saving of nearly 240–300 mg of iron in the form of menstrual blood. Thus, total iron requirements during pregnancy are 600–700 mg (6–7 mg of daily requirement of elemental iron for about 100 days). The average diet in the US provides 5–14 mg of elemental iron per day, out of which nearly one-tenth is absorbed (0.5–1.5 mg). During pregnancy, there is an additional requirement of about 2–5 mg iron every day. If the woman wants to fulfill these iron requirements solely from diet, she needs to consume about 20–50 mg of dietary iron as 10% of elemental iron is absorbed from the diet. This is practically impossible in India and other developing countries because an average vegetarian diet contains not more than 5–14 mg of iron. Also, in developing countries, majority of women enter pregnancy in an already iron-depleted condition and may be consuming an iron-deficient diet. Iron depletion can be attributed to young age of childbearing and frequent occurrence of pregnancies in a woman without allowing the recovery of iron stores in the body. Moreover, in developing countries, most people consume vegetarian, low-bioavailability diet, which is low in ascorbic acid and high in biological proteins composed entirely of cereals (containing excessive iron inhibitors such as phytates), which further reduce iron absorption.

TABLE 20.3: Iron requirements during pregnancy.

Reason for iron requirement	Amount of iron required (mg)
Iron actively transferred to the fetus	270
Iron lost through various routes of excretion	170
Iron transferred to placenta and cord	90
Iron utilized due to expansion in the maternal volume of circulating erythrocytes	400–500
Total iron requirements	980–1,000

Due to the above-mentioned reasons, in most parts of the developing world including India, there is a need for routine iron supplementation to all pregnant women because the amount of iron absorbed from the diet, together with that mobilized from the stores, is usually insufficient to meet the maternal demands imposed by pregnancy. Thus, during pregnancy, there is daily requirement for an additional 20–30 mg of elemental iron. Even though the absorption of iron is increased from 1–2 mg per day to about 6 mg per day in the later part of pregnancy, in the absence of exogenous supplemental iron the hemoglobin concentration and hematocrit would fall appreciably as the maternal blood volume increases. For these reasons, supplementation with exogenous iron during pregnancy becomes essential. Hemoglobin production in the fetus is not impaired because placenta obtains iron from the mother, even when the mother has severe IDA. If iron supplements are not given to the pregnant woman, her serum iron and ferritin levels may decline, especially during the second half of pregnancy. Therefore, it is essential that the patient's hematocrit or hemoglobin during routine pregnancy be checked at 28–32 weeks to detect any significant decrease in hemoglobin levels.

The above-mentioned obligate iron requirements during pregnancy and physiological hemodilution constitute an important cause of anemia during pregnancy. Due to this and the acute blood loss accompanying childbirth and labor, prevalence of IDA during the pregnancy is quite high and has far-reaching consequences, especially with severe degrees of anemia. Though exact data on the prevalence of anemia in women is not available, it is estimated that 60 million pregnant women worldwide are anemic. Out of these, only 4 million are in developed countries; the rest of them belong to developing countries. The prevalence rate of anemia in the US is about 1.29%. On the other hand, in India, 46% of pregnant women in urban areas and 52% in rural areas are likely to have their hemoglobin levels <11 g/dL. Anemia in pregnancy has a multifactorial etiology **(Fig. 20.6)**. Various other factors responsible for anemia during pregnancy include the following:

- Prior history of menorrhagia (loss of >80 mL of blood per month)
- Multiple gestations
- Vegetarian diet, low in heme iron
  Increased frequency of blood donation
- Chronic blood loss due to hookworm infestation, schistosomiasis, etc.
- Chronic infection (e.g., malaria)
- Chronic aspirin use

Majority of women in childbearing age have deficient iron stores due to blood loss from menstruation, repeated childbirth, and chronic hookworm infection, especially in the developing countries. In multigravidas, repeated childbearing does not give time to replenish the iron stores in between the pregnancies, thereby perpetuating anemia. Deficient or defective intake of iron, folic acid, and other hematopoietic factors due to poverty, ignorance, or absorption disorders may lead to nutritional deficiency during pregnancy. Deficiency of other micronutrients (folic acid, zinc, etc.) is also commonly seen accompanying IDA. Infants born to a mother suffering from IDA may have deficient iron stores during infancy, childhood, and adolescence. This child during the period of her pregnancy may develop manifest anemia, thereby setting up a vicious cycle.

Malaria, which is endemic in certain parts of the world, causes anemia by hemolysis. The presence of chronic infections may cause anemia by impairing hematopoiesis. Genetic factors such as thalassemia, sickle cell anemia, and glucose-6-phosphate dehydrogenase deficiency can also result in anemia. With the exception of thalassemia major, which is associated with iron overload, other genetic disorders usually have concomitant iron deficiency during pregnancy. Deficiency of vitamin B_{12}, although a rare cause of anemia during pregnancy, is sometimes seen in strict vegetarians or those eating fad diets.

MICROCYTIC ANEMIA

The three most common causes of microcytic anemia are IDA, thalassemia, and anemia due to chronic infection.

Iron Deficiency Anemia

Causes for IDA are listed in **Box 20.1**. IDA has been defined as microcytic hypochromic type. This type of anemia usually develops when body iron stores become inadequate for the need of normal erythropoiesis. Body iron stores must be reduced before red cell production is reduced. Therefore, anemia occurs at a later stage of iron deficiency. Serum ferritin < 20 ng/mL is associated with IDA. The various stages involved in the development of anemia during pregnancy are as follows:

- *Depletion of iron stores:* This stage is associated with low serum ferritin levels.
- *Impaired hemoglobin production:* In this stage, there is deficiency of iron without manifest anemia. This stage is associated with low ratio of serum iron to total iron-binding capacity (iron/TIBC), low MCV, and elevated erythrocyte protoporphyrin levels. However, hemoglobin levels remain within the normal range.
- *Manifest iron deficiency:* This stage is associated with low hemoglobin levels along with additional evidence of iron deficiency including low serum ferritin levels, low ratio of serum iron to TIBC levels, low MCV, MCH and MCHC, and elevated erythrocyte protoporphyrin.

> **BOX 20.1:** Causes of iron deficiency anemia.
>
> *Nutritional causes*
> - Iron deficiency anemia (60%)
> - Dimorphic anemia due to both deficiency of iron and folic acid
>
> *Hemolytic anemia*
> - Hemoglobinopathies
>
> *Anemia due to blood loss*
> - *Acute:* Acute blood loss (antepartum hemorrhage, PPH)
> - *Chronic:* Hookworm infestation, bleeding piles, malarial infestation
>
> (PPH: postpartum hemorrhage)

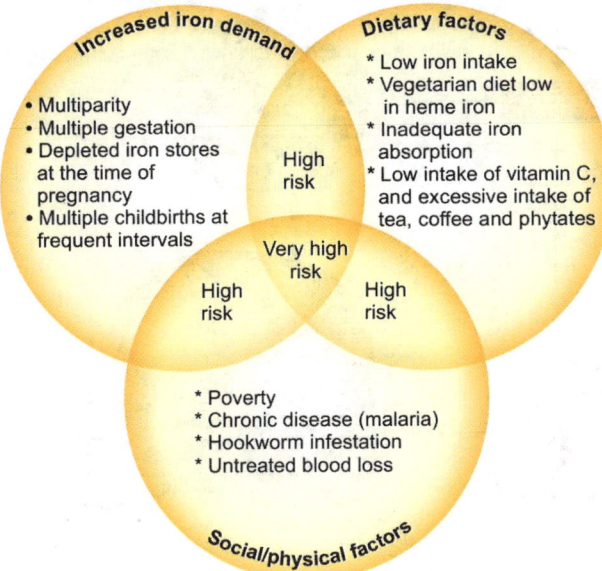

Fig. 20.6: Multifactorial etiology of anemia.

Iron is absorbed mainly from duodenum and jejunum in the ferrous form and is transported in the blood in the form of transferrin.

Thalassemia

Thalassemia includes a group of genetically inherited disorders, which are characterized by impaired or defective production of one or more normal globin peptide chains **(Fig. 20.7)**. Abnormal synthesis of globin chains can result in ineffective erythropoiesis, hemolysis, and varying degrees of anemia. Depending on whether the synthesis of alpha (α) or beta (β) chains is affected, thalassemia can be classified into two types: α-thalassemia and β-thalassemia.

Iron deficiency anemia has to be differentiated from other causes of hypochromic anemia including thalassemia **(Table 20.4)** and anemia due to chronic diseases **(Table 20.5)**.

Anemia due to thalassemia can be differentiated on the basis of erythrocyte indices. Although MCV may be reduced in thalassemia to values as low as 60–70 fL, values this low are rarely encountered in cases with IDA. Serum iron concentration is usually normal or increased in thalassemic syndromes, while it is usually low in IDA. Marrow examination and hemoglobin electrophoresis also help in differentiating between IDA and thalassemia by respectively showing normal bone marrow iron stores and increased proportions of fetal hemoglobin (HbF) and hemoglobin alpha 2 (HbA_2) in cases with thalassemia. Mentzer's index, which is calculated by diving MCV with total number of RBCs, also helps in differentiating between thalassemia and IDA based on the biological difference between the two. Lower Mentzer's index in thalassemia implies that for a given reduction of MCV, there are many more RBCs in thalassemia than in IDA.

In case the parents are carriers, accurate prenatal diagnosis in the fetus can be easily established with the help of tests such as amniocentesis and chorionic villus sampling. Women with thalassemia major and intermedia are at an increased risk of maternal complications such as cardiac failure, alloimmunization, viral infection, thrombosis, and endocrine and bone metabolism. Therefore, close

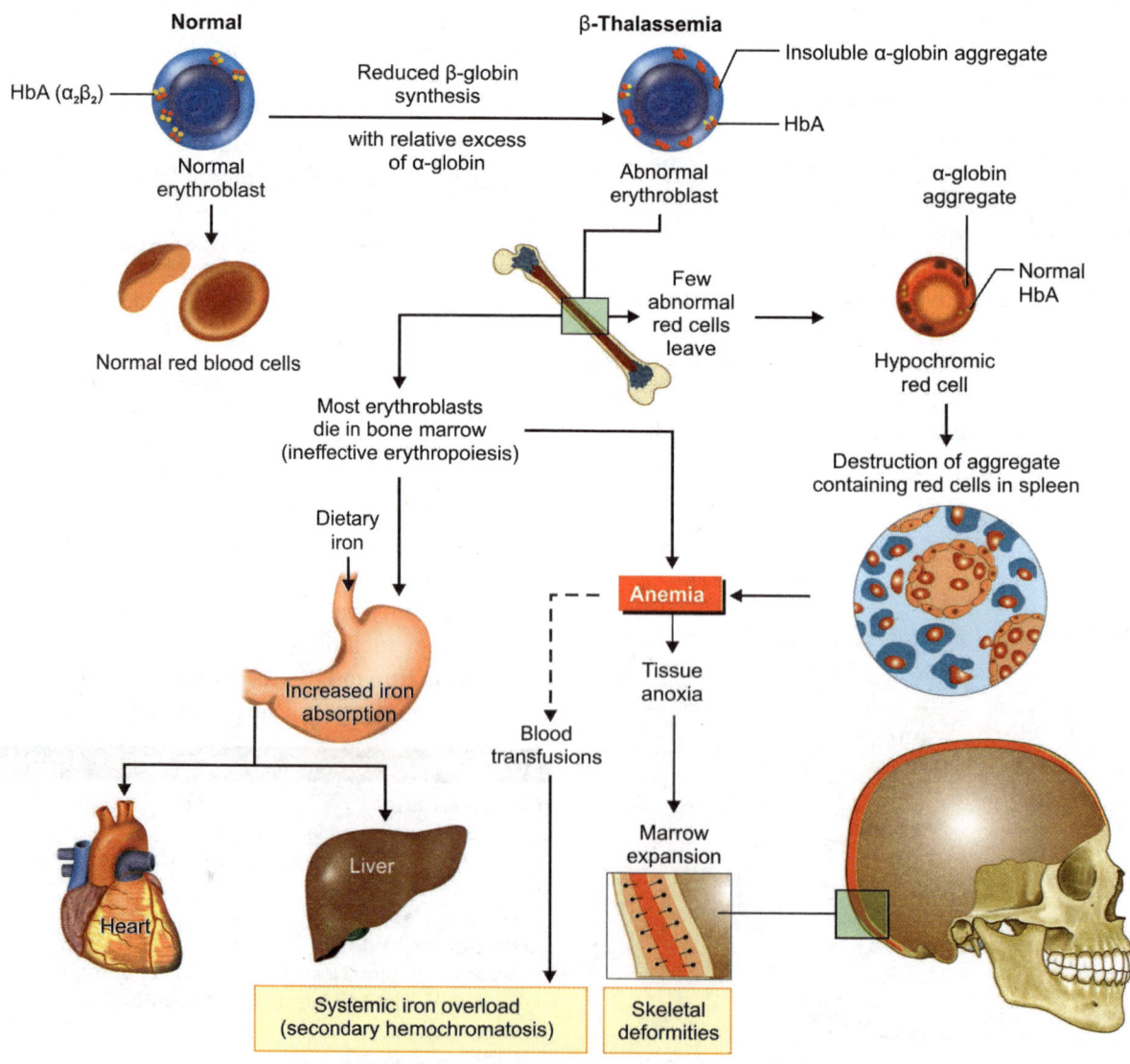

Fig. 20.7: Pathogenesis of beta thalassemia. (HbA: hemoglobin alpha)

TABLE 20.4: Differentiation between iron deficiency anemia and thalassemia.

Blood index	Iron deficiency anemia	Thalassemia
Peripheral smear	Microcytic hypochromic anemia	Microcytic hypochromic anemia
Serum iron	Reduced	Normal or high
TIBC	High	Normal
Percentage saturation	Reduced	Normal or high
Serum ferritin	Reduced	High
Hemoglobin pattern	Normal	Abnormal
HbF and HbA$_2$	Normal	High
Red cell width	High	Normal
Free erythrocyte porphyrin (normal < 35)	>50	Normal
MCV, MCHC, MCH	All reduced proportionally to the severity of anemia	All reduced to very low levels in relation to the severity of anemia
Bone marrow iron stores	Absent	Present
Mentzer's index*	>14	<11.5

Note: *Mentzer's index is calculated by dividing MCV with total number of RBCs.
(HbA$_2$: hemoglobin alpha 2; HbF: fetal hemoglobin; TIBC: total iron-binding capacity)

TABLE 20.5: Differentiation between iron deficiency anemia and anemia due to chronic diseases.

Blood index	Iron deficiency anemia	Anemia due to chronic diseases
Peripheral smear	Microcytic hypochromic anemia	Microcytic hypochromic anemia (20–30%)
Serum iron	Reduced	Normal
Total iron-binding capacity (TIBC)	High	Reduced
Percentage saturation	<16%	>16%
Serum ferritin	Reduced	Normal
MCV, MCHC, MCH	All reduced proportionally to the severity of anemia	Low/normal
Bone marrow iron stores	Absent	Present

(MCH: mean corpuscular hemoglobin; MCHC: mean corpuscular hemoglobin concentration; MCV: mean corpuscular volume)

monitoring of fetal and maternal conditions is required during pregnancy. Treatment options such as blood transfusion and postpartum prophylaxis for thromboembolism may be indicated in these cases. While iron chelation therapy is normally contraindicated during the antenatal period, it is resumed following the baby's birth, and treatment with bisphosphonates is also started.

During pregnancy, supplementation with folic acid in the dosage of 5 mg/day is required in order to reduce the risk of neural tube defects. Iron supplementation is normally not required due to the risk of iron overload. Ferritin levels of these women need to be checked to confirm if they are suffering from iron deficiency and require supplementation with iron tablets.

Iron overload due to repeated transfusions in these cases may require treatment with desferrioxamine (an iron chelator) during the preconceptional period to reduce the risk of end-organ damage. In fact, desferrioxamine is the only chelating agent which can be safely used during the second and third trimesters of pregnancy.

Chronic Iron Deficiency Anemia

Anemia can be produced due to diseases such as chronic renal insufficiency, hypothyroidism, and malignancies (hematologic malignancies, leukemia, lymphoma, myeloma, etc.). Anemia due to chronic disease is caused by a reduction in both the lifespan of existing RBCs and the number of new RBCs produced to replace dying RBCs. Cytokines, such as interleukin (IL)-1, IL-6, and tumor necrosis factor alpha, may directly reduce RBC production and survival. For example, in anemia of chronic renal failure, the kidneys do not produce sufficient erythropoietin in response to hypoxia.

The anemia due to chronic disease is usually normocytic normochromic type, but hypochromic microcytic anemia may also occur in 20–30% of patients with chronic diseases or malignancy. The differentiation between IDA and anemia due to chronic diseases is shown in **Table 20.5**. Sometimes, it may not be possible to differentiate between the two types of anemia just by the examination of the blood film. Furthermore, the serum iron concentration is usually decreased in IDA, whereas it may be normal in anemia due to chronic diseases. Also, the TIBC is usually increased in IDA, whereas it is decreased in cases of anemia due to chronic disease. In IDA, transferrin saturation is usually <16%, whereas in anemia due to chronic diseases, it is usually >16%.

 Q. Write a short note on megaloblastic anemia.

MEGALOBLASTIC (MACROCYTIC) ANEMIA

The signs and symptoms in cases of megaloblastic anemia are similar to IDA. However, nail changes do not occur normally. Megaloblastic anemia commonly occurs in multiple pregnancies (20–28 weeks), in users of oral contraceptive pills, or those consuming antiepileptic drugs. It most commonly occurs due to folate deficiency during pregnancy. The adverse effects of folate deficiency on pregnancy include increased incidence of abortion, growth retardation, abruption placentae, and preeclampsia. Deficiency of folate can also result in the development of neural tube defects, which can be prevented by periconceptional folic acid in the dosage of 0.4 mg/day in low-risk cases and 5 mg/day in high-risk women.

Megaloblastic anemia in nonpregnant women commonly occurs due to deficiency of vitamin B_{12} caused by the lack of intrinsic factor, resulting in the lack of absorption of vitamin B_{12} (**Fig. 20.8**). This, however, occurs rarely in pregnancy because deficiency of vitamin B_{12} may take months to manifest and usually causes infertility. Acquired vitamin B_{12} deficiency causing megaloblastic anemia is uncommon as the daily requirement of vitamin B_{12} is only 3.0 µg/day during pregnancy, and this can be easily met with a normal nonvegetarian diet. Vegetarians who do not eat any animal-derived substances may have a deficiency of vitamin B_{12} and should receive vitamin B_{12} supplementation in the dosage of 250 µg parenterally every month.

Investigations

- *Peripheral smear:* At least two of the following criteria must be present on the peripheral smear to establish the diagnosis of megaloblastic anemia:
  - More than 4% of neutrophil polymorphs have five or more lobes
  - Orthochromatic macrocytes having a diameter > 12 mm
  - Howell–Jolly bodies must be demonstrated.
  - Presence of nucleated red cells
  - Macropolycytes may be present.

Since the deficiency of both folate and B_{12} may result in megaloblastic anemia, it is important to differentiate between the two (**Table 20.6**) on the basis of findings of clinical examination and various investigation.

In order to prevent folate deficiency, the WHO recommends a daily folate intake of 800 µg in the antenatal period and 600 µg during lactation. Pregnant women must be advised to eat a diet rich in green vegetables (e.g., spinach and broccoli), offal (e.g., liver and kidney), etc. Treatment comprises administration of 5 mg folate per day, which must be continued for at least 4 weeks in the puerperium.

■ DIMORPHIC ANEMIA

Dimorphic anemia is characterized by deficiency of both iron and folic acid with the dominance of either one of them.

■ HEMOLYTIC ANEMIA

Hemolytic anemias may occur due to erythrocyte defects such as abnormal hemoglobin structure, metabolic disturbances, or membrane abnormalities. The lifespan of an RBC is shortened in case of hemolytic anemia due to premature destruction of red cells, which may occur extravascularly [i.e., acquired immune hemolytic anemia, inherited defects of red cell enzymes (e.g., pyruvate kinase deficiency), etc.] or intravascularly (i.e., microangiopathic hemolytic anemia of preeclampsia). Extravascular hemolysis is most commonly observed in cases of hemolytic anemia. In these cases, the RBCs are destroyed in the reticulocyte endothelial system, which when liberated get converted into bilirubin. This causes an increase in the levels of indirect bilirubin in the patient's serum. The products of bilirubin metabolism, fetal and urinary urobilinogen also increase. Erythropoiesis increases markedly and reticulocytosis also increases due to bone marrow hyperplasia. The hallmarks of extravascular hemolysis are elevated levels of unconjugated

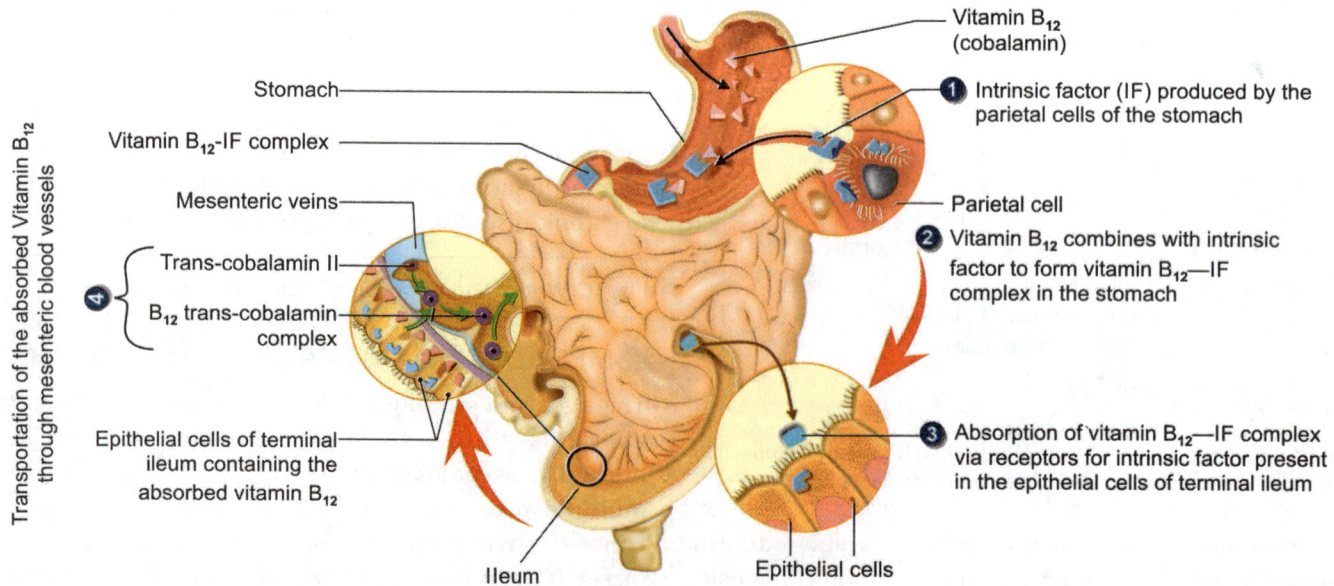

Fig. 20.8: Pathogenesis of megaloblastic anemia caused due to deficiency of intrinsic factor, resulting in impaired absorption of vitamin B_{12}.

TABLE 20.6: Differentiating between folate deficiency and anemia due to the deficiency of vitamin B_{12}.

Parameter	Anemia due to deficiency of folic acid	Anemia due to deficiency of vitamin B_{12}
Anemia	Megaloblastic	Megaloblastic
Hemoglobin/hematocrit	Reduced	Reduced
MCV	Increased	Increased
Reticulocytes	Reduced	Reduced
Neurological symptoms	Absent	Present (e.g., tingling sensation and neuropathic pain)
Color of the tongue	Lemon yellow	Magenta/red color
Serum folate levels	<3 mg/mL	Normal
Red cell folate	<150 ng/mL	Normal
Serum B_{12} levels	Normal	Reduced
Homocysteine levels	Increased	Increased
Methylmalonic acid	Normal	Increased
Formiminoglutamic acid (FIGLU) test	Positive	Negative
Schillings test	Negative	Positive (in pernicious anemia)

(MCV: mean corpuscular volume)

bilirubin, increased urinary urobilinogen levels, and reticulocytosis. The most common type of hemolytic anemia during pregnancy is intravascular microangiopathic hemolytic anemia, which is a part of HELLP (hemolysis, elevated liver enzymes, low platelet count) syndrome.

Hemolytic Anemia Associated with Hemoglobinopathy

Sickle cell disease is the most common hemoglobinopathy encountered during pregnancy. It is an autosomal recessive genetic disorder caused by the replacement of an amino acid at the sixth position, i.e., glutamic acid with valine in the β-globulin chains of hemoglobin.

This results in the development of sickle cell hemoglobin (HbS). In the oxygenated state, the solubility of HbS is similar to that of normal hemoglobin. However, in the deoxygenated state, its solubility decreases, and HbS molecules polymerize into long tube-like fibers, which cause characteristic sickling of the RBCs. These abnormal erythrocytes are removed and destroyed by the reticuloendothelial system, resulting in chronic extravascular hemolysis.

Patients with sickle cell disease do not require iron supplementation during pregnancy unless there is laboratory evidence of iron deficiency. Such patients, however, do require adequate supplementation with folate to compensate for an increased folate consumption secondary to the active process of cell replication taking place in their bone marrow.

Women with sickle cell trait should undergo preconception counseling, and the male partner must be examined to see if he carries the trait or not. If the father is a carrier, there are 25% chances of the infant having sickle cell disease. In these cases, early prenatal genetic diagnosis with the help of PCR is important to allow for the possibility of pregnancy termination.

MANAGEMENT

Q. With the help of a long essay, discuss the management of severe anemia in a grand multipara at 36 weeks of gestation.

Q. With the help of a long essay, discuss the management in case of severe anemia at 28 weeks of gestation.

Q. Write a long essay discussing the management of a primi patient with moderate anemia at 30 weeks of gestation.

Q. Discuss the management of labor in a primigravida at term with moderate anemia with the help of a long essay.

Q. With the help of a short essay, discuss investigations and management of IDA in the third trimester.

Q. With the help of a long essay, describe management and investigations in a 34-year-old G5P4L4 with hemoglobin levels 4 g% at 28 weeks of gestation. Also describe prevention of IDA.

Q. What should be the further management in the case mentioned in the beginning of the chapter?
Ans. In this case, anemia is suspected clinically. Investigations such as complete blood count (especially hematocrit and hemoglobin) with peripheral smear, blood indices, especially MCV, need to be carried out.

Q. Peripheral smear revealed presence of microcytic hypochromic type of anemia. What is the likely cause of anemia in the above-mentioned case study?
Ans. Microcytic hypochromic picture on the peripheral smear examination is suggestive of IDA. The common causes of anemia during pregnancy are: physiological causes, IDA, and anemia due to hemorrhagic causes. In this case the history revealed that the patient had yet not started taking iron supplements and gave a history of menorrhagia prior to conception. Moreover, she has three children, the oldest being 6 years old and the youngest just 1 year of age. She conceived the present pregnancy before the restoration of her already depleted iron stores. These could be reasons for her to develop IDA. Therefore, history is of paramount importance for eliciting the cause for anemia.

Q. What are the periods of pregnancy during which the mother is at an increased risk for mortality?
Ans. The periods during pregnancy when the mother is at an increased risk for mortality include the following:
- 30–32 weeks of pregnancy
- During labor
- Immediately following delivery
- Puerperium (pulmonary embolism/cardiac failure)

INVESTIGATIONS

Q. What is hematocrit value and how is it influenced by anemia?

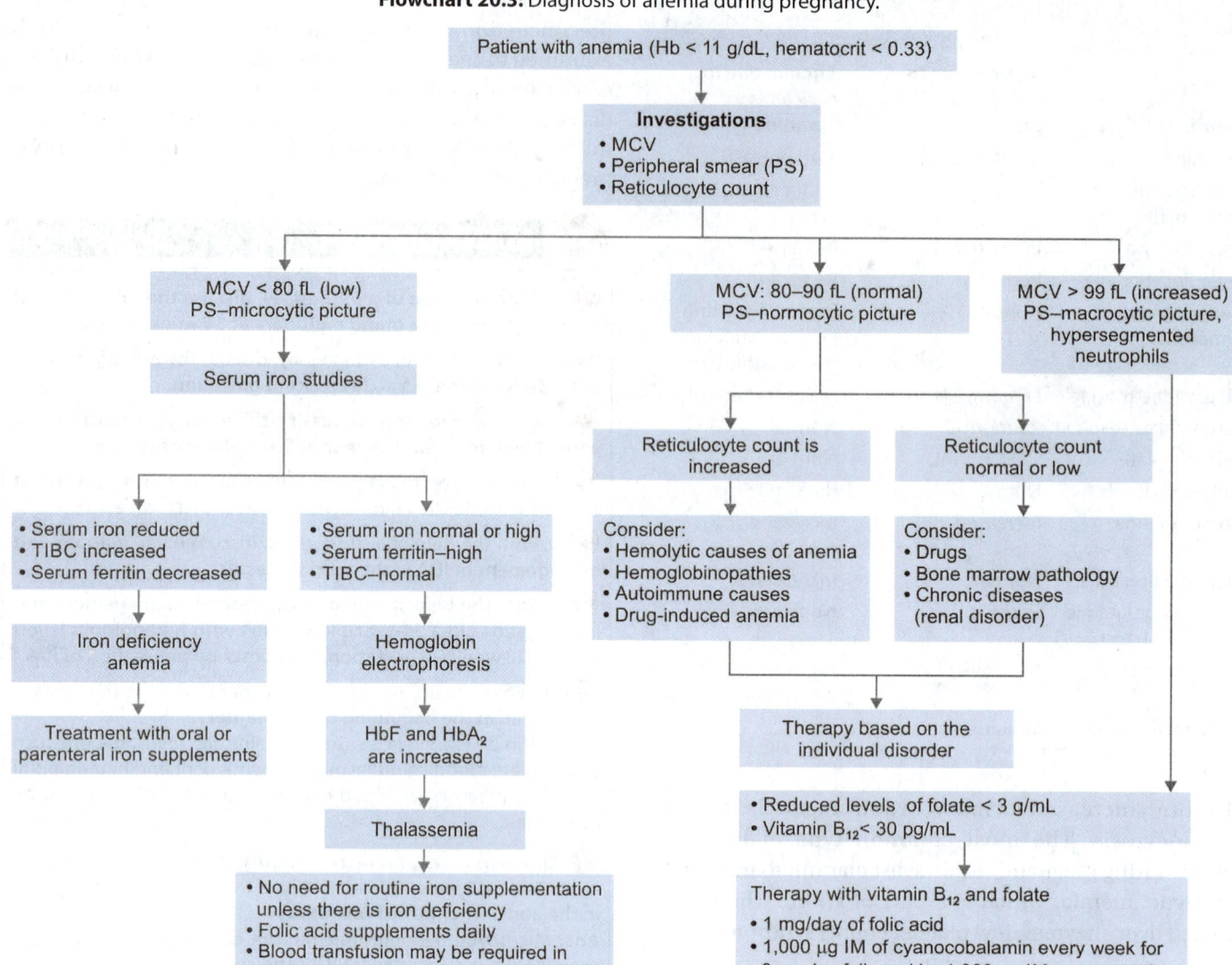

Flowchart 20.3: Diagnosis of anemia during pregnancy.

(HbA$_2$: hemoglobin alpha 2; HbF: fetal hemoglobin; IM: intramuscular; MCV: mean corpuscular volume; TIBC: total iron-binding capacity)

The algorithm for diagnosis of anemia during pregnancy is described in **Flowchart 20.3**. The following investigations need to be done.

HEMOGLOBIN AND HEMATOCRIT

Hemoglobin concentration reflects the capacity of blood to distribute oxygen from the lungs to tissues in the body. Hematocrit, on the other hand, reflects the measurement of the percentage of RBCs found in a specific volume of blood. It is sometimes also known as packed cell volume (PCV). A low hematocrit indicates a decrease in number or size of RBC mass or an increase in plasma volume. Sahli's method (**Fig. 20.9**) is most accurate and is commonly used for the estimation of blood hemoglobin levels.

The hematocrit value refers to the percentage of RBCs relative to plasma volume. In nonpregnant women hematocrit can range from 38% to 45%. However, in pregnant women, due to hemodilution, normal values can be much lower, e.g., 34% in single and 30% in twin or multiple pregnancy even with normal stores of iron, folic acid, and vitamin B$_{12}$. The lower range of hematocrit during pregnancy is probably due to "the physiologic hemodilution of pregnancy" and does not indicate a decrease in oxygen-carrying capacity or true anemia. Hematocrit level < 33% is considered iron deficient and should be treated.

BLOOD CELLULAR INDICES

Abnormalities in various blood indices with IDA are described in **Table 20.7**. Some of these indices are mentioned in the following text.

Mean Corpuscular Volume

Mean corpuscular volume indicates the morphology of the RBCs, which could be microcytic, normocytic, or macrocytic.

$$MCV = \frac{\text{Packed cell volume}}{\text{Red cell count per liter}} \times 10^{15} \text{ fL}$$

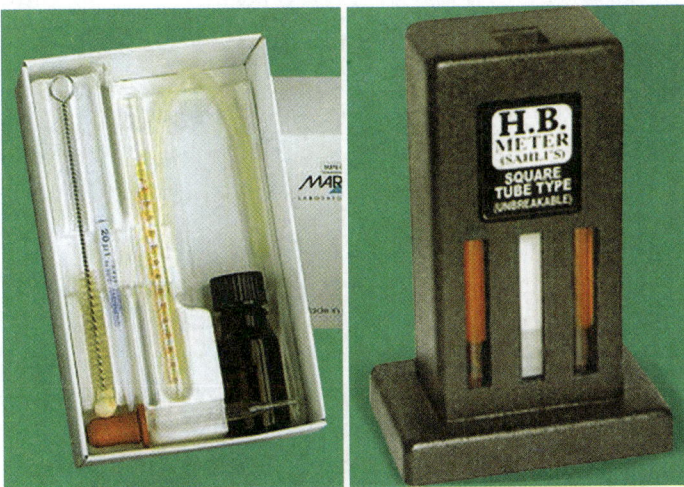

Fig. 20.9: Sahli's apparatus used for estimation of hemoglobin.

TABLE 20.7: Abnormalities in blood indices with iron deficiency anemia.

Blood index	Normal value	Value in iron deficiency anemia
MCH	26.7–33.7 pg/cell (average 30.6 pg/cell)	<26.7 pg/cell
MCHC	32–36 g% (average 33.9 g%)	<30 g%
MCV	83–97 fL (average 90 fL)	<76 fL
Hemoglobin	12.1–14.1 g/dL	<11 g/dL in first and third trimesters and <10.5 g/dL in second trimester
Hematocrit	36.1–44.3%	<36.1%
Red cell count	3.9–5.0 × 10^6 cells/µL (average 4.42 × 10^6 cells/µL)	<3.9 × 10^6 cells/µL or normal
Red cell distribution index	31–36%	<31%

(MCH: mean corpuscular hemoglobin; MCHC: mean corpuscular hemoglobin concentration; MCV: mean corpuscular volume)

Mean Corpuscular Hemoglobin

Mean corpuscular hemoglobin indicates the average weight of hemoglobin in RBC. MCH is reduced in cases of microcytosis and hypochromia. MCH alone, however, cannot distinguish between microcytosis and hypochromia.

$$MCH = \frac{Hb \text{ in gm/dL}}{Red \text{ cell count (million/mm}^3)} \times 10 \text{ pg}$$

Mean Corpuscular Hemoglobin Concentration

Mean corpuscular hemoglobin concentration represents the weight of hemoglobin/volume of cells. Since this index is independent of cell size, it is more useful than MCH in distinguishing between microcytosis and hypochromia. A low MCHC always indicates hypochromia, as a microcyte with a normal hemoglobin concentration will have a low MCH but a normal MCHC.

$$MCHC = \frac{Hb \text{ in gm\%}}{PCV} \times gm\%$$

Out of the various indices used, MCV and MCHC are the two most sensitive indices of iron deficiency.

Red Cell Distribution Width

Red cell distribution width indicates the variation in the size of RBCs. Thus, it is elevated in anemias resulting from iron deficiency.

RETICULOCYTE COUNT

Reticulocyte count helps in measuring the percentage of reticulocytes, which are slightly immature RBCs in blood. Normally, the development and maturation of the reticulocytes take place in the red bone marrow, and then they circulate for about a day in the blood stream before developing into mature RBCs. Thus, by measuring the reticulocyte count, clinician gets an idea regarding the rate of synthesis of reticulocytes by the marrow and their release into the blood stream. Normally, about 1–2% of the RBCs in the blood are reticulocytes. The reticulocyte count may rise when there is excessive blood loss or in certain diseases such as hemolytic anemia in which RBCs are destroyed prematurely.

PERIPHERAL SMEAR

Peripheral smear examination is another simple method for diagnosis of anemia. Examination of the peripheral smear is an important part of the workup of patients with anemia.

Peripheral Smear in Iron Deficiency Anemia

Figures 20.10A and B show, respectively, the normal blood smear and peripheral smear in case of IDA. Peripheral blood smear in case of iron deficiency shows microcytic and hypochromic picture. There is presence of pale-looking RBCs with large central vacuoles (hypochromic RBCs). Other findings on peripheral smear are as follows:

- *Anisocytosis (abnormal size of cells):* The RBCs are small and deformed (microcytosis). Microcytosis is apparent in the smear long before the MCV is decreased after an event producing iron deficiency.
- *Poikilocytosis (abnormal shape of cells):* Presence of pencil cells and target cells
- Presence of ring or pessary cells with central hypochromia (large central vacuoles)
- RBC osmotic fragility is slightly reduced.
- Radiochromium-51Cr studies show reduced RBC lifespan.

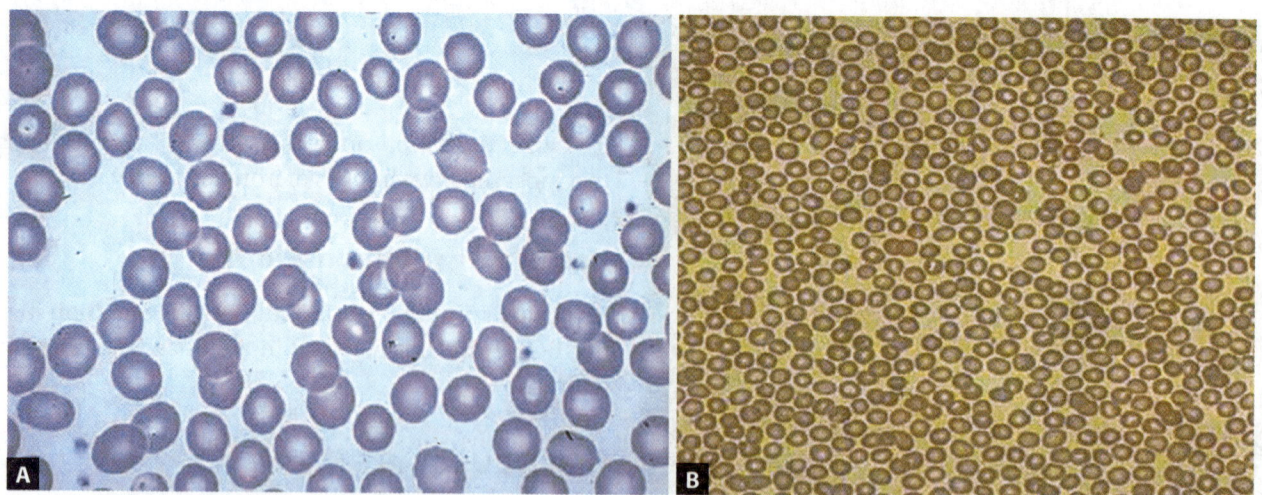

Figs. 20.10A and B: (A) Normal blood smear; (B) Peripheral smear in case of iron deficiency anemia.

Peripheral Smear in Megaloblastic Anemia

- Presence of macrocytes and megaloblasts
- Hypersegmentation of neutrophils (**Fig. 20.11**)
- Fully hemoglobinized RBCs

Peripheral Smear in Hemolytic Anemia

Peripheral smear in cases of thalassemia and sickle cell anemia is shown in **Figures 20.12A and B**, respectively. In thalassemia there is the presence of polychromatic, stippled, and target cells (**Fig. 20.12A**). Peripheral smear in case of sickle cell anemia shows the presence of crescent-shaped target cells. There may be presence of characteristic sickle-shaped cells (**Fig. 20.12B**). If the person is asplenic, there may be presence of RBCs containing nuclear material (Howell–Jolly bodies).

Peripheral Smear in Combined Folate and Iron Deficiency

Peripheral smear in these cases reveals a population of macrocytes mixed among the microcytic hypochromic cells. This combination can normalize the MCV.

> Q. Write a long essay on iron metabolism and management of severe anemia in pregnancy.

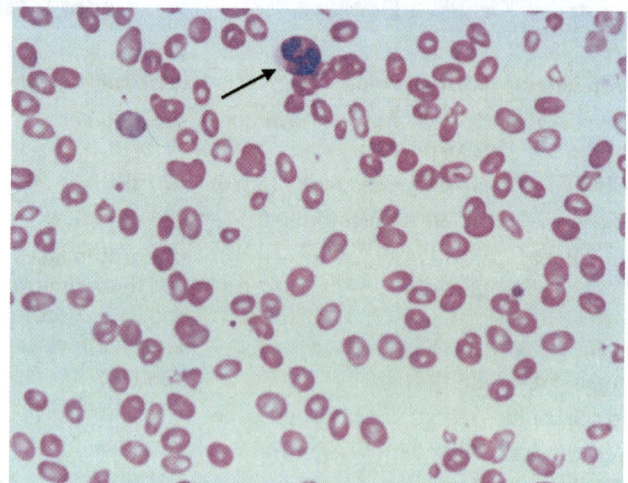

Fig. 20.11: Peripheral smear in case of megaloblastic anemia (the arrow is pointing toward hypersegmented neutrophil).

SERUM IRON STUDIES

Normal iron metabolism in the body is shown in **Figure 20.13**. A low serum iron and ferritin with an elevated TIBC is diagnostic of iron deficiency. Transferrin delivers iron to bone marrow and storage sites. Circulating transferrin is normally only about 30% saturated with iron. The remaining 70% is unbound and represents the TIBC. The finding of a low serum iron and a high TIBC is highly indicative of IDA (**Table 20.8**).

Ferritin is storage form of iron, whose concentration in the serum is proportional to total iron stores. Low serum ferritin levels are virtually diagnostic of iron deficiency as they are decreased only in IDA (**Table 20.9**). In IDA, iron stores are depleted prior to anemia; therefore, the earliest change usually observed is reduced ferritin levels (<20 ng/mL). Categorization of women using ferritin and hemoglobin estimations is described in **Table 20.9**. IDA is also associated with the elevation of erythrocyte protoporphyrin levels as there is no iron available to form hemoglobin.

STOOL EXAMINATION

Stool examination for ova and cysts (three consecutive samples) can help in determining if the cause of anemia can be attributed to parasitic infestation. Testing the stools for the presence of hemoglobin is useful in establishing gastrointestinal bleeding as the etiology of IDA. Usually, chemical testing that detects >20 mL of blood loss daily from the upper gastrointestinal tract is employed. Severe IDA can

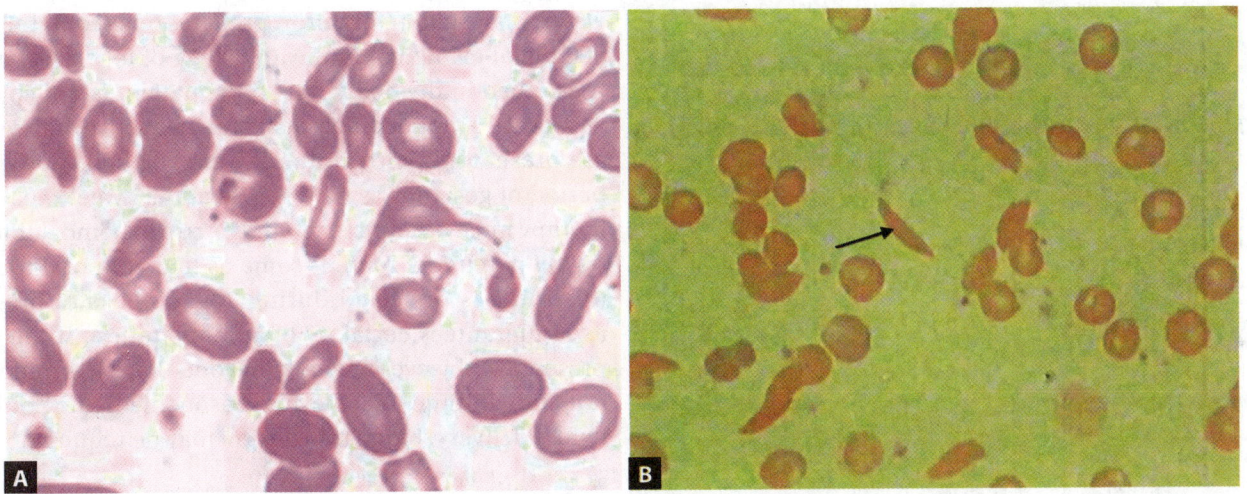

Figs. 20.12A and B: Peripheral smear in case of hemolytic anemia. (A) Thalassemia; (B) Sickle cell anemia (arrow points toward a sickle-shaped cell).

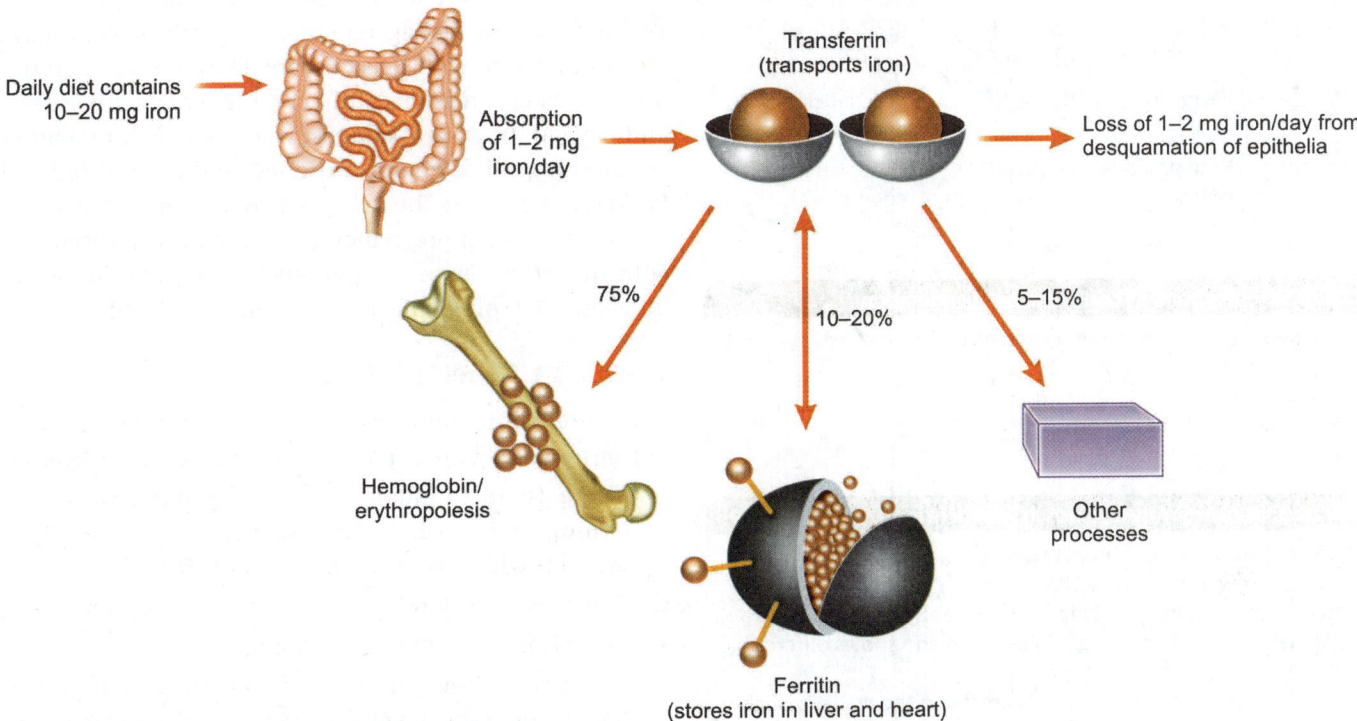

Fig. 20.13: Normal iron metabolism in the body.

occur in patients with a persistent loss of <20 mL/day. From an Indian perspective, most common worm infections associated with cases of anemia include *Ascaris lumbricoides* (round worm), *Ancylostoma duodenale* (Old World hookworm), and *Necator americanus* (New World hook worm).

URINE ROUTINE/MICROSCOPY

Urine routine/microscopy helps in detecting the presence of pus cells/occult blood or schistosomes.

HEMOGLOBIN ELECTROPHORESIS

Hemoglobin electrophoresis and measurement of HbA_2 and HbF are useful in establishing either β-thalassemia or hemoglobin C or D as the etiology of microcytic anemia. Unfortunately, simple tests do not exist for α-thalassemia in most laboratories, and it is a diagnosis of exclusion.

BONE MARROW EXAMINATION

A bone marrow aspirate stained for iron (Perls stain) can be diagnostic of iron deficiency. While the performance of bone marrow examination for the diagnosis of iron deficiency has largely been displaced by the performance of serum iron, TIBC, and serum ferritin, the absence of stainable iron in a bone marrow aspirate reflects absent iron stores. The indications of bone marrow examination have been enumerated in **Box 20.2**. It is diagnostic in identifying

TABLE 20.8: Changes in serum iron studies with iron deficiency anemia.

Blood parameter	Normal value	Value in iron deficiency anemia
Serum transferrin levels	200–360 mg/dL	>360 mg/dL
Serum iron concentration	60–175 µg/dL	<60 µg/dL
Transferrin saturation	25–60%	<25%
Ferritin levels	50–145 ng/mL	<20 ng/mL
Serum protoporphyrin	30–70 µg/dL	>70 µg/dL

TABLE 20.9: Categorization of women using ferritin and hemoglobin estimations.

Categories	Serum ferritin levels	Hemoglobin	Diagnosis
Category I	Within the normal range	Within the normal range	Normal, iron deficiency excluded
Category II	Reduced	Within the normal range	Storage iron depletion
Category III	Reduced	Reduced	Iron deficiency anemia
Category IV	Within the normal range	Reduced	Other causes of anemia

BOX 20.2: Indications of bone marrow examination.

- No response to any treatment even after 4 weeks
- Suspected aplastic anemia
- Kala-azar
- Sideroblastic anemia

BOX 20.3: Bone marrow findings in iron deficiency anemia.

- Micronormoblastic erythroid hyperplasia
- Bone marrow iron is reduced or absent
- Intermediate normoblasts are predominantly seen
- Cytoplasm of the normoblasts is reduced and shows differential staining
- Cytoplasm matures slowly in comparison to the nucleus, such that the cytoplasm is still polychromatic, while the nucleus has become pyknotic

the sideroblastic anemia by showing the presence of ringed sideroblasts **(Box 20.3)**. Occasionally, it is useful in differentiating patients with the anemia of chronic disorders or α-thalassemia from patients with iron deficiency. It also serves as the investigation of choice in cases where anemia is related to aplastic anemia.

TREATMENT/OBSTETRIC MANAGEMENT

Treatment of the patient diagnosed with iron deficiency basically depends on the period of gestation as described in **Flowchart 20.4**. If the period of gestation is <30 completed weeks of gestation, oral iron preparations (containing 200–300 mg of elemental iron with 500 µg of folic acid) must be prescribed in divided doses. If the patient is not compliant with oral therapy or other causes for ineffective oral treatment are present, parenteral therapy may be considered. If the period of gestation is between 30 and 36 weeks, parenteral therapy must be administered. The rise in hemoglobin levels by the parenteral route is same as that with oral route, but this route is preferred during 30–36 weeks of pregnancy as it guarantees certainty of administration. If the patient presents with severe anemia beyond 36 weeks and there is not enough time to achieve a reasonable hemoglobin level before delivery, blood transfusion may be required.

PATIENT PRESENTING WITH SEVERE ANEMIA IN LATE PREGNANCY (AFTER 36 WEEKS)

Women with severe anemia presenting late in pregnancy should ideally be managed in hospital settings. They may or may not present with heart failure. However, they all need urgent admission and require complete rest with sedation and oxygen. In case of congestive cardiac failure, patients should be given digitalis, diuretics, and packed red cells. Packed red cells are the preferred choice for severe anemia in the later part of pregnancy. This should be infused along with diuretics. Once the patient is stabilized, total dose infusion (TDI) of iron dextran may be considered.

BLOOD TRANSFUSION

Indications of blood transfusion for correction of anemia during pregnancy are as follows and are listed in the **Box 20.4**:

- There is not enough time to achieve a reasonable hemoglobin level before delivery, e.g., the patient presents with severe anemia beyond 36 weeks.
- There is acute blood loss or associated infections.
- Anemia is refractory to iron therapy.
- In all the above-mentioned cases, packed red cell transfusion must be given with meticulous care so as to prevent severe circulatory overload, pulmonary edema, and development of any transfusion-related reactions.

RESPONSE TO IRON THERAPY

Much before the treatment causes an improvement in the degree of anemia and hematological indices, there occurs an improvement in subjective symptoms such as fatigue and lassitude. Epithelial changes may also revert to normal. Response to treatment is shown by the indicators mentioned in **Box 20.5**.

The earliest hematological response to treatment is reticulocytosis. Initially, there is an increase in reticulocytes by 4–6 days, which peaks by 9–12 days. Hemoglobin levels usually start rising at the rate of 2 g/dL after 3 weeks. The plasma iron will gradually increase, and the initially elevated

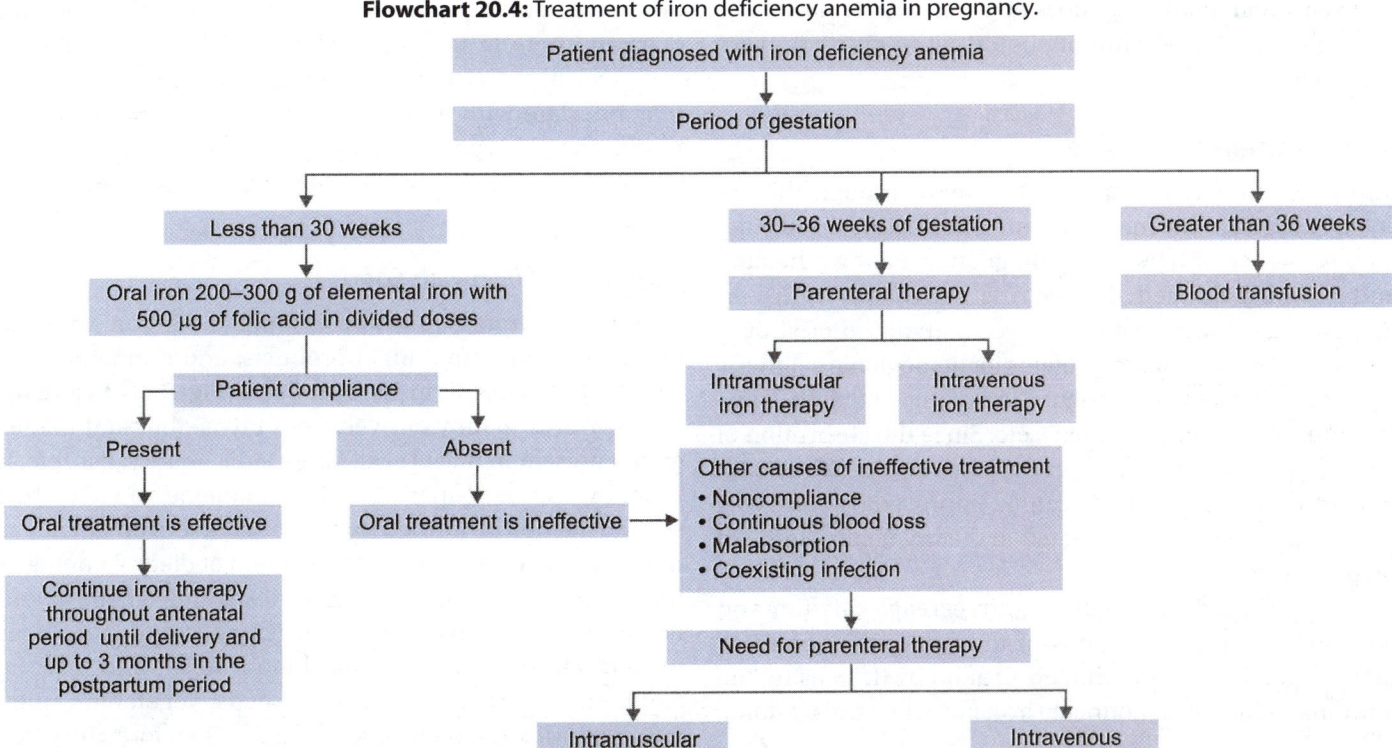

Flowchart 20.4: Treatment of iron deficiency anemia in pregnancy.

BOX 20.4: Indications for blood transfusion during pregnancy.

- Micronormoblastic erythroid hyperplasia
- There is not enough time to achieve a reasonable hemoglobin level before delivery, e.g., the patient presents with severe anemia beyond 36 weeks
- There is acute blood loss or associated infections
- Hemoglobin levels < 6 g%
- Moderate and severe anemia in patients with known heart disease or severe respiratory infections
- Symptomatic anemia not responding to conventional therapy
- Placenta previa with hemoglobin levels < 10 g/dL
- Patients developing side effects or no response to both oral and parenteral iron therapy

BOX 20.5: Indicators for showing response to iron therapy.

- Increase in the reticulocyte count (2–16%)
- Increase in hemoglobin levels
- Epithelial changes (especially in tongue and nails) revert to normal

BOX 20.6: Causes of failure of oral iron therapy.

- Incorrect diagnosis (presence of noniron deficiency microcytic anemia)
- Faulty absorption of iron
- Presence of chronic infection
- Loss of iron from the body
- Lack of patient compliance
- Persistent blood loss (hookworm, bleeding piles, etc.)
- Ineffective release of iron from a particular preparation
- Concomitant folate deficiency

TIBC will return to normal in about 1 month. Blood ferritin levels return to normal in about 4–6 months. If the predictable rise in hemoglobin does not occur after oral iron therapy, the clinician must try to find out the possible reasons. Some of the reasons are listed in **Box 20.6**.

PREVENTION OF IRON DEFICIENCY ANEMIA

As previously explained, in most parts of the developing world including India, there is a need for routine iron supplementation to all pregnant women in order to build up their iron stores. It is also advisable to build up iron store before a woman marries and becomes pregnant. This can be achieved by taking the following steps:

1. Routine determination of hemoglobin or hematocrit, starting from the time of adolescence
2. Routine screening for anemia and provision of supplements to adolescent girls, starting right from the school days
3. Encouraging consumption of diet containing iron rich foods
4. Fortification of widely consumed food with iron
5. Management of endemic infection (e.g., malaria)

Routine Determination of Hemoglobin or Hematocrit

Hemoglobin or hematocrit should be routinely determined at the time of first prenatal visit in order to detect any preexisting anemia. Anemia accompanied by ferritin levels < 20 ng/mL can also be presumed to be due to iron deficiency.

Even when the woman does take iron supplements, her hemoglobin and hematocrit should be monitored every 2–3 months.

Dietary Changes

Improving nutritional status of women through dietary changes is one of the most important strategies for reducing the prevalence of IDA during pregnancy. Eating a healthy and a well-balanced diet during pregnancy helps in maintaining the iron stores. A good quality diet should contain not only sufficient proteins for hemoglobin synthesis but also various micronutrients, including vitamin A, zinc, calcium, riboflavin, vitamin B_{12}, etc. Since the absorption of dietary iron can be affected by numerous factors **(Box 20.7)**, iron absorption in the body can be improved by observing some simple precautions related to dietary habits. Some of them are listed in **Box 20.8**.

Phytates present in whole-grain cereals, calcium and phosphorus in milk, tannins in tea, and polyphenols in many vegetables inhibit iron absorption by decreasing the intestinal solubility of nonheme iron from the meals. Adding lime juice or orange juice, both of which are rich in vitamin C, would help in increasing the absorption of nonheme iron. On the other hand, drinking excessive tea or coffee may interfere with iron absorption. All iron preparations inhibit the absorption of tetracyclines, sulfonamides, and trimethoprim. Thus, iron should not be given together with these agents.

Examples of Iron-rich Foods

Two types of iron are present in food: heme iron, which is principally found in animal products, and nonheme iron, which is found mainly in plant products **(Figs. 20.14A and B)**. Heme iron is mainly derived from myoglobin and hemoglobin present in meat (beef, lamb, etc.), poultry, fish, etc. It is better absorbed (up to 35%) than nonheme iron but forms smaller fraction of the diet. During the course of pregnancy as the iron stores decrease, the absorption of dietary nonheme iron increases. Nonheme iron is mostly in ferric form and needs to be reduced to ferrous form for absorption. Sources of heme iron include animal blood, flesh, and viscera. Nonheme iron includes cereals, seeds, vegetables, milk, and eggs. Milk is a poor source of iron. Therefore, breastfed babies may require iron supplementation.

- *Animal products:*
  - *Red meat:* Beef, pork, lamb (liver should be avoided due to high content of vitamin A)
  - *Poultry:* Chicken, duck, turkey
  - *Fish:* Shellfish (clams, mussels, sardines, anchovies, and oysters)
  - *Eggs:* One large egg (70–80 mg) contains about 1 mg of iron.
- *Plant products:*
  - *Dried fruits:* Half a cup of walnuts (125 mg) contain approximately 3.75 mg of iron, half a cup of cashew nuts approximately 2.65 mg, half a cup of raisins 2.55 mg, and half a cup of peanuts approximately 1.55 mg of iron.
  - *Green leafy vegetables:* Spinach, broccoli, kale, turnip greens, and collard greens are a good source of iron. Half-cup spinach contains nearly 2.4 mg iron.
  - Pulses, cereals, jaggery
  - Legumes, such as lima beans and green peas, dry beans, and peas
  - Yeast-leavened, whole-wheat bread and rolls
  - Iron-enriched white bread, pasta, rice, and cereals
  - Since folate deficiency has been found to commonly coexist with that of iron deficiency, diet rich in both iron and folic acid must be encouraged. Dietary sources of folate include the following:
    - Leafy, dark green vegetables
    - Dried beans and peas
    - Citrus fruits and juices, and most berries
    - Fortified breakfast cereals
    - Enriched grain products

BOX 20.7: Factors reducing the absorption of dietary iron.

- Phytates present in whole-grain cereals, legumes, nuts, seeds, etc.
- Calcium and phosphorus in milk
- Tannins in tea (a cup of tea taken with meals can inhibit iron absorption by 11%)
- Polyphenols present in many vegetables
- Increased gastric pH due to the presence of antacids or reduced gastric acidity
- High phenol content of some fruits, e.g., strawberries and melon
- Cow's milk with high content of calcium and casein inhibits iron absorption

---

BOX 20.8: Methods for improving iron absorption in the diet.

- Adding lime juice, which is a good source of vitamin C, to one's food
- Avoiding the intake of substances such as tea, coffee, and milk with the meals
- Cooking food in iron vessels
- Taking iron tablets with orange juice or water rather than with milk, tea, or coffee
- Avoiding the use of antacids with iron as lower gastric acidity reduces absorption of iron
- Eating fermented food aids iron absorption by reducing the phytate content of diet
- Increasing the intake of food containing ascorbic acid such as citrus food, broccoli, and other dark green vegetables
- Foods containing muscle protein enhance iron absorption due to the effect of cysteine-containing peptides released from the partially digested meat, which reduces ferric to ferrous salts and forms soluble iron complexes
- Cereal milling to remove bran reduces its phytic acid content by 50%

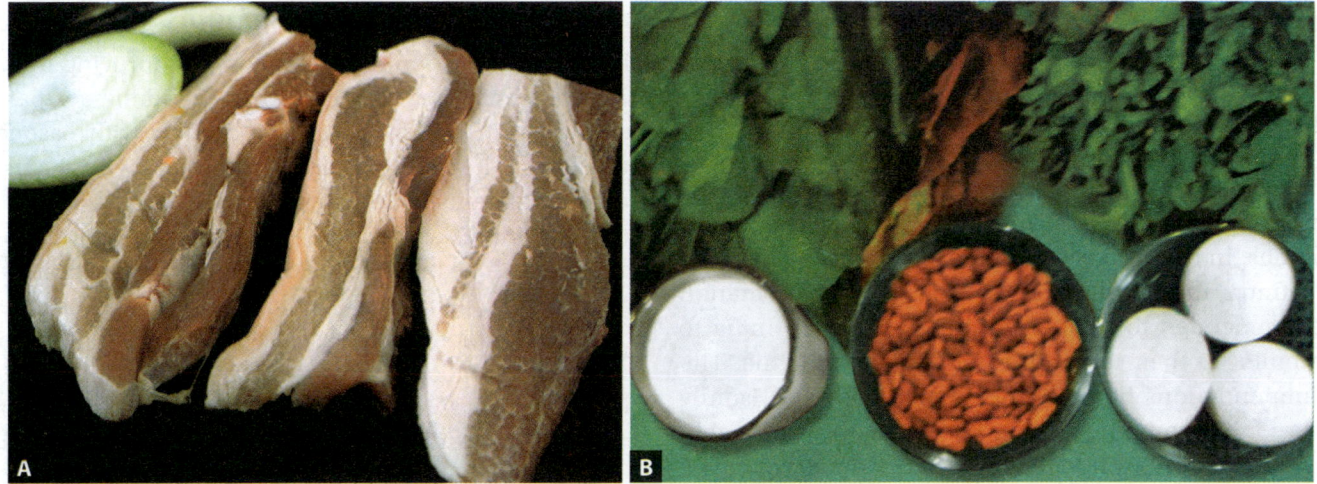

Figs. 20.14A and B: Components of healthy diet for prevention of iron deficiency anemia. (A) Sources of heme iron in the diet; (B) Sources of nonheme iron in the diet.

Fortification of Food with Iron

Fortification of the food with iron and folic acid is being tried in some countries and has been found to be one of the most effective, inexpensive, and simple strategies for ensuring adequate supply of iron to large segments of the population in both developed and developing countries. Fortification of cereal grain products was introduced in 1941 in the US when iron and three vitamins, thiamin, riboflavin, and niacin, were added to flour and bread. Ready-to-eat cereals were fortified at about the same time. Food fortification is done with iron salts such as ferrous sulfate, ferrous gluconate, ferrous fumarate, ferrous succinate, or chelated iron compounds such as bovine hemoglobin concentrate and sodium ferric ethylenediaminetetraacetate (Fe-Na-EDTA). These fortifications have contributed to an increased dietary iron intake and reductions in IDA in the US. Fortification of food has been tried in other countries as well, e.g., fortification of rice in Philippines with ferrous sulfate and fortification of wheat flour with metallic iron in European countries including Sweden, the UK, etc. There have been proposals regarding fortification of common salt with iron salts on a large scale.

Management of Endemic Infection

Malaria and hookworm infection are the major factors responsible for causing anemia in pregnancy by causing hemolysis and chronic blood loss, respectively. The preferred drug for treating malaria in pregnancy is chloroquine. Malaria prophylaxis should also be given to pregnant women in areas where malaria is endemic. Also, anthelminthic drugs such as albendazole or mebendazole are recommended to all pregnant women after the first trimester of pregnancy. These drugs would help in treating hookworm infestation. To prevent recurrence of infection, patients should be advised to take certain precautions including the use of proper footwear, improvement of sanitation, and maintenance of personal hygiene.

Exogenous Iron Supplementation

> **Q. Write a short note on national anemia prophylaxis program.**

Iron supplementation has presently become the most common strategy currently used for controlling iron deficiency in developing countries. As described previously, pregnancy results in development of physiological anemia. Also, in order to fulfill the iron requirement related to pregnancy, there is requirement for exogenous iron supplementation. The WHO recommends universal iron supplementation for pregnant women, comprising 120 mg elemental iron daily and 2,800 µg (2.8 mg) of folic acid provided weekly throughout pregnancy, beginning as soon as possible after conception in countries with prevalence of anemia < 40% and an additional 3 months postpartum in countries where prevalence is >40%.

Along with this, iron-rich diets and diets which enhance iron absorption must be encouraged as well. Iron supplementation leads to increased hemoglobin concentration, resulting in improved oxygen-carrying capacity, which acts as a buffer against increased blood loss that might occur during delivery.

In developing countries, routine iron supplementation during pregnancy is practiced, regardless of the fact whether the mother is anemic or not. In India, the Ministry of Health and Family Welfare, Government of India (2013) has recently recommended that all pregnant ladies must be given iron–folic acid supplementation (amounting to 100 mg elemental iron and 500 µg of folic acid) every day for at least 100 days, starting after the first trimester, at 14–16 weeks of gestation. This must be followed by the same dose for 100 days in postpartum period. In addition to this, all women in the reproductive age group in the preconception period and up to the first trimester of the pregnancy must be prescribed 400 µg of folic acid tablets daily to reduce the incidence of neural tube defects in the fetus. In a woman seen late in pregnancy, 120 mg of elemental iron daily is recommended during pregnancy and puerperium.

Even women belonging to reproductive age groups in the developing countries are at an increased risk of anemia because of chronic iron depletion during the menstrual cycle, inadequate dietary intakes, and recurrent infections. In lieu of the severe intensity of the problem in the country, intermittent iron–folic acid supplementation is recommended to all menstruating women in India to help build up their iron stores and prevent anemia. The recommendations by the Ministry of Health and Family Welfare (Government of India, 2013) for iron–folic acid supplementation in children, adolescents, women belonging to reproductive age groups, and pregnant women have been summarized in **Figure 20.15**.

However, presently there is not enough evidence to demonstrate with certainty that routine daily or intermittent iron or iron–folic acid supplementation in pregnancy improves functional and health outcomes for women and babies. Also, the routine iron supplementation during pregnancy to all women (regardless of their iron status) in developed countries where anemia is not prevalent is still debatable.

TREATMENT

> Q. Write a long essay on newer iron preparations available for treatment during pregnancy.
>
> Q. Write a short essay on iron sucrose.
>
> Q. With the help of a short essay, discuss parenteral iron therapy.
>
> Q. With the help of a long essay, discuss the management of postpartum anemia.

Treatment with Iron Supplements

The use of iron supplements helps in improving the iron status of the mother during pregnancy and the postpartum period, even in women who enter pregnancy with reasonable iron stores. The main problems associated with the use of iron supplements is occurrence of side effects **(Box 20.9)** including anorexia, diarrhea, epigastric discomfort, nausea, vomiting and constipation, passage of dark greenish or black-colored stools, temporary staining of teeth, etc. The enteric-coated and prolonged-release preparations are not favored as these preparations dissolve poorly in the acidic milieu of the duodenum, where maximum absorption of iron occurs. Since iron is absorbed in ferrous form, only ferrous salts must be used. Iron must be taken orally in 3–4 doses, 1 hour prior to meals. Oral iron therapy must be continued for at least 12 months after the anemia has been corrected in order to replenish the depleted iron stores. Although associated with gastrointestinal side effects, oral iron supplements are not associated with the anaphylaxis that can occur with parenteral iron preparations.

The amount of elemental iron present in different types of oral preparations varies from one another. While prescribing a dose of iron supplements to a patient, it is important to distinguish between the amount of iron compound and the equivalent amount of elemental iron in the preparation. Thus, 300 mg of hydrated ferrous sulfate, which contains 20% iron by weight, would provide 60 mg of elemental iron, while 300 mg of ferrous gluconate, which contains 12% iron by weight, would provide 36 mg of elemental iron, and 200 mg of ferrous fumarate would provide 64 mg of elemental iron **(Table 20.10)**. However, none of the iron preparations have shown superiority over the others in different studies.

Since oral iron preparations are associated with numerous previously mentioned side effects, slow-release

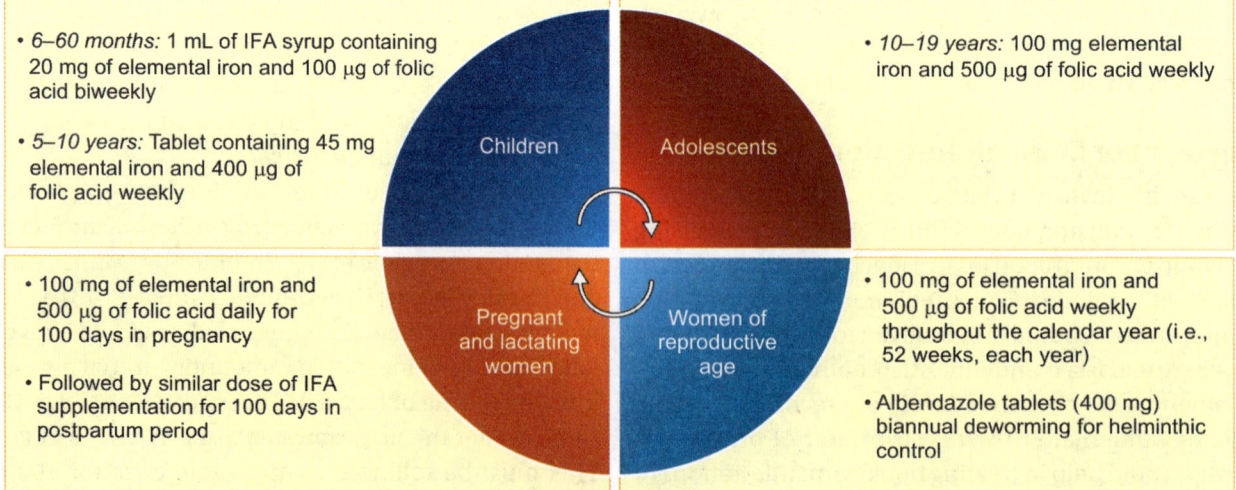

Fig. 20.15: Iron–folic acid (IFA) supplementation program by the Ministry of Health and Family Welfare (Government of India, 2013).
Source: Ministry of Health and Family Welfare, Government of India. (2013). Guidelines for control of iron deficiency anemia. [online] Available from https://www.nhm.gov.in/images/pdf/programmes/child-health/guidelines/Control-of-Iron-Deficiency-Anaemia.pdf. [Last accessed November, 2013].

Anemia in Pregnancy

BOX 20.9: Possible side effects associated with iron medication.

- Epigastric discomfort, nausea, diarrhea, or constipation
- Feces may turn black
- Interaction with various drugs, e.g., inhibition of absorption of antibiotics such as tetracyclines, sulfonamides, and trimethoprim
- Temporary staining of teeth
- Epigastric pain is likely to result from a combination of high-dose vitamin C supplements with iron tablets

TABLE 20.10: Amount of elemental iron in different iron formulations.

Molecular iron formulation	Dose of the salt (mg)	Elemental iron per tablet (mg tablet)
Hydrated ferrous sulfate	300	60
Ferrous sulfate (anhydrous)	200	74
Ferrous fumarate	200	64
Ferrous gluconate	300	36
Ferrous glycine sulfate	225	45
Ferrous succinate	100	35
Ferrous sulfate (dry)	200	65
Iron polysaccharide	140	140

supplements were introduced with the objective of reducing the occurrence of side effects. However, the efficacy of some of these slow-release preparations in terms of amount of iron absorbed is still not known for sure. Thus, only those slow-release preparations whose absorption efficacy is known should be used. Moreover, iron tablets are absorbed more completely when given in between rather than with meals because dietary factors are likely to interfere with iron absorption.

Most symptoms of iron intolerance are related to the dose of elemental iron rather than the actual prescription. Therefore, starting a smaller dose and gradually increasing it may help reduce the side effects and improve compliance. Patients who are unable to tolerate the iron tablets can be given iron in the form of syrup. Iron syrup should be preferably taken by a straw to prevent the staining of teeth.

Stoffel et al. (2017) have shown that following oral supplementation with iron, there may be an acute rise in the hepcidin levels. This may be the reason for poor absorption from the afternoon/evening dose of oral iron when iron supplements are provided daily as divided doses. Therefore, offering iron supplements on alternate days and in the form of single daily dose is likely to optimize iron absorption. According to the researchers, this must be the preferable dosing regimen in women with IDA.

How to Select the Oral Iron Salt?

There are many iron preparations available in the market, and a clinician is often confused as to which iron preparation should be advised to the patient. Ferrous sulfate is the least expensive and best absorbed form of iron. If for some reasons this is not tolerated, then ferrous gluconate or fumarate are the next choices for iron therapy. Newer iron formulations such as carbonyl iron and polymaltose iron are claimed to produce fewer side effects. Carbonyl iron has been proposed as an alternative to other commonly used iron salts, on the assumption that it can be administered in large doses with minimal side effects. This iron preparation is composed of metallic iron powder, having a particle size of <5 μm. Since it is insoluble, it is not absorbed until it is converted into ionic form. The bioavailability of carbonyl iron has been estimated to be about 70% of that of an equivalent amount of ferrous sulfate. Oral doses as high as 600 mg three times a day have not been found to be associated with any side effects. However, presently there is no good evidence available to prove this fact. Besides, these newer iron formulations are much more costly than the previously available ones.

The iron salt to be prescribed to the patient should be selected on the basis of patient compliance, tolerance, side effects, clinical situation of the patient, and availability of a particular salt. In order to build up the iron stores, oral iron must be continued for 3–6 months after hemoglobin has come to normal levels. Some of the methods of reducing side effects associated with oral iron therapy are listed in **Box 20.10**.

Though intake of iron with food would result in reduction of side effects related to gastrointestinal tract, this is controversial in the Indian settings where the staple diet consists of cereals containing phytic acid, which is supposed to interfere with iron absorption.

Parenteral Forms of Iron

The two main types of parenteral iron preparations, which were previously being used in India, were iron dextran (imferon), which could be used both intramuscularly and intravenously, and iron sorbitol citrate, which could be used only by IV route. Over the last few years, there has been a decline in the use of IM iron preparations for treatment of IDA due to safety of IV preparations in view of a much lower risk of anaphylactic reactions. Some of the indications for parenteral iron therapy are mentioned in **Box 20.11**. Sometimes, pregnant women with severe anemia present after 30–32 weeks of pregnancy. Though the rate of improvement in hemoglobin production by both oral and parenteral routes is similar, parenteral iron is preferred over oral forms during this time of pregnancy due to the certainty of administration of parenteral form of iron.

The iron preparations which are commonly being used nowadays in India include the second-generation IV

> **BOX 20.10:** Methods of reducing side effects associated with oral iron therapy.
>
> - Starting with one tablet daily and increasing the dosage every 3–5 days can sometimes help patients tolerate oral iron better than immediately starting with three-times-daily dosing
> - Avoiding the use of high-dose vitamin C supplements with iron tablets, as this would result in increased epigastric pain
> - Taking iron supplements with meals, even though this results in reduced iron absorption; the frequency of side effects is reduced as well
> - Administration of iron supplements at bedtime
> - Use of iron formulations containing reduced amount of elemental iron

> **BOX 20.11:** Indications for the use of parenteral iron therapy.
>
> - Intolerance to oral form of iron
> - When iron deficiency is not correctable with oral treatment
> - *Noncompliance on part of the patient:* The patient repeatedly fails to heed instructions or is incapable of following them
> - Patient is suffering from inflammatory bowel disease (e.g., ulcerative colitis) in which the symptoms may get aggravated by oral iron therapy
> - The patient is unable to absorb iron orally
> - Patients near term (32–36 weeks of pregnancy)
> - Rapid rise in the hemoglobin and iron stores is required
> - Nonresponse to oral iron therapy

iron preparation, iron sucrose and the third-generation preparation, ferric carboxymaltose (FCM).

Iron Sucrose

Iron sucrose is a second-generation IV iron preparation, available under a variety of names such as ferric hydroxide sucrose, ferric oxide, and iron (III) hydroxide–sucrose complex. Iron sucrose is a complex of polymolecular iron-ferric hydroxide in sucrose. This preparation of iron is available under the brand name Venofer. It contains 20 mg of elemental iron per mL of solution. Following IV injection, iron is cleared from the plasma with an initial half-life of 30 minutes, following which the half-life increases to 6 hours. The recommended dose of Venofer by the manufacturer is 200–300 mg/day to be repeated every 3–4 days. Total dose must not exceed 600 mg/week. It effectively increases the serum ferritin levels and is a relatively safe drug having fewer side effects. Some side effects which can occur include metallic taste, nausea, fever, hypotension, shivering, anaphylactoid reaction, etc. The risk of serious anaphylactic reactions is almost negligible. No test dose is required, and it is administered only via the IV route. The desired dose must be diluted in 0.9% saline prior to administration. 200 mg of sucrose is added to 100 mL of normal saline and infused over 30 minutes. In case 300 mg of iron sucrose is to be administered, it is also diluted using 100 mL of normal saline. However, in this case the solution must be infused over 1.5 hours, preferably using a volumetric infusion pump.

On the completion of infusion, 50 mL of normal saline is infused to ensure that the drug is flushed completely.

Though very few side effects have been reported with the use of this drug, brown–black staining of skin due to leakage at the site of injection has been sometimes reported. The woman must be asked to report immediately in case she experiences side effects such as local discomfort, burning, or swelling. The patient must be observed for side effects for at least half an hour following the completion of infusion. Fetal heart rate must be assessed at the time of admission and prior to discharge.

Third-generation IV Iron

Newer third-generation preparations of IV iron include FCM, ferumoxytol, and iron isomaltoside. Test dose prior to administration of these preparations is not required since the risk of serious anaphylaxis is quite low.

Ferric Carboxymaltose

Ferric carboxymaltose has been approved by the Food and Drug Administration (FDA). A maximum single dose of 1,000 mg or 20 mg/kg, whichever is lesser, is required. The rest of the total calculated dose can be administered after 1 week. For the purpose of IV infusion, maximum dose of 1,000 mg must be diluted in 100 mL of saline, and dilution must not be lower than 2 mg/mL. This solution must be infused over a period of minimum 15 minutes. Infusion of 50 mL normal saline must be done following completion of infusion to flush the drug completely. The drug is generally well tolerated and may result in side effects such as nausea, headache, abdominal pain, dizziness, constipation, diarrhea, reactions at the injection site, rash, and rarely anaphylactic reactions. FCM is generally well tolerated, and its safety profile is comparable to that of iron sucrose. One of the major advantages of FCM over iron sucrose is that a much higher dose of FCM can be given at one time, thereby reducing the requirement for repeated infusions.

A randomized controlled trial by Jose et al. (2019), comparing FCM and iron sucrose, has shown that the group receiving FCM was associated with significantly higher rise in hemoglobin levels at 12 weeks in comparison to the group receiving iron sucrose. No serious adverse events were noticed in either group.

Side Effects Associated with Parenteral Iron

The main drawbacks of IM iron are the pain and staining of the skin at the site of injection, development of fever, chills, myalgia, arthralgia, injection abscess, etc. **(Table 20.11)**. The most serious side effect associated with the use of IV iron is the risk of anaphylactic reactions, which can occur in about 0.7% of patients taking IV iron dextran. These reactions usually occur within the first few minutes of administration

TABLE 20.11: Complications associated with the use of parenteral iron.	
System affected	**Symptoms produced**
Cardiovascular	Chest pain, tightness in the chest, hypotension, tachycardia, flushing, arrhythmias, etc.
Dermatologic	Urticaria, purpura, rash, cyanosis
Gastrointestinal	Abdominal pain, nausea, vomiting, diarrhea, etc.
Musculoskeletal/soft tissue	Arthralgia, arthritis, myalgia, cellulitis, brownish discoloration/staining of underlying tissues and skin
Respiratory	Dyspnea, bronchospasm, wheezing, respiration arrest
Hematologic/lymphatic	Leukocytosis, lymphadenopathy, etc.
Neurologic	Convulsions, seizures, syncope, headache, weakness, paresthesia, dizziness, disorientation, numbness, unconsciousness, etc.

of the test dose. The earlier a reaction appears after start of infusion, the more severe it will be. These allergic reactions are generally considered to be type I hypersensitivity reactions [immunoglobulin (IgG)-related]. Allergic reactions can be particularly more common in individuals with previous history of multiple drug allergies. Therefore, before administering parenteral iron, it is important to elicit history regarding allergies to any drugs in the past. Also, parenteral iron preparations must be administered in settings where there are facilities for treatment of possible anaphylactic reactions (e.g., availability of norepinephrine, oxygen, and steroids).

It has been argued that a single iron infusion with IV iron is less likely to elicit an immune response in comparison to multiple injections given over a period of several weeks. If any adverse effect is noted, injection must be terminated at once and appropriate countermeasures must be taken. A syringe containing solution of epinephrine should be immediately available for treatment of anaphylaxis, in case this potentially fatal condition occurs.

Prior to the administration of parenteral iron, iron deficiency must be confirmed using serum ferritin levels. Caution should be observed in case the woman is suffering from asthma, eczema, or other atopic allergies.

Calculation of TDI

The total iron requirement reflects the amount of iron needed to restore hemoglobin concentration to normal or near normal levels plus an additional allowance to provide adequate replenishment of iron stores in most individuals with moderately or severely reduced levels of hemoglobin. It should be remembered that IDA will not appear until essentially all iron stores have been depleted. Thus, therapy should aim at not only the replenishment of hemoglobin iron but also the iron stores. Total dose for iron infusion is calculated through any of the following formulae:

$$\text{Total dose (mL)} = [\text{patient's weight (kg)} \times 2.3 \{14 - \text{patient's observed Hb (g/dL)}\}] + 500\text{–}1000 \text{ mg}$$

or

$$\text{Total dose (mg)} = [15 - \text{patient's Hb (g/dL)}] \times \text{body weight (in kg)} \times 3$$

Precautions Before Administration of IV Iron

Precautions to be taken before administration of IV iron include the following:

- Prior to receiving the therapeutic dose, all patients should be given an IV test dose of 0.5 mL. The test dose should be administered slowly over the time period of at least 30 seconds (IM route) or 1 minute (IV route). Flushing and hypotension may occur from too rapid injections by the IV route.
- Severe/fatal anaphylactic reactions characterized by respiratory difficulty or cardiovascular collapse have been reported with the use of iron dextran injections. Therefore, the drug should be given only when resuscitation techniques and facilities for treatment of anaphylactic and anaphylactoid shocks are readily available.
- Epinephrine should be immediately available in case there is development of acute hypersensitivity reactions. Usual adult dose of epinephrine is 0.5 mL of a 1:1,000 solution, administered through subcutaneous or IM route.
- Though most anaphylactic reactions following IV iron administration are usually evident within a few minutes, it is recommended that the patient must be observed for at least 1 hour before the administration of remainder of the therapeutic dose. If no adverse reactions are observed, iron can be administered until the calculated total amount of total iron has been administered.
- The clinician should regularly observe the patient to evaluate the occurrence of side effects such as difficulty in breathing, dizziness, development of rash, and itchy skin.
- Oral iron must be stopped at least 24 hours prior to starting injectable iron therapy. Oral iron must also be withheld while the woman is on injectable iron as well as 4 weeks after the last IV iron dose. During this period, folic acid and vitamin therapy, however, must be continued.
- Some contraindications related to the use of parenteral iron are listed in **Box 20.12**.

Assessing the Response to Iron Therapy

- *Reticulocyte count:* Increase in the count of reticulocytes is the first response to iron therapy.

> **BOX 20.12:** Contraindications related to the use of parenteral iron.
> - First trimester
> - Known hypersensitivity to IM or IV iron
> - Hemochromatosis
> - Acute systemic infection

- *Globin levels:* A rise in hemoglobin levels of 1 g/dL can be seen at the end of 2 weeks and 2 g/dL at the end of 4 weeks.

In the absence of the above-mentioned responses to iron therapy, complete investigations including bone marrow biopsy are required.

The rate of response to iron therapy is same whether it is administered orally or parenterally. The main benefit of using paternal iron is that it helps in saving critical time in case of nonresponders during late pregnancy.

Management of Anemic Patients During Intrapartum Period

Precautions to be taken during the time of labor and delivery are as follows.

First Stage of Labor

- Patient's blood grouping and crossmatching need to be done.
- Though ideally the patient must be placed in a propped-up position, the woman can be placed in any position which is comfortable to her.
- Adequate pain relief must be provided.
- Oxygen inhalation through face mask must be provided.
- Digitalization may be required, especially if the patient shows a potential to develop congestive heart failure.
- Antibiotic prophylaxis must be given as the anemic women are prone to develop infections.
- Strict asepsis needs to be maintained at the time of delivery or while performing procedures like artificial rupture of membranes.
- In case of preterm labor, β-mimetics and steroids must be administered cautiously in order to prevent pulmonary edema.

Second Stage of Labor

In order to shorten the duration of second stage of labor, forceps or vacuum can be applied prophylactically.

At the Time of Delivery

The following precautions must be taken during the time of labor and delivery in order to reduce the amount of blood loss at the time of delivery:

- Oxytocics (methergine, oxytocin, etc.) should be routinely administered during delivery in order to reduce blood loss.
- Late clamping of cord at the time of delivery prevents anemia in infancy and should be employed as a routine practice in all babies. This simple practice helps in transferring 80 mL of blood with 50 mg of iron to the baby.
- Breastfeeding for first 6 months after delivery reduces maternal iron loss by producing amenorrhea. Maternal iron and folic acid supplementation should also be continued in postpartum period.

Third Stage of Labor

- Active management of third stage of labor
- PPH to be managed aggressively
- Advice regarding contraception must be given (e.g., barrier contraception).
- Postpartum sterilization may be offered to these women if the family is complete.

COMPLICATIONS

Anemia in pregnancy can have numerous adverse effects on the mother and the fetus. Some of these include the following.

MATERNAL COMPLICATIONS

Adverse effects of anemia on the mother include the following:

- *High maternal mortality rate:* In India, 16% of maternal deaths are due to anemia.
- Cerebral anoxia, cardiac failure
- Increased susceptibility to develop infection
- Inability to withstand even slight blood loss during pregnancy or delivery
- Abortions, preterm labor

Maternal risk during antenatal period: Poor weight gain, preterm labor, pregnancy-induced hypertension, placenta previa, accidental hemorrhage, eclampsia, premature rupture of membranes, etc.

Maternal risk during intranatal period: Dysfunctional labor, intranatal hemorrhage, shock, anesthesia risk, cardiac failure, etc.

Maternal risk during postnatal period: Postnatal sepsis, subinvolution, embolism etc.

FETAL COMPLICATIONS

Fetal adverse effects include the following:
- Preterm, low birth weight, and intrauterine growth-restricted babies

- Fetal and neonatal distress requiring prolonged resuscitation and low APGAR scores at birth
- Impaired neurological and mental development
- Anemia can result in hypertrophy of placenta and cause increased placental:fetal ratio, which has been suggested to be a predictor for development of diabetes and cardiovascular diseases later in life.
- Reduction in fetal iron stores may extend into the first year of life. This may result in a higher tendency of infants to develop IDA and other associated adverse consequences on infant development related to this condition.
- Infants with anemia have higher prevalence of failure to thrive, poorer intellectual developmental milestones, and higher rates of morbidities and neonatal mortalities in comparison to the infants without anemia.

EVIDENCE-BASED CLINICAL TRIALS

List of references can be scanned through QR code to enable the readers gain deeper insight of the subject by referring to the entire article or its abstract.

CHAPTER 21

Heart Disease During Pregnancy

CASE STUDY

A 34-year-old primigravida patient gives a history of having valve prosthesis 1 year back and presently is on warfarin. She presents for the first time in the antenatal clinic at 28 weeks of gestation. Presently, she is asymptomatic.

INTRODUCTION

Pregnancy is a physiological condition that places considerable burden on the heart, forcing it to work harder during the entire period of gestation. While a normal heart is quite capable of taking this extra workload right in its stride, a diseased heart may not be able to cope. Therefore, the preexisting cardiac lesions should be evaluated with respect to the risk imposed due to the stress of pregnancy. Confidential inquiry into the causes of maternal death in the United Kingdom (2006–2008) has shown maternal cardiac disease to be the most important indirect cause for the greatest number of maternal deaths. Thus, it is of prime importance for any obstetrician to be aware about the consequences of the presence of underlying cardiac disease in a pregnant woman.

■ EFFECT OF PREGNANCY ON HEART DISEASE

- *Increased chances of heart failure/cardiac decompensation:* During pregnancy, heart failure may be precipitated by increased cardiac output, especially in association with anemia. During labor, chances of heart failure increase due to bearing down efforts, stress of labor, and increased venous return. After delivery, there is a sudden increase in venous return (10–20%) with exhausted cardiac reserve or massive embolization.
- Rheumatic activity may cause further damage to the valves during pregnancy.
- Pregnancy-induced low vascular resistance may improve the symptoms of mitral regurgitation, aortic regurgitation, and mitral valve prolapse.
- The obstetrician needs to be aware regarding the major cardiac drug classes, especially those used for treatment of hypertension and heart failure, which are contraindicated during pregnancy. Treatment of congestive heart failure during pregnancy is summarized in **Box 21.1**.
- Anticoagulation during pregnancy presents unique challenges because of the maternal and fetal side effects of warfarin, unfractionated heparin (UFH), and low-molecular-weight heparin (LMWH).

Pregnancy is associated with significant hemodynamic changes that can aggravate valvular heart disease and increase the risk of thromboembolic events. These normal physiological changes pose a substantial demand on cardiac function in patients with valvular heart disease and may require the initiation or titration of cardiovascular medications to manage volume overload, hypertension, or arrhythmias. Furthermore, pregnancy is a state of relative hypercoagulability, which clearly increases the risk of thromboembolic events.

BOX 21.1: Treatment of congestive heart failure during pregnancy.

- Consultation with the physician/cardiologist is usually required
- Recognition of the underlying cardiac disease is essential
- Rapid correction of a precipitating cause such as anemia and respiratory tract infection must be done
- Administration of β-sympathomimetic drugs for tachyarrhythmia
- Bed rest to decrease cardiac work
- *Precautions against the development of thromboembolic complication:* Exercises in bed and wearing compression stockings are of help; heparin anticoagulation may also be required
- *Diuretics to reduce the preload:* IV furosemide and chlorothiazide (25–50 mg/day) may be administered. Changes in the hematocrit and electrolytes should be monitored if the diuretics are used for a prolonged duration of time
- Administration of digoxin to improve cardiac contractility. Digoxin is usually administered orally in a loading dose of 1.0–1.5 mg over 24 hours. This must be followed by a maintenance dose of 0.125–0.375 mg/day
- Sublingual nitroglycerine is the vasodilator of choice to reduce the systemic vascular resistance

EFFECT OF HEART DISEASE ON PREGNANCY

> Q. With the help of a long essay, describe the cardiovascular functions in pregnancy with mitral valve disease.
>
> Q. Describe the physiological changes in the cardiovascular system. What are the implications of heart disease complicating pregnancy?
>
> Q. Discuss the cardiovascular changes related to rheumatic heart disease in pregnancy.
>
> Q. Describe the physiological changes occurring in the cardiovascular system during pregnancy and management of a patient with mitral stenosis during late pregnancy and labor.

The various adverse effects on pregnancy caused by the presence of heart disease are given in **Box 21.2**.

Hemodynamic Changes Occurring During Pregnancy

The following hemodynamic changes occur during pregnancy (**Fig. 21.1** and **Table 21.1**):

- There is a 30–50% increase in cardiac output. Normally the cardiac output starts increasing by around 5th week and increases rapidly until the 34th week of gestation, following which it plateaus or continues to increase slightly. The increase in cardiac output is achieved by three factors:
    1. An increase in preload because of greater blood volume. Blood volume increases by 40–50% during normal pregnancy. The increase in plasma volume is greater than the increase in red blood cell mass, contributing to the fall in hemoglobin concentration (i.e., the "Anemia in Pregnancy", see Chapter 20). The cause of underlying blood volume increase is related to an estrogen-mediated stimulation of the renin-angiotensin system, which results in sodium and water retention.
    2. Reduced afterload due to reduction in systemic vascular resistance
    3. Rise in the maternal heart rate by 10–15 beats/min
- Stroke volume increases during the first and second trimesters but declines in the third trimester due to the compression of inferior vena cava by the uterus.
- Both plasma and interstitial colloid osmotic pressures decrease throughout pregnancy. There is an accompanying increase in the capillary hydrostatic pressure. Increase in capillary hydrostatic pressure or decrease in colloid osmotic pressure is likely to cause edema.
- Decline in systemic arterial pressure begins to occur during first trimester, reaches a nadir in midpregnancy, and returns toward pregestational level before term. Blood pressure typically falls by about 10 mm Hg below baseline by the end of the second trimester because

BOX 21.2: Adverse effects on pregnancy caused by the presence of heart disease in the mother.
- Intrauterine growth restriction
- Preterm labor
- Intrauterine fetal death
- Abortion
- Fetal polycythemia
- Perinatal mortality (up to 20%)
- Increased incidence of fetal congenital heart disease (CHD) if the mother herself has CHD

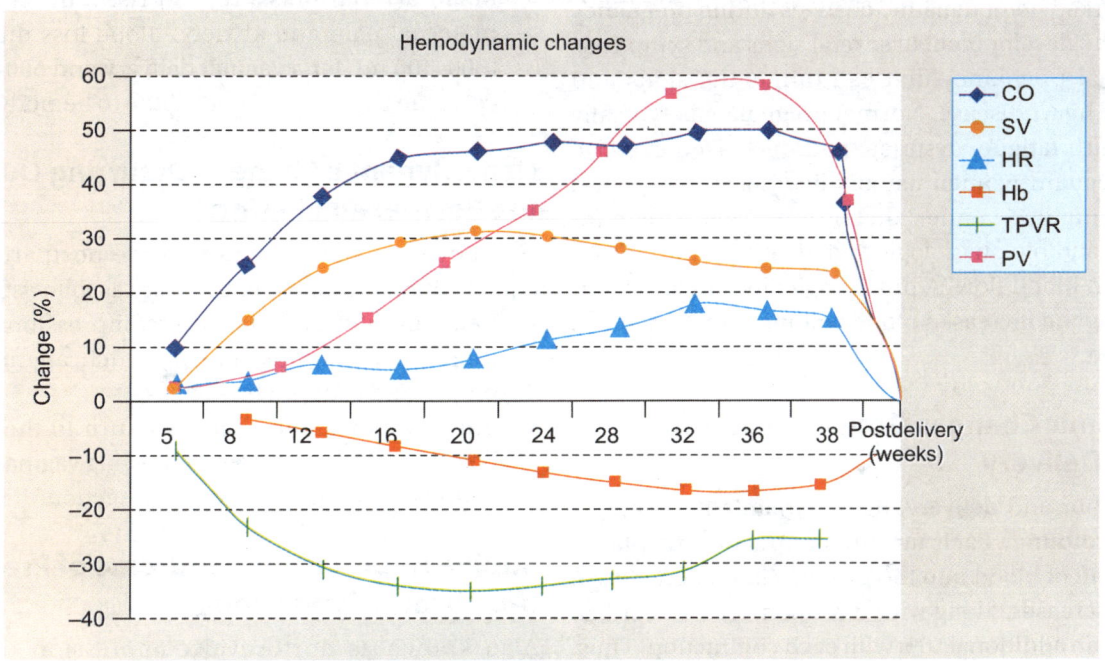

Fig. 21.1: Normal physiologic changes during pregnancy. (CO: cardiac output; Hb: hemoglobin; PV: plasma volume; SV: stroke volume; TPVR: total peripheral vascular resistance)

TABLE 21.1: Normal hemodynamic changes during pregnancy.

Hemodynamic parameter	Change during normal pregnancy	Change during labor and delivery	Change during postpartum
Blood volume	Increases by 40–50%	Increases	Decreases (auto-diuresis)
Heart rate	Increases by 10–15 beats/min	Increases	Decreases
Cardiac output	Increases by 30–50% above the baseline	Additional increase by 50%	Decreases
Blood pressure	Decreases by 10 mm Hg	Increases	Decreases
Stroke volume	Increases during first and second trimesters; decreases during the third trimester	Additional increase of 300–500 mL with each uterine contraction	Decreases
Systemic vascular resistance	Decreases	Increases	Decreases

of reduction in systemic vascular resistance and the addition of new blood vessels in the uterus and placenta. These physiological changes begin early in the first trimester, peak during the second trimester, and continue throughout the gestation and into the early postpartum period. **Figure 21.2** summarizes the changes in cardiac output with increasing duration of pregnancy. During labor, there is further increase in cardiac output, heart rate, blood pressure, and systemic vascular resistance due to the stress and anxiety of labor and delivery and uterine contractions. Moreover, there is a sudden increase in the cardiac output in the immediate postpartum period due to autotransfusion of approximately 600–800 mL of uteroplacental blood into the peripheral circulation. Cardiac output also increases during labor due to squeezing out of blood from uterus at the time of uterine contractions. Therefore, while preparing a woman for labor and delivery, it is important to anticipate that there will be important changes in maternal hemodynamic parameters.

These marked hemodynamic changes during pregnancy account for the development of several signs and symptoms during normal pregnancy that can mimic the signs and symptoms of heart disease. Normal pregnancy is typically associated with fatigue, dyspnea, and decreased exercise capacity. Pregnant women usually have mild peripheral edema and jugular venous distention. Most pregnant women have audible physiologic systolic murmurs, created by augmented blood flow. A physiologic third heart sound (S3), reflecting the increased blood volume, can sometimes be auscultated.

Hemodynamic Changes Occurring During Labor and Delivery

- During labor and delivery, hemodynamic fluctuations can be profound. Each uterine contraction displaces 300–500 mL of blood into the general circulation. Stroke volume increases, along with a resultant rise in cardiac output by an additional 50% with each contraction. Thus, it is possible for the cardiac output during labor and delivery to be 75% above baseline.

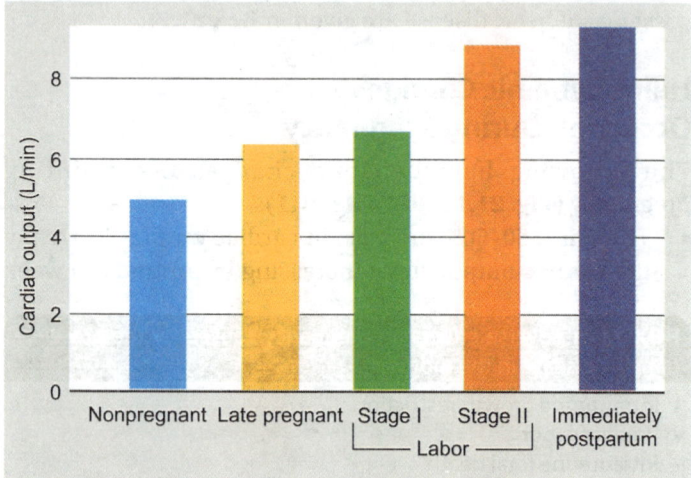

Fig. 21.2: Changes in cardiac output with increasing duration of pregnancy.
Source: Sakala EP. Obstetrics and Gynecology, 2nd edition. Philadelphia: Lippincott Williams and Wilkins; 2000.

- Mean arterial pressure also rises, in part because of maternal pain and anxiety. Blood loss during delivery (300–400 mL for a vaginal delivery and 500–800 mL for a cesarean section) can contribute to hemodynamic stress.

Hemodynamic Changes Occurring During the Postpartum Period

Hemodynamic changes during the postpartum state are equally dramatic. Some of these are as follows:
- Relief of inferior vena caval compression results in an increase in venous return, which augments cardiac output and causes a brisk diuresis.
- The hemodynamic changes return to the prepregnant baseline within 2–4 weeks following vaginal delivery and within 4–6 weeks after cesarean section.

Supine Hypotensive Syndrome of Pregnancy (Aortocaval Syndrome)

Also known as aortocaval compression or uterocaval syndrome, supine hypotension syndrome refers to the development of sudden hypotension in a pregnant woman

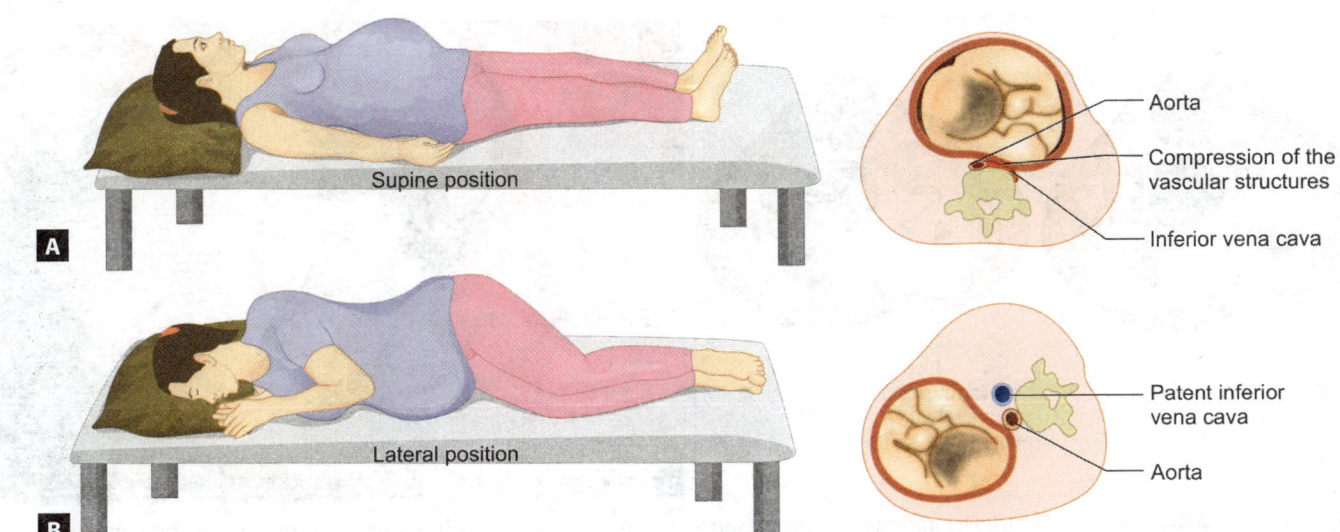

Figs. 21.3A and B: Pathogenesis of supine hypotension syndrome.

who lies flat on the bed. When the woman assumes a supine position while lying down, uterine contents of the gravid uterus press upon the inferior vena cava and aorta, thereby partially occluding them **(Figs. 21.3A and B)**. This may result in the development of hypotension and symptoms such as pallor, reduced heart rate, sweating, dizziness, and loss of consciousness. Supine hypotension syndrome can be prevented by advising the patient to assume a left lateral position while lying down rather than lying flat on a surface. In case the woman accidently lies flat on a surface and experiences symptoms suggestive of supine hypotension syndrome, she should be advised to immediately assume left lateral position. Change to left lateral position and simple reassurance explaining the benign nature of the condition seem to work in most of the cases.

CONGENITAL OR ACQUIRED CARDIAC LESIONS

Specific congenital or acquired cardiac lesions encountered during pregnancy are as follows.

Low-Risk Lesions

Mitral Regurgitation

Chronic mitral regurgitation, most commonly encountered as a result of rheumatic heart disease, is usually well tolerated during pregnancy. However, new-onset atrial fibrillations or severe hypertension can precipitate hemodynamic deterioration. Pulmonary edema and life-threatening cardiac decompensation can be produced as a result of acute mitral regurgitation (e.g., from rupture of chordae tendineae). Women with severe mitral regurgitation and signs of cardiac decompensation before pregnancy are advised to undergo mitral valve repair before conception.

Aortic Regurgitation

Aortic regurgitation, similar to mitral regurgitation, is generally well tolerated during pregnancy. Aortic regurgitation may be encountered in women with rheumatic heart disease, a congenitally deformed bicuspid aortic valve, infective endocarditis, or in the presence of connective tissue disease. Women with bicuspid aortic valves are at increased risk for aortic dissection. Therefore, it is important to follow-up such patients to assess if they develop signs and symptoms of this complication. Ideally, women with severe aortic regurgitation and signs of cardiac decompensation should undergo operative repair before conception.

Congestive heart failure resulting from mitral or aortic regurgitation can be treated with digoxin, diuretics, and vasodilators (e.g., hydralazine). Angiotensin-converting enzyme (ACE) inhibitors are teratogenic and therefore are contraindicated during pregnancy. Though the use of β-blockers may be at times associated with fetal bradycardia and growth retardation, β-blockers are generally considered safe during pregnancy.

Moderate-Risk Lesions

Mitral Stenosis

The most common valvular heart disease encountered during pregnancy is mitral stenosis **(Figs. 21.4A and B)**. In mothers with rheumatic heart valve disease, the fetus develops almost normally. The only difference noted may be mild growth retardation. The hypervolemia and tachycardia associated with pregnancy may aggravate the pressure and volume gradient across mitral valve. Elevated pressure of left atrium as a result of mitral stenosis may cause atrial fibrillations and pulmonary edema. This can sometimes precipitate heart failure and cause rapid cardiac decompensation, primarily due to an uncontrolled ventricular rate. Pulmonary edema

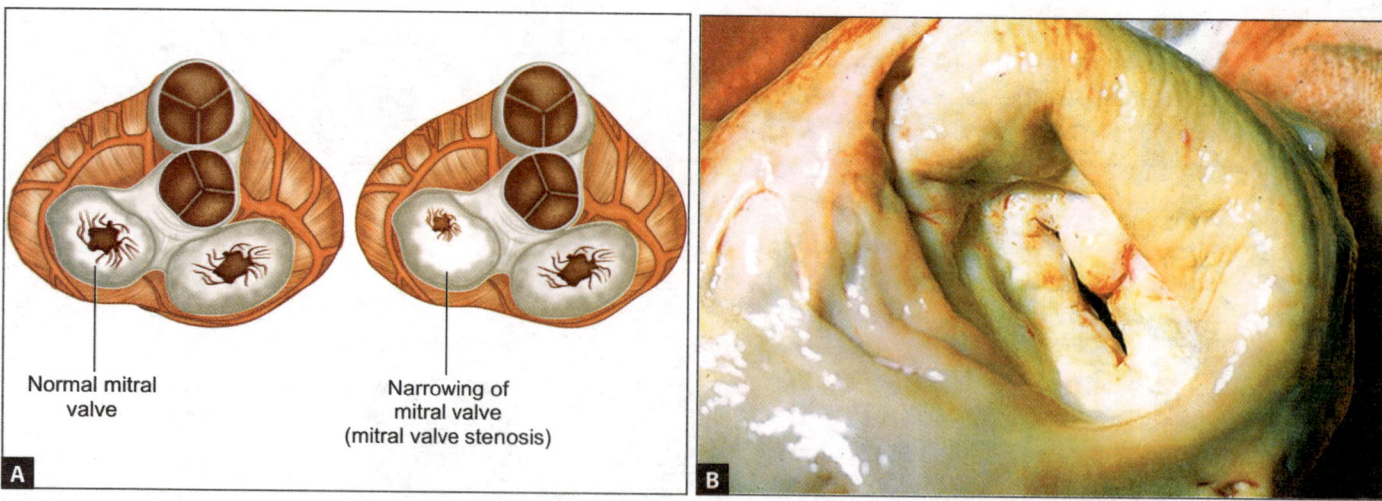

Figs. 21.4A and B: Mitral stenosis. (A) Diagrammatic representation of mitral stenosis; (B) Photograph showing stenosed mitral valves.

> **BOX 21.3:** Treatment of pulmonary edema.
> - Propping up the patient to semi-sitting position
> - Oxygen by a face mask or nasal prong
> - Furosemide (Lasix) IV 10–40 mg
> - Morphine 5 mg IV slowly. If hypotension does not occur, 10 mg can be given 15 minutes later

is common with mitral stenosis and most likely to develop immediately in the postpartum period. Treatment of pulmonary edema is summarized in **Box 21.3**. Even patients with only mild-to-moderate mitral stenosis (who have no symptoms before pregnancy) may develop atrial fibrillation and heart failure during the antepartum and peripartum periods. Patients with moderate-to-severe mitral stenosis often experience hemodynamic deterioration during the third trimester or during labor and delivery. Additional displacement of blood volume into the systemic circulation during contractions makes labor particularly hazardous.

Mild mitral stenosis can often be managed with careful medical therapy during pregnancy.

Drugs such as digoxin and β-blockers can be used to reduce heart rate, and diuretics can be used to reduce the blood volume and left atrial pressure. With development of atrial fibrillations and hemodynamic deterioration, electrocardioversion can be performed safely. Anticoagulation must be initiated with the onset of atrial fibrillations in order to reduce the risk of stroke. Patients with moderate-to-severe mitral stenosis should be referred to a cardiologist.

Severe mitral stenosis is associated with a high likelihood of maternal complications (including pulmonary edema and arrhythmias) or fetal complications (including premature birth, low birth weight, respiratory distress, and fetal or neonatal death). As a result, these women may require corrective surgery via surgical valve repair or replacement or percutaneous mitral balloon valvotomy before conception or during pregnancy **(Flowchart 21.1)**.

Heart surgery may be necessary when medical treatment fails to control heart failure or symptoms remain intolerable to the patients despite medical therapy. In case the clinician anticipates the requirement of an open heart surgery due to the associated volume load, the most reasonable approach would be to consider prepregnancy intervention. Open heart surgery during pregnancy is associated with considerable risks to the fetus. Therefore, this procedure can be justified only if the cardiac lesion would prove to be harmful to the mother, if left untreated. Such conditions would include life-threatening pulmonary edema, which cannot be managed by medical treatment. Open heart surgery is rarely indicated for congenital heart disease (CHD) in pregnancy.

While open heart surgery should not be undertaken lightly during pregnancy because of the risks to the fetus, closed mitral valvuloplasty (CMV) is a relatively safe procedure. CMV is usually done in cases of severe pulmonary congestion unresponsive to drugs, profuse hemoptysis, and any episode of pulmonary edema before pregnancy (because there is a high chance of a recurrent attack during the present pregnancy). While the second trimester of pregnancy is usually the preferred time for any heart surgery, CMV can be safely performed at any stage of pregnancy, if required. During pregnancy, percutaneous valvotomy is usually postponed to the second or third trimesters to avoid the chances of radiation exposure to the fetus during the first trimester.

Most patients with mitral stenosis can undergo vaginal delivery. However, patients with symptoms of congestive heart failure or moderate-to-severe mitral stenosis may require close hemodynamic monitoring during labor, delivery, and for several hours into the postpartum period.

Aortic Stenosis

The most common cause of aortic stenosis in women of childbearing age is congenital bicuspid valve. Mild-to-moderate aortic stenosis with preserved left ventricular (LV)

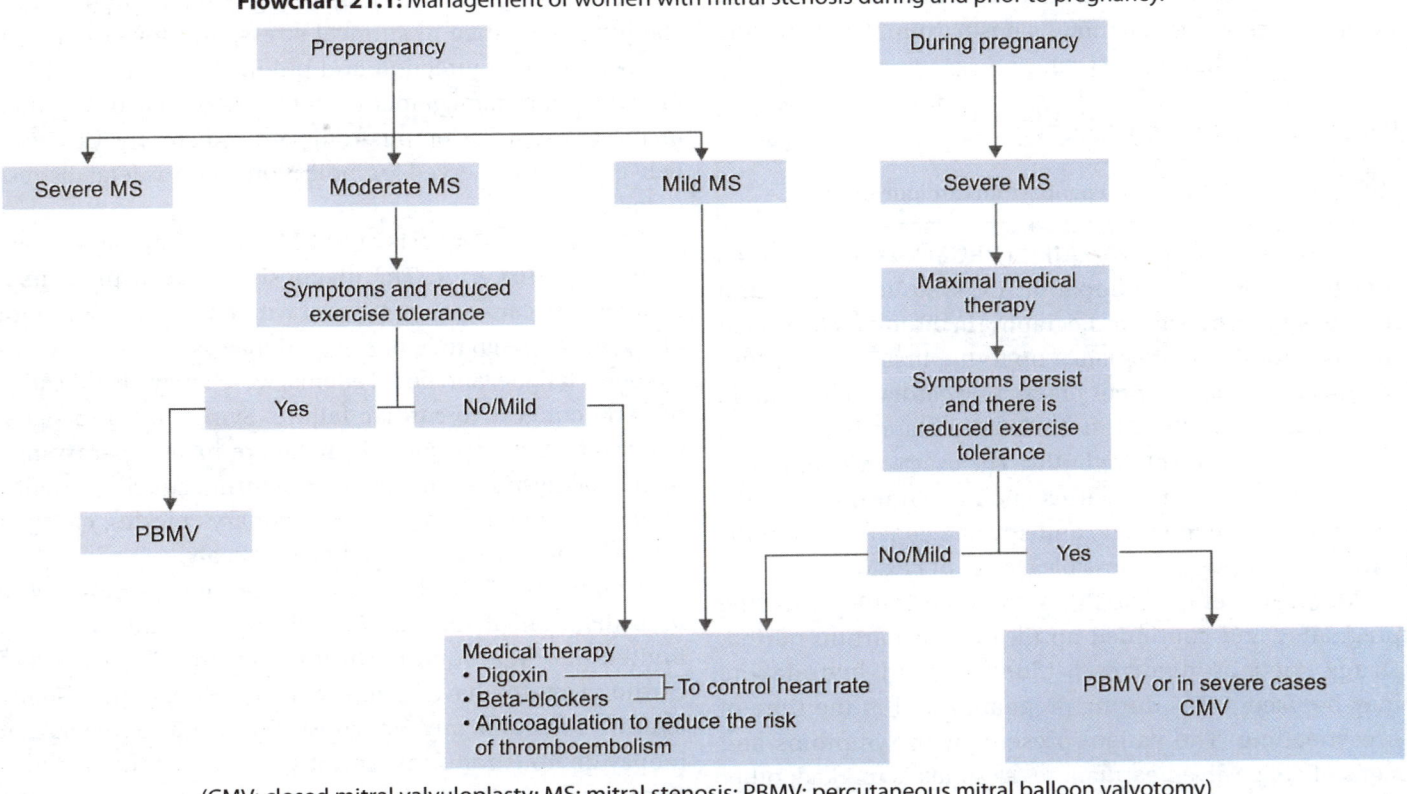

Flowchart 21.1: Management of women with mitral stenosis during and prior to pregnancy.

(CMV: closed mitral valvuloplasty; MS: mitral stenosis; PBMV: percutaneous mitral balloon valvotomy)

function is usually well tolerated during pregnancy. On the other hand, severe aortic stenosis (aortic valve area <1.0 cm^2) may be associated with a high risk of maternal morbidity. Symptoms such as dyspnea, angina pectoris, or syncope usually become apparent late in the second trimester or early in the third trimester. Women with known severe aortic stenosis should be referred to a cardiologist. Ideally, they should undergo correction of the valvular abnormality before conception. Treatment options include surgical repair, surgical valve replacement, and percutaneous balloon valvotomy.

When severe symptomatic aortic stenosis is diagnosed during pregnancy, maximal medical therapy is preferred over any intervention. However, if a patient has refractory symptoms and hemodynamic deterioration, despite maximal medical therapy, percutaneous balloon valvotomy may be performed. Similar to the cases with mitral stenosis, hemodynamic monitoring must be performed during labor and delivery in the cases of aortic stenosis.

High-Risk Lesions

The high-risk conditions are associated with an increased maternal and fetal mortality. Pregnancy is not advisable in these cases. However, if pregnancy does occur, the risks of maternal mortality and morbidity must be assessed on an individual case basis. If the maternal risk appears to be extremely high, the option of medical termination of pregnancy may be considered in order to safeguard maternal health. If the pregnancy is continued, these patients are best managed with the help of a cardiologist and maternal–fetal medicine specialist at a tertiary care center with high-risk ICU facilities and a level three neonatal unit.

Acquired Cardiovascular Disorders During Pregnancy

Maternal Placental Syndromes

A group of disorders, collectively known as maternal placental syndromes (MPS), have been associated with an increased maternal risk of premature cardiovascular disease. In the CHAMPS (Cardiovascular Health After Maternal Placental Syndromes) study, MPS was defined as the presence of preeclampsia, gestational hypertension, placental abruption, or placental infarction during pregnancy. There has been growing body of evidence, which shows close association between cardiovascular risk factors, MPS, and future development of cardiovascular disease. It is possible that an underlying abnormal vascular health that predates pregnancy manifests in the form of MPS during pregnancy or as chronic cardiovascular disease later in life. Women with MPS have been shown to be twice as likely to experience a hospital admission or revascularization procedure for coronary, cerebrovascular, or peripheral vascular disease in comparison to women without MPS. The risk of premature cardiovascular disease is higher after a MPS, especially in the presence of fetal compromise.

Peripartum Cardiomyopathy

 Q. Write a short note on peripartum cardiomyopathy.

Peripartum cardiomyopathy (PPCM) is defined as the development of idiopathic LV systolic dysfunction (demonstrated by echocardiography) in the interval between the last months of pregnancy up to the first 5 postpartum months in women without preexisting cardiac dysfunction. The incidence of PPCM in the United States is estimated to be 1 in 3,000–4,000 live births. The exact cause of PPCM is unknown, although causes such as viral myocarditis, autoimmune phenomena, and specific genetic mutations have been proposed as possible causes of PPCM.

Medical therapy for PPCM may be initiated during pregnancy and continued up till the postpartum period. Drugs such as digoxin, β-blockers, and hydralazine may be used safely during pregnancy and at the time of breastfeeding. The patient presents with symptoms and signs of congestive heart failure. Dyspnea is marked; other symptoms are orthopnea, precordial pain, and cough. The hallmark finding is marked cardiomegaly; ECG confirms increased end-diastolic dimensions. Therapy usually comprises digitalization, diuretics, low-dose heparin, and salt restriction. Diuretics help in decreasing pulmonary congestion and volume overload. In patients with systolic dysfunction, afterload is usually reduced with vasodilators. β-blockers may improve LV function in patients with cardiomyopathy. Though β-blockers are considered safe during pregnancy, there have been case reports of fetal bradycardia and growth retardation. ACE inhibitors, angiotensin receptor blockers, and aldosterone antagonists are contraindicated during pregnancy. Most ACE inhibitors can however be initiated during the postpartum period, even in women who breastfeed. Anticoagulation can be considered for select patients with severe LV dilation and dysfunction. When conventional medical therapy becomes unsuccessful, women with PPCM may require intensive IV therapy, mechanical assist devices, or even cardiac transplantation. More than 50% of the women with PPCM completely recover normal heart size and function, usually within 6 months of delivery. Women with PPCM and persistent LV dysfunction who attempt subsequent pregnancy face a high risk of maternal morbidity and mortality. These women should be counseled against subsequent pregnancies.

The mode of delivery for patients with PPCM is generally based on obstetric indications. After stabilization of the maternal condition, in most cases induction and vaginal delivery can be attempted in consultation with consultant obstetrician and anesthetic staff. The advantages of vaginal delivery are minimal blood loss, greater hemodynamic stability, avoidance of surgical stress, and lower chances of postoperative infection and pulmonary complications. Effective pain management is a necessity to avoid further increases in cardiac output from pain and anxiety. Cesarean delivery is best reserved for indications such as fetal distress or failure to progress.

The clinical diagnosis of PPCM is based on parameters enlisted in **Box 21.4**. The diagnosis of PPCM presents a challenge because many normal women in the last month of a normal pregnancy may experience symptoms such as dyspnea, fatigue, and pedal edema, which may be indicative of early congestive cardiac failure. Symptoms and signs, which raise the suspicion of heart failure, include paroxysmal nocturnal dyspnea, chest pain, nocturnal cough, presence of new regurgitant murmurs, pulmonary crackles, elevated jugular venous pressure, and hepatomegaly.

Diagnosis of PPCM rests on the echocardiographic identification of new LV systolic dysfunction during a limited period around parturition, when other causes of cardiomyopathy have been excluded. All patients usually exhibit cardiomegaly on chest X-ray. Endomyocardial biopsy demonstrates myocarditis in >70% of the patients. Persistence of symptoms for >6 months postpartum and the presence of a significantly reduced LV ejection fraction is associated with a bad prognosis.

Coronary Artery Disease

Acute myocardial infarction (AMI) during pregnancy is rare, occurring in 1 in 35,000 pregnancies. Independent predictors of AMI during pregnancy include chronic hypertension, maternal age, diabetes, and preeclampsia. Most myocardial infarctions occur during the third trimester in women older than 33 years who have had multiple prior pregnancies. Medical therapy for AMI must be modified in the pregnant patient. Percutaneous coronary intervention using both balloon angioplasty and stenting with the use of lead shielding to protect the fetus has been successfully performed in pregnant patients with AMI. Coronary angiography should be done only in cases in which coronary angioplasty or bypass surgery may be indicated during pregnancy.

Concentration of biochemical markers such as myoglobin, creatine kinase, and creatine kinase-MB has

---

BOX 21.4: Clinical definition of peripartum cardiomyopathy.

- Heart failure within last month of pregnancy or 5 months postpartum
- Absence of prior heart disease
- No determinable cause
- Strict echocardiographic indication of left ventricular dysfunction
- Ejection fraction <45% and/or fractional shortening < 30% or end-diastolic dimension >2.7 cm/m^2 body surface area

been found to be increased by two-folds, 30 minutes after delivery. On the other hand, levels of troponin I are likely to remain below the cutoff value; therefore, measurement of troponin levels must be done for diagnosing myocardial infarction after delivery.

Management

Administration of morphine sulfate can cause neonatal respiratory depression when given shortly before delivery because it has the propensity to cross the placenta. Thrombolytic therapy does not cause teratogenic effect but is associated with a risk of maternal hemorrhage, especially when given at the time of delivery. Their use may be permitted in situations where facilities for cardiac catheterization are not available. β-blockers are safe and are the drugs of choice. Organic nitrates and calcium antagonists should be administered cautiously to prevent development of maternal hypotension and potential fetal distress. While low-dose aspirin is safe to use, high-dose aspirin is reported to cause fetal growth restriction and bleeding in the neonate and the mother. Short-term heparin administration has not been found to be associated with increased maternal or fetal adverse effects. ACE inhibitors and statins are contraindicated during pregnancy. Hydralazine and nitrates may be used as substitutes for ACE inhibitors. Antiplatelets such as clopidogrel and glycoprotein IIb/IIIa receptor inhibitors have been used safely in individual pregnant patients.

Management should focus on reducing cardiovascular stress during pregnancy and the peripartum period. Termination of pregnancy may be required in patients with intractable ischemia or heart failure in the early phase of gestation. Elective cesarean section should be used in patients with active ischemia or hemodynamic instability despite adequate medical therapy.

Arrhythmias in Pregnancy

Premature atrial or ventricular complexes, or both, are the most common arrhythmias during pregnancy. They are not associated with adverse maternal or fetal outcomes and do not require antiarrhythmic therapy. Supraventricular tachyarrhythmia (SVT) is also common. Pregnancy is associated with an increased incidence of arrhythmias in women both with and without structural heart disease. Evaluation is indicated to rule out treatable cause, e.g., presence of thyroid disease.

Patients with SVT should be instructed about the performance of vagal maneuvers. Additionally, β-blockers or digoxin, or both, can be used for controlling the ventricular rate. Adenosine and direct current cardioversion are both safe during pregnancy and can be used to treat SVT. Antiarrhythmic drug therapy is initiated only if the arrhythmia persists and is symptomatic, hemodynamically important, or life-threatening. The smallest therapeutic dose of drugs known to be safe for the fetus should be used. Catheter ablation procedures should be performed, if possible, after delivery because of the unpredictable exposure to ionizing radiation.

Congenital Heart Disease in Pregnancy

The most common birth defects seen during pregnancy include patent ductus arteriosus (PDA), atrial septal defects (ASDs), and ventricular septal defects (VSDs). Other less common causes include pulmonary valve stenosis, tetralogy of Fallot (TOF), and coarctation of aorta (CoA). While the TOF may carry a maternal mortality risk of 4–20% at the time of pregnancy, ASDs can be considered as the safest of all birth defects during pregnancy.

In mothers with CHD, pregnancy is almost normal in diseases without cyanosis. However, in cyanotic mothers (e.g., TOF), many problems such as severe growth retardation and higher abortion rates may arise. Since the maternal blood has very low oxygen content in these cases, there is a lower oxygen exchange across the placenta, and the fetus gets lesser oxygen than normal. As a result, the fetus may be growth retarded, may die, or may be delivered prematurely. CoA is another special condition in which fetal loss is higher than normal as a result of lower blood flow to the placenta due to the narrowed aorta. In uncorrected CoA, the recommended management options include medical termination of pregnancy or surgical repair of the CoA before delivery. In case the pregnancy does occur in cases with uncorrected CoA, cesarean delivery is usually preferred in order to avoid the risk of dissection that might be brought on by the mother straining in labor. Also, the risk of CHD in such pregnancies is 2–4%, which is twice the incidence of heart disease in the general population. In pregnancy, the fall in systemic vascular resistance and increase in blood volume and cardiac output can cause functional deterioration in certain conditions. A minimally symptomatic woman with good ventricular function, normal oxygen saturation, and no left heart obstruction would be able to tolerate pregnancy well. Women with pulmonary hypertension or dilated aortic root (prereplacement) should be counseled against pregnancy and given appropriate contraceptive advice.

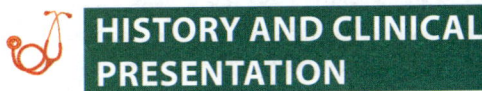

HISTORY AND CLINICAL PRESENTATION

Women with preexisting cardiac dysfunction usually experience cardiac deterioration during the end of the second trimester. Typical signs and symptoms include fatigue, dyspnea on exertion, orthopnea, nonspecific chest pain, peripheral edema, and abdominal discomfort and distention. It is important to elicit the history of the following symptoms.

DYSPNEA

> **Q. What are the causes of breathlessness during pregnancy? Write a long essay on the management of rheumatic heart failure at 34 weeks' gestation.**

Though some amount of exertional dyspnea or breathlessness can commonly occur during normal pregnancy, severe dyspnea, especially that occurring at rest or while sleeping or that resulting in inability to perform normal activities, may be suggestive of heart disease. Dyspnea can commonly result from LV failure (LVF), pulmonary embolism, etc. Pulmonary embolism is associated with acute onset of dyspnea and pleuritic chest pain. While taking the history of dyspnea, it is important to inquire the circumstances under which the patient experiences breathlessness. The dyspnea can be graded into four categories **(Table 21.2)**, depending on whether it occurs during exertion, while doing daily activities, or at rest. The history of orthopnea or shortness of breath while sleeping at night can be elicited by asking about the number of pillows the patient uses at night in order to prevent breathlessness. Paroxysmal nocturnal dyspnea can be diagnosed if the patient gives history of waking up at night, gasping for breath.

PERIPHERAL EDEMA

Pulmonary embolism is associated with acute onset of dyspnea and pleuritic chest pain. In cases with clinical suspicion for pulmonary embolism, history about various risk factors associated with DVT also needs to be taken.

PALPITATION

Palpitation may be due to ectopic beats, atrial fibrillations, supraventricular and ventricular tachycardias, thyrotoxicosis, anxiety, etc. The obstetrician must take the history about previous episodes of palpitations, precipitating/relieving factors, duration of symptoms, and the presence of associated symptoms such as chest pain, dyspnea, or dizziness.

TABLE 21.2: Medical Research Council classification of dyspnea.

Grade	Description
I	No dyspnea at rest; dyspnea is present only while doing strenuous exercise (e.g., walking up the hill)
II	Shortness of breath when walking with the people of same age group on ground level
III	Limitation of walking pace (slower than others) as a result of dyspnea. The Individual has to stop in between to catch breath
IV	The individual needs to stop to catch her breath after walking nearly every 100 m on level ground
V	Severe degree of dyspnea, which severely limits the individual's activities of daily living and prevents her from leaving her house

CHEST PAIN

Acute history of chest pain radiating to shoulders/neck may be suggestive of myocardial infraction. Chest pain in association with headache, dysarthria, limb weakness, etc., may be indicative of CNS causes.

LIGHT-HEADEDNESS OR FAINTING

Owing to the normal pregnancy-related cardiovascular changes (described previously), many healthy pregnant women may show symptoms mimicking those of cardiac disease, including fatigue, dyspnea, light-headedness, etc. Even in normal pregnancy, numerous abnormal findings suggestive of cardiac abnormalities may be observed on physical examination, ECG, and echocardiography. Some of these are described in **Table 21.3**. The woman must be best re-assured in these cases.

On the other hand, clinical indicators of heart disease during pregnancy are enlisted in **Box 21.5**.

GENERAL PHYSICAL EXAMINATION

VITAL SIGNS

- *Pulse:* The pulse rate is important. A rapid heart rate is almost always an indication that the patient is anxious or ill. The pulse must be recorded in both the upper limbs. Abnormalities in pulse pattern may be suggestive of underlying cardiac disease. The presence of radio-femoral delay could be suggestive of CoA.
- *Blood pressure:* The correct method of measuring blood pressure has been fully described in Chapter 18.
- *Respiratory rate:* Look for any signs which suggest that the patient has difficulty in breathing (dyspnea).
- *Finger clubbing:* Clubbing of fingers may be associated with diseases of the heart or lungs.
- *Cyanosis:* It is bluish discoloration of the skin and mucous membranes due to the presence of at least 5 g% of deoxygenated hemoglobin in the blood. The presence of cyanosis suggests that arterial saturation is <85%. The places to look for peripheral cyanosis are the fingertips, including underneath the nail beds. The places to look for central cyanosis are the lips and tongue.
- *Features indicative of infective endocarditis:* Features such as splinter hemorrhages (areas of hemorrhage under the fingernails or toenails), Janeway lesions (small, nontender, erythematous or hemorrhagic macular or nodular lesions, occurring most commonly on the palms and soles including the thenar and hypothenar eminences), and Osler's nodes (tender, transient nodules commonly present in the pulp of fingers; at times they may also be present in the sole of the feet)

TABLE 21.3: Normal findings in pregnancy suggestive of heart disease.

Clinical examination

Symptoms:
- Fatigue, tiredness
- Dyspnea, orthopnea
- Syncope
- Reduced exercise capacity
- Palpitations, light-headedness

Physical findings:
- Peripheral edema, hyperventilation
- Displaced apical impulse
- Distended neck veins with prominent a and v waves and brisk x and y descent
- Widely split first and second heart sounds
- Soft ejection systolic murmur
- Increased intensity of S_1, persistent splitting of S_2
- Pulmonary basilar rales

Investigations

Chest X-ray	ECG	Echo
• Straightening of left upper cardiac border • Horizontal position of the heart • Increased lung markings • Small pleural effusions in the early postpartum period	• Right or left axis deviation • Small Q waves and inverted p wave in lead III • ST-segment depression • t-wave changes • Sinus tachycardia and higher incidence of arrhythmias • Premature atrial or ventricular ectopic beats • Increased R/S ratio in leads V2 and V1	• Small pericardial effusion • Functional tricuspid, pulmonary, and mitral regurgitation • Mild increase in left ventricular systolic and diastolic dimensions • Unchanged or slightly improved left ventricular systolic function • Preservation of ejection systolic volume • Moderate increase in size of right atrium, right ventricle, and left atrium

BOX 21.5: Clinical indicators of heart disease during pregnancy.

Symptoms:
- Progressive dyspnea or orthopnea
- Nocturnal cough
- Hemoptysis
- Syncope
- Chest pain

Signs:
- Cyanosis
- Clubbing of fingers
- Persistent distension of the neck veins
- Systolic murmur grade ≥3/6
- Diastolic murmur
- Cardiomegaly
- Persistent arrhythmia

BOX 21.6: Characteristics of a functional murmur.

- It is midsystolic
- It is soft, not louder than grade 2/6
- It is ejection in character
- It does not radiate
- It is usually heard best over the mitral or aortic areas
- It is usually asymptomatic

Auscultation

Upon auscultation of the precordial area, normal heart sounds (S1 and S2) can be heard. Upon auscultation, it is important to note whether or not an additional sounds (e.g., murmur, opening snap, click, and third or fourth heart sounds) are present. The cardiac areas, which are most commonly auscultated, include the following:

- *Mitral area (at the point of cardiac apex):* Corresponds to the left fifth intercostal space and is 1 cm medial to the midclavicular line
- *Tricuspid area:* The lower left parasternal border is the tricuspid area.
- *Pulmonary area:* The left second intercostal space
- *Aortic area:* The right second intercostal space
- *Second aortic area or the Erb's area:* The left third intercostal space

Functional murmurs are frequently heard during pregnancy due to the increased cardiac output and do not require further investigation or management. The functional murmur needs to be distinguished from a pathological one. The characteristics of a functional murmur are enumerated in **Box 21.6**. The characteristics of some commonly encountered pathological murmurs are described in **Table 21.4**.

- *Hepatomegaly:* Presence of hepatomegaly or ascites on abdominal examination could be due to congestive heart failure.
- *Peripheral edema:* Presence of edema in the feet or sacral edema could occur due to congestive cardiac failure.

SPECIFIC SYSTEMIC EXAMINATION

EXAMINATION OF CARDIOVASCULAR SYSTEM

Palpation

In normal individuals, the cardiac apex is normally palpated in the left fifth intercostal space, 1 cm medial to the midclavicular line. The cardiac apex may be shifted downward and outward in cases of LV enlargement.

TABLE 21.4: Characteristics of some common pathological murmurs.

Type of lesion	Location	Character	Shape	Duration	Radiation
Mitral stenosis	Mitral area	Low-pitched, rough, and rumbling	Plateaus with presystolic accentuation	Mid-diastolic and presystolic	–
Tricuspid stenosis	Tricuspid area	Low-pitched, rumbling	Plateaus	Mid-diastolic	–
Mitral regurgitation	Apex	High-pitched	Plateaus	Holosystolic	Radiates to axilla
Tricuspid regurgitation	Tricuspid area	High-pitched	Plateaus	Holosystolic	–
Ventricular septal defect	Lower left sternal border	High-pitched	Plateaus	Holosystolic	Heard across the sternum
Aortic stenosis	First aortic area	High-pitched, harsh, or musical	Crescendo–decrescendo	Midsystolic	Radiates to carotids
Pulmonary stenosis	Pulmonary area	High-pitched, harsh, or musical	Crescendo–decrescendo	Midsystolic	–
Aortic regurgitation	Second aortic area	High-pitched, blowing	Decrescendo	Early diastolic	Towards apex
Pulmonary regurgitation	Pulmonary area and one interspace below	High-pitched, blowing	Decrescendo	Early diastolic	–

A detailed examination of the cardiovascular system is beyond the scope of this book. The reader needs to refer to a standard medical textbook for that.

ABDOMINAL EXAMINATION

Palpation of abdomen in pregnant women with heart disease is unlikely to show any abnormality related to the heart disease per se, except for organomegaly or ascites as previously described.

MANAGEMENT

In a woman with heart disease, the following areas must be considered at the time of pregnancy or while considering pregnancy:
- Prepregnancy management
- Antepartum management
- Peripartum management.

TREATMENT/OBSTETRIC MANAGEMENT

Q. With the help of a long essay, describe the next line of management in the case study mentioned in the beginning of the chapter.

Q. Write a long essay describing the management of 30-year-old primi patient with heart disease complicating pregnancy.

Q. With the help of a long essay, discuss the antenatal, intrapartum, and postpartum management of a woman with rheumatic heart disease during pregnancy.

Q. Using a short essay, discuss the New York Heart Association (NHYA) classification. Also discuss the management of the NHYA class 2 mitral stenosis.

Q. Are all valve lesions problematic, or are there specific conditions where you may have to focus on the pregnant woman?

Q. Write a long essay on the management of rheumatic heart failure at 34 weeks' gestation.

PREPREGNANCY MANAGEMENT

Management of women with heart disease should be preferably by a multidisciplinary team involving the obstetrician and cardiologist. The impact that her heart condition is likely to have on the pregnancy must be discussed well in advance before the patient becomes pregnant. The various issues, which need to be discussed at this time, are described below:
- *Risk assessment:* A careful cardiac examination and assessment of functional capacity is required to determine the likelihood that patient would be able to tolerate the increased hemodynamic burden of pregnancy, labor, and delivery, and the risk of complications during gestation. Patients with heart disease who are planning pregnancy must have their risk assessed by performing the following tests:
  • Thorough cardiovascular history and examination
  • 12-lead ECG
  • Transthoracic echocardiogram
  • Arterial oxygen saturation measurement
  • Percutaneous oximetry
- *Risk stratification:* The New York Heart Association (NYHA) functional classification of heart disease is shown in **Table 21.5**. Patients can be classified into various NYHA classes based on their underlying functional cardiac status. Patients with NYHA class III

TABLE 21.5: New York Heart Association functional classification of heart failure.

Class	
Class I	Patients with cardiac disease, but without resulting limitations of physical activity. Ordinary physical activity does not cause fatigue, palpitations, dyspnea, or anginal pain
Class II	Patients with cardiac disease, resulting in slight limitation of physical activity. They are comfortable at rest. Ordinary physical activity results in fatigue, palpitations, dyspnea, or anginal pain
Class III	Patients with cardiac disease, resulting in marked limitation of physical activity. They are comfortable at rest. Less than ordinary physical activity results in fatigue, palpitations, dyspnea, or anginal pain
Class IV	Patients with cardiac disease, resulting in an inability to carry on any physical activity without discomfort. Symptoms of cardiac insufficiency may even be present at rest. If any physical activity is undertaken, discomfort is increased

and IV are at a higher risk. Depending on the type of heart disease diagnosed, patients can be stratified into low risk, intermediate risk, or high risk **(Box 21.7)**. In women who have only milder forms of heart disease with no underlying hemodynamic problems, nothing special needs to be done. However, in patients belonging to high-risk category and having potential or real hemodynamic problems (signs of heart failure or low cardiac output), important decisions including the need for medical termination of pregnancy may be required. Indications for medical termination of pregnancy in patients with heart disease are enumerated in **Box 21.8**. In these cases, other alternatives of motherhood including options such as surrogacy or adoption can be considered.

- *Risk associated with the use of anticoagulant drugs:* Women who have prosthetic heart valves and are of childbearing age should be counseled about the potential issues that might arise, including the development of thrombosis. If these individuals are prescribed anticoagulant drugs, there could be risks associated with the use of these drugs during pregnancy.
- *Women undergoing assisted reproductive techniques (ARTs):* Women with heart disease undergoing any procedure related to ARTs are often at an increased risk. The multidisciplinary team should discuss the matter before initiating any such treatment.
- *Cardiac surgical interventions:* Any cardiac surgical interventions in women of childbearing age should take into account the effect these may have on pregnancy. For e.g., due to the increased risk of thrombosis associated with the use of prosthetic mechanical valves during pregnancy, consideration should be given toward using tissue valves for valve replacement.
- *Medical/surgical correction:* Associated medical disorders such as anemia, diabetes, and thyroid disorders must

BOX 21.7: Risk stratification of patients depending upon the underlying cardiac disease.

Low-risk lesions:
- Atrial septal defect, ventricular septal defect, patent ductus arteriosus
- Small left-to-right lesions
- Repaired lesions without residual cardiac dysfunction
- Bicuspid aortic valve without stenosis
- Mild–moderate pulmonic stenosis
- Valvular regurgitation with normal ventricular systolic function
- Isolated mitral valve prolapse without significant regurgitation
- Mitral regurgitation with normal LV function and NYHA class I or II
- Aortic regurgitation with normal LV function and NYHA class I or II
- Asymptomatic aortic stenosis with low mean gradient (<50 mm Hg) and normal LV function (EF >50%)

Intermediate-risk lesions:
- Mitral stenosis
- Large left-to-right shunts
- Uncorrected CoA
- Unrepaired cyanotic congenital heart disease
- Moderate aortic stenosis
- Prosthetic valves
- Severe pulmonary stenosis
- Moderate-to-severe systemic ventricular dysfunction
- Marfan syndrome with a normal aortic root
- Moderate or severe MS

High-risk lesions:
- Eisenmenger's syndrome
- NYHA (class III or IV symptoms)
- Patients with significant pulmonary hypertension
- Marfan syndrome with aortic root or major valvular involvement (diameter of aortic root >4.0 cm)
- Peripartum cardiomyopathy with residual LV systolic dysfunction
- Complex cyanotic heart disease (TOF, Ebstein's anomaly, TA, TGA)
- Severe AS with or without symptoms
- Aortic or mitral valve disease, or both (stenosis or regurgitation), with moderate or severe LV dysfunction (EF <40%)

(AS: aortic stenosis; CoA: coarctation aorta; EF: ejection fraction; LV: left ventricular; MS: mitral stenosis; NYHA: New York Health Association; TA: tricuspid arteries; TGA: transpositioning of great arteries; TOF: tetralogy of Fallot)

BOX 21.8: Indications for medical termination of pregnancy in patients with heart disease.

- Primary pulmonary hypertension
- Eisenmenger's syndrome
- Pulmonary veno-occlusive disease
- Severe lung disease with pulmonary hypertension—some cases of cardiomyopathy with NYHA class III or IV symptoms
- Marfan syndrome with an abnormal aorta
- History of PPCM
- Severe uncorrected valvular stenosis

(NYHA: New York Health Association; PPCM: peripartum cardiomyopathy)

be managed or corrected prior to pregnancy. Surgical correction when indicated (e.g., commissurotomy or mitral valve replacement for mitral stenosis, coronary bypass for ischemic heart, or correction of cyanotic heart diseases) must be done prior to pregnancy.

- *Advice regarding contraception:* In women with severe heart disease, preconception counseling (including advice regarding contraception) should be started right from adolescence. Advice regarding contraception should be given taking into account any increased risks of thrombosis or infection associated with the various contraceptive methods and their interaction with various heart lesions. The parameter of key importance regarding contraception in these patients is its efficacy. The consequences of contraceptive failure in women with severe heart disease can prove fatal. Barrier methods are safe for all cardiac patients and clearly have the added benefit of providing protection against sexually transmitted diseases. Subdermal progestogen implants and progestogen-loaded intrauterine devices are efficacious and are a safe method for most women with significant heart disease. Combined oral contraceptive pills are relatively contraindicated in women with heart disease because the estrogen component of the combined oral contraceptive confers an increased risk of thrombosis. It is therefore contraindicated in pregnant woman with heart disease who already has a high thrombotic risk. These women must also be educated regarding the importance of emergency contraception in case they do have an unprotected sexual intercourse. Sterilization by tubal ligation may be appropriate for women in whom pregnancy would be at high risk.
- Prenatal folic acid must be administered in the dosage of 400–500 µg/day.
- Woman's rubella immunization status must be checked. Immunization must be considered if the patient is not immune.
- In anticipation of pregnancy, drugs with potential harm to the fetus (e.g., ACE inhibitors having a potential to cause fetal renal dysgenesis, if administered during pregnancy) should be discontinued.

ANTENATAL MANAGEMENT

Investigations

Noninvasive testing in a patient with heart disease may include an ECG, chest radiograph, and echocardiogram. The ECG may reveal a leftward shift of the electrical axis, especially during the third trimester, when the diaphragm is pushed upward by the uterus. Routine chest radiography should be avoided, especially in the first trimester, due to the risk of radiation exposure to the fetus. Echocardiography is an invaluable tool for the diagnosis and evaluation of suspected cardiac disease in the pregnant patient.

Antenatal Care

Advice for patients with heart disease during the antenatal period is enlisted in **Table 21.6**.

- *Prevention of risk factors:* The focus of care early in pregnancy must be to avoid risk factors including infection, high blood pressure, obesity, multiple pregnancies, anemia, arrhythmia, etc. Since these risk factors are likely to exacerbate the symptoms related to heart disease, they must be identified as soon as possible and treated aggressively.
- *Treatment of heart failure:* If heart failure develops during the antenatal period, the woman must be preferably admitted to the hospital. Drugs such as digoxin and diuretics form the cornerstones of therapy. Once heart failure is brought under control, most women can be discharged from hospital.
- *Fetal surveillance:* Strict fetal surveillance may be required during the antenatal period. When the patient is stable, no special treatment is needed. However, when there are signs of hemodynamic compromise, careful fetal monitoring is required. IUGR and fetal asphyxia are the major concerns. Clinical and ultrasound examinations are most commonly performed. Ultrasonographic

TABLE 21.6: Advice for patients with heart disease during pregnancy.

Patients with class I and II disease during pregnancy	Patients with class III and IV disease during pregnancy
• *Bed rest:* At least 10 hours each night and half an hour after each meal	• If seen early enough in pregnancy (<13 weeks of gestation), termination may be considered
• Light housework and walking is permitted, but no heavy work must be done	• If the woman chooses to continue pregnancy, prolonged hospitalization or bed rest may be required
• Weight gain during pregnancy must not exceed 12 kg	• Strict adherence to advice and medical treatment must be followed
• She should be advised to avoid contact with persons who have respiratory tract infections including common cold and flu condition. Pneumococcal and influenza vaccines are usually recommended	• Cesarean section is poorly tolerated in these cases; therefore, vaginal delivery is preferred (in the absence of any obstetric indications)
• Cigarette smoking is prohibited	
• Anemia should be treated actively during pregnancy; hemoglobin levels should be preferably kept at or above 12 g/dL throughout pregnancy	
• Tachycardia with mitral stenosis can be treated with β-blockers such as propranolol so as to keep the heart rate within 80 beats/min	

examination is very helpful and helps in the assessment of the following parameters:
- Considering termination of pregnancy in highly complex cases
- Providing maternal reassurance that everything is fine
- Confirming gestational age
- Assessing the amniotic fluid volume.

To rule out fetal anomalies in cases of CHD, other tests that might be required in special circumstances are as follows:
- Cardiotocography to measure fetal heart rate
- Color Doppler flow studies to measure fetal and maternal placental blood flow
- Fetal blood sampling to detect low oxygen content
- *Fetal echocardiography:* Women with CHD are at a relatively increased risk of having a baby affected with CHD and should be offered fetal echocardiography.

- *Management by a multidisciplinary team:* Like the preconceptional period, these women with heart disease must be assessed clinically as soon as possible in the antenatal period by a multidisciplinary team comprising a cardiologist, obstetrician, anesthetists, midwives, neonatologists, etc. Delivery should be planned to take place at a tertiary unit, which would be able to provide combined obstetric, cardiological, and surgical care for a woman with heart disease.
- *Use of β-blockers:* In women on β-blockers (for e.g., for the treatment of systemic hypertension or to reduce the risk of arrhythmia), there is a small increased risk of IUGR. Therefore, in these cases fetal growth should be monitored regularly, using ultrasound measurement of fetal abdominal circumference. Empirical therapy with β-blocker is advisable in patients with aortic coarctation, Marfan syndrome, and ascending aortopathy for other reasons (e.g., a bicuspid aortic valve).

  Severity levels of mitral and aortic stenosis that are not problematic in nonpregnant women may be poorly tolerated in pregnancy. Reduction of heart rate is often the key to successful management, especially in cases of stenosis of the mitral valve. β-blockers are useful in this context. β-blockers rather than digoxin should be used to control the heart rate for patients with functionally significant mitral stenosis.
- *Bed rest:* According to the guidelines by the American College of Cardiology/American Heart Association (ACC/AHA) (2006), the importance of simple interventions, such as bed rest, limitation of activities, and avoidance of the supine position, should not be overlooked. Restricted activity helps in avoiding tachycardia, improving renal perfusion, and promoting elimination of water by inducing diuresis. At rest, blood flow to several organs (especially skeletal muscles) reduces greatly, thereby reducing the workload on heart.
- *Dietary salt restriction:* Moderate dietary salt restriction of 4–6 g/day is sufficient to prevent excessive retention of water and sodium.
- *Diuretics:* Administration of loop diuretics may be required if salt restriction is not sufficient to limit the intravascular volume expansion. Diuretics must be used judiciously because they may compromise placental perfusion and inhibit fetal growth by reducing placental volume.
- *Digoxin:* Its use may be required in patients showing symptoms of heart failure despite optimal medications. Digoxin acts by improving the contractility of heart and providing relief from symptoms such as easy fatigability, orthopnea, and weakness. It may also be used for controlling ventricular rate in atrial arrhythmias.
- *Increased frequency of antenatal visits:* In general, prenatal visits should be scheduled every month in women with mild disease and every 2 weeks in women with moderate or severe disease, until 28–30 weeks and weekly thereafter until delivery.
- *Use of various cardiac interventions:* Percutaneous catheter interventions are safe and effective in the treatment of coronary disease and mitral and pulmonary valve stenosis. In contrast, balloon dilation for aortic valve disease should only be considered for highly selected cases as it carries a higher risk and a lower success rate. Such interventions in pregnancy should only be performed by experienced operators, and radiation exposure should be minimized. If cardiac surgery requiring the use of cardiopulmonary bypass does need to be performed, consideration should be given to early delivery of the fetus if it is viable. The standard technique of cardiopulmonary bypass is often associated with deep hypothermia and low perfusion pressure, which carries nearly 30% risk of fetal mortality. Therefore, in order to protect the fetus, hypothermia should be avoided as far as possible, and perfusion pressures must be kept as high as possible. In pregnancy, if there is clinical evidence of acute coronary insufficiency or myocardial infarction, coronary angiography is appropriate. The radiation exposure to the fetus is not sufficient so as to contraindicate this essential diagnostic procedure.
- *Use of antiarrhythmic medicines during pregnancy:* Premature atrial or ventricular beats are common in normal pregnancy. These usually are not treated. However, in patients with preexisting arrhythmias, their frequency and hemodynamic severity may be exacerbated due to pregnancy. Pharmacologic treatment is usually reserved for patients with severe symptoms or in the presence of sustained episodes, which are poorly tolerated. Sustained tachyarrhythmias, such as atrial flutter or atrial fibrillation, should be treated promptly.

If possible, all antiarrhythmic drugs should be avoided during the first trimester and those known to be teratogenic should be avoided throughout pregnancy. Based on their safety profiles, preferred drugs during pregnancy include digoxin, β-blockers (possibly excluding atenolol), and adenosine. Sometimes antiarrhythmic drugs such as quinidine, sotalol, lidocaine, flecainide, and propafenone can also be considered. However, presently there is lack of evidence regarding the use of appropriate drugs during pregnancy. Amiodarone is generally regarded as contraindicated in pregnancy, although it has been described as successful in certain case reports. It is not teratogenic but may cause neonatal hypothyroidism. Electrical cardioversion is considered to be relatively safe during pregnancy.

Intrapartum Care

- *Multidisciplinary team:* Management of intrapartum care should be supervised by a multidisciplinary team experienced in the care of women with heart disease as described previously. A clear plan for management of labor and the puerperium in women with heart disease should be established well in advance. The steps which must be taken for class I and II patients during labor are enlisted in **Box 21.9**.
- *Reduction of additional load:* The main objective of management should be to minimize any additional load on the cardiovascular system from delivery and the puerperium. This is usually best achieved with the help of the following:
    - Aiming for spontaneous onset of labor
    - Providing effective pain relief with low-dose regional analgesia
    - Assisting vaginal delivery with instruments such as the ventouse or forceps
    - Limiting or even avoiding active maternal bearing down ("pushing").

Vaginal delivery over cesarean section is the preferred mode of delivery for most women with heart disease, whether congenital or acquired. Cesarean section is considered only in the presence of specific obstetric or cardiac considerations. Some of the indications for cesarean section are described in **Box 21.10**.

Induction of labor may sometimes be more appropriate, especially in order to optimize the timing of delivery in relation to anticoagulation or due to the deteriorating maternal cardiac function. However, it should be recognized that induction of labor before 41 weeks of gestation, especially in nulliparous women with an unfavorable cervix, increases the likelihood of cesarean section.

- *Effective pain relief:* Pain control should be offered with epidural anesthesia and adequate volume preloading. Control of pain helps in reducing tachycardia, myocardial workload, and cardiac output. IM or IV labor analgesia may be used in the early stages of labor. Epidural blockade is the preferred mode for analgesia in the later stages of labor, provided that the patient is not on anticoagulants. Administration of epidural narcotics is preferred over epidural anesthetics.
- *Administration of IV fluids:* IV fluids must be administered at a rate of not more than 75 mL/h in order to keep the patient on the dry side.
- *Continuous monitoring with pulse oximetry:* Mild degree of desaturation may be corrected by administration of oxygen via nasal prongs rebreathing mask.
- *Proper position:* Positioning the patient on the left lateral side helps in reducing the associated hemodynamic fluctuations.
- *Proper hemostasis:* If any surgical intervention is undertaken (e.g., episiotomy), meticulous attention must be paid to hemostasis in order to avoid hemorrhage. Even a minor degree of hemorrhage can cause marked cardiovascular instability in pregnant women with reduced cardiac reserve.
- *Intrapartum antibiotic prophylaxis:* There is currently no evidence that prophylactic antibiotics are necessary to prevent endocarditis in cases of uncomplicated vaginal

BOX 21.9: Steps to be taken for class I and II patients during labor.

- Patient must be placed in a semirecumbent position with lateral tilt
- Vital signs must be monitored every 15–20 minutes during the first stage and every 10 minutes during the second stage
- Pulse rates >100 beats/min and respiratory rates >24/min may be indicative of impending heart failure
- Oxygen may be administered by face mask
- Pulse oximetry may be done
- IV fluids must be restricted to about 75 mL/h
- Straining during the second stage of labor must be avoided as far as possible
- Outlet forceps or ventouse delivery can be used to shorten the second stage of labor
- No bolus oxytocin must be administered because it can result in sudden hypotension. Ergot alkaloids (Methergine) must also be avoided due to the risk of sudden hypertension
- Prophylaxis for bacterial endocarditis (mainly for *Streptococcus viridans*) must be administered in patients with rheumatic heart disease, valvular prosthesis, previous endocarditis, cardiac surgery, and cyanotic heart disease
- Thromboprophylaxis may be required in patients with mitral stenosis, heart failure, valvular prosthesis, and other general risk factors

BOX 21.10: Indications for cesarean section.

- Marfan syndrome with dilated aortic root
- Aortic aneurysm
- Women with a mechanical Björk–Shiley mitral valve who have opted for warfarin anticoagulation should also be considered for elective section to reduce the time off warfarin
- Taking warfarin within 2 weeks of labor

delivery. The European Cardiology Society guidelines (2015) as well as the AHA (2007) do not recommend the routine use of endocarditis prophylaxis for cesarean section delivery or for uncomplicated vaginal delivery without infection. However, in developing countries prophylactic antibiotics are usually given in all cases of operative delivery and to women at increased risk, such as those with mechanical valves or a history of previous endocarditis. Prophylactic antibiotic cover should also be given in case any intervention is likely to be associated with the risk of significant or recurrent bacteremia. Also, some centers do administer endocarditis prophylaxis at the time of vaginal delivery in women with structural heart disease, as an uncomplicated delivery cannot always be anticipated. Preventive antibiotics generally recommended for patients, who are at the highest risk of developing infective endocarditis, include the following:
- Prosthetic heart valve
- Valve repair with prosthetic material
- Previous history of infective endocarditis
- Many congenital heart abnormalities, such as single ventricle states, transposition of the great arteries, and TOF.

Such women must be prescribed antibiotic prophylaxis before undergoing oral, dental, or upper respiratory tract procedure.

Recommended antibiotic prophylaxis for high-risk women with heart disease undergoing oral, dental, or upper respiratory tract procedures is described in **Table 21.7**.

Use of Various Cardiovascular Drugs During Pregnancy

Commonly used cardiovascular drug classes and their potential adverse effects during pregnancy are shown in **Table 21.8**.

Management of the Third Stage of Labor

- *Control of postpartum hemorrhage:* At the time of management of the third stage of labor in women with heart disease, bolus doses of oxytocin can cause a fall in systemic vascular resistance, thereby resulting in severe hypotension. Therefore, this should be avoided. Low-dose oxytocin infusions are safer and may be equally effective. Ergometrine is best avoided in most cases as it can cause vasoconstriction and acute hypertension. Misoprostol may be safer, but it can cause problems such as hyperthermia. Presently, the evidence regarding the use of misoprostol in patients with heart disease is largely limited. It should be used only if the benefits outweigh any potential risks. At the time of cesarean section, uterine compression sutures may be effective in controlling postpartum hemorrhage due to uterine atonicity.

TABLE 21.7: Recommended antibiotic prophylaxis or high-risk women with heart disease undergoing oral, dental, or upper respiratory tract procedures.

Category	Drug and dosage
High-risk patient who can take oral medicine	2 g of amoxicillin (If enterococcal infection is of concern, vancomycin may also be given)
High-risk patient who is unable to take oral medicines	Ampicillin, in the dosage of 2 g IM or IV or Cefazolin or ceftriaxone in the dosage of 1 g IM or IV
High-risk patient who has (oral) penicillin allergy	2 g cephalexin* or 600 mg clindamycin IV or 500 mg of azithromycin or clarithromycin
High-risk patient who is allergic to penicillins and is unable to take oral medication	Cefazolin or ceftriaxone* in the dosage of 1 g IM or IV or 600 mg IM or IV clindamycin

Note: *Cephalosporins should not be used in an individual with a history of anaphylaxis, angioedema, or urticaria with penicillins.
Source: Wilson W, Taubert KA, Gewitz M, Lockhart PB, Baddour LM, Levison M, et al. Prevention of infective endocarditis: guidelines from the American Heart Association: a guideline from the American Heart Association Rheumatic Fever, Endocarditis, and Kawasaki Disease Committee, Council on Cardiovascular Disease in the Young, and the Council on Clinical Cardiology, Council on Cardiovascular Surgery and Anesthesia, and the Quality of Care and Outcomes Research Interdisciplinary Working Group. Circulation. 2007;116(15):1736-54.

- *Prevention of thromboembolic complications:* There is approximately 2% risk for development of thromboembolic complications in patients with rheumatic heart disease. To prevent this complication, it is necessary to initiate ambulation shortly after delivery, use compression bandages for lower extremities, and administer prophylactic LMWH during labor, delivery, and immediate postpartum period.

- *Prevention of pulmonary edema immediately after delivery:* Immediately after delivery, there is a sudden transfusion of blood from the lower extremities and uteroplacental circulation into the systemic circulation as a result of the loss of obstructive effect of the uterus on venous return. This may result in the increase in blood volume to an extent where it exceeds the pumping ability of heart, resulting in pulmonary edema. To prevent the occurrence of pulmonary edema, the patient must be placed in a sitting position following delivery, because this posture allows a more gradual adaptation to the postpartum hemodynamic changes by increasing venous pooling in the lower extremities and thereby reducing venous return to the heart.

Also, if the patient is under the effect of epidural anesthesia, the anesthesiologist must raise the level of anesthesia and sympathetic blockade.

TABLE 21.8: Cardiovascular drugs used during pregnancy.

Drug	Use	Potential side effects	Safety during pregnancy	Safety during breastfeeding
Adenosine	Arrhythmia	None reported	Yes	No data available
β-blockers	Hypertension, arrhythmias, MI, ischemia, HCM, hyperthyroidism, mitral stenosis, Marfan syndrome, cardiomyopathy	Low birth weight, hypoglycemia, respiratory depression, prolonged labor	Yes	Yes
Digoxin	Arrhythmia, CHF	Low birth weight, prematurity	Yes	Yes
Diuretics	Hypertension, CHF	Reduced uteroplacental perfusion	Unclear	Yes
Lidocaine	Arrhythmia, anesthesia	Neonatal CNS depression	Yes	Yes
Low-molecular-weight heparin	Mechanical valve hypercoagulable state, DVT, AF, Eisenmenger's syndrome	Hemorrhage, unclear effects on maternal bone mineral density	Limited data	Limited data
Nitrates	Hypertension	Fetal distress with maternal hypotension	Yes	No data
Procainamide	Arrhythmia	None reported	Yes	Yes
Unfractionated heparin	Mechanical valve hypercoagulable state, DVT, AF, Eisenmenger's syndrome	Maternal osteoporosis, hemorrhage, thrombocytopenia, thrombosis	Yes	Yes
Warfarin	Mechanical valve hypercoagulable state, DVT, AF, Eisenmenger's syndrome	Warfarin embryopathy, fetal CNS abnormalities, hemorrhage	Yes, after 12 weeks of gestation	Yes

(AF: atrial fibrillation; CHF: chronic heart failure; CNS: central nervous system; DVT: deep vein thrombosis; HCM: hypertrophic cardiomyopathy; MI: myocardial infarction)

Postpartum Care

Since the hemodynamic parameters may not return to baseline for many days after delivery, patients at intermediate or high risk may require monitoring for at least 72 hours postpartum. Close monitoring of the patient should be continued during the puerperium mainly to prevent or detect development of early complications such as infection, hemorrhage, and thromboembolism.

Patients with Eisenmenger's syndrome are at risk of death for up to 7 days postpartum and therefore require close observation for a longer period of time, postpartum. Unstable cardiac conditions such as pulmonary hypertension or cardiomyopathy and conditions like Eisenmenger's syndrome, which are at a high risk of death in the postpartum period, may require surveillance for up to 2 weeks. The cases at high risk should be assessed by a multidisciplinary team, as a minimum, at 6 weeks after delivery. In cases where there are continuing concerns, another assessment can take place at 6 months. Following these assessments, the woman should return to her periodic cardiac outpatient care.

- If any pregnant or postpartum woman has unexpected and persistent dyspnea or is noted to be unusually tachypneic or tachycardic and the possibility of pulmonary embolism has been excluded, she may have PPCM. She should be investigated further by echocardiography.
- ACE inhibitors are safe to use in breastfeeding mothers.
- Due to an increased risk of postpartum hemorrhage in women with heart disease who are on anticoagulation therapy, the introduction or reintroduction of warfarin should be delayed until at least 2 days postpartum. Meticulous monitoring of anticoagulation is essential.

PREGNANCY IN THE PRESENCE OF PROSTHETIC HEART VALVE

Q. Describe the management of pregnant women with heart disease having a prosthetic mitral valve.

Q. Discuss the peripartum management of thromboprophylaxis in a pregnant patient with prosthetic heart valves.

Several conditions such as the use of mechanical valves, certain prothrombotic conditions (antiphospholipid antibody syndrome, atrial fibrillation, etc.), prior episode of venous thromboembolism, acute DVT, or thromboembolism during pregnancy require the initiation or maintenance of anticoagulation during pregnancy. The use of prosthetic heart valves in patients at the time of pregnancy is likely to be associated with an increased risk of thrombosis. Besides thrombosis, other risks associated with pregnancy in women with prosthetic valves are related to increased hemodynamic burden and untoward fetal effects caused by cardiovascular drugs and anticoagulants. Women with bioprosthetic valves typically do not require anticoagulation unless there are other thromboembolic risk factors. However, bioprosthetic valves have a significantly higher incidence of valve failure in comparison to mechanical valves. Newer generation mechanical valves are associated with a lower thromboembolic risk in comparison to older mechanical valves. Other factors that increase thromboembolic risk include previous history of thromboembolic event, atrial fibrillation, prosthesis in the mitral position, multiple prosthetic valves, etc.

One of the most important concerns in pregnant patients with heart disease is the state of hypercoagulability that exists throughout pregnancy, which is likely to put women at higher than usual risk of thromboembolism, especially in women with prosthetic heart valves. As a result, there is a requirement to use anticoagulant drugs throughout the pregnancy. The three most common agents considered for use during pregnancy are: UFH, LMWH, and warfarin. However, at present, no anticoagulation strategy has been found to be equally safe for both the mother and the fetus.

When therapeutic anticoagulation is administered during pregnancy, there is the risk of pregnancy-specific bleeding related to delivery of baby and placenta. The risk of unexplained hemorrhage or antepartum hemorrhage due to placenta previa or abruption appears to be increased in women with mechanical valves on therapeutic anticoagulation. The patient should also be informed that the risk of life-threatening thromboembolic events and a thrombotic stroke exists regardless of the anticoagulant regimen utilized. Discussion of these risks as well as the type of anticoagulant regimen to be used should be included in prepregnancy counseling in such patients.

Oral therapy with warfarin is effective but has the potential of causing congenital embryonic abnormalities because of its potential to cross the placenta. Women taking warfarin preconceptionally should be advised to continue oral anticoagulation until they are pregnant because the risk of warfarin embryopathy (defects in cartilage and bone) is low in the first 6 weeks of gestation. Women of reproductive age should closely monitor their menses and if it is delayed, they must undergo a pregnancy test immediately. Warfarin exposure early in pregnancy (after 6 weeks) is likely to cause a specific embryopathy affecting cartilage and bone (chondromalacia punctata, with stippled epiphyses and nasal and limb hypoplasia). However, some studies show that a dosage of 5 mg of warfarin per day may not be teratogenic. The incidence of warfarin embryopathy has been estimated to be between 4% and 10%; the risk is highest when warfarin is administered during 6–12 weeks of gestation. When administered during the second and third trimesters, warfarin has been found to be associated with fetal CNS abnormalities, probably related to the development of microhemorrhages in the neuronal tissues. However, the use of warfarin has been found to be safe during breastfeeding. Moreover, regular use of warfarin throughout the pregnancy is associated with the risk of fetal intracranial bleeding, particularly during vaginal delivery, unless warfarin is stopped before labor.

On the other hand, heparin (both UFH and LMWH) are not associated with any teratogenic defects as they do not cross the placenta. However, they may cause side effects such as maternal osteoporosis, hemorrhage, thrombocytopenia, thrombosis or heparin-induced thrombocytopenia and thrombosis (HITT) syndrome, and a high incidence of thromboembolic events with older generation mechanical valves. Also, their efficacy is lower in comparison to warfarin for preventing thrombosis in patients with prosthetic heart valves. Moreover, heparin may require twice-daily SC injections and is associated with higher rates of maternal valve thrombosis.

However, nowadays LMWHs are increasingly becoming the preferred treatment modality over UFH in several countries because of their improved pharmacokinetics and bioavailability, and their reduced side-effects profile. Increasing evidence suggests that therapeutic LMWH may serve as an acceptable alternative even to warfarin for many women as it provides better protection than UFH against thrombotic risk and is associated with improved fetal outcomes in comparison to warfarin.

Unfractionated heparin may be administered parenterally or subcutaneously throughout pregnancy; when used subcutaneously for the anticoagulation of mechanical heart valves, the recommended starting dose is 17,500–20,000 U twice daily. The appropriate dose adjustment of UFH is based on peak (taken 4–6 hours after drug ingestion) activated partial thromboplastin time (aPTT) of 2.0–3.0 times the control level. High doses of UFH may be required during pregnancy to achieve the target aPTT because of the hypercoagulable state associated with pregnancy. Lower doses of UFH may be appropriate for anticoagulation in certain cases, such as the prevention of venous thromboembolism during pregnancy.

Low-molecular-weight heparin produces a more predictable anticoagulant response than UFH and is less likely to cause side effects like HITT. The 2020 ACC/AHA guidelines recommend maintaining peak antifactor Xa levels between 0.8 and 1.2 U/mL when therapeutic LMWH is used.

Direct thrombin inhibitors, such as dabigatran, should not be considered an alternative to therapy with either warfarin or heparin in patients with prosthetic valves during pregnancy. Evidence is lacking on the efficacy and safety of dabigatran in patients with prosthetic valves.

Women with mechanical prosthetic valves require anticoagulation throughout the pregnancy. The following regimens can be used:

- *Low-dose warfarin:* As per the European Society of Cardiology (ESC, 2021) guidelines, the best anticoagulation regimen to be used in pregnant patients with prosthetic heart valves is low-dose warfarin in the dosage <5 mg daily throughout pregnancy with the monitoring of ionized normalized ratio (INR) of 3.0 (range 2.5–3.5). Concerns about warfarin embryopathy are quite rare with the dosage <5 g/day.
- *Warfarin along with targeted replacement using heparin:* Added to the regimen of therapy with oral anticoagulants during pregnancy is the targeted replacement with parenteral heparin (continuous IV, dose-adjusted SC UFH, or dose-adjusted SC LMWH) during the first

trimester (6–12 weeks) and late third trimester (beyond 36 weeks). Warfarin (in the dosage >5 mg) should be stopped by the sixth week of gestation to reduce the risk of fetal defects. This regimen is however associated with an increased risk of thrombotic complications and maternal mortality.

Warfarin can then be restarted from 13th week of pregnancy and continued up to week 36 of pregnancy. Warfarin must be discontinued and continuous UFH be administered till about 2–3 weeks before the date of planned delivery or at about 36th week. In women with prosthetic valves at high risk of thromboembolic complications, addition of low-dose aspirin should also be considered. Although high-dose aspirin may promote premature duct closure, low-dose aspirin is considered as a safe option during pregnancy.

If labor begins while the woman is receiving warfarin, anticoagulation should be reversed and cesarean delivery should be performed. Since the fetus is also therapeutically anticoagulated, if the patient had been taking warfarin continuously, cesarean delivery is preferred to reduce the risks of fetal trauma and hemorrhage. If emergent delivery is necessary, fresh frozen plasma (FFP) should be administered prior to cesarean delivery in sufficient amount to reach a target INR of 2.0. Depending upon timing and dose, the administration of vitamin K to the mother prior to delivery can also reverse the effect of warfarin in the fetus and therefore reduce the risk of fetal hemorrhage. If the mother was not fully reversed at the time of delivery, the newborn may also be administered FFP and vitamin K. If heparin is administered during pregnancy, it should be discontinued at least 12 hours before induction, or reversed with protamine if spontaneous labor develops.

Following delivery, IV UFH, or SC LMWH must be resumed 4–6 hours after delivery in the absence of any complications. Heparin must be resumed at a prophylactic dose, gradually increasing the dose to achieve therapeutic anticoagulation over the coming 24–72 hours. Warfarin therapy may be resumed the night after delivery if no bleeding complications occur. After an uncomplicated vaginal delivery, warfarin can be resumed the same day. However, if the woman has had a cesarean section, this should be delayed for 1–2 days.

COMPLICATIONS

MATERNAL COMPLICATIONS

Q. What are the chances that a fetus of the mother with congenital heart disease will also develop congenital heart disease?

A validated cardiac risk score which helps in predicting a woman's chance of having adverse cardiac complications during pregnancy is enlisted in **Table 21.9**. Each risk factor has been given a value of 1 point. The probability of mother to experience adverse cardiac event is 5%, 27%, and 75%, respectively, for the points of 0, 1, and higher than 1.

Cardiac disease during pregnancy can cause considerable maternal morbidity. Pregnant women with heart disease are at an increased risk for cardiac complications such as heart failure, arrhythmias, and stroke. The diseases which are associated with the highest risk to the mother during pregnancy are enumerated in **Box 21.11**. However, few women with heart disease actually die during pregnancy.

The high-risk exceptions, which are associated with high mortality rate, include women with Eisenmenger's syndrome, pulmonary vascular obstructive disease, or Marfan's syndrome with aortopathy. Pregnant women with congenital heart lesions are at an increased risk for heart failure, arrhythmia, stroke, neonatal complications, and even death in some conditions.

Eisenmenger's syndrome can cause severe pulmonary hypertension as a consequence of a long-standing, left-to-right shunt lesion such as ASD, VSD, or PDA. In these cases, the risk of maternal mortality can be as high as 30–50%. Among the CHDs, TOF carries a 4–20% risk of mortality in the mother. ASDs are perhaps the safest of all birth defects. Rheumatic heart valve disease is another risk, with patients having mitral stenosis associated with a 1% chance of developing pulmonary edema during pregnancy.

TABLE 21.9: Predictors of maternal risk for cardiac complications.

Criteria	Example	Points
Prior cardiac events	Heart failure, stroke before current pregnancy, etc.	1
Prior arrhythmia NYHA III or IV or cyanosis	Symptomatic sustained tachyarrhythmia or bradyarrhythmia requiring treatment	1
Valvular and outflow tract obstruction	Aortic valve area <1.5 cm^2, mitral valve area <2 cm^2, or LV outflow tract peak gradient >30 mm Hg	1
Myocardial dysfunction	LVEF <40%, restrictive cardiomyopathy, or hypertrophic cardiomyopathy	1

(LV: left ventricular; LVEF: left ventricular ejection fraction; NYHA: New York Health Association)

BOX 21.11: Heart diseases associated with an increased risk for cardiac complications.

- Eisenmenger's syndrome
- Primary pulmonary hypertension
- Marfan's syndrome with aortopathy
- Cor pulmonale
- Congenital heart diseases (tetralogy of Fallot)
- Rheumatic heart valve disease (mitral stenosis)
- Connective tissue disorders (e.g., Ehlers–Danlos syndrome)

The risk of CHD in the fetus of pregnant women with CHD is about 2–4%, which is about twice the incidence of heart disease in the general population. This risk also varies with different conditions. For instance, it is 3% in parents with TOF, but almost 18% in those with aortic stenosis. These defects are usually concordant, i.e., the defect in the child is usually the same one as that of the mother.

Connective tissue disorders such as Ehlers–Danlos syndrome (a disorder of the connective tissue of the body resulting in loose skin and lax joints) can cause a higher risk of bleeding from major blood vessels that might rupture during pregnancy.

FETAL COMPLICATIONS

In most mothers with cardiac disease, the fetus develops almost normally. However, some cardiac conditions may be associated with adverse neonatal outcomes during pregnancy **(Box 21.12)**. For e.g., patients with rheumatic heart valve disease may suffer mild growth restriction, with babies born being lighter by around 200 g.

In cyanotic mothers, many problems such as severe growth restriction and higher abortion rates may arise. In these conditions, the maternal blood has very low oxygen content, due to which there is a lower oxygen exchange across the placenta. As a result, the fetus gets lesser supply of oxygen than normal, which can cause fetal death or premature delivery. Another condition, which is associated with high rates of fetal loss due to reduced blood flow to the placenta as a result of narrowing of aorta, includes CoA.

> **BOX 21.12:** Predictors for adverse neonatal outcomes during pregnancy.
> - NYHA III or IV or cyanosis during the baseline prenatal visit
> - Maternal LV dysfunction
> - Anticoagulation during pregnancy
> - Maternal smoking
> - Multiple gestation
>
> (LV: left ventricular; NYHA: New York Health Association)

EVIDENCE-BASED CLINICAL TRIALS

List of references can be scanned through QR code to enable the readers gain deeper insight of the subject by referring to the entire article or its abstract.

PART II: GYNECOLOGY

SECTION 4

Normal and Abnormal Menstruation

22. Normal Gynecological Examination
23. Abnormal Uterine Bleeding due to Endometrial Cancer
24. Heavy Menstrual Bleeding due to Leiomyoma
25. Menopause

CHAPTER 22

Normal Gynecological Examination

CASE STUDY

A 55-year-old G4P4 lady visits the clinic for routine gynecological checkup. She attained menopause 5 years ago. There is no significant family history or past treatment history.

She underwent myomectomy for symptomatic uterine fibroids 10 years ago. On examination, her blood pressure was 120/80 mm Hg and pulse rate was 84 beats/min. There were no signs and symptoms of anemia and no lymphadenopathy. The patient does not have any problem and has just presented for a routine gynecological checkup.

INTRODUCTION

There are many aspects to women's health which are related to gynecological care. Some such gynecological problems commonly encountered in clinical practice include abnormal menstrual bleeding, abdominal mass, gynecological cancers, pelvic pain, infertility, etc. Some such common gynecological problems would be discussed in detail in the following chapters. For being able to diagnose the abnormal gynecological complaints, it is important for the clinician to be able to perform a normal gynecological examination. Since taking an adequate history and performing a complete pelvic examination is of utmost importance for detection of underlying pathology, this would be discussed in detail in this chapter.

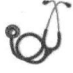

HISTORY AND CLINICAL PRESENTATION

History must be taken in a nonjudgmental, sensitive, and thorough manner. Detailed history and clinical vaginal examination form an important aspect of a normal gynecological checkup. Importance must be given toward maintenance of patient–physician relationship. It is important for the gynecologist to maintain good communication with the patient in order to elicit proper history and to be accurately able to recognize her problems. The manner of speaking, words used, tone of speaking, and body language are important aspects of the patient–physician interaction. Kindness and courtesy must be maintained at all times. These aspects are especially important in case of male gynecologists because the gynecological history entails asking some private and confidential questions from the female patients. Also, the women may be reluctant while telling the history regarding her menstrual cycles to the male gynecologist. It is important for a male gynecologist to take the history and perform the vaginal examination in the presence of a third party or a chaperone (a female nurse or the patient's female relative or friend). A chaperone must also be present while a female gynecologist is performing the clinical examination.

The gynecologist must begin taking the history, starting with open-ended questions to help alleviate the woman's anxiety. The woman should be encouraged to describe the problems in her own wordings. The gynecologist must attentively listen to the woman's history without making frequent interruptions. Adoption of certain tacts by the gynecologist such as maintaining eye contact with the patient, nodding, and brief clarification of important points help in conveying the gynecologist's attention toward the woman's problems. This would help the woman develop confidence in her healthcare provider.

The clinician must adopt both an empathetic and an inquisitive attitude toward the patient. The patient's privacy must be respected at all costs. The gynecologist must refrain from asking personal questions until appropriate patient confidence has been established. The gynecologist needs to listen more and talk less while taking the patient's history. The clinician must avoid interrupting, commanding, and lecturing while taking history. If any serious condition (e.g., malignancy) is suspected, the diagnosis must not be disclosed to the patient until it has been confirmed by performing investigations. Bad news must preferably be told to the patient when she is being accompanied by someone (relative, friend, or spouse). The seriousness and urgency of the situation must be explained to the patient without causing undue alarm and fright to the patient. The clinician must never give false reassurance to the patient. Honest advice and opinion must always be provided.

■ HISTORY OF PRESENTING COMPLAINTS

Asking the age of the patient is especially important. Risk factors related to a particular pathology in question (e.g., postmenopausal bleeding) need to be asked. Some common gynecological problems with which the patient may present are described below.

Abnormal Menstrual Bleeding

For detailed history and examination in cases presenting with abnormal uterine bleeding (AUB), please refer to Chapter 23.

Abdominal Pain

Pain in the abdomen is one of the most common clinical complaints in medical practice. Besides gastrointestinal pathology, underlying gynecological pathology is also a common cause of pain per abdomen. Gynecological problems such as pelvic tuberculosis, PID, and endometriosis may be commonly associated with chronic pain. Acute lower abdominal pain may occur in association with gynecological abnormalities such as ectopic pregnancy, torsion or rupture of an ovarian cyst, and chocolate cyst. The following points need to be asked while taking history of pain:

- *Exact site of pain*: Pain of ovarian or tubal origin is usually felt in the lower abdomen, above the inguinal ligament. Pain of uterine origin is diffusely present in the hypogastric region.
- *Radiation of pain*: Pain of uterine origin is often referred to the inner aspect of the thighs, but does not usually extend beyond the knees. Pain due to appendicitis may initially start in the right iliac region and later radiate to the umbilicus.
- *Nature of pain*: The nature of the pain, whether burning, gnawing, throbbing, aching, or excruciating in nature, needs to be determined.
- *Intensity of pain*: The degree of severity of pain, whether mild, moderate, or severe, needs to be determined. Pain of severe intensity may interfere with sleep and work.
- *Aggravating and relieving factors for pain*: The history of various relieving and aggravating factors for pain must be taken.
- *Relationship of other factors with pain*: Relationship of pain to other factors such as menstruation (dysmenorrhea), coital activity (dyspareunia), micturition (dysuria), defecation (dyschezia), posture, and movement needs to be determined.
- *Dysmenorrhea or pain associated with menstruation can be of two types*: Spasmodic and congestive dysmenorrhea. Spasmodic dysmenorrhea usually has no cause and is seen on day 1 or 2 of menstruation. On the other hand, pain due to congestive dysmenorrhea is usually due to some underlying pathology (endometriosis, PID, etc.). This pain may be premenstrual, menstrual, or postmenstrual in origin. In case of dysmenorrhea due to PID, the pain improves with menstruation, whereas in case of endometriosis, the pain worsens after menstruation due to ectopic menstruation. Dysmenorrhea during the menstrual periods could be due to fibroids or adenomyosis. Dysmenorrhea during the three phases of menstrual cycle (premenstrual, menstrual, and postmenstrual) is typical of endometriosis.

Abdominal Lump

History and examination for lump in the abdomen has been described in detail in Chapter 31.

Infertility/Amenorrhea

For taking detailed history regarding infertility and amenorrhea, refer to Chapters 34 and 35, respectively.

Hirsutism

Hirsutism refers to increased or excessive growth of hair in women. This is usually related to increased androgen production in the body.

Urinary Problems and Sexual Dysfunction

Women may often present to the gynecology clinic with the main complaints of urinary problems such as urinary incontinence (stress or urge incontinence), dysuria (related to urinary tract infection, etc.), voiding difficulties (due to pelvic prolapse, etc.), or sexual dysfunction (e.g., low sexual desire, reduced libido, sexual arousal disorders, orgasmic disorders, sexual pain disorders, and vaginismus).

Vaginal Discharge

History suggestive of pelvic, vaginal, or vulvar infections, e.g., vaginal discharge, vulvar or vaginal lesions, fever, pelvic pain, abnormal bleeding of the genital tract, and previous history of having sexually transmitted infections or PID, also needs to be asked. For detailed information regarding various causes of vaginal discharge, please refer to Chapter 26.

Pelvic Organ Prolapse

For detailed information related to history and clinical presentation in cases of pelvic organ prolapse, kindly refer to Chapter 29.

■ PAST MEDICAL HISTORY

Past history of medical illnesses such as hypertension, hepatitis, diabetes mellitus, cancer, heart disease, pulmonary disease, and thyroid disease needs to be taken. The patient's previous medical and surgical problems may have a bearing on her present complaints. For e.g., a history of longstanding diabetes could be responsible for development of genital candidiasis and associated pruritus. A patient with previous medical history of severe anemia or cardiovascular heart disease may require special anesthetic preparation (e.g., correction of anemia or treatment of cardiovascular pathology) before undergoing a major gynecological surgery (e.g., hysterectomy).

Triad of diabetes, hypertension, and obesity is associated with an increased risk of endometrial carcinoma. A history of sexually transmitted disease (especially infection with chlamydia) may have a direct bearing on future infertility. Previous history of PID or puerperal sepsis could be responsible for producing gynecological complaints such as menstrual disturbances, lower abdominal pain, congestive dysmenorrhea, and infertility. The presence of endocrinological disorders (e.g., thyroid dysfunction) could be responsible for producing menstrual irregularities.

Previous history of undergoing abdominal surgery such as cesarean section, removal of appendix, excision of ovarian cyst, and myomectomy may result in the development of pelvic adhesions. These may not only make any subsequent surgery difficult but also be the cause of common gynecological problems such as pelvic and abdominal pain, infertility, menstrual disturbances, and dyspareunia.

FAMILY HISTORY

Certain gynecological cancers (e.g., cancer of the ovary, uterus, and breast) have a genetic predisposition. A woman may be at a high risk of development of such cancers in the future if there is a positive family history of such cancers in her first-degree relatives (especially mother and sister). Menstrual patterns, including age of menarche, frequency and regularity of cycle, associated dysmenorrhea, and age of attaining menopause, tend to be similar amongst the family members. Common gynecological problems such as premature menopause, menorrhagia, and premenstrual tension have been observed to run within families. Other medical disorders, such as thyroid dysfunction, allergic diathesis, and coagulation disorders, which may be responsible for development of gynecological complaints, are often familial in nature.

MARITAL AND SEXUAL HISTORY

Details of the woman's marital life including her age at the time of marriage, how long she has been married, and sexual history need to be asked. Details of the woman's sexual history are particularly important. Some such details include her age at the time of first sexual intercourse; her current sexual activities (vaginal, oral, anal, and manual), frequency of her sexual intercourses, is she currently seeking a pregnancy, is she presently using any method of contraception (if yes, the type of contraception used), is she or her partner experiencing any sexual dysfunction (frigidity in the woman or impotence or premature ejaculation in the male or problems with libido, arousal, lubrication, or orgasm in both males and females), current frequency of her sexual activities, past sexual activities, number of sexual partners (currently and in the past), sexual preferences (heterosexual, homosexual, or both), pain at the time of sexual intercourse (dyspareunia), etc. History regarding the use of any contraception (both in the past and in the present) needs to be asked. History related to sexual abuse also needs to be elicited.

OBSTETRIC HISTORY

Details of every pregnancy conceived irrespective of their ultimate outcome need to be recorded. Number of previous live births, stillbirths, deaths, miscarriages (both spontaneous and induced), history of recurrent miscarriages if any, medical termination of pregnancies, and number of children living at present need to be noted. The ages of the youngest and eldest children also need to be inquired. The mode of delivery of each baby (normal vaginal delivery or cesarean section) and details of any obstetric complications encountered, e.g., puerperal or postabortal sepsis, PPH, obstetrical interventions (use of forceps, vacuum, etc.) and other obstetric or gynecological complications (soft-tissue injuries such as cervical tears, an incompetent cervical os, genital fistulae, complete perineal tear, genital prolapse, and stress urinary incontinence), and chronic backache also need to be inquired from the patient. Severe degree of PPH and obstetric shock may lead to pituitary necrosis and Sheehan syndrome or postpartum hypopituitarism. This could be the cause of amenorrhea or hot flushes in a young woman who had recently suffered from massive PPH at the time of delivery. It is a good idea to ask the names of the patients' children at the time of taking history. It helps in reducing patients' anxiety and increasing the confidence in her healthcare provider.

PAST TREATMENT HISTORY

History of Previous Surgery

The patient should be asked about any surgery she has undergone in the past. The reason for undergoing surgery, particularly of abdominal or pelvic origin, type of incision (laparoscopy or laparotomy), and any history of postoperative complications need to be inquired.

Past Medication History

In the medication history, the patient should be asked about the various medicines she has been consuming. The details of various medicines including their dosage, route of administration, frequency, and duration of use need to be asked. The patient must be specifically asked about the various medicines she has been taking including prescription drugs, over-the-counter (OTC) drugs, herbal drugs, and any therapy related to alternative medicine.

History of allergy to any medication also needs to be asked.

GYNECOLOGICAL HISTORY

Previous Gynecological History

History of other gynecologic problems in the past, such as previous history of ovarian cysts, uterine fibroids, infertility, endometriosis, polycystic ovarian syndrome, pelvic organ prolapse, and urinary or anal incontinence, needs to be asked. She also needs to be inquired if any treatment for these problems was instituted in the past. History of undergoing some gynecologic procedure (e.g., endometrial biopsy, laparoscopy, and hysterectomy) in the past must be asked. Screening for intimate partner violence also needs to be done.

Screening for Gynecological Malignancy

History of screening tests done for screening gynecological malignancy, especially Pap test, needs to be asked. History related to the date and results of the last test, diagnosis, and follow-up of abnormal Pap smears must also be taken. For details related to screening for cervical pathology, kindly refer to Chapter 27.

MENSTRUAL HISTORY

The menstrual history needs to be taken in detail. The following details need to be recorded: age of menarche, date of last menstrual period, cycle length, whether regular or irregular, number of days the bleeding takes place, amount of bleeding (in terms of pads soaked), and the presence of any associated symptoms, such as cramps, bloating, or headaches.

Detailed menstrual history which needs to be asked in cases of AUB has been described in Chapter 23.

NORMAL MENSTRUAL CYCLE

> Q. Write a long essay discussing the physiology of menstruation.

The events of the normal menstrual cycle are shown in **Figure 22.1**. The first day of a typical menstrual cycle (day l) corresponds to the first day of menses. The menstrual phase usually lasts for 5 days and involves the disintegration and sloughing of the functionalis layer of the endometrium. Interplay of various prostaglandins (e.g., prostaglandin F2-alpha and prostaglandin E2) is involved in the regulation of menstrual cycle. Prostaglandin F2-alpha causes myometrial contractions and vasoconstriction, whereas prostaglandin E2 causes vasodilatation and muscle relaxation. A typical menstrual cycle comprises 28 days. Ovulation occurs in the middle of the menstrual cycle, i.e., day 14 of a typical cycle.

The first 14 days of the cycle, before the menstruation occurs, form the proliferative phase, while the next 14 days of the cycle form the secretory phase. During the follicular phase of normal ovarian cycle (equivalent to the proliferative phase of endometrial cycle), there is an increase in the blood levels of the hormone estrogen. During this phase, the maturation of the dominant follicle takes place. At the midpoint of the cycle, ovulation occurs. Following the process of ovulation, the ruptured ovarian follicle gets converted into corpus luteum (CL), the main hormone produced by CL being progesterone. During the luteal phase of the ovarian cycle (corresponding to the secretory phase of endometrial cycle) as the CL matures, the main hormone produced is progesterone. The endometrium during this phase gets transformed for implantation of conceptus in anticipation of the pregnancy. If pregnancy occurs, the rising levels of human chorionic gonadotropin (hCG) stimulate and rescue the endometrium. In case the pregnancy does not occur, the CL undergoes regression. As a result, the levels of estrogen and progesterone rapidly decline, causing withdrawal of the functional support of the endometrium. This results in menstrual bleeding, marking the end of one endometrial cycle and the beginning of the other.

Role of Various Hormones in Regulation of Menstrual Cycles

Initial follicular development is independent of hormonal influence. However, soon FSH takes control and stimulates a cohort of follicles, encouraging them to develop into preantral stage. FSH causes aromatization of the androgens present in the theca cells into estrogen in the granulosa cells. Out of the various follicles, only one single follicle is destined to develop into a dominant follicle, which undergoes ovulation. Estrogen exerts a negative feedback effect on FSH as a result of which growth of all the follicles except dominant follicle is inhibited. Estradiol levels derived from the dominant follicle increase rapidly and exert a negative feedback effect on FHS release. While causing a decline in FHS levels, the mid-follicular rise in estradiol levels exerts a positive feedback influence on LH secretion. The presence of LH in the follicle prior to ovulation is important for optimal follicular development, which ultimately results in formation of a healthy oocyte. A surge of LH takes place just prior to ovulation. Its levels rise steadily during the late follicular phase. It initiates luteinization and progesterone production in the granulosa layer. A preovulatory rise in progesterone facilitates the positive feedback action of estrogen and may be required to induce the midcycle FSH peak. Ovulation occurs about 10–12 hours after the LH peak and 24–36 hours after the peak estradiol levels have been

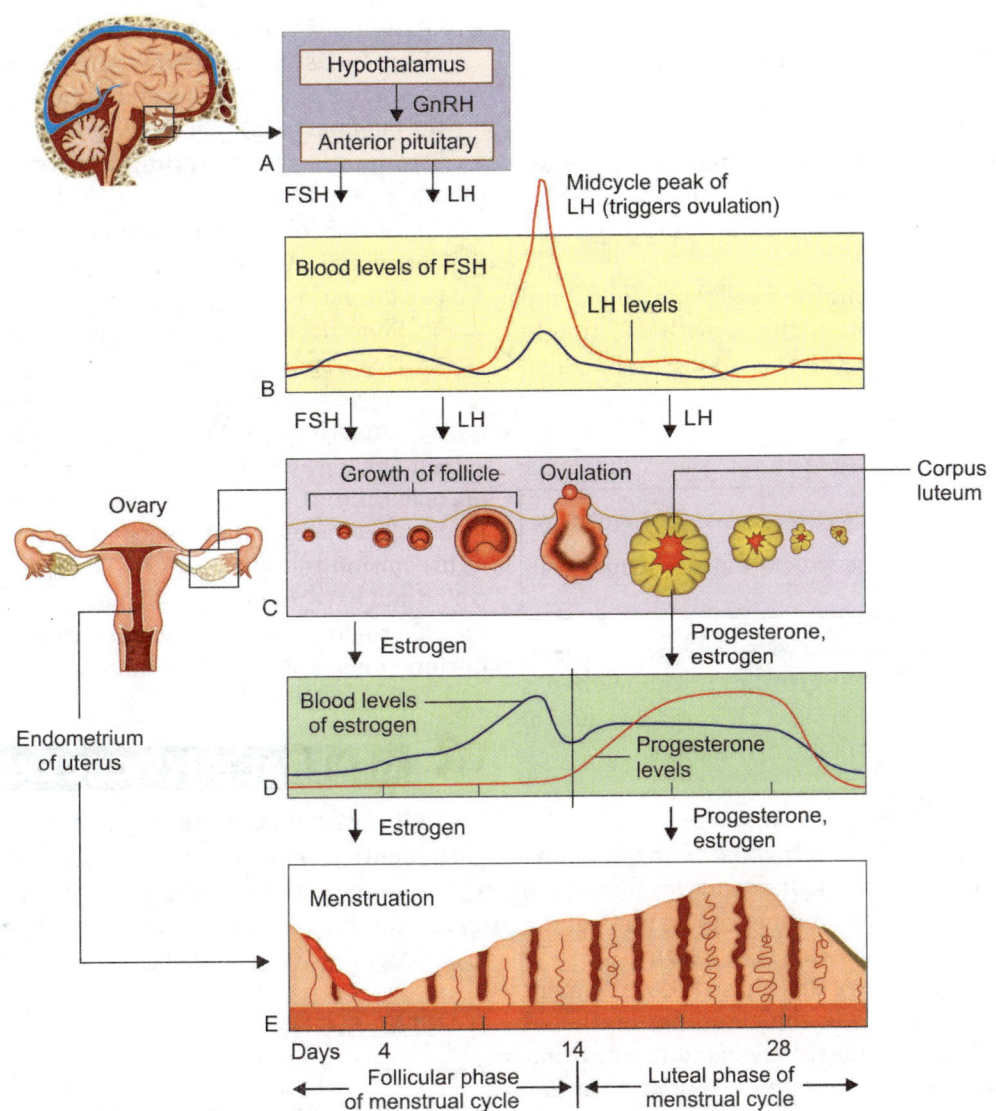

Fig. 22.1: Normal menstrual cycle.

attained. The onset of LH surge is the most reliable indicator of impending ovulation. The various phases of menstrual cycle are described next.

Proliferative (Follicular) Phase

The proliferative (follicular) phase extends from day 5 to day 14 of the typical cycle. In this phase, endometrial proliferation occurs under estrogen stimulation. Estrogen is produced by the developing ovarian follicles under the influence of FSH. This causes marked cellular proliferation of the endometrium and an increase in the length and tortuosity of the spiral arteries. Endometrial glands develop and contain some glycogen. This phase ends as ovulation occurs. The following changes take place during the proliferative phase (Fig. 22.2):

- Functional and basal layers of endometrium become well defined. Proliferation mainly occurs in the functional layer. The basal layer measures 1 mm in thickness, while the functional layer reaches a maximum thickness of about 3.5–5 mm by 14th day.

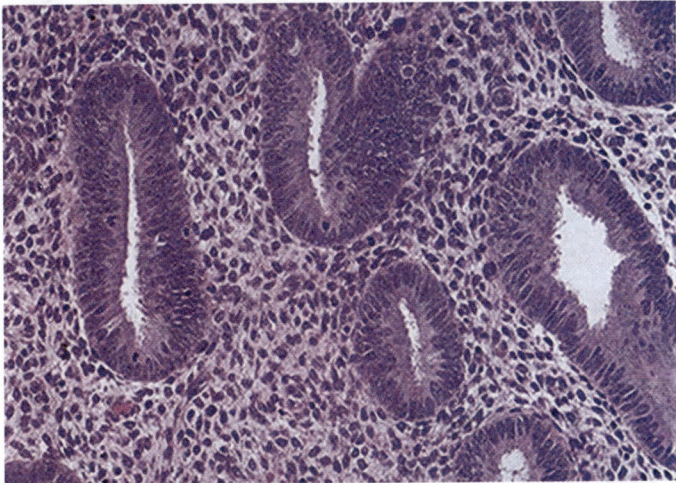

Fig. 22.2: Proliferative endometrium.

- Glands become elongated and slightly sinuous and the columnar epithelium lining them becomes taller. In the beginning, the glands are narrow and tubular, lined by low

columnar epithelial cells. Mitosis becomes prominent, and the areas of pseudostratification are observed.
- There is an increase in ciliated and microvillous cells in the endometrial glands.
- Endometrial stroma becomes edematous with wide separation of the individual cells. The stroma gets infiltrated with numerous cells including macrophages, leukocytes, etc.
- In the initial phase, the spiral vessels are uncoiled and unbranched. However, soon the growth of straight vessels occurs so that they start becoming more coiled and spiraled.

Ovulation

> **Q.** Write a long essay discussing the physiology of ovulation.
>
> **Q.** Write a short note on the structure and functions of a mature Graafian follicle.

The events preceding ovulation are as follows: estrogen production peaks (must be >200 pg/mL for >24 hours) and is responsible for triggering the FSH and LH surge. Rupture of the ovarian follicle follows, resulting in ovulation.

Secretory (Luteal) Phase

Secretory phase is marked by production of progesterone and less potent estrogens by the CL. It extends from day 15 to day 28 of the typical cycle. The endometrial features of the secretory phase include the following **(Fig. 22.3)**:
- Most characteristic feature of this phase is development of subnuclear vacuolation in the glandular epithelial cells. In this, the glycogen-filled vacuoles develop between the nuclei and the basement membrane (by day 17–18). This is the first evidence that ovulation has taken place.
- Endometrium measures about 8–10 mm in the secretory phase. The secretory phase reaches its peak activity by the 22nd day of the cycle, after which no growth occurs.

- Glands become crenated and tortuous to assume a characteristic corkscrew-shaped appearance. The corkscrew pattern of the glands becomes saw-toothed in the later part of the secretory phase.
- Stroma of the functional layer further becomes edematous.
- Spiral arterioles become prominent.
- Functional layer of the endometrium can be divided into two layers:
  1. Superficial or compact layer
  2. Deep, spongy layer

If pregnancy occurs, the placenta produces hCG to replace progesterone. As a result, the endometrium (and the accompanying pregnancy) are maintained. If pregnancy does not occur, the estrogen and progesterone levels cause negative feedback at the hypothalamus, resulting in a fall in the levels of the hormones FSH and LH. The spiral arteries become coiled and have reduced blood flow. At the end of this period, they alternately contract and relax, causing disintegration of the functionalis layer and eventually menses.

GENERAL PHYSICAL EXAMINATION

General physical examination involves the observation of the patient's general appearance; orientation in time, place, and person; nutritional status; and the patient's demeanor (calm, anxious, or aggressive). The following features need to be observed at the time of general physical examination.

VITAL SIGNS

The patient's vital signs such as temperature, blood pressure, pulse, respiratory rate, height, and weight need to be taken.

HEIGHT AND WEIGHT

Height of the patient (in meters) and her weight (in pounds) can be used for calculation of BMI. Classification of the woman as underweight, normal weight, and obese has been described in **Table 22.1**. Calculation of BMI is especially important in women who appear underweight or overweight. Underweight women may commonly suffer from amenorrhea and other menstrual irregularities, whereas overweight women are at an increased risk for endometrial cancer.

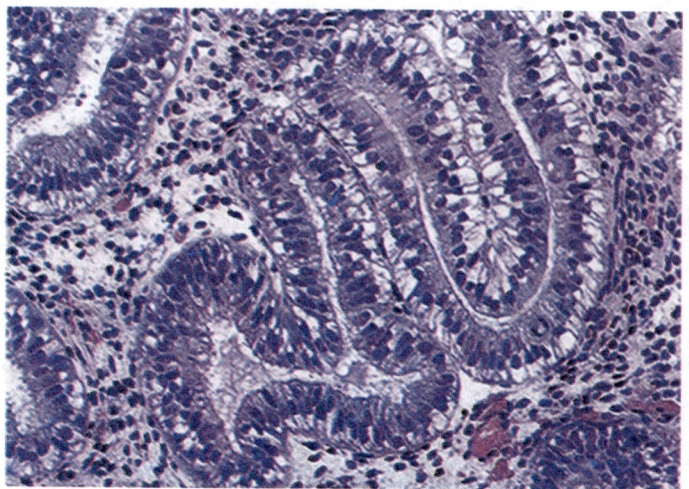

Fig. 22.3: Secretory phase endometrium.

TABLE 22.1: Classification of weight according to BMI.

Weight for height status	BMI
Very low	<16.5
Low	16.5–19.8
Normal	19.8–25.9
High	26.0–29.9
Very high	>30.0

(BMI: body mass index)

ANEMIA, DEHYDRATION

Excessive blood loss may result in the development of anemia.

SIGNS SUGGESTIVE OF HYPERANDROGENEMIA

Signs suggestive of hyperandrogenemia such as hirsutism (presence of facial hair) and deepening of voice may be related to the presence of androgen-secreting tumors or chronic anovulatory states (polycystic ovarian disease).

BLOOD PRESSURE

Blood pressure that is persistently ≥140 mm Hg (systolic) or ≥90 mm Hg (diastolic) is considered as elevated. Patients with hypertension are at an increased risk for the development of endometrial cancer.

NECK EXAMINATION

Local examination of the neck may reveal enlargement of thyroid gland or lymph nodes of the neck. Neck examination should also involve palpation of cervical and supraclavicular lymph nodes.

LYMPHADENOPATHY

Lymphadenopathy could be a sign of advanced metastatic disease associated with malignancy. The neck, axilla, and groins must also be palpated for the presence of enlarged lymph nodes.

THYROID EXAMINATION

It is important to examine the thyroid gland because menstrual abnormalities may be commonly associated with thyroid dysfunction. While hypothyroidism is commonly associated with oligomenorrhea, hyperthyroidism may be responsible for producing menorrhagia. Various signs and symptoms associated with hypothyroidism and hyperthyroidism are described in detail in Chapter 13.

BREAST EXAMINATION

Examination of the breasts should be carried out in three positions: with the patient's hands on her hips (to accentuate the pectoral muscles), with her arms raised, and then in supine position. Both the breasts must be inspected for symmetry, skin or nipple retraction, presence of any obvious growth or mass, and skin changes such as dimpling, retraction, crusting, or peau d'orange appearance. Both the breasts must be then palpated bilaterally for the presence of lumps, masses, and tenderness. The nipples are assessed for the presence of discharge. Axillary and supraclavicular regions are palpated for the presence of any lymphadenopathy. The following points need to be particularly observed on examination of breast:

- Breast examination may reveal changes indicative of early pregnancy. This is especially important in cases where pregnancy is not suspected, for e.g., in young unmarried girls.
- *Staging of breast development*: This could be important in women who have yet not attained sexual maturity. For details related to the Tanner stages of breast development, kindly refer to Chapter 35.
- In all women and especially those above the age of 30 years, breasts must be routinely palpated to exclude tumor formation.
- Bilateral milk discharge from the nipples may indicate galactorrhea due to hyperprolactinemia. Ruling out the presence of galactorrhea is especially important in cases that are infertile and suffer from oligomenorrhea or amenorrhea.
- Unilateral bloody nipple discharge could be associated with an intraductal papilloma, which is a benign lesion.

EXAMINATION OF BACK AND SPINE

Back must be assessed for symmetry, tenderness, or masses. Flanks must be assessed for pain on percussion as it could be indicative of renal disease.

SPECIFIC SYSTEMIC EXAMINATION

ABDOMINAL EXAMINATION

Inspection

The patient must be advised to breathe normally and relax. The examiner must stand on the right side of the patient. The following points need to be noted on inspection of the abdomen:

- *Abdominal shape*: The clinician must note for abdominal shape, whether symmetrical or asymmetrical.
- *Umbilical eversion or inversion*: In normal women, umbilicus is usually inverted (sunken) even if abdomen is distended due to obesity. Umbilical eversion can occur as a result of increased intra-abdominal pressure in conditions such as pregnancy, ascites, and intra-abdominal tumors.
- *Abdominal enlargement*: The specific region of abdominal distention (ascites, intra-abdominal lump) needs to be noted. The different abdominal quadrants are shown in **Figure 22.4**.
- *Organomegaly*: Very large spleen or liver arising from left or right hypochondriac regions, respectively, can be identified on abdominal inspection. Gross enlargement of the liver may produce a bulge in the right upper quadrant, whereas gross enlargement of the spleen may be seen as a bulge in the left upper quadrant.
- *Presence of dilated veins and varicosities*: Presence of prominent veins over the abdomen is abnormal and

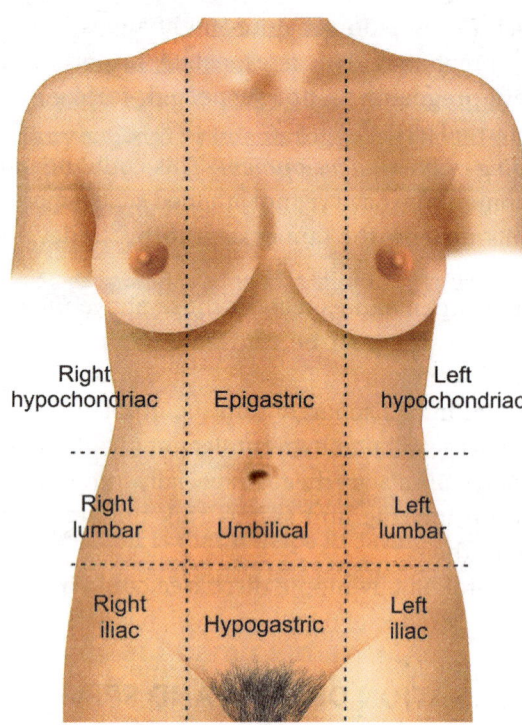

Fig. 22.4: Abdominal quadrants.

may be due to inferior cava obstruction or portal hypertension.
- *The mobility of abdominal wall with breathing:* If the abdominal mass moves up and down while breathing, it is likely to be intra-abdominal in origin. In case of a pelvic mass, the movements of the lower abdominal wall may be restricted.
- *Presence of striae or scar marks over the abdomen:* Abdominal striae (stripes over the abdomen) may be often present in parous women. The presence of striae could be indicative of previous pregnancies in the past or recent weight loss. Scars over the abdomen may indicate previous surgical operations and deserve further inquiry.
- *Signs of intraperitoneal and retroperitoneal hemorrhage:* The following signs are indicative of intraperitoneal and retroperitoneal hemorrhages:
  • *Grey Turner's sign:* This is the sign which is associated with discoloration (bruising) at the flanks.
  • *Cullen's sign:* This is the sign which is associated with periumbilical bruising.

Palpation

Normal abdomen should be soft and nontender, with no masses. It is important that the clinician warms his/her hands before palpating the patient's abdomen. The patient should be instructed to flex her hips and knees, which helps in relaxing the abdominal musculature, thereby making palpation easier.

If the patient does not relax sufficiently, the clinician may find it difficult to elicit relevant findings during the abdominal examination. Adequate relaxation can be achieved by making the patient comfortable and gaining her confidence. Asking the patient to take slow deep breaths can also help. The clinician must place his/her palm flat over the patient's abdomen.

Palpation must be done gently, while applying pressure by flexing the fingers in unison at the metacarpal–phalangeal joints. The following points must be noted while palpating the abdomen:
- *Tone of abdominal muscles:* It can be assessed upon palpation. When muscle tone is increased, there may be resistance to depression of the abdominal wall by the palpating hand. This hypertonia is commonly accompanied with the presence of tenderness. Reduced tone of the abdominal muscles, on the other hand, could be associated with divarication of rectus muscles.
- *Abdominal tenderness:* There must be no tenderness or rebound tenderness present on abdominal palpation. Rebound tenderness refers to pain upon removal of pressure and may be indicative of localized peritonitis or appendicitis. Tenderness must be recorded on a scale of 1–4, where 1 corresponds to mild and 4 to most severe type of pain.
- *Organomegaly:* In the absence of any pathology, most abdominal organs are not palpable in normal people. Palpation of all the abdominal quadrants for the presence of any mass, firmness, irregularity, or distention must be performed. The clinician should preferably adopt a systemic approach while palpating the abdomen. He/she must start from the right upper quadrant and systemically palpate all the quadrants while moving down in a clockwise direction. Though a grossly enlarged organ (especially spleen and liver) can be visualized on inspection of the abdomen, organomegaly can be better appreciated on palpation. The normal edge of liver is sharp, smooth, soft, and flexible. The liver can descend for up to 3 cm on deep inspiration. In some normal subjects, its edge can be palpable just below the right costal margin without being enlarged. The normal spleen in a healthy subject is not palpable.
- *Abdominal mass:* If an abdominal mass is felt on abdominal palpation, the following need to be determined:
  • *Location of the mass and its shape, size, and texture:* Location of the mass in relation to the various abdominal quadrants needs to be determined. Shape of the mass (round, oval, irregular, etc.) and its size (in cm) also need to be determined. The surface texture of the mass, whether smooth, nodular, regular, or irregular, needs to be determined.
  • *Margins of the mass:* The clinician must try to locate the margins of the mass. In case of the mass arising

from the uterus, it may not be possible to localize the lower margin of the mass. Margins of a malignant tumor may be irregular and may not be well defined.

- *Consistency of the mass*: Consistency of the mass whether hard, firm, rubbery, soft, fluctuant, indentable, or pulsating needs to be determined. Masses like leiomyomas usually have a firm consistency unless they have undergone degeneration. On the other hand, ovarian masses may have cystic consistency. In case of a malignant ovarian tumor, there may be variegated consistency. Furthermore, a malignant mass may be associated with indistinct margins, fixed or restricted mobility, and the presence of ascites. The pregnant uterus is soft in consistency and hardens with contractions. A full bladder may present as a tense and tender mass in the hypogastric region.
- *Mobility of the mass*: The mobility of the mass, whether free or fixed to adjacent tissues, and its movement in relation to respiration need to be determined. While a benign tumor is freely mobile, the malignant tumor may be fixed or have a restricted mobility.
- *Unilateral or bilateral mass*: Tumorous masses arising from both the ovaries are more likely to be malignant in comparison to the unilateral masses arising from a single ovary.
- *Tenderness on palpation*: Benign masses such as fibroids and benign ovarian cysts are usually nontender on palpation. Tenderness upon palpation may be associated with conditions such as ectopic pregnancy, PID, twisted ovarian cysts, and red degeneration of fibroids. In conditions like acute peritonitis, there may be guarding, rigidity, and rebound tenderness of the lower abdomen.
- *Differentiating the intra-abdominal masses from those arising from abdominal wall*: Masses arising from the abdominal wall can be distinguished from those inside the abdomen by asking the patient to tighten her abdominal wall muscles. The patient can tighten her abdominal wall muscles by lifting her head off the pillow and looking at her toes. When the patient tightens her abdominal wall muscles, the masses arising from the abdominal wall will remain palpable, while the intra-abdominal masses would no longer be palpable.

Percussion

For percussion, the fingers of the clinician's left hand are spread slightly. He/she then places the palmar surface of the middle phalanx of middle finger flat over the area he/she wishes to percuss. The two distal phalanges of the middle finger of the clinician's right hand must be then flexed and its tip used to strike perpendicularly the middle phalanx of middle finger of left hand (already placed in an area wished to be percussed) **(Fig. 22.5)**. The striking finger must be

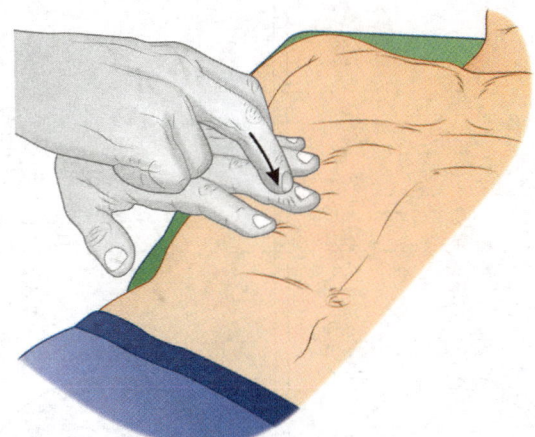

Fig. 22.5: Technique of percussion.

withdrawn as soon as the stroke is delivered. Delivery of the stroke is through flexion of the wrist and the finger at the metacarpophalangeal joint and not through any actions in the elbow or shoulder.

The percussion sound note is tympanitic when the site is over an area of air-filled bowel, whereas it is dull in the presence of fluid. Shifting dullness on percussion can be used to determine whether the abdominal distention is due to the presence of fluid (ascites) or an intra-abdominal tumor.

Percussion of the abdomen is valuable in the diagnosis of tumor and in distinguishing it from ascites and in deciding whether it is intraperitoneal or retroperitoneal. Most intraperitoneal tumors arising from the pelvic organs are dull to percussion, whereas a retroperitoneal tumor usually has one or more loops of bowel adherent to it in front, which may give a tympanitic note on percussion. Percussion also helps in differentiating between a large ovarian cyst and ascites. In case of an ovarian cyst, the tumor is dull on percussion, whereas both the flanks are tympanitic due to the presence of intestines. In case of ascites, on the other hand, the abdomen is tympanitic in the midline due to the presence of intestines, whereas both the flanks are dull on percussion **(Figs. 22.6A and B)**. The technique of percussion also helps in the detection of the following:

- *Liver dullness*: Measurement of liver dullness
- *Presence of ascites*: Ascites is commonly associated with malignant tumors. However, all malignant tumors may not be associated with ascites, because only epithelial ovarian malignancies produce ascites. Some benign conditions, which may also be associated with ascites, include tubercular peritonitis and pseudo-Meigs syndrome. The presence of ascites is basically detected by two tests: fluid thrill and shifting dullness. Dullness in the flanks upon percussion and shifting dullness indicates the presence of free fluid in the peritoneal cavity.

Shifting Dullness

Presence of dullness in both flanks when the patient is supine and dullness only in the dependent flank when the

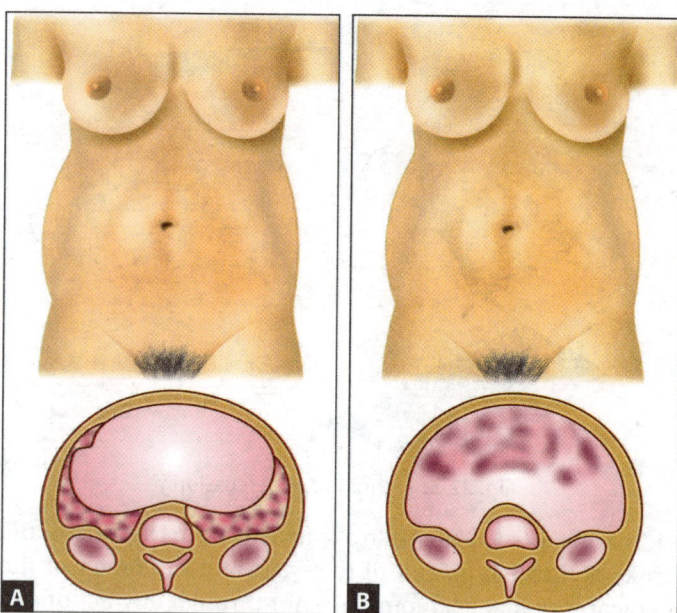

Figs. 22.6A and B: Shifting dullness. (A) Shows presence of an ovarian or uterine tumor, whereas (B) shows ascites. Dullness is indicated by light pink areas, whereas resonance is shown in dark pink.

patient is on her side indicate the presence of ascites. The ability to demonstrate shifting dullness increases with the volume of ascitic fluid. Shifting dullness may be absent if the volume of ascitic fluid is only small. This test comprises the following steps:

1. The patient is laid supine and the clinician starts percussing from the midline of the abdomen toward one of the flanks. The level at which the percussion note changes from tympanitic to dull is noted, and then the patient is instructed to turn to the side opposite to the one where the percussion is being done. In normal individuals (without the presence of any intra-abdominal mass), gas-filled bowels float on top of the ascitic fluid when the patient is in supine position, whereas fluid gravitates in the flanks. This is responsible for producing tympanitic note in the midline of abdomen and a dull note in the flanks.
2. The patient is then turned to her side and allowed time so that the fluid gravitates to the side of dependent flank.
3. Now the clinician performs the percussion once again.
4. The dependent flank where the fluid had gravitated would sound dull to percussion, while the nondependent flank would be tympanitic.
5. The patient is then turned to the other side and the above-mentioned steps are again repeated.

Fluid Thrill

Another test for ascites is the demonstration of fluid thrill. The test comprises the following steps **(Fig. 22.7)**:
1. Patient is laid supine, and the clinician places one hand flat against her flank on one side.
2. An assistant (e.g., a nurse) or the patient herself is asked to place the ulnar aspect of her hand firmly in the midline of the abdomen.

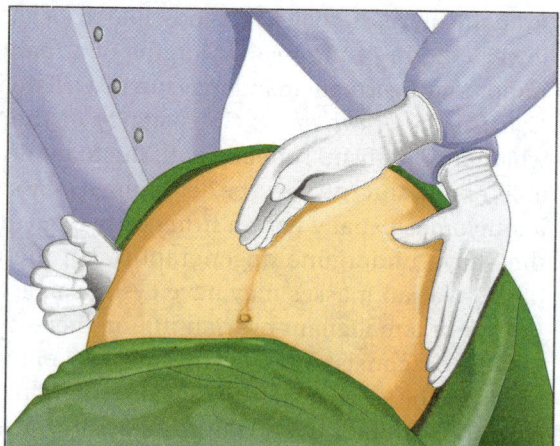

Fig. 22.7: Fluid thrill.

3. Without crossing arms, the gynecologist taps the opposite flank of the abdomen with his/her other hand. In case the ascitic fluid is present, the impulse generated by the tap will be transmitted to the clinician's other hand on the flank. The hand on the abdomen helps in preventing the transmission of the impulse over the abdominal wall. Fluid thrill is demonstrable only if a large volume of ascitic fluid is present. The absence of shifting dullness or fluid thrill or both does not rule out the presence of a small-volume ascites.

Auscultation

Auscultation does not form an important part of abdominal examination. The purpose of auscultation of the abdomen is mainly to listen for bowel sounds produced by peristaltic activities and vascular sounds. The presence of bowel sounds in the abdomen of the patient who had undergone surgery is indicative of recovering bowel activity in the postoperative period.

CARDIOVASCULAR SYSTEM EXAMINATION

Routine examination of cardiovascular system involves palpation of cardiac impulse and auscultation of the heart at the apex for the presence of any sounds, murmurs, clicks, etc.

Detailed examination of the cardiovascular system is required in cases of past history of cardiovascular disease or complaints suggestive of a possible cardiovascular pathology while taking history.

EXAMINATION OF THE PULMONARY SYSTEM

Examination of the pulmonary system may be required to detect the presence of wheezes, rales, rhonchi, and bronchial breath sounds.

PELVIC EXAMINATION

Pelvic examination forms an important aspect of the gynecological checkup of a woman. The anatomy of female

Normal Gynecological Examination **475**

external and internal genitalia is shown in **Figures 22.8 and 22.9A and B**, respectively. According to the current recommendations by the American Congress of Obstetricians and Gynecologists (2011), annual pelvic examination must be performed for women aged 21 years and older. In case the patient is asymptomatic, she needs to decide whether she should have a pelvic examination or not. Annual screening for chlamydial and gonorrheal infection is advised for women who are at high risk for infection (e.g., history of having a new sexual partner, multiple sexual partners, and sexual partner having multiple sexual contacts).

Before starting a pelvic examination, the clinician must take verbal consent from the patient. Written consent is not required, except in cases of examination under anesthesia. In case of adolescents and children, parental consent is

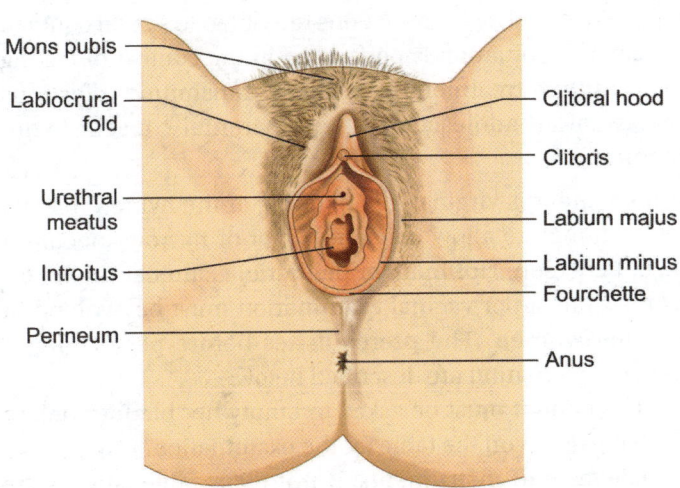

Fig. 22.8: Normal anatomy of female external genitalia.

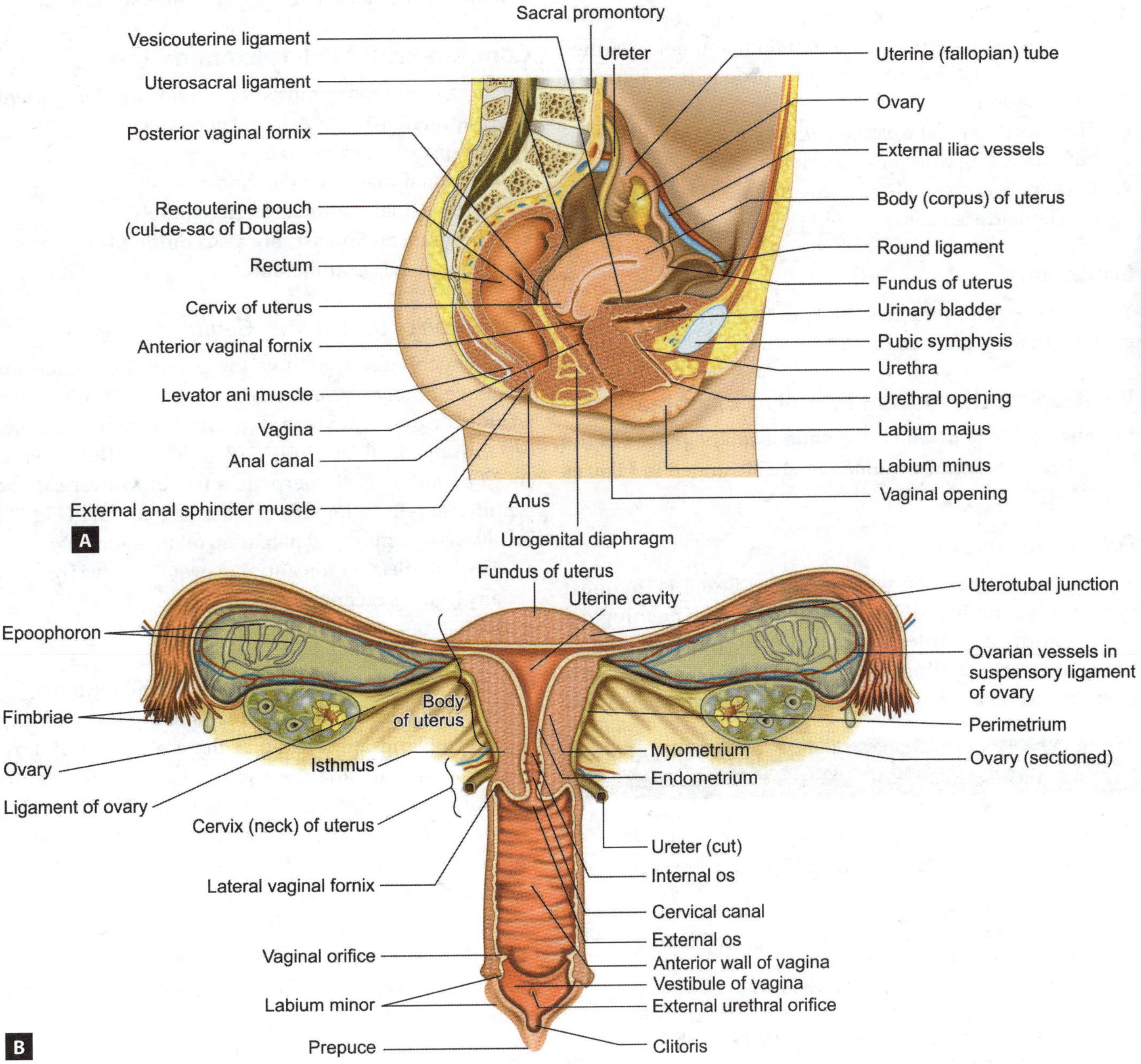

Figs. 22.9A and B: Normal anatomy of female internal genitalia. (A) Midsagittal view; (B) Coronal view.

required for pelvic examinations unrelated to sexual contact. If pelvic examination is performed in the context of testing or instituting treatment for sexually transmitted infections in case of an adolescent patient, parental consent is not required.

If the patient is virginal, the opening of the hymen may be wide enough to allow only one finger or narrow speculum (e.g., Pederson, Huffman, or pediatric) examination. As far as possible, a per vaginal examination must be avoided in virginal women. The prerequisites before performing a pelvic examination are described below:

- The patient must be asked to empty her bladder before lying down on the table for the examination.
- Gloves and instruments, if not disposable, should be sterilized by autoclaving before reuse.
- Since this is an intimate examination, it requires the patient's full cooperation. The patient must be described the procedure of pelvic examination, and her informed consent must be taken before proceeding with the examination.
- The clinician must wear nonsterile gloves on both hands before starting with the examination.
- Both male and female examiners should be chaperoned by a female assistant.

Equipment

The basic equipment required for performing a pelvic examination are given in **Box 22.1**.

Positioning the Patient for Pelvic Examination

Various positions in which the patient can be placed at the time of gynecological examination are illustrated in **Figures 22.10A to C**.

Full Dorsal Position

The full dorsal position with the knees flexed is the most commonly employed position used for gynecological examination in clinical practice. This position allows adequate per speculum and vaginal examinations. This position also enables the clinician to inspect the vagina and cervix for taking vaginal swabs and cervical smears. However, this examination does not allow adequate exposure of the lateral vaginal walls. The examiner stands to the right of the patient. The patient can be made to relax by partly covering her knees and thighs with a sheet. Elevating the head of the table 30–45° enables the woman to relax, thereby facilitating bimanual examination.

Lithotomy Position

Lithotomy position involves the use of stirrups to hold the flexed lower limbs and the movement of the patient to the edge of table. This position may be uncomfortable and awkward for the patient.

Though this position is not commonly used for clinical examination, it is often used at the time of vaginal surgeries and for examination of the patient under anesthesia.

Components of Pelvic Examination

Pelvic examination comprises the following components:
- Examination of the external genitalia
- Per speculum examination
- Bimanual vaginal examination
- Rectovaginal examination (if required)
- Abdomen and breasts are also commonly examined as a part of pelvic examination.

Inspection of the External Genitalia

The gynecologist examines the external genitalia for the presence of any obvious lesions or signs of inflammation. Examination of external genitalia reveals areas of discoloration, ulceration, and redness. Ulcerative areas could be indicative of herpetic infection, vulvar carcinoma, syphilis, etc. Examination of external genitalia **(Fig. 22.11)** involves inspection and palpation of the following:
- The hair distribution and skin over the vulva (presence of any lesions, ulcers, etc.)
- Labia minora and majora
- Perineal body
- Clitoris, urethral meatus, vestibule, and introitus

Bartholin and paraurethral glands (the openings of Bartholin gland are located at the 4 o'clock and 8 o'clock positions just outside the hymenal ring). The glands are normally not palpable when healthy. The paraurethral glands lie adjacent to the distal urethra. If the glands appear enlarged or tender, an attempt should be made to express exudate, which could be suggestive of infection.

Per Speculum Examination

Speculum examination of the vagina and cervix involves inspection of external genitalia, vagina, and cervix. Per speculum examination may reveal normal vaginal wall rugosities or smoothness of vaginal epithelium, which

> **BOX 22.1:** Equipment required for performing a pelvic examination.
>
> - An examining table
> - Good light source (preferably cold light)
> - Speculum of appropriate size (narrow speculums for virginal patients)
> - Materials for obtaining cervical cytology
> - Cotton swabs for obtaining samples of vaginal discharge
> - pH indicator paper
> - Dropper bottles of saline and potassium hydroxide for performing wet slide preparations
> - Water-soluble lubricant, disposable gloves, materials for draping the patient

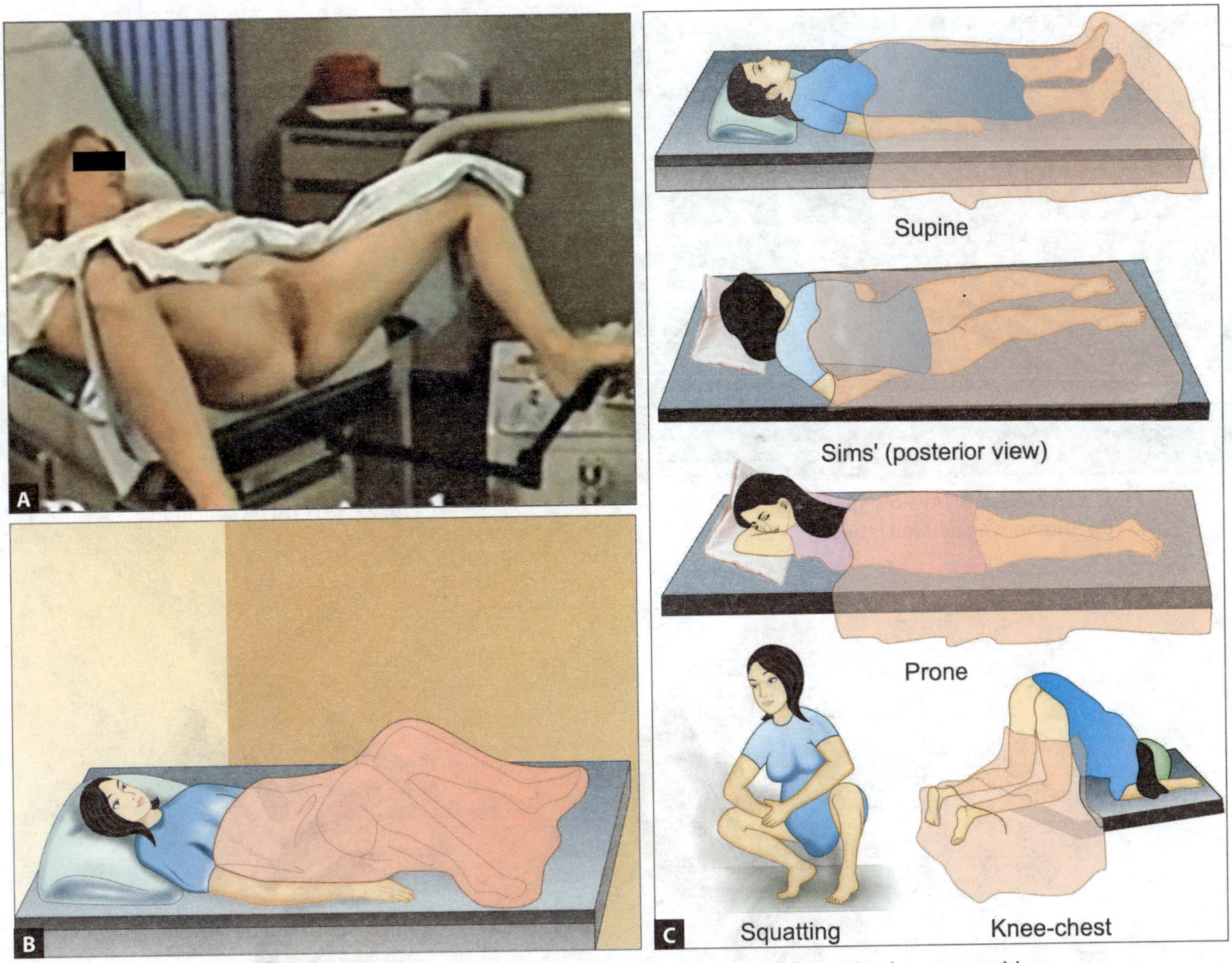

Normal Gynecological Examination **477**

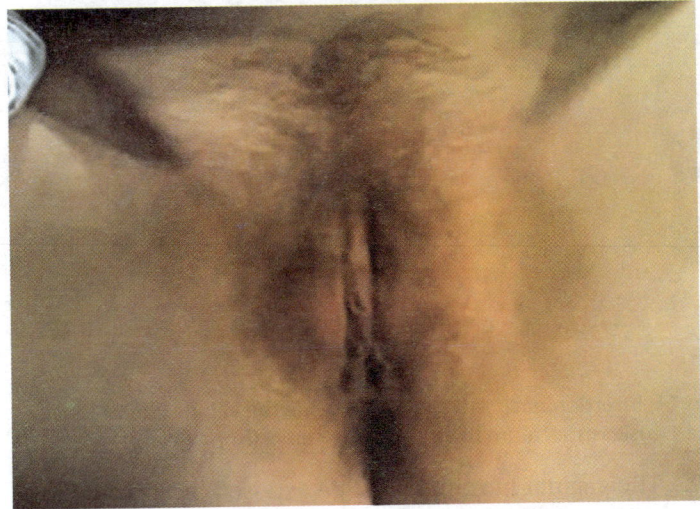

Figs. 22.10A to C: Patient's position for gynecological examination. (A) Lithotomy position; (B) Dorsal recumbent position; (C) Other positions sometimes used for gynecological procedures.

Fig. 22.11: Inspection of female external genitalia.

could be suggestive of atrophic vaginitis. The presence of masses, vesicles, or any other lesions can also be assessed on per speculum examination. This examination should ideally precede the bimanual examination. This is primarily because the vaginal discharge can be seen and removed for examination before it gets contaminated with the lubricant used for vaginal examination; moreover, the cellular debris from the cervix and uterus remains undisturbed and can be obtained for cytological studies at the time of per speculum examination. Also, many superficial vaginal lesions may start bleeding following the vaginal examination and may not allow an optimal per speculum examination. The types of speculum which can be used are described below.

Examination using Sims' speculum: Cervical examination can also be performed using a Sims' vaginal speculum **(Fig. 22.12A)** and an anterior vaginal wall retractor **(Fig. 22.12B)**. This speculum allows the assessment of vaginal walls and evaluation of the presence of uterine prolapse such as cystocele or rectocele. However, cervical inspection using Sims' speculum is associated with two main disadvantages: the gynecologist needs to bring the patient to the edge of the table. Also, help of an assistant may be required while conducting a per speculum examination using a Sims' speculum.

Examination using Cusko's speculum: A self-retaining, bivalve speculum such as Cusko's speculum **(Fig. 22.13)** serves as ideal equipment for vaginal examination. This speculum allows appropriate vaginal exposure so as to

478 Normal and Abnormal Menstruation

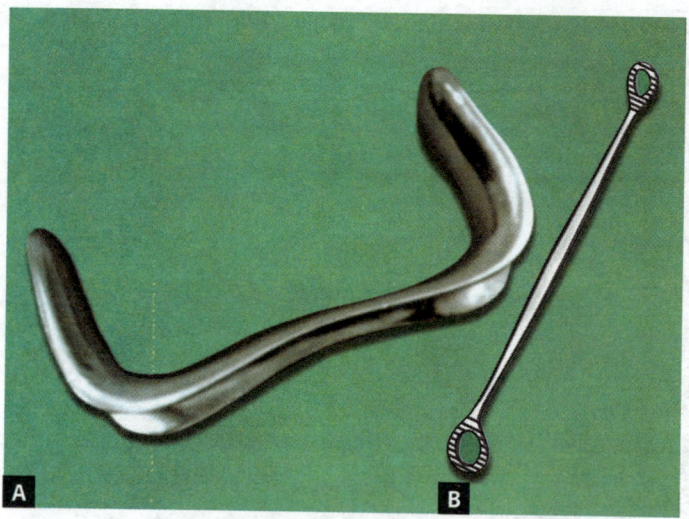

Figs. 22.12A and B: (A) Sims' speculum; (B) Anterior vaginal wall retractor.

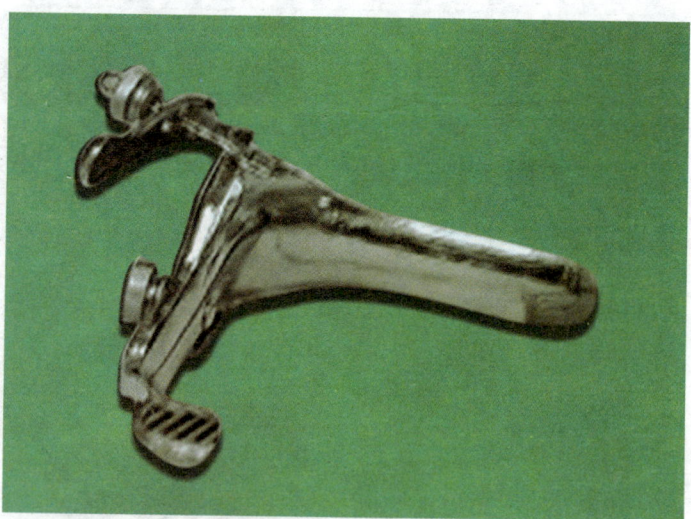

Fig. 22.13: Cusko's speculum.

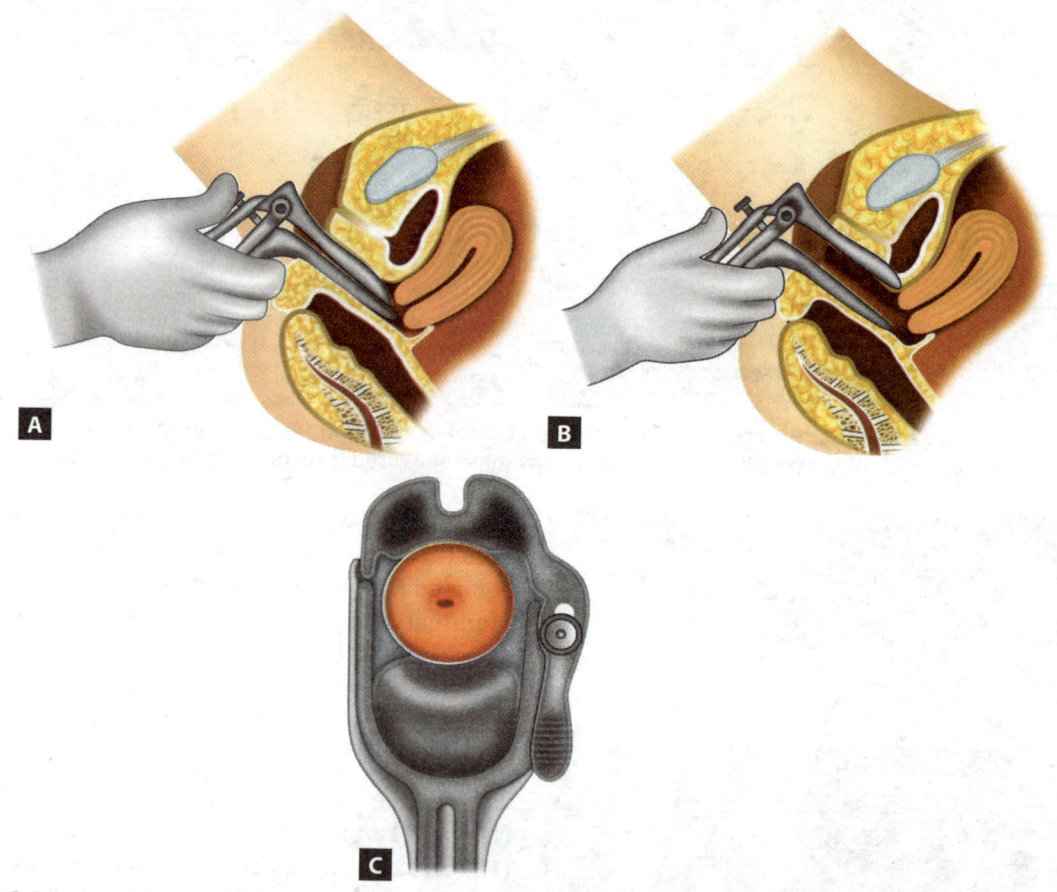

Figs. 22.14A to C: Per speculum examination using a Cusko's speculum. (A) Insertion of closed speculum inside the vaginal; (B) Gradually opening the speculum to visualize the cervix; (C) Fully opened Cusko's speculum to visualize the cervix (front view).

ensure adequate vaginal inspection (**Figs. 22.14A to C**). The presence of cervical lesions (ectropion, polyps, cervical erosions, etc.) can be visualized. Cervical inspection using this speculum also permits the gynecologist to take Pap smear at the time of per speculum examination.

Procedure of insertion of Cusko's speculum:
1. The gynecologist must firstly warm and lubricate the speculum by holding it under running tap water.
2. The vaginal introitus must be exposed by spreading the labia from below using the index and middle fingers of the left hand.
3. The Cusko's bivalve speculum must then be inserted at an angle of 45°, pointing slightly downward. Contact with any anterior structures must be avoided.
4. Once past the introitus, the speculum must be rotated to a horizontal position and insertion continued until its handle is almost flush with the perineum.

5. The blades of the speculum are opened up for a distance of approximately 2–3 cm using the thumb lever in such a way that the cervix "falls" in between the blades.
6. The speculum can be secured in its position by using the thumb nut in case of a metal speculum. The speculum must not be moved while it is in a locked position.
7. The cervical and vaginal walls must be observed for the presence of lesions or discharge. Specimens for culture and cytology must also be obtained.
8. While removing the speculum, it must be withdrawn slightly to clear the cervix. As the cervix gets cleared off, the speculum must be loosened and its blades allowed to fall together. The speculum must then be rotated to an angle of 45° and continued to be withdrawn.

Bimanual Vaginal Examination

Following the per speculum examination, a bimanual vaginal examination must be performed. First one and then two fingers (usually the index and middle fingers) are inserted into the vaginal introitus, following which a bimanual vaginal examination is done **(Figs. 22.15A and B)**.

Bimanual vaginal examination is usually more informative than per speculum examination and can be performed in most women.

Procedure: The bimanual vaginal examination comprises the following steps:
1. A water-based, soluble, nongreasy lubricant must preferably be used. A water-soluble jelly is the best and if that is not available, cetrimide solution must be used.
2. The labia are separated with the thumb and index finger of left hand.
3. Following this, the two fingers of right hand, first one finger and then the second finger, are inserted into the vagina only when the patient relaxes the muscles around the vagina and when it is clear that a two-finger examination would be possible without causing any pain.
4. Cervical shape, size, position, mobility, consistency, and tenderness caused by pressure or movement need to be assessed. The position and direction of the cervix are the guides to the position of the body of the uterus. If the cervix is pointing in the downward and backward direction, the anterior lip of the cervix would be encountered first on the vaginal examination. This indicates the anteverted position of the uterus. On the other hand, if the cervix is pointing in the upward and forward directions, the posterior lip of cervix would be encountered first on the vaginal examination. This indicates the retroverted position of the uterus.

A nonpregnant healthy cervix is usually firm in consistency. The cervix tends to soften during pregnancy. Under normal circumstances, the movement of cervix in any direction must not be painful. However, pain upon moving the cervix (also known as cervical motion tenderness) is a common symptom of PID (salpingo-oophoritis) and ectopic pregnancy.

In clinical scenario, the vaginal examination is immediately followed by a bimanual examination **(Figs. 22.16A to C)** without removing fingers from the vaginal introitus.

5. While the fingers of the examiner's right hand are still inside the vaginal introitus, the palm of his/her left hand is placed over the abdomen. The success of bimanual examination primarily depends on the ability of the examiner to use the abdominal hand more often than the vaginal fingers.
6. To feel the uterus, the vaginal fingers should move the cervix as far backward as possible to rotate the fundus downward and forward. The abdominal hand is then placed just below the umbilicus and gradually moved lower until the fundus is caught and pressed against the fingers in the anterior fornix.

The following points are noted on bimanual examination: size of the uterus, its position (anteverted or retroverted, anteflexed or retroflexed), and mobility (restricted mobility or fixed uterus). If there is a mass felt, its relation to the uterus is noted, like whether the mass is felt separate to the uterus or is continuous with it. When the mass is felt separate from the uterus, the origin of the mass is most likely from the adnexa or broad ligament. However, if the mass is continuous with the uterus, it probably arises from the uterus, like a fibroid.

Size of the uterus: Bulky uterus corresponds to a 6-week pregnant size and is slightly larger than the normal. When the uterus appears to be filling all the fornices, it corresponds to 12-week size. The in-between size could be between 8 and 10 weeks. Both the adnexa must then be palpated between the vaginal fingers in the lateral vaginal fornices and the abdominal hand to look for the presence of any mass or abnormality.

Rectovaginal Examination

Combined rectal and vaginal examination is done when required. Similar to the bimanual exam, the examiner inserts a lubricated, gloved finger into the rectum to feel for tenderness and masses, while the other finger remains inside the vagina. Per rectum examination will help reveal masses in the posterior pelvis. Rectovaginal examination allows optimal palpation of the posterior cul-de-sac and uterosacral ligaments, as well as the uterus and adnexa. The presence of nodularity in the pouch of Douglas and tenderness of uterosacral ligaments are signs of endometriosis. If a rectovaginal examination is performed, anorectal findings

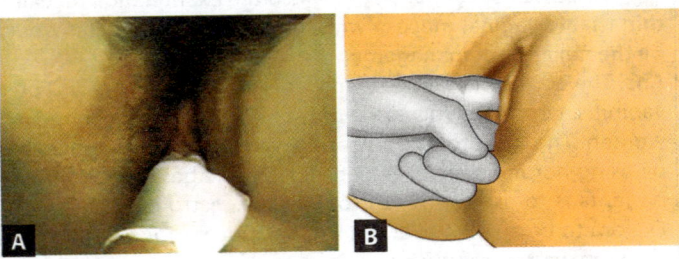

Figs. 22.15A and B: Two-finger vaginal examination.

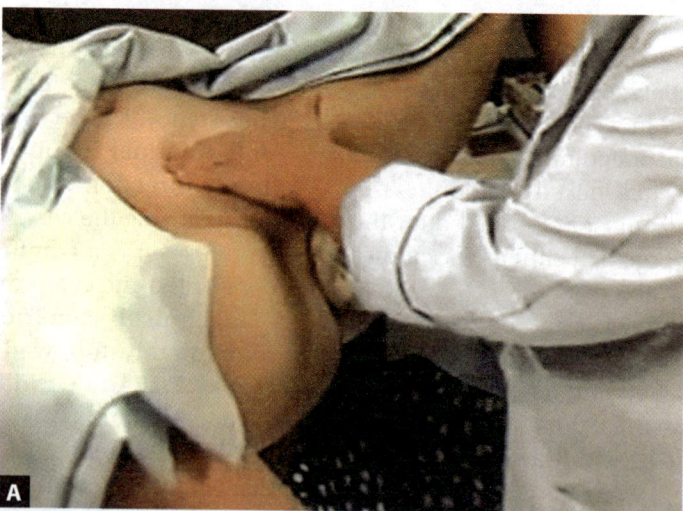
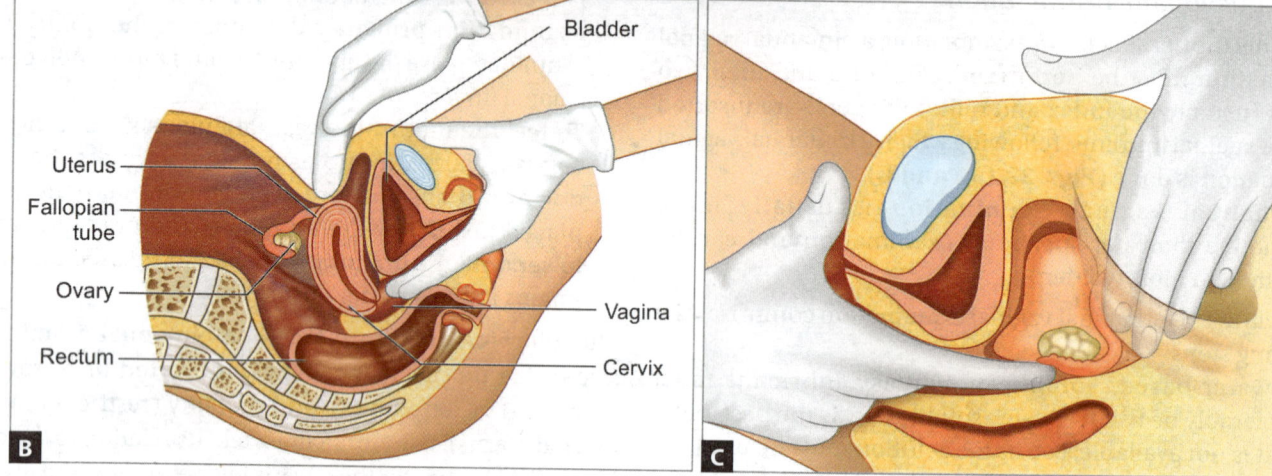

Figs. 22.16A to C: Bimanual vaginal examination. (A and B) Procedure of bimanual examination; (C) Examination of adnexa on bimanual examination.

should also be documented (e.g., hemorrhoids and rectal mass) in the gynecologist's notes. At the time of rectovaginal examination, the same finger should not be used to examine both the vagina and rectum to avoid transmission of human papillomavirus or contamination with blood. Some practitioners include rectovaginal examination as part of the routine pelvic examination, while others do this procedure only in specific cases.

 ## MANAGEMENT

Q. What would be the next line of management in the case study described in the beginning of the chapter?
Ans. Since the patient does not give history of any gynecological problem and the clinical examination is essentially within normal limits, there is no requirement for any gynecological intervention. However, a routine Pap smear and mammography are indicated in this patient because the patient is >40 years of age. The detailed description about Pap smear examination has been given in Chapter 27. The routine mammography had been previously recommended by the United States Preventive Services Task Force (USPSTF) at an interval of every 1–2 years for women aged 40 and older up to the age of 50 years. However, according to the latest recommendations by the USPSTF (2009), there is no requirement for routine screening of women between the ages of 40 and 50 years. After 50 years of age, 2-yearly mammograms are recommended. Screening mammography is usually not required after the age of 75 years. On the other hand, according to the National Health Service (NHS) Breast Screening Program, free breast screening is done every 3 years for all women in the UK aged 50 years until the age of 70 years. The recommendations for annual Pap smear examination are described in Chapter 27.

Q. In case the vagina on per speculum examination revealed thin friable vaginal mucosa with loss of rugosities, what would be the next line of management?
Ans. The above-mentioned symptoms are indicative of atrophic vaginitis, which may be commonly encountered in menopausal women. The symptoms of atrophic vaginitis can be prevented by using hormone replacement therapy. The best option in such patients is to use topical estrogens, e.g., estrogen cream (e.g., Evalon) to be applied over the vaginal mucosa for a few months until the symptoms subside.

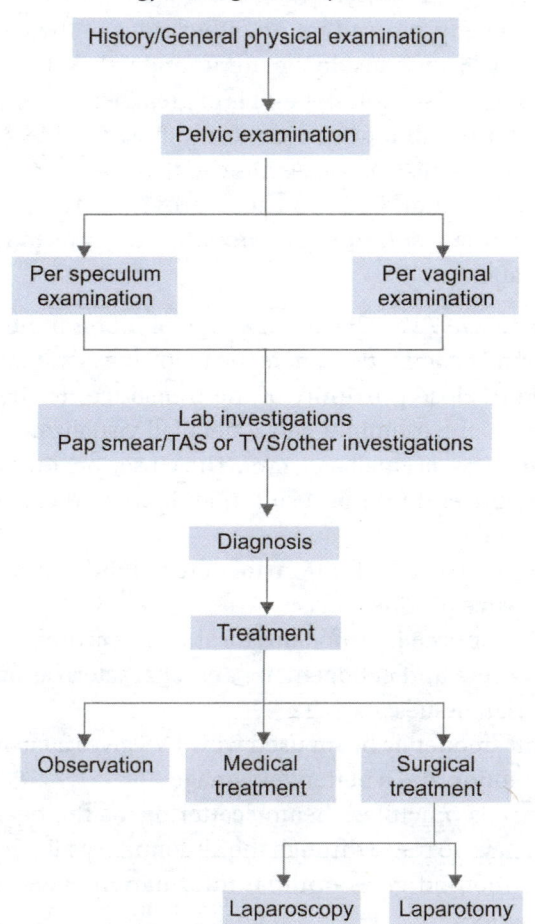

Flowchart 22.1: Management of the patient presenting with gynecological complaints.

(TAS: transabdominal sonography; TVS: transvaginal sonography)

Management of a patient presenting with gynecological complaints is summarized in **Flowchart 22.1**. The aims of management are as follows:
- Making and confirming the patient's diagnosis
- Assessing the severity or stage of the disease
- Rendering treatment based on the stage of the disease
- Following up the patient's response to treatment

INVESTIGATIONS

ULTRASOUND EXAMINATION

Introduction

It has been over 35 years since ultrasound was first used on pregnant women. Nowadays, besides obstetric indications, ultrasound is commonly being used for gynecological patients. Ever since its introduction in the late 1950s, ultrasonography has presently become a very useful diagnostic tool in both obstetrics and gynecology. Ultrasound examination has presently been considered to be a safe, noninvasive, accurate, and cost-effective investigation for evaluation of gynecological pathology. Ultrasound waves, which are very-high-frequency sound waves ranging

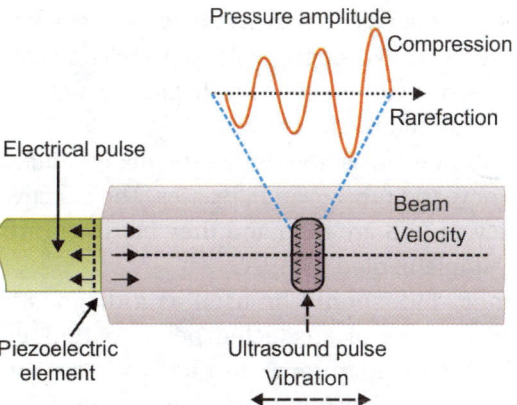

Fig. 22.17: Principle of ultrasound.

between frequencies of 2.5 and 7.0 MHz, are generally used for this purpose.

Principle of Ultrasound

Ultrasound is a procedure which uses high-frequency sound waves to view internal organs. Ultrasound imaging uses the principles of sonar developed for ships at sea, or radar detection for speedy cars. The ultrasound probe has piezoelectric crystals in it, which convert the electric current into sound waves. These sound waves pass through the mother's abdomen as the clinician moves the transabdominal transducers over the mother's abdomen after application of water-soluble gel, which acts as a coupling agent. As these sound waves pass through the internal structures and hit various body structures, they get reflected back, which can be used to identify distance between body parts and their size and shape **(Fig. 22.17)**. When the sound waves hit a high-density structure such as a bone, they are reflected back in the form of high-velocity waves, giving a white appearance on the screen. However, when these sound waves hit a less dense structure, reflected waves are of a lower velocity. These waves give a black appearance on the screen. These reflected waves are picked up by the piezoelectric crystals inside the transducer and get converted into electric signals, which are then displayed on the screen. Repetitive arrays of ultrasound beams from the transducer scan the pelvic structures in thin slices and are reflected back onto the same transducer. The information obtained from different reflections is recomposed back into a picture on the monitor screen.

Uses of Ultrasound Examination in Gynecological Diseases

Ever since ultrasonography has been discovered, it has been playing an immense role as a diagnostic tool in medical sciences. The field of obstetrics and gynecology is no exception to it. Ultrasound, both transabdominal and transvaginal, is widely used in clinical practice. TVS alone and also when supplemented with TAS could detect many clinically missed cases of pelvic masses or suspected pelvic pathology on provisional diagnosis made clinically. TVS acts as an effective complementary diagnostic aid in evaluation of many gynecologic conditions such as leiomyomas, AUB, endometriosis, ovarian cysts, malignancies, ectopic pregnancy, and tubo-ovarian masses. The effectiveness and accuracy of TVS are high and they increase further when TVS is supplemented with TAS.

Hence, TVS should be used as a diagnostic tool for any pelvic mass or suspected pelvic pathology prior to laparoscopy or laparotomy. Its diagnostic capabilities may reduce the need for other invasive procedures and aid in clinical decision-making. This being a noninvasive and an outpatient department procedure has resulted in a high amount of patient compliance. Also, the cost incurred in laboratory investigations and hospital stay for laparoscopy or laparotomy can be avoided, and individual organs and fine structures are seen better transvaginally. However, the regional survey offered by the transabdominal full bladder approach remains necessary to provide anatomic orientation, particularly when the patient has not been studied previously.

In some patients TAS is required, especially when the mass has extended beyond the true pelvis or has dimensions > 10 cm. However, there is no doubt about the fact that ultrasonography, especially TVS, seems to be an important armamentarium and adjunct to the clinical acumen in day-to-day gynecological practice, especially in the tertiary center.

Types of Ultrasound

Ultrasound for the purpose of diagnosis of gynecological pathology is primarily done by two ways: TVS and TAS. Recently, Doppler ultrasound is also increasingly being used. The different probes used for performing TAS and TVS examination are respectively shown in **Figures 22.18A and B**.

Transvaginal Ultrasound

While doing a TVS examination, a specially designed transducer, covered with a well-lubricated condom, is placed inside the vagina, after having the women empty her bladder **(Fig. 22.19)**. The transducer is then moved around the vagina and pressed up on either sides of the cervix, to allow visualization inside the uterus and pelvis. TVS is most useful in the first trimester and is of great help in fat women and in those with retroverted uterus, in whom TAS may not be able to visualize pelvic details clearly.

Transvaginal examination provides images with much better resolution as compared to transabdominal examination.

Advantages of TVS: The use of a vaginal probe at the time of ultrasound examination offers the following advantages:

- Due to close proximity of the transducer to the pelvic organs, the examiner gets a detailed visualization of the structures as small as 1 mm. The closer proximity of the transducer does not result in an increased exposure or risk.
- One can use palpation to detect tenderness or the presence of adhesions.
- TVS is an excellent modality for assessment of endometrial thickness and echogenicity and characterization of the ovarian tissues.
- High-frequency beam used with TVS gives a far superior resolution and a better field image.
- There is much less beam scattering, as the beam does not have to travel through the abdominal wall. Therefore, this method gives optimal information even in obese patients.
- TVS avoids interference from the interposed bowel loops as in the case of abdominal scanning.
- TVS is a totally noninvasive, nontraumatic, and nontoxic procedure. At the present time, there is no information regarding the influence of TVS on the embryo, fetus, neonate, or child's development. Till date, there have been no reports of any damage due to transvaginally guided procedures, or after scanning the patients.
- Since the transvaginal procedure does not require full bladder, it can be performed immediately, especially during emergencies. It spares the patient the inconvenience of the full bladder. Therefore, it affords

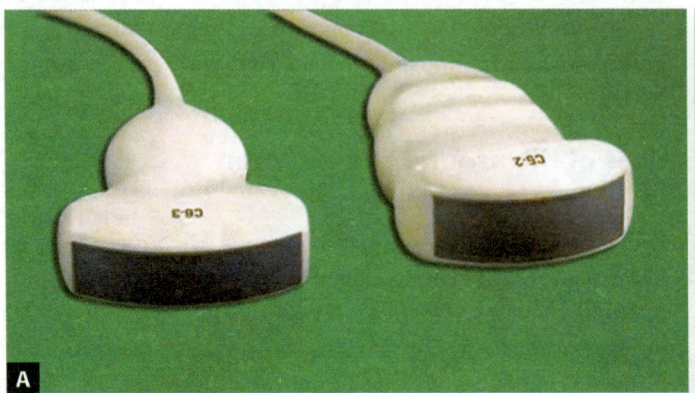
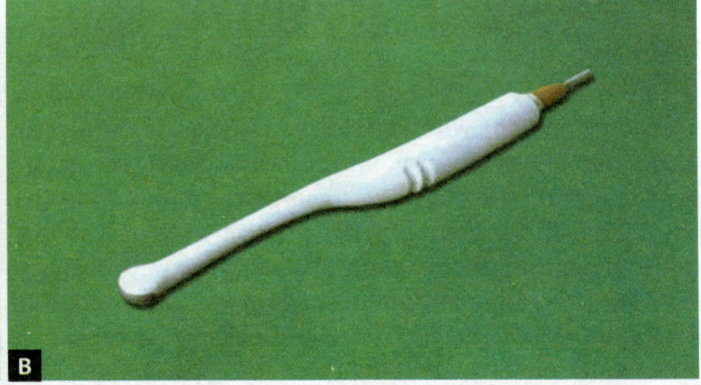

Figs. 22.18A and B: Ultrasound probes. (A) TAS probe; (B) TVS probe.

good patient acceptance without the discomfort of a full bladder.
- Physician can incorporate the procedure into the overall examination while the patient is still in the lithotomy position at the time of the bimanual examination.

Disadvantages of TVS: Some of the following disadvantages can be associated with the use of TVS:
- There is a limited field of view due to limited depth of sound penetration, caused by a higher frequency transducer. Therefore, findings larger than 7–10 cm or those outside the true pelvis are difficult to scan with the vaginal probe.
- Considerable experience is required both to obtain a satisfactory image and to interpret them.
- Uterine length, which is a routine measurement by TAS, is difficult to be measured by TVS.
- TVS cannot be done in cases of vaginal stenosis or intact hymen.
- There is an inability to image the highly placed ovaries.
- Large probe caliber renders the examination difficult for some elderly postmenopausal women. In elderly patients the vagina has less elasticity, and this limits the maneuverability of the probe.

Transabdominal Sonography

Unlike the TVS examination, which is performed after having the patient empty her bladder, TAS gives a clearer visualization of pelvic details when the patient's bladder is full. Therefore, the patient should be advised to drink plenty of fluids before examination so as to have a full bladder. This allows the uterus to be lifted out of the pelvis during examination for obtaining better image. After application of a lubricant over the patient's abdomen, the transducer is then placed in contact with the patient's abdomen and moved around over it in order to visualize the uterine cavity, endometrium, and adnexa **(Figs. 22.20A and B)**.

Normal Pelvic Anatomy as Visualized by Transvaginal Ultrasound

Figures 22.21A to E illustrate the normal pelvic anatomy as visualized on ultrasound examination.
- *During menses (day 1–4)*: In the menstrual phase, the endometrium appears as a thin, broken, central interface, measuring approximately 2–3 mm in thickness. Blood and tissue in the endometrial cavity produce a central anechoic area. During the first day or so of menstruation, the endometrial complex consists of a thick hyperechoic density surrounding the anechoic menstrual debris with the presence of posterior enhancement. With the progression of menstruation, the hypoechoic central echo representing blood, tissue, and thickened hyperechoic endometrium will disappear.

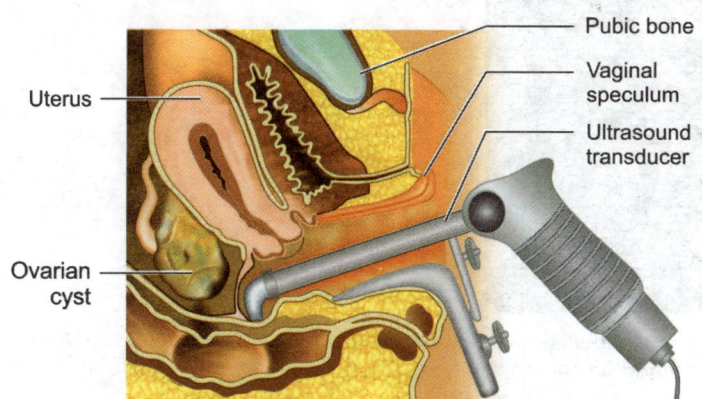

Fig. 22.19: Technique of TVS.

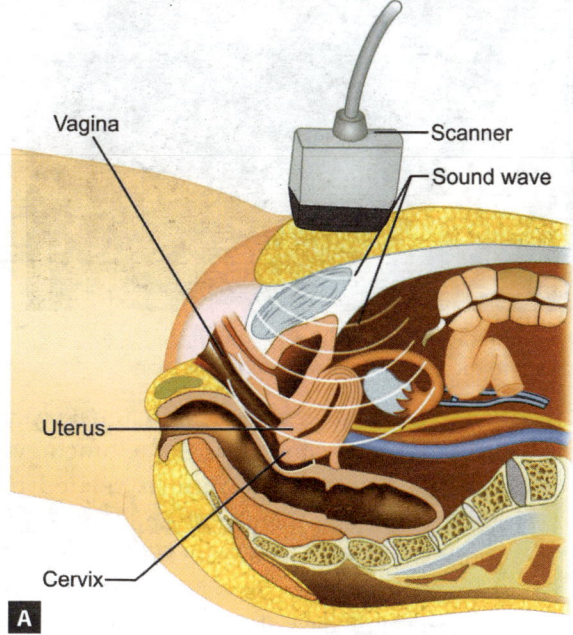

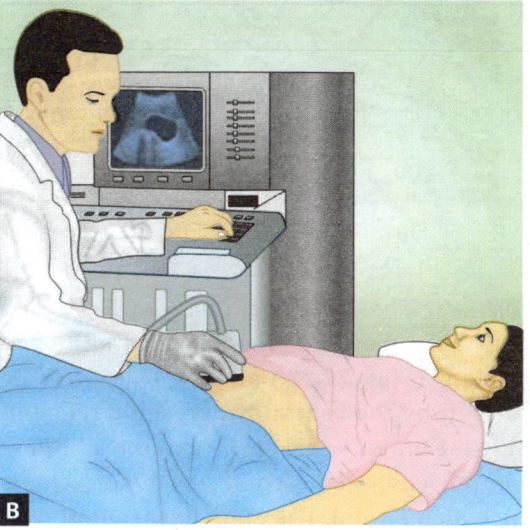

Figs. 22.20A and B: Technique of doing TAS.

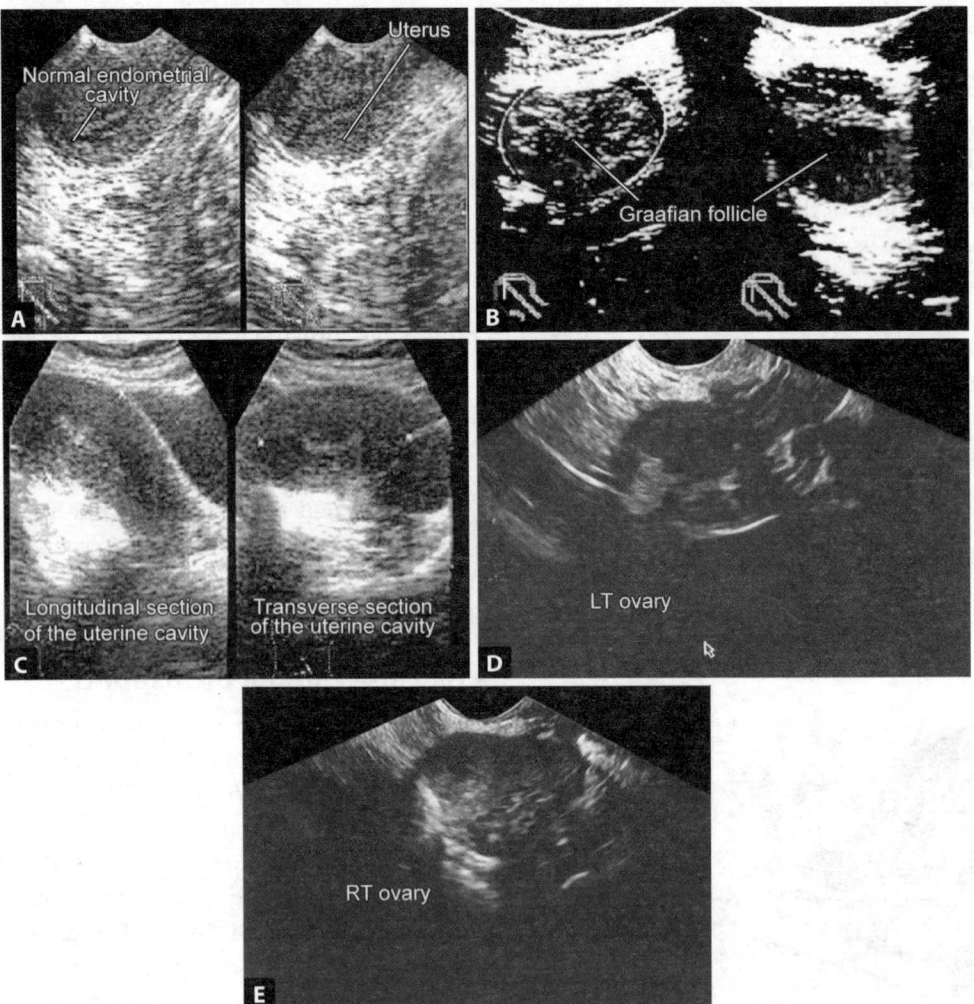

Figs. 22.21A to E: Normal pelvic anatomy as visualized on ultrasound examination. (A) Normal transvaginal scan of the uterus; (B) Normal transvaginal scan of the ovary; (C) Normal uterus as visualized on transabdominal scan; (D) Normal left-sided ovary as visualized on the transvaginal scan; (E) Normal right-sided ovary as visualized on the transvaginal scan. (LT: left; RT: right)

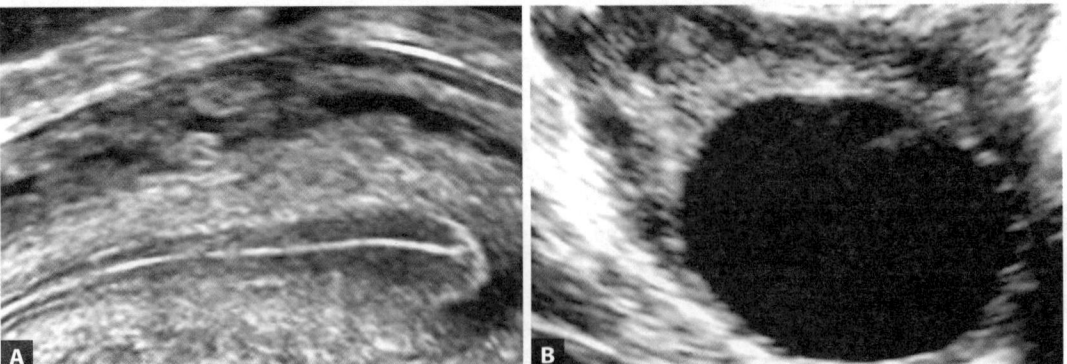

Figs. 22.22A and B: (A) TVS of the uterus in the proliferative phase, showing the presence of a well-defined "three line sign"; (B) Ovary showing the presence of a dominant follicle.

- *Early proliferative phase endometrium (day 5–9):* In the proliferative phase, there is a presence of a well-defined "three line sign" **(Figs. 22.22A and B)**. The "three line sign" is formed by the central hyperechoic reflection representing the endometrial cavity and the additional hyperechoic reflections representing the thin developing layer of the endometrium. The outer lines represent the interface between endometrium and myometrium. There is a hypoechogenic functional layer. The general hypoechogenic character of the functional layer of the proliferative endometrium is related to the simple configuration of the glands and blood vessels. There is minimal or absent posterior acoustic enhancement.

- *Late proliferative phase (day 10–14):* Periovulatory endometrium has a thickness between 6 and 8 mm and is moderately echogenic. There is a continued thickening of the endometrial echo complex during this phase. The halo is still present; the three line sign is also present, but the outer lines may begin to thicken. The total endometrial thickness may increase up to 10 mm or greater.

- *During the luteal phase:* In the immediate pre- and postovulatory period (2 days postovulation), an additional inner hyperechogenicity of variable thickness, which corresponds to a relatively high fluid content of these inner functional layers, could be seen with TVS. A small amount of fluid (1–2 mL) can be seen in some individuals within the lumen of the endometrium, resulting in the halo sign. Since linear measurement of endometrial thickness really represents two layers of endometrium, i.e., the anterior and posterior wall, some researchers have suggested that such measurements must be divided by two. The total double layer thickness in the luteal phase ranges from 4 to 12 mm with an average of 7.5 mm. The luteal phase endometrium tends to be hyperechoic and maximum in thickness. There is a presence of posterior acoustic enhancement, and three line sign is also absent.

COMPUTED TOMOGRAPHY EXAMINATION

Computed tomography examination is usually not performed during pregnancy due to the risk of radiations. It may however be useful in gynecological cases diagnosed with abdominal or pelvic masses. CT examination may also help in delineating the enlarged lymph nodes and other retroperitoneal pathologies. It is usually indicated in the presence of malignancy.

MAGNETIC RESONANCE IMAGING EXAMINATION

Though MRI examination does not expose the patient to ionizing radiations, its high cost prevents its routine use in obstetrics and gynecology practice. MRI examination helps in identification of soft-tissue planes and diagnosis of adenomyosis, Müllerian defects such as vaginal agenesis and uterine didelphys, ureteral stones, and urethral obstruction.

HYSTEROSALPINGOGRAPHY

Hysterosalpingography (HSG) is a radiological procedure, which involves injection of a radiopaque material into the uterine cavity through the cervical canal, followed by fluoroscopy with image intensification in order to investigate the shape of the uterine cavity and the shape and patency of the fallopian tubes. HSG helps in detecting intrauterine abnormalities such as submucous fibroids and intrauterine adhesions and checking the patency of the fallopian tubes (tubal obstruction, hydrosalpinx, pyosalpinx, etc.). The detailed procedure of HSG has been described in Chapter 34.

PAP SMEAR (PAPANICOLAOU TEST)

Pap smear has been described in detail in Chapter 27.

POSITRON EMISSION TOMOGRAPHY

Positron emission tomography (PET) is an imaging modality, which uses radioactive drug (tracer) to help delineate the metabolic or biochemical function of the body's tissues and organs. It appears to be a promising tool for diagnosis of recurrent and metastatic diseases as well as lymph nodal involvement in case of malignancy, particularly ovarian and cervical cancers.

TREATMENT/GYNECOLOGICAL MANAGEMENT

Gynecological diagnosis is made after careful analysis of the positive findings related to the history and clinical examination. Based on the results of various investigations, the clinician should form a list of likely differential diagnosis in his/her mind. The correct diagnosis can be confirmed on the basis of findings of the various investigations. After ascertaining the diagnosis, the next step is to establish the severity of the disease. In case of malignancy, cancer staging must be done. Treatment is decided based on the diagnosis of disease and its severity. This is especially important in case of malignancy where treatment would change depending on the stage of malignancy. The duty of the gynecologist does not end once the treatment has been dispensed; the duty of the clinician is also to assess the patient's response to the treatment by calling her for follow-up visits. Before the patient leaves the clinic, the future plans regarding management must be discussed with her. Patient information brochures and handouts must be provided to the patient. She should also be advised about the next follow-up visit. Treatment options for various gynecological complaints such as abnormal bleeding patterns, pelvic organ prolapse, pelvic pain, and infertility would be discussed in detail in the successive chapters of this book.

EVIDENCE-BASED CLINICAL TRIALS

 List of references can be scanned through QR code to enable the readers gain deeper insight of the subject by referring to the entire article or its abstract.

CHAPTER 23

Abnormal Uterine Bleeding due to Endometrial Cancer

CASE STUDY

A 45-year-old nulliparous woman, married since last 15 years, presented to the gynecological emergency with a severe episode of bleeding following a period of amenorrhea since past 7 months. The patient does not give any positive family history of cancer. She gives a history of undergoing treatment in the past which she was supposed to take on the first 5 days of the cycle. According to the patient, this was for treatment of her infertility. She also had been prescribed treatment for her excessive facial hair and advised to reduce her weight. However, she took no heed of the advice. She was unable to conceive despite of taking treatment. At the time of general physical examination, her BMI was 27 (obese range) and blood pressure was 150/90 mm Hg.

INTRODUCTION

> Q. Write a long essay discussing the FIGO classification system for abnormal uterine bleeding (AUB).

It can be seen that the above-mentioned case study has been formulated to simulate the situation of a patient presenting with AUB probably due to an anticipated malignancy. Heavy menstrual bleeding (HMB) is a type of AUB which has been described in detail in Chapter 24. This chapter would primarily focus around AUB related to endometrial malignancy.

Abnormal uterine bleeding can be defined as any deviation in the normal frequency, duration, or amount of menstrual blood loss in a woman belonging to the reproductive age group. AUB is inclusive of HMB or mistimed bleeding. AUB can be acute or chronic:

- *Acute AUB:* This can be defined as an episode of heavy bleeding which in the opinion of the clinician is of sufficient quantity to require immediate intervention for prevention of further blood loss.
- *Chronic AUB:* This can be defined as the bleeding from uterine corpus that is abnormal in duration, volume, regularity, and/or timing. This abnormality must have been present for majority of time during the past 6 months. This type of bleeding does not require immediate medical attention.

There has been general inconsistency in the nomenclature used for describing AUB in the women of reproductive age group and there is a plethora of potential causes. Previously used nomenclature such as dysfunctional uterine bleeding (DUB), menorrhagia, oligomenorrhea, metrorrhagia, etc., has been revised. The term metrorrhagia has been replaced by the term intermenstrual bleeding, which denotes bleeding occurring between clearly defined cyclic and predictable menses. This may occur randomly or at a regular time in each cycle. In order to harmonize the definitions of normal and abnormal bleeding symptoms and to classify and subclassify underlying potential causes of AUB in the women belonging to the reproductive age groups, the Menstrual Disorders Committee of FIGO (2011), devised two systems:

1. *FIGO AUB system 1:* This is for nomenclature and definition of symptoms of normal and AUB in the reproductive years and,
2. *FIGO AUB system 2:* This system is for the classification of causes of AUB in reproductive age group based on the findings of clinical examination and imaging.

FIGO AUB SYSTEM 1

This nomenclature system is based on four components related to normal menstruation:
- Duration of flow
- Frequency
- Regularity
- Volume of blood loss

Some changes were made in the nomenclature system in 2018 and are described in **Table 23.1**.

FIGO AUB SYSTEM 2

> Q. Describe in detail the PALM-COEIN classification of AUB.

Abnormal Uterine Bleeding due to Endometrial Cancer

TABLE 23.1: FIGO (2018) system 1 for nomenclature of symptoms of normal and abnormal uterine bleeding.

Characteristic	AUB
1. Duration of blood flow	Normal ≤ 8 days Prolonged > 8 days
2. Frequency	Normal—24–38 days Frequent < 24 days Infrequent > 38 days Amenorrhea—absent (no periods or bleeding)
3. Cycle to cycle variation (regularity)	Regular variation (shortest to longest ≤ 9 days) Irregular (shortest to longest 10+ days)
4. Volume of blood loss	Heavy, normal, light Acceptance of the definition of heavy menstrual bleeding as described by NICE (bleeding volume sufficient to interfere with the woman's quality of life)

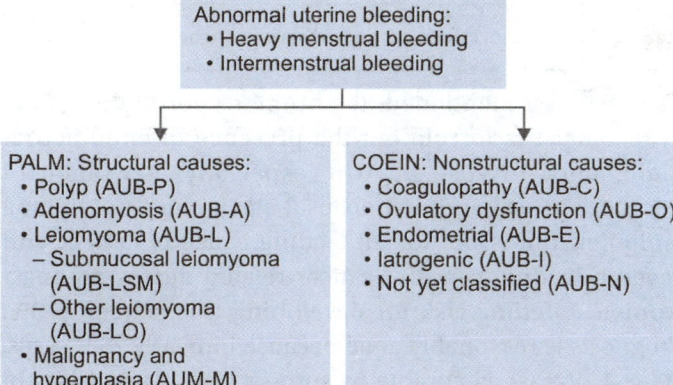

Flowchart 23.1: Basic PALM-COEIN classification system.

(*Source:* Munro MG, Critchley HO, Broder MS, Fraser IS, FIGO Working Group on Menstrual Disorders. FIGO classification system (PALM-COEIN) for causes of abnormal uterine bleeding in nongravid women of reproductive age. Int J Gynaecol Obstet. 2011;113:3-13.)

FIGO (2011) has approved a new classification system (PALM-COEIN) for causes of AUB in nongravid women of reproductive age **(Flowchart 23.1)**. Of the nine categories in the new FIGO classification system (PALM-COEIN), the first four are defined as visually objective structural criteria (PALM), the pathologies that can be measured visually with imaging techniques, such as sonography and/or histopathology testing. The next four are unrelated to structural abnormalities (COEI: coagulopathy, ovulatory dysfunction, endometrial, and iatrogenic), which are the nonstructural entities that are not defined on imaging or histopathology testing. In these cases, clinical assessment with detailed history-taking, physical examination, and lab investigations helps the clinician to arrive at the diagnosis of AUB. The "iatrogenic" category refers to AUB associated with the use of exogenous gonadal steroids, intrauterine systems (IUSs) or devices, or other systemic or local agents. The final category stands for the entities that are not yet classified (N). This classification system for the causes of AUB is likely to facilitate clinical care and treatment of such patients. Taking the patient's medical history should be guided by the PALM-COEIN classification system to exclude various pathologies and reach a specific diagnosis regarding the cause for AUB. In 2018, some changes were made in the FIGO AUB system for causes and are described in **Table 23.2**.

Documentation of AUB using the PALM COEIN classification system: If any component is present, it is represented by 1. If absent, it is represented by 0. Therefore, AUB due to leiomyomas can be represented by: $P_0 A_0 L_1 M_0 C_0 O_0 E_0 I_0 N_0$ or simply AUB-L.

Postmenopausal Bleeding

Q. Discuss in detail the causes of PMB as well as its diagnosis and management.

TABLE 23.2: Summary of changes to FIGO AUB system 2: Causes or contributors to AUB in the reproductive years (PALM-COEIN).

AUB-A	Refined sonographic diagnostic criteria
AUB-L	Inclusion of type 3 as a submucous leiomyoma Type definitions and distinctions Distinction between types 0 and 1; 6 and 7 Distinction between types 2 and 3; 4 and 5
AUB-C	This category no longer includes AUB associated with pharmacologic agents which impair blood coagulation. This type of AUB is now included in AUB-I
AUB-I	Now includes AUB associated with all iatrogenic processes including the use of pharmacological agents used for anticoagulation as well as those thought to interfere with ovulation
AUB-O	This category no longer includes ovulatory disorders associated with drugs known or those suspected to interfere with ovulation
AUB-N	The name of the category has been changed from "Not Yet Classified" to Not Otherwise Classified There is a brief discussion regarding a potential new cause of AUB the so-called uterine "niche" or isthmocele following lower segment cesarean section

Source: Munro MG, Critchley HOD, Fraser IS; FIGO Menstrual Disorders Committee. The two FIGO systems for normal and abnormal uterine bleeding symptoms and classification of causes of abnormal uterine bleeding in the reproductive years: 2018 revisions. Int J Gynaecol Obstet. 2018;143(3):393-408.

Postmenopausal bleeding (PMB) can be defined as bleeding occurring 1 year after cessation of menses in women at the age of climacteric. Some likely causes for PMB are described in **Table 23.3**.

Patients with AUB/PMB in whom diagnosis of endometrial cancer needs to be excluded are summarized in **Box 23.1**.

Endometrial Cancer

 Q. Write a short note on endometrial cancer

As previously mentioned, the prime responsibility of the gynecologist is to rule out the presence of endometrial malignancy in case of AUB, especially in women of perimenopausal and menopausal age groups. Carcinoma endometrium is the fourth leading cause of cancer and seventh leading cause of cancer-related deaths amongst women. Lifetime risk for developing this cancer is 3%. Prognosis is reasonably good because in nearly 75% cases, stage 1 disease is curable by surgery only. Most cases of endometrial cancer are histologically of adenomatous type.

The endometrioid type of adenocarcinoma accounts for about 80% of endometrial cancers. The endometrial cancers can be of different grades (G1, G2, and G3) based on the degree of cellular differentiation, anaplasia, and glandular architecture, with higher grade of tumor associated with a worse prognosis. Traditionally, Bokhman (1983) has introduced a classical dualistic model which classifies endometrial carcinoma into two histological subtypes: type I (endometrioid) and type II (serous) tumors. Difference between the two is described in **Table 23.4**.

HISTORY AND CLINICAL PRESENTATION

CLINICAL PRESENTATION

Abnormal perimenopausal and PMB should always be taken seriously and properly investigated, no matter how minimal or nonpersistent. Detailed history for assessing the nature of blood loss needs to be taken from the patient by elucidating the patient's clinical presentation. Some of these questions are described below.

Nature of Bleeding

The clinician needs to ask questions to determine the pattern of bleeding—amount of bleeding; the time of bleeding (the days in the menstrual cycle during which the bleeding occurs); intermenstrual intervals (between the episodes of bleeding); and cycle regularity (whether the bleeding pattern is regular or irregular). This would help in ruling out bleeding due to other causes such as cervical cancer, rectal bleeding, etc.

Amount of Bleeding

Initially, the clinician needs to establish whether the woman is having heavy, light, or moderate amount of blood loss.

TABLE 23.3: Causes of postmenopausal bleeding.

Likely cause	Percentage of cases
Atrophic vaginitis: Vaginal atrophy, senile vaginitis	30%
Exogenous estrogens	30%
Endometrial carcinoma	10–15%
Endometrial or cervical polyps	10%
Endometrial hyperplasias	5–10%
Miscellaneous	10%

BOX 23.1: Women in whom it is essential to rule out the diagnosis of endometrial cancer.

- All patients with postmenopausal bleeding
- Postmenopausal women with pyometra (pyometra may be present in women with senile endometritis or those with endometrial carcinoma)
- Women in whom pap smear show atypical endometrial cells
- Perimenopausal women with intermenstrual bleeding or HMB
- Premenopausal women with AUB, particularly if there is a history of anovulation

(AUB: abnormal uterine bleeding; HMB: heavy menstrual bleeding)

TABLE 23.4: Difference between type 1 and type 2 endometrial cancers.

Parameter	Type 1	Type 2
Tumor grade	Constitute grade 1 or grade 2 endometrioid tumors	Constitute grade 3 endometrioid or nonendometrioid histology (clear cell, serous subtypes, etc.)
Mutations	The likely mutations include PTEN and KRAS mutations	P53 mutations are commonly encountered
Dependence on estrogen	These tumors are estrogen dependent and usually begin as endometrial hyperplasia	These tumors are estrogen independent and usually arise in the background of atrophic endometrium
Degree of differentiation	These tumors are better differentiated	These tumors are less well differentiated
Total number of cases	Constitute 80% of total cases	Constitute 20% of total cases
Risk factors	Combined oral contraceptive pills and smoking are protective factors	Smoking is not protective
Age group	Occurs in younger, perimenopausal, nulliparous, obese women	Occurs in older, postmenopausal, multiparous, thin patients
Race	White	Black
Prognosis	Good prognosis, less aggressive tumor	Poor prognosis, more aggressive tumor

Estimating the quantity of blood loss is a very subjective issue when considering vaginal bleeding. Accurate assessment of the menstrual blood loss may not be possible and best estimates of menstrual blood loss are the only source clinicians have to consider commonly.

Total number or pads or tampons used by the patient during the heaviest days of her bleeding can give a rough estimation of the amount of bleeding. However, the number of pads used for the same amount of bleeding may vary from woman to woman depending on their hygienic preferences. Some questions which the obstetrician can ask in order to assess the amount of blood loss are as follows:

- How frequently does she require changing her pads during the day?
- Does she have to use double protection? (e.g., simultaneous use of a tampon and pad or use of double pad. For the purpose of calculating the amount of blood loss, it can be assumed that an average tampon holds 5 mL and the average pad holds 5–15 mL of blood).
- Does she have to get up in the night to change her protection?
- Is there any history of passage of blood clots? Normally, the blood lost from the vessels in the endometrial lining forms small clots and this helps in reducing the blood flow. Under normal circumstances, these blood clots are broken down by fibrinolysins, present in the endometrial cavity, and the menstrual blood loss is in form of a fluid. However, in case of very heavy bleeding, the blood is extruded too quickly for the clots to lyse within the uterus. In this situation, the blood clots in the vagina and the menstrual flow include blood clots.
- Does she stain her bedding or clothes despite wearing tampons and pads?
- Does she ever experience "flooding" or sudden rushing out of a large quantity of blood?
- Does she have to stay at home or take time off work during the episode of bleeding?
- How long do her periods last?
- Is the amount of bleeding so much as to interfere with the patient's lifestyle?
- Is there constant pain in the lower abdomen during menstrual periods?
- Are the menstrual periods irregular?
- Does she experience tiredness, fatigue, or shortness of breath (symptoms of anemia)?
- The type of sanitary protection being used by the patient is also important since the patient may be required to less frequently change the newer absorbent pads in comparison to the home-made cloth-based sanitary protection.
- *History of nocturnal change of pads*: This is indicative of HMB/AUB affecting her quality of life requiring her to wake up from her sleep to change her pads.

Pictorial blood loss assessment chart (PBAC): Objective assessment of blood loss can be done using PBAC **(Fig. 23.1)**. In this method, number of tampons and sanitary pads used per day during the period are marked by placing a tally mark under the day next to the box **(Fig. 23.1)**. This must be representative of the amount of bleeding noted each time the pad is changed. Presence of blood clots must be indicated based on their approximate size (size of a dime or a quarter). The total score is then calculated by multiplying the total number of tallies in each row by the multiplying factor at the end of each row. The row totals are then added to calculate the actual score. Count of >100 on PBAC is suggestive of HMB.

Duration of Bleeding

Bleeding occurring for >8 days at a stretch can be considered as prolonged.

Day	Day 1	Day 2	Day 3	Day 4	Day 5	Day 6	Day 7	Day 8	Day 9	Day 10	Total tallies	Multiplying factors	Row total
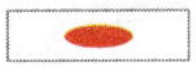 (pad - small spot)												X1	
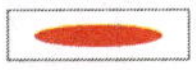 (pad - medium)												X5	
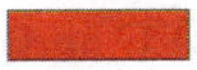 (pad - soaked)												X20	
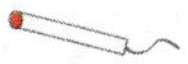 (tampon - small)												X1	
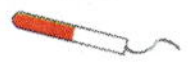 (tampon - medium)												X5	
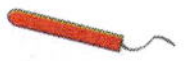 (tampon - soaked)												X10	
Small blood clots (= Dime)												X1	
Large blood clots (≥ Quarter)												X5	
Menstrual accidents												X5	
Total score (sum of rows)													

Fig. 23.1: Pictorial blood loss assessment chart.

Pattern of Bleeding

Sudden change in the bleeding pattern, for example, excessive bleeding at regular intervals, which suddenly becomes irregular, must be regarded with caution. In these cases, investigations must be undertaken to discover the exact pathology. She must be also asked about the intermenstrual intervals between the episodes of bleeding: number of days following which the bleeding occurs and cycle regularity.

Smell

Presence of a foul-smelling vaginal discharge points toward the presence of infection or a necrotic malignant growth. Malignant growths often undergo necrosis in the areas of reduced blood supply.

Relation of Bleeding to Sexual Intercourse

Bleeding following sexual intercourse is usually related to the lesions of cervix or vagina. Simple vaginitis (e.g., candidal infection and bacterial vaginosis) may cause intermenstrual bleeding, while gonorrhea and chlamydia may present with heavier bleeding attributed primarily to the copious discharge mixed with the blood. If a woman presents with the history of postcoital bleeding, cervical cancer must be specifically ruled out.

Other temporal associations of the bleeding episode, whether postpartum or postpill, also need to be asked.

Differentiating between Ovulatory and Anovulatory Bleeding

In most women with true anovulatory bleeding, the cause of bleeding can be established by taking history itself. Characteristics of ovulatory and anovulatory menstrual cycles which can be determined by taking appropriate history are enlisted in **Table 23.5**.

Features Indicative of Presence of Endometrial Malignancy

The pointers in the history of bleeding, indicative of underlying malignancy in case of AUB include the following:
- Sudden change in the bleeding pattern
- Irregular bleeding
- Intermenstrual bleeding
- Postcoital bleeding
- Dyspareunia, pelvic pain
- Lower extremity edema, which could be secondary to metastasis.

Patient's Age

Patient's age can provide important pointer toward the diagnosis of underlying pathology.

TABLE 23.5: Characteristics of ovulatory and anovulatory menstrual cycles.

Ovulatory menstrual cycles	Anovulatory menstrual cycles
Regular cycle length	Unpredictable cycle length
Regular bleeding pattern	Unpredictable bleeding pattern: Frequent spotting, infrequent heavy bleeding
Biphasic temperature curve	Monophasic temperature curve
Presence of premenstrual symptoms such as dysmenorrhea, breast tenderness, change in cervical mucus, Mittelschmerz, etc.	No premenstrual molimina
Ovulatory cycles may be painful	Anovulatory cycles are painless
Positive result from use of luteinizing hormone (LH) predictor kit	Negative result

Women Belonging to Postmenopausal Age Group

The risk of developing endometrial cancer increases with age, with 90% cases occurring in postmenopausal women. This risk of endometrial cancer is 1% at 50 years of age, which increases to about 25% at 80 years of age. 8% of cases may occur amongst premenopausal women and 3% cases may show familial association. The endometrial cancer peaks in the age group of 55–70 years, with mean age being 62 years. Thus, the American College of Obstetricians and Gynecologists recommends endometrial evaluation in women aged 35 years and older who have AUB.

Though endometrial cancer can be asymptomatic in nearly 10% cases, the most common clinical symptom associated with endometrial cancer is abnormal or irregular uterine bleeding. Therefore, in case a postmenopausal woman presents with AUB, she should receive an immediate workup for endometrial cancer. Presence of endometrial hyperplasia/malignancy must be ruled out in all postmenopausal women presenting with bleeding, especially those having risk factors for endometrial malignancy

Women of Reproductive Age Group

The most common cause of abnormal bleeding patterns in women belonging to the reproductive age group is pregnancy-related complications. Since pregnancy-related bleeding must be considered as the first differential diagnosis in the women of childbearing age who present with AUB, it is important to take history of the period of amenorrhea preceding the episode of blood loss or having a positive pregnancy test during that period. Potential causes of pregnancy-related bleeding include spontaneous miscarriage, ectopic pregnancy, placenta previa, abruptio placentae, trophoblastic disease, etc. Uterine leiomyomas are a common cause for menorrhagia in the women belonging to reproductive age group. Uterine leiomyomas have been discussed in details in Chapter 24.

Young Patients

The most common etiology in a young patient having irregular menses since menarche is anovulation.

Other questions which need to be asked while taking history in such patients include the following:

- Sexual activity/history of vaginal infection
- *History of chronic anovulation [e.g., that associated with polycystic ovarian syndrome (PCOS)]:* It is associated with unopposed estrogen stimulation. Presence of hirsutism or excessive growth of facial hair, obesity, and acne point toward PCOS. PCOS is associated with unopposed estrogen stimulation, elevated androgen levels, and insulin resistance and is a common cause of anovulation. Women with feminizing ovarian tumors are associated with unopposed estrogen production, which acts as a risk factor for endometrial cancer.
- *History of galactorrhea or secretion of milk from breasts:* Any patient complaining of a milky discharge from either breast (while not pregnant, postpartum, or breastfeeding) needs estimation of prolactin levels to rule out the presence of a pituitary tumor. Galactorrhea could be related to underlying hyperprolactinemia, which can cause oligoovulation or eventual amenorrhea.
- *History of any eating disorder, stress, etc.:* It is important to elicit the history of any eating disorders/stress, etc. Hypothalamic suppression secondary to eating disorders, stress, or excessive exercise may induce anovulation, which sometimes manifests as irregular and HMB or amenorrhea.
- *History of foul-smelling discharge per vaginum:* This could be related to the presence of sexually transmitted diseases or carcinoma cervix. Age is an important consideration in these cases because women in reproductive age groups are more likely to suffer from sexually transmitted diseases while diagnosis of cervical cancer is more likely in older women. Presence of vaginal discharge could also be suggestive of pyometra.
- *Presence of pressure symptoms:* This could be related to the presence of a large pelvic mass (uterine or adnexal mass) pressing upon the bladder or rectum resulting in pressure symptoms like increased urinary frequency and/or rectal symptoms such as constipation and tenesmus.
- *Plans regarding future fertility and contraception:* It is important to take the patient's history regarding her plans for future fertility and child bearing in order to decide appropriate patient management, e.g., decision for hysterectomy must be avoided as far as possible in a young women desiring future fertility.
- *Symptoms suggestive of pregnancy:* Symptoms suggestive of pregnancy, e.g., morning sickness, breast changes, etc., also need to be enquired from the patient.

- *Previous papanicolaou (Pap) smears:* History of undergoing Pap smears in the past needs to be elicited. Previous normal Pap smears help in ruling out cervical malignancy.
- Sexual activity/history of vaginal infection
- *History of genital trauma:* Genital trauma may result in bleeding from the vagina or rectum. It is especially important to rule out sexual abuse in young girls, presenting with bleeding who have yet not attained menarche.
- Symptoms suggestive of coagulopathies
- History of symptoms suggestive of premenstrual molimina (breast tenderness, edema, mood swings, etc.), and other symptoms such as dyspareunia, dysmenorrhea, and dyschezia. Vaginal irritation or dyspareunia could also be related to atrophic vaginitis.
- Presence of underlying systemic illnesses (renal, hepatic failure, etc.)

History of Pain in the Abdomen

Pain in the abdomen could be indicative of underlying malignancy. Typical pain associated with carcinoma endometrium is known as Simpson's pain. This pain usually referred to the hypogastrium or both the iliac fossa. It is related to pyometra and may be present in 15% patients. It usually occurs at the same time in a day and subsides on its own.

Past Treatment/Drug History

- *History of drug intake:* Intake of drugs such as anticoagulants (e.g., warfarin), hormones (e.g., unopposed estrogens, tamoxifen, etc.), selective serotonin reuptake inhibitors, antipsychotics, and corticosteroids may typically cause bleeding. Thus, the patient should be asked if she had been prescribed any of the above-mentioned medicines in the past. Since herbal substances, such as ginseng, ginkgo, and soy supplements, may also cause menstrual irregularities, history of intake of such products must also be taken.
- *History of contraceptive use [intrauterine device (IUD) or hormones]:* Commonly, an IUD causes increased uterine cramping and menstrual flow.
- *Use of unopposed estrogens without combination with progesterone (in form of oral contraceptive pills or HRT):* Use of unopposed estrogens (without combination of progesterone) may predispose the woman to develop endometrial hyperplasia or cancer in future. Chronic proliferation of the endometrium may cause adenomatous hyperplasia, which may result in the development of atypical adenomatous hyperplasia, eventually leading to the development of endometrial carcinoma.

Menstrual History

The history of menstrual cycles before the occurrence of episode of abnormal bleeding, including features such as duration of bleeding, the cycle length, whether cycles were regular or irregular, whether there was pain during cycles, etc. needs to be enquired. The age of menarche and that at which menopause was attained also needs to be asked. Endometrial cancer is also more common in women who have had early menarche and late menopause. These factors are likely to result in a prolonged or unopposed exposure of the endometrium to estrogen, which may result in an increased risk for development of endometrial cancer.

Obstetric History

Eliciting the patient's obstetric history is particularly important because certain pathological conditions (e.g., endometrial malignancy and uterine leiomyomas) are more likely to develop in nulliparous women. Since nulliparity acts as a risk factor for the development of both endometrial carcinoma and uterine leiomyomas, the two are frequently observed to coexist together. On the other hand, conditions like cervical malignancy are more likely to develop in multiparous women.

Past Medical History

- *Past history of chronic illness:* The patient should be asked about the past history of any chronic medical illness like diabetes mellitus, hypertension, coronary artery disease (CAD), etc., and obesity. This is especially important because the triad of obesity, hypertension, and diabetes is associated with an increased risk of endometrial cancer.
- *Symptoms of thyroid dysfunction:* The alteration of the hypothalamic-pituitary axis may result in either amenorrhea (hyperthyroidism) or menorrhagia (hypothyroidism). For signs and symptoms suggestive of hypothyroidism and hyperthyroidism, kindly refer to Chapter 13.
- *Corpus cancer syndrome:* Triad of obesity, hypertension, and diabetes mellitus is likely to be associated with an increased risk of endometrial cancer.
- *Hepatic/renal failure:* History suggestive of systemic illnesses, including hepatic/renal failure needs to be asked. The disorders of these organs are likely to result in bleeding abnormalities.
- *History of excessive bruising or known bleeding/coagulation disorders:* History related to initial screening for detecting an underlying disorder of hemostasis in patients with excessive bleeding is described in **Box 23.2**. Patients having positive history at the time of initial screening should be considered for further evaluation including consultation with a hematologist and assessment for diseases such as Von Willebrand's disease (Von Willebrand factor and ristocetin cofactor) and hemophilia.

Family History

Personal or family history of endometrial, ovarian, or breast cancer is another predisposing factor for development of endometrial cancer. Two important hereditary cancer syndromes which may be involved with development of endometrial cancers are Lynch syndrome II or HNPCC syndrome (hereditary nonpolyposis colorectal cancer), and Cowden syndrome **(Table 23.6)**. Most common cancers

BOX 23.2: Clinical screening for detecting an underlying disorder of hemostasis in patients with AUB.

- Heavy menstrual bleeding since menarche
- One of the following conditions:
  - Postpartum hemorrhage at time of childbirth
  - Excessive bleeding at the time of surgery
  - Excessive bleeding at the time of dental procedures
- Two or more of the following conditions:
  - Excessive bruising with mild trauma, one or two times per month
  - Epistaxis, one or two times per month
  - Frequent gum bleeding
  - Family history of bleeding symptoms

Source: Kouides PA, Conard J, Peyvandi F, Lukes A, Kadir R. Hemostasis and menstruation: appropriate investigation for underlying disorders of hemostasis in women with excessive menstrual bleeding. Fertil Steril. 2005;84(5):1345-51. doi: 10.1016/j.fertnstert.2005.05.035.

TABLE 23.6: Hereditary endometrial cancer syndromes.

Hereditary syndromes	Gene mutation	Inheritance pattern	Tumor phenotype	Endometrial cancer (lifetime risk)
Lynch syndrome II (HNPCC)	Germline mutations in DNA mismatch repair gene, EPCAM, which affects the genes: *MLH-1, MSH-2, MSH-6,* and *PMS-2*	Autosomal dominant	Cancer colon, endometrium, ovary, stomach, small bowel, and urinary tract	25–60%
Cowden syndrome	PTEN	Autosomal dominant	• Breast cancer • Hamartoma • Glioma • Endometrial cancer	5–10%

(EPCAM: epithelial cell adhesion molecule; HNPCC: hereditary nonpolyposis colorectal cancer; MLH: mutL homolog; MSH: mutS homolog; PTEN: phosphatase and TENsin homolog)

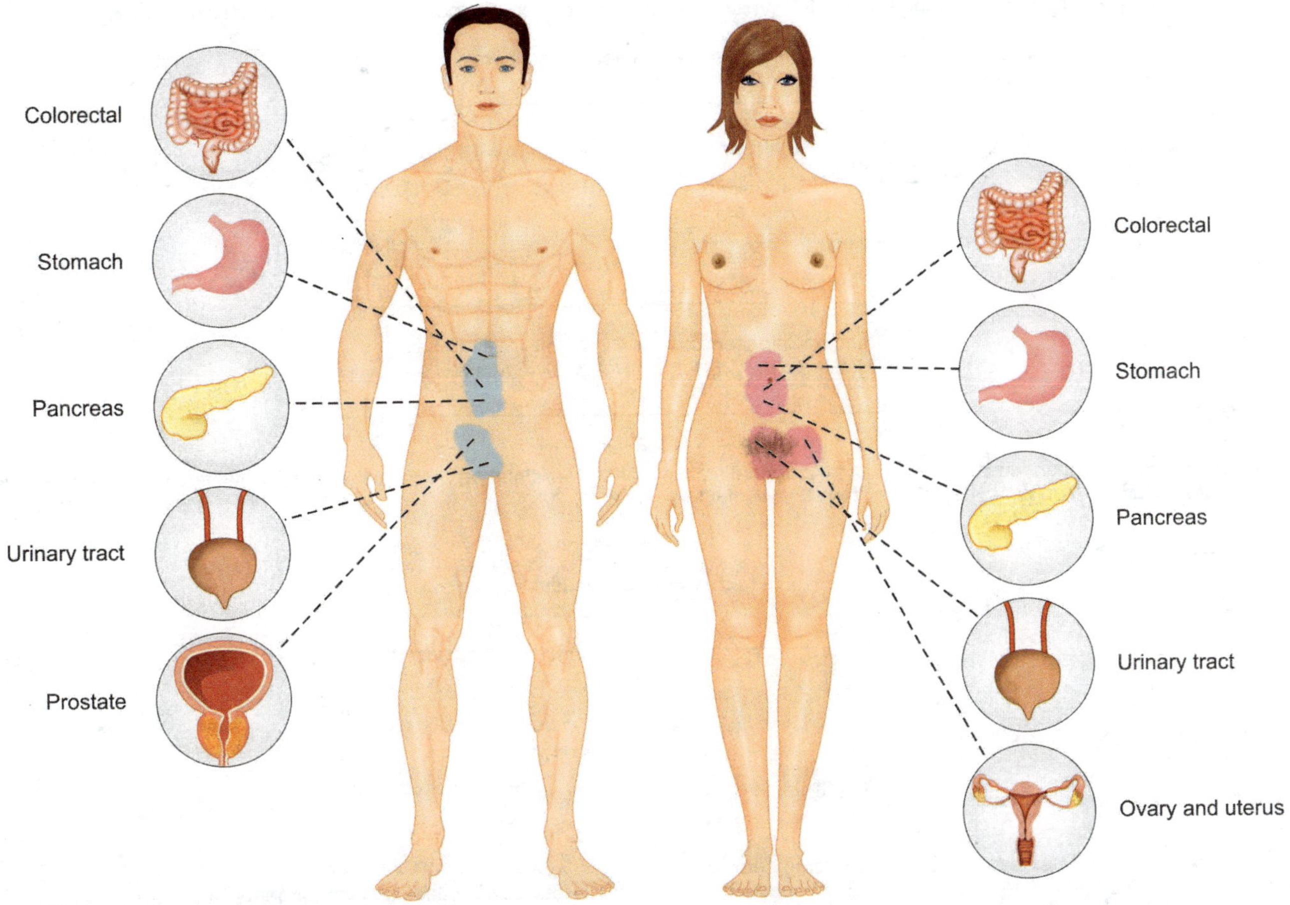

Fig. 23.2: Most common* cancers in men and women with Lynch II syndrome.
*Other rare cancers associated with Lynch syndrome 2 include hepatobiliary tract cancers, small bowel cancers, brain cancers, and skin cancers (sebaceous neoplasms).

> **BOX 23.3:** Recommendations for genetic screening of Lynch syndrome II.
>
> - Patients with endometrial or colorectal carcinoma and tumor with microsatellite instability [indicative of defects in the DNA mismatch repair system (MMR)]
> - First degree relatives of patients with endometrial or colorectal carcinoma diagnosed before the age of 60 years or other rare cancers* are at an increased risk of lynch syndrome II based on personal and medical history
> - First or a second degree relative with a known DNA MMR mutation
>
> *Other rare cancers associated with Lynch syndrome 2 include hepatobiliary tract cancers, small bowel cancers, brain cancers, and skin cancers (sebaceous neoplasms).

encountered in men and women with lynch syndrome are described in **Figure 23.2**. Recommendations for genetic screening for lynch syndrome are tabulated in **Box 23.3**. **Flowchart 23.2** demonstrates the protocol for screening the women with endometrial cancer for lynch syndrome using molecular markers. **Table 23.7** shows the lifetime cancer risk comparison amongst the women with lynch II syndrome versus the general population.

■ RISK FACTORS

Risk factors for endometrial cancer which need to be elicited at the time of taking history are tabulated in **Box 23.4**.

There are some factors which can reduce the risk for endometrial cancer, which are tabulated in **Box 23.5**.

GENERAL PHYSICAL EXAMINATION

General physical examination should focus on signs related to excessive blood loss (tachycardia and hypotension), symptoms related to endocrinopathies, including polycystic ovary disease (such as obesity and hyperandrogenism: acne, hirsutism, and deepening of voice), hyperprolactinemia, and hypothyroidism. The following points should be typically looked at the time of general physical examination.

■ BODY MASS INDEX

Obese women (with increased BMI) are more likely to be suffering from endometrial malignancies. Obesity increases

Flowchart 23.2: Screening for Lynch II syndrome using the molecular markers for endometrial carcinoma.

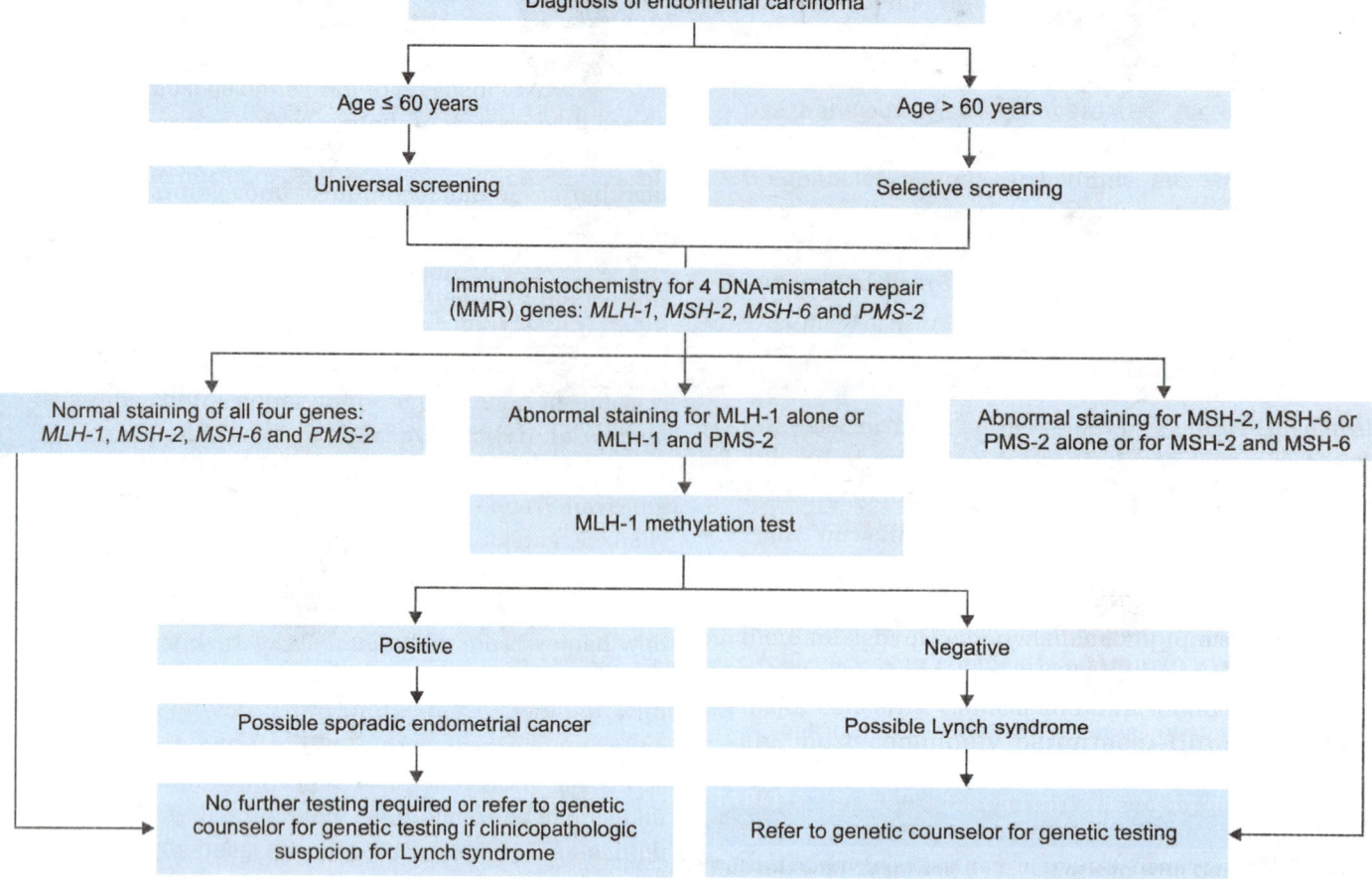

TABLE 23.7: Lifetime cancer risk comparison.				
	Colorectal cancer	*Endometrial cancer*	*Ovarian cancer*	*Stomach cancer*
Individuals with Lynch syndrome	<80%	<60%	<24%	<13%
General population	5%	2.8%	1.2%	<1%

BOX 23.4: Risk factors for endometrial cancer.

- Age between 55 and 75 years (mean age 63 years)
- White race
- Prolonged unopposed exposure to high-dose estrogens [exposure to both exogenous (tamoxifen, HRT, etc.) and endogenous estrogen sources (obesity, granulosa cell tumors, PCOS, etc.)]
- Obesity
- High socioeconomic status
- Early menarche, late menopause
- *Nulliparity or low parity:* Nulliparous women are likely to have two to four times more risk in comparison to multiparous women
- Anovulatory cycles/infertility
- Postmenopausal estrogen therapy
- Estrogen secreting ovarian tumors
- Tamoxifen therapy (in high cumulative doses)
- *Lynch syndrome II (HNPCC):* Mutations in the mismatch repair gene (MLH-1, MSH-2, MSH-6, and PMS-2): 24–60% cases of endometrial or colorectal cancer
- *Mutations:* PTEN, p53, and BRCA-1 gene mutations
- Higher education and income levels
- *Corpus cancer syndrome:* Combination of diabetes, obesity, and hypertension with carcinoma endometrium

(HNPCC: hereditary nonpolyposis colorectal cancer; HRT: hormone replacement therapy; MLH-1: mutL homolog; MSH: mutS homolog; PCOS: polycystic ovarian syndrome; PTEN: phosphatase and TENsin homolog)

> **BOX 23.5:** Protective factors for endometrial cancer.
> - Multiparity
> - Long-term use of oral contraceptives (2-year use is likely to reduce the risk by 50%; use for 5 years can further extend the protective effect over 15–20 years)
> - Smoking (helps in reducing estrogen levels early and predispose the women to attain early menopause)
> - *Postpartum sterilization:* Likely to reduce the risk of cancer spread to the ovaries
> - *Dietary factors:* Red meat consumption is not protective

> **BOX 23.6:** Causes of mass in the abdomen in association with postmenopausal bleeding.
> - Endometrial cancer (uterine enlargement)
> - Pyometra (could be due to endometrial or cervical malignancy)
> - Estrogen-secreting tumor of ovary (e.g., granulosa cell tumor)
> - Uterine fibroid (rarely)

the levels of free estrogen in the body by decreasing the levels of serum hormone binding proteins. Moreover, aromatization of the androgen, epiandrostenedione to estrone occurs in peripheral fat.

BLOOD PRESSURE

Increased blood pressure could be related with an increased risk for endometrial cancer.

PALLOR

Pallor could be related to anemia caused by excessive blood loss.

ENDOCRINOPATHY

The clinician must look for following signs in order to rule out presence of an endocrinopathy:
- Signs of hyperthyroidism and hypothyroidism.
- *Galactorrhea:* This could be related to increased prolactin production.
- *Blood sugar:* Type 2 diabetes could be associated with an increased risk for endometrial cancer.

SPECIFIC SYSTEMIC EXAMINATION

PER SPECULUM EXAMINATION

Per speculum examination helps in identifying any trauma or bleeding causing lesions of vagina, cervix, etc.

ABDOMINAL EXAMINATION

Abdominal examination to detect the presence of hepatic and splenic enlargement or presence of any abdominal mass has been described in Chapter 22. **Box 23.6** describes causes for mass in the abdomen in association with PMB.

PELVIC EXAMINATION

Pelvic examination is unnecessary and must not be done in young girls presenting with the history of menorrhagia, who are not sexually active. Pelvic examination may be particularly useful in women belonging to reproductive age group, presenting with AUB. The pelvic examination has been described in detail in Chapter 22 and may reveal enlargement due to uterine fibroids, adenomyosis, or endometrial carcinoma. An enlarged uniformly shaped uterus in a postmenopausal patient with bleeding suggests endometrial cancer until proven otherwise.

Clinical findings most encountered in cases of early-stage endometrial cancer are a normal examination of vagina, uterus, and cervix, although advanced disease may be associated with an enlarged uterus or pelvic mass. Cervical and vaginal metastasis can cause cervical stenosis, pyometra, or a mucosanguineous vaginal discharge. Regional metastasis may present in form of a bladder or rectal mass.

The specific indicators which point toward the cause of bleeding on pelvic examination include the following:
- *Per speculum examination:* Inspection of the vagina and cervix helps in detecting presence of visible lesions [polyps, erosions, tears, malignancy, pregnancy-related complications (expulsion of products of conceptions) or infection]. Signs of excessive blood loss must also be noted on per speculum examination. The actual site of bleeding can also be assessed through a per speculum examination. Presence of vaginal/cervical discharge on per speculum examination indicates the presence of infection.
- Careful inspection of the lower genital tract must be done to detect the presence of lacerations, vulvar or vaginal pathology, and cervical lesions or polyps.
- *Vaginal and bimanual examination:* Size, shape, position, and firmness of the uterus should also be examined. Identification of uterine enlargement or irregularity, which may be associated with some structural cause of acute AUB (e.g. leiomyoma, etc.) may also be detected.

BREAST EXAMINATION

Breast examination in cases of AUB should specifically aim at the following:
- *Detection of a breast lump:* Detection of a tumorous mass could be an indicator of breast malignancy. History of treatment with tamoxifen (anti-cancer drug, commonly used in cases of breast malignancy) needs to be enquired in such patients. Patients with breast cancer (BRCA-1 or 2 positive) on tamoxifen therapy are likely to be associated with 2–4 folds increased risk for endometrial cancer. Therefore, AUB in women under treatment with tamoxifen could be related to endometrial hyperplasia, thereby warranting prompt investigation and careful follow-up.

> **BOX 23.7:** Differential diagnosis of abnormal uterine bleeding.
>
> *Postmenopausal women*
> - Cervical cancer, cervicitis
> - Atrophic vaginitis, endometrial atrophy
> - Submucous fibroids, endometrial hyperplasia, and endometrial polyps
> - Hormone replacement therapy
>
> *Premenopausal women*
> - *Complications of pregnancy:* Intrauterine pregnancy, ectopic pregnancy, spontaneous abortion, gestational trophoblastic disease, placenta previa
> - *Infection, trauma:* Cervicitis, PID, endometritis, laceration, abrasion, foreign body, IUCD
> - *Benign pelvic pathology:* Cervical polyp, endometrial polyp, leiomyoma, adenomyosis, etc.
> - *Malignancy, neoplasm:* Cervical, endometrial, or ovarian malignancy
> - *Premalignant lesions:* Cervical lesions, endometrial hyperplasia
> - *Trauma:* Foreign bodies, abrasions, lacerations, sexual abuse or assault
> - *Medications/iatrogenic:* Intrauterine device, hormones (oral contraceptives, estrogen, progesterone), anovulatory cycles, hypothyroidism, hyperprolactinemia, Cushing's disease, polycystic ovarian syndrome, adrenal dysfunction/tumor, stress (emotional factors, excessive exercise)
> - *Systemic diseases:* Hepatic disease, renal disease, coagulopathy, thrombocytopenia, von Willebrand's disease, leukemia
>
> (IUCD: intrauterine contraceptive device; PID: pelvic inflammatory disease)

- *Presence of galactorrhea:* Hyperprolactinemia is an important cause of amenorrhea and infertility.

DIFFERENTIAL DIAGNOSIS

The specific diagnostic approach in the case of AUB should be based on patient's age, i.e., whether the patient belongs to the premenopausal, perimenopausal, or postmenopausal age groups **(Box 23.7)**. In premenopausal women, belonging to the reproductive age group, having normal findings on physical examination, the most likely diagnosis is AUB secondary to anovulation.

Abnormal uterine pathology, particularly endometrial carcinoma, is common in postmenopausal or perimenopausal women presenting with AUB. Therefore, in the women belonging to perimenopausal and menopausal age groups, endometrial biopsy (EB), and other investigations for detecting endometrial hyperplasia or carcinoma must be considered early during the course of investigations.

Women receiving HRT may often present with abnormal bleeding. Most sources recommend evaluation of abnormal bleeding, if it lasts >6–9 months after initiation of HRT.

MANAGEMENT

> **Q.** Discuss the diagnosis and management of AUB in women of reproductive age group.

Management of AUB in women belonging to reproductive age groups and in perimenopausal age groups has been described in **Flowcharts 23.3 and 23.4**, respectively.

INVESTIGATIONS

Aim of diagnosis in cases of AUB is to assess the nature and severity of bleeding. In case of severe acute bleeding, the aim of management is to stabilize the patient by maintaining the airway, breathing, and circulation (ABC). In cases of severe bleeding, the emergency control of bleeding can be done through administration of conjugated estrogens. Once the bleeding has been controlled, steps must be taken to identify the underlying organic causes. The following investigations need to be undertaken.

BLOOD INVESTIGATIONS

Complete Blood Count

Estimation of the patient's hemoglobin levels with blood counts would help in determining the patient's degree of anemia. Chronic blood loss related to AUB may often result in the development of anemia.

Urine Human Chorionic Gonadotropin Levels

Pregnancy remains the most common cause of AUB in patients of reproductive age group. Bleeding could be related to pregnancy complications including threatened abortion, incomplete abortion, or ectopic pregnancy. Therefore, pregnancy should be the first diagnosis to be excluded before instituting further testing or medications.

Study of Coagulation Factors

Tests involving study of coagulation factors include prothrombin time, partial thromboplastin time, bleeding time, platelet count, assessment of Von Willebrand factor, etc. These tests are not routinely ordered because they are expensive and the bleeding disorders are rarely encountered. However, these studies may be required in case any bleeding disorders [e.g., Von Willebrand disease, idiopathic thrombocytopenic purpura (ITP), hemophilia, etc.] are suspected from history or if the platelet count is reduced.

Thyroid Function Tests

Though thyroid dysfunction can result in menorrhagia, thyroid function should not be routinely carried out on women with HMB. While menorrhagia may result due to hyperthyroidism, oligomenorrhea is more likely to result due to hypothyroidism. Thyroid testing should only be carried out when the patient shows signs and symptoms, suggestive of thyroid disease.

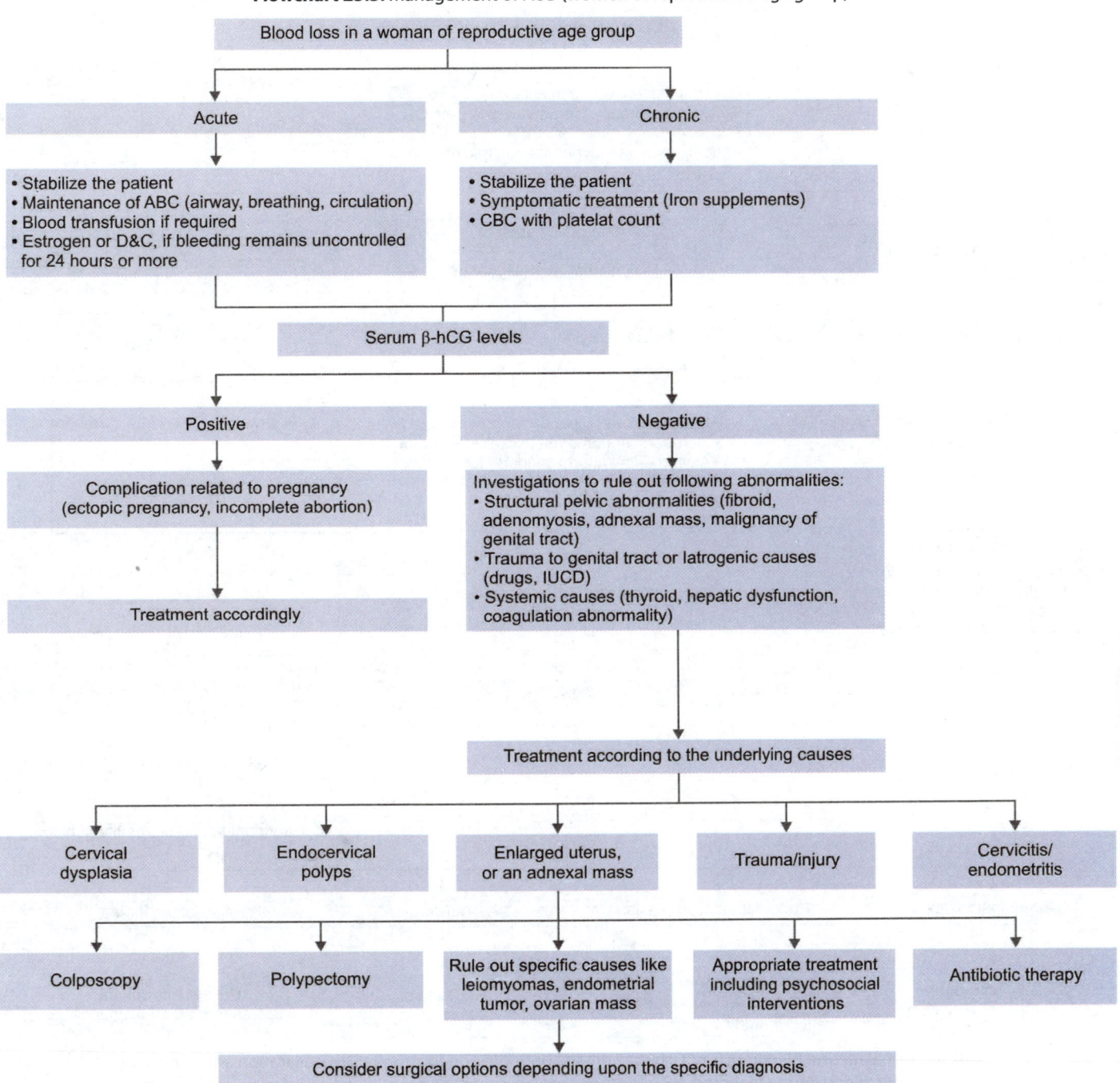

Flowchart 23.3: Management of AUB (women of reproductive age group).

(β–hCG: beta-human chorionic gonadotropin; AUB: abnormal uterine bleeding; CBC: complete blood count; D&C: dilatation and curettage; DUB: dysfunctional uterine; IUCD: intrauterine contraceptive device)

Liver Function and/or Renal Function Tests

Dysfunction of either organ can alter coagulation factors and/or the metabolism of hormones resulting in abnormal bleeding patterns. Liver function tests are ordered when liver disease is suspected, such as in persons with alcoholism or hepatitis. Liver function tests involve study of liver enzymes like serum glutamic oxaloacetic transaminase (SGOT), serum glutamic pyruvate transaminase (SGPT), alkaline phosphatase, etc., whereas tests like blood urea nitrogen (BUN) and creatinine levels assess renal functioning.

Hormone Assays

Measurement of luteinizing hormone (LH), follicle stimulating hormone (FSH), and androgen levels helps in diagnosing patients with suspected PCOS.

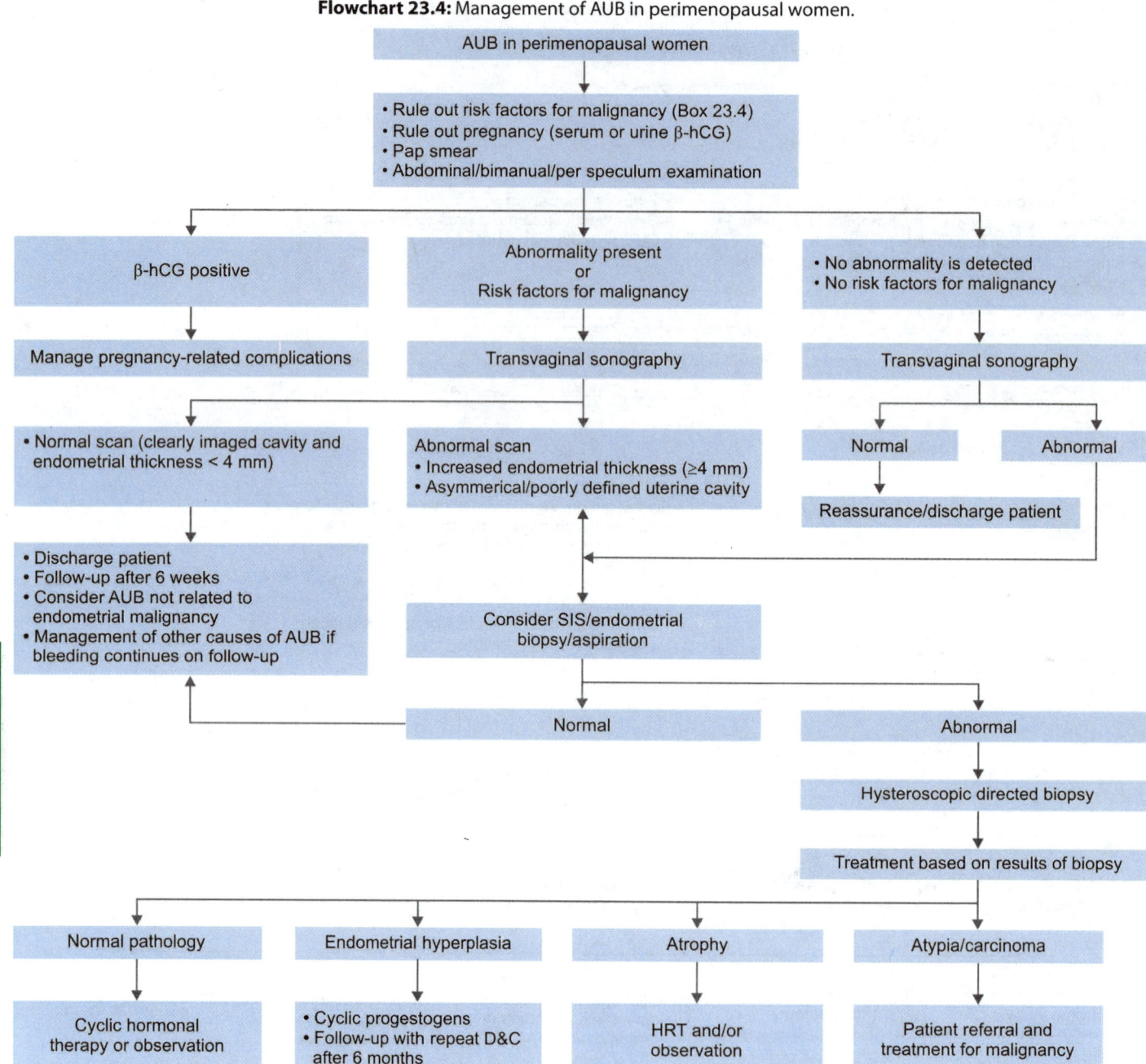

Flowchart 23.4: Management of AUB in perimenopausal women.

(AUB: abnormal uterine bleeding; β-hCG: beta-human chorionic gonadotropin; D&C: dilatation and curettage; DUB: dysfunctional uterine bleeding; HRT: hormone replacement therapy; SIS: saline infusion sonography;)

Iron Studies

This includes assessment of serum iron levels, total iron binding capacity, and ferritin levels.

■ IMAGING STUDIES

Ultrasound Examination

Pelvic ultrasound is the best noninvasive imaging investigation to assess uterine shape, size, and contour; endometrial thickness and adnexal areas. Imaging studies help in detection of small, focal, irregular, or eccentrically located endometrial lesions. Imaging should be undertaken if any of the conditions described in **Box 23.8** are suspected. Ultrasound examination can be performed through two routes: transabdominal and transvaginal. Both transabdominal and transvaginal ultrasound examinations help in inspecting the uterus, endometrium, and/or adnexa.

Transabdominal Ultrasound

Transabdominal sonography (TAS) helps in excluding pelvic masses, and various pregnancy-related complications. It helps in delineating the presence of an enlarged uterine cavity and/or presence of cystic/solid spaces within the uterine cavity Transvaginal sonography (TVS) complemented by Doppler ultrasonography may be more informative than TAS **(Figs. 23.3 to 23.5)**.

> **BOX 23.8:** Indications for imaging in case of abnormal uterine bleeding (AUB).
>
> - The uterus is palpable abdominally
> - Vaginal examination reveals a pelvic mass of uncertain origin
> - Pharmaceutical treatment fails
> - Bleeding in perimenopausal or postmenopausal women
> - AUB in a women over the age of 40 years, having a weight > 90 kg
> - AUB in women having any of the risk factors for development of endometrial cancer including infertility, nulliparity, family history of colon or endometrial cancer, and exposure to unopposed estrogens

Transvaginal Ultrasound

Transvaginal ultrasound is especially indicated in the women at high risk for endometrial cancer. Features suggestive of endometrial cancer on ultrasound examination are enlisted in **Box 23.9**.

Measurement of endometrial thickness on transvaginal ultrasound has become a routine investigation in patients with AUB, especially those belonging to the postmenopausal age groups. If the endometrial thickness on TVS is ≥4 mm, an endometrial sample should be taken to exclude endometrial hyperplasia. Increased endometrial thickness on transvaginal ultrasound examination is an indication for further follow-up by saline infusion sonography (SIS) or hysteroscopic-guided EB. Histopathological examination is especially important in these cases to rule out endometrial hyperplasia, atypia, and carcinoma. Endometrial sampling is not usually required in case the endometrial thickness is <4 mm. In premenopausal women with suspected endometrial neoplasia, sonographic measurement of endometrial thickness is not used as an alternative to endometrial sampling.

Normal Ultrasound Examination of the Uterus

On ultrasound imaging the normal myometrium should have a homogeneous echodensity. The bladder should be anechoic. Uterine measurements of 5 cm width, 4 cm anterior posterior plane thickness, and 8 cm length are taken as the general upper limits of a normal uterus.

The normal endometrium as visualized by TVS is described in Chapter 22. As described previously, the endometrial thickness and appearance changes during the various phases of the menstrual cycle.

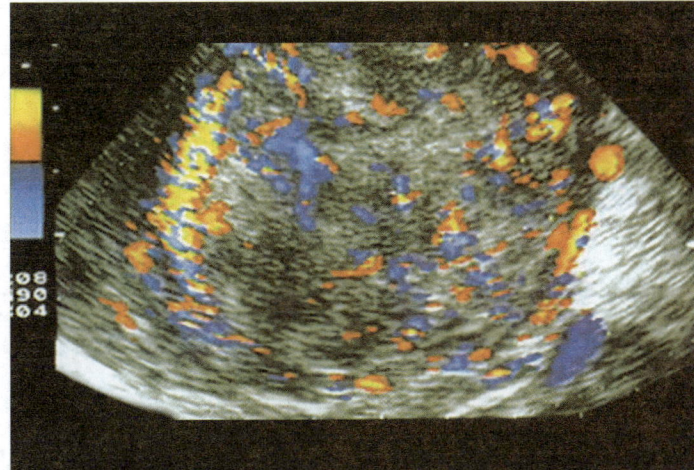

Fig. 23.3: Doppler ultrasound in a patient with endometrial carcinoma; there were prominent peripheral and central vascular signals on ultrasound, which revealed presence of an advanced stage III endometrial adenocarcinoma.

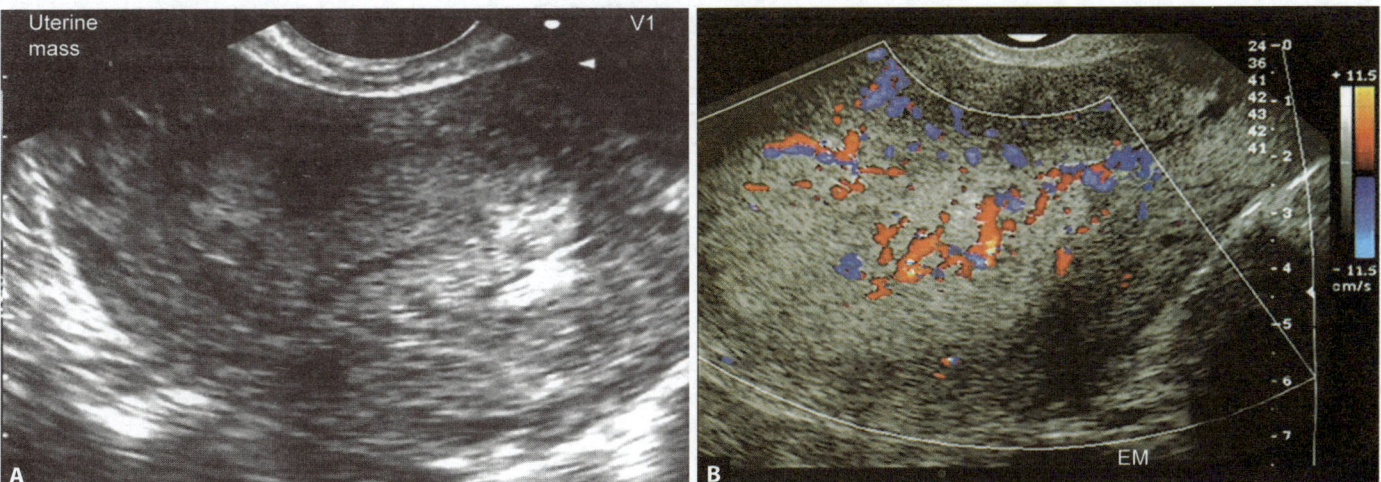

Figs. 23.4A and B: (A) Transvaginal ultrasound in a 52-year-old menopausal patient with the complaints of irregular bleeding and offensive vaginal discharge since 2–3 months. Ultrasound revealed the presence of a heterogeneous mass within the endometrial cavity, which was observed to be replacing the normal endometrial stripe; (B) Doppler ultrasound in the same patient showing increased vascular flow. Hysteroscopic-guided biopsy revealed the diagnosis of advanced stage endometrial cancer.

500 Normal and Abnormal Menstruation

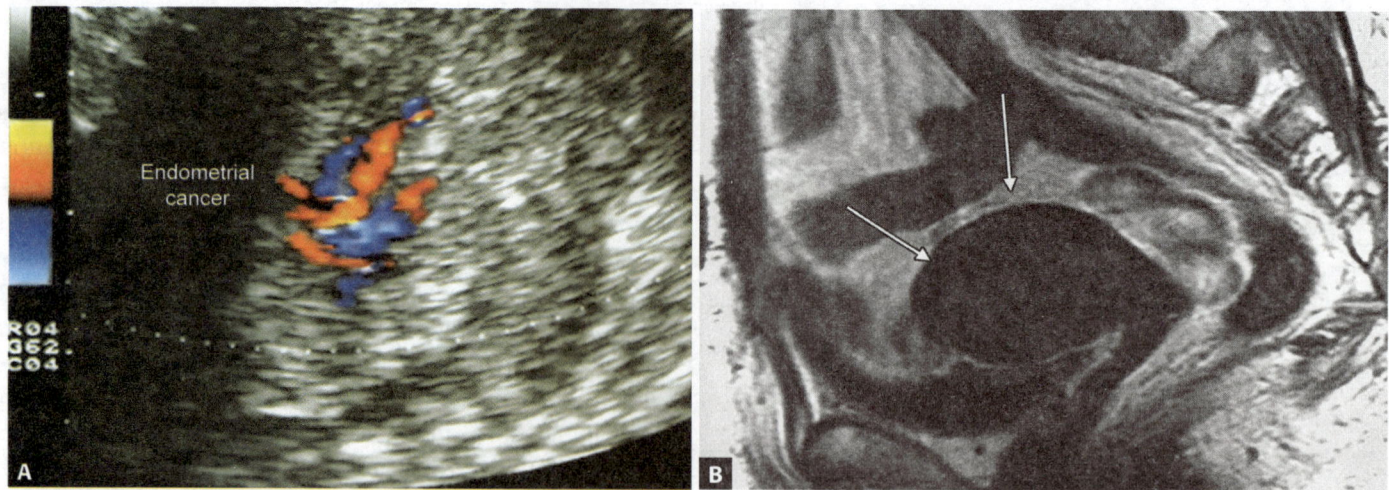

Fig. 23.5A and B: (A) Color Doppler examination in a 58-year-old postmenopausal patient presenting with irregular bleeding and abdominal pain since 1 month. Color Doppler ultrasound examination revealed thick heterogeneous endometrium with proliferation of blood vessels. A diagnosis of advanced stage endometrial cancer was made; (B) Magnetic resonance imaging scan showing endometrial adenocarcinoma in the same patient as described in (A). T1-weighted images on MRI examination revealed a large tumor of low-signal intensity, expanding within the uterine cavity. There was no spread to distant body organs. On the basis of findings of clinical and radiological examination, the disease was classified as stage III endometrial cancer.

> **BOX 23.9:** Features suggestive of endometrial cancer on transvaginal sonography.
>
> - Heterogeneous and irregular endometrial thickening
> - Polypoid mass lesion
> - Intrauterine fluid collection
> - Frank myometrial invasion
> - Disruption of subendometrial halo on ultrasound may also be suggestive of myometrial involvement

SALINE INFUSION SONOGRAPHY

Saline SIS serves as an alternative to hysteroscopy. This technique employs the use of sterile saline solution as a negative contrast medium in conjunction with traditional transvaginal ultrasound **(Fig. 23.6)**. Thus, besides imaging the uterine cavity, this technique also helps in evaluating the patency of the fallopian tubes. The advantage of SIS over hysteroscopy is that this technique also helps in scanning the ovaries, pelvis, and peritoneal cavity, while imaging the uterine cavity. While abdominal or transvaginal ultrasound can identify myomas and thickened endometrium, these imaging techniques are unable to differentiate between the various potential etiologies of thickened endometrium, e.g., polyps, submucous myomas, homogenously thickened endometrium, etc. Sonohysterography helps in differentiating between these intracavitary lesions and focal or diffuse endometrial abnormalities and helps in determining whether an abnormality is endometrial or subendometrial in origin **(Figs. 23.7A and B)**. SIS is able to clearly delineate the masses or defects inside the uterine cavity. SIS helps in differentiating between focal lesions (polyps and submucosal myomas) and global endometrial thickening. SIS can be used as a second-line diagnostic procedure in women with AUB when findings from transvaginal ultrasound are nonconclusive.

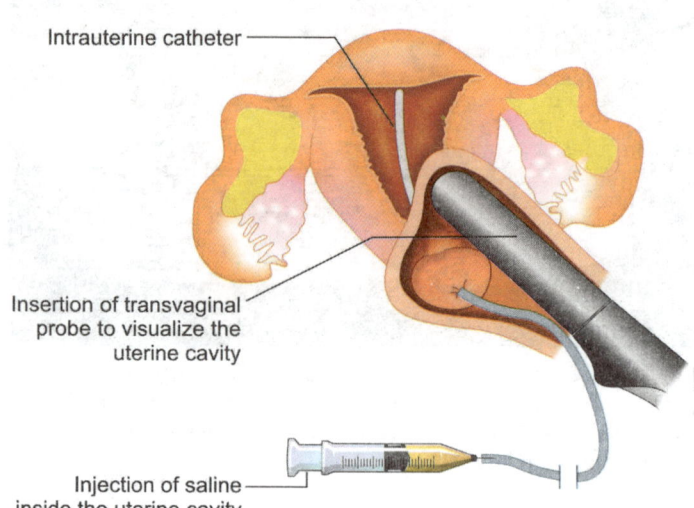

Fig. 23.6: Procedure of doing saline infusion sonography.

Saline SIS is associated with minor side effects like pelvic discomfort (cramping or menstrual like pain). Complications like severe pain and infection can occur, but are relatively rare. SIS has been observed to have high sensitivity rate of 94.9% and specificity rate of 89.3%. Thus, this would help in avoiding hysteroscopy in nearly 40% cases. There is a theoretical possibility of propulsion of cancer cells from the uterine cavity into the peritoneal cavity. This can be prevented by using low pressure infusion in women at risk for cancer.

Procedure

The procedure of SIS involves the following steps:
1. The patient is asked to empty her bladder.
2. A speculum is used to expose the cervix, which is cleansed with a betadine swab.

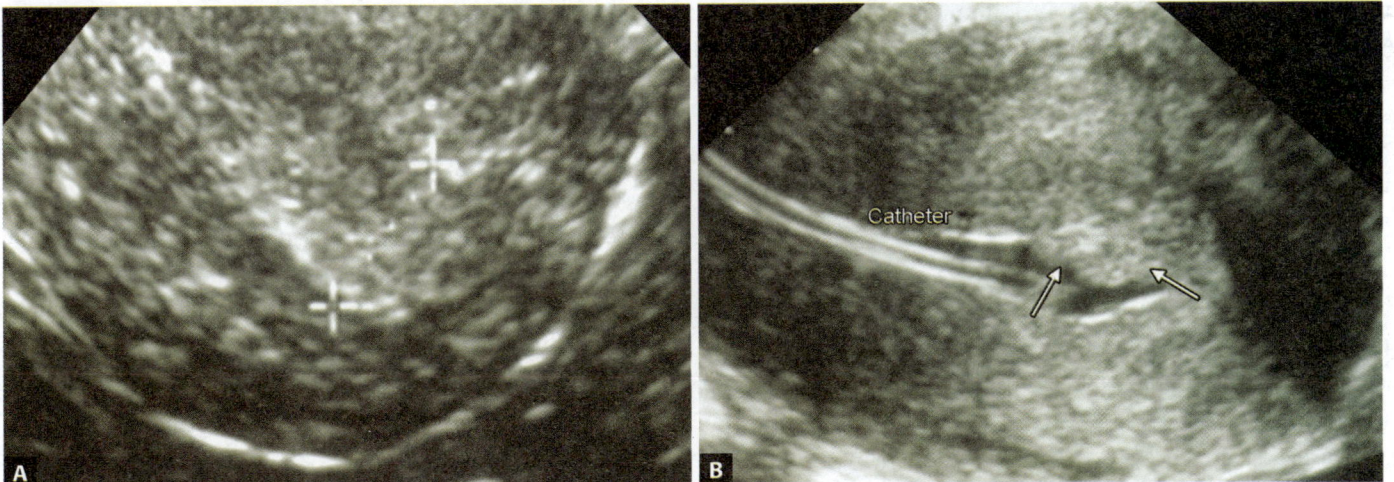

Figs. 23.7A and B: (A) Presence of thickened endometrium on TVS in a patient with AUB; (B) Saline infusion sonography of the same patient, as mentioned in (A), revealing presence of an endometrial polyp.

3. A catheter is then inserted inside the uterine cavity. Various catheters may be used, including: 5-F urinary catheter, with or without an occlusive balloon; pediatric feeding tubes; insemination catheters, etc.
4. It is important to flush the catheter with sterile saline solution before inserting it inside the uterine cavity in order to prevent the introduction of echogenic air bubbles.
5. Advancement of the catheter inside the uterine cavity can be assisted by grasping the end of the catheter 2–3 cm from the tip with a ring forceps and gently feeding it through the cervical os so as to position the tip beyond the endocervical canal.
6. After the correct placement of the catheter, the speculum is carefully removed while the catheter is left in place. Following the correct placement of the catheter, sterile saline solution is instilled inside the uterine cavity. Only about 2–5 mL of sterile solution is required to produce an adequate distension.
7. While the sterile saline solution is being instilled inside the uterine cavity, a covered transvaginal probe is inserted into the vagina and continuous scanning in the sagittal and coronal or transverse planes is performed.
8. There is no contraindication to SIS in nonpregnant, noninfected women who are bleeding.
9. The procedure can cause vagal episodes, particularly in nulliparous women who have not had any children in the past. In such cases, premedication with nonsteroidal antiinflammatory drugs (NSAIDs) such as ibuprofen or naproxen is recommended.

CT SCAN

Computed tomography scan in cases of endometrial carcinoma helps the surgeon in assessing the distant metastasis. Otherwise, CT scan is likely to be more useful in cases of ovarian malignancy for the primary assessment of the tumor rather than the endometrial one.

MRI SCAN

Magnetic resonance imaging examination is recommended for assessing the extension of optimal disease and is usually considered superior to CT scan for local staging. Contrast-enhanced MRI imaging further improves the accuracy in detecting myometrial invasion or cervical involvement. Both in cases of cervical and endometrial malignancy, MRI offers the best diagnostic accuracy for staging, assessing lymphadenopathy, defining advanced disease, planning radiation ports, monitoring response to treatment as well as post treatment surveillance to detect relapse.

ENDOMETRIAL STUDIES

In case the endometrial thickness is > 4 mm on transvaginal ultrasound examination, endometrial studies should be done in order to exclude endometrial hyperplasia. Endometrial sampling is usually performed with an office EB, which can be performed in an outpatient setting, most commonly using a pipelle device, without any requirement for anesthesia and is a noninvasive approach.

ENDOMETRIAL BIOPSY

Endometrial biopsy is the most commonly used diagnostic test for AUB, which helps in providing histopathological examination of the endometrium. It helps in providing an adequate sample for diagnosis of endometrial problems in nearly 90–100% of cases. However, it may fail to detect the presence of small masses including polyps and leiomyomas. The indications for EB are listed in **Box 23.10**. Perimenopausal and menopausal women with bleeding following a period of amenorrhea must also have an EB because these women are at a high risk for development of endometrial carcinoma, polyps, or hyperplasia in future. Other patients who are at an increased risk of development of endometrial malignancy include patients with triad of hypertension, diabetes, and obesity and those with chronic anovulation (e.g., PCOS), atypical glandular cells (AGUS) on Pap smear, new-onset menorrhagia, etc. EB can be performed as an outpatient investigation and does not require general anesthesia as is required for D&C. Thus, this procedure has superseded D&C and has presently become the gold standard for obtaining endometrial tissue and for detecting endometrial diseases.

Histological Findings on Endometrial Biopsy

Identifying the underlying endometrial histopathology is important for the gynecologist in order to initiate correct treatment for AUB. While most cases of hyperplasia without atypia are likely to regress on their own, atypical hyperplasia/endometrioid intraepithelial neoplasia is likely to progress to malignancy in 25–33% cases. Details related to endometrial hyperplasia have been described later in the text.

BOX 23.10: Indications for endometrial biopsy.
- Endometrial thickness on TVS is ≥ 4 mm (in postmenopausal women)
- Persistent intermenstrual bleeding
- AUB in a woman > 35 years of age
- AUB in postmenopausal women
- Treatment failure or ineffective treatment
- Patients having high risk factors for the development of endometrial cancer
- There is a pelvic mass and the uterus is > 10 weeks gestation in size
- There is a pelvic mass and no facility for urgent ultrasound scan is available
- Patient with the history of unopposed exposure to estrogens
  - Clinical history suggestive of long-term estrogen exposure even in the presence of normal endometrial thickness
  - Endometrial thickness >12 mm despite of low-clinical disease suspicion

(AUB: abnormal uterine bleeding; TVS: transvaginal sonography)

Procedure of Endometrial Sampling/Biopsy

Endometrial sampling is performed without any prior cervical dilatation and comprises of the following steps:

- Firstly, the patient is placed in the lithotomy position and then a bimanual examination is conducted in order to assess the uterus (size, position, presence of masses, etc.).
- The cervix is then visualized with help of a Sim's speculum and a tenaculum (which is applied over the anterior lip of cervix). The cervical os is cleaned with help of betadine solution.
- A uterine sound is then inserted gently through the cervical os until the sound passes easily to the fundus. The distance from the fundus to the external cervical os can be measured with the help of gradations on the uterine sound and is usually equal to 6–8 cm. This helps in assessing the position and size of the uterine cavity and minimizing the risk of perforation.
- When the position and size of the uterine cavity have been assessed, the EB curette **(Figs. 23.8A and B)** is inserted gently inside the uterine cavity until any significant resistance is felt **(Fig. 23.9A)**. The EB curette is a narrow metal cannula having serrated edges with side openings on one end and a syringe can be attached for suction at the other end.
- While inside the uterine cavity, the cannula is rotated several times in order to scrape off the endometrial lining **(Figs. 23.9B and C)**.
- This procedure should be repeated at least four times and the device rotated by 360° to ensure adequate coverage of the area.
- These endometrial scrapings are then sucked into the syringe.
- When adequate amount of endometrial curetting have been obtained, the curette is removed and samples are sent for microscopic examination.

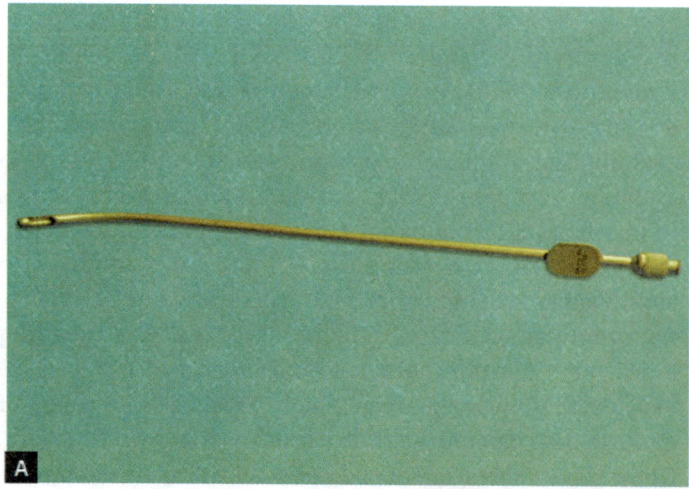
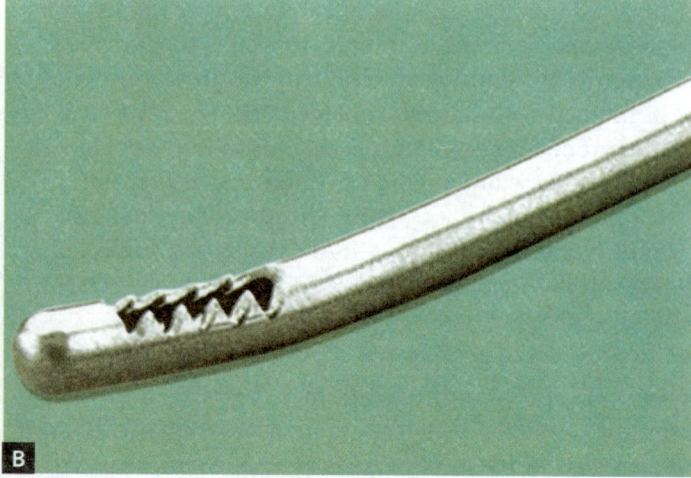

Figs 23.8A and B: Endometrial biopsy curette. (A) Photograph showing endometrial biopsy curette; (B) Magnified view showing the upper end of the biopsy curette with serrated edges.

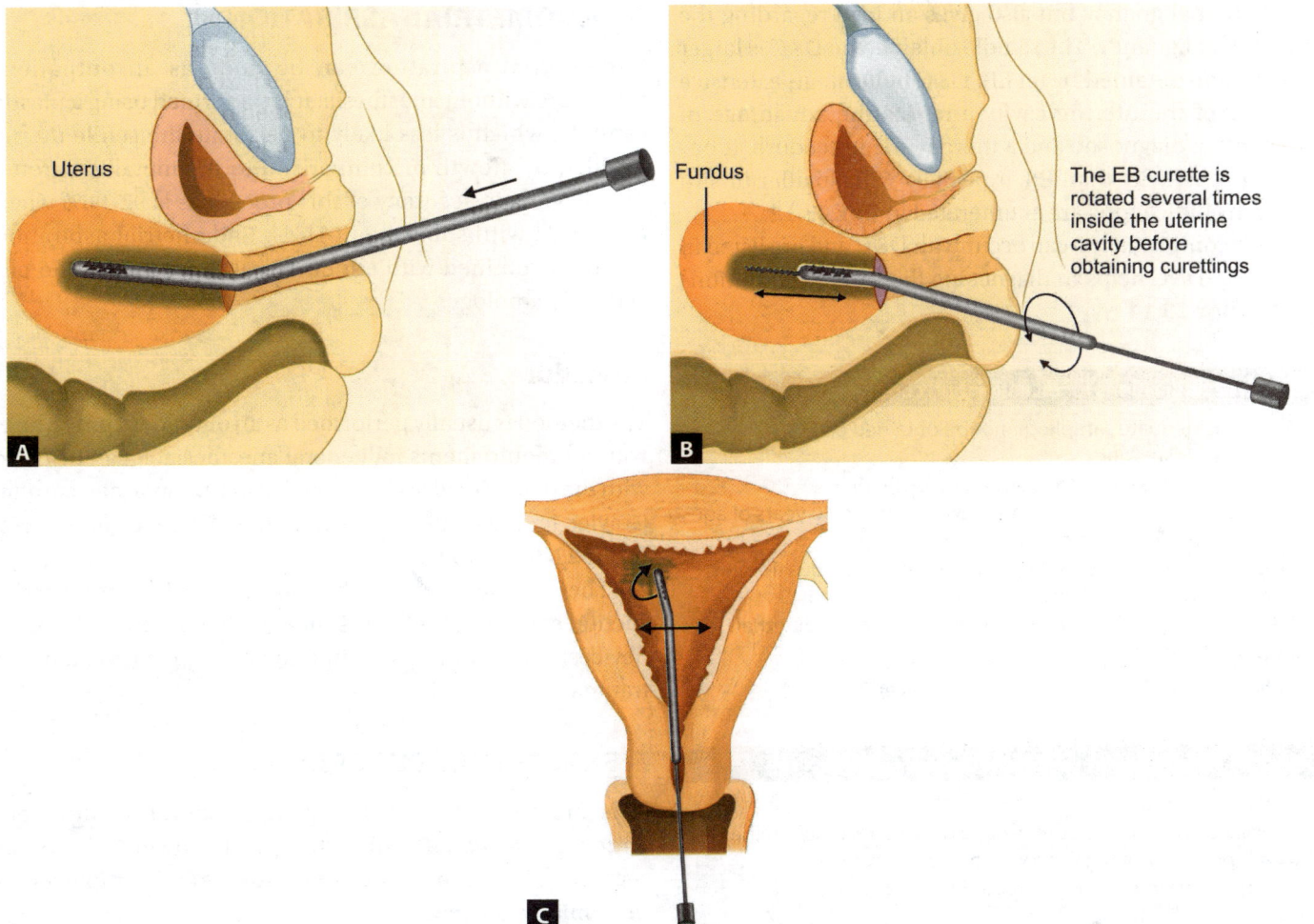

Figs. 23.9A to C: (A) Placement of the EB curette inside the uterine cavity; (B) Before obtaining the endometrial curettings, the EB curette is rotated several times inside the uterus; (C) Transverse section of endometrial cavity showing the EB curette.

- One set of sample is sent in normal saline for assessment of acid-fast bacilli (AFB). Other set of sample is sent in acetone for assessment of histopathology. Normal endometrial tissue may be described as proliferative or preovulatory (under the effect of hormone estrogen) and secretory or postovulatory endometrium (under the effect of hormone progesterone).
- Endometrial biopsy should not be performed in the presence of a normal or ectopic pregnancy. All patients with the potential for pregnancy should be considered for pregnancy testing prior to the performance of the procedure.

Complications

Though EB is largely a safe procedure, it can be associated with certain complications which are tabulated in the **Box 23.11**.

DILATATION AND CURETTAGE

Though this procedure was frequently done in the past for AUB, it is rarely done nowadays. Some surgeons may choose to perform D&C as the initial procedure in some women.

> **BOX 23.11:** Complications of endometrial biopsy.
> - Prolonged bleeding
> - Infection, bacteremia, sepsis, and acute bacterial endocarditis
> - Uterine perforation
> - Intraoperative and postoperative cramping

This may include the women who cannot tolerate an office biopsy, those with heavy bleeding (D&C serves as a both therapeutic and diagnostic procedure in these cases) and women who are at a high risk of developing endometrial cancer (e.g., those with Lynch syndrome). Women having insufficient endometrial cells with EB may undergo D&C. Evaluation with D&C may be required in case of persistent or recurrent bleeding, even after office EB reveals benign findings.

The procedure of D&C involves obtaining scrapings from the endometrium and the cervix and is usually performed under general anesthesia. The procedure involves gradual dilatation of the cervix to <8 cm under general anesthesia, followed by the use of small sharp curette for systematic, thorough, gentle sampling of all parts of the uterine cavity including tubal osteal areas. Not only does it help in detecting the site of malignancy but also gives an idea regarding the spread of malignancy. The sample obtained on D&C is larger than the one obtained by an EB. D&C helps in an extensive sampling of the uterine cavity and has the advantage of being both a diagnostic and a therapeutic procedure. It has a higher sensitivity than EB, especially with smaller in-situ lesions. Its indications are enumerated in **Box 23.12**.

A few complications can occur with D&C and are listed in **Box 23.13**. D&C helps in diagnosing the various conditions listed in **Box 23.14**.

> **BOX 23.12:** Indications for dilatation and curettage.
>
> - When an adequate sample cannot be obtained on EB
> - Cervical os is stenotic
> - Medical treatment fails to control severe bleeding
> - Persistent or recurrent bleeding between 20 and 40 years of age and the clinical suspicion of malignancy is high
> - Diagnosis of endometrial polyps, intrauterine mucous fibroids, areas of endometritis, hyperplasia or cancer, or lost IUDs
> - Bleeding recurs following a negative report on endometrial biopsy/aspiration
>
> (EB: endometrial biopsy; IUD: intrauterine device)

> **BOX 23.13:** Complications of dilatation and curettage.
>
> - Uterine perforation
> - Cervical damage due to use of large dilators, resulting in the development of cervical incompetence in future
> - Postoperative infection or intrauterine adhesions

> **BOX 23.14:** Advantages of dilatation and curettage.
>
> - Diagnosis of organic disease, e.g., tuberculosis
> - Diagnosis of uterine pathology, e.g., endometritis, polyp, carcinoma, fibroids, etc.
> - *Diagnosing the type of endometrial histopathology:* Hyperplastic, proliferative, secretory, irregular ripening, irregular shedding, atrophic endometrium, etc.
> - Therapeutic effect (controversial)
> - Arrest of severe or persistent bleeding, particularly that associated with hyperplastic endometrium

ENDOMETRIAL ASPIRATION

Endometrial aspiration can be done as an outpatient procedure without anesthesia. It is performed using a plastic cannula, which is less likely to perforate the senile uterus invaded by growth in comparison to the metallic curette. The diagnostic accuracy of this procedure is 92–98% when compared with subsequent D&C. Endometrial aspiration is often combined with endocervical curettage to rule out cervical pathology.

Procedure

The method is usually performed as an outpatient procedure, without requirements for general anesthesia. It can be done with the help of devices like, pipelle curette, Sharman curette, Gravlee jet washer, Isaacs cell sampler, Vabra® aspirator, etc. **(Figs. 23.10A and B)**.

The sample produced by the newer slim endometrial suction curettes (pipelle) is similar to that produced by older devices, while at the same time causing much less pain and trauma.

FRACTIONAL CURETTAGE

This method involves taking three samples, one from endocervical canal, and others from lower and upper segments. This procedure is nowadays rarely employed in the clinical practice.

CERVICAL CULTURES AND PAPANICOLAOU SMEAR

Cervical cultures and a Pap smear are appropriate initial steps to evaluate for the presence of sexually transmitted diseases or cervical dysplasia. Examination of cervical cytology is not a very sensitive test for detection of endometrial cancer and is presently not recommended for the screening of endometrial cancer.

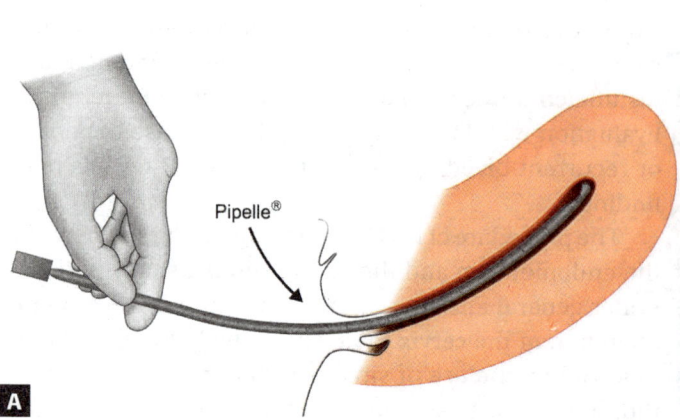
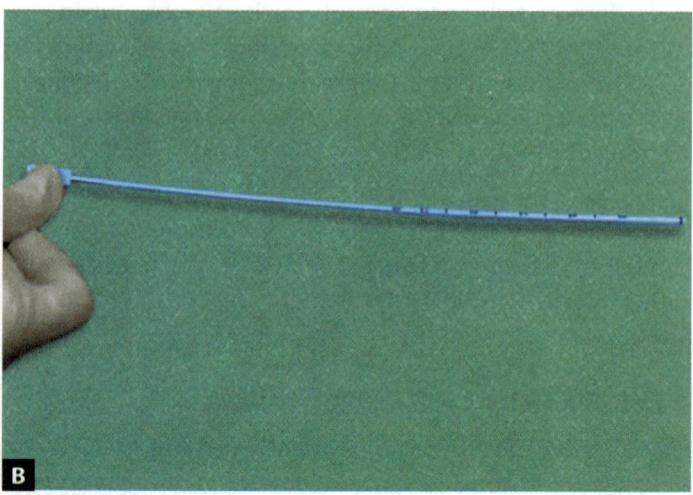

Figs. 23.10A and B: (A) Diagram showing endometrial aspiration; (B) Pipelle® endometrial sampler for doing endometrial aspiration.

Abnormal Uterine Bleeding due to Endometrial Cancer

HYSTEROSCOPY

Nowadays, hysteroscopy with biopsy can be regarded as the "gold standard" investigation for the diagnosis of AUB. Hysteroscopy with biopsy provides the most comprehensive evaluation of the endometrium and is recommended for use in any woman with equivocal or suspicious findings on biopsy or ultrasonography **(Fig. 23.11)**. Some of the indications for use of hysteroscopy are described in **Box 23.15**. Hysteroscopy allows for direct visualization of the endometrial cavity along with the facility for directed biopsy. Therefore, it serves as a better option in comparison to D&C alone. Some of the advantages of hysteroscopy over D&C are described in **Box 23.16**.

However, there are the following disadvantages associated with the use of hysteroscopy: It is a more invasive procedure, is associated with significant financial cost, as well as more physical discomfort in comparison to EB or D&C. Also, hysteroscopy may not be always available, especially in the primary setup.

SCREENING FOR ENDOMETRIAL CANCER

Presently, routine screening of women for endometrial cancer is not recommended. The only exception to this is the women with Lynch syndrome who are at a markedly high risk for developing endometrial cancer and therefore must undergo screening. Strategies for screening and prevention of endometrial cancer in these women include endometrial sampling and risk-reducing hysterectomy. Presently, there are no recommendations for routine screening for asymptomatic patients on tamoxifen. However, any abnormal bleeding in a patient on tamoxifen needs to be further evaluated.

ENDOMETRIAL HYPERPLASIA

> **Q. Write a long essay discussing the classification and management of endometrial hyperplasia.**

Chronic proliferation of the endometrium results in the development of hyperplasia (first simple hyperplasia, followed by atypical hyperplasia), leading to the development of endometrial carcinoma in future. Endometrial hyperplasia usually results from unopposed estrogen production, regardless of the etiology. If a woman takes unopposed estrogen (without progesterone), her relative risk of developing endometrial cancer is 2.3 compared to that of nonusers and increases to 9.5, if unopposed estrogens are taken for 10 years or longer.

As per the WHO (1994), endometrial hyperplasia was traditionally classified into four groups based on glandular complexity as simple (cystic) or complex (adenomatous), with or without cytological atypia as follows:

1. Simple hyperplasia (cystic without atypia)
2. Complex hyperplasia (adenomatous without atypia)
3. Simple hyperplasia (cystic with atypia)
4. Complex hyperplasia (adenomatous with atypia)

Endometrial intraepithelial neoplasia (EIN) classification was subsequently proposed by the endometrium Collaborative group in 2000 and included two categories:

- Endometrial hyperplasia (benign)
- Premalignant lesion (endometrial intraepithelial neoplasia)

The premalignant lesion could progress into malignancy (well-differentiated endometrial adenocarcinoma) over the long run. As per the ACOG, the EIN classification was considered superior to WHO (1994) classification system.

Subsequently, in 2014 WHO proposed a new classification system **(Table 23.8)**, which is accepted by the international society of gynecological pathologists and divided endometrial hyperplasia into two categories **(Figs. 23.12A to C)**:

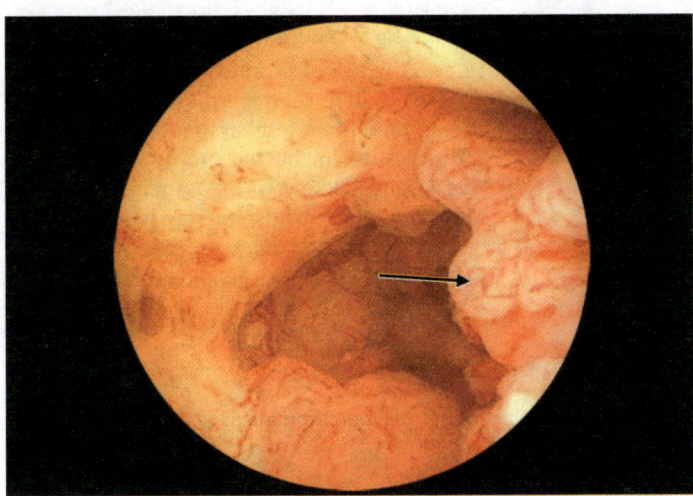

Fig. 23.11: Hysteroscopic appearance of an exophytic endometrial cancer growth (indicated by arrow)

BOX 23.15: Indications for hysteroscopy and biopsy.

- Women with erratic/irregular menstrual bleeding
- Medical therapy has failed to control the bleeding
- Transvaginal ultrasound suggestive of intrauterine pathology such as polyps or submucous fibroids.

BOX 23.16: Advantages of hysteroscopy over dilatation and curettage.

- Diagnosis of polyps, submucous fibroids, hyperplasia, etc.
- The whole uterine cavity can be visualized with hysteroscopy; very small lesions such as polyps can be identified and biopsied or removed at the time of hysteroscopy
- Biopsy of the suspicious areas can also be carried out
- Hysteroscopy is more sensitive than D&C, especially at diagnosing polyps and submucosal leiomyomas
- In combination with EB, hysteroscopy has almost 100% accuracy in diagnosing endometrial dysplasia and cancer
- Bleeding from ruptured venules and ecchymoses can be readily identified

(D&C: dilatation and curettage; EB: endometrial biopsy)

TABLE 23.8: Classification of endometrial hyperplasia proposed by WHO (2014).

New term	Synonyms	Genetic changes	Progression to invasive endometrial carcinoma	Treatment
Hyperplasia without atypia	Benign endometrial hyperplasia; simple nonatypical endometrial hyperplasia; complex nonatypical endometrial hyperplasia; simple endometrial hyperplasia without atypia; complex endometrial hyperplasia without atypia	Low level of somatic mutations in scattered glands with morphology on histopathological examination staining showing no changes	<5% over 20 years (majority of cases will regress spontaneously during follow-up)	Since majority of cases are likely to regress on their own, observation alone is likely to be successful. Progestogen treatment may be required in women who do not retreat following observation alone and in symptomatic women with AUB. The LNG-IUS (for a minimum of 6 months) acts as the first-line medical treatment. Second line therapy comprises of using continuous progestogens (medroxyprogesterone 10–20 mg/day or norethisterone 10–15 mg/day) for a minimum of 6 months in women who decline LNG-IUS. Use of cyclical progestogens should be avoided. Women should be advised to retain the LNG-IUS for up to 5 years especially if the adverse effects are tolerable and fertility is not desired, because this is likely to reduce the risk of future relapse
Atypical hyperplasia/ endometrioid intraepithelial neoplasia	Complex atypical endometrial hyperplasia; simple atypical endometrial hyperplasia; endometrial intraepithelial neoplasia	Many of the genetic changes typical for endometrioid endometrial cancer are present, including: micro satellite instability; PAX2 inactivation; mutation of PTEN, KRAS and CTNNB1 (β-catenin)	25–33%	Due to the risk of progression to malignancy in cases of atypical hyperplasia such women should undergo a total hysterectomy. Laparoscopic route for hysterectomy is preferred because it is likely to be associated with a shorter duration of hospital stay, reduced post-operative pain, and quicker recovery time

(AUB: abnormal uterine bleeding; KRAS: Kirsten rat sarcoma viral oncogene homolog; LNG-IUS: levonorgestrel-releasing intrauterine system; PTEN: phosphatase and TENsin homolog)

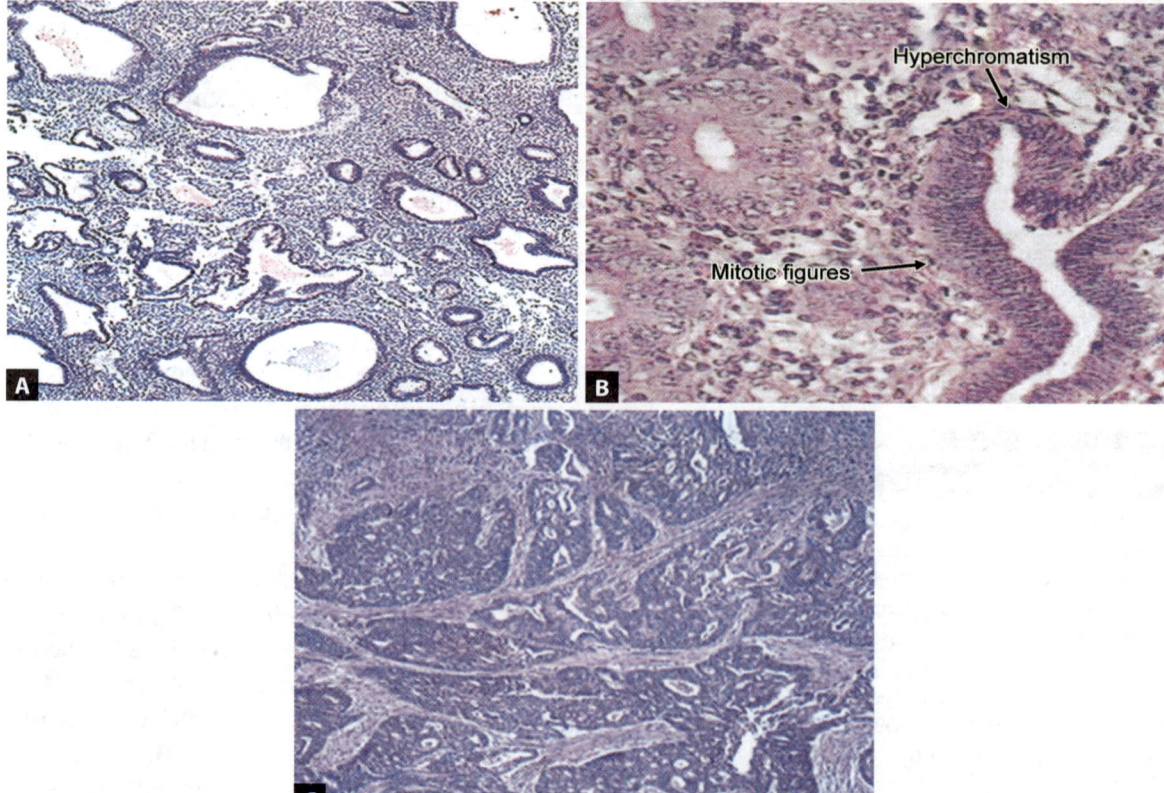

Figs. 23.12A to C: Histopathological appearance of various endometrial changes. (A) Benign endometrial hyperplasia; (B) Histopathological appearance of endometrioid intraepithelial neoplasia; (C) Histopathological appearance of frank adenocarcinoma endometrium.

- Hyperplasia without atypia
- Atypical hyperplasia or endometrioid intraepithelial neoplasia

This new classification by WHO (2014) is likely to be more successful in identification of precancerous lesions amongst women at risk of progression to malignancy in future.

Management of Endometrial Hyperplasia

Management algorithm in cases of endometrial hyperplasia is described in **Flowchart 23.5 and Table 23.8**.

Women with endometrial hyperplasia, who are on HRT, should avoid using systemic estrogen-only HRT, especially

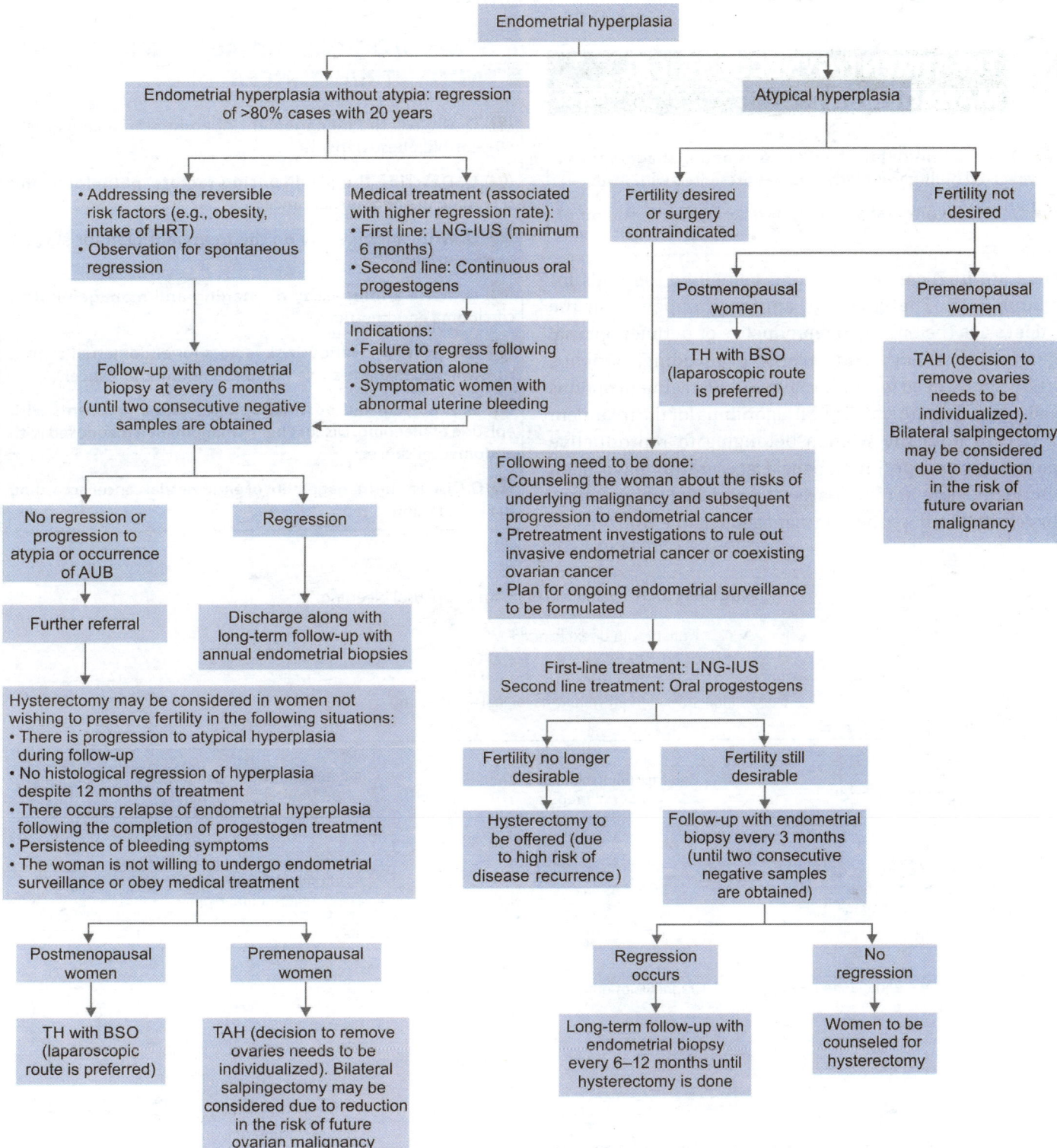

Flowchart 23.5: Management of endometrial hyperplasia.

(AUB: abnormal uterine bleeding; BSO: bilateral salpingo-oophorectomy; HRT: hormone replacement therapy; LNG-IUS: levonorgestrel-releasing intrauterine system; TAH: total abdominal hysterectomy; TH: total hysterectomy)

if their uterus is intact. They should be encouraged to start using a combined HRT preparation. They should also be advised to immediately report any unscheduled vaginal bleeding. Women already taking a sequential combined HRT preparation, and wishing to continue using HRT, should be encouraged to change to a source of continuous progestogen replacement using the levonorgestrel-releasing IUS (LNG-IUS) or a continuous combined HRT preparation.

℞ TREATMENT/GYNECOLOGICAL MANAGEMENT

 Q. Discuss in detail the diagnosis and management of 38 years old multiparous lady who has presented with AUB.

Q. Discuss alternatives to hysterectomy for treatment of AUB.

There are medical, surgical, and combined methods for treating AUB. The choice of approach depends on the patient's age (belonging to reproductive or perimenopausal age group), etiology and severity of bleeding, patient's fertility status, need for contraception, and treatment options available at the care site. Typical algorithms for the treatment of AUB in both the women belonging to reproductive age groups and perimenopausal age groups have been described before in **Flowcharts 23.3 and 23.4**, respectively. **Flowchart 23.6** describes the management of PMB.

Medical treatment is the option of choice in young women (<20 years of age) presenting with atypical bleeding. This has been described in detail in Chapter 24. Surgical options used for treatment of AUB can be of two types—(1) uterine conservative surgery (endometrial ablation) and (2) hysterectomy. Both the treatment options in presence of benign uterine pathology have also been discussed in detail in Chapter 24.

GYNECOLOGICAL MANAGEMENT OF ENDOMETRIAL CANCER

Q. Discuss the management of endometrial cancer in a 40-year-old obese patient.

Q. Describe the predisposing factors, pathology, and screening of endometrial cancer.

Q. Write a long essay on the treatment plan for stage 1 endometrial cancer.

Q. Write a long essay on staging and management of carcinoma endometrium.

Q. Discuss the various risk factors for endometrial cancer. How will you manage stage1 grade 3 endometrial cancer?

Q. A 60-year-old postmenopausal woman presents with episode of bleeding. Discuss her management if diagnosed with endometrial cancer.

Q. Discuss the management of endometrial cancer according to FIGO staging.

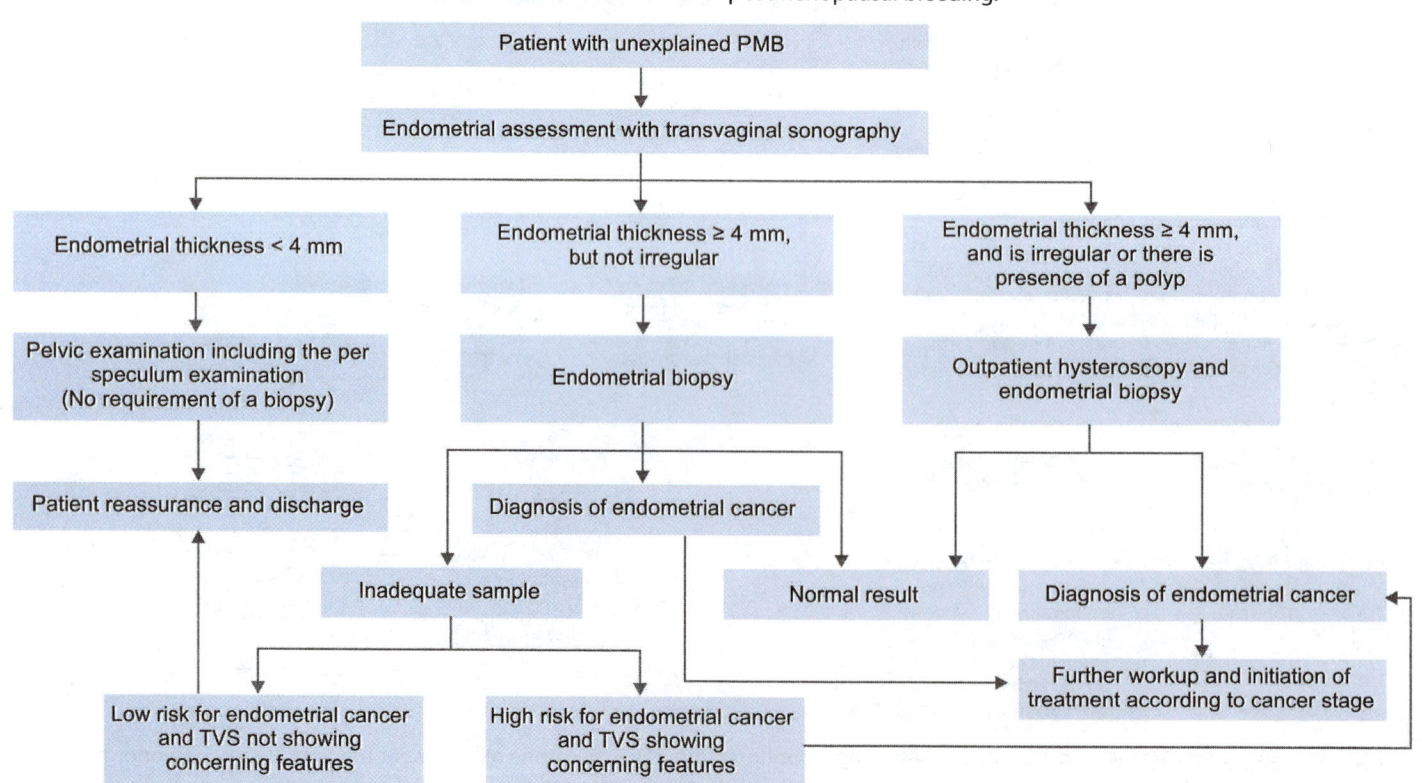

Flowchart 23.6: Evaluation of postmenopausal bleeding.

> **Q.** What should be the likely management plan in the case study mentioned in the beginning of the chapter?
>
> **Q.** In the above-mentioned case study, what does the patient's history suggest? How is it significant regarding her current situation?
>
> **Ans.** The history of the patient suggests that she most probably suffered from chronic anovulation as a result of polycystic ovarian disease. She was most probably prescribed clomiphene citrate for ovulation induction. Chronic anovulation is likely to cause unopposed endometrial stimulation with estrogen, resulting in development of endometrial hyperplasia and/or cancer in the long run. There are also other factors in the patient's history such as nulliparity, high BMI, high blood pressure and the patient belonging to perimenopausal age group, which point towards a high risk for development of endometrial malignancy.

The most serious concern in postmenopausal and perimenopausal women with AUB is endometrial carcinoma. Investigations in these cases must be mainly directed toward ruling out endometrial cancer. This mainly involves the assessment of endometrial thickness using TVS and study of endometrial cytology using EB, aspiration, D&C, or hysteroscopic guided biopsy.

STAGING OF ENDOMETRIAL CANCER

FIGO and TNM Staging of endometrial cancer are described in the **Table 23.9**. Total extrafascial hysterectomy with bilateral salpingo-oophorectomy (BSO) with pelvic and para-aortic lymph node dissection is the standard procedure used for staging endometrial cancer. If metastases are evident, cytoreduction may be performed. While staging is commonly performed via laparotomy or robot-assisted laparoscopy, vaginal or conventional approaches may be used for some women. Surgery alone is curative for women who are at a low risk of disease persistence or recurrence. Women with intermediate or high-risk disease may require adjuvant therapy.

Most patients with endometrial cancer must undergo surgical staging. Complete surgical staging involves—total hysterectomy, BSO, pelvic, and para-aortic lymph node dissection. Omentectomy, peritoneal biopsies, and peritoneal washings are less routinely performed and considered mostly in nonendometrioid endometrial cancer (NEEC) patients. Lymphadenectomy may be omitted in patients with negligible risk of lymphatic spread. Detection of occult, microscopic metastases upstages patients. This provides important prognostic information to the gynecologist, enabling them to plan the adjuvant treatment accordingly.

Degree of Differentiation

Based on the degree of differentiation of cells present on histopathological examination, endometrial carcinoma can be classified into three grades—grade 1 (G1), grade 2 (G2), and grade 3 (G3). These are described in **Box 23.17**.

TABLE 23.9: Staging of endometrial cancer.

TNM staging	FIGO stage	Characteristics
Tx		Primary tumor cannot be assessed
T0		No evidence of primary tumor
T1	Stage I[a]	Tumor confined to the corpus uteri[a]
T1a	Stage IA[a]	No or less than half myometrial invasion
T1b	Stage IB	Invasion equal to or more than half of the myometrium
T2	Stage II	Tumor invades cervical stroma, but does not extend beyond the uterus
T3	Stage III	Local and/or regional spread of the tumor
T3a	Stage IIIA	Tumor invades the serosa of corpus uteri and/or adnexa
T3b	Stage IIIB	Vaginal and/or parametrial involvement
T3c	Stage IIIC	Metastasis to pelvic and/or para-aortic lymph nodes[b]
N1	Stage IIIC1	Metastasis to pelvic lymph nodes
N2	Stage IIIC2	Positive para-aortic nodes with or without positive pelvic lymph nodes
	Stage IV	Tumor invades bladder and/or bowel mucosa and/or distant metastasis
T4[c]	Stage IVA	Tumor invasion of the bladder and/or bowel mucosa
M1	Stage IVB	Distant metastasis including intra-abdominal metastasis and/or inguinal lymph nodes

[a]Endocervical glandular involvement alone should be considered stage I.
[b]Positive cytology must be reported separately without affecting the stage.
[c]The presence of bullous edema is not sufficient evidence to classify as T4.
Source: Pecorelli S. Revised FIGO staging for carcinoma of the vulva, cervix and endometrium. Int J Gnecol Obstet. 2009;105:103-4. doi: 10.1016/j.ijgo.2009.02.012.
Brierley JD, Gospodarowicz MK, Wittekind C. TNM classification of malignant tumours. 8th edition. Oxford and Hoboken: Wiley; 2017.

Prognostic Risk Groups of Endometrial Cancer Patients

Prognostic risk groups of endometrial cancer patients according to the joint guidelines (2020) by the European Society of Gynaecological Oncology (ESGO), the European SocieTy for Radiotherapy and Oncology (ESTRO), and the European Society of Pathology (ESP) are described in **Table 23.10**.

- *Low risk:* Women with grade 1 endometrial cancer with endometrioid histology, confined to the endometrium. This can be considered as a subset of stage 1 A disease where endometrial-myometrial junction is intact. This category includes stage 1 A G1 and G2. Overall probability

> **BOX 23.17:** Degree of differentiation of endometrial cancer.
>
> - *G1:* Presence of 5% or less of a nonsquamous or nonmodular solid growth pattern
> - *G2:* Presence of 6–50% or less of a nonsquamous or non-modular solid growth pattern
> - *G3:* Presence of >50% of a nonsquamous or nonmodular solid growth pattern. All types of nonendometrioid growths such as papillary serous, clear cell, and carcinosarcomas can be considered as high-grade growths

TABLE 23.10: Prognostic risk groups of endometrial cancer patients according to the joint guidelines (2020) by the ESGO, the ESTRO, and the ESP.

Risk group	Tumor characteristics
Low risk	Stage IA EEC G1, G2 without substantial LVSI
Low-intermediate risk	Stage IB EEC G1 and G2 without substantial LVSI or stage IA EEC G3 without substantial LVSI or stage IA NEEC without myometrial invasion
High-intermediate risk	Stage I EEC with substantial LVSI regardless of grade and depth of invasion or stage IB EEC G3 regardless of LVSI status or stage II tumors
High risk	Stage III–IVA with no residual disease or stage I–IVA NEEC with myometrial invasion, and with no residual disease
Advanced metastatic	Stage III-IVA with residual disease or stage IVB

(EEC: endometrioid endometrial cancer; LVSI: lymph-vascular space invasion; NEEC: nonendometrioid endometrial cancer)
Source: Concin N, Matias-Guiu X, Vergote I, Cibula D, Mirza MR, Marnitz S, et al. ESGO/ESTRO/ESP guidelines for the management of patients with endometrial carcinoma. Int J Gynecol Cancer. 2021;31(1):12-39. doi: 10.1136/ijgc-2020-002230.

of recurrence is very low following surgical treatment alone.
- *Intermediate risk:* Women with endometrial cancer where myometrium is invaded (stage 1 A G3 or 1B G2 and G3 disease) or there is occult cervical stromal disease (stage 2). This group can be further divided into two subgroups: low-intermediate risk and high-intermediate risk based on following prognostic factors:
  - Outer one-third myometrial invasion
  - *Grade of differentiation:* G2 or G3
  - Lymph vascular space invasion

  This further classification into low- and high-intermediate groups has clinical significance because adjuvant therapy is not required in the low-intermediate risk group, whereas it would be required in the high-intermediate risk group. As a result, the low-intermediate risk group is likely to be associated with reduced morbidity.
- *High risk:* High-risk endometrial carcinoma includes women with stage 3 or higher stage of endometrial cancer, regardless of their histology or grade. This category also comprises uterine papillary serous carcinoma (UPSC), which includes serous and clear cell carcinomas. Women with such cancers are deemed to be at a high-risk irrespective of their stage. Therefore, these women are at high risk of relapse and death.

TCGA Molecular Classification for Endometrial Cancer

> **Q.** Write a short note on The Cancer Genome Atlas (TCGA) classification of endometrial cancer.
>
> **Q.** Write a short note on endometrial cancer.

Endometrial cancer has been observed to share genomic features with serous ovarian cancer, the basal-like subtype of breast cancer, and colorectal cancer. TCGA has devised the molecular classification of endometrial cancer using combined immunohistochemistry (ICH) and mutation analysis. All endometrial cancer histotypes are represented in all four molecular subgroups, despite some specific overlap. The Proactive Molecular Risk Classifier for Endometrial Cancer (ProMisE) is a recently developed tool which helps in identifying these following four distinct molecular subgroups of endometrial cancer:

1. Polymerase epsilon exonuclease domain mutated (POLE EDM)/POLE ultramutated,
2. Mismatch repair deficient (MMRd)/microsatellite instability hypermutated
3. Nonspecific molecular profile or copy number low (NSMP/p53wt or p53 wild strain)
4. p53-mutated/copy-number-high (p53 abn or p53 abnormal)

While the MMRd and p53 mutations can be reliably tested by ICH compared to sequencing, POLE mutation status is presently dependent on targeted sequencing of the POLE exonuclease domain. ProMisE algorithm for assessing a new endometrial cancer sample with help of these molecular markers is shown in **Figure 23.13**. When confronted with a new sample from a case of endometrial cancer, firstly, MMR-deficiency against MSH 6, and PMS2 proteins are evaluated using ICH. Secondly, POLE exonuclease domain is tested by sequencing exons 9-14. Lastly, ICH for p53 is performed. This helps in determining patients with normal expression (IHC score 1+) versus complete loss/null (IHC score 0) or accumulation (IHC score 2+). p53 IHC (1+) is indicative of p53 wild strain, while p53 IHC (0 or 2+) is indicative of p53 abn.

The clinical significance of these molecular markers with respect to the management-related decisions is described in **Table in 23.11**. Patients with POLE EDM or p53-mutated markers have significantly altered prognosis/outcome compared to patients allocated to the MMR deficient (MMRd) or p53 wt groups. Therefore, such patients may require a modified adjuvant treatment decision.

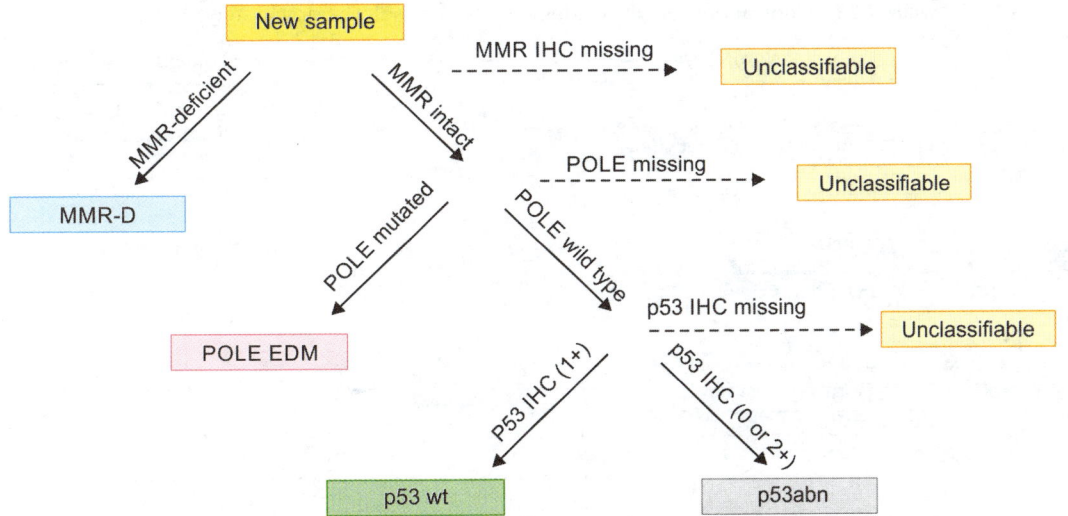

Fig. 23.13: The Proactive Molecular Risk Classifier for Endometrial Cancer (ProMisE) Algorithm to assess a new endometrial cancer sample.

TABLE 23.11: Clinical significance of the molecular markers.	
Type of mutation	**Management-related significance**
POLE EDM	Must be given options in immunotherapy (for rare recurrence or advanced disease unresponsive to conventional therapy)
MMRd	Patient must be referred for hereditary cancer counseling and testing options in immunotherapy
p53 wt (wild strain)	Lower likelihood of metastatic disease: hysterectomy/BSO managed in the community
P53 abn (abnormal stain)	Fertility sparing treatment not recommended; complete/aggressive surgical staging must be done; high likelihood of requiring chemoradiation

TABLE 23.12: Surgical management of endometrial cancer.	
Cancer stage	**Treatment**
Stage IA (G1-G2)	Type 1 hysterectomy and bilateral salpingo-oophorectomy. Lymphadenectomy not required.
Stage 1A G3/1B (G1-G3)	Type 1 hysterectomy and bilateral salpingo-oophorectomy with or without bilateral pelvic-para-aortic lymphadenectomy
Stage II tumors	Radical (type III) hysterectomy with bilateral salpingo-oophorectomy with bilateral pelvic/para-aortic lymphadenectomy
Stage III tumors	Maximal surgical cytoreduction with a good performance status
Stage IV A tumors	Anterior and posterior exenteration
Stage IV B tumors	Systemic therapeutic approach with palliative surgery

■ MANAGEMENT OF ENDOMETRIAL CANCER

Management of endometrial hyperplasia has been previously shown in **Flowchart 23.5**. The surgical management of endometrial cancer has been summarized in **Table 23.12**. For patients with stage I and II A, the treatment of choice is type 1 hysterectomy and BSO with lymph node sampling. Removal of a vaginal cuff is usually not required in these cases. The removed tumor specimen is examined for tumor size, depth of myometrial invasion and extension into the cervix. Lymphadenectomy may be done in selective cases of stage 1 disease **(Flowchart 23.7)**. Surgery alone may serve as an appropriate treatment option for patients with stage IA (G1 and G2) tumors in whom there is no evidence of invasion of the lymphovascular space, cervix, or isthmus, peritoneal cytology is negative and there is no evidence of metastasis. In all the other patients, some form of adjuvant radiotherapy is indicated **(Table 23.13)**. This method helps in bringing about a significant reduction in the incidence of vaginal vault/pelvic recurrence and in improving the disease-free survival.

Stage II and III cancers are also treated with surgery followed by adjuvant radiotherapy or chemoradiation. Stage IV cancers are usually nonoperatable and treatment needs to be individualized. Usually, a combination of surgery, radiotherapy, hormone therapy, or chemotherapy is required. Chemotherapy regimens mainly comprise of combination therapy using carboplatin and paclitaxel. Alternatively, a triplet regimen comprising of paclitaxel/doxorubicin/cisplatin (TAP regimen) is also being used.

Adjuvant Therapy for Endometrial Cancer

Table 23.13 describes the requirement for adjuvant therapy based on the cancer stage. Decision for administration of adjuvant therapy for endometrial cancer is based on stage, the histological grade of differentiation, histological subtype,

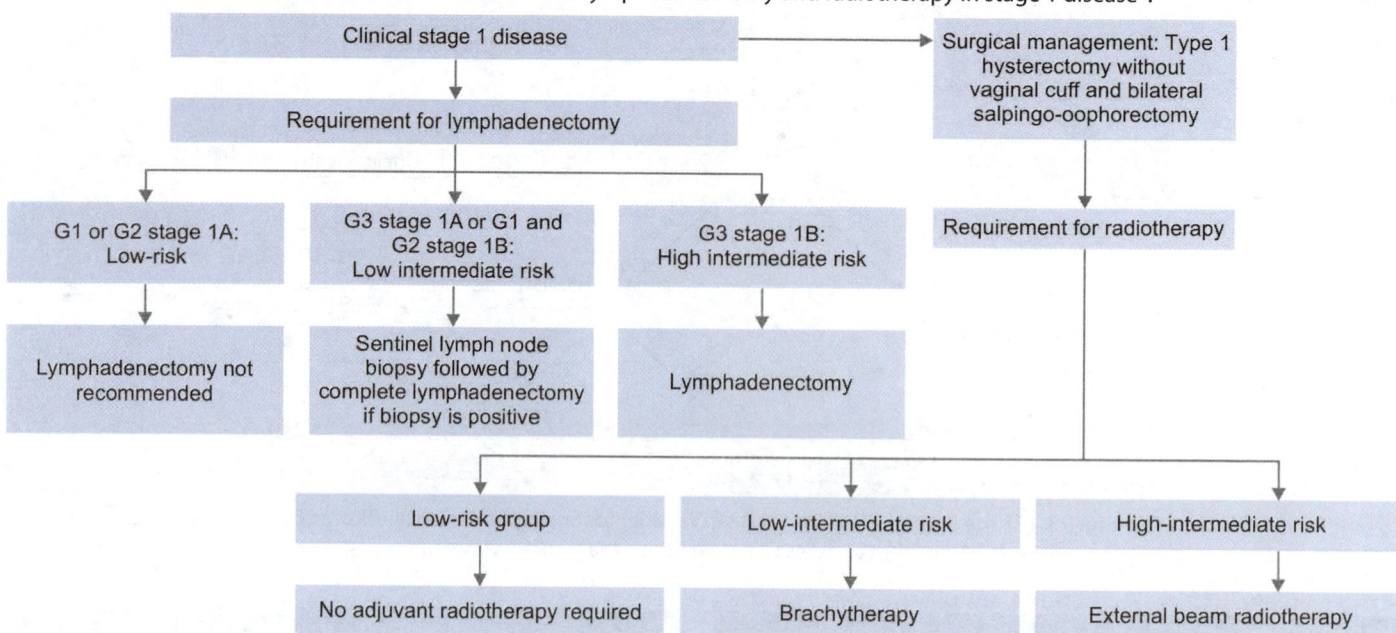

Flowchart 23.7: Indications for lymphadenectomy and radiotherapy in stage 1 disease*.

*Both pelvic and paraortic lymph nodes are removed

TABLE 23.13: Adjuvant therapy in cases of endometrial cancer.	
Cancer stage	**Adjuvant therapy**
Stage 1A (G1–G2)	Observation
Stage 1A (G3)/ 1B G1–G2	Observation or vaginal brachytherapy. In case of negative prognostic factors, pelvic radiotherapy and/or adjunctive chemotherapy can be considered
Stage 1 B (G3)	Pelvic radiotherapy. In case of negative prognostic factors, a combination of radiation and chemotherapy (chemoradiation) can be considered
Stage II	Pelvic radiotherapy and vaginal brachytherapy. In presence of negative prognostic factors, chemoradiation may be considered
Stage III/IV	Chemotherapy: • If positive nodes, sequential radiotherapy • If metastatic disease, chemoradiation for palliative therapy

and few molecular markers. As previously discussed, the ProMisE has identified four risk groups of endometrial cancer patients using a combination of ICH and mutation analysis: POLE EDM, MMRd, p53 wild type, and p53-mutated. Patients allocated to the POLE or abnormal p53 expression subtype may be associated with a significantly altered outcome. Therefore, there may be a requirement for a modified adjuvant treatment decision in these patients.

Lymphadenectomy

Bilateral pelvic and para-aortic lymphadenectomy may be required in the presence of the following:
- Evidence of an extrauterine disease
- Tumor that is FIGO grade 3
- Nonendometrioid type endometrial cancer
- Tumor invasion >50% of the myometrial thickness

The levels of lymph node dissection are as follows:

Level 1: Internal and external iliac group of lymph nodes

Level 2: Common iliac and the presacral lymph nodes

Level 3: Aortic inframesenteric

Level 4: Aortic infrarenal

Boundaries of Pelvic Lymph Node Dissection

Boundaries of pelvic lymph node dissection are tabulated in **Table 23.14**.

Boundaries of Para-aortic Lymph Node Dissection

This should include all lymph nodes below the bifurcation of aorta, superiorly. The inferior boundary of dissection is the left renal vein. The area of dissection is divided by the inferior mesenteric artery into two:

1. Supramesenteric area which lies above the inferior mesenteric artery
2. Inframesenteric area which lies below the inferior mesenteric artery

TABLE 23.14: Boundaries of pelvic lymph node dissection.	
Boundary	**Landmark structure**
Lateral	Psoas major on which lies the ilioinguinal nerve
Medial	Obliterated hypogastric artery (continuation of the internal iliac vessel)
Anterior	Anterior circumflex iliac vein
Superior	Bifurcation of the common iliac artery
Inferior	Obturator nerve

Sentinel Lymph Node Biopsy

 Q. Write a short essay on sentinel lymph node biopsy.

Lymph node metastasis is one of the most common routes for the spread of gynecological malignancies. Status of lymph nodes plays a vital role in the management and planning of these tumors. In these cases, biopsy of the sentinel lymph node assumes importance. Sentinel lymph node can be described as the first lymph node draining the lymphatic flow from the cancer site. Thereby, it has the highest possibility of involvement. In case sentinel node is negative, rest of the lymph nodes are unlikely to be involved. In these cases, lymphadenectomy can be omitted. On the other hand, if sentinel lymph node is found to be positive on frozen section, lymphadenectomy can be directly performed during the surgery.

Follow-up

Following complete treatment, initially the follow-up must be every 3 monthly for 2 years. Next 3 years, the follow-up should be 6-monthly. Following this, there should be an annual follow-up. During each follow-up visit, complete history must be taken followed by physical examination. Vault smear is usually not required in absence of symptoms. In case of suspected recurrence on history and physical examination, USG, MRI, and PET scan may be required.

Fertility-sparing Treatment

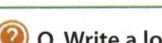 Q. Write a short note discussing the fertility sparing therapy in cases of carcinoma endometrium.

Fertility sparing treatment option may work for young women who have yet not completed their family and has grade 1 stage 1A tumor. Some prerequisites for using fertility-sparing treatment are mentioned in **Box 23.18.** In these cases, surgery may be postponed, and progestin therapy may be used for treating the cancer. High dose progestogens (e.g., medroxyprogesterone acetate can be used). Due to high incidence of side effects with oral therapy, LNG IUS is preferred. However, this therapy is still in its experimental stage and warrants strict patient monitoring while on this

> **BOX 23.18:** Prerequisites for fertility sparing treatment.
> - Patient has been counseled that this treatment is not the standard therapy
> - Patient is compliant with follow-up protocol
> - Patient has a strong desire to preserve reproductive function
> - Stage 1A grade 1 tumor
> - Endometrial-myometrial junction is not involved
> - Diagnosis is based on histopathological analysis of the tumor specimen
> - MRI documents the absence of myometrial invasion
> - Absence of any suspicious lymph nodes or metastatic disease on imaging
> - Absence of synchronous ovarian tumors on imaging
> - No evidence of Lynch II syndrome (on IHC for MMR proteins)
> - There is no contraindication to medical treatment with progestogens or pregnancy
> - Evaluation by the reproductive endocrinology and infertility team strongly recommends this mode of therapy

therapy. An EB should be done every 3–6 months. If there's still no cancer after 6 months, the woman can be advised to plan a pregnancy. However, she needs to be continuously monitored every 6 months to detect development of a recurrence. Since the chances of cancer recurrence are high in these cases, she should be recommended TH/BSO, once her childbearing is complete.

Prognosis

Q. Write a long essay discussing the factors which influence the treatment of carcinoma endometrium.

Some important adverse prognostic variables in case of endometrial cancer are as follows:

- *Age:* Patients > 70 years of age or < 40 years of age are associated with poor survival rates.
- *Histologic type:* Nonendometrioid cancers (UPSC) are likely to be associated with poor prognosis. Also, grade 1 endometrioid cancers are associated with a better prognosis, whereas grade III histology is likely to be associated with a poor prognosis.
- *Tumor size:* Tumor size > 2 cm is likely to be associated with > 15% chances of lymph node invasion, thereby resulting in a poor prognosis.
- *Hormone receptor status:* Tumors positive for estrogen or progesterone receptors are likely to be associated with a better prognosis, including the survival rate and survival time.
- *Myometrial invasion:* Deep myometrial invasion is likely to be associated with poorer prognosis.
- *Lymphovascular space invasion:* Involvement of the lymph nodes is likely to be associated with a poorer prognosis.
- *Cervical and isthmus extension:* Extension of the cancer to the cervix and/or uterine isthmus is likely to be

associated with a poor prognosis, lymph node metastasis, and intraperitoneal spread.

- *DNA ploidy:* Patients with diploid tumors are likely to have a better survival rate in comparison to the aneuploid tumors.
- *Metastasis to the lymph nodes:* This can be considered as one of the most important prognostic factors with the survival reducing by nearly 50% with lymph nodal involvement.
- *Adnexal involvement:* Involvement of adnexa is likely to be associated with a poorer prognosis.
- *Positive peritoneal cytology:* Positive peritoneal cytology in absence of other poor prognostic factors is not of much significance related to survival unless the tumor is extrauterine or belongs to the UPSC system.
- *Molecular tumor markers:* Loss of the tumor marker, PTEN, can be considered as an independent prognostic factor for favorable survival in cases of endometrial cancer.

EVIDENCE-BASED CLINICAL TRIALS

List of references can be scanned through QR code to enable the readers gain deeper insight of the subject by referring to the entire article or its abstract.

CHAPTER 24

Heavy Menstrual Bleeding due to Leiomyoma

CASE STUDY

A 33-year-old G2P1 patient presented with complaints of excessive menstrual bleeding since last 6 months. Despite of heavy bleeding during the periods, the periods were otherwise regular. The patient was prescribed mefenamic acid, but did not show any response to treatment. A D&C was done a month ago which revealed benign pathology. Pelvic examination revealed an irregularly enlarged uterus (about 6 weeks in size). The mass was contiguous with the cervix and could not be moved away from the cervix. An ultrasound examination was done, which showed presence of a submucous fibroid about 4 cm in diameter.

INTRODUCTION

A normal menstrual cycle is 21–35 days in duration in which the bleeding lasts for an average of 7 days (ranging between 4 days and 10 days), with flow varying between 25 mL and 80 mL. Heavy menstrual bleeding (HMB) is defined as excessive blood loss interfering with physical, social, emotional, or marital quality of life. It may be excessive in amount (>80 mL) and/or duration of flow (>5 days), but the cycle remains unaltered. As per the recommendations by FIGO (2011), previously used terminologies such as menorrhagia, metrorrhagia, menometrorrhagia, polymenorrhea, and dysfunctional uterine bleeding (DUB) are no longer used. Instead, FIGO has recommended the use of terminologies such as HMB, prolonged bleeding, infrequent or frequent bleeding, and irregular bleeding. HMB can occur due to several causes **(Table 24.1)**. In this chapter, special emphasis would be given to HMB resulting due to uterine fibroids.

UTERINE MYOMAS

Myomas (fibromyomas, leiomyomas, or fibroids) are well-circumscribed benign tumors developing from uterine myometrium, most commonly encountered among women of reproductive age group (30–45 years), with their prevalence ranging between 20% and 40%. The chances of having uterine fibroids increases until 50 years of the age and then declines sharply. Fibroids usually shrink to about half their original size after menopause. Combined HRT, particularly use of transdermal estrogen, can cause growth of the myomas following menopause.

TABLE 24.1: Causes of heavy menstrual bleeding.

Organic causes	Endocrinologic causes	Anatomic causes	Iatrogenic causes
• Genitourinary infections • Bleeding disorders • *Organ dysfunction:* Hepatic or renal failure • Sexual abuse resulting in bleeding from urethra or rectum • Coagulation disorders like von Willebrand's disease; factor II, V, VII, and IX deficiencies; prothrombin deficiency; idiopathic thrombocytopenic purpura; and thrombasthenia	• *Thyroid dysfunction:* Hypothyroidism and hyperthyroidism • Adrenal gland dysfunction • Prolactin producing tumors of the pituitary gland • PCOS • Obesity • Vasculature imbalance	• Uterine fibroids • Endometrial polyps • Endometrial hyperplasia • Pregnancy complications (miscarriages) • Adenomyosis • Cancer (uterine, ovarian and cervical cancer)	• IUDs (copper T 380A/ParaGaurd) • *Steroid hormones:* Medroxyprogesterone and other progestins (when stopped), prednisone • Chemotherapy agents (paclitaxel, docetaxel, etc.) • Medications (e.g., anticoagulants like aspirin, warfarin, heparin, etc.)

(IUD: intrauterine device; PCOS: polycystic ovarian syndrome)

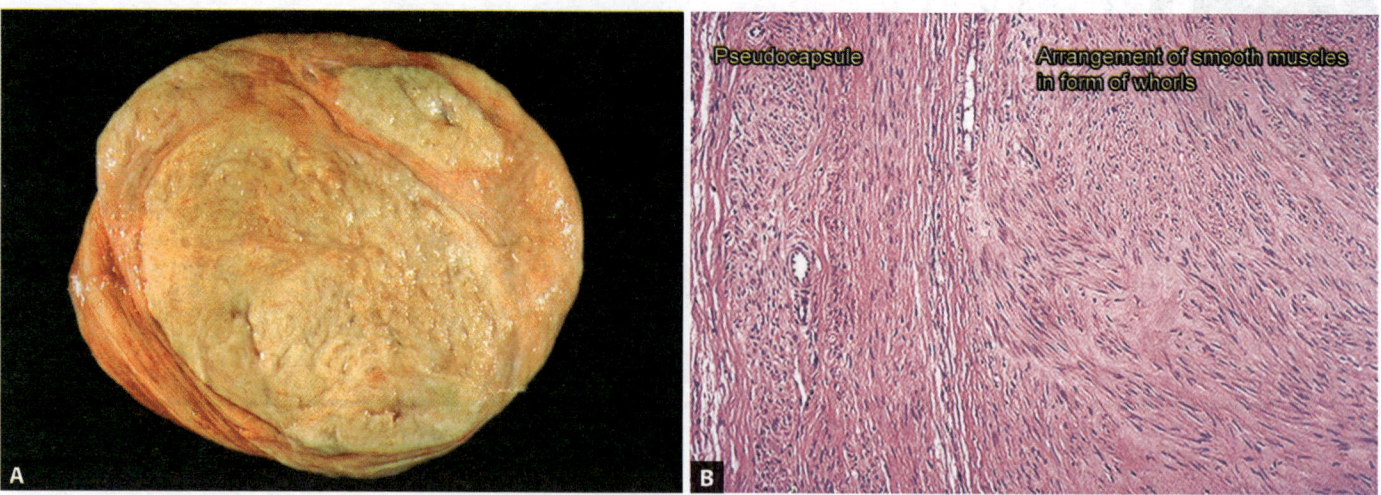

Figs. 24.1A and B: (A) Macroscopic appearance of a leiomyoma appearing as a pale, firm, rubbery, well-circumscribed mass; (B) Histological appearance of a fibroid showing presence of interlacing smooth muscle fibers surrounded by varying amount of connective tissue.

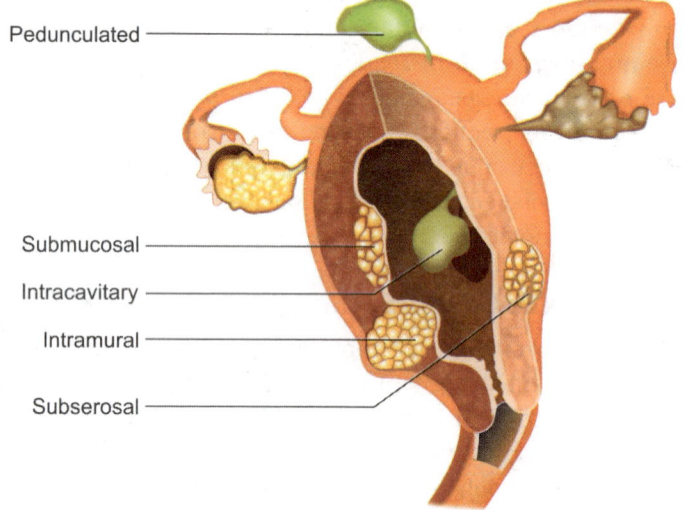

Fig. 24.2: Different types of leiomyomas.

A typical myoma is a pale, firm, rubbery, well-circumscribed mass distinct from neighboring tissues and has a whorled appearance due to presence of interlacing fibers of myometrial muscle, separated by varying amount of connective tissue fibers **(Figs 24.1A and B)**. The fibroid is surrounded by a connective tissue capsule, which helps in fixing the tumor to the myometrium. The vessels supplying blood to the tumor lie in the capsule and send radial branches into the tumor. As a result, the central portion of the fibroid receives the least blood supply and is the first to undergo degeneration. On the other hand, the calcification usually starts at the periphery and extends inward along the blood vessels. Fibroids can be single or multiple and may range in size from that of a small seedling to that of bulky masses which can distort and enlarge the uterus. Small fibroids often remain undiagnosed as they rarely produce any symptoms. Though most leiomyomas are situated in the body of the uterus, they may be confined to the cervix, specially the supravaginal portion in nearly 1–2% cases. The characteristic symptom of leiomyomas is menorrhagia; the duration of menstrual period may be normal or prolonged, and the blood loss is usually heaviest on 2nd and 3rd day. The nearer the leiomyomas are to the endometrial cavity, the more likely are they to produce menorrhagia. Normally, a woman with leiomyomas would never experience amenorrhea even of short duration, unless she is pregnant or past the menopause. In fact, women with fibroid are likely to have a late menopause.

TYPES OF FIBROIDS

Fibroids can be classified as submucosal, intramural, or subserosal based on their location within the uterine wall **(Fig. 24.2)**. Of the different types of fibroids, the most common are intramural (interstitial) fibroids, which are present in nearly 75% cases, followed by submucous (15%) and subserous fibroids (10%).

Submucosal fibroids, also known as subendometrial fibroids, grow beneath the uterine endometrial lining. This type of fibroid is thought to be primarily responsible for producing prolonged, HMB. Submucosal fibroids are most likely to cause distortion of the endometrial cavity.

FIGO CLASSIFICATION OF FIBROIDS

The FIGO(2018) classification of fibroids according to their location between submucous, subserous, and interstitial layers in the uterus is described in **Table 24.2** and **Figure 24.3**. This system was developed to describe and classify the fibroids in more uniform and consistent manner.

MECHANISM OF PRODUCTION OF HMB BY THE FIBROIDS

The mechanism by which endometrial polyps or fibroids cause HMB is not well understood. Some of the factors

TABLE 24.2: FIGO classification system of uterine fibroids.

Location of fibroid	Type of fibroid	Description
Submucosal	0	Pedunculated intracavitary
	1	<50% intramural
Intramural	2	≥50% intramural
	3	Contact with the endometrium, 100% intramural
	4	Intramural
	5	Subserosal, ≥50% intramural
Subserosal	6	Subserosal, <50% intramural
	7	Subserosal pedunculated
	8	Others (cervical, intraligamentous)
Hybrid		Two numbers are listed separated by a hyphen. By convention, the first refers to the relationship with the endometrium while the second refers to the relationship to the serosa. One example is given below (2–5)
Hybrid (example)	2–5	Submucous and subserous, each with less than half the diameter in the endometrial and peritoneal cavities, respectively

Source: Munro MG, Critchley HOD, Fraser IS; FIGO Menstrual Disorders Committee. The two FIGO systems for normal and abnormal uterine bleeding symptoms and classification of causes of abnormal uterine bleeding in the reproductive years: 2018 revisions. Int J Gynaecol Obstet. 2018;143:393-408. doi: 10.1002/ijgo.12666.

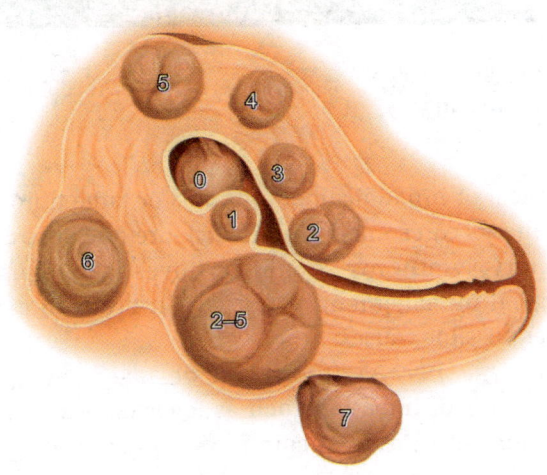

Fig. 24.3: FIGO classification of fibroids.

associated with fibroids which may be responsible for producing HMB are as follows:
- Increased size of endometrial cavity resulting in an increased bleeding surface area (normal surface area is 15 cm²)—especially in cases of submucous fibroids
- Associated endometrial hyperplasia, hyperestrogenism, pelvic congestion, etc.
- Probable interference with contractions of the uterine muscles—especially in cases of intramural fibroids
- Stasis and dilatation of venous plexus which may be due to imbalance in production of various vasodilators and vasoconstrictors. There may also be impaired endometrial hemostasis.
- Alteration in the ratio of prostaglandins and thromboxane, affecting the uterine milieu.

HISTORY AND CLINICAL PRESENTATION

Q. Write a long essay on clinical presentation and management of a case of fibroids in a 30-year-old woman.

- *Heavy menstrual bleeding:* As previously mentioned, one of the important causes of HMB in women belonging to the reproductive age group is leiomyomas (provided that any pregnancy-related complication has been ruled out). The main symptoms attributable to leiomyomas are excessive or prolonged menstrual bleeding. Questions which need to be asked regarding the nature of bleeding, amount of bleeding, duration of bleeding, pattern of bleeding, and timing of bleeding have already been described in **Chapter 23**. Amount of blood loss can be assessed by taking a count of how many pads or tampons (lightly stained/partially stained or fully stained), she needs to change during each day of her menstrual cycle.
- *Passage of clots:* Passage of clots is suggestive of heavy blood flow. Menstrual blood does not normally clot due to presence of high fibrinolytic activity. Therefore, presence of clots indicates that blood flow exceeds the intrinsic fibrinolytic activity. Passage of clots (>1 inch in diameter) or changing of pads every 3 hours has been correlated with blood loss >80 mL during menses (Warner et al, 2004). Blood loss can be assessed based on the number of pads or clothes, partially or fully soaked, which the woman changes during her periods. Objective assessment of blood loss can be done using PBAC. Kindly refer to Chapter 23 for details. This chart is associated

with sensitivity of 80% and specificity of 100%. Count of >100 on PBAC is suggestive of HMB.

- *Anemia:* Excessive bleeding, if remains untreated over a long period of time, can result in the development of anemia. Anemia can manifest itself by producing symptoms such as palpitations, breathlessness, fatigue, lassitude, and loss of weight. Symptoms of anemia usually manifest at hemoglobin levels <7 g%.
- *Intermenstrual bleeding:* Irregular bleeding is usually not a characteristic symptom of myomas. Therefore, in cases with irregular bleeding, endometrial disease must be ruled out. Causes of intermenstrual bleeding in cases of fibroids are listed in **Box 24.1**.

The association between endometrial cancer and leiomyomas is real, though not direct. The same type of the patient may be subject to both the diseases because both the diseases are related to hyperestrogenism. Therefore, every women suffering from leiomyomas who has continuous or irregular bleeding should be subjected to endometrial aspiration to rule out the presence of endometrial cancer before her treatment is planned.

- *Pain:* Dysmenorrhea may often accompany HMB in cases of fibroid uterus. Spasmodic dysmenorrhea may result when expulsion of a pedunculated submucous tumor stimulates uterine contractions. Congestive dysmenorrhea may also occur due to associated pelvic congestion. Interruption of local growth factors within fibroids is likely to result in altered pain sensation. Presence of fibroids in the cornual region is also likely to result in spasmodic pain due to increased concentration of prostaglandin F2alpha (PGF2α) in the uterine environment.

Even in absence of bleeding, pain may sometimes be present in patients with leiomyomas. It could be acute **(Box 24.2)** or chronic. Chronic pain is usually caused by large fibroids, stretching the uterosacral ligaments resulting in chronic heaviness and pain.

- *Pressure symptoms:* Other symptoms related to leiomyomas include symptoms related to pressure on adjacent organs. These may include symptoms such as backache (due to the pressure on spinal nerves); urinary symptoms, such as increased diurnal frequency and urgency (due to bladder irritability); bowel dysfunction (due to pressure on intestines); and rectal tenesmus and constipation (due to pressure on rectum).

Urinary symptoms are common with anterior wall and cervical fibroids. Retention of urine can also occur when fibroid in the posterior wall gests incarcerated in the pouch of Douglas, causing a change in UV angulation. In case a woman with fibroids presents with urinary retention, she must be catheterized. Continuous bladder drainage may be required if the residual urine volume is >120 mL.

> **BOX 24.1:** Causes of intermenstrual bleeding in cases of fibroids.
> - Pedunculated submucous myomas, protruding through the vagina, which become infected or ulcerated
> - Presence of sarcomatous changes in the leiomyoma
> - A coincidental pregnancy state
> - Coincidental carcinoma of the uterus or an endometrial/cervical polyp

> **BOX 24.2:** Causes of acute pain in cases of fibroids.
> - Red degeneration of fibroids
> - Torsion of pedunculated fibroids
> - Extrusion of fibroid polyp
> - Sarcomatous changes
> - Adhesions with other organs
> - Associated endometriosis/pelvic inflammatory disease, etc.
> - Spasmodic dysmenorrhea
> - Infection
> - Expulsion of pedunculated submucous tumors through cervix
> - When the fibroid outgrows its blood supply, thereby causing necrosis (rarely)

> **BOX 24.3:** Causes of fever or discharge per vaginum in cases of fibroids.
> - Associated PID
> - Infected fibroid polyp
> - Red degeneration

- Cervical or broad ligament fibroids or large fibroids on the uterus can sometimes produce ureteric obstruction. Urinary symptoms should be investigated prior to surgical management of fibroids in order to exclude other possible causes.
- *Discharge per vaginum and/or fever:* Symptoms suggestive of infection such as fever or discharge per vaginum are rarely encountered in cases of fibroids **(Box 24.3)**.
- *Loss of appetite or weight loss:* May be rarely present in cases of fibroids where there is an associated endometrial or ovarian carcinoma or in case of sarcomatous change in the fibroid.
- *Secondary polycythemia:* Secondary polycythemia in a patient with fibroid can cause her face to appear pink and flushed. This may be due to the myomatous erythrocytosis syndrome which is a rare phenomenon because most patients with fibroids are likely to present with anemia rather than erythrocytosis. Secondary polycythemia in these cases could be due to the following causes:
    - Fibroids pressing on ureter may stimulate kidneys to produce erythropoietin.
    - Fibroid may itself be erythropoietic with the islands of extramedullary hematopoiesis.

This symptom is likely to disappear with the removal of fibroids.

- *Asymptomatic:* Despite of the above-mentioned symptoms, majority of the fibroids may be asymptomatic.

  Therefore, in suspected cases of fibroids, detailed history regarding the nature of bleeding, presence of any pressure symptoms, infertility and any complications during pregnancy related to the presence of fibroids need to be elicited. Other details which must be elicited while taking history include the following:
- *Patient's age:* As previously mentioned, patient's age can provide important pointer toward the diagnosis of underlying pathology. Uterine leiomyomas are typically more common during fourth or fifth decades of life. Incidence of leiomyomas at 45–50 years is 20 times more than at 25–30 years, with the incidence being nearly 70% in the white population and 80% in the black population at the age of 50 years.
- *Obstetric history:* Uterine fibroids are more common in nulliparous women in comparison to the multiparous women. Parity reduces the risk of fibroids by three- to fivefold.
- *History of contraceptive use:* Commonly, contraception such as an intrauterine device causes increased uterine cramping and menstrual flow. On the other hand, use of OCPs is likely to be associated with a reduced risk. Risk of fibroids is reduced by nearly 50% with the history of OCP use for greater than 14–15 months. However, use of OCPs in very young age (13–16 years) is likely to be associated with an increased risk.
- *Presence of any coagulation-related disorder:* It is important to rule out the presence of any coagulation-related disorders by taking the history of excessive bruising or bleeding on minor trauma and family history of known bleeding disorders. This is especially important in a young patient who does not stop bleeding during her first menses. This is a very common presentation for an undiagnosed bleeding disorder (e.g., Von Willebrand's disease) in a young girl.
- *Symptoms of thyroid dysfunction:* The alteration of the thyroid function may produce menstrual abnormalities like amenorrhea or oligomenorrhea (hypothyroidism) or menorrhagia (hyperthyroidism).
- *History of intake of any medications:* Intake of drugs like hormones or anticoagulants may typically cause bleeding.
- *Plans regarding future fertility and contraception:* These should be ascertained in order to decide appropriate patient management.
- History of undergoing pap smears in the past.

RISK FACTORS

History related to risk factors which can result in the development of fibroids also needs to be taken. Some of these are described next.

Heredity

Genetic factors are likely to play an important role in the pathogenesis of fibroids. Patient with a positive family history of fibroid, especially in the first-degree relatives (mother or sister) is especially at an increased risk of developing fibroids. Many chromosomal abnormalities have been detected in cases of leiomyomas, the most common being translocation between the long arms of chromosomes 12 and 14, with others being, trisomy 12, rearrangement of short arm of chromosome 6 and long arm of chromosome 10, and deletion of chromosomes 3 and 7.

Multiple uterine and cutaneous leiomyomatosis (MUCL): MUCL, also known as Reed's syndrome, is an autosomal dominant genetic condition. Families with MUCL are likely to have a mutation in the fumarate hydratase gene. Affected women are at an increased risk of developing benign smooth muscle tumors (leiomyomas) in the skin and uterus. A MUCL variant, hereditary leiomyomatosis and renal cell cancer (HLRCC) is associated with hereditary leiomyomatosis and renal cell carcinoma in affected individuals.

Race

Black women are more likely to have fibroids than the women of other racial groups. Furthermore, fibroids occur in black women at a younger age and tend to be larger and more numerous.

Dietary Factors

Women who consume red meat are likely to have a three times higher incidence of having fibroids in comparison to the women who are vegetarian. However, the incidence of having fibroids in women who consume fish is similar to that in vegetarians.

Body Mass Index

Incidence of fibroids is higher amongst obese women. 10% increase in BMI is likely to be associated with an 18-fold increase in the risk of fibroids.

High Estrogen Levels

High estrogen levels predispose a woman to develop fibroids. Some factors which may be responsible for an increased risk of fibroids related to hyperestrogenism are as follows:
- Exposure to OCPs at the age of 13–16 years is associated with a high risk for development of uterine fibroids. However, use of OCPs in middle age group acts as a protective factor. Presently, there is no evidence that use of low-dose oral contraceptives causes benign fibroids to grow, thus uterine fibroids are not a contraindication to their use.
- Obesity increases the risk probably due to higher levels of endogenous estrogens.

- Smoking reduces the risk of fibroids by decreasing the levels of endogenous estrogens.
- Childbearing during the reproductive years (25–29) provides greatest protection against myoma development by producing amenorrhea (thereby reduced estrogen levels) during pregnancy.

There is a positive association between fibroids and the pelvic inflammatory disease.

GENERAL PHYSICAL EXAMINATION

Signs of anemia: Abnormal blood loss, if allowed to continue over a long period of time can result in the development of anemia.

SPECIFIC SYSTEMIC EXAMINATION

An abdominal and pelvic examination should be performed in women presenting with HMB. Pelvic examination should be preferably avoided in the women under the age of 20 years.

ABDOMINAL EXAMINATION

Abdominal distension in cases of fibroids could be suggestive of following:

- *Large fibroid:* Large fibroid may be palpable per abdomen. However, a leiomyoma has to attain the size of approximately 12–14 weeks before the abdominal swelling becomes palpable per abdomen. It may be difficult to detect the leiomyomas smaller than this on abdominal examination.
- *Pseudomeig's syndrome:* This syndrome is associated with a triad of fibroids, ascites, and right-sided pleural effusion. Disparity between the growth of fibroids and vascularity is likely to result in inflammation and fluid exudation.

In case of uterine fibroids, the mass usually appears to be arising from the pelvis, i.e., it may be difficult to get below the mass. The mass is usually well defined, having a firm consistency and a smooth surface. It is usually movable from side to side, but not from above downward. If the fibroid has undergone cystic degeneration, it may appear soft and cystic in consistency, rather than hard. Presence of multiple fibroids can result in an irregular appearance of the mass. The mass is nearly always dull to percussion because the intestines usually lie behind and besides the mass. The mass is rarely tender on touch. In case of a single subserous leiomyoma with a long pedicle, it may be difficult to recognize its connection with the uterus. In such cases, it might be difficult to distinguish the fibroid from an ovarian tumor.

Palpation

In cases with fibroids, bilateral renal angles must be palpated for presence of any mass/tenderness, etc., because large fibroids can compress the ureters, causing hydronephrosis.

PELVIC EXAMINATION

The method of conducting the pelvic and bimanual examination has been discussed in details in Chapter 22. Bimanual examination helps in assessment of uterine size, shape, and contour. Presence of an enlarged, irregularly shaped, nontender, and mobile uterus with firm consistency is suggestive of fibroids in women aged 30–50 years. On bimanual examination, it is found that the tumor either replaces the uterus or is attached to the cervix. A uterine mass can be differentiated from an adnexal mass on the basis of parameters as described in **Table 24.3**.

This is an important point because if the mass was lateral or moved apart from the cervix, the most likely diagnosis would have been presence of an adnexal mass.

Cervix may be sometimes pulled up, because when the uterus is enlarged to a size > 24 weeks, the uterus may rest on pubic symphysis causing the cervix to appear pulled up.

DIFFERENTIAL DIAGNOSIS

PREGNANCY

Pregnancy must always be ruled out in a woman of reproductive age group, presenting with an abdominal lump. A urine pregnancy test and an ultrasound examination help in confirming the diagnosis of pregnancy.

TABLE 24.3: Differentiating between uterine and an adnexal mass.		
Parameter	Uterine mass	Adnexal mass
Separation of mass from uterus	Mass cannot be separated from the uterus	Mass is separate from the uterus
Transmitted mobility	Uterus moves with the movement of the mass	Uterus does not move with the movement of mass
Presence of a groove	No groove felt between the mass and the uterus	Groove felt between the mass and the uterus
Hingorani's sign*	Absent	Present

*Hingorani's sign is elicited by placing the patient in Trendelenburg's position. This position is likely to result in upward displacement of mass due to which one can easily elicit a groove between the uterus and the mass.

ADENOMYOSIS

Adenomyosis is a condition associated with presence of endometrial tissue within the uterine myometrium. In cases of diffuse adenomyosis, the uterus is symmetrically enlarged to the size between 12 and 14 weeks. Cases of focal adenomyosis are associated with asymmetrical uterine enlargement. In these cases, it may be difficult to differentiate adenomyosis from uterine fibroids. Adenomyosis is often associated with pain and uterine tenderness. Therefore presence of menorrhagia along with dysmenorrhea is more suggestive of adenomyosis in comparison to fibroids. MRI helps in establishing the exact diagnosis and differentiating between fibroids and adenomyosis.

BENIGN OVARIAN TUMOR

At times, it may become particularly difficult to differentiate between a subserous fibroid and a solid benign ovarian mass. Furthermore, a subserous fibroid may not be associated with menorrhagia. The two can be differentiated from each other on a pelvic examination as explained in Chapter 31.

BICORNUATE UTERUS

One horn of a bicornuate uterus may often be mistaken for a myoma. Ultrasound examination may help confirm the diagnosis.

MALIGNANCY

Sometimes malignancies like endometrial carcinoma and uterine sarcomas may produce a mass indistinguishable from a myoma. Ultrasound may help in distinguishing between the two.

MANAGEMENT

Q. Discuss in detail the role of conservative management and hysterectomy in a woman with multiple uterine fibroids.

Q. Discuss the various conservative management procedures in a 30-year-old multiparous woman with fibroid uterus.

Q. Write a long essay discussing recent trends in the management of fibroid uterus.

Q. Briefly describe recent trends in the management of fibroids.

Q. What would be the best treatment option in the case study described in the beginning of the chapter?
Ans. Since the age of woman in the above-mentioned case study is 33 years and she desires future fertility, myomectomy appears to be the best treatment option. The route for myomectomy needs to be determined based on many factors including the type of myomas, degree of myometrial invasion, and number of myomas. The severity of the problem and its duration must be taken into account. In this case, the woman has a submucosal fibroid of size 4 cm on the ultrasound, having <50% myometrial invasion. Therefore, the best option appears to be hysteroscopic resection.

Q. What are the possible medicolegal pitfalls associated with the case of menorrhagia?
Ans. Following are the possible medicolegal pitfalls associated with the cases of menorrhagia:
- *Ruling out pregnancy:* If the patient with menorrhagia belongs to the reproductive age group, pregnancy should be ruled out by performing a pregnancy test in order to rule out any pregnancy-related complication (threatened or incomplete abortion, ectopic pregnancy, or retained products of conception) as the cause of bleeding.
- After ruling out pregnancy, imaging studies should be ordered.
- *Ruling out malignancy:* Every high risk or postmenopausal patient with uterine bleeding must be first evaluated for endometrial or other gynecological malignancy.
- *Risk of pregnancy with use of GnRH agonists:* When treating patients with progestin therapy or with GnRH therapy, the women must be informed that pregnancy may still be possible since these drugs are not a form of birth control. Since the safety of these drugs on pregnancy is not known, an effective form of contraception must be used in these cases.

Presently, the main modality of curative treatment in a patient with leiomyomas is surgery. Medical therapy does not help in curing myomas. It can just provide symptomatic relief and help in reducing the size of the tumor by decreasing its blood supply. The management plan of a patient diagnosed with fibroid uterus, presenting with menorrhagia is described in **Flowchart 24.1**.

INVESTIGATIONS

Only investigations which are required in a case of leiomyomas are described next. Investigations which may be required to be carried out in the case of AUB based on history and clinical examination are described in Chapter 23.

COMPLETE BLOOD COUNT ALONG WITH PLATELET COUNT AND A PERIPHERAL SMEAR

CBC with platelet count must be conducted to rule out presence of anemia.

IMAGING STUDIES

Imaging modalities such as ultrasound (both transabdominal and transvaginal ultrasound) and MRI are noninvasive investigations, which play an important role in the management of patients with leiomyomas.

Ultrasound Examination

Nowadays, ultrasound examination (both transvaginal and transabdominal ultrasound) has become the investigation of choice for diagnosing myomas. The advantages of ultrasound imaging are good patient tolerance, noninvasive nature of the investigation, relatively low cost, easy availability, and high

Flowchart 24.1: Management plan of a patient with fibroid uterus presenting with HMB.

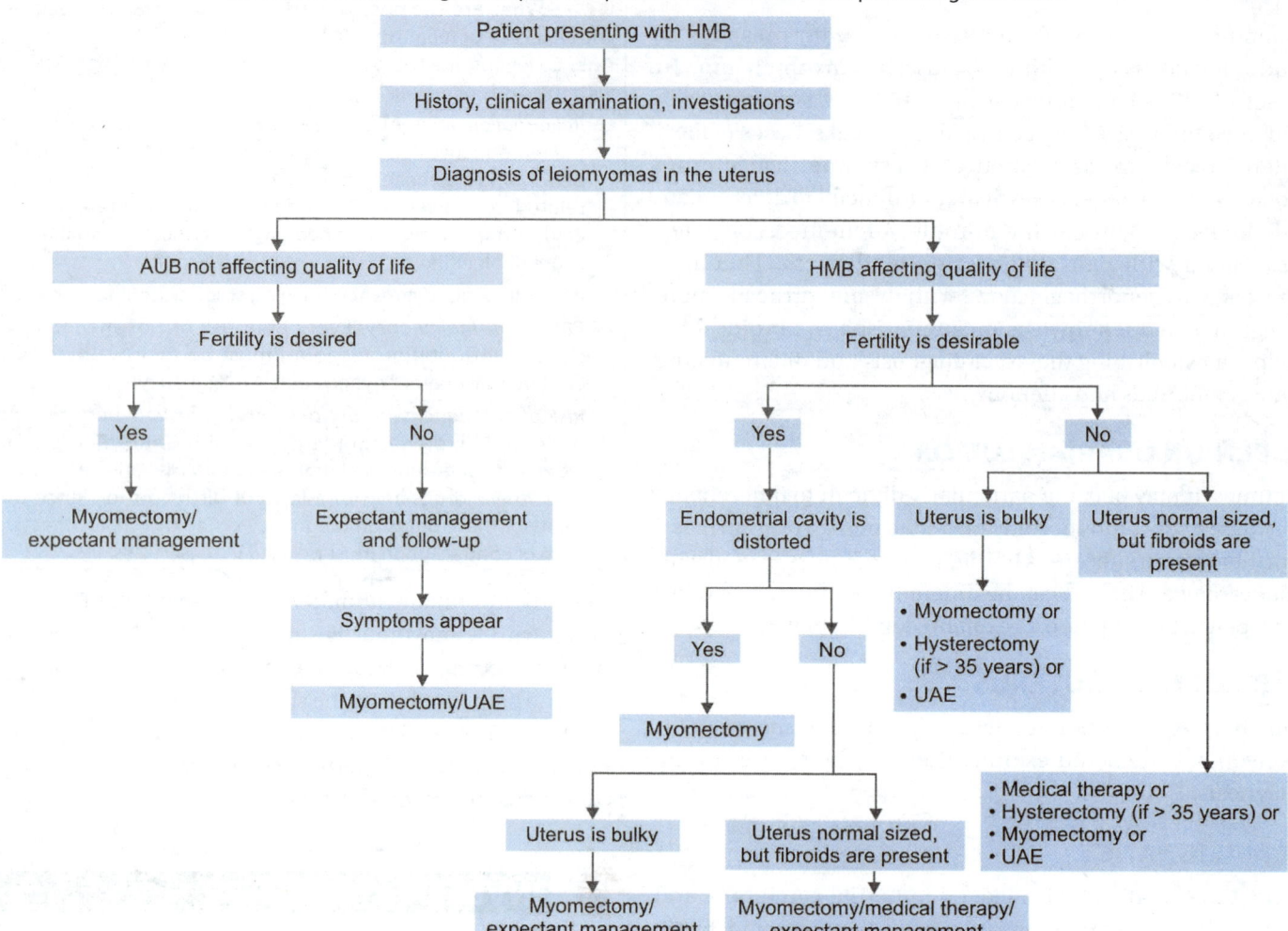

(HMB: heavy menstrual bleeding; UAE: uterine artery embolization)

accuracy rates. Ultrasound examination helps in assessing the overall uterine shape, size, and contour; endometrial thickness, adnexal areas and presence of hydronephrosis. It helps in detection of small, focal, irregular, or eccentrically located endometrial lesions. It also helps in detecting if there is any protrusion of the fibroid into the endometrial cavity or if there is any distortion of the uterine outline. Presence of any degenerative changes in fibroids can also be identified on ultrasound, e.g., irregular central anechoic areas seen in in cystic degeneration; bright echogenic areas with distal shadowing in cystic degeneration, etc. Preoperative finding on sonography can guide the gynecologist while performing surgery, hysteroscopy, laparoscopy, etc. Ultrasound examination can help in assessing the size, location, and number of uterine fibroids. Any associated pathology such as adnexal mass, associated adenomyosis, and hydronephrosis can also be delineated on ultrasound examination. It may be sometimes very difficult to differentiate between submucous myomas and endometrial polyps on ultrasound examination. In these cases, the investigations such as saline infusion sonography (SIS) and hysteroscopy help in arriving at the correct diagnosis.

Color flow Doppler can help distinguish between a malignant and nonmalignant lesion by showing high vascular flow in a malignant mass.

Though MRI is an investigation which helps in accurately establishing the definitive diagnosis of myomas, the high cost associated with its use, prevents its widespread use in clinical practice. Presently, ultrasound examination forms the most commonly used investigation modality for initial evaluation.

Transvaginal Ultrasound

Transvaginal sonography (TVS) can help in detecting myomas as small as 2.5 cm within the uterus **(Figs. 24.4A to D)**. Most new transvaginal probes offer variable frequency transducers with frequencies between 5.0 MHz and 7.5 MHz. The higher the frequency used, the better is the resolution of the image. However, with the use of higher frequency ultrasound probes, the field of view largely gets restricted. As the uterus enlarges, a lower-frequency transducer must be used to visualize the organ. The 7.5 MHz vaginal probe works best with a normal or minimally enlarged uterus. The 5.0 MHz vaginal probe usually images

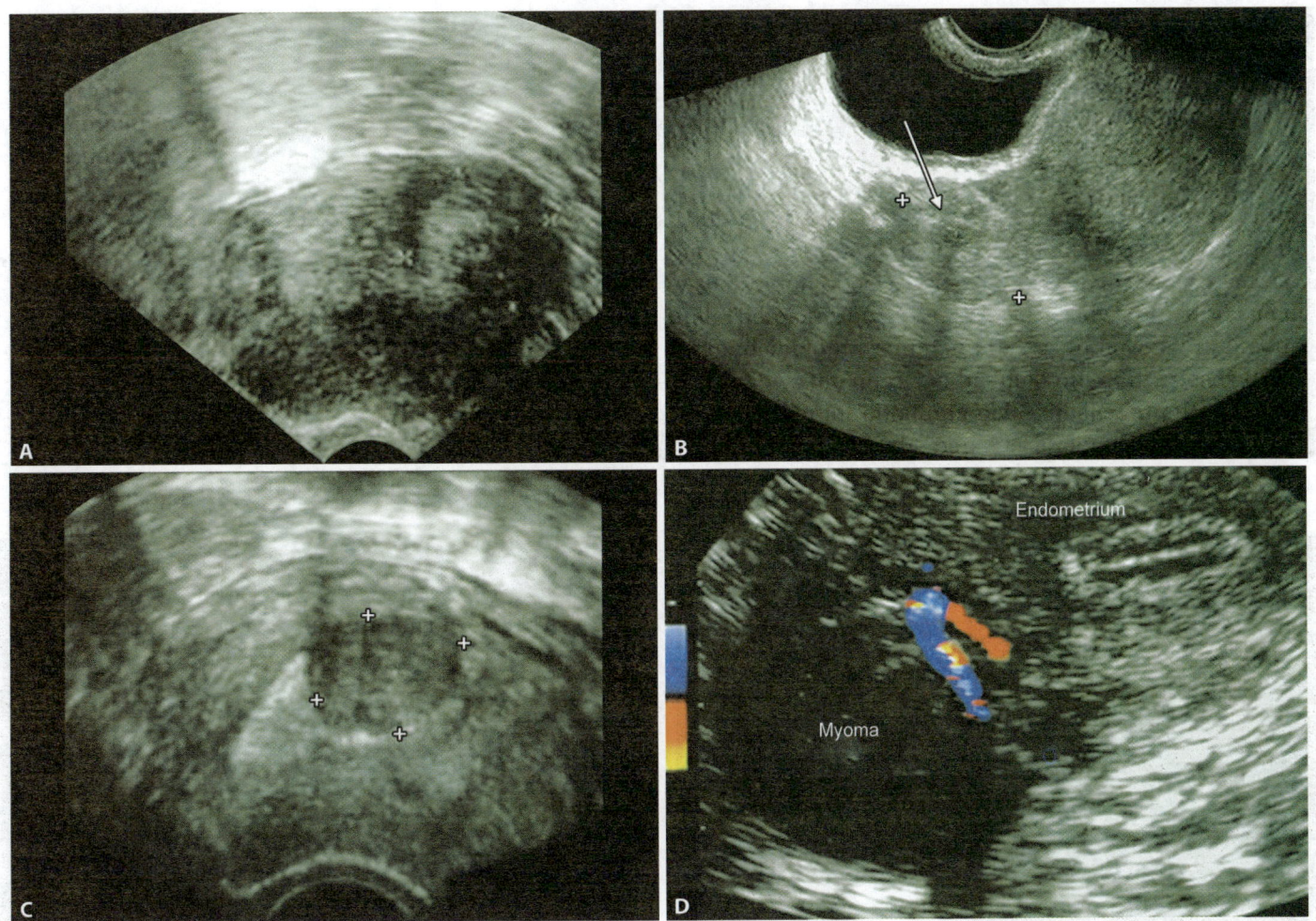

Figs. 24.4A to D: Ultrasound appearance of fibroids. (A) Intramural fibroid; (B) Pedunculated fibroid having a diameter of 3.74 cm (shown with the help of an arrow); (C) Submucous fibroid protruding inside the endometrial cavity; (D) Color Doppler showing presence of subserosal fibroid with peripheral vascularization.

a uterus up to the size of 12 weeks of gestation. If the uterus is larger than this, transabdominal imaging with a 2.5 or 3.5 MHz probe is required.

Various studies have found the sensitivity of TVS in detection of leiomyomas to range from 90% to 100% and specificity to range from 80% to 94%.

Though transvaginal ultrasonography is associated with higher resolution in comparison to transabdominal sonography (TAS), it may not always be useful in distinguishing between a submucosal fibroid, endometrial polyp, and adenomyosis. A newer technique, called SIS or sonohysterography, uses saline infusion into the endometrial cavity to enhance the detection of fibroids and polyps.

Sonohysterography (Saline Infusion Sonography)

Saline infusion sonography involves infusion of fluid inside the endometrial cavity in order to enhance the evaluation of endometrial cavity and adnexa at the time of ultrasound examination. As previously described, one of the major advantage of sonohysterography is its ability to differentiate polyps from submucous leiomyomas. SIS has been demonstrated to cause improved evaluation of the endometrial cavity and assessment of tubal patency. SIS also helps in detection of endometrial pathology such as uterine synechiae, endometrial polyps (**Figs. 24.5 A and B**), and submucous leiomyomas. One of the major limitations of sonohysterography has been the assessment of tubal patency. The procedure of SIS has been described in Chapter 23.

Magnetic Resonance Imaging

Though the use of MRI is not routinely recommended, it is useful in mapping the size and location of leiomyomas (**Figs. 24.6 and 24.7**) and in accurately identifying adenomyosis. Though MRI gives images with better resolution, due to its high cost, MRI is usually reserved for only special cases. MRI is usually performed in cases in which the diagnosis is not clear on ultrasound examination. Other pelvic pathology such as ovarian neoplasms can also be identified on MRI. MRI is preferable to CT for imaging myomas as it does not expose the patients to ionizing radiations.

Magnetic resonance imaging is a highly accurate technique for evaluating uterine leiomyomas, adenomyosis,

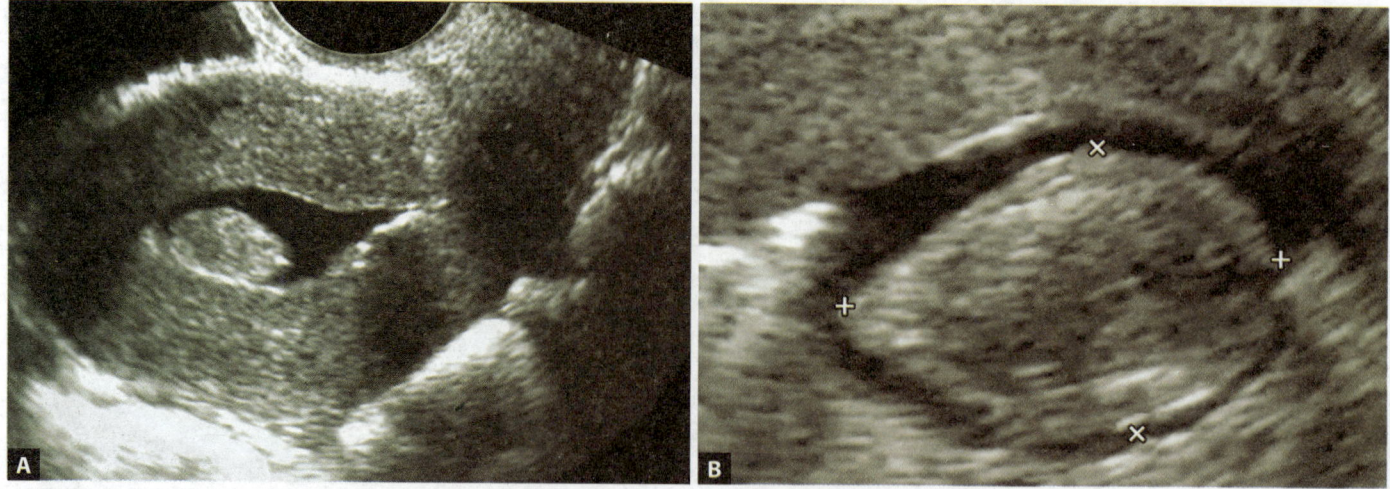

Figs. 24.5A and B: (A) Saline infusion sonography (SIS) demonstrating a uterine polyp; (B) Visualization of intracavitary fibroid on SIS.

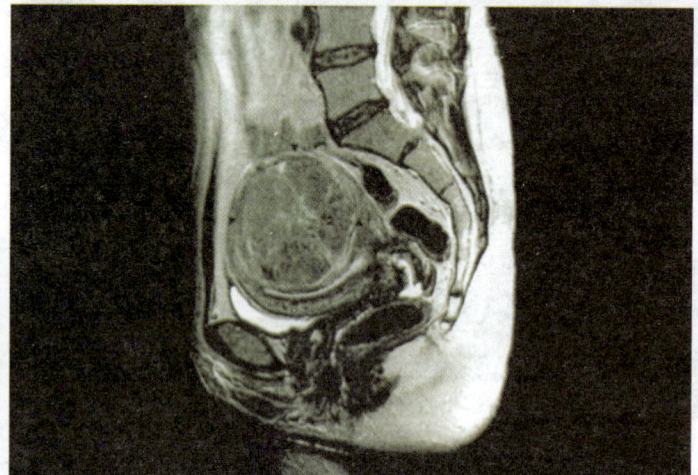

Fig. 24.6: T1-weighted magnetic resonance image showing an intramural fibroid of size 8 cm.

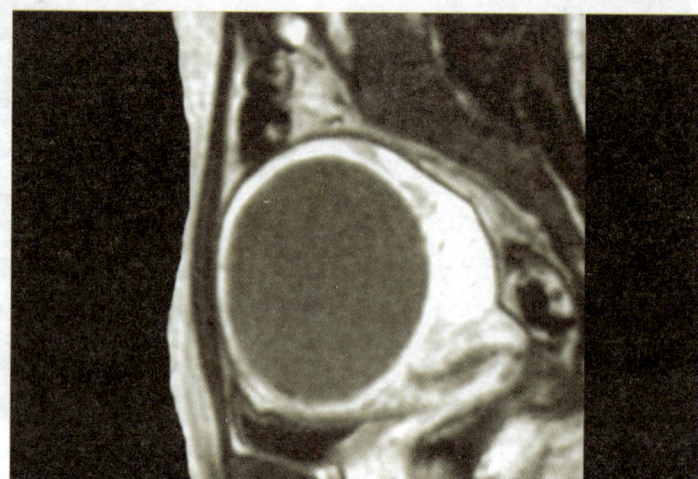

Fig. 24.7: A 43-year-old woman with large submucosal fibroid. Enhanced T1-weighted magnetic resonance image obtained 4 months after uterine artery embolization shows that uterine fibroid decreased to 9 cm in maximum diameter (46% tumor volume reduction) and was not enhancing. Muscular layer of the uterus is enhanced.

and uterine anomalies. Magnetic resonance images clearly delineate the myometrium, junctional zone, and endometrium, allowing highly accurate mapping of the size, location, and degree of myometrial involvement of uterine leiomyomas **(Figs. 24.6 and 24.7)**. It is much more accurate in identifying and mapping adenomyosis. The major limitation of MRI is the high cost involved.

PAP Smear

In case the patient has risk factors for endometrial cancer or she is in the perimenopausal age group or gives history of intermenstrual and postcoital bleeding, endometrial biopsy (endometrial aspiration and endocervical curettage) and Pap smear are required to rule out carcinoma endometrium and carcinoma cervix, respectively.

Intravenous Pyelography

In case of large subserous, cervical or lower segment or broad ligament fibroids, which appear to be pressing upon the ureters, intravenous pyelography may be required to rule of hydronephrosis or ureteronephrosis.

PAC Work-up

Investigations for preanesthetic work up such as blood sugar levels, Kidney function test (KFT), LFT, X-ray chest, ECG, and urine routine/microscopy may be done in cases where surgery is required.

TREATMENT/GYNECOLOGICAL MANAGEMENT

Specific treatment for menorrhagia is based on a number of factors including:
- Overall health and medical history
- Extent of the condition and symptoms produced
- The effects of menorrhagia on the patient's lifestyle
- Personal preference
- Patient's age
- Desire for future fertility

- Uterine size and rate of growth of the uterus
- Duration and severity of the heavy bleeding
- Underlying cause of the condition

In case the patient is diagnosed with fibroid uterus, the ultimate treatment depends on factors such as the number of fibroids, size of fibroids, the proximity of the fibroids to the endometrial cavity, and severity of symptoms caused by them. The closer the fibroids are to the endometrial cavity, the more they are likely to be symptomatic. Even if the diagnosis of fibroids has been made, it does not necessarily imply that they are the cause of bleeding. The menstrual periods may be heavy even if the fibroids were not present. Since abnormal uterine bleeding can result from other causes, such as endometrial cancer and hormonal problems, it is important that women with fibroids, especially the women in the perimenopausal age group, who experience abnormal vaginal bleeding receive a thorough evaluation for endometrial cancer.

The various treatment options which can be used in a woman with fibroid uterus are enumerated in **Table 24.4** and described in **Flowchart 24.2**. In the properly selected woman with symptomatic fibroids, the result from the selected treatment should be an improvement in the quality of life. In case of uterine fibroids, skilled judgment is required to decide whether surgical treatment options such as myomectomy or hysterectomy would be required or use of medical treatment options like tranexamic acid would be appropriate. Medical management should be tailored toward alleviation of symptoms like bleeding and pain.

Various treatment options in a woman with fibroid uterus based on the patient's age and desire for future childbearing is described in **Flowchart 24.3**. If the woman has completed her family and does not wish to preserve her uterus, hysterectomy can be done. Myomectomy is an option for women, who desire future pregnancy or wish to preserve their uterus. Removal of fibroids that distort the uterine cavity may be indicated in infertile women, where no other factors have been identified, and in women about to undergo IVF treatment. However, the women undergoing myomectomy should be counseled regarding the chances of occurrence of massive bleeding during myomectomy

TABLE 24.4: Treatment options for uterine myomas in women with fibroids.

Management	Indication
Conservative management	Asymptomatic women with small fibroids
Medical management	As an alternative to surgery in following cases: • Perimenopausal women • Women medically unfit for surgery • Women unwilling for surgery
Surgical management (myomectomy and hysterectomy)	Definitive treatment
Destruction of fibroids (myolysis, uterine artery embolization, uterine artery ligation, and focused ultrasound)	Limited evidence as these procedures are still under research stage

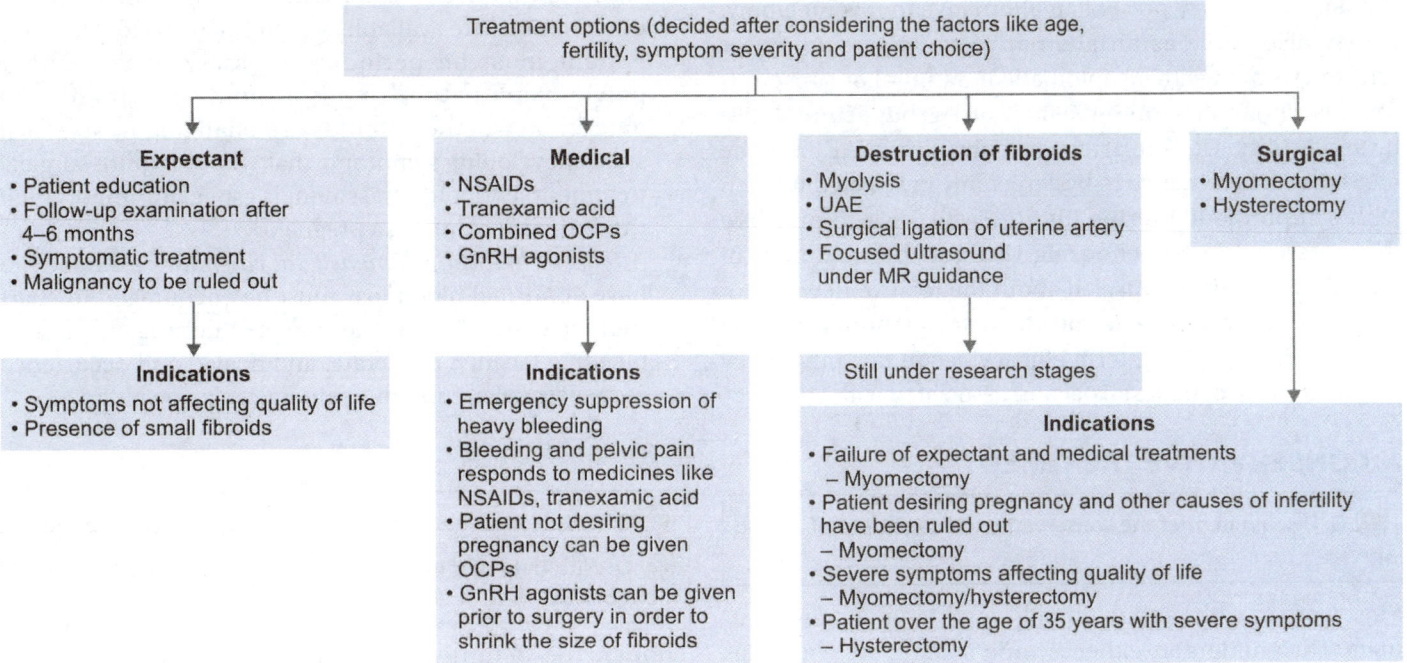

Flowchart 24.2: Treatment options for a patient diagnosed with fibroid uterus.

(GnRH: gonadotropin-releasing hormone; MR: magnetic resonance; NSAIDs: nonsteroidal anti-inflammatory drugs; OCP: oral contraceptive pill; UAE: uterine artery embolization)

Flowchart 24.3: Various treatment options in a woman with fibroid uterus based on the patient's age and desire for future childbearing.

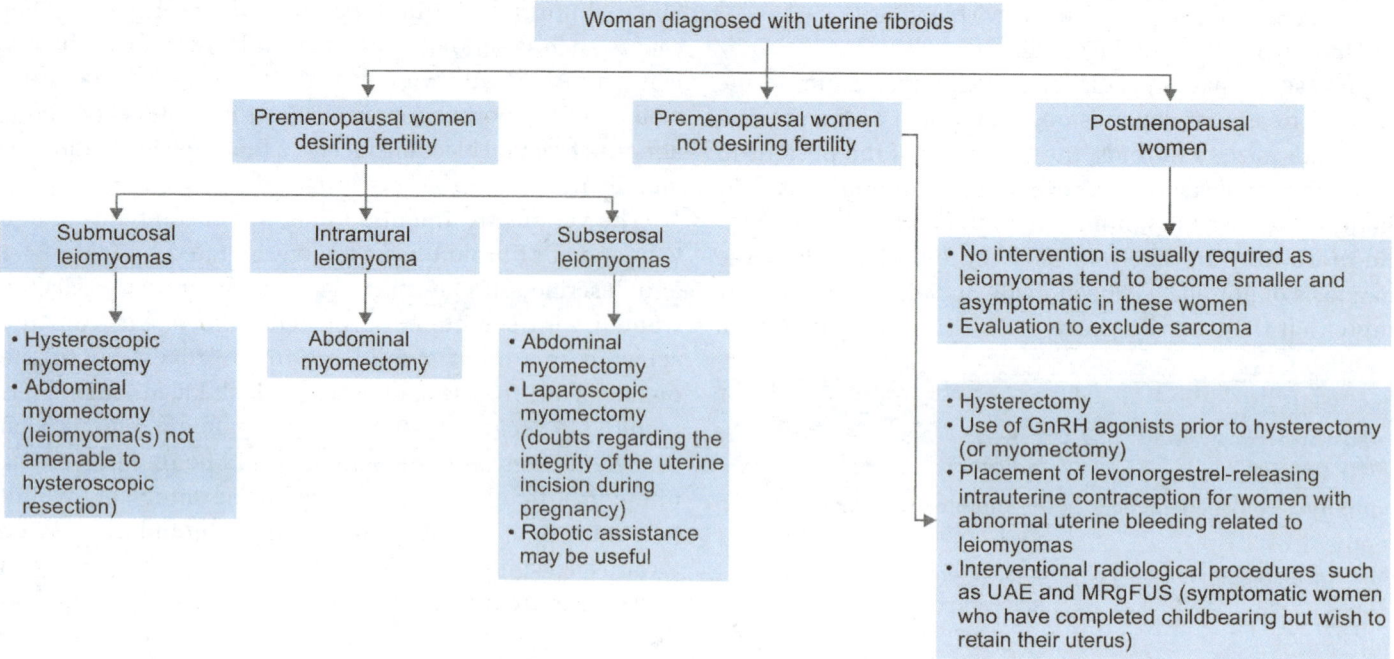

(GnRH: gonadotropin-releasing hormone; MRgFUS: magnetic resonance guided focused ultrasound; UAE: uterine artery embolization)

and the risk for conversion to hysterectomy at the time of surgery. Once the decision regarding myomectomy has been taken, the next step is deciding the route of myomectomy: hysteroscopic, laparoscopic, or abdominal. Hysteroscopic myomectomy should be considered as first-line conservative surgical therapy for the management of symptomatic intracavitary or submucosal fibroids. A hysteroscopic myomectomy is usually preferred in cases of submucosal fibroids showing minimal myometrial involvement. Laparoscopic myolysis (destruction of myoma via diathermy) may present an alternative to myomectomy. It may also serve as an alternative to hysterectomy for selected women with symptomatic intramural or subserous fibroids who wish to preserve their uterus but do not desire future fertility. Uterine artery embolization (UAE) may be offered as an alternative to hysterectomy in selected women with symptomatic uterine fibroids who wish to preserve their uterus. Women choosing UAE for the treatment of fibroids should be counseled about the relative newness of the procedure and absence of adequate literature regarding the possible risks, long-term efficacy, fecundity, pregnancy outcomes, and patient satisfaction associated with UAE.

CONSERVATIVE TREATMENT

> Q. Discuss in brief the conservative management of fibroid uterus.

Most women with uterine fibroids do not require any treatment. Their tumors are either asymptomatic or the symptoms (such as pelvic pain or menorrhagia) can be controlled with common medications such as over-the-counter pain medication for control of pain and iron supplements in presence of symptoms related to anemia. Patient counseling and education form an important component of the conservative management and comprises the following:

- The patient must be reassured that the bleeding related to fibroids is a common, benign cause of bleeding and nothing to worry about.
- Patient must be provided information regarding various treatment options, including the probable expectations and adverse effects. Patient must be reassured that in case she experiences failure with one treatment option, other options are available, which can be used.
- Patient must be periodically assessed with either pelvic examination or ultrasound examination to determine whether fibroids are changing in size or if she is developing symptoms that would require surgical treatment. Periodic assessment is especially important if the patient is planning a pregnancy.
- *Advice to maintain a menstrual calendar:* Women who have abnormal blood loss must be encouraged to chart their menstrual blood loss every month. Amount of bleeding (scanty, moderate, and heavy) and occurrence of menstrual cramps and pain must also be noted.

MEDICAL TREATMENT

> Q. Write a short essay on medical management of fibroids.
>
> Q. With help of a long essay, discuss the medical management of AUB.

Though the definitive treatment for uterine fibroids is surgery, medical therapy is sometimes instituted with the following aims:

Aims of Medical Management

- Alleviation of symptoms
- Improvement of hemoglobin status before surgery
- Emergency suppression of heavy bleeding
- Minimizing the size and vascularity of uterine fibroids prior to surgery.
- To facilitate laparoscopic surgery or allow the use of transverse incision.

Acute menorrhagia requires prompt medical intervention. Emergency suppression of an episode of heavy prolonged menstrual bleed can be achieved by norethisterone 15 mg/day or medroxyprogesterone acetate in a dose of 30 mg/day for 3 weeks. Conjugated equine estrogens are also used for emergency control of bleeding. Medical therapy must be tailored according to each individual, taking into consideration factors such as the patient's age, coexisting medical diseases, family history, and desire for fertility. For more details regarding medical therapeutic options for control of AUB, refer to Chapter 23. Medical therapeutic options for control of HMB in a patient with leiomyomas are described in **Box 24.4**.

Prostaglandin Synthetase Inhibitors

Nonsteroidal anti-inflammatory drugs (typically mefenamic acid) may be particularly useful when bleeding is associated with pelvic pain and dysmenorrhea. Various NSAIDs including mefenamic acid have been shown to significantly reduce menstrual blood loss by inhibiting the enzyme prostaglandin synthetase, which is involved in production of prostaglandins. Imbalance between various levels of prostaglandins is thought to be responsible for the pathogenesis of menorrhagia. Side effects associated with their use include nausea, vomiting, gastric discomfort, diarrhea, and dizziness. Rarely, it can cause hemolytic anemia or thrombocytopenia. However, mefenamic acid has been observed to be less effective than hemostatic agents (tranexamic acid) in reducing the amount of blood loss (20% vs. 54%), but in general it has a lower side effect profile. Mefenamic acid is administered in the dose of 500 mg TDS during menses. Other analgesic drugs belonging to the class of NSAIDs, including drugs like naprosyn, ibuprofen, indomethacin, and diclofenac may also prove to be effective in reducing pelvic pain and dysmenorrhea.

Hemostatic Agents

Tranexamic acid: Under normal circumstances, clotting of blood requires conversion of fibrinogen into fibrin. Fibrinolytic substances (fibrinolysins) in the blood are responsible for breakdown of blood clot, resulting in prolonged bleeding. Hemostatic agents like tranexamic acid help in reducing the blood loss by inhibiting this fibrinolytic activity, thereby sealing the bleeding vessels. The tranexamic acid is administered in the intravenous dosage of 10–15 mg/kg body weight two to three times a day or 0.5–1 g per day orally in divided doses, leading to a total of 3–6 g/day for the first 3 days of the cycle. Side effects due to tranexamic acid are dose related and may include symptoms such as nausea, vomiting, diarrhea, and dizziness. Rarely, there may be transient color vision disturbance or intracranial thrombosis. This drug has now been approved by the US Food and Drug Administration (FDA) for treatment of heavy bleeding. In the UK, tranexamic acid is used in preference to NSAIDs for the first-line management of patients with fibroids having HMB.

Ethamsylate: This drug helps in achieving hemostasis by reducing capillary bleeding. It helps in increasing the capillary wall strength and increasing platelet adhesion. It is used orally in the dosage of 250–500 mg three times a day.

Gonadotropin-releasing Hormone Agonists

Gonadotropin-releasing hormone agonists can be considered as the most effective medical therapy for uterine myomas.

Mode of action: GnRH is produced by the hypothalamus and stimulates the release of the gonadotropins like FSH and luteinizing hormone (LH) by the pituitary gland. These hormones then trigger the ovary to secrete hormones like estrogen and progesterone, which in turn stimulate ovarian follicular development. Administration of GnRH agonists simulates the action of GnRH in the body. However, continuous exposure to GnRH agonists desensitizes the pituitary gonadotrophs resulting in loss of gonadotropin release thereby causing a reduction in estrogen production. Therefore, following an initial gonadotropin release associated with rising estradiol levels, gonadotropin levels eventually fall off to castrate levels, with resultant hypogonadism. Therefore, due to the use of GnRH agonists, medical oophorectomy or medical menopause is produced. Most women with fibroids will develop amenorrhea, improvement in anemia (if present) and a significant reduction in uterine size within 3 months of initiating this therapy.

BOX 24.4: Medical options available for treatment of menorrhagia.

- *Antispasmodic agents:* NSAIDs, buscopan (menstruating days only)
- *Hemostatic agents:* Ethamsylate, tranexamic acid (menstruating days only)
- Combined oral contraceptive pills (day 5–25)
- Progestogens [e.g., norethisterone, primolut N, dydrogesterone (duphaston), and medroxyprogesterone (provera) (day 5–25)]
- Hormone replacement therapy
- *Androgens:* Danazol, GnRH therapy (daily continuous therapy)
- Mirena (levonorgestrel intrauterine system)

(GnRH: gonadotropin-releasing hormone; NSAIDs: nonsteroidal anti-inflammatory drugs)

As previously described, estrogen helps in promoting the growth of fibroids. As a result, treatment with GnRH agonists, by reducing estrogen production may cause nearly 50% reduction in the initial volume of the myoma within 3 months of therapy. Maximum fibroid shrinkage usually occurs after 3 months of treatment. Therefore, GnRH agonist treatment should be restricted to a 3–6 months interval. GnRH agonists are at times prescribed before surgery for uterine fibroids. They help in reducing the blood loss at the time of surgery by shrinking the tumor size, thereby eliminating the need for blood transfusions at the time of surgery. Use of GnRH agonists in woman of childbearing age can help to shrink the size of fibroid tumors, thereby eliminating the need for a hysterectomy, thus preserving fertility. Alternatively, their use may allow a simpler surgical procedure like laparoscopic hysterectomy, thereby avoiding abdominal surgery. GnRH agonists must not be used preoperatively before every myoma surgery, rather it must be used with a particular endpoint in the mind, volume reduction, resolution of anemia, or both.

Dosage and some commonly used formulations **(Table 24.5)**: GnRH agonists are available in various forms including nasal spray, subcutaneous injections, slow release intramuscular injections, and subdermal pellets. Some of the commonly used preparations of GnRH agonists include leuprolide acetate, Goserelin (zoladex), buserelin, nafarelin, triptorelin, etc.

Side effects: GnRH agonists are usually used on a short-term basis due to high costs and severe adverse effects. Side effects associated with GnRH agonists are common to menopause and may include side effects like hot flashes, mood swings, depression, weight gain, headaches, and vaginal dryness. These side effects are usually reversible upon cessation of treatment. The most important side effect of concern in the women using GnRH agonists is osteoporosis. A prolonged hypoestrogenic state associated with their use leads to bone demineralization resulting in osteoporosis. Moreover, there is a rapid resumption of menses and pretreatment uterine volume after discontinuation of GnRH agonists. Therefore, these women should not be prescribed these drugs for >6 months. Certain approaches which may be used to protect the women against osteoporosis include the following:

- *Use of add-back therapy:* In this therapy, estrogen and progestin are added in a dosage, which is high enough to maintain bone density, but too low to counter-balance the beneficial effects of the GnRH agonists.
- Addition of a bone-protective drug like bisphosphonates, calcium supplements, etc. can also be considered.

Since the use of GnRH agonists does not result in sterility, the danger of conception, although rare, is present. Furthermore, if a woman becomes pregnant during their use, there is some risk for birth defects. Therefore, the women should be advised to use barrier contraception during the entire course of GnRH agonist therapy. GnRH agonists are not indicated in women who are pregnant or are trying to become pregnant while using the drug.

Before using these drugs, the gynecologist should be certain that there is no underlying malignancy, particularly leiomyosarcoma, endometrial cancer, etc. The use of these drugs can delay the detection and treatment of the malignancy and can result in some severe complications.

Gonadotropin-releasing Hormone Antagonists

Gonadotropin-releasing hormone antagonists (ganirelix) compete with endogenous GnRH for pituitary binding sites. The advantage of using antagonists over agonists is the rapid onset of clinical effects without the characteristic initial flare-up response observed with GnRH agonist treatment. However, treatment of leiomyomas using these agents is cumbersome due to the requirement of daily injections. Treatment, however, is accompanied by hypoestrogenic symptoms. When long-acting compounds are available, GnRH antagonists might be considered for medical treatment before surgery.

Exogenous Progestins and Oral Contraceptive Agents

Use of exogenous progestins is not likely to bring about a reduction in the size of fibroids. Exogenous progestins, however, may help in providing relief against the HMB associated with leiomyomas, especially if administered continuously for 21 out of 28 days. Progestogen-releasing intrauterine devices [levonorgestrel-releasing intrauterine system (LNG-IUS)] may be beneficial for controlling HMB associated with fibroids. However, there is an associated risk of expulsion with the use of this device. The LNG-IUS is described in details later in the text. Long-term use of depot medroxyprogesterone acetate is likely to provide some protection against the development of fibroids. However, its role in the protection against fibroid-associated

TABLE 24.5: Some commonly used GnRH agonists in gynecological practice.

Name of the GnRH agonist	Route of administration	Dosage of GnRH agonist
Buserelin	Intranasal	900–1,200 µg per day
Leuprorelin (leuprolide acetate depot)	Subcutaneous Intramuscular	• 0.1–1.0 mg/day • 3.75 mg/month • 11.25 mg implant every 3 months
Nafarelin	Intranasal	400–800 µg/day
Goserelin (zoladex)	Subcutaneous	3.6 mg/month or 10.6 mg subcutaneous implant every 3 months
Triptorelin	Intramuscular	2–4 mg/month
Histrelin	Subcutaneous	10 µg/kg/day

HMB presently remains unclear. Some studies continue to suggest that estrogen-progestin contraceptive pills are contraindicated in women with uterine leiomyomas because these pills are likely to cause uterine enlargement. However, most clinicians feel that use of OCPs can partially suppress estrogen stimulation, reducing the growth of uterine fibroids resulting in long-term protection.

It is difficult to determine the effectiveness of both exogenous progestins and OCPs in the treatment of leiomyoma-associated symptoms. This might serve as a useful option for women with fibroids desiring contraception.

Levonorgestrel Intrauterine System

Progestogen-releasing intrauterine devices (LNG-IUS or Mirena®) were initially developed as a highly effective and reversible method of contraception. However, its use has also been observed to provide excellent reduction in the amount of menstrual blood loss. LNG-IUS helps in reducing the amount of menstrual blood loss by causing the local release of the progestogen, levonorgestrel, within the uterine cavity. However, use of LNG-IUS is likely to be associated with a high expulsion rate (6–13%) in comparison to the rate of 3% in the general population. Women should be warned about this risk before they start using LNG-IUS. The device contains 52 mg of levonorgestrel, a progestin, which is released at the rate of approximately 20 μg/day. This dose of progesterone helps in thinning the endometrial lining, thereby helping in considerably reducing the volume of menstrual blood loss. Menstrual bleeding may eventually stop while the IUS is in place. The device has now been approved by the FDA for control of HMB. Another added advantage of using IUS is that it provides effective contraception for a period of 5 years and must be removed or replaced after the expiry of this period. However, IUS should not be used in presence of large uterine fibroids (>3 cm), which cause distortion of the uterine cavity. Use of IUS can result in the development of side effects like change in menstrual bleeding pattern such as frequent, prolonged, or heavy bleeding; spotting, light, scanty bleeding, irregular bleeding, or cessation of bleeding; development of ovarian cysts; weight gain; edema; headache; depression and nervousness; mood swings; nausea; pain including lower abdominal pain, back pain, breast pain, and dysmenorrhea; acne; and vaginal discharge including cervicitis, genital infections, etc. Other side effects related to the use of IUS include the following:

- Breakthrough bleeding in the first few cycles
- About 20% develop amenorrhea within 1 year
- Presence of functional ovarian cysts
- High risk of expulsion.

Antiprogestins and Progesterone Receptor Modulators

Since progesterone appears to be capable of stimulating growth of the uterine fibroids, antiprogestins like mifepristone and progesterone receptor modulators can help in reducing fibroid growth. Mifepristone is a selective antagonist of progesterone and is thought to cause a reduction in the size of leiomyomas comparable to that caused by GnRH. Mifepristone is administered in the dose of 5–50 mg once a day for a period of 3–6 months and is not currently approved by the USFDA for the treatment of myomas. The main impediment to its off-label use is that currently available doses (200 mg) are not appropriate. The primary concern with the use of both these agents is the potential for an increased risk for endometrial cancer or hyperplasia.

Progesterone Receptor Modulators

Selective progesterone receptor modulators (SPRMs), e.g., ulipristal acetate (UA), can also cause a reduction in the uterine size in cases of fibroid uterus. It acts by inhibiting ovulation but has little impact on serum estradiol levels. It is also likely to induce apoptosis in uterine fibroid cells and prevents multiplication of cells. Results from PEARL I study show that treatment with UA in the dosage of 5 and 10 mg for 13 weeks is likely to help reduce the size of fibroids in comparison to placebo. It is also able to effectively control the excessive bleeding occurring due to the presence of uterine fibroids in >90% patients.

PEARL II study has revealed that intake of UA in the dosage of both 5 mg and 10 mg is likely to be better than once-monthly dosage of a GnRH analog (e.g., leuprolide acetate) in controlling uterine bleeding. Moreover, UA was better tolerated, was able to control bleeding rapidly, and was significantly less likely to cause hot flashes in comparison to leuprolide acetate.

PEARL III and extension trials were performed to assess the effect of long-term use of UA with repeated treatment cycles. In the PEARL III trial, 10 mg of UA was administered for a period of 12 weeks. In PEARL III extension trials, 10 mg of UA was administered for four courses along with norethisterone acetate between the courses of UA. Repeated 3-month course of UA has been shown to effectively control bleeding and shrink fibroids in patients with symptomatic fibroids. The results in this trial are similar to that with PEARL I and PEARL II.

The use of UA in the dosage of 5 mg for uterine fibroids was temporarily suspended in March 2020 due to the risk of serious liver damage (injury and failure) with some cases even requiring liver transplantation. As per medicines and healthcare products regulatory agency (MRHA, 2021), though this suspension has been lifted, this medication must only be used for intermittent treatment of moderate-to-severe symptoms of uterine fibroids before menopause only when surgical procedures (including UAE) are not acceptable to the woman, have failed or are not suitable (because the risk outweighs the benefits). UA should no longer be prescribed for controlling symptoms of uterine fibroids while waiting for surgical treatment (RCOG, 2018).

Selective Estrogen Receptor Modulators (e.g., Raloxifene)

Some studies have shown that the use of selective estrogen receptor modulators (SERMs) helps in reducing the size of fibroids and improving clinical outcomes. However, well-designed, randomized studies in future are required to establish definite evidence regarding the benefit of SERMs in treating women with uterine fibroids.

Danazol

This is an androgenic agonist, with strong antigonadotropic activity, due to which it can inhibit LH and FSH. As a result, it can suppress fibroid growth, but is also associated with a high rate of adverse effects such as weight gain, acne, hirsutism, edema, hair loss, deepening of voice, flushing, sweating, vaginal dryness, etc. and is thus often less acceptable to patients. For detailed description regarding danazol, refer to Chapter 30. Another androgenic drug, gestrinone decreases myoma volume and induces amenorrhea in women with leiomyomas. An advantage of this drug is that there is a carryover effect after it is discontinued. Gestrinone, however, is not available in the United States. It is marketed in Europe, Australia, and Latin America. It is also available in India.

Conjugated Equine Estrogen (Premarin)

Conjugated equine estrogens are effective in controlling acute, profuse bleeding. This drug helps in controlling bleeding by exerting a vasospastic action on capillary bleeding by increasing the level of various clotting factors in the blood including fibrinogen, factor IV and factor X, and improving platelet aggregation and capillary permeability. Estrogen also induces formation of progesterone receptors, making subsequent treatment with progestins more effective.

This drug helps in controlling acute bleeding, but does not treat the underlying cause. Therefore appropriate long-term therapy should be administered depending on the underlying pathology, once the acute episode has been controlled. These agents are administered intravenously in a dose of 25 mg every 4 hourly in patients with acute bleeding, for a maximum of 48 hours. If the bleeding slows down, the patient is followed-up with estrogen-progestin therapy for 7 days. This may be followed-up with OCPs for 3 months.

A D&C procedure may be necessary if no response is noted within 24 hours following the use of premarin. D&C should not be routinely used for treatment of menorrhagia because it provides only short-term relief, typically lasting for about 1–2 months. This procedure is used best in conjunction with hysteroscopy to evaluate the endometrial cavity for pathology. For detailed description of the procedure of D&C, refer to Chapter 24.

ENDOMETRIAL ABLATION

Endometrial ablation does not have much role in controlling bleeding related to leiomyomas uterus. Endometrial ablation, with or without hysteroscopic myomectomy, also may be sometimes considered in women who do not desire future childbearing. While large intrauterine myomas serve as a contraindication for these procedures, a woman with small fibroids (<3 cm) can be treated using endometrial ablation. These techniques may be also useful in controlling HMB in the women wishing to conserve their uterus. This technique has been described in further details later in this chapter. Since intramural and subserosal leiomyomas are not affected by this procedure, bulk or pressure symptoms are unlikely to improve. In case of presence of submucous leiomyomas, microwave ablation is possible if the leiomyoma is <3 cm, and resection of the leiomyoma with rollerball ablation is indicated if the leiomyoma is >3 cm in size.

SURGICAL OPTIONS

Surgery forms the definite treatment modality for uterine leiomyomas. The three main surgical options, which can be used in the women with leiomyoma uterus include— (1) myomectomy, (2) hysterectomy, and (3) more recently UAE. Women should be informed that having a UAE or myomectomy would potentially allow them to retain their uterus. Some indications, when the gynecologist needs to resort to surgery in case of a woman with leiomyomas in the uterus are enumerated in the **Box 24.5**.

Besides acting as a definitive cure for myomas, surgical management is also used in the following circumstances:

- Control of excessive uterine bleeding
- Control of pain and symptoms related to excessive pelvic pressure
- History of infertility or recurrent pregnancy loss with distortion of endometrial cavity or tubal occlusion
- Menorrhagia not responding to conservative or other medical treatment modalities
- There is a high clinical suspicion of malignancy
- Growth of fibroid continues even following the menopause
- Menorrhagia results in severe iron deficiency anemia

BOX 24.5: Indications for surgery in patients with myomas.

- Presence of large fibroids (>3 cm in diameter)
- Severe bleeding, having a significant impact on a woman's quality of life, which is refractory to drug therapy
- Persistent or intolerable pain or pressure
- Urinary or intestinal symptoms due to presence of a large myoma
- History of infertility and future pregnancy is desired
- History of recurrent spontaneous abortions and future pregnancy is desired
- Rapid enlargement of a myoma (especially after menopause) raising the suspicion of leiomyosarcoma (a rare cause)

- Recurrent pregnancy losses (all the other causes have been ruled out and uterine fibroids appear to be the most likely cause of recurrent miscarriages).

Hysterectomy

Hysterectomy, a major surgical operation involving the removal of the woman's uterus helps in providing definitive cure for uterine leiomyomas **(Fig. 24.8)**. Hysterectomy can be performed in several ways: abdominally, vaginally, and in some cases laparoscopically. Robotic hysterectomy is also being done nowadays. Recovery time varies from 2 to 6 weeks. Hysterectomy is more expensive and is associated with greater mortality and morbidity in comparison to other surgical procedures (myomectomy, UAE, etc.). The mortality rate for hysterectomy ranges from 0.1 to 1.1 cases per 1,000 procedures.

The morbidity rate usually is 40%. The main advantage of hysterectomy over other invasive interventions is that it eliminates both current symptoms and the chance of recurrent problems due to leiomyomas. Hysterectomy should be considered only when any of the indication mentioned in **Box 24.6** occurs.

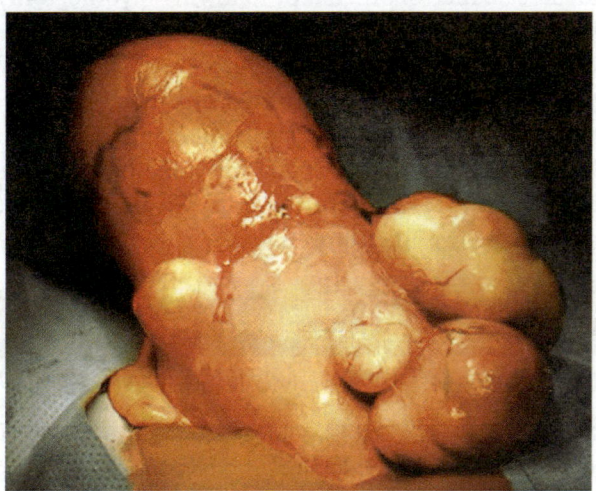

Fig. 24.8: Hysterectomy specimen showing presence of multiple subserosal fibroids.

BOX 24.6: Indications for hysterectomy.

- Woman with acute hemorrhage who does not respond to other therapies
- The woman no longer wishes to retain her uterus and fertility or may be at an increased future risk of other diseases such as cervical intraepithelial neoplasia, endometriosis, and adenomyosis which could be eliminated by hysterectomy
- Patient wishes for amenorrhea
- Other treatment options (medical, myomectomy, UAE, etc.) have failed or are contraindicated
- Rapidly enlarging fibroids or there are concerns of leiomyosarcoma (in case of rapidly enlarging fibroids) even in otherwise asymptomatic cases

(UAE: uterine artery embolization)

As mentioned before, hysterectomy is a major surgery, which is associated with numerous complications including high rates of morbidity and mortality. Some other disadvantages of hysterectomy are enumerated in **Box 24.7**. One of the important complications associated with hysterectomy is damage to the surrounding structures such as ureters. Risk of ureteric injury during hysterectomy could be associated with the fibroids at the following locations—cervical (anterior, central, or posterior), broad ligament and retroperitoneal fibroids. Preoperative management in case of suspected ureteric obstruction comprises of intravenous pyelography or stenting the ureters, especially with illuminant stents. In case of suspicion during surgery, the following can be done: observation of the peristalsis of ureters, cystoscopy, or transurethral stenting and repair cystostomy.

The removal of the uterus can frequently result in significant physical strain and psychological stress. Thus, prior to the decision of hysterectomy, the gynecologist should have detailed discussion with the patient regarding the advantages and disadvantages of the surgical procedure, its impact on sexual feelings, fertility and bladder function, probable treatment complications, the woman's expectations, and issues related to menopause and their psychological impact. Removal of healthy ovaries should not be routinely undertaken during the surgery.

Removal of ovaries should only be undertaken with the express wish and consent of the woman. Removal of the ovaries at the time of hysterectomy may be considered in the women with a significant family history of breast or ovarian cancer or those suspected of developing future ovarian malignancy. Women should be informed about the risk of possible loss of ovarian function and its consequences, even if their ovaries are retained during hysterectomy. The women should be counseled regarding the possible requirement for HRT following oophorectomy.

Next step is to decide the route of surgery—vaginal route (vaginal hysterectomy), abdominal route (abdominal hysterectomy), or laparoscopic route [laparoscopic hysterectomy or laparoscopic-assisted vaginal hysterectomy (LAVH)]. Usually, vaginal hysterectomy is preferred over abdominal hysterectomy. Compared with abdominal hysterectomy, vaginal hysterectomy is associated with reduced rate of morbidity (shorter hospital stay and faster recovery) and other complications. Laparoscopic hysterectomy or LAVH is also associated with reduced rates of morbidity and complications (postoperative pain, hospital stay, and recovery period) in comparison with abdominal

BOX 24.7: Disadvantages of hysterectomy.

- High risk of complications (risk of intraoperative hemorrhage, damage to other abdominal organs, etc.)
- Requirement of general or regional anesthesia
- The recovery time varies from 2 to 8 weeks
- Early onset of menopause
- Possible requirement for hormone replacement therapy in future

hysterectomy. However, LAVH may not be widely available as its performance requires specific laparoscopic training and skills. Various factors must be taken into consideration before deciding the route of surgery. Some of the factors, which need to be taken into account, are listed in **Box 24.8**.

When abdominal hysterectomy is decided upon, then both types of abdominal hysterectomies—(1) the total method (removal of the uterus and the cervix) and (2) subtotal method (removal of the uterus and preservation of the cervix) should be discussed with the woman.

Hysterectomy with Central, Cervical Fibroids

> Q. Write a short essay on cervical fibroids
>
> Q. Discuss briefly the technique of hysterectomy in case of cervical fibroids.

Following precautions may be required during hysterectomy in these cases:

- In these cases, the bladder may be pulled up so caution must be observed while opening the peritoneum.
- Wherever possible, enucleation of cervical fibroid is preferred to correct the anatomy prior to the placement of uterine clamps.
- Uterine vessels must be clamped under direct vision.
- Clamps should be placed as closed and parallel to the lateral borders of the cervix.
- Bisection of the uterus and enucleation of the myoma is preferred prior to the application of clamps to the parametrium.
- During laparoscopic surgery, thermal injury is most likely. Therefore, extreme caution must be observed with application of cautery or lasers to the tissues near or over the ureter.

Myomectomy

> Q. Write a long essay on myomectomy.
>
> Q. Discuss in brief about myomectomy: methods, indications, and prevention of complications.
>
> Q. Write a short essay discussing the controversies in myomectomy.
>
> Q. write a short essay describing the principles of myomectomy.
>
> Q. With help of a short essay discuss myomectomy.

Surgical removal of myomas from the uterine cavity is termed as myomectomy. Although myomectomy allows preservation of the uterus, present evidence indicates a higher risk of blood loss and greater operative time with myomectomy in comparison to hysterectomy. Numerous techniques are used nowadays for performing myomectomy. These include the following—performing a myomectomy through an abdominal incision, vaginal incision, with help of a laparoscope, or with help of a hysteroscope. Removal of the myoma relieves symptoms in >75% of women. Summary of ACOG practice bulletin (2021) regarding the management of leiomyomas is enumerated in **Box 24.9**.

Patient Counseling

There are times, when myomectomy is associated with uncontrollable bleeding and thus needs to be converted into an abdominal hysterectomy during the time of planned surgery. Therefore, if myomectomy is selected as the therapeutic option, the women should be counseled about small risk of reoperation and the risk of conversion to hysterectomy in nearly 1–5% cases. The woman undergoing myomectomy also needs to be counseled regarding the following:

- 40–60% chance of pregnancy following myomectomy
- 30–50% chances of recurrence or persistence of fibroids following myomectomy
- 20–25% risk of relaparotomy after myomectomy
- 1–5% risk of persistence of HMB following myomectomy

Some of the indications for myomectomy are listed in **Box 24.10**. Myomectomy is a viable therapeutic alternative to hysterectomy in women with symptomatic

---

BOX 24.9: Summary of ACOG practice bulletin (2021) for management of leiomyomas.

Evidence level A (based on well designed, randomized controlled trials):
- Hysterectomy is the definitive cure for symptomatic leiomyomas; however, abdominal myomectomy is a safer and more effective option in women who wish to become pregnant
- Use of GnRH agonists and vasopressin preoperatively at the time of myomectomy helps in reducing the amount of blood loss

Evidence level C (based on evidence from expert committee reports or opinions and/or clinical experience of respected authorities):
- Safety of laparoscopic myomectomy has yet not been established in women planning pregnancy
- Hysteroscopic myomectomy is an effective option for women with submucous fibroids

---

BOX 24.8: Factors to be taken into consideration before deciding the route of surgery.

- Presence of other gynecological conditions or diseases
- Uterine size, and location, number and size of uterine fibroids
- Mobility and descent of the uterus
- Size and shape of the vagina
- History of previous abdominal surgery

BOX 24.10: Indications for myomectomy.

- Women with symptomatic myomas, desiring fertility
- Large myomas (especially the submucosal or intramural type)
- Any symptomatic fibroid (which causes menometrorrhagia) also needs to be treated
- When in vitro fertilization is indicated (especially if the myoma results in the distortion of the uterine cavity)

myomas, who desire fertility. If the myoma (especially the submucosal or intramural type) is large in size (>5 cm), most studies recommend that it must be removed. Large submucosal or intramural myomas may not only cause distortion of endometrial cavity, they may also result in menometrorrhagia. Both these factors have been shown to result in reduced fertility. Large myomas may also result in complications for the future pregnancies (miscarriage, preterm delivery, etc.).

Any symptomatic myoma (e.g., myoma which causes menometrorrhagia) also needs to be treated. However, finding of a small asymptomatic leiomyoma in an infertile woman is not an indication for immediate myomectomy.

Success rate of IVF is most significantly affected by presence of intramural or submucosal fibroids which distort the uterine cavity. Therefore, presence of intramural or submucous myomas which distort the endometrial cavity in a woman undergoing IVF is also an indication for myomectomy. However, if the myoma does not distort the endometrial cavity, the indications for myomectomy are not so clear. The available evidence does not support myomectomy before assisted reproductive technology in patients with asymptomatic myomas that do not significantly distort the uterine cavity or cause abnormal uterine bleeding.

Due to a high rate of myoma recurrence, a myomectomy is generally not recommended for women who have completed childbearing, yet continue to suffer from excessive heavy menstrual periods, pelvic pressure, and pain due to fibroids.

Risks Associated with Myomectomy

Risks associated with myomectomy are enumerated in **Box 24.11**. Since there are numerous risks associated with myomectomy, the expected benefits of myomectomy must be weighed against the risks associated with the procedure, before carrying out this surgery. The most important complication associated with myomectomy is intraoperative blood loss. The following precautions must be taken to reduce/prevent blood loss:

- Four-units cross-matched blood must be made available for transfusion.
- Anemia must be corrected before performing the elective myomectomy.
- Use of GnRH agonists/misoprostol prior to surgery may help in preventing anemia by reducing the blood loss related to HMB.

> **BOX 24.11:** Risks associated with myomectomy.
> - Increased postoperative blood loss
> - Hysterectomy may be required during the surgery, if myomectomy appears dangerous or difficult
> - Increased risk of uterine rupture at the time of delivery
> - Need for mandatory cesarean section in case the patient achieves pregnancy
> - Increased risk for postoperative adhesions
> - Recurrence of myoma postoperatively

- Before performing myomectomy, it is important to counsel the patient regarding the possibility that intraoperative findings may contraindicate myomectomy and require that hysterectomy be performed instead.
- During surgery, uterine artery occlusion may be done with help of a tourniquet or Bonney's myomectomy clamp.
- Dilute vasopressin can be injected prior to surgery to prevent the blood loss.

If pregnancy is desired, there is a risk of uterine rupture after myomectomy during delivery. This can occur irrespective of the route for myomectomy (abdominal, laparoscopic, or hysteroscopic myomectomy) due to excessive dissection of myometrial muscles during the surgery.

Development of postoperative adhesions following myomectomy is an important complication of myomectomy. This complication has been shown to occur more with laparoscopic as compared to the abdominal procedure. In order to reduce the risk of development of postoperative intestinal adhesions, incisions over the peritoneal aspect of the posterior uterine wall must be avoided during surgery.

Recurrence of myomas postoperatively is another complication associated with myomectomy (more with laparoscopic as compared to the abdominal procedure). A small myoma at the time of surgery may get overlooked and not get removed. This may result in future recurrence of myoma postoperatively.

Deciding the Type of Myomectomy to be Performed

Myomectomy can be performed via abdominal, laparoscopic, hysteroscopic, or robotic routes. If myomectomy is being performed to regain fertility, the next question, which requires to be answered is, what type of myomectomy would be associated with best pregnancy outcome—abdominal, laparoscopic, hysteroscopic or robotic? These various options are discussed below:

Abdominal myomectomy: The advantage of abdominal myomectomy is that large fibroids can be quickly removed. The surgeon is able to feel the uterus, which is helpful in locating myomas that may be deep in the uterine wall or are very small in size. The disadvantage of a laparotomy is that it requires an abdominal incision. The main complication of myomectomy is that it weakens the uterine musculature. As a result, a woman who becomes pregnant after a myomectomy may require a cesarean delivery to prevent rupture of the uterus at the myomectomy site. Blood loss during myomectomy is also a potential problem. It can be limited by the use of tourniquets or vasoconstrictive agents (e.g., vasopressin). The use of intravascular vasopressin injections should be avoided and patients should be monitored carefully.

Steps: After inspecting the uterus to determine the number and position of the fibroids, the uterine endometrium overlying the fibroid is cut, following which the fibroids are separated and removed from the normal uterine muscle (**Figs. 24.9A to J**). After the removal of the fibroids, normal uterine muscle can be sewn back together.

Bonney's approach is often used for posterior myomas by creating a functional anterior incision, at the same time avoiding a posterior defect and the various complications, which may be associated with it. In this approach, an elliptical incision is made transversely across the posterior fundal region, taking care to avoid the interstitial portion of the fallopian tube. After the primary tumor is removed, other leiomyomata can also be removed through the same incision. Excessive myometrium needs to be trimmed away. Interrupted sutures in layers are then used to obliterate the dead space, approximate the myometrium, and accomplish satisfactory hemostasis. The posterior flap of myometrium is draped over the fundus and fixed to the anterior surface of the uterus with the help of fine sutures. This is known as the Bonney's hood (**Fig. 24.10**).

Myomectomy with cesarean section: Though myomectomy can be performed at the time of cesarean delivery, it should be best avoided due to the risk of excessive bleeding due to increased vascularity related to fibroids. Preferably removal of only pedunculated fibroids must be considered at the time

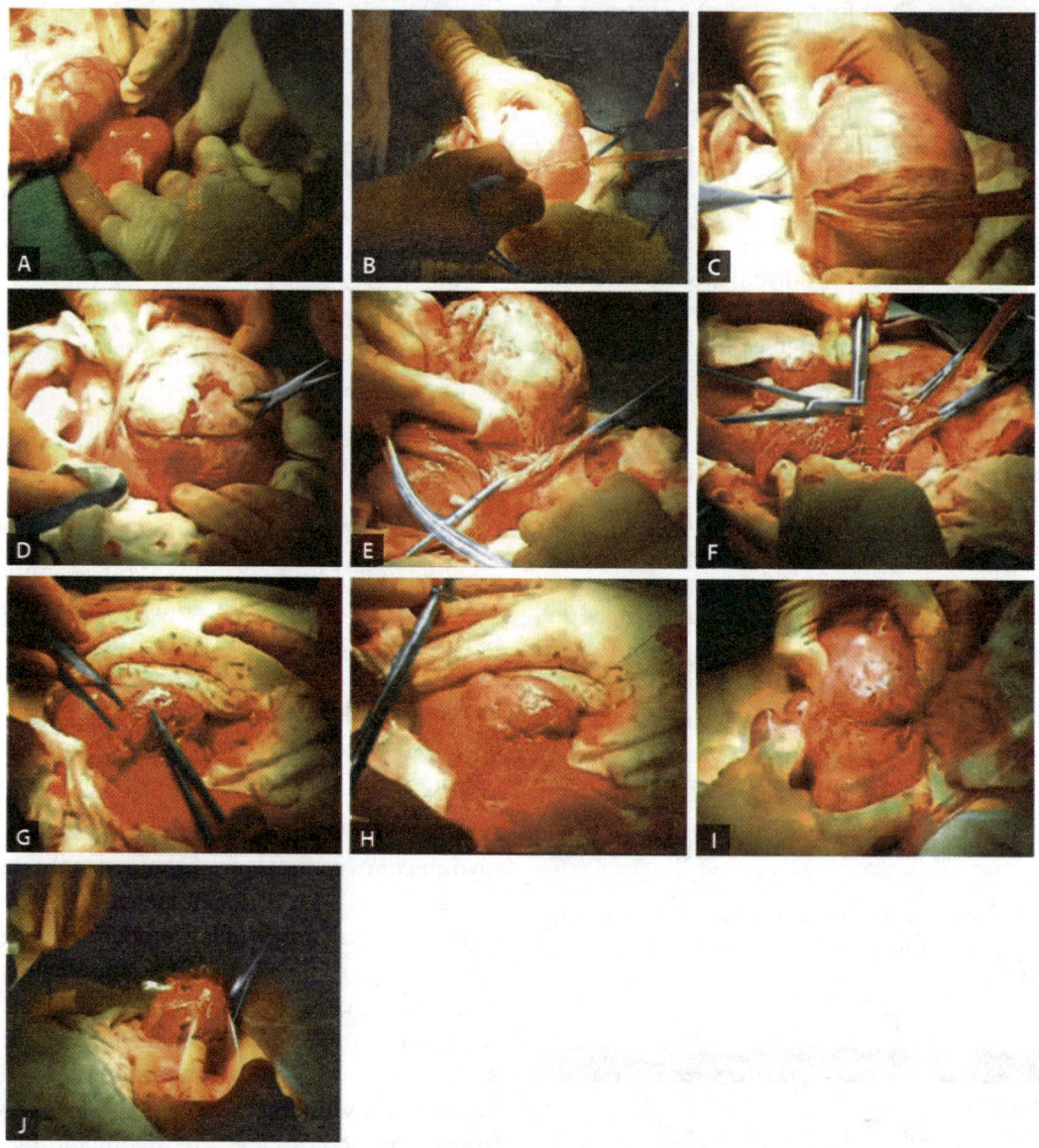

Figs. 24.9A to J: Abdominal myomectomy. (A) Uterus containing multiple fibroids is visualized; (B) A horizontal uterine incision is given over the anterior surface of the uterus, avoiding a posterior incision wherever possible; (C) The incision is extended through the pseudocapsule to expose the myoma; (D and E) The plane of cleavage is developed between the myoma and the myometrium with the help of blunt and sharp dissection by which the myoma is enucleated and delivered outside the uterus; (F) Stitching of the myoma bed once the fibroid has been enucleated out; (G and H) The uterine myometrium is being approximated using layered interrupted delayed-absorbable sutures; (I) Suturing of the uterine incision is complete; and (J) Placement of an adhesion barrier over the suture line to prevent development of adhesions.

of cesarean delivery. Also decision of removing fibroids at the time of cesarean delivery best depends upon the surgeon's expertise and facilities for blood transfusion.

Laparoscopic myomectomy: Fibroids can also be removed by laparoscopy. The challenges of this surgery rest with the surgeon's ability to remove the mass through a small abdominal incision and to reconstruct the uterus. Concerns have been raised regarding the surgeon's ability to suture the uterus with an adequate multilayer closure laparoscopically. The choice of surgical approach is largely dependent on surgical expertise of the surgeon.

Though use of morcellators has permitted the removal of larger myomas, there is a danger of injury to surrounding organs.

Laparoscopic myomectomy is most commonly used for removing subserosal fibroids. The steps for removal of a subserosal myoma are shown in **Figures 24.11A to H**. Once the fibroids are removed, they are cut into pieces and removed from abdomen via laparoscopic, abdominal, or vaginal route. This process is known as morcellation and can be performed with help of a morcellator or a knife. Morcellation may be associated with an increased risk of peritoneal dissemination. Therefore, it must be preferably performed using an endobag to avoid spillage. Also, caution must be maintained if there is a suspicion of sarcomatous changes in the myoma.

Advantages of laparoscopic myomectomy: Advantages of laparoscopic myomectomy are described in **Box 24.12**. Since laparoscopic myomectomy is a less invasive procedure

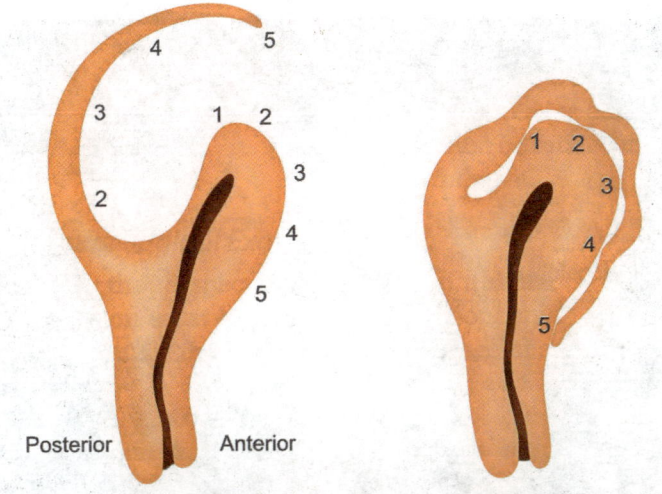

Fig. 24.10: Bonney's hood approach.

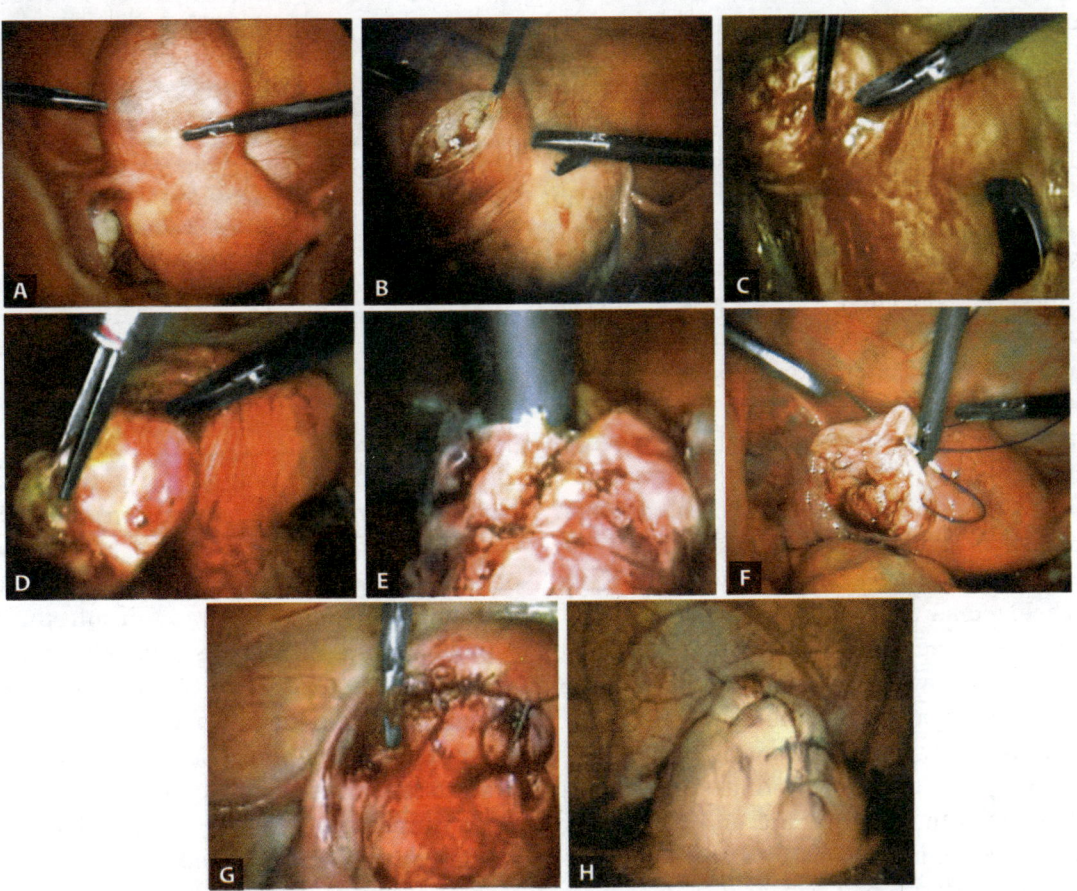

Figs. 24.11A to H: Laparoscopic myomectomy. (A) Presence of a subserous fibroid, which is handled laparoscopically; (B) An incision given over the surface of fibroid; (C) The myoma is gradually shelled out from the underlying myometrium; (D) The myoma has been shelled out completely; (E) The large fibroid is morcellated and removed from the body; (F) Following the removal of myoma the small raw area left after removal is stitched together with Vicryl sutures; (G) The closure of uterine myometrium is almost complete; (H) The myometrial suture line following the completion of surgery.

BOX 24.12: Advantages of laparoscopic myomectomy.

- Less invasive procedure
- Fewer operative and postoperative complications (postoperative adhesions, blood loss, paralytic ileus, infection, etc.)
- Reduced surgical morbidity resulting in improved postsurgical outcomes
- Significantly reduced hospital stay and quick recovery
- May be performed as an outpatient surgery under general or regional anesthesia

BOX 24.13: Complications of laparoscopic myomectomy.

- Development of uterine rupture during pregnancy (most commonly third trimester)
- Development of postoperative adhesions
- Recurrence of myoma after myomectomy
- The procedure requires more level of skill and training in comparison to the abdominal surgery

in comparison to the conventional abdominal myomectomy, it is associated with fewer complications in the operative and postoperative periods, compared to that of the abdominal procedure. Laparoscopic myomectomy results in significantly reduced hospital stay following surgery, reduced surgical morbidity, and improved patient outcome and recovery. Blood loss during surgery is significantly less with laparoscopy.

Complications of laparoscopic myomectomy: Complications of laparoscopic myomectomy are listed in **Box 24.13**. The most important complication following myomectomy is the development of adhesions postoperatively.

Development of these postoperative adhesions is particularly important as these adhesions can trap the adnexa, resulting in tubal blockage, etc. Hence, this can impair the woman's fertility, resulting in further problems in women desiring future fertility. Development of adhesions postoperatively is less commonly associated with laparoscopic myomectomy in comparison to abdominal myomectomy. There has been a recent advancement in laparoscopic surgery, associated with the use of special substances, called adhesion barriers, which help prevent the formation of scar tissue after surgery. Small sheets of cloth-like material can be wrapped around the raw areas from surgery and this material prevents nearby tissue from adhering to the site of surgery **(Fig. 24.12)**. After a few weeks, the material dissolves, leaving the newly healed surgery sites fairly free of adhesions. While the use of these barriers may not be completely perfect in preventing adhesions, they have been shown to help reduce the formation of adhesions.

As previously mentioned, the operative and postoperative complications associated with laparoscopic myomectomy are much less in comparison to abdominal myomectomy. One of the most important complications associated with any type of myomectomy is the risk of uterine rupture during pregnancy. Though both laparoscopic and abdominal myomectomies can result in uterine rupture, the timing of this drastic complication varies between the two procedures. While, uterine rupture following abdominal myomectomy commonly occurs during labor that following laparoscopic myomectomy commonly occurs during the third trimester of pregnancy (after 36 weeks).

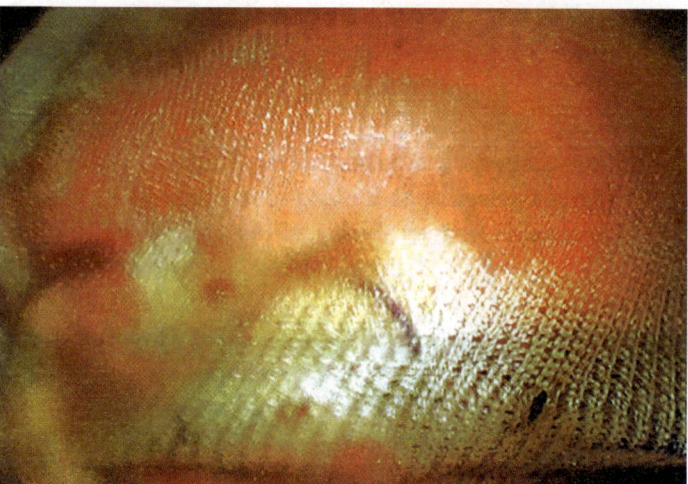

Fig. 24.12: Use of adhesion barriers for prevention of postoperative adhesions.

BOX 24.14: Possible reasons for uterine rupture following laparoscopic myomectomy.

- Natural tendency of the uterus to undergo hyperplasia and hypertrophy during pregnancy
- Less perfect reconstruction of uterine tissues
- Proper repair of the uterine wall may not be possible (especially with large, numerous, or deeply embedded uterine myomas)
- Presence of a hematoma over scar tissue
- Wide use of electrosurgery for obtaining hemostasis during laparoscopic surgery

Some possible reasons for the uterus to rupture following laparoscopic myomectomy are listed in **Box 24.14**.

Laparoscopic myomectomy is associated with less perfect reconstruction of uterine tissue in comparison to abdominal myomectomy. As a result, the risk of uterine rupture is more with laparoscopic procedure in comparison to abdominal procedure. Also, when the myomas are deeply embedded in the myometrium or are large in size or numerous, proper repair of the uterine wall may not be possible with laparoscopic procedure. Wide use of electrosurgery for obtaining hemostasis during laparoscopic surgery may be another factor involved in reducing the scar strength. Use of electrosurgery may result in poor vascularization, tissue necrosis, and adverse effects on scar strength. Excessive bleeding during the surgery can result in hematoma formation, which can weaken the uterine walls by resulting in the formation of fibrous tissue.

During myomectomy, extensive manipulation of uterine tissue is performed. The uterine muscles have an ability to regenerate slowly. If the edges of the wound are accurately sutured, the healing of the uterine wound takes place through regeneration of myometrial muscles. This results in strengthening of the uterine walls. On the other hand, if the edges of the wound are not approximated properly, healing occurs by secondary intention, thereby resulting in the formation of fibrous tissue, which considerably weakens the postoperative scar. Thus, in order to avoid scar rupture during pregnancy, precautions to be taken are listed in **Box 24.15**.

Hysteroscopic myomectomy: Hysteroscopic myomectomy forms the procedure of choice for completely submucosal myomas or those myomas having <50% extension into the myometrium **(Fig. 24.13)**. Some of the indications for hysteroscopic myomectomy are listed in **Box 24.16**. Besides the submucous leiomyomas, other most common lesions found during diagnostic office hysteroscopy include cervical and uterine polyps, uterine septa, intrauterine adhesions, endometrial hyperplasia, endometrial cancer, etc.

If fertility is not desired and abnormal uterine bleeding related to the presence of submucosal myomas is the main symptom for its hysteroscopic removal, concomitant endometrial ablation, or resection may provide better resolution of abnormal bleeding in comparison to myomectomy alone.

Hysteroscopic myomectomy can be performed as a simple outpatient procedure where a hysteroscope is placed into the uterine cavity and the leiomyomas are resected out **(Figs. 24.14A to C)**. The technique of hysteroscopic resection of submucous leiomyomas was first described by Neuwirth and Amin in 1976. Since the use of hysteroscope requires instillation of fluid inside the uterine cavity, it is important to monitor ongoing fluid balance carefully during hysteroscopic removal of fibroids. According to the European Society of Hysteroscopy, submucous leiomyomas have been classified into three categories depending on the degree of myometrial invasion **(Fig. 24.15)**. T-0 corresponds to pedunculated submucous leiomyomas. T-I represents submucous leiomyomas with <50% invasion into the myometrial wall and T-II are those with >50% invasion. Removal of myomas belonging to the categories T-0 and T-I should be attempted using a hysteroscope. However, hysteroscopic resection should not normally be attempted in

> **BOX 24.15:** Precautions to be taken to prevent scar rupture after laparoscopic myomectomy.
> - Proper approximation of the edges of the incision (inverting the edges of the myometrium)
> - One must never use radiofrequencies to achieve hemostasis during surgery
> - Long time interval must be planned between surgery and pregnancy (>1 year)
> - Elective cesarean section in these patients before 36 weeks

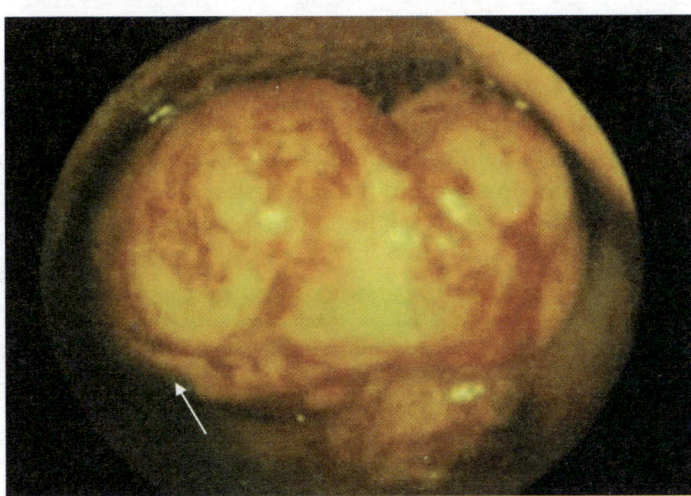

Fig. 24.13: Appearance of submucosal myoma on hysteroscopy (indicated by arrow).

> **BOX 24.16:** Indications for hysteroscopic myomectomy.
> - Infertility (submucosal fibroids per se may be responsible for producing infertility or reducing the pregnancy rate in women undergoing in vitro fertilization)
> - Repeated pregnancy losses
> - Abnormal uterine bleeding

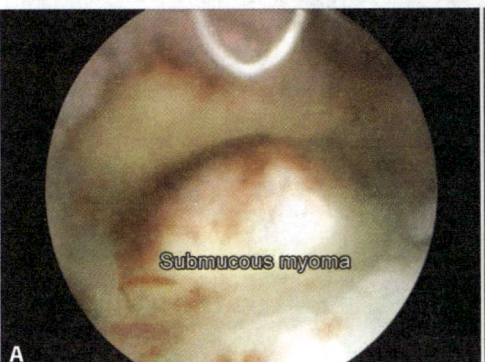 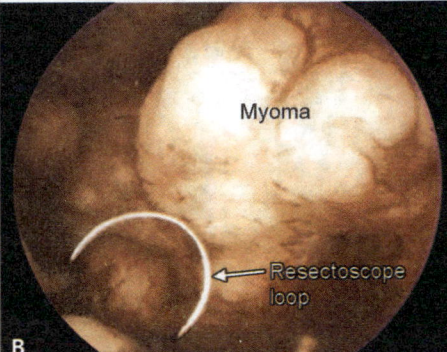 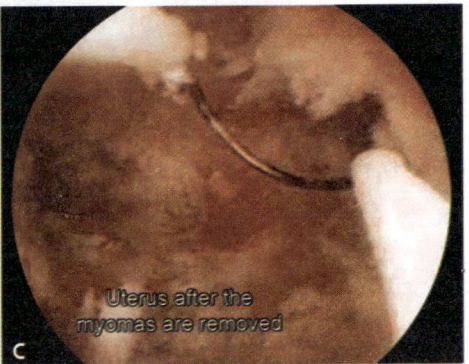

Figs. 24.14A to C: (A) Hysteroscopic view showing presence of a submucous fibroid; (B) Beginning of the hysteroscopic resection of submucous fibroid; (C) Completion of the hysteroscopic resection of submucous fibroid.

fibromyomas belonging to T-II category. This is so because, when submucous myomas have intramural extensions >50%, hysteroscopic resection may be associated with a higher rate of complication, including increased rate of conversion to laparotomy, higher rates of intravascular extravasation of distending media, prolonged operating times, and increased requirement for repeat surgery. Therefore, endoscopic removal of intramural or submucosal leiomyomas > 5 cm in diameter or with myometrial involvement >50% should be attempted only by very experienced endoscopists. Hysteroscopic myomectomy has been associated with significant complications some of which are listed in **Box 24.17**.

Robotic myomectomy: A new minimally invasive surgical procedure for gynecological patients, which has nowadays been commonly employed, is robotic surgery using da Vinci® robotic surgical system. The first robot, the da Vinci® Surgical System (Intuitive Surgical, Inc., Sunnyvale, CA) was first approved by the USFDA for gynecologic applications in April 2005. The da Vinci® surgical robot is a major advancement in the field of gynecological surgery which enables the surgeon to operate accurately through small incisions and allows comprehensive reconstruction of the uterine wall, irrespective of the location of the tumor. This system takes surgical precision and technique beyond the human hand and allows for rapid and precise suturing, dissection, and tissue manipulation.

In this minimally invasive procedure, several small incisions are made along the abdomen and the surgical tools are inserted through these incisions **(Fig. 24.16)**. The movement of each instrument and each surgical maneuver is controlled by the surgeon, who sits on a console slightly away from the site of surgery.

The da Vinci® surgical system can offer numerous benefits over traditional open surgery. Some of these include—shorter duration of hospital stay, reduced pain, faster recovery, reduced amount of blood loss, requirement for fewer transfusions and reduced risk of infection, risk of scar formation, and overall improved quality of life.

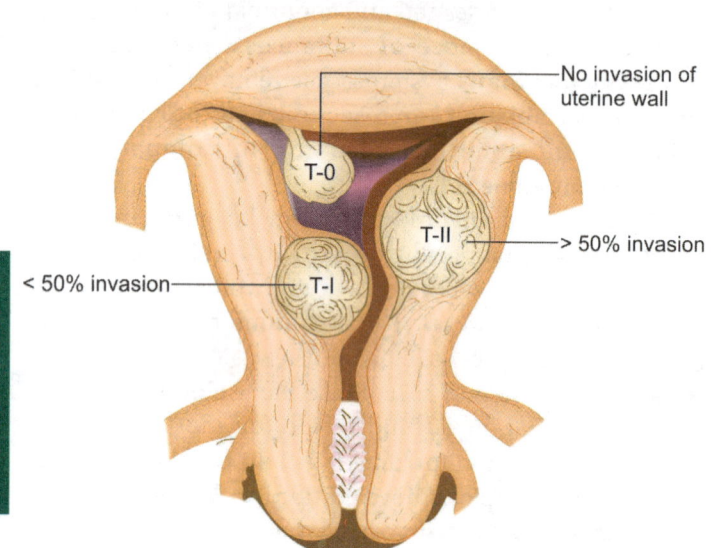

Fig. 24.15: European Society of Hysteroscopy classification of myomas.

> **BOX 24.17:** Complications related to hysteroscopic myomectomy.
> - Severe intraoperative bleeding, requiring an emergency hysterectomy
> - Electrical burns to the genital tract, bowel, etc.
> - Hyponatremia, blindness, coma, and death from excessive absorption of irrigant fluid have also been reported
> - Fluid imbalance may occur with prolonged surgical procedures
> - The fertility and pregnancy outcomes following hysteroscopic myomectomy appear to be similar to those following laparoscopic and abdominal myomectomies

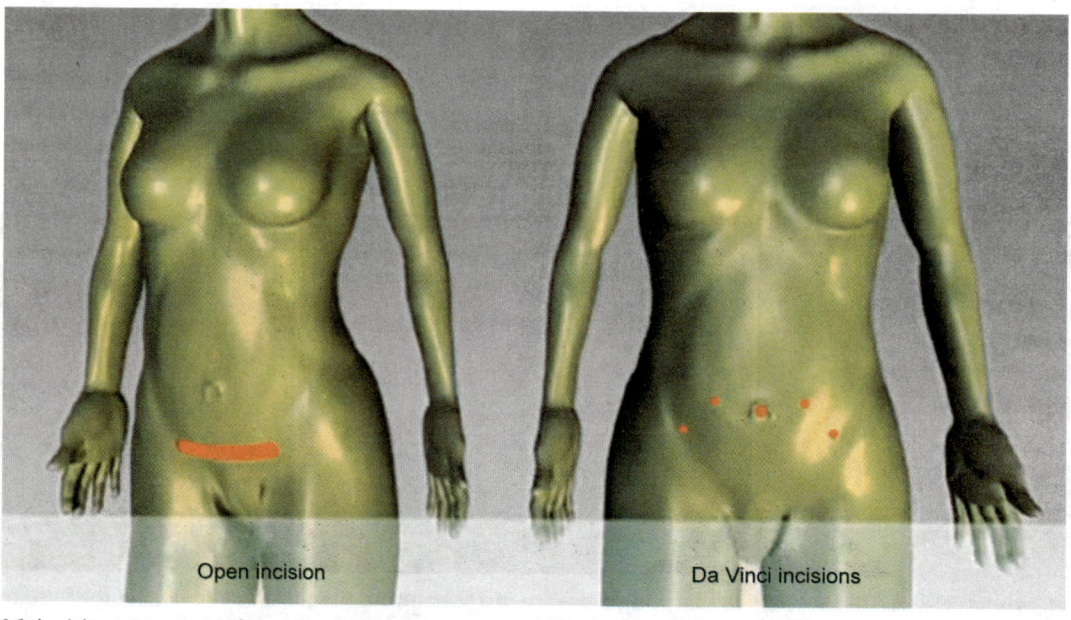

Fig. 24.16: Incision given in traditional open surgery compared to the minimal small incisions given in the robotic surgery.

The use of robot helps in improving the dexterity, thereby enabling the surgeon to manipulate and dissect tissue in a delicate, controlled fashion. This helps in improving the efficiency, accuracy, ease, and comfort associated with the performance of laparoscopic operations. Patients undergoing robotic-assisted laparoscopic myomectomy (RALM) are likely to be associated with significantly decreased estimated blood loss, complication rates, and length of stay. Advantages of robotic technology over abdominal myomectomy and conventional laparoscopy have been enumerated in **Boxes 24.18 and 24.19**, respectively.

Robotic myomectomy is presently performed in patients with any single myoma smaller than 15 cm and with fewer than 15 myomas in total. Preoperative MRI is very useful for defining the myoma size, number and locations, and for ruling out adenomyosis. Some contraindications for performing robotic myomectomy are as follows:

- Uterine fundus is palpable above the umbilicus.
- Presence of diffuse adenomyosis on MRI
- Uterine cavity cannot be clearly visualized by MRI.

The integrity of the scar following robotic myomectomy has yet not been tested because there have been small reports of pregnancy occurring following robotic-assisted myomectomy.

Operative procedure:

- *Operative setup:* The basic robotic setup consists of the patient-side robot, a vision cart and the robotic master console (**Figs. 24.17 and 24.18**)
- *Steps of surgery:* Using a combination of hand controls and foot pedals, the robotic surgeon operates from the remote master console (**Figs. 24.19 and 24.20**).
- *Patient positioning:* The patient is placed in a position identical to that during conventional laparoscopy, i.e., in

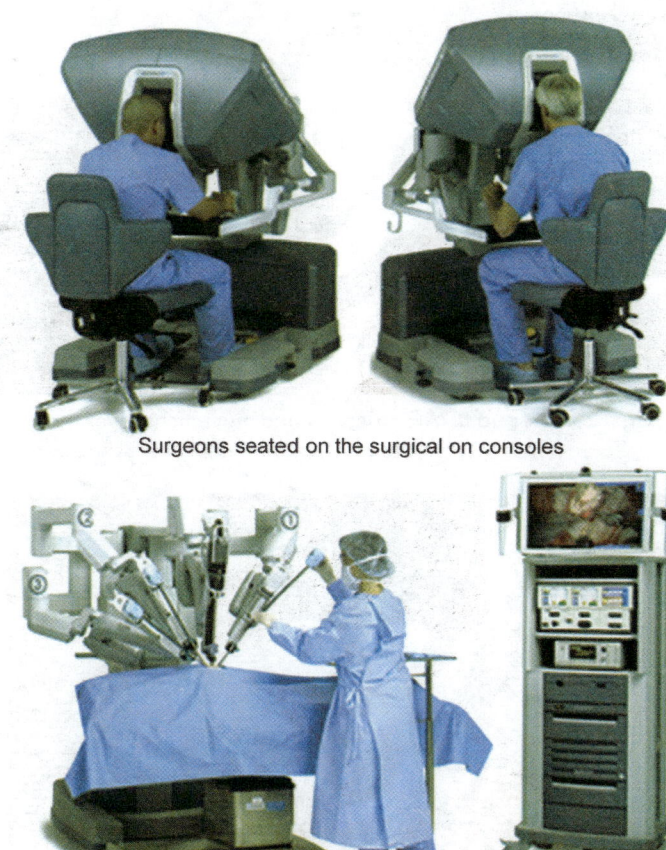

Fig. 24.17: Full da Vinci® Si HD surgical system with two surgical consoles both with surgeons seated; one patient cart; one female nurse attending vision cart (© 2012 Intuitive Surgical, Inc.)

BOX 24.18: Advantages of robotic-assisted laparoscopic myomectomy (RALM) in comparison with abdominal myomectomy.

- Shorter duration of hospital stay
- Reduced blood loss
- Quicker return to daily activities
- Reduced scarring
- Fewer postoperative complications
- Reduced blood loss (110 mL with RALM vs. 176 mL with abdominal myomectomy)

(RALM: robotic-assisted laparoscopic myomectomy)

BOX 24.19: Advantages of robotic technology over conventional laparoscopy.

- Absence of tremor
- Procurement of a three-dimensional image
- Superior instrument articulation
- Downscaling of movements
- Increased comfort for the surgeon
- A faster operator learning curve with the robotic system

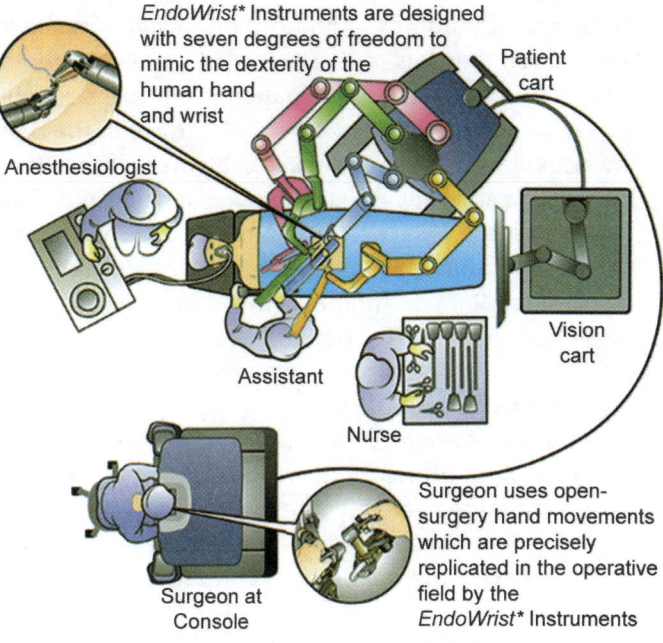

Fig. 24.18: Set up of the operating room (© 2012 Intuitive Surgical, Inc.)

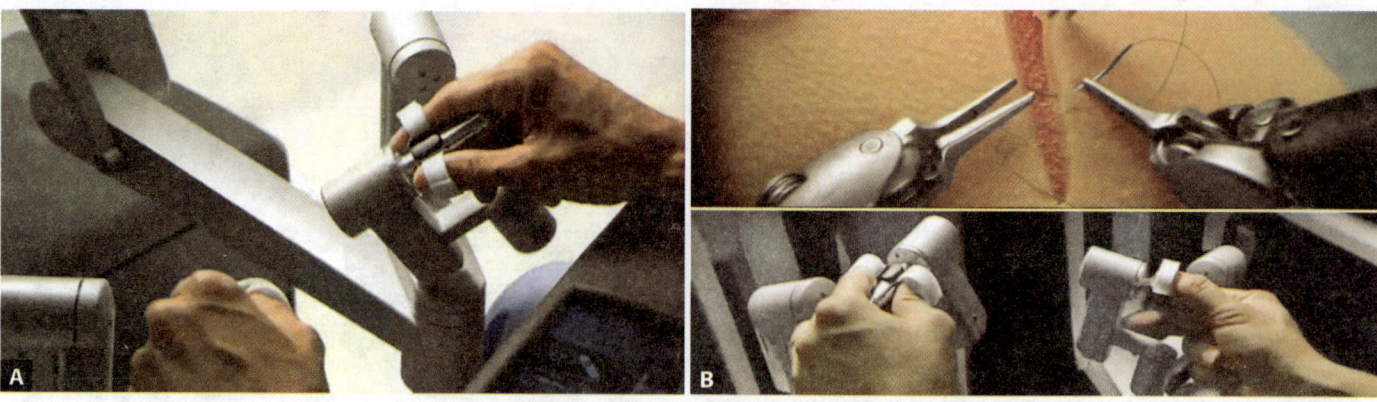

Figs. 24.19A and B: (A) Surgeon's hand movements over the surgical console; (B) Surgeon's fingers controlling the movements of the robotic equipment to stitch the abdominal incision (© 2012 Intuitive Surgical, Inc.).

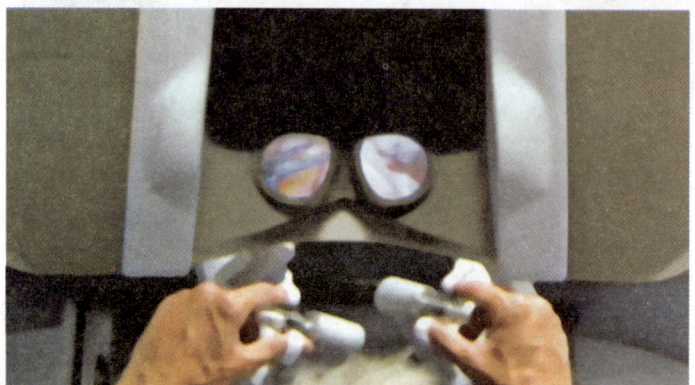

Fig. 24.20: Cameras of the robotic system which help in providing magnified, three-dimensional, high-definition view of the operating field (© 2012 Intuitive Surgical, Inc.).

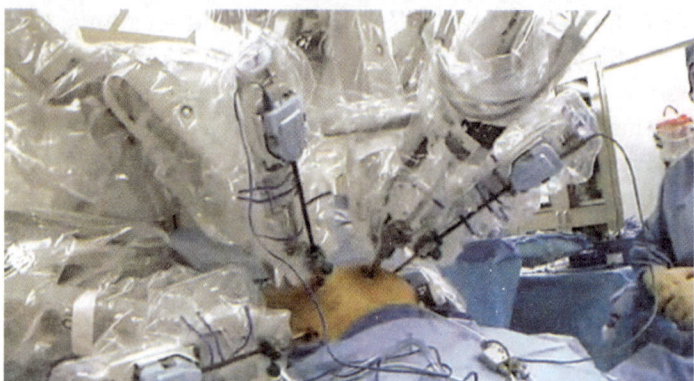

Fig. 24.21: Robotic operating equipment after being inserted into the patient's abdomen (© 2012 Intuitive Surgical, Inc.).

dorsal lithotomy position with feet in Allen stirrups, and the arms padded and tucked.

- *Trocar placement:* Placement of trocars is shown in **Figure 24.21**.
- *Docking:* After trocar placement, the patient is placed in Trendelenburg position and the process of docking undertaken. For this, the patient-side cart with robotic arms is brought between the patient's legs. Each robotic arm is then connected to a trocar. The trocar in the right lower quadrant is left undocked. This trocar is used by the bedside assistant as a conventional laparoscopic port for the purpose of suction/irrigation, passage of needles, tissue retraction, and morcellation. The exchange of instruments on the robotic arms is also done by the bedside assistant. The steps of robotic myomectomy following the insertion of trocars are described in **Figures 24.22A to F**.
- *Myoma location and removal:* Once the uterus is visualized, a dilute concentration of vasopressin is injected into the myometrium surrounding the myoma after localizing the fibroid on the uterine surface based on the MRI examination performed preoperatively.
- *Incision over the uterine surface:* Using the robotic harmonic shears, a horizontal or longitudinal hysterotomy incision is made over the surface of fibroid **(Fig. 24.22A)**.
- *Enucleation of myoma:* The myoma is enucleated in a fashion identical to open/laparoscopic myomectomy with help of robotic tenaculum and/or a bipolar coagulator **(Figs. 24.22B to D)**. Following removal, the removed myomata are placed in the posterior cul-de-sac or in the paracolic gutters for retrieval and morcellation at the end of the case.
- *Hysterotomy closure:* Once each myoma is completely enucleated out, the hysterotomy incision is then closed with help of a multilayer closure using sutures and suturing techniques identical to those used in an open/laparoscopic myomectomy **(Figs. 24.22E and F)**. The deeper layers are closed using interrupted or running sutures of 0 polyglactin 910. The uterine serosa is closed with a baseball-stitch technique using 2-0 poliglecaprone 25.
- *Morcellation:* Following hysterotomy closure, the specimens are morcellated and retrieved through the accessory port. This is usually done after the robot itself has been undocked.

It is very likely that these different techniques, open, laparoscopic, robotic, and robot-assisted myomectomy will continue to co-occur in the future, and which technique

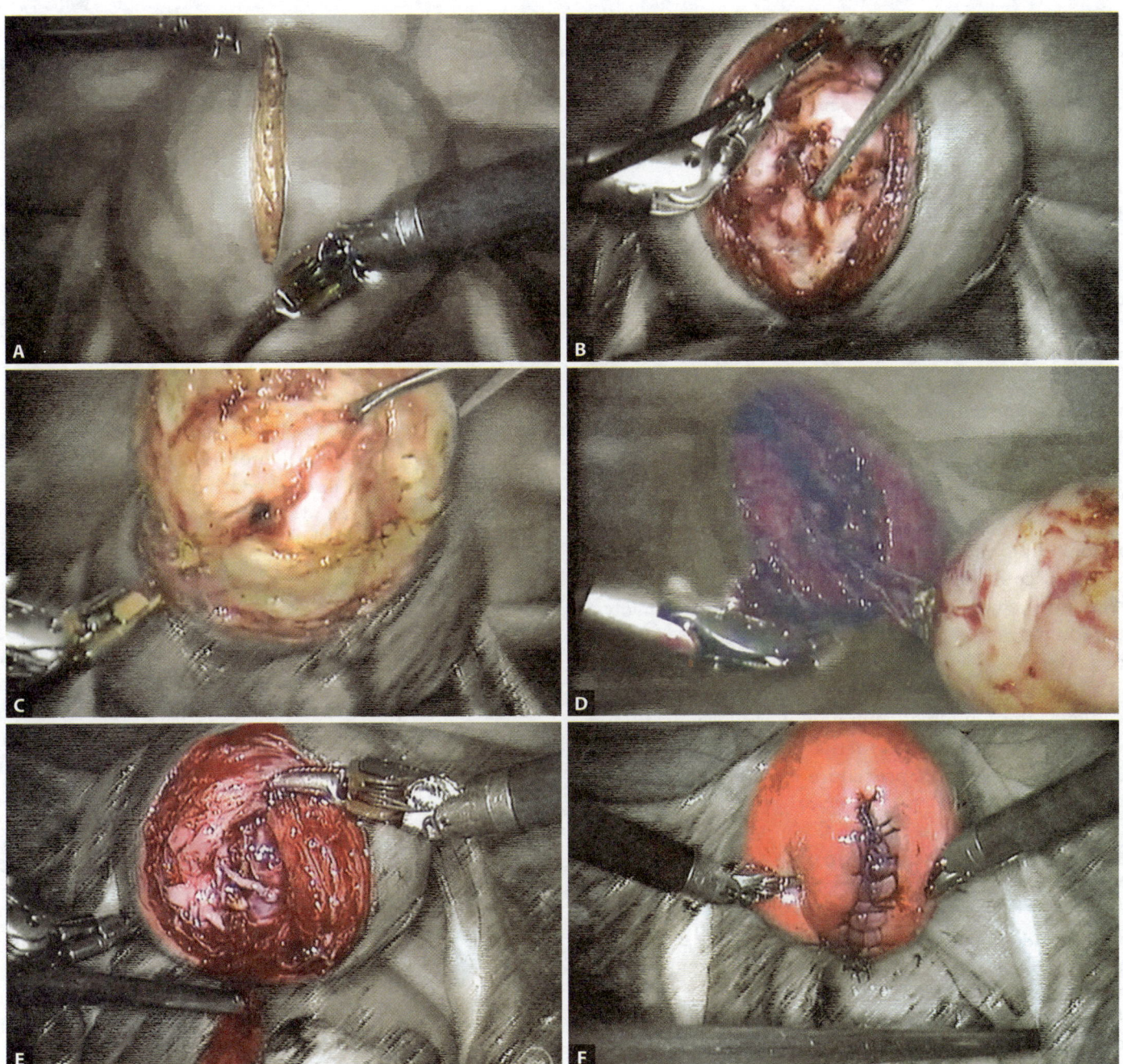

Figs. 24.22A to F: Robotic myomectomy. (A) Using the robotic harmonic shears, a hysterotomy is made over the myoma; (B and C) Shelling out of myoma; (D) Myoma has been completely removed from the myoma bed; (E) A multilayer closure is performed employing sutures and suturing techniques that are identical to those of an open myomectomy; and (F) Suturing of the uterine surface is complete. (*Source:* Computerized generation of images)

would be given preference over the other would be based on the clinical scenario and surgeon expertise. More research is needed to define preoperative factors to label one approach better than the other for a given clinical situation, both in terms of patient outcomes and cost effectiveness.

DESTRUCTION OF THE FIBROIDS

Several procedures have been designed to treat the myomas by destroying their blood supply instead of removing them. Some of these are described next.

MYOMA COAGULATION (MYOLYSIS)

Myoma coagulation, also known as myolysis, is a laparoscopic procedure which helps in shrinking the fibroids without removing them. The procedure is performed laparoscopically, in which either a laser or a cryo needle is passed directly into the fibroid to destroy both the fibroid tissue and the blood vessels feeding it. This technique is easier to master than myomectomy, because no suturing is required. The destroyed fibroid tissues are eventually absorbed by the uterus. Presently, myoma coagulation is not recommended for women desiring future fertility because the procedure is thought to result in the formation of scar tissue, which is likely to weaken the strength of the uterine wall. Due to this, there are high chances of uterine rupture during the pregnancy in case the woman conceives following myolysis. Although some women who underwent the procedure have conceived and have been uneventfully delivered by cesarean section, the fertility and pregnancy outcomes after laparoscopic myolysis remain unknown. Presently, however, the patients undergoing myolysis are advised not to attempt to conceive following the procedure. The indications for myolysis include symptomatic patient presenting with menorrhagia, pelvic pain, or pressure symptoms due to fibroids pressing upon the adjacent organs; presence of four or fewer myomas with a size of <5 cm; or the size of the largest subserosal myoma is <10 cm in diameter. Other concomitant laparoscopic pelvic surgery, such as adhesiolysis, excision of endometriosis or adnexal surgery, can be carried out at the same time. Sometimes, concomitant hysteroscopic endometrial ablation is performed at the end of laparoscopic myolysis to further assist in the treatment of menorrhagia. Complications associated with myolysis include pelvic infection, bacteremia, bleeding, adhesion formation, etc. Thus, laparoscopic myolysis may present an alternative to myomectomy or hysterectomy for selected women with symptomatic intramural or subserous fibroids who wish to preserve their uterus, but do not desire future fertility. However, this procedure is infrequently used in current practice.

Uterine Artery Embolization

> **Q. With help of a long essay discuss UAE.**
>
> **Q. Write a short essay discussing the role of UAE in obstetrics and gynecology.**

Uterine artery embolization is a relatively new, novel technique for treatment of uterine fibroids, which was first performed by Ravina, a French Gynecologist in 1995. UAE is a nonhysterectomy surgical technique, which helps in reducing the size of the uterine fibroids by shrinking them, without actually removing them. Besides uterine fibroids, the technique of embolization has been used to treat various other medical pathologies like inoperable cancers, brain aneurysms, arteriovenous shunts in the lung, etc.

Preoperative Preparation

The following must be done before performing the surgical procedure:

Patient counseling: Before undergoing UAE, all women should be counseled that this procedure is relatively new, and presently its long-term effects and durability, including fertility and pregnancy outcomes, are not yet known. Many interventional radiologists advise against the use of this procedure for women contemplating pregnancy in the future. History and physical and pelvic examination must be done prior to the procedure to rule out any contraindication for UAE **(Box 24.20)**.

Investigations

- The investigations, which must be done prior to the procedure, include CBC, serum electrolyte level, renal function tests, and coagulation profile.
- Routine cervical cytology and endometrial sampling should be performed.

Procedure

The procedure of UAE itself lasts between 1 to 2 hours. Though anesthesia is usually not required, the procedure is usually performed under sedation. The interventional radiologist introduces and manipulates a catheter through the femoral artery into the internal iliac and uterine arteries **(Fig. 24.23)**.

Once the fibroids are visualized on X-ray, an embolizing agent [gelatin microspheres (trisacryl gelatin) or polyvinyl alcohol] is injected, which helps in blocking both the uterine arteries, thereby cutting off the blood supply to the fibroids **(Figs. 24.24 and 24.25A and B)**. Compared to normal uterine cells, fibroid cells are much more sensitive to low oxygen saturation. Thus, due to the lack of sufficient blood supply, the fibroids become avascular and shrink,

BOX 24.20: Contraindications of uterine artery embolization.
- Active genital infection
- Genital tract cancer
- Compromised immune status
- Severe vascular disease limiting access to the uterine arteries
- Allergy to intravenous contrast
- Impaired renal function

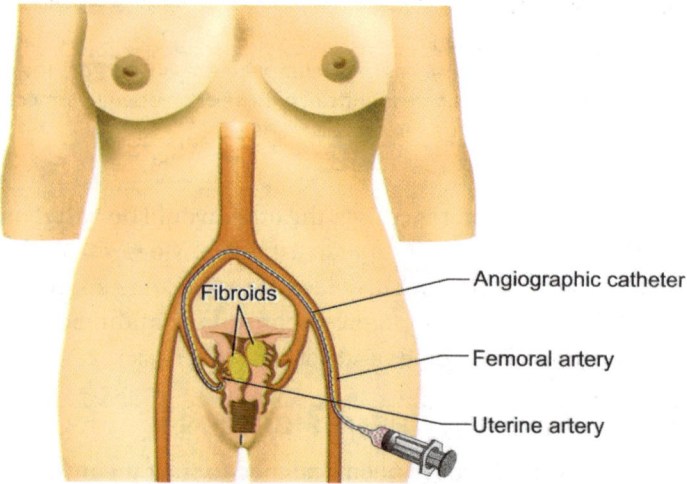

Fig. 24.23: Passing the catheter through femoral artery into the uterine artery.

ultimately resulting in cell death, their degeneration and eventual absorption by the myometrium. The normal myometrium, on the other hand, receives new blood supply from vaginal and ovarian vasculature. As fibroids begin to undergo necrosis, any active bleeding commonly subsides. The dying cells of the fibroids may release toxins, which may cause irritation to the surrounding tissues, thereby causing pain and inflammation in the first few days following the procedure. Though the rate of recovery usually varies from one woman to the other, it usually takes a few months for the fibroids to fully shrink and the full effect of the procedure to be evident.

Uterine artery embolization has been found to be associated with numerous fertility-related complications including increased rate of miscarriage and abnormal placentation during pregnancy.

Uterine artery embolization can be an effective treatment for uterine fibroids, especially in women whose symptoms are sufficiently bothersome to warrant myomectomy or hysterectomy.

Presently, the estimated mortality rate of 1 per 10,000 women for UAE is lower than the mortality rate of approximately 3 per 10,000 women for hysterectomy. The worldwide success rate of the procedure in producing improvement of symptoms has been considered to be approximately 85%. UAE may be the right treatment choice for women in whom the symptomatic relief may be obtained by shrinking the fibroids to a little more than half their present size. However, UAE may not be very helpful for women with extremely large fibroids because they may not shrink enough to make a significant difference in the symptoms. 3–6 months following UAE, the uterus and fibroids are likely to have decreased by about 40% in size. About 90% of women who were symptomatic due to the large size of their fibroids would experience a significant improvement in their symptoms. About 10–15% of women who have UAE may continue to suffer from menorrhagia and may require some other treatment modality.

Systematic review of randomized trials have shown that the procedure of UAE is associated have a reduced duration of hospital stay, reduced pain following surgery, and earlier return to work in comparison to hysterectomy or myomectomy. However, the procedure has been found to be associated with more complications such as number of unscheduled visits and rate of readmission. The women with larger uteri and/or more number of leiomyomas are likely to be associated with high failure rates.

Complications

Total radiation exposure following UAE is similar to that of one to two CT scans or barium enemas. Management of pain following the procedure may require a 1-day hospital stay, followed by 1–2 weeks of medications with NSAIDs. Most women return to normal activity within 1–3 weeks.

- *Major complications:* Major complications such as pulmonary embolism, arterial thrombosis, groin

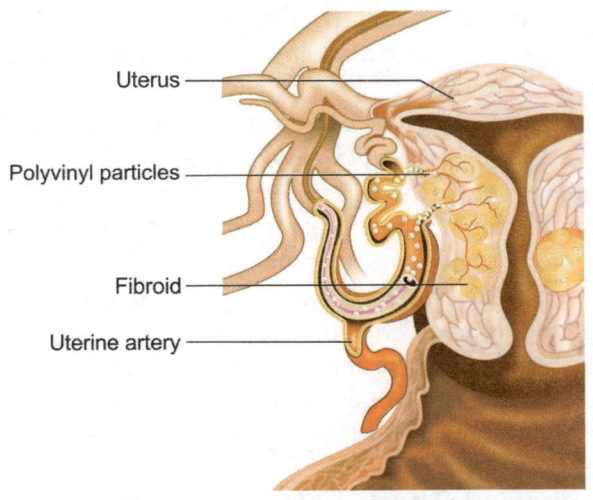

Fig. 24.24: Blocking the blood supply of fibroids.

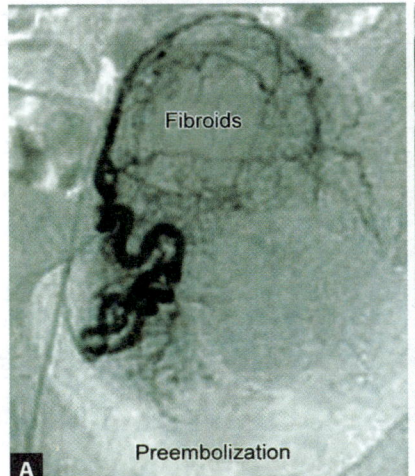
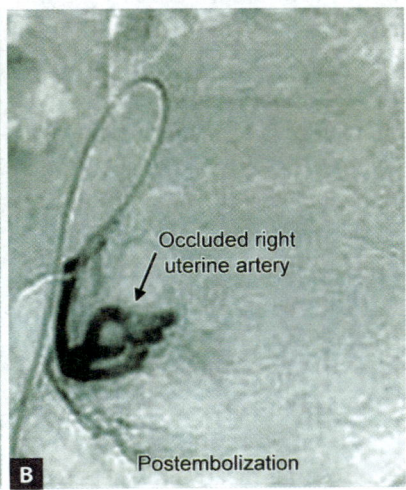

Figs. 24.25A and B: Arteriogram showing embolization of the right uterine vessels: (A) Preembolization arteriogram showing increased blood supply to the fibroids; (B) Postembolization arteriogram showing occluded blood supply to the fibroids (indicated by the arrow).

hematomas, local infections, guidewire perforation of arteries, allergic reaction to contrast medium, endometritis, ischemia of pelvic organs, sepsis, and death are rare events with UAE. These may occur in approximately 0.5% cases of embolization performed for symptomatic fibroids.

- *Early acute abdominal pelvic pain:* Nearly all women may experience some degree of acute pain within the first few weeks, often requiring hospitalization with intensive pain management protocols and monitoring. The pain is thought to be due to nonspecific ischemia of the uterus and fibroids. It often responds to pain control with analgesics like opiates and NSAIDs.
- *Postembolization syndrome:* Following UAE, some women may develop low-grade fever, leukocytosis, increasing pelvic pain, and a vaginal discharge. Many of these women may also experience malaise, nausea, and exhaustion.

  The combination of these symptoms is known as postembolization syndrome and is probably related to transient fibroid degeneration and uterine ischemia. The condition is usually self-limiting and symptoms may last from few days to weeks; the patient may be hospitalized for antibiotic therapy. The postembolization syndrome normally regresses over time. However, if the symptoms seem to worsen over the period of time, an examination and evaluation for infection is important. In presence of severe infection, hysterectomy may be required.
- *Misembolization:* Since the particles that are used for embolization are very small, in a few instances, the particles may travel through blood vessels to areas besides the fibroid tissue, where they are actually intended to go. This is termed as misembolization.
- *Infection:* The incidence of febrile morbidity and sepsis following embolization has been reported to be between 1.0 to 1.8%. Some of the infections, which can occur, include pyometra with endomyometritis, bilateral chronic salpingitis, tubo-ovarian abscess, and infection of the myomas. The most frequent pathogen that has been isolated is *Escherichia coli*. Though some women may respond to antibiotic therapy, others may require prolonged hospitalization, intensive therapy, and sometimes even hysterectomy. Prophylactic antibiotics have not been shown to be effective and should be used only in women at higher risk of infection.
- *Effect on fertility:* The ovaries may stop functioning in about 5% of the women following embolization and early menopause may result. This may be a particularly devastating complication for young patients who wish to conceive in future. The ovarian function may cease due to reduced blood supply. The blood supply to the ovaries may be blocked off due to misembolization or as a result of the blockage of uterine artery in women in whom the main blood vessels supplying the ovaries branches off from the uterine artery. As a result, if the uterine artery is blocked, the blood supply to the ovary is also blocked off and the ovaries may cease functioning.
- *Pregnancy outcomes:* Though this procedure helps in preserving the uterus, pregnancies following UAE have been reported to be at higher risk in comparison to the general population. Women becoming pregnant following UAE may be at significantly increased risk for postpartum hemorrhage, preterm delivery, cesarean delivery, malpresentation, and uterine rupture.

  Presently, however there is limited evidence regarding the pregnancy outcomes following UAE. As a result, the women who wish to conceive in future are not recommended to use UAE as treatment option for their fibroids. Better evidence in form of future well-designed, randomized studies is required before UAE can be confidently recommended to the women with fibroids desiring future fertility.
- *Risk of underlying malignancy:* Similar to myolysis, no samples are sent for biopsy in UAE; therefore, any underlying malignancy is likely to remain undetected. However, this is unlikely to cause any problem because the chances of malignancy in cases of fibroids are extremely low.
- *Persistent or chronic pain:* In 5–10% of women, the pain persists for >2 weeks. Presence of uterine infection should be ruled out in these cases. Persistent pain in the absence of infection or pain lasting longer than 2–3 months may require surgical intervention.
- *Transcervical fibroid tissue passage:* Overall, transcervical fibroid tissue passage may occur in approximately 2.5% of the patients. This may be associated with severe pain, infection, or bleeding and is one of the most common complications requiring hospitalization.

Laparoscopic Uterine Artery Ligation

Gynecologists have recently created a surgical technique to surgically ligate off the uterine arteries using the laparoscope rather than blocking them with embolization agents. The advantages of the surgical uterine artery ligation over UAE are that there is a little risk of misembolization to other areas and there is no theoretical risk of premature menopause that may accompany UAE. If, however, some women have a branch of the uterine artery as the only blood supply to the ovaries, then surgical ligation of the uterine artery may cut off blood supply to the ovaries, resulting in an early menopause for these women. Presently, however, UAE is preferable to laparoscopic uterine artery occlusion.

Focused Ultrasound (MRgFUS) for Treatment of Fibroids

This is another new technique for destruction of fibroids, which is still under the research stages. In this technique, ultrasound energy, which uses high-frequency energy in the form of sound waves, is used for destroying fibroids. This energy can be focused on a single point inside a patient's body (for example on a fibroid) so that the heat created by the energy is able to destroy the fibroid cells by causing coagulative necrosis **(Fig. 24.26)**. Since the technique uses MRI to focus the ultrasound waves, hence the term "magnetic resonance-guided focused ultrasound (MRgFUS)" is used to describe this technique. Still in its early stages of development, focused ultrasound is a noninvasive alternative to treat fibroids. The use of focused-ultrasound is associated with very low risk and rapid recovery. However, presently there is limited evidence regarding the safety and efficacy of the procedure; therefore, it is not recommended for women desiring future fertility. In future, with the improvement in technology, MRgFUS would probably serve as a proven alternative for women with symptomatic fibroids.

ExAblate 2000 System

This is a new device, approved by the FDA, based on MRgFUS technique which serves as a noninvasive method for treating fibroids, while retaining the uterus. The procedure involves repeated targeting and heating of fibroid tissue, using ultrasound energy while the patient is under continuous MRI. The focused ultrasound energy can be used to generate sufficient heat so as to cause protein denaturation and cell death. In this device, MRI is used for visualizing patient anatomy, mapping the volume of fibroid tissue to be treated, monitoring the temperature of the uterine tissue after heating, and monitoring the focused ultrasound beam that heats and destroys the fibroid tissue using high-frequency, high-energy sound waves. The procedure can last as long as 3 hours. While many fibroids can be treated with this device, fibroids close to sensitive organs such as the bowel or bladder and those outside the image area cannot be treated. This system is also not indicated for leiomyomas which can be removed with help of a hysteroscope or those fibroids which are heavily calcified. This treatment option can be, however, used in women considering future pregnancy following counseling.

Though the device has been shown to successfully treat fibroid-related menorrhagia in nearly 70% of the women within 6 months of treatment, the remaining 30% have been observed to require an alternative surgical treatment for fibroids within a year. This implies that while the ExAblate treatment may succeed in reducing the symptoms from the treated fibroids, there may be a recurrence of fibroids in some women, thereby requiring an additional treatment either with ExAblate or an alternative treatment modality. The device labeling indicates that no more than two treatments should be performed in a 2-week period. The maximum size of fibroids that can be treated with this method is not yet known. Symptomatic improvement is observed within the first 3 months following this procedure and this improvement has been found to be maintained at least through 24–36 months follow-up. Increasing amount of experience with this method has been found to be associated with a lower incidence of adverse events. The procedure is time consuming and costly, but short-term morbidity is low and recovery is rapid. Good quality trials are required in the future to determine long-term outcome and optimal candidates for this procedure.

CONSERVATIVE MANAGEMENT OF AUB-E: ENDOMETRIAL ABLATION

> Q. Discuss elaborately the current status of endometrial ablative techniques.
>
> Q. Write a short essay on the latest trends in endometrial ablative techniques.
>
> Q. Write a short essay on transcervical resection of the endometrium (TCRE).
>
> Q. Write a short essay on endometrial ablation.
>
> Q. Write a long essay discussing the various procedures related to endometrial ablation.

Endometrial ablation is defined as a minimally invasive procedure to alleviate AUB/HMB in women who do not desire removal of their uterus. The ideal patient undergoing endometrial ablation must have AUB-E as determined by the FIGO classification system (Chapter 23). AUB-E can be described as abnormal uterine bleeding due to primary endometrial disorder. In these cases, there is an absence of any structural cause, ovulatory dysfunction, coagulation disorder or iatrogenic cause of bleeding. Moreover, the uterus should not be enlarged, with length of the cavity being no >11 cm and uterine contour must be regular. As discussed previously, please note that endometrial ablation is not usually used in cases of HMB related to leiomyomas. It is just discussed here for the sake of completion.

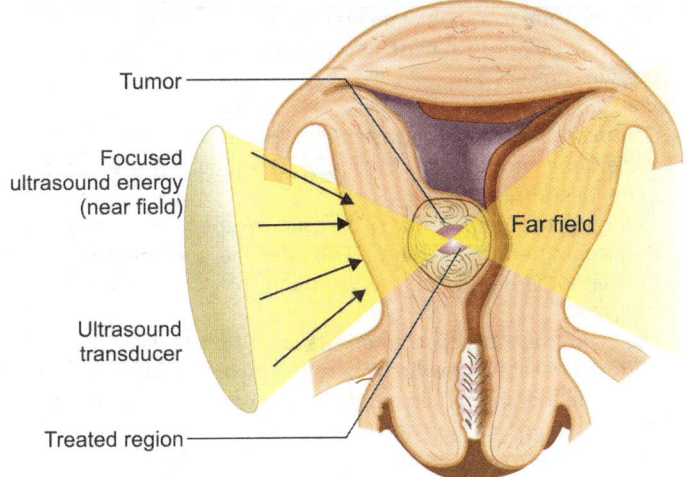

Fig. 24.26: Focused ultrasound (MRgFUS) for treatment of fibroids.

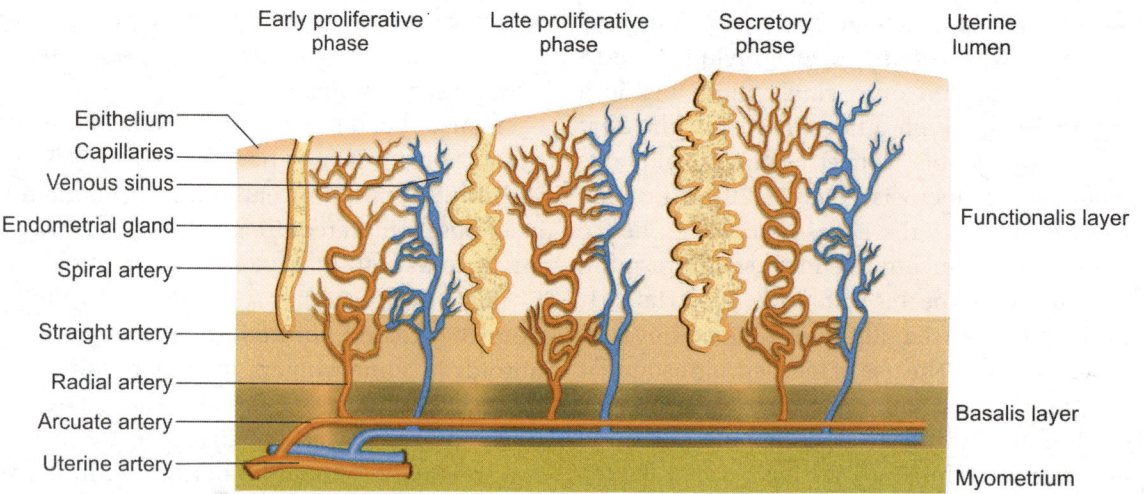

Fig. 24.27: Layers of endometrium during the various phases of menstrual cycle.

BOX 24.21: Indications for endometrial ablation.

- AUB due to ovulatory causes in premenopausal women
- AUB in hemodynamically stable women in whom medical therapy is contraindicated or unsuccessful
- Women with chronic menorrhagia
- Woman does not desire future fertility
- Failure of medical treatment
- AUB due to endometrial dysfunction
- Menorrhagia is unresponsive to hormonal or pharmacological therapy
- Malignant disease of the cervix and/or endometrium has been ruled out
- Uterine size < 10 weeks; submucous fibroids < 5 cm
- Endometrium is normal with no risk of hyperplasia

(AUB: abnormal uterine bleeding)

BOX 24.22: Patient preparation for endometrial ablation.

Preoperative evaluation:
- Taking informed consent after adequate counseling
- Urine pregnancy test (to rule out pregnancy)
- Performing cervical cultures (to rule out infection)
- Uterine evaluation:
  – Endometrial sampling (to exclude endometrial hyperplasia or cancer)
  – Assessment of the uterine cavity for the presence of intra-cavitary myomas, endometrial polyps, or other abnormalities (e.g., uterine septum), using saline infusion sonography (SIS) or office hysteroscopy to assess the uterine cavity
  – Sounding of the uterus (<10 weeks in size)
  – Removal of an intrauterine contraceptive device (IUCD) (if present)
  – Endometrial preparation using GnRH agonists initiated 30–60 days prior to the procedure (to be used only with nonresectoscopic ablation devices with the exception of thermachoice device and NovaSure)

Operative setup:
- *Antibiotic prophylaxis:* Not routinely administered prior to endometrial ablation
- *Anesthesia:* Resectoscopic ablation may be performed with regional or general anesthesia. Nonresectoscopic endometrial ablation can be performed using local, regional, or general anesthesia
- *NSAIDs:* Administration of an oral nonsteroidal anti-inflammatory drug at least 1 hour preoperatively to inhibit uterine contractions

Follow-up:
- *Counseling regarding contraception:* Women who have undergone endometrial ablation must be counseled about the need for contraception
- *Exclusion of endometrial neoplasia:* Women with recurrent abnormal uterine bleeding (AUB) after the procedure must be evaluated with endometrial sampling to exclude endometrial neoplasia
- *Use of postmenopausal hormone therapy:* Women with endometrial ablation who want to use postmenopausal hormone therapy should be prescribed progestins along with estrogen for protection against development of endometrial cancer in the residual tissue

(GnRH: gonadotropin-releasing hormone)

Endometrial ablation involves surgical destruction of the endometrium. In this method, the endometrium is destroyed to the level of the basalis layer of myometrium **(Fig. 24.27)**, which is approximately 4–6 mm deep, depending upon the stage of the menstrual cycle. The procedure may help in controlling the amount of bleeding. In some women, menstrual bleeding may not completely stop, but is reduced to normal or lighter levels. In most cases, women with heavy bleeding are treated first with medication. The women whose bleeding does not respond to hormonal or pharmacological therapy and who want to conserve their uterus must be offered endometrial ablation. If ablation does not control heavy bleeding, further treatment or surgery may be required. Some indications for endometrial ablation are described in **Box 24.21**. The preparation of the patient prior to the procedure of endometrial ablation is described in **Box 24.22**.

Endometrial ablation may be offered as an initial treatment for AUB after full discussion with the woman regarding the risks and benefits associated with the procedure and of other available treatment options. The outcome of these techniques would be better if these are performed when the endometrial lining is thin. Endometrial ablation should

BOX 24.23: Contraindications for use of endometrial ablation techniques.

- Presence of endometrial carcinoma or premalignant change of the endometrium (e.g., adenomatous hyperplasia)
- Patient with any anatomic or pathologic condition associated with weakness of the myometrium (e.g., history of previous classical cesarean sections or transmural myomectomy)
- A patient with active genital or urinary tract infection at the time of procedure (e.g., cervicitis, vaginitis, endometritis, salpingitis, or cystitis)
- A patient with an intrauterine device (IUD) currently in place
- A patient who is pregnant or who wants to become pregnant in the future
- Postmenopausal women
- Women having congenital uterine anomalies (e.g., bicornuate uterus)
- A uterine cavity length that is >10–12 cm

BOX 24.24: Procedures for endometrial ablation.

First-generation procedures:
- Hysteroscopic laser ablation
- Transcervical resection of the endometrium **(Figs. 24.29A and B)**
- Roller ball ablation of the endometrium **(Figs. 24.30A and B)**

Second-generation procedures:
- Cryoablation
- Hydrothermal ablation
- Laser thermoablation
- Microwave ablation
- Thermal balloon ablation
- Electrosurgical ablation
- Photodynamic ablation
- Radiofrequency-induced thermal ablation
- NovaSure (bipolar radiofrequency ablation) **(Figs. 24.31A to E)**

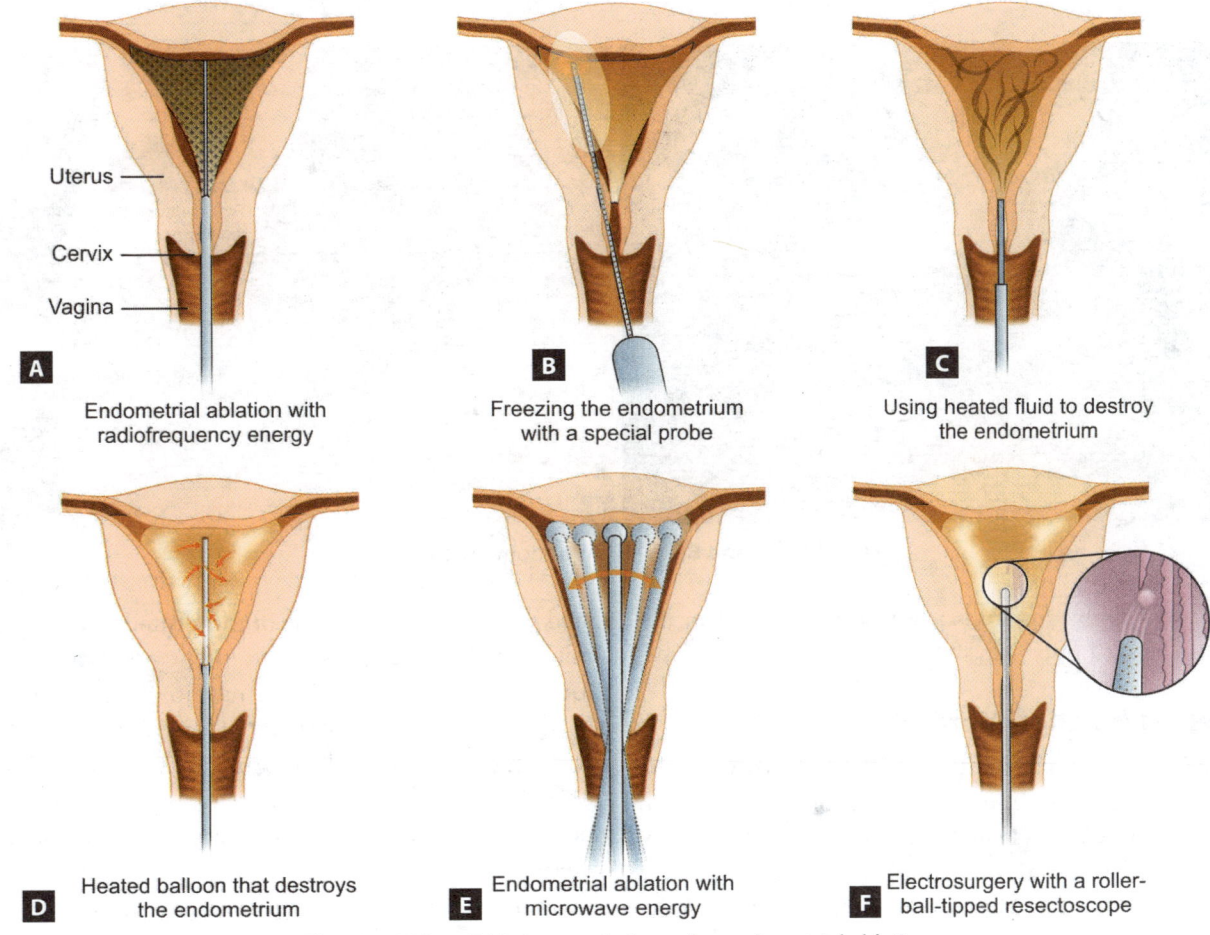

Figs. 24.28A to F: Various techniques for endometrial ablation.

be considered in women who have a structurally normal uterus, which is <10 weeks in size. It can also be sometimes offered to the women having small uterine fibroids (<3 cm in diameter). Some contraindications for not performing endometrial ablation are listed in **Box 24.23**. Endometrial ablation should not be done in women past menopause or in cases suspected to be suffering from various disorders of the endometrium including endometrial hyperplasia, endometrial cancer, and current or recent infection of the uterus. An endometrial aspiration must be preferably carried out to rule out any malignancy before doing this procedure.

Even though endometrial ablative techniques help in conservation of uterus, these must not be offered to the women planning future pregnancy. Women must be advised to avoid subsequent pregnancy and to use effective contraception, if required, following endometrial ablation.

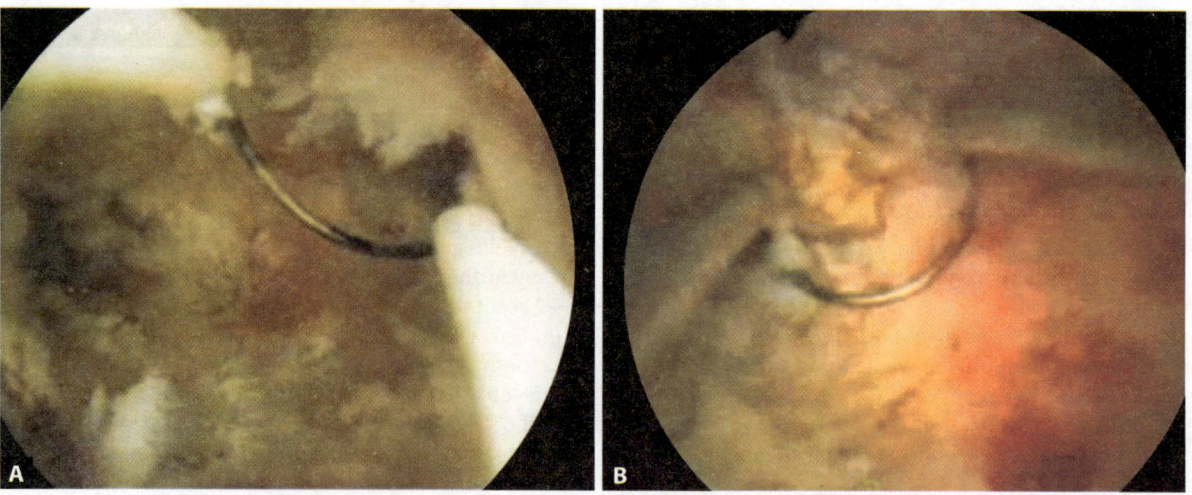

Figs. 24.29A and B: Transcervical resection of the endometrium. (A) Wire loop touching the endometrial surface; (B) Wire loop resecting out the endometrium.

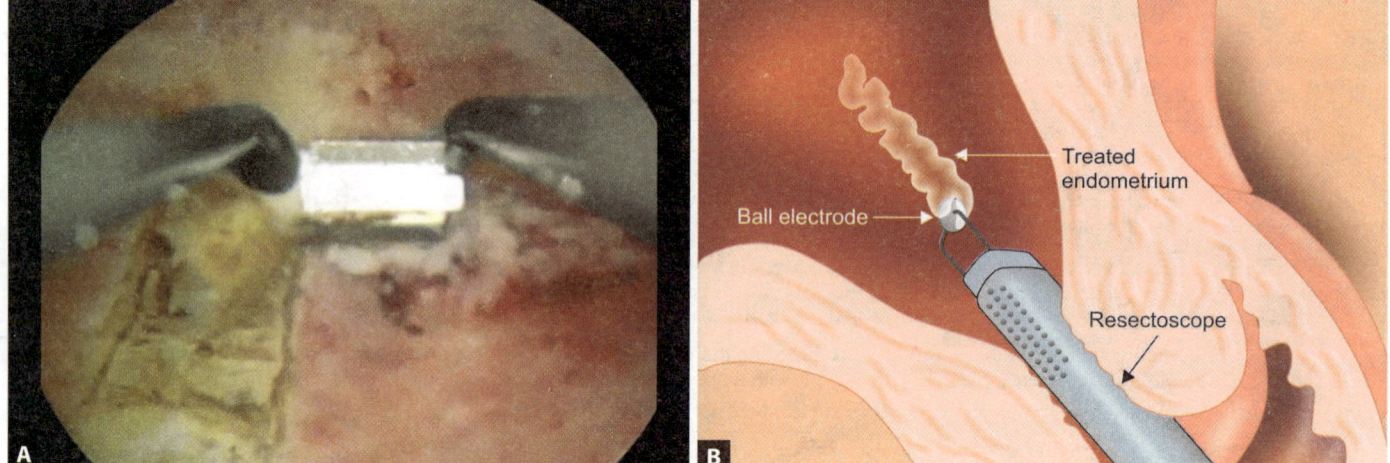

Figs. 24.30A and B: Roller ball endometrial ablation.

Endometrial ablation must also not be performed in the women who have Copper-T in situ.

Endometrial Ablation Methods

These methods help in treating DUB by destroying the endometrial lining. These methods for endometrial ablation are mainly of two types—(1) first-generation (hysteroscopic) methods and (2) second-generation (nonhysteroscopic) methods **(Box 24.24 and Figs. 24.28A to F)**. Hysteroscopic methods include laser and electrosurgical resection (roller ball and TCRE). Electrosurgical method that uses the wire loop to resect out the endometrial lining is called transcervical resection of endometrium (TCRE). The wire loop is around 6 mm long and is attached at an angle to a pencil-shaped handle. On the other hand, electrosurgical technique that uses the heated roller ball to burn away the endometrial tissue is called roller ball ablation. The roller ball is a ball about 2 mm wide that rotates freely on its handle. Some nonresectoscopic (second generation) technologies, which have been approved for use in the United States by the FDA include using bipolar radiofrequency (NovaSure device), hot liquid filled balloon (ThermaChoice), cryotherapy (Her Option), circulating hot water (Hydro ThermAblator), etc. Nonresectoscopic endometrial ablation techniques are more widely practiced than resectoscopic ablation, since they require less specialized training and often have a shorter operative time.

Though the use of endometrial ablation helps in avoiding hysterectomy, there is nearly 12% probability that endometrial resection would not be able to control AUB, thereby resulting in the future requirement of hysterectomy within the next 4 years. Endometrial resection/ablation can cause side effects like uterine perforation, fluid overload, hemorrhage, infection, etc. **(Box 24.25)**. Despite this, the rate of occurrence of complications is less than that associated with hysterectomy. Endometrial resection/ablation also helps in avoiding possible ovarian dysfunction, psychological effects, and other side effects related to

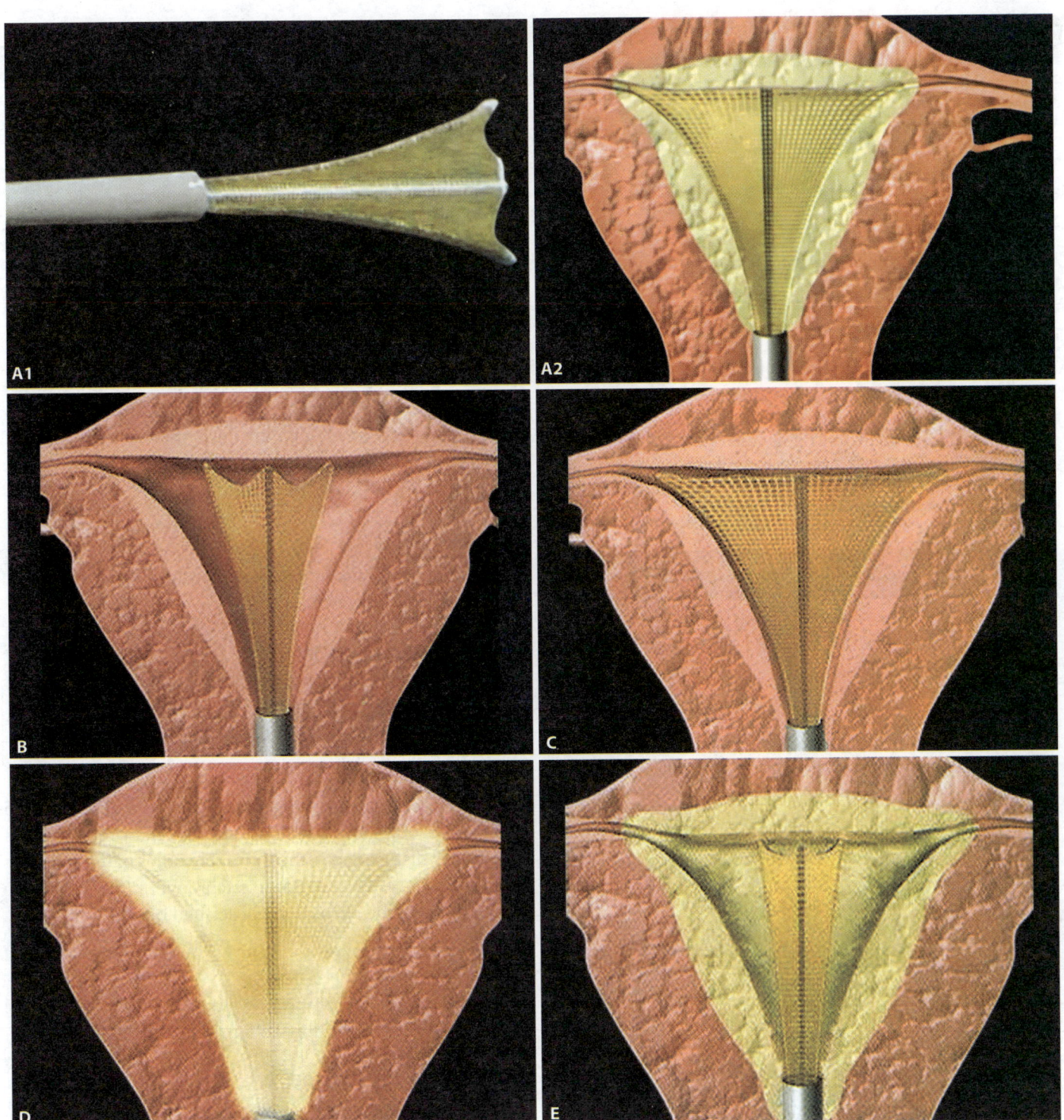

Figs. 24.31A to E: Procedure of endometrial ablation using the NovaSure device. (A) The NovaSure device, triangular, mesh-like; (B) Insertion of the device inside the uterine cavity; (C) Expansion of the mesh-like device, conforming to the uterine dimensions; (D) Delivery of electrical energy through the mesh for approximately 90 seconds; (E) The mesh-device is retracted back into the wand, following which it is removed from the uterus.

hysterectomy. However, hysterectomy is preferable over endometrial resection if the patient has a large uterus, or some underlying uterine pathology like fibromyomas or severe endometriosis. Presently, hysterectomy remains the most absolutely curative treatment for AUB-E. The comparison between abdominal hysterectomy and endometrial resection is shown in the **Table 24.6**.

Endometrial Ablation in Women Desiring Pregnancy

Endometrial ablation is intended for use only in women who do not desire future pregnancy because the likelihood of pregnancy is significantly decreased following this procedure. Since the procedure does not result in absolute sterility, there have been occasional reports of pregnancy

BOX 24.25: Complications which can occur due to endometrial ablation.

Commonly occurring complications:
- Cramping
- Vaginal discharge

Rare complications:
- Uterine perforation
- Hemorrhage
- Hematometra
- Pelvic infection
- Excessive fluid absorption (in the hysteroscopic methods)
- Urinary tract injuries
- Bowel injuries
- Burn injuries to the vagina and perineum (due to circulating hot water)
- Perioperative hysterectomy
- Carbon dioxide embolism
- Necrotizing fasciitis and death
- Uterine cavity occlusion, cervical stenosis
- Postablation tubal sterilization syndrome (cyclic or intermittent pelvic pain in women who have undergone tubal ligation prior to endometrial ablation)

TABLE 24.6: Abdominal hysterectomy versus endometrial resection.

	Abdominal hysterectomy	Endometrial resection
Duration of hospital stay	Longer theater times and hospital stay	Day-stay or overnight procedure
Rate of complications	Higher complication rate (45%)	Lower rate of complications (0–15%)
Mortality and morbidity rates	Higher	Lower
Time for resumption of normal activities	2–3 months	2–3 weeks
Overall health care costs	Higher healthcare costs because of longer theater time and duration of hospital stay	Lower healthcare costs because of shorter theater time and duration of hospital stay

following the procedure. However, the pregnancies following the ablative procedures can be dangerous for both mother and fetus.

Furthermore, patients undergoing endometrial ablation procedures who had previously undergone tubal ligation are at an increased risk of developing postablation-tubal sterilization syndrome, which can even require hysterectomy. This can occur as late as 10 years following the procedure. Postablation-tubal sterilization syndrome is believed to be related to the regeneration of endometrium in the cornual areas of the uterus. Blood from these glands can flow back into the proximal fallopian tubes in cases where the lower uterine segment is extensively scarred. As a result, the proximal oviduct distends and may also be associated with cyclic pelvic pain.

COMPLICATIONS

Various complications related with uterine myomas include the following:

TORSION

Torsion of the pedicle of a subserous pedunculated leiomyoma may interfere first with venous, then with the arterial supply. This may result in an initial extravasation of blood followed by the eventual development of gangrene.

ASCITES/PSEUDO-MEIGS SYNDROME

Very mobile pedunculated subserous tumors may produce ascites by causing mechanical irritation of the peritoneum. Sometimes, ascites may be accompanied by a right-sided hydrothorax, resulting in the development of a condition known as pseudo-Meigs syndrome.

INFECTION

A submucous leiomyoma may sometimes become infected and ulcerated at its lower pole.

SECONDARY CHANGES (DEGENERATION)

> Q. Write a short essay on red degeneration.
> Q. Discuss briefly about degeneration of fibroids and its effect on management.

Certain degenerative changes can occur in a fibroid, when the fibroid outgrows its blood supply. As a result of the circulatory disturbances, the tumor becomes painful, tender, softened, and enlarged. Some such degenerative changes taking place in the fibroids are described here.

Atrophy

Shrinkage of the fibroid can occur as a result of reduced blood supply of the fibroid, usually following menopause.

Hyaline Degeneration

This is the most common type of degeneration in which the fibrous tissue cells are replaced by a homogeneous substance which stains pink with eosin. The bundles of muscle fibers become isolated and die off causing large areas of the tumor to become structureless. Eventually, the liquefaction of hyaline material occurs, leaving behind ragged cavities filled with colorless or blood-stained fluid.

Calcification

This type of degeneration may initially occur with the presence of fatty deposits within the leiomyomas. At a later stage in this process, there is deposition of phosphates and carbonates of calcium along the course of blood vessels. Calcification usually begins at the periphery of the fibroid and can be identified with the help of radiography. At a later stage, there may be widespread deposition of calcium throughout the tumor resulting in "wombstone" appearance or a peripheral distribution resulting in an "egg-shell" appearance.

Myxomatous/Cystic Degeneration

This type of degeneration is characterized by the presence of complex cystic spaces filled with gelatinous fluid.

Red/Carneous Degeneration

This type of degeneration of uterine fibroid usually develops during pregnancy. It may be associated with constitutional symptoms such as malaise, nausea, vomiting, fever, and severe abdominal pain. The myoma may become soft and necrotic in the center and is diffusely stained red or salmon pink in color. Though the pathogenesis of the condition is not yet clear, it is believed that the purple-red color of the myoma is probably due to the thrombosis of blood vessels supplying the tumor. The myoma may also develop a peculiar fishy odor due to infection by the coliform organisms. Although the patient may develop mild leukocytosis and a raised erythrocyte sedimentation rate, the condition is essentially an aseptic one. It needs to be differentiated from other conditions including appendicitis, twisted ovarian cyst, accidental hemorrhage, etc. Ultrasound examination usually helps in establishing the correct diagnosis. On ultrasound examination, the tumor shows a mixed echodense and echolucent appearance. Red degeneration occurring during pregnancy must be managed conservatively. The patient must be advised bed rest and prescribed analgesics to relieve the pain. The acute symptoms subside gradually within the course of 3–10 days and pregnancy then proceeds uneventfully.

Sarcomatous Change

Fibroids are benign uterine growths and usually do not turn malignant. Occurrence of malignant changes in a leiomyoma is an extremely rare occurrence. According to Jeffcoate, sarcomatous changes are found in only 0.2% of tumors. The average rate of malignancy in a fibroid uterus is about 0.5%. Also, the rate of occurrence of uterine leiomyosarcomas is extremely low, with the incidence being about 0.67/1,000 women per year. The average age of women who develop fibroids is 38 years. Although sarcomas can rarely occur in young women, the average age of a woman who develops a sarcoma is 63 years. So, in a young woman (<40 years) with fibroids, there is not much risk of malignancy. According to a recent study, diagnosis of uterine sarcoma can be reliably made using a combination of a contrast (enhanced) MRI and a blood measurement of lactate dehydrogenase (LDH-3). At the time of the MRI, a liquid dye called gadolinium is injected into the blood vessel. Since the sarcoma contains more blood vessels than normal uterine muscle, an enhanced image would be produced on gadolinium-enhanced MRI. On the other hand, LDH is an enzyme made in muscle cells. The sarcoma is supposed to produce LDH isoenzyme 3 in high quantities. Therefore, presence of an abnormal image on contrast MRI and increased LDH-3 levels can imply that a sarcoma is present. However, these tests are still in the research stages, and they need to be confirmed by further well-designed studies in future before they can be given total acceptance in clinical practice.

A suspicion of malignancy must be kept in mind in case of sudden increase in the size of fibroid, sudden development of pain or tenderness in the myoma, systemic upset, and pyrexia or postmenopausal bleeding. Macroscopically, a sarcomatous tumor appears grayish in color with areas of necrosis and hemorrhage (Figs. 24.32A to D). The consistency of sarcoma is soft and friable and not firm like that of a fibroid. The malignant process usually begins at the center of the tumor and the diagnosis is made on the histopathological examination of the removed myoma specimen. Therefore, leiomyosarcomas present with masses, which tend to be softer in comparison to their surroundings due to tissue necrosis and, internal cystic degeneration and hemorrhage. It is, however, difficult to separate the leiomyosarcomas from the surrounding myometrium at attempted myomectomy because of their invasive nature. Investigations such as cervical cytology, endometrial sampling, and ultrasound, especially color Doppler have not been found to be totally reliable. MRI helps in distinguishing between benign and malignant tumors. Sarcomas with a malignant behavior usually have 10 or more mitoses per high power yield, are nonencapsulated and therefore may rapidly spread via the bloodstream and lymphatics. They can spread to the adjacent structures and from there to abdomen and lungs. Tumor with <5 mitosis per high power field is likely to behave in a benign manner. The index of suspicion for malignancy should increase with patient's age and a past history of pelvic irradiation. Intraoperative or postoperative diagnosis of leiomyosarcoma warrants an oncologic consultation.

Leiomyosarcomas are usually associated with a poor prognosis and have a 5-years survival rate of approximately 30%.

If the patient's fibroids are observed to be growing, she should be called for a repeat pelvic examination after every 1–3 months. If the fibroid suddenly becomes symptomatic or increases in size, then surgery may be considered. Since, the incidence of sarcomas is so low, it is not clinically justifiable to believe that a growing fibroid indicates malignancy. However, if the patient is postmenopausal, any growth in the uterus may be a cause for concern. In these cases, endometrial carcinoma must be ruled out first.

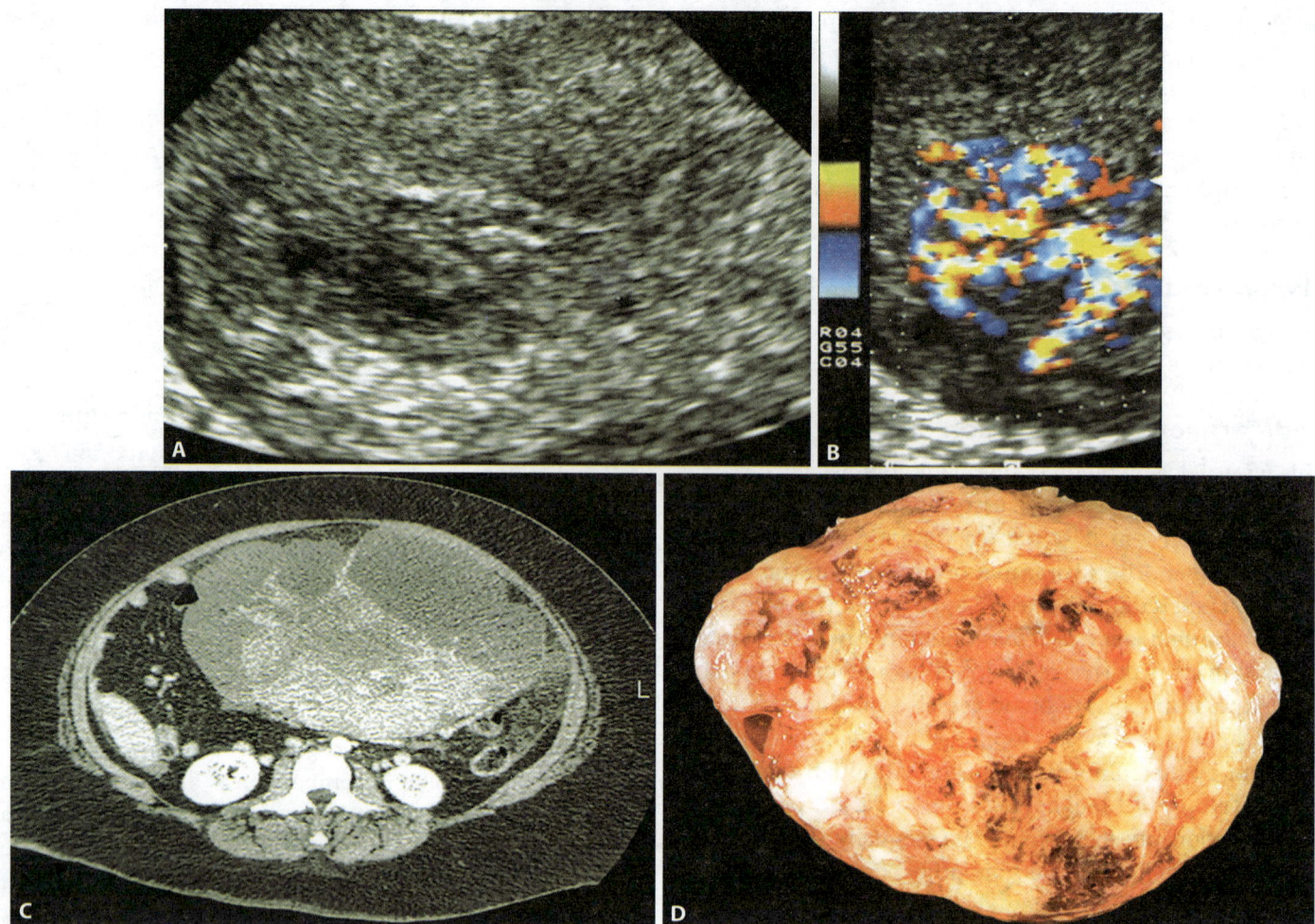

Figs. 24.32A to D: Leiomyosarcoma: (A) Ultrasound examination revealed presence of a hypoechogenic mass; (B) Doppler ultrasound showing presence of a highly vascular mass in the same patient as described in Figure 24.32A; (C) Computed tomography scan in the same patient showed a uterine mass with hemorrhagic and necrotic areas; (D) Gross specimen of leiomyosarcoma as obtained upon hysterectomy.

Cellular Fibroids

These fibroids are likely to be more cellular than the usual types because the smooth muscle content is likely to more in these fibroids. Therefore, they may sometimes mimic leiomyosarcomas. However, they can be differentiated from sarcomas due to the absence of nuclear atypia in them.

STUMP

STUMP can be defined as the smooth muscle tumors with uncertain malignant potential. These tumors can have either of the following histopathological findings:

- 5–10 mitoses per 10 high-power fields without nuclear atypia or giant cells
- 2–10 mitoses per 10 high-power fields with nuclear atypia or giant cells.

These tumors assume importance because they require regular follow-up as they are associated with a high risk of recurrence.

ASSOCIATED PATHOLOGIES

Some likely gynecological pathologies which may be present along with the fibroids due to resemblance of their etiopathogenetic mechanism, include the following:

- Anovulation and multiple follicular cysts
- Endometrial hyperplasia
- Endometrial carcinoma (3%)
- Endometriosis/ adenomyosis (30%)
- Salpingo-ophoritis (15%)
- Infertility (2–3%)

FIBROIDS AND INFERTILITY

The relationship between myomas and infertility is still controversial and has been a subject of extensive debate. Presently, it is not yet known for sure whether infertility is the cause or the effect of leiomyomas. 30% of women with infertility may have fibroids. Also, in women with fibroids, 5–10% are infertile and in nearly 2–3% women, infertility may be solely due to fibroids.

Mere presence of myomas in an infertile patient should not be considered as a cause of her infertility. Firstly, she should be investigated for all the other common causes of infertility (including the tubal factor, the ovarian factor, male factor, etc.). Only after all the other common causes of infertility in a woman have been ruled out, presence of myomas may be considered as the cause for infertility in a woman. The extent to which presence of myomas can influence fertility in a woman depends upon the position of fibroids inside the uterus, the number of fibroids, and their size. Nearly 40% women conceive following myomectomy in cases of submucous fibroids, but rarely with intramural fibroids. The effect of uterine fibroids on the woman's fertility pattern has been discussed in detail in Chapter 34. Uterine fibroids could be responsible for infertility through the mechanisms listed in **Box 24.26**.

FIBROIDS AND PREGNANCY

Possible Effects of Fibroids on Pregnancy

Majority of fibroids remain unchanged in size during pregnancy. Most fibroids remain uncomplicated during pregnancy. However, they may show an invariable enlargement during pregnancy due to presence of congestion, edema, and degeneration; they usually return back to their original size afterward. Presence of fibroids during pregnancy can result in an increased risk of the following pregnancy-related complications, especially if the placenta implants over or in close proximity to a myoma:

- Miscarriage
- First trimester bleeding
- Abruption (large fibroids, usually > 20 cm in diameter are more likely to cause abruption and abdominal pain)
- Prelabor rupture of membranes or preterm labor
- Intrauterine growth restriction
- Prolonged/obstructed labor
- Very large-sized uterine myomas can cause respiratory embarrassment and urinary retention
- Fibroids located in the lower uterine segment may be associated with an increased likelihood of the following complications:
  - Fetal malpresentation (breech presentation)
  - Cesarean section, cesarean hysterectomy
  - Postpartum hemorrhage
  - Myomectomy should not be performed in pregnant women because of the increased risk of uncontrolled bleeding. The exception to this may be presence of symptomatic subserous fibroids on a pedicle <5 cm thick.

> **BOX 24.26:** Causes for the potential subfertility related to fibroids.
> - Dysfunctional uterine contractility (may interfere with gamete transport and implantation of the fertilized ovum)
> - Distortion of the endometrial cavity (due to submucous fibroids)
> - Disturbances of ovulation
> - Focal endometrial vascular disturbance
> - Endometrial inflammation
> - Secretion of vasoactive substances
> - Enhanced endometrial androgen environment
> - Submucous fibroids are more likely to cause subfertility
> - Interference with the ascent of sperms in cases of cervical fibroids
> - Fibroids > 5 cm, and those close to the cervix or tubal ostia, are also thought to be more problematic

EVIDENCE-BASED CLINICAL TRIALS

List of references can be scanned through QR code to enable the readers gain deeper insight of the subject by referring to the entire article or its abstract.

CHAPTER 25

Menopause

CASE STUDY

A 52-year-old patient presented to the gynecological clinic with complaints of hot flushes and vaginal dryness since last 15 days. She has two children, both grown up and married and do not live with her. Since last 15 months, she has not experienced any periods. One year prior to this, she had been experiencing periods irregularly with gradual diminishment of the blood flow. She had taken this to mean that she had attained menopause. She arrives in the clinic appearing irritable and depressed. She has read on the Internet that use of hormones may help her deal with menopausal symptoms. So, she is requesting the doctor to prescribe her hormones to help her deal with the condition. She is otherwise healthy and has not suffered from any health-related problems in the past.

INTRODUCTION

Q. Write a short essay on menopause.

Menopause can be defined as the cessation of ovarian function resulting in permanent amenorrhea (lasting for at least 1 year). The woman can be considered as menopausal, if she has not had any menstrual bleeding for at least 12 months. The onset of menopause involves physical, sexual, and psychological adjustments. Therefore, this is a retrospective diagnosis, which can be established only after 12 months of amenorrhea in the appropriate age group. Though menopause usually occurs as a natural process of aging, it can also be surgically induced by bilateral oophorectomy, ovariotoxic chemotherapy, or radiations. Menopause normally occurs between the age of 45 and 55 years, with the average age being about 51 years. In India, women are likely to attain menopause at a younger age, varying between 42 and 50 years.

Climacteric (perimenopause or the menopausal transition) is the phase of waning ovarian activity, which may begin 2–3 years before menopause and may continue 2–5 years after it. This can be regarded as the phase of transition between the active and inactive ovarian function. The period of menopausal transition varies from 2 to 8 years.

The period following menopause is known as postmenopause. The first 4 years following menopause are the early postmenopause and the later years are the late postmenopause.

Hormone therapy is generally prescribed for treating troublesome menopausal symptoms such as hot flushes or vaginal dryness. Menopausal hormone therapy (MHT) or the hormone therapy or the previously used term HRT refers to the intake of supplements of hormones such as estrogen alone or estrogen in combination with progesterone (progestin in its synthetic form). Short-term use of hormones (<5 years) is usually not associated with an increased risk of complications (e.g., increased risk for breast cancer). MHT is not prescribed to all menopausal women. The hormones must be consumed for the shortest period of time possible. They must be selectively prescribed to women who are at high risk for menopausal abnormalities. Indications for the use of MHT are as follows:

- *Menopausal and postmenopausal patients:* Symptomatic patients suffering from vasomotor, urinary symptoms, or symptoms related to genital atrophy, such as dryness, itching, dysuria, and dyspareunia require MHT. Individuals at high risk for cardiovascular diseases, osteoporosis, Alzheimer's disease, etc., may also require MHT. Estrogen exerts a cardioprotective effect by maintaining high levels of high-density lipoprotein (HDL) and lowering the levels of low-density lipoprotein (LDL).

Q. Write a short essay on premature menopause.

- *Premature menopause:* Cessation of menses in a woman aged 40 years or younger is called premature menopause. Women suffering from premature menopause, such as premature ovarian failure, or those who have undergone surgical oophorectomy must be prescribed HRT.

ETIOLOGY

> Q. Describe in detail the alterations which are likely to take place in the levels of estrogen during menopause.
>
> Q. Discuss briefly the endocrinological changes occurring during menopause.

Menopause occurs due to a decline in ovarian activity resulting in a gradual depletion in the number of oocytes produced by the ovary. As a result, there is a decline in the levels of hormones, estrogen and inhibin. There is nearly 50% reduction in androgen production and approximately 90% reduction in estrogen production at the time of menopause. Estrogen levels may become as low as 10–20 pg/mL. There is failure of ovulation, failure of formation of corpus luteum, and failure of secretion of progesterone by the ovaries. Estrogenic activity is reduced and there occurs endometrial atrophy, resulting in amenorrhea. Initially, there is a rebound increase in the secretion of follicle-stimulating hormone (FSH) and luteinizing hormone (LH) by the anterior pituitary due to the removal of negative feedback inhibition of gonadotropin production, resulting in an increase in the levels of FSH [>40 international units (IU)/mL] and LH (>20 IU/mL). However, with further advancing years, the gonadotropic activity of pituitary glands also ceases and a fall in FSH levels eventually occurs **(Fig. 25.1)**.

The cycles eventually become anovulatory and there is no progesterone production. The ovarian stroma does continue to produce estrogens and androgens. The adrenal androgen production also continues though at a lower level. These androgens are converted into estrone in the peripheral tissues. Unopposed action of estrone on the endometrium eventually results in proliferative changes, hyperplasia and sometimes even carcinoma.

HISTORY AND CLINICAL PRESENTATION

- *History of presenting complaints:* At the time of presentation, it is important to ask the patient's age at the time of her presenting complaints as well as at the time of menopause. She needs to be asked about the type of menopause, whether spontaneous or iatrogenic. Besides the detailed history of presenting symptoms and clinical presentation (described next), it is also important to elicit the following histories:
- *Family history:* Family history of osteoporosis, coronary heart disease (CHD), and breast cancer needs to be enquired. This history may be important at the time of taking decision for starting HRT.
- *Patient's lifestyle:* Detailed history related to the patient's lifestyle such as dietary intake of calcium and vitamin D, exposure to sunlight, exercise, smoking, and alcohol needs to be asked.

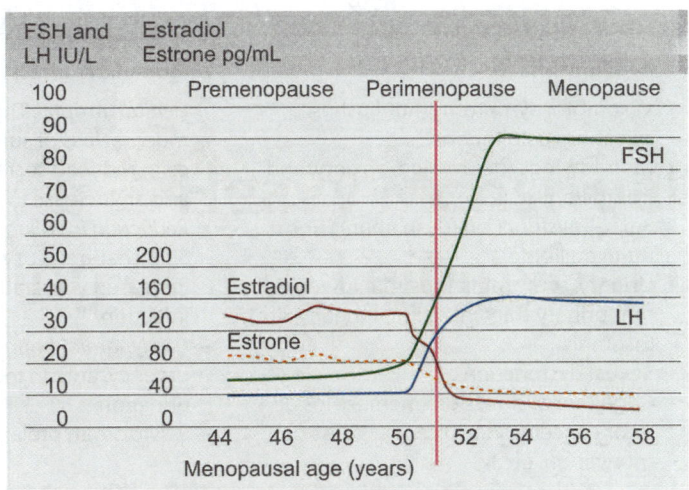

Fig. 25.1: Changes in the levels of various hormones at the time of menopause.

- *Medical history:* Previous history of medical problems such as diabetes, hypertension, and dyslipidemia must be taken. History of intake of drugs (e.g., corticosteroids, thyroxine, etc.) which may act as a risk factor for osteoporosis also needs to be asked.

CLINICAL PRESENTATION

> Q. Describe in detail the clinical features likely to occur in the women during menopause.

Menopause is a hypoestrogenic state, which can result in the various effects enlisted in **Table 25.1**. History of all these effects needs to be elicited.

Anatomical Changes

Anatomical changes occurring during menopause include atrophy and retrogression of the genital organs. Moreover, there are aberrations in the endocrine balance maintained during the child-bearing period.

Symptoms

Nearly 60–70% of women remain asymptomatic; others may experience various symptoms, which are described next. These need to be elicited at the time of taking history.
- *Vaginal dryness:* Signs and symptoms of vaginal dryness include dryness, itching, burning, pain, or light bleeding with sexual intercourse, increased urinary frequency or urgency.
- *Cessation of periods:* This could be a sudden cessation or gradual diminution in the amount of blood loss for each successive menstrual period, until the menstrual flow eventually ceases.
- *Hot flushes:* Hot flushes and sweating commonly occur as a result of vasomotor disturbances and may be present in nearly 85% of women. These may be preceded by a headache. Hot flush can be defined as an acute sensation

TABLE 25.1: Various effects of menopause.

Immediate effects	Intermediate effects	Long-term effects
• Vasomotor symptoms (hot flushes, sweating, palpitations) • Mood swings (depression, anxiety, and irritability) • Sexual dysfunction (dyspareunia and reduced libido) • Urinary symptoms (dysuria, lower recurrent urinary tract infection, urgency, etc.) • Insomnia • Sexual dysfunction • Cognitive dysfunction (memory loss, poor concentration, tiredness, loss of motivation, etc.)	• *Genital atrophy:* Thinning of the vaginal mucosa, loss of superficial keratinized cells, reduced secretions from the glands, and an increase in the vaginal pH • *Reduction in collagen support and atrophy:* Skin changes, easy bruising, and an increased vulnerability to trauma and infection • *Urodynamic changes:* Stress incontinence, urgency, and an increased frequency of urination • Pelvic organ prolapse	• *Osteoporosis:* It is due to estrogen deficiency and affects the trabecular bone • Cardiovascular effects • Dementia

of heat and skin changes, which may be associated with profuse perspiration. Skin changes may be in form of reddening of the skin over neck, chest, and head accompanied by an increase in heart rate and a feeling of intense body heat. It is mediated by noradrenaline and serotonin. There is an increase in core body temperature and vasodilatation during hot flushes.

- *Osteoporosis:* There is likely to be a reduction in bone mineral mass, resulting in osteopenia and/or osteoporosis, which may predispose to fracture development.
- *Mental symptoms:* Mental depression may occur due to disturbed sleep and inability to cope up with the body changes. There may also be irritability and loss of concentration. Pseudocyesis (fear of pregnancy) and cancer phobia may develop in some women.
- *Neurological symptoms:* These may include paresthesias (sensation of pins and needles).
- *Libido:* Although many women experience reduced libido, some women may also experience an increase in libido due to riddance of menstruation and fear of pregnancy.
- *Urinary symptoms:* These may include symptoms such as dysuria, stress, and urge incontinence and recurrent vaginal infections. Genital symptoms, such as dryness of vagina, dyspareunia, genital prolapse, and urinary and/or fecal incontinence may also occur.
- *Long-term effects:* In the long term, menopause is likely to result in complications such as arthritis, osteoporosis, fracture, cerebrovascular accidents, ischemic heart disease, myocardial infarction (MI), atherosclerosis, stroke, skin changes, and Alzheimer's disease.

GENERAL PHYSICAL EXAMINATION

The various physical changes which may be observed on general physical examination at the time of menopause are illustrated in **Figure 25.2** and are described as follows:

- *Hair:* The hair may become thinner and lose its luster.
- *Teeth:* Teeth may loosen and gums may recede.
- *Skin:* Skin and mucous membranes become drier and skin develops a rough texture.
- *Breasts:* The breasts may droop and flatten.
- *Spine:* Changes in the spine, e.g., kyphosis, may be present.

Measurement of blood pressure and body mass index is also important in these patients.

SPECIFIC SYSTEMIC EXAMINATION

PER SPECULUM EXAMINATION

The following findings are observed on per speculum examination:

- *Vulva:* Atrophic changes in vulva are natural sequelae of estrogen deficiency characterized by loss of normal architecture and thinning of the skin. Vulvar atrophy may also occur.
- *Vagina:* There may be loss of thick keratinized mucosa and reduction in the amount of glycogen produced by the vaginal epithelium. There is an increase in the vaginal pH. A vaginal pH of >4.5 is almost always associated with estrogen deficiency. These changes are clinically visible in the form of thinning of the vaginal walls, loss of rugae, and narrowing of the vaginal orifice, and may result in symptoms such as dyspareunia.
- *Features suggestive of atrophy:* There may be thinning of the skin of labia minora and vestibule, and reduction in the amount of fat in labia majora. There is also reduction of pubic hair. Red patches around the urethra and introitus caused by senile vulvulitis may occur.
- *Pelvic organ prolapse:* Cystocele or rectocele may be detected on a per speculum examination. For detailed information related to examination in case of pelvic organ prolapse, kindly refer to Chapter 29.

PER VAGINAL EXAMINATION

The following findings are observed on per vaginal examination:

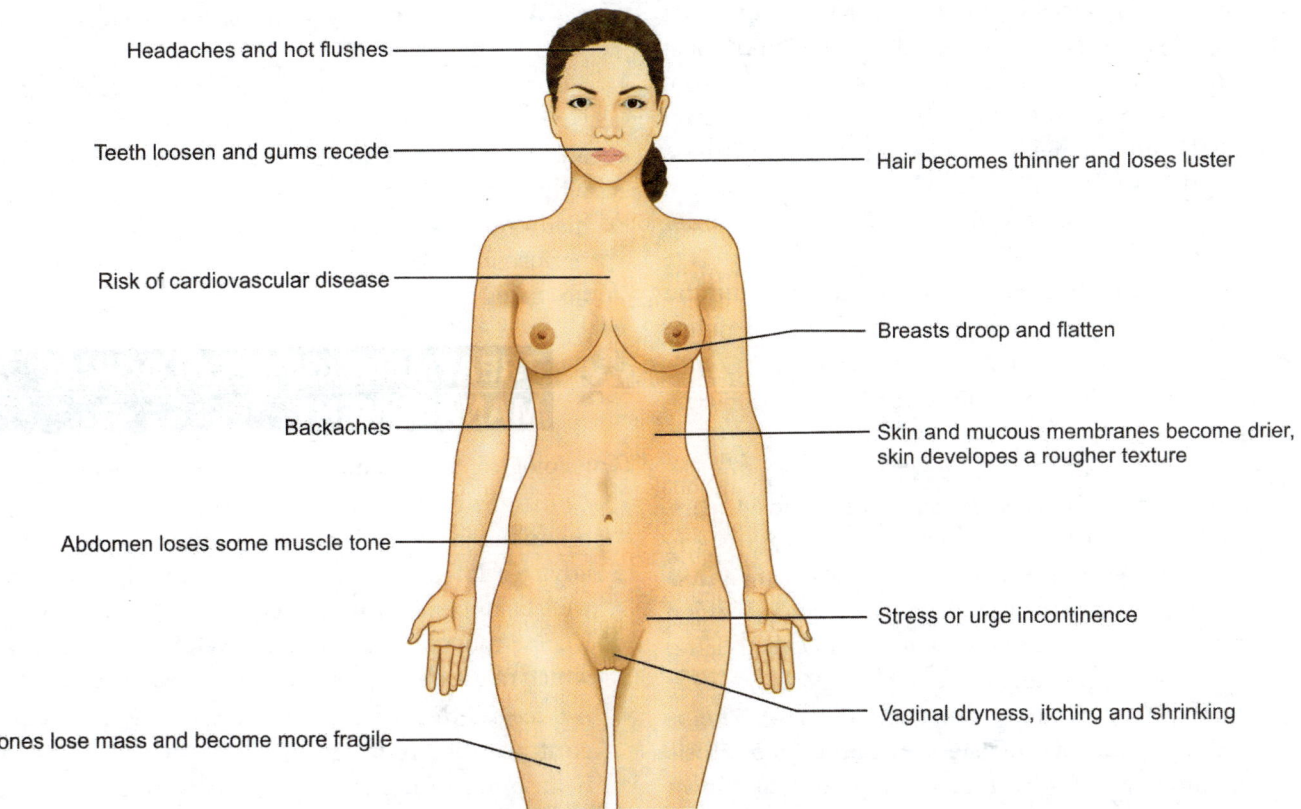

Fig. 25.2: Effects of menopause on the female body.

- *Uterus:* There is reduction in the size of the fundus relative to the cervix, a decrease in myometrial thickness, and thinning of the endometrium. Laxity of the pelvic cellular tissues and ligaments predispose to the development of uterovaginal prolapse.
- *Ovaries:* The postmenopausal ovary decreases in size even during use of HRT and should not be palpable on routine pelvic examination. Any enlargement of the ovary should be considered as malignancy until proven otherwise in postmenopausal women.

MANAGEMENT

Management comprising of investigations and definitive obstetric management is discussed next.

INVESTIGATIONS

CLINICAL PRESENTATION

Menopause can be easily diagnosed on the basis of clinical presentation (e.g., amenorrhea, night sweats, hot flushes, etc.), when the patient is at least 1 year postmenopausal. A triad of hot flushes, amenorrhea for 1 year, and raised serum FSH levels >40 IU/L helps in establishing the diagnosis of menopause. In a woman belonging to menopausal age group, with amenorrhea of >1 year or irregular menstrual cycles, determination of serum FSH levels for confirmation of menopause is not required. Serum FSH levels may be, however, required in the following cases:
- Young age
- Posthysterectomy (without oophorectomy)
- Atypical symptoms (irregular bleeding, etc.)

In menopausal women, while both serum FSH and LH levels are >40 IU/L, serum estradiol levels are <20 pg/mL

Prior to the initiation of MHT, the following investigations need to be performed:
- *History and physical examination:* A complete history and physical examination including blood pressure measurement, assessment of breasts, and pelvic and rectal examination must be done.
- *Routine investigations:* These include estimation of blood sugar, lipid profile, serum calcium and phosphorus levels, levels of alkaline phosphatase (could be elevated in women with osteomalacia, which needs to be treated before initiating therapy for osteoporosis), serum 25-hydroxy vitamin D3 levels and electrocardiogram.
- *Endometrial sampling and/or biopsy:* This may be required in cases with high-risk factors for endometrial cancer (e.g., morbid obesity and diabetes), history of abnormal uterine bleeding, and history of polycystic ovary disease or prior use of estrogenic medications. Continuous bleeding, AUB, or irregular bleeding during the perimenopausal or menopausal period must be considered as abnormal and warrants investigations to rule out any potential malignancies. As previously

described, endometrial evaluation (TVS or endometrial aspiration in case of endometrial thickness >4 mm) must be definitely performed in these cases. Endometrial sampling/biopsy helps in ruling out endometrial hyperplasia and malignancy. Also presence of chronic vulvar pruritus or irritation, which does not respond to estrogen therapy, requires complete evaluation in order to rule out underlying malignancy.

If endometrial aspiration is unable to evaluate the uterine cavity or if the uterus is not normal on pelvic examination (it is enlarged and irregular), a D&C with hysteroscopy can be performed to arrive at an accurate diagnosis.

- *Pap smear examination:* As previously described in Chapter 27, in women between the age of 30 and 64 years, routine Pap smear is recommended at every 3 yearly interval in the age group between 25 and 49 years and at every 5 yearly interval between 50 and 64 years. In women above the age of 65 years, no screening is necessary after adequate negative previous screening results.
- *Dual energy X-ray absorptiometry (DEXA):* DEXA helps in determining the level of osteopenia and osteoporosis and the propensity for fracture development. As shown in **Figure 25.3**, DEXA technique measures bone density at three sites—(1) lumbar spine, (2) hip, and (3) femoral neck. Using a DEXA scan, the patient's bone density is compared to the average bone density in young adults of same sex and race. The score is called the T-score and it expresses the bone density in terms of standard deviations (SDs) below the peak young adult bone mass. According to National Osteoporosis Foundation Guidelines, there are several groups of people who must be considered for DEXA scan. These are as follows:
  - All postmenopausal women below the age of 65 years who have risk factors for osteoporosis.
  - Women aged 65 years and older
  - Postmenopausal women with fractures
  - Women having any of the conditions associated with osteoporosis.
- *Hormone levels:* Measurement of levels of estrogen and FSH help in deciding the requirement for HRT.
- *Mammography:* Mammography is mandatory in women with high-risk factors for breast cancer (e.g., family history of breast cancer). Mammography must also be performed before starting HRT in those women who are not being annually screened with mammography.

℞ TREATMENT/GYNECOLOGICAL MANAGEMENT

Gynecological management comprises the following steps:
- *Counseling:* This involves explaining the normal menopause-related changes to the patient, giving her advice related to contraception, and asking her to eat a well-balanced nutritious diet (rich in vitamin A, C, D, and E). She must be advised to do weight-bearing exercises, which may help to prevent or delay osteoporosis.
- *Advice related to contraception:* Low-estrogen oral contraceptive (containing 20 μg of ethinyl estradiol) is an option for perimenopausal women who require relief of menopausal symptoms, and who also desire contraception at the same time. When perimenopausal women taking a low-dose oral contraceptive during perimenopause reach the age 50 or 51 years or achieve menopause, either the pill must be stopped altogether, or postmenopausal estrogen regimen must be started if required for the control of menopausal symptoms.
- *Antidepressants or antianxiety agents:* These may be prescribed to relieve the woman of her anxiety and depression.
- *Lifestyle modifications:* These help in reducing the risk of osteoporosis and in improving the quality of life. Some of the strategies for lifestyle modification are as follows:
  - Weight-bearing exercises (walking, jogging, etc.)

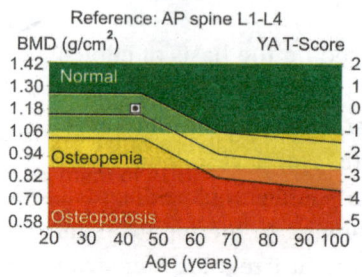
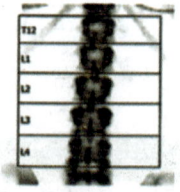
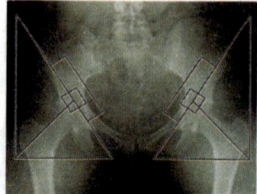
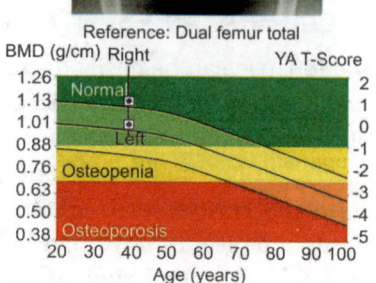

Fig. 25.3: Process of bone densitometry.

- Exposure to sunlight
- *Increasing the intake of food rich in calcium and vitamin D:* These women must receive 1–1.5 g of elemental calcium and 1,000–1,500 IU of vitamin D daily.
- *Menopausal hormone therapy:* MHT helps in providing relief from immediate postmenopausal symptoms. This therapy has been described in detail later in the chapter.
- *Alternative therapy:* This may involve the use of naturally available substances such as black cohosh, phytoestrogens, red clover, oil of evening primrose, and vitamin E. These are described in detail later in the chapter.
- *Treatment of hot flushes:* Low doses of certain antidepressants [selective serotonin reuptake inhibitors (SSRIs), e.g., paroxetine, fluoxetine, citalopram, etc., and serotonin and norepinephrine reuptake inhibitors (SNRIs), such as venlafaxine, desvenlafaxine, etc.] may decrease hot flushes. Though unlicensed, both SSRIs and SNRIs have been found to be more effective than placebo in reducing the symptoms of hot flushes. Drugs, such as gabapentin (Neurontin) and clonidine (a centrally acting α-agonist), can also be used for the treatment of hot flushes. Clonidine is a licensed nonhormonal treatment for vasomotor symptoms such as hot flushes.
- *Transdermal skin patches:* Their use helps in avoiding first-pass effect and liver metabolism. Hormonal implants and Mirena have also been recently introduced in MHT.
- *Osteoporosis treatment:* Medicines, such as bisphosphonates (etidronate, tiludronate, etc.), hormones, such as estrogen, and selective estrogen receptor modulators (SERMs) (e.g., raloxifene) play an important role in osteoporosis treatment.
- *Tibolone:* This is a synthetic derivative of 19-nortestosterone, which has weak estrogenic, progestogenic, and androgenic action. In the dosage of 2.5 mg daily, tibolone is cardioprotective, helps in improving bone resorption, and relieving vasomotor symptoms. This drug may, however, cause irregular bleeding in nearly 15% of individuals. Short period of therapy over 3–5 years is advocated. Reduction in dosage must be done as soon as possible. Estradiol levels must be maintained at 100 pg/mL.
- *Other treatment options:* These include nonhormonal alternatives such as SERMs, selective tissue estrogen activity regulator (STEAR), etc. These are also described in detail later in the chapter.

MENOPAUSE HORMONE THERAPY

> Q. Write a long essay on menopause and modern trends in HRT therapy.
>
> Q. Write a long essay, describing the physiology of menopause and its management.
>
> Q. With help of a long essay discuss the physiological changes occurring during menopause. Discuss the use of MHT for dealing with the problems related to menopause.
>
> Q. Discuss in detail the indications and different regimens of MHT.
>
> Q. Discuss in brief the treatment of menopause.
>
> Q. Discuss the management of postmenopausal symptoms.
>
> Q. Write a short essay on MHT.
>
> Q. What is the next step of management in the case study described in the beginning of this chapter?
>
> Ans. Estrogen therapy remains the gold standard for relief of menopausal symptoms, in particular, hot flushes, and therefore is a reasonable option for this case. HRT should be preferably avoided in those with a history of breast cancer, CHD, a previous venous thromboembolic event, stroke, etc. In an otherwise healthy woman, the absolute risk of an adverse incident is particularly low. Both conjugated estrogen and 17-beta estradiol (oral or transdermal) appear to be equally effective for the treatment of hot flushes. The most commonly used dosage of estrogens include conjugated estrogen 0.625 mg, 1 mg micronized 17-beta-estradiol, or 50 μg/day transdermal 17-beta-estradiol. Low-dose preparations in general contain one-half the standard dose. Although it is not known if lower doses of estrogen or progestin have less of an effect on the breast and cardiovascular system, low-dose estrogen treatment for short term (2–3 years) is preferred whenever possible and can be considered as the treatment of choice for postmenopausal women with moderate-to-severe vasomotor symptoms having no contraindications for estrogen use.

Menopausal hormone therapy or the hormone therapy or HRT, HRT (older terminology, previously used) refers to a woman taking supplements of hormones such as estrogen alone or estrogen in combination with progesterone (progestin in its synthetic form). MHT can be taken in the form of a pill, patch, gel, vaginal cream, or slow-releasing suppository, which can be placed in the vagina (**Fig. 25.4**).

Figure 25.5 shows pills of MHT displayed in a circular dispenser. HRT pills contain synthetic hormones such as

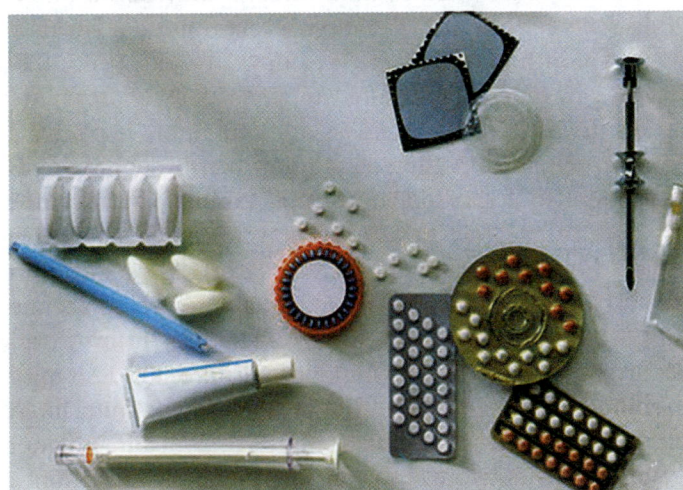

Fig. 25.4: Different types of preparations for hormone replacement therapy.

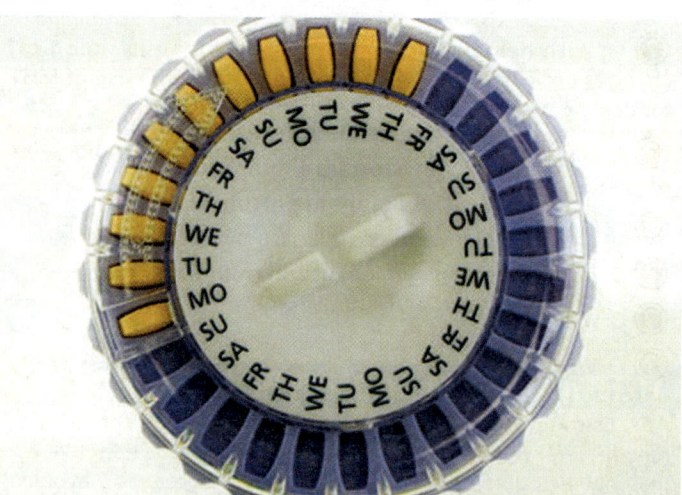

Fig. 25.5: Pills of hormone replacement therapy in a circular dispenser.

estrogen and progestogen, and these are arranged in the slots of a circular dispenser. The slots are marked by days of the month so that the woman is reminded to take them on a regular basis. The color of the pills may change depending on the composition of its constituents.

Different Types of MHT Preparations

There are three routes of estrogen administration available—(1) oral, (2) transdermal, and (3) vaginal. HRT can be taken in the form of a pill, patch, gel, vaginal cream, or slow-releasing suppository which can be placed in the vagina. Some commonly available HRT preparations are as follows:

- *Pills containing conjugated estrogen and progesterone:* One of the most commonly used brands of conjugated estrogens is Premarin®, manufactured from the urine of pregnant horses (mares). Most clinicians recommend starting with a low dose of oral conjugated estrogen, i.e., 0.45 mg or 0.625 mg. Low-dose conjugated estrogen in the dosage of 0.3 mg daily is unlikely to be associated with any side effects. Dose interval may be modified as daily for initial 2–3 months, every other day for next 2–3 months, and every third day for next 2 months. Therapy must be thereafter stopped if the symptoms are controlled. If the lowest dose does not improve patient's symptoms, a higher dose option can be considered. Natural equine conjugated estrogen must be prescribed in the dosage of 0.625 mg or micronized estradiol (in the dose of 1–2 mg/day) for days 1–25 each month and progestogen, such as medroxyprogesterone acetate (5–10 mg), dydrogesterone (5–10 mg), micronized progesterone (100–500 mg), norethisterone N (2.5 mg), norethindrone, or norgestrel must also be administered daily for days 13–25 each month in order to prevent endometrial hyperplasia and/or cancer. No hormones are given during the remainder of the month. Most patients demonstrate withdrawal bleeding during the hormone-free interval. To prevent withdrawal bleeding, these hormones can also be prescribed continuously. Many patients may have irregular bleeding, but 95% are likely to become amenorrheic within 1 year. In case of women with hysterectomy, progestins are not required. To reduce the inherent risks related to hormone therapy, lowest effective dose of MHT must be prescribed for the shortest amount of time. All types of estrogen can provide relief from the menopausal symptoms. Birth control pills containing very low-dose estrogen can be considered as a good option for women in their 40s who experience troublesome symptoms of climacteric (e.g., hot flushes, irregular bleeding, etc.) and who still require a dependable form of contraception. However, birth control pills are generally not recommended for postmenopausal women because the dose of estrogen is higher than that required to provide relief against hot flushes.
- *Vaginal estrogen preparations (creams, ring, and tablets):* Very low doses of vaginal estrogen in form of vaginal creams, vaginal ring, or vaginal estrogen tablets can be used for treating women with vaginal dryness. Such low-dose vaginal estrogens do not usually require concurrent use of a progestin pill. Estrogen vaginal cream (Ovestin cream containing the active hormone estriol) can be used in the dosage of 1–2 g every day for days 10–12 each month, for a period of 3–6 months until the symptoms disappear.
- *Transdermal skin patches:* Estrogen patches, containing 3.2 mg of 17-β estradiol, release about 50 μg of estradiol daily. These patches are effective for increasing bone density and treating menopausal symptoms. Women with an intact uterus who use an estrogen patch must also take progestins simultaneously to reduce the risk of uterine cancer. Estrogen patch treatment may be associated with fewer complications in comparison to treatment with oral estrogen preparations. These patches are applied below the waistline and changed twice weekly.
- *Subdermal implants:* Hormone-containing subdermal implants having estradiol are licensed for use. These implants are inserted subcutaneously over the anterior abdominal wall, using local anesthesia. Estradiol implants may be available in formulations containing 25, 50, or 100 mg of estradiol. They can a kept for a period of 6 months and help in maintaining the ratio of E2 to E1.
- *Mirena:* Use of LNG IUS has been recently introduced in MHT.

USES OF MHT

Aims of using MHT are listed in **Box 25.1**. Various uses of MHT are enlisted in **Table 25.2**. Currently, estrogen therapy is not considered to be a first-line therapy for

> **BOX 25.1:** Aims of using menopausal hormone therapy.
> - To overcome short-term and long-term consequences of estrogen deficiency
> - Relief of menopausal symptoms, e.g., vasomotor symptoms, urogenital atrophy, etc.
> - Prevention of osteoporosis and increase in bone mineral density (reduction in the risk of vertebral and hip fractures)
> - To maintain the quality of life

TABLE 25.2: Various uses of menopausal hormone therapy (HRT).

Menopausal symptoms	Treatment
Depression	Estrogen therapy with or without antidepressants
Sleep problems	Estrogen therapy
Migraine headaches	Continuous hormone regimens should be used. Cyclic regimens must be avoided to prevent initiating the estrogen withdrawal headaches
Moderate-to-severe vasomotor symptoms without any history of breast cancer or cardiovascular disease	Short-term estrogen therapy
Vaginal atrophy	Vaginal estrogens can be used in almost all postmenopausal women with symptoms of vaginal atrophy except for those with a history of breast cancer
Mild urogenital atrophy	Vaginal moisturizing agents on a regular basis and vaginal lubricants at the time of intercourse
Moderate-to-severe urogenital atrophy	Low-dose vaginal estrogen

prevention of osteoporosis. Presently, bisphosphonates and/or raloxifene have been recommended as the first-line treatment for prevention of osteoporosis.

Estrogen therapy is also no longer indicated for the prevention of CHD in postmenopausal women. This recommendation initially made by the American Heart Association (AHA) in 2001 has been further strengthened by the results of the Women's Health Initiative (WHI) and Heart and Estrogen/Progestin Replacement Study (HERS)-II trials. The emerging evidence suggests that the risk of CHD events with HRT is majorly limited to older postmenopausal women, with younger postmenopausal women at very low risk for CHD-related events. In older women, HRT may be associated with an increased risk of CHD, venous thromboembolism, and stroke. This increase is more in women having pre-existing risk factors for cardiovascular disease. The same risk does not occur in younger menopausal women.

Based on the results of WHI study, MHT should also not be prescribed after the age of 65 years for prevention of dementia.

Estrogen therapy is not recommended for women with a personal history of breast cancer due to the increased risk of breast cancer recurrence with estrogen therapy as observed in the Hormonal replacement therapy after Breast Cancer—Is It Safe? (HABITS) trial. This trial had to be terminated midway in the year 2003 due to an unacceptable risk of breast cancer for the women (having a previous history of breast cancer) exposed to HRT.

Senile Vaginal Atrophy

> **Q.** What is vaginal atrophy and what are the various management options in menopausal women with vaginal atrophy?
>
> **Q.** Write short essay on senile vaginitis.

The epithelial lining of the vagina and urethra is extremely sensitive to estrogen, and estrogen deficiency results in thinning of the vaginal epithelium. This leads to vaginal atrophy (atrophic vaginitis), causing symptoms of vaginal dryness, itching, dyspareunia, abnormal vaginal discharge, vaginal discomfort, etc. Both systemic HRT and vaginal estrogen therapy are effective for genitourinary atrophy symptoms. However, vaginal estrogen treatment (cream, tablets, or ring) may be more effective for providing relief from genitourinary symptoms without causing toxicity related to high systemic levels. This option must be used for nearly all postmenopausal women with symptoms of vaginal atrophy except for those with past history of breast cancer. Besides vaginal estrogens, other treatment modalities for vaginal dryness include vaginal moisturizers or lubricants; vaginal estrogen and a medication called ospemifene (brand name Osphena). All these treatment modalities are temporary. The vaginal dryness usually returns when the treatment is stopped. Vaginal lubricants and moisturizers do not contain any hormones and therefore have no side effects. These various therapies are described as follows:

Hormone Replacement Therapy

Hormone therapy is useful for treating vaginal atrophy and other menopausal symptoms such as hot flushes. Since the use of hormone therapy is likely to result in systemic side effects, local vaginal estrogen treatments are preferable over systemic therapy due to reduced incidence of side effects.

Vaginal Lubricants and Moisturizers

Lubricants help in reducing friction and discomfort from dryness during sexual intercourse. The lubricant is applied inside the vagina or on the penis just before sexual intercourse. Some such vaginal lubricants and moisturizers include Astroglide®, petroleum jelly (Vaseline®), K-Y Silk-E Vaginal Moisturizer® or KY Liquibeads Vaginal Moisturizer®, Feminease®, etc. Moisturizers must be applied into the vagina three to four times a week. These should not be used immediately before sexual intercourse because they may cause irritation of vaginal tissues. Oil-based lubricants, such as petroleum jelly may be harmful to the latex condoms and/or diaphragms, thereby reducing their efficacy in preventing pregnancy or sexually transmitted infections. Polyurethane condoms can be used with oil-based lubricants. Moreover, water or silicone-based lubricants can be used with latex condoms and diaphragms. Application of betadine solution externally or use of hot Seitz bath is also likely to provide protection from vaginal pain and irritation. Hand and body lotions should not be used over vaginal tissues because they are likely to cause irritation.

Vaginal Estrogens

Several types of vaginal estrogen products are available:
- *Estrogen cream:* Estrogen cream preparations (e.g., Premarin®, Estrace®, and Evalon® cream) are initially inserted into the vagina every day for 2–3 weeks, and then one or two times weekly. Though use of estrogen cream is associated with minimal side effects, its application can at times be messy; it can be difficult to measure the amount of cream accurately and to insert it into the vagina.
- *Vaginal estrogen tablet:* The vaginal estrogen tablet (Vagifem®) is a small tablet, which can be inserted inside the vagina with the help of a disposable applicator. It is initially inserted every day for 2 weeks and then on twice weekly basis.
- *Vaginal estrogen ring:* Vaginal estrogen ring, e.g., Estring®, is a flexible plastic ring which is to be worn inside the vagina at all times and is replaced at the interval of every 3 months. Estring® is different from Femring® (another vaginal ring) which is used for the purpose of HRT and releases a much higher dose of estrogen in the body in order to provide relief from the menopausal symptoms.

Oral Tablet of Ospemifene

Ospemifene has been described in detail later in the text.

Guidelines for Use of Menopausal Hormone Therapy during Menopause

 Q. Write a short essay on present guidelines on MHT.

The following guidelines must be followed before prescribing MHT to menopausal women:
- Before prescribing MHT, women must be informed about the risks and benefits of prescribing MHT.
- Dose and duration of MHT should be consistent with the patient's treatment goals and safety issues, and need to be individualized.
- Menopausal hormone therapy can be considered as the best treatment option for vasomotor symptoms, mood changes, and vaginal symptoms.
- Bisphosphonates are considered as the treatment of choice in the prevention of osteoporosis amongst the postmenopausal women.
- Menopausal hormone therapy can be considered as an effective and appropriate therapy for prevention of osteoporosis-related fractures in women at high risk (provided they are <60 years of age or <10 years of menopause).
- Risk of cardiovascular events related to MHT is largely limited to the elderly postmenopausal women (>60 years of age or >10 years menopausal).
- As per the Clinical Practice Guidelines (2015) by the Endocrine Society, prior to the prescription of MHT, women need to be screened for the risk of cardiovascular disease and breast cancer. The most appropriate therapy must be recommended based on risk-benefit considerations.
- For women at moderate risk of cardiovascular disease, transdermal rather than oral estrogen is preferred. For women with an intact uterus, micronized progesterone rather than synthetic progestins such as medroxyprogesterone acetate must be prescribed.
- Low-dose vaginal estrogen and ospemifene provide effective therapy for the genitourinary symptoms of menopause. Prescription of nonhormonal therapies (e.g., vaginal moisturizers and lubricants) must be considered for symptomatic women who are at a high risk for cardiovascular disease.
- In women with premature ovarian insufficiency, systemic MHT is recommended at least until the average age of natural menopause.
- Risk of breast cancer attributable to MHT is small and further decreases after the cessation of treatment. However, the current safety data does not support the use of MHT in breast cancer survivors.
- Risk of venous thromboembolism and ischemic stroke increases with oral MHT. However, the absolute risk is rare below the age of 60 years.

Contraindications

Some absolute contraindications to MHT are described in **Box 25.2**.

BOX 25.2: Contraindications for consuming menopausal hormone therapy.

- Undiagnosed genital tract bleeding
- Current or past history of breast cancer
- Family history of breast cancer
- Coronary heart disease
- Thromboembolism, heart attack, or stroke
- Hypertriglyceridemia
- Familial hyperlipidemia
- Undiagnosed genital bleeding
- Active intrinsic liver disease
- Gallbladder disease
- Estrogen-dependent tumors
- History of uterine cancer

ALTERNATIVE THERAPY

Alternative therapy may be required for symptomatic women who do not wish to take HRT or have some contraindications for the use of HRT. Nonhormonal alternatives, such as black cohosh, phytoestrogens (soy preparations or isoflavones), red clover, oil of evening primrose, vitamins (e.g., vitamins E and C), minerals (e.g., selenium), ginseng, liquorice, dong quai, etc. can also be used. There is little scientific evidence regarding the clinical effectiveness of various complementary and alternative therapies to help alleviate menopausal symptoms.

Phytoestrogens (Soy Preparations or Isoflavones)

Phytoestrogens are plant substances that have effects similar to those of estrogens and comprise two important groups, isoflavones and lignans. The major isoflavones are genistein and daidzein. The isoflavone daidzein is metabolized extensively in the human gut into a more estrogenic secondary metabolite equol. The major lignans are enterolactone and enterodiol. Isoflavones are found in food stuffs such as soybeans, chick peas, red clover, and some legumes such as beans and peas. Lignans are found in oil seeds such as flaxseed, cereal bran, whole cereals, vegetables, legumes, and fruits. Phytoestrogens have been shown to cause a reduction in hot flushes, vaginal symptoms, and an improvement in bone mineral density (BMD).

Soy products may serve as a suitable alternative for women with breast cancer or those do not want to take hormone therapy for relief of menopausal symptoms. These products can be considered as SERMs because they may exert estrogen agonist effects on certain tissues and antiestrogenic effects at certain other tissues. Long-term risks and potential adverse effects of phytoestrogens have yet not been fully characterized. For example, some researchers have shown that long-term use of phytoestrogens in postmenopausal women is likely to result in endometrial hyperplasia, which can serve as a precursor for endometrial cancer. Further research is required for fully characterizing the safety and potential adverse effects of phytoestrogens.

Vitamin E

It has been reported that the intake of vitamin E supplements is likely to provide relief from mild hot flushes. Presently, there is lack of well-designed randomized trials proving the clinical effectiveness of vitamin E in relieving hot flushes. Some studies have shown that consumption of vitamin E in the dosage >400 IU may be associated with some adverse effects, typically cardiovascular disease risk.

Oil of Evening Primrose

Evening primrose oil is rich in gamma-linolenic acid. Though oil of evening primrose may not be effective for treating hot flushes, there is some evidence regarding its efficacy for treatment of breast tenderness and/or premenstrual syndrome.

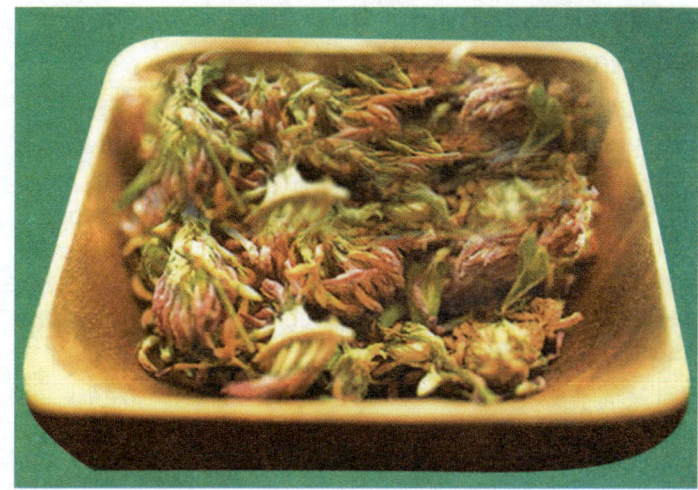

Fig. 25.6: Black cohosh, natural remedy for the treatment of menopause.

Dong Quai

Dong quai is commonly used in traditional Chinese medicine. It has not been found to be superior to placebo for treatment of menopausal symptoms.

Black Cohosh

Black cohosh is a herb (*Actaea racemosa*), member of buttercup family **(Fig. 25.6)**. This is a perennial plant, which is native to North America. It is a commonly prescribed nonhormonal natural preparation for hot flushes and other menopausal symptoms.

Commercial preparations of black cohosh are commonly made from its roots and rhizomes. Presently, there is no definite evidence available in literature regarding its efficacy. As of now, the effect of black cohosh is not thought to be any better than that of placebo. According to the opinion by ACOG (2001), black cohosh must be used for 6 months or less in women with menopausal symptoms. Presently, the North American Menopause Society also recommends the use of black cohosh for treating menopausal symptoms, for a period of up to 6 months, because of its relatively low incidence of side effects when used over the short term. The mode of action of black cohosh is probably related to its estrogenic activity. According to the US Pharmacopoeia, women using black cohosh must discontinue using it and consult their healthcare practitioners in case they experience symptoms of liver dysfunction.

Presently, there is on-going research for evaluating the effectiveness and safety of black cohosh. There is some apprehension regarding the potential estrogenic effect of black cohosh on the breast. Therefore, presently black cohosh is not recommended as a safe therapy for women with breast cancer or who have some risk factors for breast cancer.

OTHER TREATMENT OPTIONS

Selective Estrogen Receptor Modulators

Selective estrogen receptor modulators (e.g., raloxifene) may prevent osteoporosis, but have no beneficial effects on genitourinary or vasomotor symptoms. These agents show high affinity toward estrogen receptors and have estrogen agonist and antagonist properties. These drugs have selective actions on the specific target tissues. New agents are being developed which produce desirable actions without the unwanted side effects.

Raloxifene

This drug does not cause endometrial proliferation, but produces a favorable response in the bones and on lipid profile. While there has been no evidence of reduction in the evidence of wrist or hip fractures, it causes nearly 50% reduction in the incidence of vertebral fractures. The main side effect associated with the use of raloxifene is an increase in the incidence of venous thromboembolism. Raloxifene, therefore, can be considered as a treatment option for prevention of osteoporosis-related spinal fractures. This must be accompanied by periodic evaluation of bone density in the hips. If bone loss occurs, another treatment option can be considered.

Arzoxifene

It is an estrogen agonist-antagonist similar to raloxifene. While it is an estrogen agonist in bone and on lipids, it is an estrogen antagonist in the endometrial and breast tissues.

Ospemifene

Ospemifene is another SERM, which is recently been used for the treatment of vaginal dryness. It is administered in the dosage of 60 mg/day orally for the treatment of vaginal and vulvar atrophy. It is a prescription medication that is similar to estrogen, but is not estrogen. In the vaginal tissue, it acts similarly to estrogen. In the breast tissue, it acts as an estrogen antagonist. The medication may cause hot flushes as a side effect. This medication may be associated with an increased risk for thromboembolism or endometrial cancer. Further research is required for evaluation of the risk of these complications.

Drugs in Development

There are many newly discovered SERMs (droloxifene, lasofoxifene, ormeloxifene, etc.), which are still under research stages. These drugs have the potential for prevention and treatment of osteoporosis.

Selective Tissue Estrogen Activity Regulators

Selective tissue estrogen activity regulators (e.g., tibolone) are effective against all menopausal symptoms and also provide protection against osteoporosis. However, the cardiovascular effects of these agents are still controversial.

Tibolone

 Q. Write a short essay on tibolone.

This drug is being marketed as post-MHT in many countries, including the European continent, but not in the US. It is available under the brand names of Livial, and Liviella (in the dosages of 1.25–2.5 mg) and is used for prevention of osteoporosis. The standard dose of tibolone was 2.5 mg, but now with emerging evidence doses as low as 1.25 mg have also been shown to be effective. Tibolone has been shown to have a beneficial effect on treatment of hot flushes and vaginal dryness. The use of this drug has been found to be associated with an increase in libido and an improvement in sexual response. It also has a protective action on the bones. There is no evidence of an increase in adverse effects such as coronary artery disease, risk of venous thromboembolism or risk of breast cancer. It has also not been found to be associated with endometrial proliferation.

Other Therapeutic Modalities for Control of Vasomotor Symptoms

In women with moderate to severe vasomotor symptoms, other drugs such as clonidine and SSRIs, e.g., fluoxetine, venlafaxine, gabapentin, etc., can also be used.

COMPLICATIONS

OSTEOPOROSIS

Q. Write a long essay discussing prevention and management of postmenopausal osteoporosis.

Q. Write a short essay on bone health in menopausal women.

Q. Discuss in detail the diagnosis, prevention, and complications of osteoporosis in postmenopausal women.

Osteoporosis is defined as a disease characterized by reduced bone mass and microarchitectural deterioration of bone tissue, resulting in enhanced bone fragility and an increased fracture risk. Osteoporotic fractures are a significant cause of mortality and morbidity in the UK. Estrogen appears to control the function of both osteoclasts and osteoblasts in bone, and this influences the rate of absorption and deposition of calcium. Remodeling of bone continues throughout life.

However, following menopause, due to estrogen deprivation, the osteoclastic activity far exceeds the osteoblast's ability to lay down calcium. Low levels of natural estrogen around and after menopause diminish the body's ability to absorb calcium and to metabolize vitamin D. This results in the thinning of trabecular bone and eventually osteoporosis. Various other risk factors for the occurrence of osteoporosis are enumerated in **Box 25.3**.

Low levels of vitamin D are highly prevalent amongst women with osteoporosis. Vitamin D also plays an important role in normalizing Parathyroid hormone (PTH) levels. Deficiency of vitamin D is associated with an increased risk of falls and fractures and can be treated by prescribing 60,000 IU vitamin D sachets or injection vitamin D in the dosage of 6 lac units. Administration of vitamin D is likely to improve calcium absorption, raise bone marrow density, and reduce the risk of falls as well as that of fractures.

The risk of fractures due to osteoporosis depends on the bone mass at the time of menopause and rate of bone loss following menopause. Peak bone density in women normally occurs at about 25 years of age, following which the bone loss starts to occur. After the age of 35 years, men and women normally lose 0.3–0.5% of their bone density per year as a part of normal aging process **(Fig. 25.7)**.

Menopause results in falling estrogen levels, which may result in the development of primary osteoporosis. As the regulatory effect of estrogen on bone resorption is lost, it is accelerated and not adequately balanced by compensatory bone formation.

Osteopenia is a condition characterized by the reduced protein and mineral content of the bone, but is less severe than that in osteoporosis.

The fractures most commonly occurring with osteoporosis include compression fractures in vertebral bones, hip, radius, etc. **(Fig. 25.8)**. These fractures are responsible for considerable pain, decreased quality of life, loss of workdays, and disability. During menopause, there is likely to be deterioration of the bones of vertebral column resulting in a stooped posture or kyphosis. This is also known as "dowager's hump". Due to osteoporotic changes in the vertebral bones, they are likely to become weaker and thinner. The intervertebral disks also lose their fluid content, undergo degeneration, and become compressed. As a result, the spine loses its normal S-shape and becomes kyphotic **(Fig. 25.9)**.

An approach combining the assessment of BMD and estimation of the patient's clinical risk factors for fracture development with use of the fracture risk assessment tool (FRAX) is likely to improve the evaluation of patients with osteoporosis.

Assessment of BMD using DEXA is the gold standard for the diagnosis of osteoporosis. Using a DEXA scan, the patient's bone density is compared to the average bone density in young adults of same sex and race. The score is called the T-score and it expresses the bone density in terms of SDs below the peak young adult bone mass. Osteoporosis can be defined as the bone density score of –2.5 SD or below.

Osteopenia, on the other hand, can be defined as a bone density T-score between –1 SD and –2.5 SD amongst all women who are aged 65 years or older. Severe osteoporosis is used to describe those patients who have a T-score below –2.5 SD and have suffered a fragility fracture. Normal BMD is defined as a T-score between +2.5 SD and –1.0 SD. For every decrease in T-score by a value of one, the risk of fractures is likely to double.

For younger women, interpretation of bone density measurement is done using another score known as the Z-score. This score is calculated by comparing the patient's bone density with the average bone density in adults of same age, sex, and race. Z-score lower than –2 requires diagnostic evaluation for causes other than postmenopausal bone loss.

The FRAX tool developed by the WHO helps in assessing an individual's 10 years risk for developing fractures (spine, forearm, hip, or shoulder). This tool is accessible online. It incorporates 11 risk factors and femoral neck raw BMD in g/cm^2. This helps in calculating the 10 years fracture risk probability. This tool also helps in identifying the patients who may benefit from pharmacotherapy.

> **BOX 25.3:** Risk factors for development of osteoporosis.
> - Female gender
> - *Genetic predisposition:* Family history of osteoporosis
> - Age > 65 years
> - Vertebral compression fractures
> - Fragility fractures after the age of 40 years
> - Caucasian or Asian race
> - Thin or small body frames (low body mass index)
> - Multiparity
> - Excessive alcohol consumption, cigarette smoking
> - Lack of exercise, sedentary lifestyle
> - Diet low in calcium and vitamin D (poor exposure to sunlight)
> - Low estrogen levels, amenorrhea, etc.
> - Drugs [corticosteroids, anticonvulsants (phenytoin), etc.]
> - Other endocrine disorders (Cushing's syndrome, hyperparathyroidism, hyperthyroidism, etc.)
> - Rheumatoid arthritis

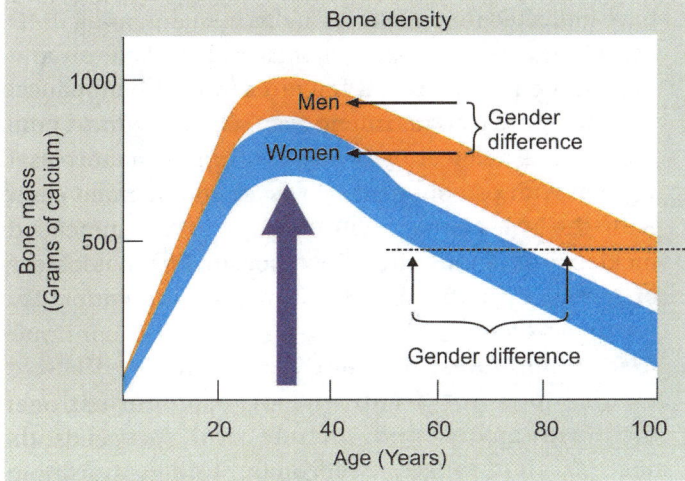

Fig. 25.7: Changes in bone marrow density with age and gender.

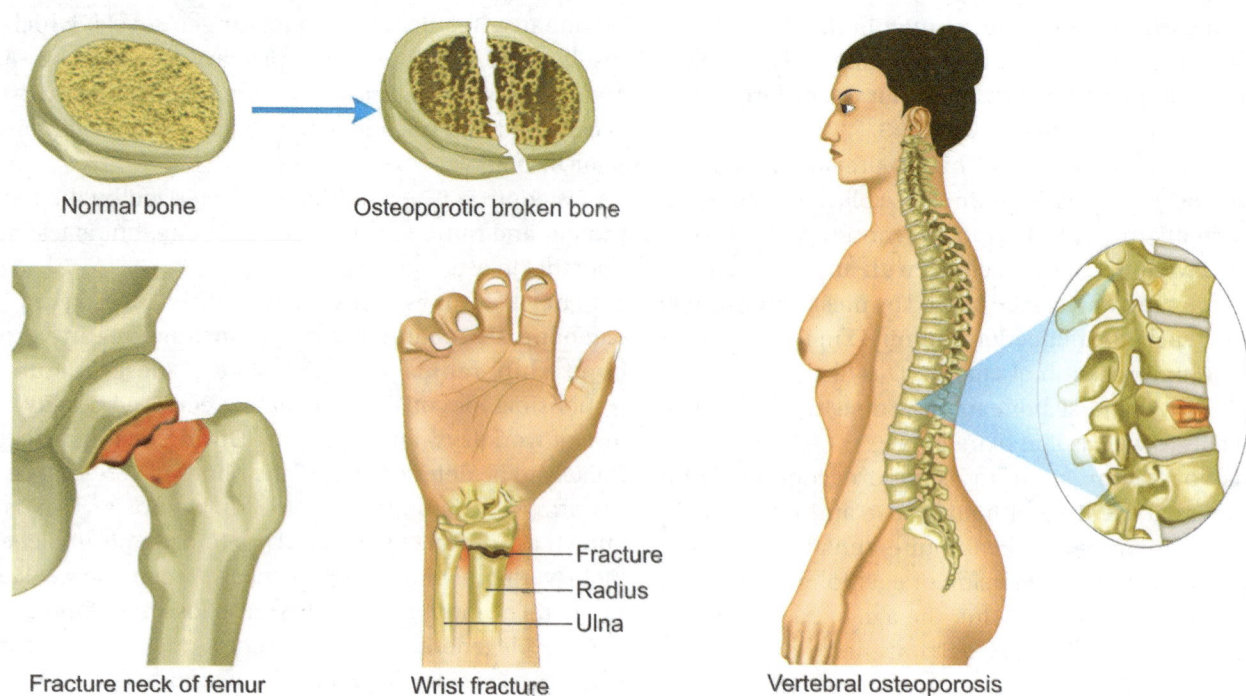

Fig. 25.8: Fractures due to osteoporosis.

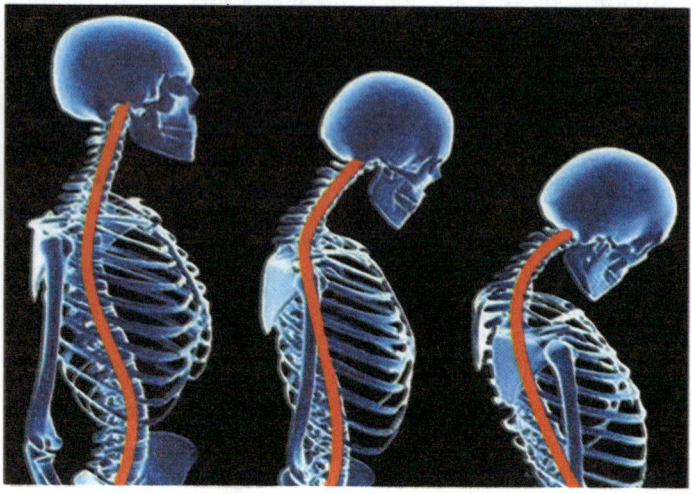

Fig. 25.9: Changes in vertebral column due to osteoporosis.

In order to reduce the risk for development of osteoporosis later in life, lifestyle modifications such as regular weight-bearing exercises, and high intake of vitamin D and calcium must begin during adolescence. For prevention of osteoporosis-related fractures, the following therapeutic options are available:

- *Menopausal hormone therapy:* While MHT helps in preventing the onset of osteoporosis, it has little effect in the treatment of established osteoporosis. MHT provides additional hormones, which help in locking the receptors on cell surface and repairing the balance between the minerals absorbed and minerals retained in the bloodstream **(Fig. 25.10)**. Due to lack of estrogen, minerals such as calcium are not retained inside the bone. As a result, the bone is not able to retain its strength and it wastes away. Various mechanisms which through which estrogen therapy helps prevent the occurrence of osteoporosis are listed in **Box 25.4**. Calcium supplementation is valuable in elderly postmenopausal women. However, it may be less effective in younger, physically active patients. Physical exercise is also likely to be important in prevention of the osteoporotic fractures mainly through improvement of posture, mobility, and muscular functioning.
- *Selective estrogen receptor modulators:* SERMs such as raloxifene (Evista) have been approved by the United States Food and Drug Administration (USFDA) for the prevention and treatment of osteoporosis in postmenopausal women. Results from the MORE (Multiple Outcomes of Raloxifene Evaluation) study have indicated that raloxifene helps in maintaining BMD by acting as an estrogen agonist in the skeleton and preventing new vertebral fractures in postmenopausal women. Moreover, raloxifene also helps in reducing the risk of breast cancer by nearly 65% in postmenopausal women with osteoporosis. However, the main concern with the use of raloxifene therapy is the increased incidence of venous thromboembolism. Previous history of venous thromboembolism is a contraindication for use of raloxifene.
- *Bisphosphonates:* Presently, the most effective medications for treatment of osteoporosis are bisphosphonates and include oral formulations such as alendronate, risedronate, and ibandronate and intravenous formulations such as pamidronate

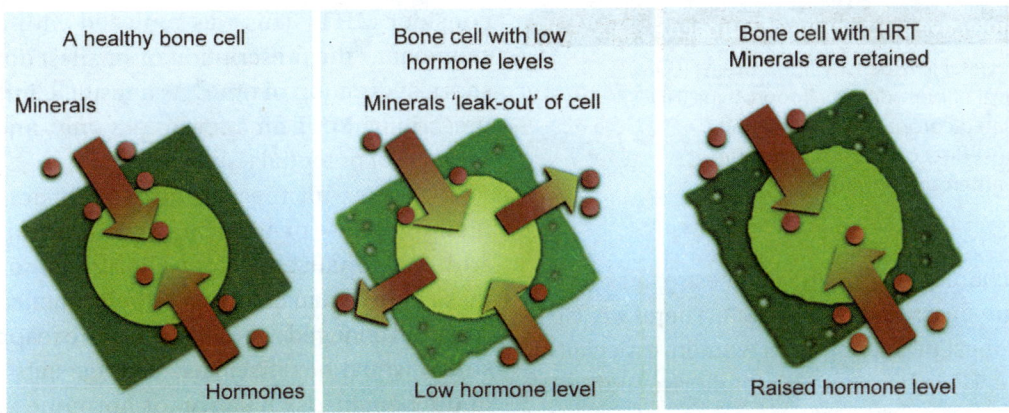

Fig. 25.10: Effect of hormone replacement therapy on osteoporosis.

> **BOX 25.4:** Mechanisms for prevention of osteoporosis.
> - Inhibition of osteoclastic resorption
> - Increase in intestinal calcium absorption
> - Increase in 1,25-dihydroxyvitamin D_3 which increases calcium absorption
> - Increased renal conversion of calcium
> - Increased survival and support of osteoblasts

TABLE 25.3: Dosage of some commonly used bisphosphonates.

	For prevention	For treatment
Alendronate	5 mg daily 35 mg daily	10 mg daily 70 mg weekly
Risedronate	5 mg daily 35 mg weekly 150 mg monthly	5 mg daily 35 mg weekly 150 mg monthly
Ibandronate	2.5 mg daily	2.5 mg daily 150 mg monthly
Zoledronic acid	5 mg IV every 2 years	5 mg IV every year

and zoledronic acid. These drugs reduce the risk of fracture development by suppressing bone resorption by osteoclasts. They, however, do not reduce osteoblast formation. Bisphosphonates can be used both for prevention and treatment of osteoporosis. It can be considered as the drugs of choice for treatment of established osteoporosis. This can be in the form of weekly alendronate, monthly ibandronate, or yearly IV zoledronic acid. Dosages of some commonly used bisphosphonates are enlisted in **Table 25.3**.

This medication must be taken empty stomach and calcium must be consumed after 4 hours of taking bisphosphonates. Longest duration for which therapy with bisphosphonates can be tried is 5 years.

- *Tibolone:* This drug has been described in detail previously in the text.
- *Novel therapies:* New therapeutic agents such as calcitonin nasal spray (useful for treatment of painful vertebral crush fractures), injectable recombinant PTH, and a monoclonal antibody (denosumab) have also been approved for the treatment of osteoporosis.
- *Denosumab:* This is human monoclonal antibody to receptor activator of nuclear factor kappa-B ligand (RANKL). RANKL is secreted by osteoblasts and binds to its receptor RANK on the surface of osteoclasts, thereby stimulating its activity. Denosumab binds with great affinity to RANKL, thereby preventing the activation of RANK. Thus, it prevents both the maturation and survival of osteoclasts as well as active bone resorption by osteoclasts. Denosumab administered in the dosage of 60 mg S/C injection in upper arm, upper thighs, or abdomen, every 6-monthly for 36 months, is likely to be associated with reduced risk of vertebral, nonvertebral, and hip fractures in postmenopausal women with osteoporosis. All patients should simultaneously also receive 1,000 mg of calcium and 400 IU of vitamin D daily. Discontinuation of denosumab therapy should be followed by the administration of antiresorptive therapy such as bisphosphonates, HRT, and SERMS to prevent rebound bone loss.
- *Teriperatide:* Teriperatide is a portion of natural human parathormone, comprising of amino acid sequence 1 through 34 of the complete PTH molecule. First 34 amino acids in teriperatide is the bioactive portion of the hormone. Once daily injection of this drug is likely to have a net effect of stimulating new bone formation resulting in an increased bone density. This therapy is approved for use in US and Europe. It is administered in the dosage of 20 µg daily via subcutaneous route. Therapy is usually administered over a period of 24 months.

CARDIOVASCULAR DISEASE

Premenopausal women are likely to be protected against cardiovascular heart diseases in comparison to the men belonging to the same age groups. This could be partly related to high HDL and low LDL levels in premenopausal women.

> **BOX 25.5:** Cardioprotective mechanisms of estrogen.
> - Decrease in the level of low-density lipoproteins (LDLs)
> - Increase in the level of high-density lipoproteins (HDLs)
> - Nitric oxide mediated coronary vasodilatation
> - Direct vasodilatory effect on the endometrium
> - Reduction in the atheroma volume

Various other mechanisms through which estrogen exerts a protective effect are described in **Box 25.5**. Therefore, CHD is uncommon amongst premenopausal women, especially if they do not smoke. However, there is a rapid rise in the risk of CHD following menopause and presently cardiovascular disease has become a leading cause of death amongst postmenopausal women in the UK.

Initially, it was believed that prescription of MHT is likely to result in protection against the development of cardiovascular heart diseases. There had been lack of clear guidelines regarding the use of post-MHT since the past decade. However, now estrogen replacement therapy is no longer indicated for the prevention of cardiovascular heart diseases in postmenopausal women.

This recommendation initially made by the AHA in 2001 had been further strengthened by the results of the WHI and HERS (HERS and HERSII) trials. WHI was initiated in 1991 by the US National Institute of Health and comprised of three clinical trials and an observation study, which were directed to address the major health-related problems causing mortality and morbidity amongst postmenopausal women. This was one of the largest trials comprising of more than 16,000 women, who were randomized to receive either continuous combined MHT or placebo. The WHI (estrogen plus progestin trial) was stopped in July 2002, after investigators found that the combination hormone therapy resulted in health risks, which outweighed the benefits. Participants were followed for an average of 5.6 years. The results of WHI study (2002) showed that the use of MHT did not cause any cardiovascular benefits. Moreover, the results of this study also showed that the use of MHT might also be associated with an increased risk of stroke, venous thromboembolism, and breast cancer. These conflicting findings have raised speculation regarding the effect of MHT on the woman's cardiovascular risk.

Before 2002, prior to the publication of results of this study, use of MHT was characterized as providing significant cardiovascular and skeletal benefits, with minimal or no adverse effects. The results of WHI study were interpreted in various ways; many societies and health organizations now started claiming that MHT was dangerous. Some health authorities started recommending that MHT must be prescribed only in cases where the vasomotor symptoms were severe and could not be managed with alternative therapies. This led to holdup of the previous consensus, which stated, "all menopausal women should consider MHT". This was replaced with a new consensus statement, "the prescription of smallest dose of MHT for the shortest duration of time". As a result, clinicians now started prescribing MHT for a few weeks only, and then stopping it because of potential risks.

However, all the authorities did not accept the conflicting results of WHI study. The European Menopause and Andropause Society (EMAS) stood firmly against these conceptual changes in their practical guidelines. The situation changed again following the reappraisal of the WHI study, which has disclosed that age acts as a major factor in the benefit-risk balance for hormone users. Subsequent analysis of the WHI study published in 2007 identified that the timing of administration of MHT is likely to be significant. Little cardiovascular harm is observed when MHT is commenced in the immediate postmenopausal period in comparison to the administration of MHT many years after menopause.

In contrast to the results of the WHI study (2002), outcomes of the RCT (published in the BMJ, 2012), which took its data from the Danish Osteoporosis Prevention Study (DOPS), have shown that continued use of MHT amongst the menopausal women for a period of 10 years has been found to be associated with a significant reduction in the risk of MI, heart failure, or death with no increased risk of venous thromboembolism or stroke. According to the authors of this study, long-term use of MHT, when started soon after menopause for a prolonged duration of time, does not increase the risk of adverse cardiovascular events.

Moreover, in this study, synthetic 17-β-estradiol was used, while in the WHI study, conjugated equine estrogens were used. This difference in medication, along with variations in patient characteristics, probably was the cause of disparity in the results between this study and the WHI study.

Present evidence indicates that the benefits outweigh the risks of the MHT treatment started for most women near the menopause. For such women, MHT not just provides relief from hot flushes, night sweats, and vaginal dryness, but also helps in reducing the risks for heart disease and fracture. The results of WHI study are now interpreted as high risk of cardiovascular disease due to MHT in older women who are on an average 10–12 years past menopause. The emerging evidence suggests that the risk of cardiovascular heart diseases events with MHT is majorly limited to older postmenopausal women, with younger postmenopausal women at very low risk for cardiovascular heart diseases-related events. This increase is more in women having pre-existing risk factors for cardiovascular disease.

COMPLICATIONS DUE TO MENOPAUSAL HORMONE THERAPY

Complications related to the use of MHT in menopausal women are listed in **Box 25.6** and described in detail next.

BOX 25.6: Complications due to menopausal hormone therapy.
- Endometrial cancer
- Breast cancer
- Venous thromboembolism
- Coronary heart disease
- Gallstones
- Dementia
- Alzheimer's disease

Breast Cancer

Women's Health Initiative trial and the Million Women study have shown that there is a small increased risk of breast cancer in women who take combined estrogen–progestin therapy in comparison to those taking estrogen-only preparations or tibolone. A critique of the Million Woman study has shown that this study could have suffered from detection bias because the women participating in this study were recruited from the National Breast Screening Programme.

Early menopause often occurs in women undergoing treatment for breast cancer. In these women, hormone therapy (estrogen only or combined estrogen and progestogens) by any route is not recommended. The hormones could increase the chance of the cancer recurrence. These recommendations are based on the results from the WHI and the HABITS trial. The HABITS trial had to be terminated midway in the year 2003 due to an unacceptable risk of breast cancer or the women (having a previous history of breast cancer) exposed to MHT.

Even if MHT is prescribed for short term, mammograms and breast examinations must be routinely performed. According to the recommendations by the USFDA, labels describing the warnings related to the possible risk of heart disease, stroke, and cancer must be added to all estrogen and estrogen–progestin-containing MHT preparations.

Dementia

Based on the results of WHI study, post-MHT should also not be prescribed after the age of 65 years for prevention of dementia. However, some clinicians feel that estrogen treatment might be helpful in preventing dementia, if prescribed in the early years after menopause.

Stroke

Women's Health Initiative trial has shown that the combination of estrogen with progestins increases the risk of ischemic stroke in generally healthy postmenopausal women. This increased risk does not appear to be related to the timing of the initiation of MHT. On the other hand, HERS, the first large RCT examining the effect of hormone therapy on risk of strokes, has not indicated any significant association between post-MHT and risk of stroke among postmenopausal women followed up for a mean of 4.1 years.

Endometrial Hyperplasia and Endometrial Cancer

Unopposed estrogen therapy at any dose and duration between 1 and 3 years is likely to increase the risk for endometrial hyperplasia and endometrial cancer. WHI trial has shown that hormone therapy with estrogens alone is likely to result in an increased risk of endometrial cancer. Cancer can occur even after 6 months of unopposed estrogen therapy in women having an intact uterus. In such women, progestin preparations, either sequentially or in a low-dose regimen, should be added along with estrogens. Women who have undergone hysterectomy do not require progestins. In women who have undergone subtotal hysterectomy, it is important to establish that there is no residual endometrium before prescribing estrogen only MHT.

EVIDENCE-BASED CLINICAL TRIALS

List of references can be scanned through QR code to enable the readers gain deeper insight of the subject by referring to the entire article or its abstract.

SECTION 5

Abnormalities of the Vagina and Cervix

26. Vaginal Discharge
27. Cervical Intraepithelial Neoplasia (Abnormal Pap Smear)
28. Cancer Cervix (Postcoital Bleeding)

CHAPTER 26

Vaginal Discharge

CASE STUDY

A 23-year-old unmarried lady presented to the gynecological OPD with the complaints of vaginal discharge since last 4–5 days. She described the discharge as being white in color and curd-like in consistency. It was associated with significant itching and discomfort, which greatly interfered with her normal routine and disturbed her sleep. The patient does not give history of ever having any sexual partner or indulging in any kind of sexual activity. There is no past medical history of diabetes or any other medical disorder in the past. The patient does give history of taking a 7-day course of the antibiotic erythromycin, which was prescribed to her by a general practitioner for throat infection, a few days back.

INTRODUCTION

PATHOLOGICAL VAGINAL DISCHARGE

Vaginal discharge is one of the most common presenting complaints faced by the gynecologists in clinical practice. The most important challenge for the gynecologist is to differentiate between the pathological and physiological causes of discharge (**Table 26.1**). A normal vaginal discharge consists of 1–4 mL of fluid that is white or transparent and odorless. This physiologic discharge is formed by sloughing epithelial cells, normal bacteria, and vaginal transudate. If a pathological cause of discharge is suspected, the gynecologist needs to diagnose the exact cause for vaginal discharge. Some common causes of pathological vaginal discharge are described in **Table 26.2**. In most cases, women develop a sense of their own vaginal discharge and learn to identify what is acceptable or excessive for them. The amount of physiological vaginal discharge can vary in the same woman. Some of the factors, which can influence the amount of physiological discharge, include the following: woman's age, pregnancy, use of hormonal preparations (oral contraceptive pills, etc.), and the woman's personal habits and level of hygiene.

TABLE 26.1: Differentiating between physiological and pathological causes of vaginal discharge.

Characteristic	Physiological vaginal discharge	Pathological vaginal discharge
Discomfort to the patient	Does not usually cause any discomfort to the patient (except for hygiene problems)	Usually causes significant distress and irritation to the patient
Color of the discharge	Translucent to whitish in color	May vary in color from dirty white to yellowish-green
Association of itching	Is not associated with itching	May be associated with itching
Variations in the amount of discharge during the different phases of menstrual cycle	Amount of discharge may vary in different phases of menstrual cycle	Amount of discharge does not vary in different phases of menstrual cycle
Smell of the discharge	Not foul smelling	May be foul smelling

TABLE 26.2: Causes of pathological vaginal discharge.

Infective discharge	Other causes for discharge
• Vulvovaginal candidiasis • Vaginitis caused by *Trichomonas vaginalis, Chlamydia trachomatis* • Sexually transmitted disease (*Neisseria gonorrhoeae*) • Bacterial vaginosis • Acute pelvic inflammatory disease • Postoperative pelvic infection • Postabortal/postpartum sepsis *Less common causes* • Human papillomavirus • Primary syphilis • *Mycoplasma genitalium* • *Ureaplasma urealyticum* • *Escherichia coli*	• Retained tampon or condom • Chemical irritation • Allergic responses • Ectropion • Endocervical polyp • Intrauterine device *Less common causes* • Atrophic changes • Physical trauma • Vault granulation tissue • Vesicovaginal fistula • Rectovaginal fistula • Neoplasia (cervical, vulvar, vaginal, or endometrial)

Physiological vaginal discharge is commonly encountered among women belonging to the reproductive age group and varies in amount and consistency during the various phases of the menstrual cycle. For example, the cervical discharge becomes profuse just prior to ovulation. During this phase, the discharge is watery, transparent and can be stretched for nearly 7–8 cm between the two fingers of examining hand. Following ovulation, the amount of cervical discharge greatly diminishes in quantity, becomes thicker in consistency, yellowish-whitish in color, and loses its capacity of stretching.

VULVOVAGINITIS

Vulvovaginitis can be considered as one of the most common causes for pathological vaginal discharge, irritation, and itching in women. Vulvovaginitis commonly results due to inflammation of the vagina and vulva or changes in the normal vaginal flora and is most often caused by bacterial, fungal, or parasitic infection. Nearly 90% of cases of vaginitis are secondary to bacterial vaginosis, vulvovaginal candidiasis (VVC), and trichomoniasis. Of these different types of vaginitis, VVC is one of the most common infective causes of vaginal discharge that affects nearly 75% of women at some time during their reproductive lives. On the other hand, bacterial vaginosis, despite of being asymptomatic in most of the cases is one of the most common diagnoses in women attending genitourinary medicine clinics. The characteristic features of different types of vaginitis are summarized in **Table 26.3** and would be described in details later in the chapter. Different types of vaginal discharge are shown in **Figure 26.1**. Other important causes for vulvovaginal discharge include atrophic/contact vaginitis and sexually transmitted diseases (STDs), which have also been described later in the chapter.

Vulvovaginal itching generally is not a normal finding in healthy women; if this symptom is present, especially in presence of vaginal discharge, vulvovaginitis (especially candidal) must be specifically ruled out. In absence of vaginal discharge, other dermatologic conditions (e.g., lichen sclerosis and rarely, vulvar cancer) should also be considered.

TABLE 26.3: Features of the most common causes of vaginitis.

Basis of diagnosis	Bacterial vaginosis	Vulvovaginal candidiasis	Trichomoniasis
Signs and symptoms	• Thin, grayish to off-white colored discharge; unpleasant "fishy" odor, with odor especially increasing after sexual intercourse • The discharge is usually homogeneous and adheres to vaginal walls	Thick, white (curd like) discharge with no odor	Copious, malodorous, yellow-green (or discolored) discharge, pruritus and vaginal irritation, dysuria, no symptoms in 20–50% of affected women
Physical examination	Normal appearance of vaginal tissues; grayish-white colored discharge may be adherent to the vaginal walls	• Vulvar and vaginal erythema, edema and fissures **(Fig. 26.2)** • Thick, white discharge that adheres to vaginal walls	• Vulvar and vaginal edema and erythema, "strawberry" cervix in up to 25% of affected women **(Fig. 26.3)** • Frothy, purulent discharge
Vaginal pH (normal ≤ 4.5)	Elevated (>4.5)	Normal	Elevated (>4.5)
Microscopic examination of wet-mount and potassium hydroxide (KOH) preparations of vaginal discharge	"Clue cells" (vaginal epithelial cells coated with coccobacilli)—few lactobacilli, occasional motile, curved rods, belonging to *Mobiluncus* species	Pseudohyphae, mycelial tangles or budding yeast cells	• Motile trichomonads • Many polymorphonuclear cells
"Whiff" test (Normal = no odor)	Positive	Negative	Can be positive
Additional tests	Amsel's criteria **(Box 26.1)** is positive in nearly 90% of affected women with bacterial vaginosis	KOH microscopy, Gram stain, culture	• *Deoxyribonucleic acid (DNA) probe tests:* Sensitivity of 90% and specificity of 99.8% • *Culture:* Sensitivity of 98% and specificity of 100%

Sources: Carr PL, Felsenstein D, Friedman RH. Evaluation and management of vaginitis. J Gen Intern Med. 1998;13:335-46.doi: 10.1046/j.1525-1497.1998.00101.x.
Sobel JD. Vaginitis. N Engl J Med. 1997;337:1896-903. doi: 10.1056/NEJM199712253372607.

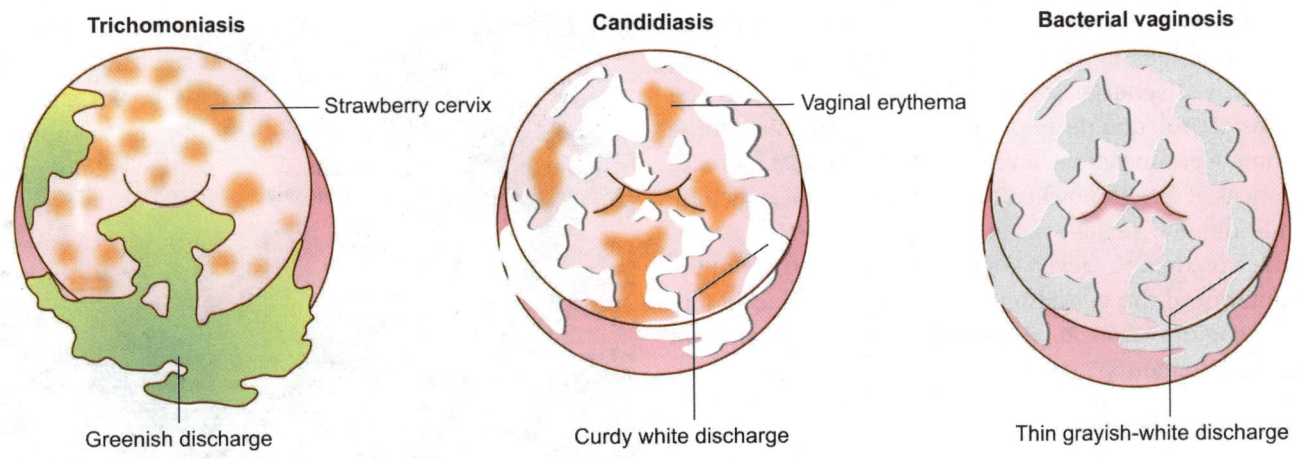

Fig. 26.1: Different types of vaginal discharge.

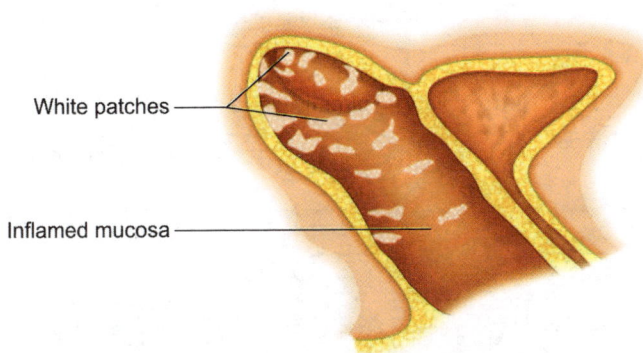

Fig. 26.2: Appearance of vulva and vagina in cases of vulvovaginal candidiasis.

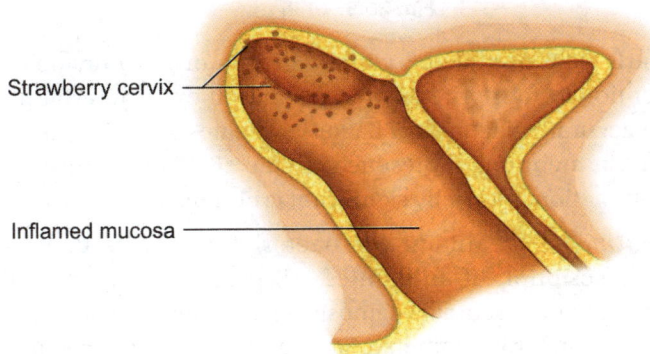

Fig. 26.3: Appearance of vulva and vagina in trichomoniasis.

BOX 26.1: Amsel's diagnostic criteria for bacterial vaginosis.
- Thin, homogeneous discharge
- Positive "Whiff test"
- Presence of "clue cells" on microscopic examination
- Vaginal pH > 4.5

Pathophysiology

The normal vaginal epithelium undergoes cornification under the influence of estrogen. This thickening of the vaginal epithelium helps in protecting women against infection. Normal vaginal epithelium is inhabited by the bacteria, *Lactobacillus acidophilus,* which produces hydrogen peroxide. This is not only toxic to the pathogens present in the vagina; it also helps in maintaining the healthy vaginal pH between 3.8 and 4.2. Vaginitis occurs either due to alteration of vaginal flora by the introduction of pathogens or due to the changes in the vaginal environment that allow pathogens to proliferate. Vaginal pH may increase with age, phase of menstrual cycle, sexual activity, hormone therapy, contraception choice, pregnancy, presence of necrotic tissue or foreign bodies, and use of hygienic products or antibiotics. This change in vaginal pH may encourage the growth of pathogenic microorganisms. Changes in the vaginal environment, such as an increase in glycogen production in pregnancy or altered estrogen and progesterone levels from the use of oral contraceptives, may also encourage the growth and development of *Candida albicans.*

Bacterial Vaginosis

Q. Write a long essay on bacterial vaginosis.

Bacterial vaginosis is one of the most important causes of vulvovaginitis. Initially, this was termed as bacterial vaginitis. However, later it was discovered that the condition was primarily caused due to the alteration of normal vaginal flora, rather than due to any specific infection. Due to the absence of inflammation, the term "vaginosis" rather than "vaginitis" is now being preferred. The normal vaginal epithelium contains numerous bacteria called *L. acidophilus*. These bacteria release hydrogen peroxide, which is toxic to other aerobic and anaerobic bacteria. Bacterial vaginosis typically is associated with a reduction in the number of the normal hydrogen peroxide-producing *Lactobacilli* in the vagina.

The resultant change in pH allows proliferation of organisms that are normally suppressed such as *Haemophilus vaginalis, Gardnerella mobiluncus, Mycoplasma hominis, Gardnerella vaginalis,* and *Peptostreptococcus* species. These organisms may produce metabolic byproducts, such as amines, that further increase the vaginal pH and cause exfoliation of vaginal epithelial cells. These amines are also responsible for the characteristic malodorous discharge in bacterial vaginosis. Bacterial vaginosis is not dangerous, but it can cause disturbing symptoms. Certain factors have been identified that increase the chances of developing bacterial vaginosis. These include multiple or new sexual partners, vaginal douching, and cigarette smoking. However, the role of sexual activity in the development of the condition is not fully understood and bacterial vaginosis can still develop in women who have not had sexual intercourse.

Clinical Presentation

Approximately 50–75% of women with bacterial vaginosis are asymptomatic. Symptomatic women with bacterial vaginosis have a broad spectrum of clinical presentations:
- The classic presentation is a vaginal discharge with its characteristic odor and a clinical examination that is otherwise normal.
- There is presence of white milky, nonviscous discharge which is adherent to the vaginal wall. pH of the discharge is >4.5.
- A fishy odor is produced when the discharge is mixed with 10% potassium hydroxide (KOH) solution due to production of amino metabolites from various organisms (amine or Whiff test).
- There is no or minimal vaginal irritation.
- *Presence of clue cells:* The epithelial cells acquire a fuzzy border due to adherence of bacteria.

Bacterial vaginosis is mainly diagnosed using Amsel's criteria, with three of the four findings required to establish its diagnosis (**Box 26.1**).

Diagnosis

Microscopic examination: Gram's staining of the vaginal discharge can be considered as the gold standard for diagnosis of bacterial vaginosis. The presence of clue cells (**Fig. 26.4**) can be considered as the single most reliable predictor of bacterial vaginosis. Clue cells are believed to be the most reliable diagnostic sign of bacterial vaginosis. Clue cells are vaginal epithelial cells, which are studded with bacteria on their surface. This results in the obscuration of their borders. In addition to clue cells, women with bacterial vaginosis have fewer of the normal vaginal bacteria, called lactobacilli. A vaginal pH > 4.5 is also suggestive of bacterial vaginosis.

Whiff Test (**Fig. 26.5**): This test is diagnostic of bacterial vaginosis and is performed using KOH solution. The test is said to be positive if there is production of a typical fishy odor when KOH comes in contact with discharge of a woman with bacterial vaginosis.

Amsel's Criteria: Amsel's criteria (**Box 26.1**) help in establishing the diagnosis of bacterial vaginosis in

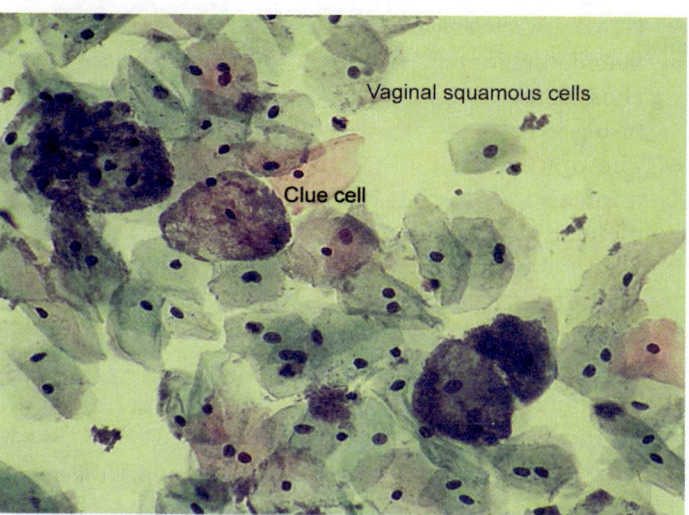

Fig. 26.4: Clue cells.

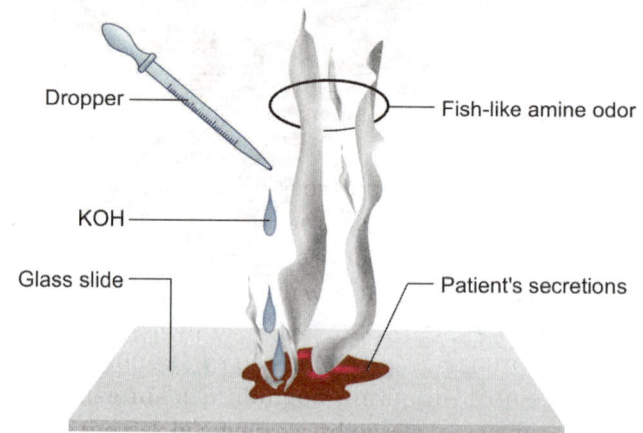

Fig. 26.5: Whiff test.

nearly 90% of affected women. Three of the previously-mentioned four criteria must be met in order to establish the accurate diagnosis of bacterial vaginosis. Of the various criteria mentioned, presence of clue cells on microscopic examination is a highly significant criterion.

Treatment: Treatment for bacterial vaginosis consists of prescription of antibiotics. All pregnant women with symptomatic bacterial vaginosis must undergo treatment to obtain relief from bothersome symptoms. While previously, some clinicians avoided the use of metronidazole in the first trimester because of its potential to cross the placenta, the CDC no longer discourages the use of metronidazole in the first trimester. Moreover, routine screening and treatment of all pregnant women with asymptomatic bacterial infection to prevent preterm birth and its consequences are not presently recommended by the ACOG, United States Preventive Services Task Force (USPSTF), and CDC.

A few of the routinely used antibiotics include the following:
- *Metronidazole:* The WHO has recommended metronidazole as the first-line therapy for the treatment of bacterial vaginosis. A 7-day course of metronidazole (500 mg BD) is effective in nearly 85% cases. Vaginal therapy with

0.75% metronidazole gel (5 g once daily for 5 days) has been found to be as effective as oral metronidazole. The choice of whether to use oral or vaginal therapy should be based upon patient preference.

- The oral metronidazole can cause some minor, but unpleasant side effects, such as anorexia, nausea, metallic taste, abdominal cramps, headache, glossitis, dryness of mouth, dizziness, rashes, and transient neutropenia. Despite of these side effects, it is believed to be the most effective treatment. Tinidazole is an antibiotic that appears to have fewer side effects than metronidazole and is also effective in treating bacterial vaginosis. Ornidazole, 500 mg vaginal tablet daily for 7 days is another effective option. Use of vaginal tablets helps in avoiding first past metabolism. Treatment of male sexual partners of affected women is not required.
- *Lincosamides:* Vaginal clindamycin cream, 2% (cleocin), or oral clindamycin, 300 mg twice daily for 7 days is also effective.
- *Ampicillin:* Ampicillin 500 mg TDS or cephalosporins 500 mg BID for 7 days is also effective.
- *Tetracyclines:* Tetracycline 500 mg four times a day or doxycycline 100 mg twice daily for 7 days is effective.

Vulvovaginal Candidiasis

> Q. Write a short note on monilial infection.
> Q. Write a short note on recurrent vulvovaginitis.

General Features

Monilial vgainitis is also termed as vaginal candidiasis. Candidal organisms are part of the normal vaginal flora. However, overgrowth of the organism can cause penetration of superficial epithelial cells, resulting in vulvovaginitis. VVC is the second most common cause of vaginitis in the United States and the most common cause of vulvovaginitis in Europe. In most of the cases (80–92%), infecting agent is the yeast *C. albicans* **(Fig. 26.6)**. Recently, due to the increasing use of over-the-counter antifungal medications, the frequency of nonalbicans species, e.g. *C. glabrata, C. tropicalis,* etc., in causation of candidal vaginitis has greatly increased. All *Candida* species produce similar vulvovaginal symptoms, although the severity of symptoms is milder with nonalbicans species such as *C. glabrata* and *C. parapsilosis*.

Clinical Features

In VVC, the discharge is usually white and thick, with no odor and a normal pH. Pruritus vulva is a cardinal feature. Women with VVC frequently complain of pruritus, vaginal irritation, dysuria, vulvar and vaginal erythema and occasionally, vulvar burning, soreness, and scaling and fissures of vulvar tissue. There may be accompanying dysuria and/or dyspareunia. Symptoms may often worsen during the week prior to menses.

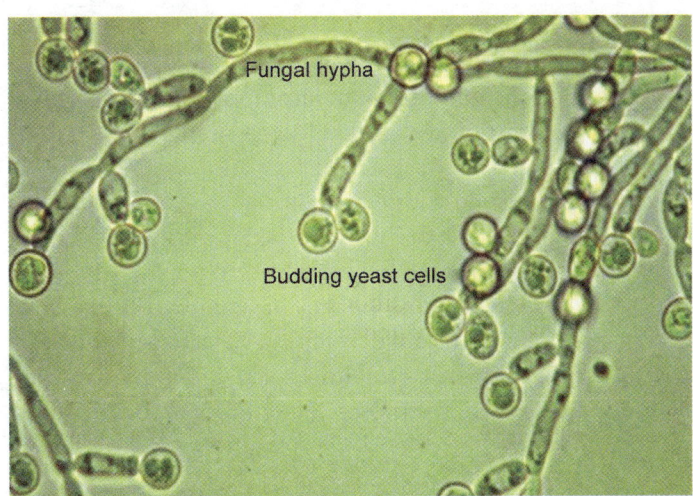

Fig. 26.6: Wet mount preparation of *Candida albicans*.

BOX 26.2: Criteria of complicated *Candida* infection.

- Severe signs/symptoms of vulvovaginitis
- Identification of *Candida* species other than *C. albicans*, particularly *C. glabrata*
- Pregnancy, poorly controlled diabetes, immunosuppression, and debilitation
- History of recurrent (≥4/year) culture-verified vulvovaginal candidiasis

Recurrent episodes of vulvovaginal candidal infection can commonly occur. Recurrent VVC can be defined as four or more episodes of symptomatic infection within 1 year. Vaginal cultures should always be obtained to confirm the diagnosis and identify less common *Candida* species, if present. Complications of VVC are rare. However, episodes of complicated *Candida* infection have been sometimes reported. Characteristics of complicated infections include one or more of the criteria mentioned in **Box 26.2**. Chorioamnionitis in pregnancy and vulvar vestibulitis syndrome has also been reported.

Candidal organisms are not transmitted sexually, and episodes of VVC do not appear to be related to the number of sexual partners. Treating the male partner is unnecessary unless he is uncircumcised or has inflammation of the glans of the penis. Recurrent VVC is defined as four or more episodes in a 1-year period. It is not clear whether recurrences are secondary to predisposing and/or precipitating factors, sexual transmission, intestinal reservoir, or vaginal persistence.

Risk Factors

Severe factors are thought to be associated with an increased risk for uncomplicated VVC. Some such factors, which are associated with an increased risk of this infection, include the following:

- Women using oral contraceptive pills or an IUCD for contraception

- Diabetes mellitus
- Antibiotic use
- Immunodeficiency or use of immunosuppressive agents
- Use of tightfitting synthetic undergarments
- Pregnancy
- Previous episode of VVC

This infection is more likely to occur during pregnancy probably because high levels of estrogen or glycogen in the vaginal secretions during pregnancy are likely to increase a woman's risk of developing VVC. Use of adequate pharmacotherapy and avoidance of risk factors can help in the resolution of symptoms related to VVC over a short period of time.

Diagnosis

Microscopic examination: Microscopic examinations of wet-mount and KOH preparations are positive in 50–70% of patients with candidal infections. In patients whose symptoms are strongly suggestive of candidal vaginitis, but the microscopic examination is negative, Gram staining or culture using Nickerson's medium or Sabouraud's dextrose agar may prove to be helpful. In candidal infections, KOH preparation may reveal budding filaments, mycelia, or pseudohyphae. A fungal culture may be used if the diagnosis is uncertain. Microscopy for candidal disease has an estimated sensitivity of 65%.

Vaginal pH: The vaginal pH in women with *Candida* infection is typically normal (4–4.5). This helps to distinguish candidial infection from trichomoniasis or bacterial vaginosis.

Treatment

Antifungals: Imidazoles and triazoles are presently the most extensively used antifungal drugs for treatment of VVC. Imidazole antifungal agents, which can be used in form of creams and pessaries for treatment of VVC, include butoconazole, clotrimazole, and miconazole. Some of these agents are freely available over the counter. Triazole agents include systemically acting agents such as fluconazole. A single dose of triazole antifungals (e.g., 150 mg of fluconazole) has also been shown to be effective in most cases.

Alternatively, topical azole antifungal agents can be applied daily for 7–14 days. Oral fluconazole in the dosage of 150 mg every 72 hours for three doses serves as an effective therapy for severe or complicated vulvovaginitis. This should be then followed by weekly doses for a few weeks. The underlying predisposing factors must be corrected to provide long-term relief. In cases of recurrent VVC, initial therapy should be with 150 mg of oral fluconazole every 72 hours for three doses, followed by maintenance dosage of fluconazole 150 mg once every week for 6 months. If oral fluconazole does not appear as a feasible option, a topical azole or an alternative oral azole (e.g., itraconazole) followed by maintenance therapy with topical antifungal agents must be instituted for 6 months.

Most clinicians prefer not to use fluconazole during pregnancy due to an increased risk of major congenital malformations. Administration of oral azoles during the first trimester is not recommended due to the risk of development of various birth defects such as abnormalities of cranium, face, bones, and heart after first trimester exposure to high-dose therapy (400–800 mg/day). Most clinicians, however, prefer to use topical formulations of imidazole (clotrimazole and miconazole) and triazole antifungals during pregnancy **(Table 26.4)**. Systemic absorption of these topical medications is minimal, posing little risk of transfer to the unborn baby. Topical nystatin is another safe alternative to azole antifungals that can be used during the first trimester of pregnancy. Since nystatin has negligible systemic absorption, there are unlikely to be any major malformations associated with the use of this drug. The recommended dose of nystatin during pregnancy is 100,000 units intravaginally once daily for 2 weeks. For symptomatic relief of redness or itching, short-term use of a low-potency topical corticosteroid is also considered as a safe option during pregnancy.

TABLE 26.4: Topical antifungal therapy for *Candida* vulvovaginitis.

Antifungal drugs	Intravaginal cream preparation
Butoconazole	2% cream: Application of 5 g/day intravaginally for 3 days
Clotrimazole	1% cream: Application of 5 g/day intravaginally for 7–14 days
Miconazole	2% cream: Application of 5 g/day intravaginally for 7 days
Tioconazole	5% ointment: Application of 5 g intravaginally in a single application
Terconazole	0.4% cream: Application of 5 g/day intravaginally for 7 days 0.8% cream: Application of 5 g/day intravaginally for 3 days
Antifungal drugs	**Intravaginal suppository**
Clotrimazole	• 100 mg vaginal tablet, one tablet per day intravaginally for 7 days • 500 mg vaginal tablet, one tablet administered intravaginally in a single dose application • Clotrimazole 100 mg vaginal tablet, two tablets per day intravaginally for 3 days
Miconazole	200 mg vaginal suppository per day for 3 days or 100 mg vaginal suppository per day for 7 days
Nystatin	1,00,000 unit vaginal tablet (Mycostatin), one tablet per day intravaginally for 14 days
Terconazole	80 mg vaginal suppository, one suppository per day for 3 days

Corticosteroids: Topical corticosteroids are commonly prescribed to alleviate symptoms such as itchiness and redness, which may commonly occur in cases of VVC.

Treatment of sexual partners: Although sexual transmission of *Candida* species can occur, the present available evidence does not support treatment of sexual partners in cases of VVC. However, in woman with recurrent vulvovaginitis, this issue presently remains controversial.

Breastfeeding women: The American Academy of Pediatrics (AAP) considers the use of fluconazole to be safe in breastfeeding infants. Also, nystatin can be used in nursing mothers because it does not enter the breast milk.

Complicated VVC: It includes recurrent or severe disease, or when there is presence of adverse factors in the host (e.g., immunocompromised host). This also includes persistent infection with species other than *Candida albicans* (e.g., *C. glabrata*, *C. tropicalis*, etc.) due to the increasing use of over-the-counter antifungal medications. By the time complicated VVC is diagnosed, the patient has already received conventional therapy with azoles and nystatin.

Culture and sensitivity is usually advised in order to isolate the involved organism. However, in case of emergency situation, if infection with *C. glabrata* is suspected, while awaiting the culture results, it is a reasonable choice to administer the patient either nystatin or, if not available, miconazole nitrate 1,200 mg on alternate days. This can be used with oral itraconazole 200 mg daily for 2 weeks. Otherwise, treatment involves use of various salvage therapies. The aim of these "salvage" therapies is to eradicate the organism from the vagina. Due to this, prolonged treatment for at least 2 weeks is necessary in most of the cases. There are, however, no randomized studies available and the optimum length of treatment presently remains unclear.

Salvage treatment: The optimal salvage therapy to be used in these patients is presently not known. One approach may be to use oral systemic fungicidal therapy in combination with topical therapy to penetrate into vaginal epithelia. The various salvage treatment options, which can be employed, are as follows:

- *First-line salvage therapy:* This therapy can be considered as the use of intravaginal flucytosine (5FC) for 2–3 weeks in combination with amphotericin or nystatin (both being polyene antibiotics).
- *Second-line salvage therapy:* Following the failure of 5FC or nystatin, the next step is the administration of intravaginalboric acid. The typical dose of boric acid in case of VVC caused by *C. glabrata* is 600 mg intravaginally per night for 14 consecutive nights. One should remember that boric acid capsules if swallowed orally can prove to be fatal. Presently, there is little evidence regarding the safety of boric acid in women at the time of pregnancy. Unless the vaginal epithelium is severely excoriated, only a limited amount of boric acid is systemically absorbed. Therefore, in most of the cases, the amount absorbed through the vaginal mucosa is minimal and risk to the unborn fetus is negligible.
- *Third-line salvage therapy:* The next treatment step presently remains unclear. Most clinicians consider a prolonged course, i.e., 4 weeks of either 5FC or nystatin or boric acid, but there is currently no strong evidence to support this.
- *Fourth-line salvage therapy:* If the patient still has persistent infection, the next step may depend on the susceptibility profile of the isolate *C. glabrata*, which will usually remain susceptible to 5FC and moderately susceptible to azoles. In case there is resistance to 5FC, it would be a wise decision to use either boric acid or vaginal pessaries containing topical imidazoles, e.g., clotrimazole 500 mg or miconazole nitrate 1,200 mg on alternate days alongside intensive oral treatment. Systemic therapy with triazoles, such as voriconazole, posaconazole, or high-dose fluconazole, can also be considered. The length of course is unclear, but this may be dictated by the patient's ability to tolerate the drug.
- *Fifth-line salvage therapy:* If the patient still remains infected, then they may be effectively incurable. Suppressive vaginal boric acid may be a useful option here. For treatment of vaginitis caused by *Candida krusei*, treatment comprises intravaginal clotrimazole, miconazole, or terconazole for 7–14 days. For treatment of vaginitis caused by all other species of *Candida*, conventional dosage of fluconazole is preferred.

Trichomoniasis

 Q. Write a short note on trichomonas vaginitis.

General Characteristics

This vaginitis is caused by the protozoa *Trichomonas vaginalis* **(Fig. 26.7)**, a motile organism affecting nearly 180 million women worldwide and currently accounting for 10–25% of vaginal infections. Trichomonads are usually transmitted sexually **(Fig. 26.8)** and may be identified in 30–80% of the male sexual partners of infected women. Trichomoniasis may commonly act as a vector for other STDs, including, the HIV.

Clinical Features

Classic manifestations of vaginal trichomoniasis include a purulent, frothy, yellow discharge with an abnormal odor, pruritus, and dysuria. The typical discharge associated with this infection is profuse, thin, creamy or slightly green in color, irritating, and frothy. Since the discharge commonly causes pruritus and inflammation of the vulva and vagina,

580 Abnormalities of the Vagina and Cervix

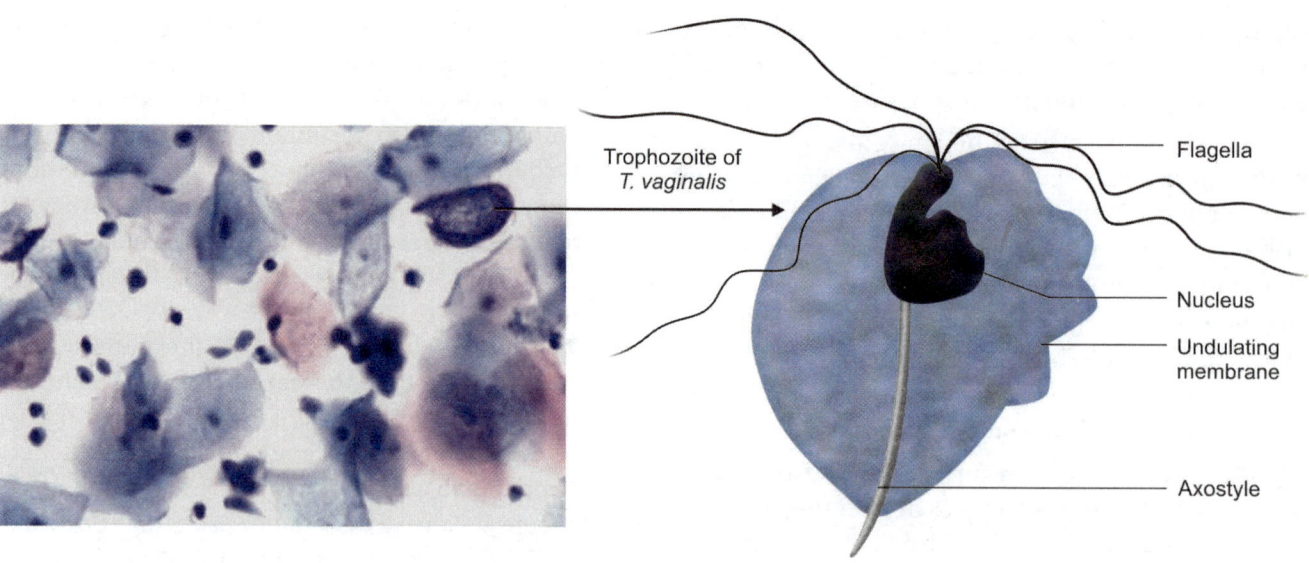

Fig. 26.7: *Trichomonas vaginalis.*

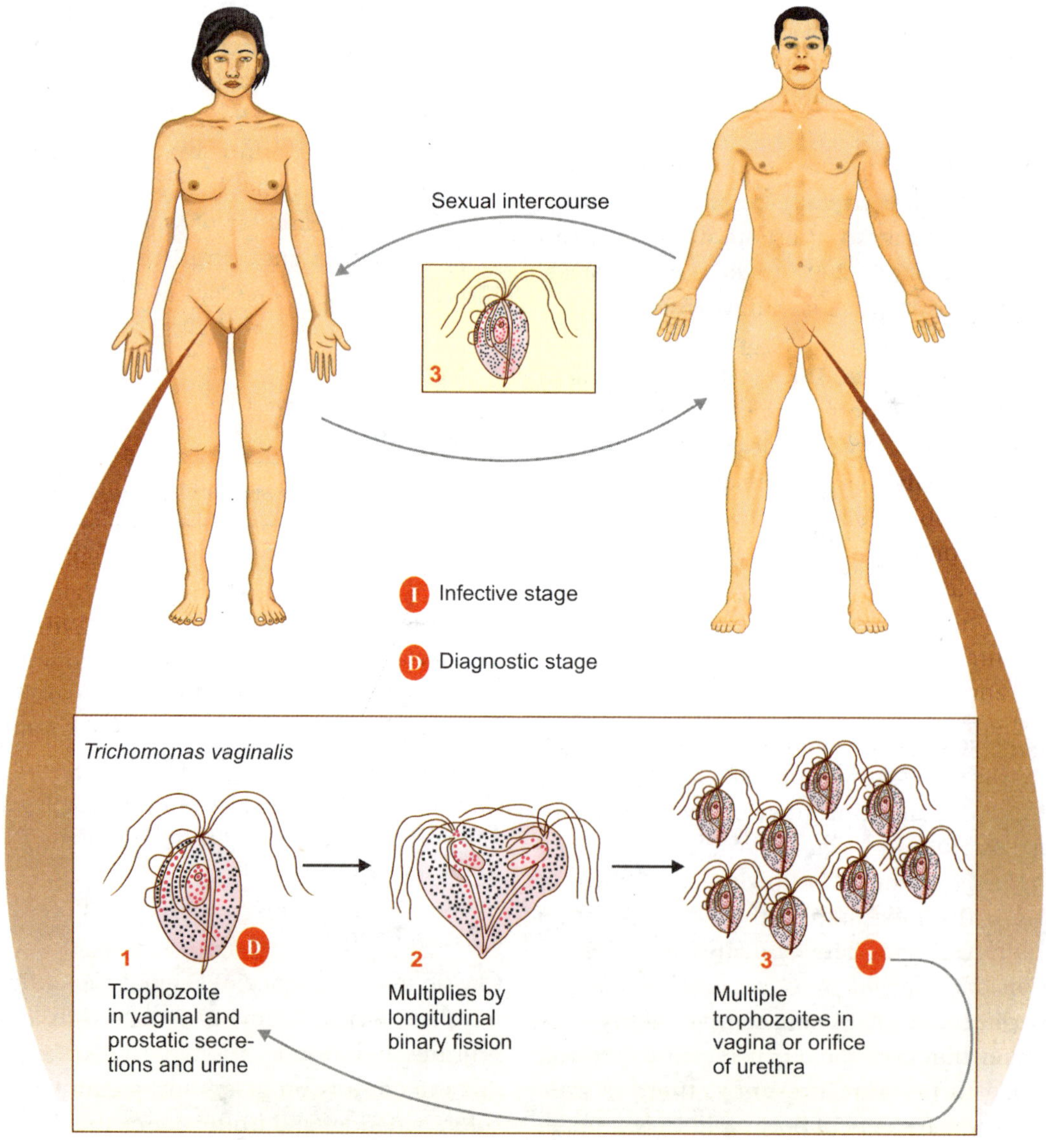

Fig. 26.8: Transmission of *Trichomonas vaginalis.*

the vaginal walls are often tender and appear angry looking. There may be presence of multiple, small, punctuate, strawberry spots on the vaginal vault, and portiovaginalis of the cervix resulting in a "strawberry vagina". The pH of the discharge is often elevated, i.e., >4.5.

Risk Factors

Risk factors for trichomoniasis include use of an intrauterine device (IUD), cigarette smoking, and having multiple sexual partners. Since trichomoniasis is a sexually transmitted disorder, both the sexual partners must be treated and instructed to avoid sexual intercourse until both partners have been cured.

Diagnosis

Microscopic examination: Motile trichomonads are usually observed on microscopic examination of wet mounts. Warming the slide and decreasing the intensity of substage lighting are ways for increasing the detection rate of trichomonads on the microscopic examination. If the index of suspicion for trichomoniasis is high and microscopic examination of the wet mount preparation reveals negative results, the microorganism may be cultured using Diamond's medium. Additionally, tests using deoxyribonucleic acid (DNA) probes and polymerase chain reaction (PCR) tests, which are associated with high rates of sensitivity and specificity, may also be performed. Another test, which is highly sensitive and specific for detection of trichomoniasis, is the latex agglutination test. In this test, a trichomonas antibody or antigen, attached to latex beads, is mixed with the speculum sample. If the protozoan is present in the discharge sample, it reacts with the latex bead complex, resulting in an agglutination reaction. The results of the test are usually available within 10 minutes to an hour. However, the high cost of this examination has largely limited the widespread use of this test in the urgent care setting.

Treatment

Metronidazole in the dose of 200 mg TDS or 375 mg BID must be prescribed to both the partners for a period of 7 days. As per the recent recommendations by the WHO (2003) and CDC (2015), a single 2 g dose of metronidazole is recommended. In case of treatment failure, CDC recommends multidose regimen involving administration of 500 mg metronidazole twice a day for 7 days, whereas WHO recommends treatment with 400–500 mg of metronidazole, twice a day for 7 days. CDC has recently changed its recommendations in case of HIV-positive women and advocates the use of multiple dose regimen rather than a single dose one.

As per the meta-analysis by Howe (2017), this recommendation must be extended to all the women. Recent research studies have also favored the use of 7-day multiple doses regimen in all the women rather than a single dose regimen due to a reduction in treatment failure rates with multiple dosage regimens.

However, as per the recommendations by CDC, a single dose of 2 g of metronidazole must be administered for management of vaginal trichomoniasis to all women who are not HIV-positive. This single dose regimen has been found to be associated with a greater cure rate varying from 90 to 95% in comparison to the week-long treatment with either 250 mg TID or 375 mg BID of metronidazole. Additionally, the single-dose regimen is more convenient to take in comparison to 7-day regimen and is associated with better patient compliance. Since trichomoniasis is largely believed to be an STD, both the partners should be advised to avoid intercourse or use a condom during the course of therapy. An alternative to metronidazole could be to prescribe tinidazole in the dose of 300 mg BD for 7 days or secnidazole in a single dose of 1,000 mg daily for 2 days. The husband should be treated simultaneously, especially if the woman develops recurrent infection. Use of metronidazole is contraindicated during pregnancy and lactation for treatment of vaginal trichomoniasis.

During early pregnancy, the following may be used: vinegar douches to lower the vaginal pH, trichofuran suppositories, and Betadine® gel.

Atrophic Vaginitis

Atrophic vaginitis is one of the most common causes for vaginal discharge in the postmenopausal women. After menopause, vaginal atrophy can result due to falling estrogen levels. Dyspareunia is common complication of atrophic vaginitis. Per speculum examination in women with vaginal atrophy may show loss of vaginal rugosity and thinning of the vaginal epithelium. This condition can be treated using topical formulations of conjugated estrogens (Premarin) in the dosage of 2–4 g intravaginally qHS.

SEXUALLY TRANSMITTED DISEASES

> Q. Write a long essay on management of sexually transmitted diseases.

Sexually transmitted diseases are infections that can be transferred from one person to another due to any type of sexual contact. Some of the STDs which would be discussed in relation to their propensity to cause vaginal discharge are chlamydial infection, genital herpes, and gonorrhea. Though these STDs are most commonly associated with vaginal discharge, other common STDs in women have also been described just for the sake of completion. Many STDs are treatable, but effective cures are lacking for others, such as HIV, herpes simplex virus (HPV), and hepatitis B and C. Condoms are commonly thought to protect against STDs. Condoms are useful in decreasing the spread of certain infections, such as *Chlamydia* and gonorrhea; however, they do not fully protect against other infections such as genital herpes, genital warts, syphilis, and acquired immunodeficiency syndrome (AIDS). Early diagnosis and treatment of infections are important for prevention of the spread of STDs infections. Some risk factors associated with STIs include the following:

- Age under 25 years
- No condom use
- Frequent change of sexual partners in past 3 months
- History of having multiple sexual contacts
- Similar symptoms (e.g., dysuria, dyspareunia, etc.) in the partner
- Previous history of sexually transmitted infection.

Chlamydial Infection

 Q. Write a long essay on chlamydial infections.

Chlamydia trachomatis is a gram-negative, aerobic, intracellular pathogen which is typically coccoid or rod shaped. However, it is different from other bacteria because it requires growing cells in order to remain viable. *Chlamydia* cannot be grown on an artificial medium because it cannot synthesize its own adenosine triphosphate (ATP) molecules. *C. trachomatis* can be considered as one of the most common causes for STD, worldwide, in association with blindness and infertility. *Chlamydia* has a very unique life cycle **(Fig. 26.9)**, which alternates between a nonreplicating, infectious elementary body (EB) and a replicating, noninfectious reticulate body (RB). The EB, which is metabolically inactive can be considered equivalent to the spore and helps in transmitting the disease. The infectious EB attaches to the host cells. Following the entry into the cell, it gets differentiated into a RB. Once inside a cell, the EB germinates as the result of interaction with glycogen and gets converted into its reticulate form. The reticulate form divides by binary fission every 2–3 hours and has an incubation period of about 7–21 days in its host. Within 40–48 hours, the RBs transform back into infective EBs, which are subsequently released from the infected cell through the process of exocytosis and infect the neighboring cells.

Clinical Features

The majority of women with chlamydial infection remain asymptomatic. However, some women may develop vaginal discharge, dysuria, abdominal pain, increased urinary frequency, urgency, urethritis, and cervicitis. Infection of the urethra is often associated with chlamydial infection of the cervix. Chlamydia is very destructive to the Fallopian tubes. If left untreated, nearly 30% of women with chlamydia may develop PID. Pelvic infection often results in symptoms such as fever, pelvic cramping, abdominal pain, or dyspareunia. Pelvic infection can often lead to infertility or even absolute sterility. Tubal destruction due to chlamydial infection may also result in an increased incidence of tubal pregnancy. PID due to *C. trachomatis* is associated with higher rates of consequent tubal infertility, ectopic pregnancy, and chronic pelvic pain in comparison with pelvic inflammatory disease (PID) caused by other infections such as gonorrhea. Occasionally, patients with chlamydial infection may develop

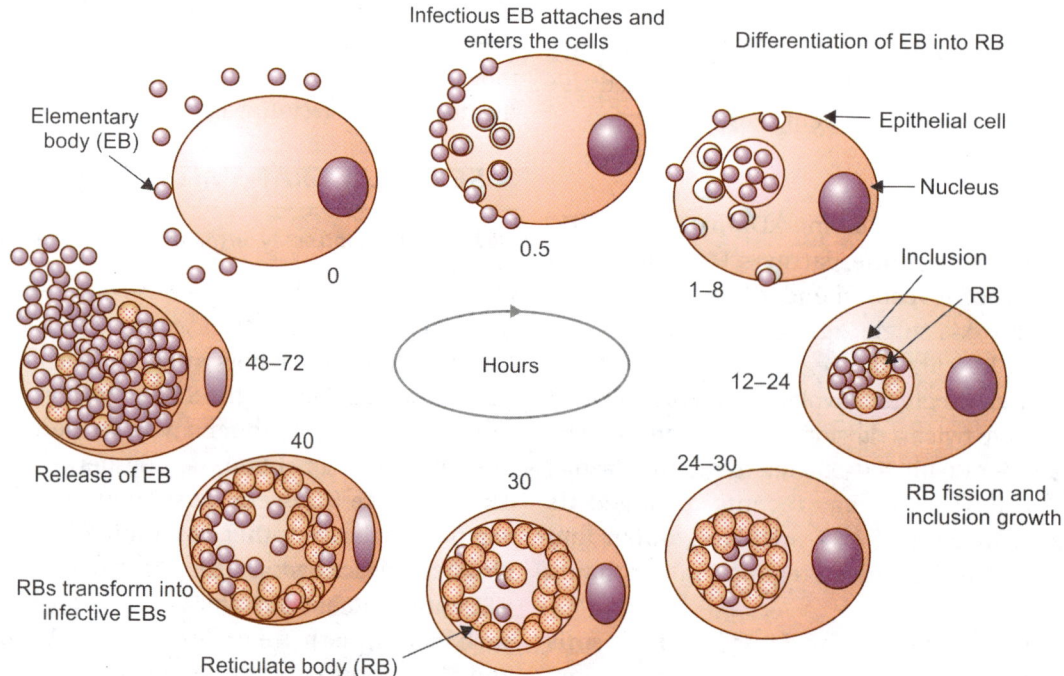

Fig. 26.9: Life cycle of *Chlamydia trachomatis*.

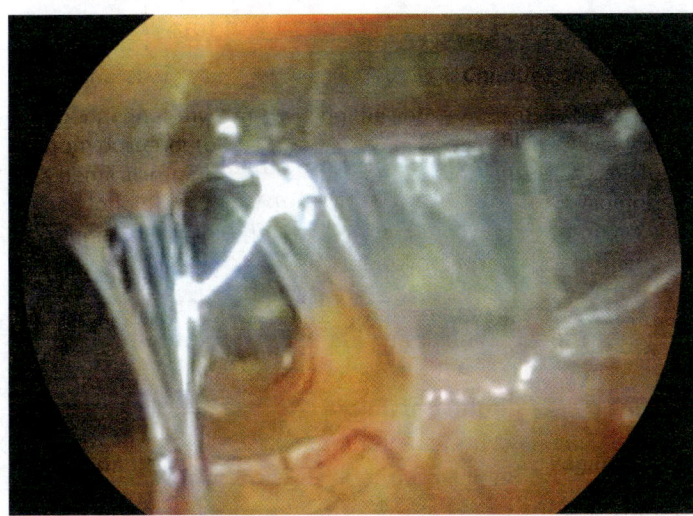

Fig. 26.10: Fitz–Hugh–Curtis syndrome.

an inflammation of the liver capsule and adjacent peritoneal surfaces resulting in perihepatitis. This is also known as Fitz–Hugh–Curtis syndrome **(Fig. 26.10)**. *Neisseria gonorrhoeae* not only causes similar clinical syndromes as *C. trachomatis* but also coexists in a significant percentage of patients with chlamydial infection. Therefore, women undergoing testing for *C. trachomatis* should also be simultaneously tested for *N. gonorrhoeae*.

Chlamydial infection, similar to gonorrhea, is associated with an increased incidence of premature births. Additionally, the organism can infect the infant during passage through the infected birth canal, leading to serious eye damage or pneumonia. Due to this, all newborns born to women infected with *C. trachomatis* must be treated with eye drops containing a broad-spectrum antibiotic (e.g., tetracycline), which kills chlamydia.

Investigations

- *Nucleic acid amplification testing (NAAT):* NAAT using either PCR or transcription-mediated amplification (TMA) of vulvovaginal swabs in women can be considered as the test of choice for establishing the diagnosis of chlamydial infection. This is a highly sensitive test (90–95% sensitivity), which can be useful in various situations, including the medicolegal cases. First-catch urine samples and endocervical swabs (if available) can also be used. If amplification techniques are unavailable, tests such as antigen detection and genetic probe methods can be applied to endocervical or urethral swabs for diagnosing chlamydial infection.
- *Polymerase and ligase chain reactions:* Newer tests such as polymerase and ligase chain reactions, DNA probe, and DNA amplification are also being used.
- *Immunoassay:* Rapid tests for chlamydia may be used for establishing the diagnosis in low-resource settings.
- Enzyme-linked immunosorbent assay (ELISA) is no longer recommended in the UK.

Management

Prevention: The National Chlamydia Screening Programme (NCSP) in the UK aims at preventing and controlling chlamydial infection through early diagnosis and treatment of asymptomatic infection. It aims at reducing the onward transmission to sexual partners and preventing the consequences of untreated infection. Under this program, all sexually active individuals under the age of 25 years are educated about chlamydia, and provided access to sexual health services to help reduce the risk of infection or transmission. It is recommended that sexually active young individuals under the age of 25 years be annually screened for chlamydial infection or whenever they change partner. If an individual test is positive for chlamydia, testing should be done again at 3 months following treatment. Screening for chlamydia should be offered as an integrated component of the existing sexual and reproductive health services including primary care-based services, community contraceptive services, abortion services, etc. There is also a provision for internet-based testing and pharmacy-based testing to ensure that young people have universal access to testing.

Under this program, home-based methods of screening involving the self-collected first-void urine specimen and vulvovaginal swabs have been found to be acceptable. These are likely to improve the universal screening rates. RCTs have demonstrated a reduction in the risk of PID amongst the women screened for *C. trachomatis*.

Medical Treatment

- Treatment of chlamydia involves the use of broad-spectrum antibiotics, with the most commonly used antibiotic being azithromycin in a single dosage of 1 g per orally. Alternatively, doxycycline can be used orally in the dosage of 100 mg BID for 7 days.
- The combination of cefoxitin and ceftriaxone with doxycycline or tetracycline also proves to be useful.
- Erythromycin or amoxicillin in TID or QID dosage may also be given during pregnancy.
- Use of protective barrier such as condoms often helps to prevent the spread of the infection.
- Chlamydial infection, similar to gonorrhea, can infect the infant during passage through the infected birth canal, leading to serious eye damage or pneumonia. Due to this, all newborns born to women infected with *C. trachomatis* must be treated with eye drops containing a broad-spectrum antibiotic (e.g., tetracycline), which kills chlamydia.
- *Follow-up:* The patient should be called for a follow-up, 6 weeks following the completion of treatment to check

for partner notification, reinforcing health education, assessing the efficacy of treatment, and exclusion of reinfection. Test of cure is usually not required unless the patient is pregnant, noncompliant or re-exposure is suspected.

- *Chlamydial infection during pregnancy:* Use of antibiotics such as quinolones and tetracyclines is usually not advised during pregnancy. Amoxicillin in the dosage of 500 mg three times a day for 7 days appears to be a reasonable alternative. Use of clindamycin and azithromycin can also be considered during pregnancy. As per the recommendations of British National Formulary (BNF), use of azithromycin during pregnancy must be restricted to only those situations where no other alternative is available.

Genital Herpes

> Q. Write a short essay on the management of genital ulcer disease.
>
> Q. Write a short essay on herpes genitalis.
>
> Q. Write short essay discussing about the HSV infection.

Genital herpes is a viral infection caused by the HSV (most commonly HSV II) which is transmitted through sexual contact. Two types of viruses are commonly associated with herpes lesions: HSV I and HSV II. HSV I is commonly responsible for causing herpes blisters in the perioral region, while HSV II is more commonly associated with lesions in the genital or the perianal area. Genital herpes is spread only by direct person-to-person contact. The virus enters through the mucous membrane of the genital tract via microscopic tears. From there the virus travels to the nerve roots near the spinal cord and settles down permanently.

Diagnosis

Clinical presentation: Diagnosis is usually based on clinical examination. Genital herpes is suspected when multiple painful blisters and vesicles are present on the external genitalia including the vulva, vagina, cervix, perianal area, or inner thigh, which ultimately develop into shallow and painful ulcers within a period of 2–6 weeks. They are frequently accompanied by itching and mucoid vaginal discharge. There may be associated vulval pain. In case of primary infection, these symptoms can be very severe, resulting in swelling, ulceration, and infection of the vulva. Ulceration may also occur in the cervix. Primary infection may also be occasionally associated with tender inguinal lymphadenopathy, which is commonly due to secondary infection.

Following the exposure to the virus, there is incubation period, which generally lasts from 3 to 7 days before development of lesions begins. Prior to this, there are no symptoms and the virus cannot be transmitted to others.

The primary infection may be associated with constitutional symptoms such as fever, malaise, vulval paresthesia, itching, or tingling sensation on the vulva and vagina followed by redness of the skin. Finally, the formation of blisters and vesicles begins, which eventually develop into shallow and painful ulcers within a period of 2–6 weeks. When the blisters break, they are usually very painful to touch. These lesions peak in 7 days and last for approximately 2 weeks. The outbreak is self-limited and usually heals without scarring.

From the beginning of itching, until the time of complete healing of the ulcer, the infection is definitely contagious. Recurrent infection, on the other hand, is less severe and self-limiting, and occasionally may be even asymptomatic.

Investigations

- *Cytological tests:* The blister fluid may be sent directly to the laboratory in the viral culture medium. However, this test is not very sensitive and may be associated with a high false negative rate of nearly 50%.
- *Immunological tests:* Immunological blood tests for detecting antibodies are not commonly used for making a diagnosis.
- *Other diagnostic tests:* Other diagnostic tests such as PCR and HSV NAAT screening tests are being used to identify HSV in some laboratories and are associated with higher sensitivity in comparison to the viral culture.
- *Biopsy:* The Tzanck smear is a rapid, fairly sensitive, and inexpensive method for diagnosing HSV infection. Smears are preferably prepared from the base of the lesions and stained with 1% aqueous solution of toluidine blue "O" for 15 seconds. Positive smear is indicated by the presence of multinucleated giant cells with faceted nuclei and homogeneously stained "ground glass" chromatin (Tzanck cells).

Management

Treatment of genital herpes helps in shortening the duration of attack, preventing the occurrence of complications, and reducing the risk of transmission. Various steps for management in these cases include the following:

- *General measures:* This involves drinking large quantity of water to dilute the urine, thereby reducing pain on micturition. Other general measures which help in reducing pain include use of saline bath analgesic drugs such as NSAIDs, etc., and use of topical anesthetic gel.
- *Oral antiviral medications:* Oral antiviral medications, such as aciclovir (200 mg five times a day), famciclovir (250 mg three times a day), or valaciclovir (500 mg twice daily), which prevent the multiplication of the virus, are commonly used. All these drugs help in reducing the

severity and duration of episodes. However, they do not alter the natural history of the disease. Local application of aciclovir provides local relief and accelerates the process of healing. In severe cases, aciclovir can be administered intravenously in the dosage of 5 mg/kg body weight every 8 hourly for 5 days.

- The couple is advised to abstain from intercourse starting right from time of experiencing prodromal symptoms until total re-epithelialization of the lesions occurs.
- Supervision of a genitourinary specialist may be required for administration of suppressive antiviral therapy in case the patient suffers more than six attacks each year.
- Although topical agents do exist, they are generally less effective than oral formulations and therefore are not routinely used. However, it is important for the clinician to remember that there is still no curative medicine available for genital herpes and the above-mentioned antiviral drugs only help in reducing the severity of symptoms and duration of outbreaks.
- Since the initial infection with HSV tends to be the most severe episode, an antiviral medication is usually recommended. Though the use of these medications can significantly help in reducing pain and decreasing the length of time until the sores heal, treatment of the first infection does not appear to provide protection against the future episodes. In contrast to a new outbreak of genital herpes, recurrent herpes episodes tend to be milder in intensity. In these cases, the benefit of antiviral medication is derived only if therapy is started immediately prior to the outbreak or within the first 24 hours of the outbreak. Thus, the antiviral drug must be provided to the patient well in advance and the patient is instructed to begin treatment as soon as she experiences the preoutbreak "tingling" sensation or as soon as the blisters appear.
- Herpes can be spread from one part of the body to another during an outbreak. Therefore, it is important to instruct the patient not to touch her eyes or mouth after touching the blisters or ulcers. She must be asked to scrupulously wash her hand. Clothing that comes in contact with ulcers should not be shared with others.
- Couples who want to minimize the risk of transmission should always use condoms if a partner is infected. Such couples must be instructed to avoid all kinds of sexual activity, including kissing, during an outbreak of herpes.

Gonorrhea

Introduction

Gonorrhea is an STD, which is derived from the Greek words "gonos" (seed) and "rhoia" (flow) implying "flow of seeds" and is caused by the bacterium *N. gonorrhoeae*. Gonorrhea is spread through contact with the penis, vagina, mouth, or anus. It can also be spread from mother to baby at the time of delivery.

Etiology

The disease is characterized by adhesion of the gonococci to the surface of urethra or other mucosal surfaces. The gonococci penetrate through the intercellular spaces between the columnar epithelial cells and reach the subepithelial connective tissue by the 3rd day of infection. Gonococci usually penetrate the columnar epithelial cells because the stratified squamous epithelium is relatively resistant to infection. In women, endocervix (columnar epithelium) is the primary site of infection. From here, the infection can spread to urethra and vagina giving rise to a mucopurulent discharge. The incubation period is 2–8 days.

Diagnosis

Clinical presentation: The disease may present as follows:

- The most common clinical presentation of the disease in men is acute urethritis resulting in dysuria and a purulent penile discharge. Lesions due to gonorrhea are summarized in **Figure 26.11**. The infection may extend along the urethra to the prostate, seminal vesicles, and epididymis, resulting in complications such as epididymitis, prostatitis, periurethral abscesses, and chronic urethritis. The infection may spread to the periurethral tissues, resulting in formation of abscesses, and multiple discharging sinuses (watering-can perineum).
- In women, the primary site of infection is the endocervix and the infection commonly extends to the urethra and vagina, giving rise to mucopurulent discharge. Symptomatic patients commonly experience vaginal discharge, dysuria, and abdominal pain. Gonorrhea can rarely cause intermenstrual bleeding or menorrhagia as a result of endometritis.
- The infection may extend to Bartholin's glands, endometrium, and fallopian tubes. The gonococci can typically ascend to the fallopian tubes at the time of menstruation or after instrumentation (for MTP) giving

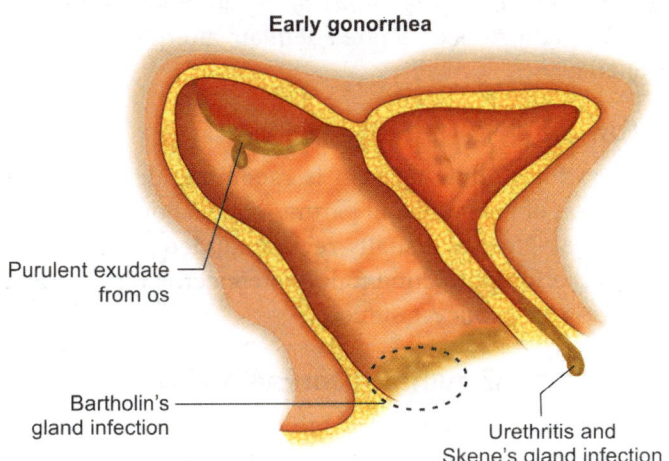

Fig. 26.11: Lesions due to gonorrhea.

rise to acute salpingitis. Acute salpingitis may be followed by PID. This may be associated with a high probability of sterility if not treated adequately. Peritoneal spread occasionally occurs and may produce a perihepatic inflammation, resulting in Fitz–Hugh–Curtis syndrome.
- Usually no abnormal findings are present on clinical examination. Men may rarely show epididymal tenderness or balanitis.

Investigations
- *Nucleic acid amplification tests:* These tests show higher sensitivity than culture in both symptomatic and asymptomatic cases of gonorrhea.
- *Culture and sensitivity:* Culture using an endocervical and urethral swab specimen provides maximum sensitivity.

Patients in whom NAAT is positive must be confirmed for gonorrhea by culture on selective medium (which has been impregnated with antibiotics).

Management
Uncomplicated anogenital infection in adults: Treatment comprises using the following antibiotics: Ceftriaxone 500 mg IM or cefixime 400 mg (oral if IM dose is contraindicated or refused) or spectinomycin 2 g IM as a single dose. Doxycycline 100 mg BID for 7 days or azithromycin 1 g PO (single dose) is usually added with a third-generation cephalosporin. This addition is recommended even if chlamydial infection is negative because its use may help delay the onset of resistance to cephalosporins. Due to emerging antibiotic resistance against *N. gonorrhoeae*, an antibiotic should be chosen in such a way that it is able to eliminate infection in at least 95% of cases in the local community.

Pregnant or breastfeeding mothers: Treatment comprises using the following antibiotics: Ceftriaxone 500 mg IM single dose with azithromycin 1 g PO or spectinomycin 2 g IM as a single dose with azithromycin 1 g PO. Use of quinolone or tetracycline antibiotics is usually not advisable during pregnancy. Use of azithromycin is advisable only under circumstances where adequate alternatives are not available.

Follow-up
At least one follow-up visit is recommended to ensure resolution of infection and partner notification. Test of cure using NAAT test is usually recommended after 2 weeks of completion of treatment due to concerns regarding the emerging antibiotic resistance.

Granuloma Inguinale (Donovanosis)
Granuloma inguinale, also known as "donovanosis" or "granuloma venereum" is a disease caused by the bacteria *Calymmatobacterium granulomatis*. The disease is characterized by occurrence of painless genital ulcers which can be sometimes mistaken for syphilitic ulcers. However, these ulcers are associated with destruction of internal and external tissue, along with leakage of mucus and blood. The disease is highly contagious and is transmitted through repeated sexual or anal intercourse. Very rarely, the infection may spread due to oral sexual activity.

Clinical Features
The disease is characterized by presence of small, painless, beefy-red nodules, which usually appear on the genitals or around the anus, after about 10–40 days of the contact with the bacteria. The skin gradually wears away and the nodules soon get converted into raised, beefy-red, velvety, open, fleshy, oozing lesions called granulation tissue. These lesions are usually painless, but bleed easily if injured. The infection often spreads, mutilating the infected tissue and continues to destroy the tissue until it is treated. The lesions occur typically on the labia or the perineum in the women and may spread to inguinal region. Rarely, the vaginal wall or cervix may also be involved.

Diagnosis
Microscopic examination of smears from the lesions shows presence of pathognomonic intracytoplasmic donovan bodies and clusters of bacteria with bipolar (safety pin) appearance.

Treatment
The standard form of therapy comprises treatment with erythromycin, streptomycin or tetracycline (500 mg QID) for 3 weeks, or treatment with ampicillin for 12 weeks.

Lymphogranuloma Venereum
Lymphogranuloma venereum (LGV) is a STD, caused by the bacteria *C. trachomatis* (L1, L2, and L3 serovars) which primarily infects the lymphatic ducts and the lymph nodes. The bacteria gain entrance into the body either through the breaks in the skin or through the epithelial cell layer of mucous membranes. From there, the organism travels via the lymphatic channels into the lymph nodes and multiplies within mononuclear phagocytes of the lymph nodes, while it passes through them. The clinical picture is termed as inguinal syndrome if the buboes or abscesses typically develop in the inguinal region where draining lymph nodes are located. The rectal syndrome arises if the infection takes place via the rectal mucosa through anal sex. It is mainly characterized by development of symptoms related to proctocolitis. Under rare circumstances, the oral sex may result in the pharyngeal syndrome, which is characterized by development of buboes in the neck region.

The LGV infection occurs in three stages—(1) primary, (2) secondary, and (3) tertiary. In majority of cases, the patients in primary and secondary stages remain undetected. Primary stage is usually characterized by self-limited painless genital ulceration at the site of contact. These signs usually appear by 3 days to a month after exposure. Primary lesion in the urethra may result in the symptoms of nonspecific urethritis. The primary stage normally heals within a few days. Erythema nodosum may occur in approximately 10% of cases.

The most common sites of primary infection in men include the coronal sulcus, frenulum, prepuce, penis, urethra, glans, and scrotum. In women, the most common sites of the primary lesion include the posterior vaginal wall, fourchette, posterior lip of the cervix, and vulva.

The secondary stage usually occurs after 10–30 days. The secondary stage is characterized by the formation of enlarged, tender regional lymph nodes known as buboes. Patients may experience constitutional symptoms, such as fever, headache, malaise, chills, nausea, vomiting, and arthralgias. The infection spreads to the lymph nodes via the lymphatic drainage pathways, resulting in lymphadenitis and lymphangitis and tender inguinal and/or femoral lymphadenopathy. Lymphangitis of the dorsal penis may also occur and resembles "string or cord". In women, the infection can result in the development of cervicitis, perimetritis or salpingitis as well as lymphangitis and lymphadenitis in the deeper nodes. With the progression of the disease, the lymph nodes enlarge and are called buboes. The buboes may be painful initially and later become painless. This is often associated with inflammation, thinning, and fixation of the overlying skin. Eventually, there occurs development of necrosis, fluctuant and suppurative lymph nodes, abscesses, fistulas, strictures, and sinus tracts. As the infection subsides and healing occurs, fibrosis may develop. This is known as the tertiary stage and can result in the development of lymphatic obstruction, chronic edema, and strictures. Tertiary stage is characterized by proctocolitis and may produce symptoms such as anal pruritus, bloody mucopurulent rectal discharge, fever, rectal pain, tenesmus, constipation, and weight loss.

Chancroid (Soft Sore)

Chancroid is a STD caused by the bacteria *Haemophilus ducreyi*, characterized by occurrence of painful sores on the genitalia. The disease is typically more common in the developing countries. Following an incubation period of 1 day–2 weeks, the disease begins with a small nodule. Within a few days, these become filled with pus and eventually rupture, leaving painful, open sores or ulcers in the genital region. These ulcers can range in size from 1 cm to 3 cm in diameter. Ulcers can bleed or ooze pus and can take weeks to heal without medication. The ulcer may range in size from 3 mm to 50 mm across and is painful. The borders of the ulcer may be either sharply defined and undermined or have irregular or ragged edges. The ulcer base is covered with a gray or yellowish-gray material and it bleeds easily on being traumatized or scraped. The patient has one or more painful genital ulcers. The combination of a painful ulcer with tender or suppurative lymphadenopathy is pathognomonic of chancroid.

While the infected men have a single ulcer, infected women frequently have multiple (four or more ulcers), with fewer symptoms. The ulcers typically appear in the fourchette and labia minora in women. "Kissing ulcers" commonly develop over the labia. These are ulcers that occur on opposing surfaces of the labia. The affected women may commonly experience dysuria and dyspareunia. The initial "soft chancre" of chancroid ulcer may sometimes be mistaken as a "hard" chancre, the typical sore of primary syphilis. Approximately one-third of the infected individuals will develop enlargement of the inguinal lymph nodes. The most commonly used antibiotics for treatment of chancroid include ciprofloxacin, trimethoprim, or erythromycin.

Syphilis

Introduction

Syphilis is an STD caused by the spirochete *Treponema pallidum*. Syphilis infection could be acquired or congenital. Though the route of transmission of acquired syphilis is almost always through sexual contact, sometimes congenital syphilis can occur via transmission from mother to child in utero. The incubation period of the disease varies between 9 and 90 days.

Diagnosis

Clinical presentation: The acquired disease comprises an early stage and a late stage of infection. Early infection is typically characterized by three phases—(1) primary, (2) secondary, and (3) early latent phase (<2 years of infection). Late stage of infection includes late latent phase (>2 years of infection) and the tertiary phase.

- *Primary phase:* Primary lesions appear approximately 10–90 days after the initial exposure. Primary lesion, also known as a chancre, often appears at the point of contact, usually the external genitalia. The chancre of syphilis is a firm, painless, relatively avascular, circumscribed, indurated, and superficially ulcerated lesion. The chancre of syphilis is often termed as "hard chancre" in order to distinguish it from the "soft sore" caused by *H. ducreyi*. The "hard chancre" of syphilis usually persists for about 4–6 weeks and heals spontaneously. In most patients, a painless regional lymphadenopathy develops within 1–2 weeks after the appearance of the chancre. As a result, the regional lymph nodes often become swollen, discrete, rubbery, and nontender.

- *Secondary phase:* Secondary syphilis occurs approximately 1–6 months after the primary infection.

This stage is typically characterized by a "flu-like" syndrome, lymphadenopathy, and the appearance of symmetrical reddish-pink nonitchy rashes on the trunk and extremities. The rash can involve the palms of the hands and the soles of the feet. In moist areas of the body, such as the anus and vagina, the rash often develops into flat, broad, whitish lesions known as condylomata lata. Mucous patches may also appear on the genitals or in the mouth. All of the lesions of secondary stage are infectious and harbor active *Treponema* organisms and therefore patients in this stage are most contagious. Other common symptoms of this stage include fever, malaise, sore throat, weight loss, headache, meningismus, enlarged lymph nodes, etc.

- *Latent syphilis:* Following the secondary stage, there often occurs a period of quiescence known as "latent syphilis". No clinical manifestations are evident during this phase and all the lesions of secondary stage have disappeared. The diagnosis during this period is possible only by serological tests. In many cases, this phase is followed by natural cure.
- *Tertiary syphilis:* In some cases, manifestations of tertiary syphilis may appear after several years. Tertiary syphilis usually occurs 1–10 years after the initial infection and is characterized by the formation of gummas, which are soft, tumor-like balls of granulomatous inflammation. Other characteristic features of untreated tertiary syphilis include neuropathic joint disease (characterized by degeneration of joint surfaces resulting in loss of proprioception), neurosyphilis, and cardiovascular syphilis.
- *Congenital syphilis:* Congenital syphilis could be either early or late. Amongst symptomatic infants, the most common clinical findings include the following: hepatomegaly, jaundice, rhinitis (nasal snuffles), rashes, generalized lymphadenopathy, skeletal abnormalities, etc. Infected infants may suffer severe sequelae, including cerebral palsy, hydrocephalus, sensorineural hearing loss, and musculoskeletal deformity. A characteristic feature of the disease is a pink-colored nasal discharge or 'bloody snuffles,' caused by syphilitic rhinitis. Syphilitic rhinitis may result in a characteristic saddle nose. Anterior bowing of the mid-tibia may be associated with the classic feature, "sabre shin".

Investigations

- Dark-field microscopy
- *Nontreponemal tests:* Kahn's test, rapid plasma regain (RPR), and Venereal Disease Research Laboratory Test (VDRL)
- *Treponemal tests:* Microhemagglutination assay for *T. pallidum* antibodies (MHA-TP), and fluorescent treponemal antibody absorption (FTA-ABS).

Management

- All women must be offered screening for other STIs including HIV.
- Primary, secondary, and early latent stages of syphilis can generally be treated with a single-dose IM injection of 2.4 million units of benzathine penicillin-G, which is unlicensed in the UK. Alternatively, a single dose of azithromycin can be administered in a single dosage as the second-line therapy. On the other hand, cases of neurosyphilis can be treated with procaine penicillin-G along with concomitant oral probenecid as the first-line therapy.
- *Management in pregnant women:* In the third trimester of pregnancy, second dose of benzathine penicillin-G must be administered 1 week after the first dose.

HISTORY AND CLINICAL PRESENTATION

The various specific symptoms on history, per speculum and per vaginal examination related to different types of vaginitis have been described previously in the text. This section provides a basic overview of clinical approach in a patient presenting with vaginal discharge.

HISTORY OF PRESENTING COMPLAINTS

- *Vaginal discharge:* Appearance of vaginal discharge is a prominent symptom of vaginitis. Since some amount of discharge may be due to physiological causes, it is important to enquire the patient about change in the volume, color, or odor of vaginal discharge, if also observed previously.

  For most patients with vaginal discharge, laboratory evaluation and investigations do not lead to an etiologic diagnosis; thus, lengthy evaluations are not indicated. The first step in the gynecological evaluation of patients with vaginal discharge is to obtain a directed history. A complete history and physical examination are all that are required in most cases. Questions regarding the type of vaginal discharge that need to be asked include the following:
  - The amount of discharge
  - Color of vaginal discharge
  - Duration of symptoms
  - Presence of any odor with the discharge
  - Association of the discharge with menstrual cycles
- *Duration of infection:* Information related to the duration of symptoms helps in establishing the diagnosis of acute or chronic disease. It is also important to know if there has been recurrence of symptoms.
- *Site of symptoms:* The site commonly involved (e.g., presence of ulcers on vulva or vagina) needs to be asked.

- *History of constitutional symptoms:* History of constitutional symptoms such as fever, pelvic or abdominal pain, and malaise may be associated with PID.
- *History of vulvar/vaginal irritation and itching:* History of any vaginal pruritus or discomfort in association with the vaginal discharge needs to be asked. While there is usually no vulvar/vaginal irritation in cases of bacterial vaginosis, vaginal irritation or pruritus is characteristically present in cases of trichomoniasis or VVC. Asking the time when the patient experiences discomfort is also important. History of pruritus and discomfort especially at night is typically suggestive of pinworm infection.
- *History of urinary symptoms:* History of urinary symptoms such as increased frequency of urination, urgency, and dysuria needs to be enquired. This is important because such symptoms may be frequently associated with vaginitis.
- *Estrogen status:* Since atrophic vaginitis is a common cause of vaginitis in a hypoestrogenic woman, the clinician needs to take the history related to estrogen status. In order to establish the estrogen status of a woman, it is important to know if she is menopausal or otherwise hypoestrogenic (e.g., taking antiestrogenic drugs).
- *Hygiene practices:* It is important to ask the patient about certain hygiene practices which may have an important role in the etiopathogenesis of her problem. Some of these habits include:
  - Habits such as vaginal douching at least once a week are associated with an increased risk of bacterial vaginosis, suggesting that daily habits may play an important role in the development of bacterial vaginosis.
  - Regular use of irritants such as soaps, baths, spermicides, perfumes, douches, and creams can also cause vulvovaginitis.
  - Tightfitting, synthetic, nylon undergarments can increase moisture, exacerbating the condition. The patient should be asked to wear loose fitting cotton undergarments.
  - Wiping the anus from posterior to anterior while using the toilet paper is likely to increase the risk for developing vaginitis.

Interpretation of the various causes of vaginal discharge based on the history is shown in **Table 26.5**.

- *History of symptoms suggestive of malignancy:* In women belonging to perimenopausal and postmenopausal age groups, malignancy (vulval, vaginal, endometrial, or cervical) is a common cause of vaginal discharge. Thus, in these women, it is important to enquire about vaginal bleeding or spotting, watery discharge, and postmenopausal or postcoital bleeding. Detailed history of symptoms related to cervical and endometrial malignancy has been described in Chapters 28 and 23, respectively. Vaginal intraepithelial neoplasia can present with vaginal discharge and/or postcoital spotting. Vulvar intraepithelial neoplasia may cause vulvar pruritus Fallopian tube cancer, though a rare type of cancer, may present with a serosanguineous vaginal discharge and pelvic pain.
- *Dysuria and dyspareunia:* History of dysuria and dyspareunia may be commonly associated with vulvovaginitis. However, both these conditions could be

TABLE 26.5: Interpretation for the various causes of vaginal discharge based on the history and examination.

Clinical elements		Bacterial vaginosis	Trichomoniasis	Vulvovaginal candidiasis
Symptoms	Color of vaginal discharge	Thin, grayish, homogeneous	Green-yellow	White, curd-like
	Consistency	Frothy	Frothy	Curdy
	Amount of discharge	Abundant	Varies	Varies
	Vaginal irritation and itching	May be present or absent	Present	Present
	Dyspareunia	Absent	Present	Absent
Signs	Vulvar erythema and strawberry cervix	*Absent*: Vaginal lining usually appears pink	*May be present or absent*: Vaginal lining is tender	*May be present or absent*: Vaginal lining is dry and red
	Bubbles in the vaginal fluid	May be present or absent	Present	Absent
Saline wet mount/potassium hydroxide (KOH)	Clue cells	Present	Absent	Absent
	Motile protozoa	Absent	Present	Absent
	Hypha/pseudohyphae	Absent	Absent	Present
	Whiff test	Positive	May be positive or negative	Negative
pH with nitrazine paper		>4.5	>4.5	<4.5

related to numerous other causes, which need to be ruled out. For example, the exact time of dysuria in relation to the flow of urine needs to be asked. Dysuria related to vaginitis is usually external and produces pain and burning sensation when urine touches the vulva. On the other hand, internal dysuria, defined as pain inside the urethra, is usually a sign of cystitis.

SEXUAL HISTORY

A detailed history related to the patient's sexual practices needs to be taken. History suggestive of a recent change in sexual partner is associated with an increased risk of acquiring sexually transmitted infections such as *T. vaginalis*, or cervicitis related to *N. gonorrhoeae* or *C. trachomatis*. Previous history of any STDs needs to be enquired. The other questions which need to be asked include the following:

- Current and previous sexual partners
- History of having protected or unprotected intercourse
- Frequent change of sexual partner in past 3 months
- History of having multiple sexual contacts
- Similar symptoms (e.g., dysuria, dyspareunia, etc.) in the partner
- Use of any oral contraceptives, or IUCDs in the past
- Presence of positive pregnancy test in the patient
- The gender of the woman's sexual partner needs to be asked. Women having sexual intercourse with other women are at an increased risk of bacterial vaginosis.

PAST MEDICAL HISTORY

- Any history of experiencing similar symptoms in the past
- Use of any antibiotics in recent past (act as a predisposing factor for development of candidal vulvovaginitis)
- History of a systemic disease that could affect the vulvovaginal area (e.g., HSV and Behçet's disease can cause vulvovaginal ulcers).
- Women with diabetes or HIV infections are prone to develop VVC.

GENERAL PHYSICAL EXAMINATION

No specific findings are present on general physical examination.

SPECIFIC SYSTEMIC EXAMINATION

PELVIC EXAMINATION

Per Speculum Examination

On per speculum examination, the following features need to be observed:

- *Identification of the site of discharge:* A per speculum examination can help identify the anatomic site of involvement (vulva, vagina, or cervix).
- *Thickness of vaginal mucosa:* Vaginal mucosa may be thin and friable with loss of folds in cases of atrophic vaginitis.
- *Signs of vaginal mucosal inflammation:* Presence of erythema, petechial spots, or ecchymoses on vaginal mucosal surface, could be related to VVC or trichomoniasis **(Table 26.5)**.
- *Type of vaginal discharge:* The pooled vaginal discharge should be assessed for color, consistency, volume, odor, and adherence to the vaginal walls. While bacterial vaginosis is typically characterized by absence of inflammation, both trichomonal and candidial infection may be associated with vulvar and vaginal erythema, edema, and excoriation. Punctate hemorrhages may be visible on the vagina and cervix. The characteristic features of different types of vaginal discharge as observed on per speculum examination are described in **Table 26.5**.
- *Presence of any lesions:* The external genitalia must be examined for the presence of inflammation, lesions or masses. There may be presence of lesions over external genitalia or foreign bodies and signs of cervical inflammation.

Bimanual Pelvic Examination

The gynecologist must assess the patient for presence of uterine or tubo-ovarian tenderness on vaginal examination. Cervical tenderness could be indicative of PID. The technique of bimanual examination has been explained in Chapter 22.

DIFFERENTIAL DIAGNOSIS

Pathological Vaginal Discharge

The diagnosis of vaginitis is based on the patient's symptoms, physical examination, the findings of microscopic examination of the wet mount and KOH preparations, and the results of the pH litmus test. The various causes of vaginal discharge based on patient's age group are listed in **Table 26.6**.

Sexually Transmitted Diseases

Presence of STDs **(Table 26.7)** is an important cause for vaginal discharge.

Infections Involving the Lower and Upper Genital Tract—PID

Pelvic inflammatory disease is characterized by the presence of following clinical features—pelvic pain, adnexal tenderness, fever, and vaginal discharge. The infection could be caused by STDs such as gonococci and *Chlamydia*. It can also occur as a sequela following spontaneous or induced abortions or delivery. In these cases, the infection is commonly polymicrobial, involving organisms such as staphylococci, streptococci, coliform bacteria, and *Clostridium perfringens*.

Vaginal Discharge

TABLE 26.6: Different causes of vaginal discharge.

Premenarchal	Childbearing age	Postmenarchal
• Poor perineal hygiene (wiping the anus from posterior to anterior) • Chemical irritants (e.g., bubble baths and lotions) • Vaginal foreign bodies • Pinworm infection • Skin conditions—eczema, psoriasis, and seborrhea	• Sexually transmitted diseases [chlamydial infection, herpes simplex virus (HSV), and gonorrheal infection] • Bacterial vaginosis, *Trichomonas* species, *Candida* species, and gonorrhea (many of these are associated with sexual abuse) • Chemical irritants	• Atrophic vaginitis • Cervicitis, cervical cancer, vulvar, vaginal, or sometimes even endometrial cancer

TABLE 26.7: Sexually transmitted diseases of the lower genital tract.

Organism	Vulva	Vagina	Cervix corpus	Adnexa
HSV	Ulcers			
Molluscum contagiosum	Molluscum lesions			
HPV	Genital warts		Intraepithelial neoplasia, cancer	
Chlamydia trachomatis			Cervicitis, endometritis	Salpingo-oophoritis
Neisseria gonorrhoeae	Skene gland adenitis		Cervicitis, endometritis	Salpingitis
Trichomonas		Cervicovaginitis		

(HPV: human papilloma virus; HSV: herpes simplex virus)

MANAGEMENT

Q. What is the likely diagnosis in the case study mentioned at the beginning of the chapter?
Ans. The patient's symptomatic history is typically indicative of candidal vulvovaginitis. The predisposing factor which led to the development of vaginitis in this case is most likely to be exposure to antibiotics.

Q. What are the likely medicolegal pitfalls associated with the case of vaginal discharge?
Ans. The possible medicolegal pitfalls associated with the case of vaginal discharge are as follows:
- Failure to consider child sexual abuse in the correct clinical context
- Failure to appreciate that endometrial and/or endocervical lesions also may be the cause of vaginal spotting after menopause.

Q. What should be offered for severe pruritus to a woman with vulvovaginal candidiasis?
Ans. A mildly sedating antihistamine at bedtime may help in relieving the nocturnal irritation and scratching (chlorpheniramine 4 mg orally).

Q. What are the most common causes for vaginal discharge in premenarchal women?
Ans. The most common cause for itching, soreness, bleeding, and foul-smelling vaginal discharge in premenarchal women has been suggested to be presence of a vaginal foreign body. Vulvovaginitis may also be secondary to sexual abuse of the premenarchal children.

BOX 26.3: General principles involved in the evaluation of a woman with vaginitis.

- Obtaining a history and performing a physical examination
- Testing for the three most common disorders causing vaginitis in premenopausal women—bacterial vaginosis, vulvovaginal candidiasis, and trichomoniasis
- If tests for evaluation of these three common causes of vaginal discharge are negative, then evaluation for less common and rare causes of vaginitis, including tests for sexually transmitted diseases need to be done

Q. Write a long essay discussing the syndromic approach to reproductive tract infections. Also, discuss the drawbacks of this method.
Ans. Syndromic management is the method of treating a patient where the clinical decisions are made on the basis of clinical signs and symptoms in the patient. This approach is typically followed while treating patients with genital ulcer or vaginal discharge.

Q. Discuss in details management of vaginal discharge.

Q. Write a long essay on vulvovaginitis.

Q. Write a long essay discussing pruritus vulvae.

The key steps involved in the evaluation of women with symptoms of vaginitis are tabulated in **Box 26.3**. Syndromic management of a patient with vaginal discharge has been shown in **Flowchart 26.1**.

INVESTIGATIONS

Due to the nonspecific nature of the symptoms, laboratory investigations for documentation of the etiology of

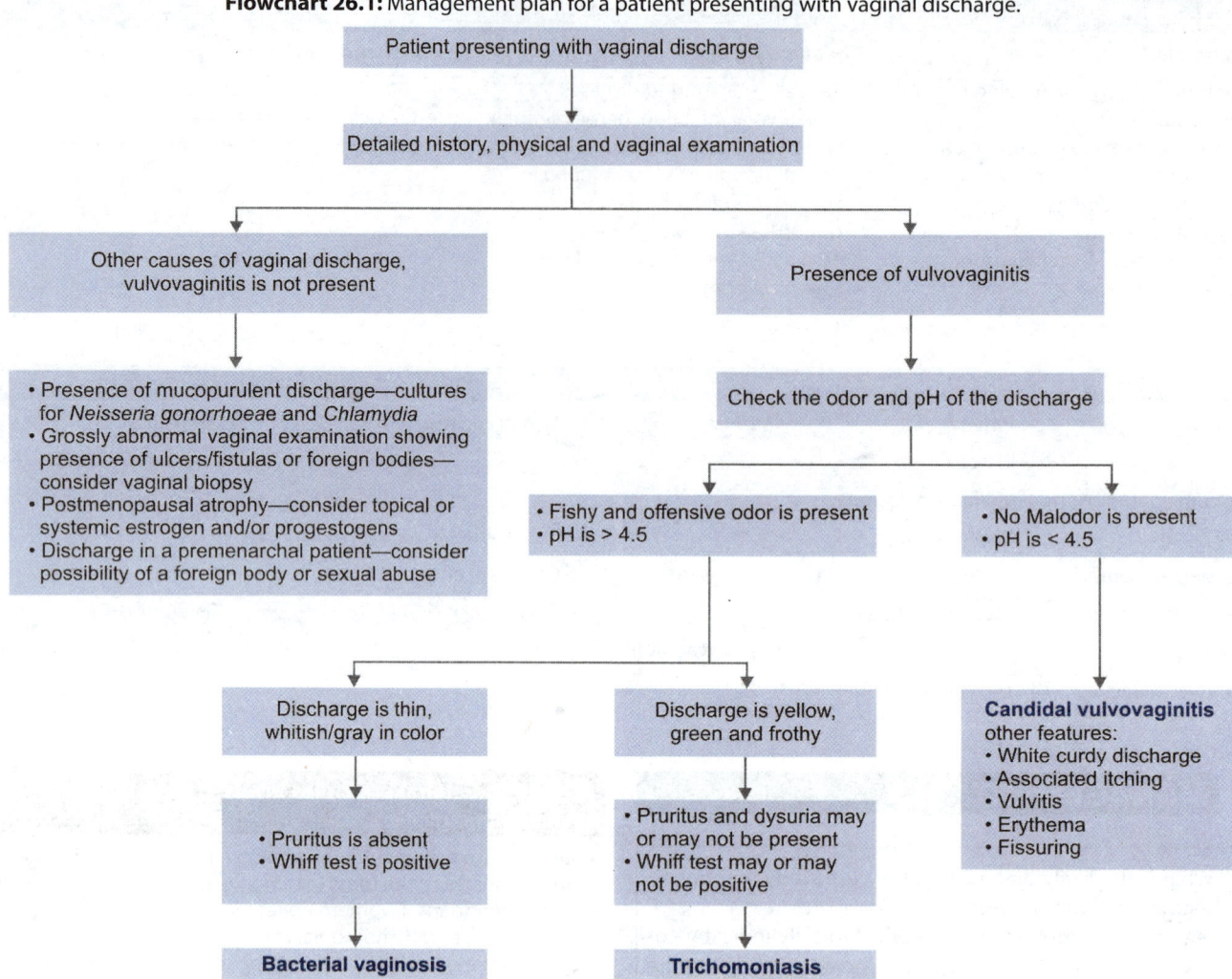

Flowchart 26.1: Management plan for a patient presenting with vaginal discharge.

vaginitis are required before initiation of therapy. In a patient presenting with vaginal discharge, the following investigations need to be carried out.

PREGNANCY TEST

Pregnancy test must be done to rule out pregnancy because certain treatment medicines might be contraindicated during pregnancy.

MICROSCOPIC EXAMINATION

If the findings of the history and/or physical examination suggest that the patient has vaginitis, a sample of the vaginal discharge should be obtained for gross and microscopic examination. Microscopic examination of normal vaginal discharge mainly shows squamous epithelial cells, polymorphonuclear leukocytes, and microorganisms related to the *Lactobacillus* species. Pathological vaginal discharge could be associated with the presence of candidal buds or hyphae in case of candidal infection or presence of motile trichomonads in case of infection with *T. vaginalis*. Clue cells (epithelial cells studded with adherent coccobacilli) may be observed in cases of bacterial vaginosis. Presence of a large number of polymorphonuclear cells without any evidence of candidal species, trichomonads, or clue cells is highly suggestive of cervicitis.

Wet Mount Preparation

The wet smear is an easy, reliable method of screening for STDs. The necessary equipment for performing a wet smear includes normal saline, slides, cover slips, and a microscope. The procedure of wet mount preparation involves the following steps (Fig. 26.12):

- A specimen of the discharge is collected from the cervix or posterior fornix of vagina with a cotton-tipped applicator at the time of per speculum examination.
- The sample is placed on the slide with a drop of saline.
- The slide is covered with a cover slip and then examined microscopically using low power (for white blood cells, red blood cells, and epithelial cells) and then under high power of microscope to look for trichomonads, clue cells, pseudohyphae, *Lactobacillus*, and white blood cells.
- The saline should be at room temperature, and microscopy should be performed within 10–20 minutes

Vaginal Discharge

level is also high in cases with atrophic vaginitis. A pH > 4.5 is found in 80–90% of patients with bacterial vaginosis and frequently in patients with trichomoniasis. VVC is normally associated with a pH of <4.5.

ALTERNATIVE OPTIONS TO MICROSCOPIC EXAMINATION

In case the microscopic examination is not available, commercial diagnostic testing methods (e.g., rapid antigen and NAAT) may be used for confirming the clinical diagnosis of bacterial vaginosis or trichomonas vaginitis. However, none of these methods are sufficiently sensitive for detecting candidal organisms. For confirming the diagnosis of candidal species, vaginal culture must be obtained.

VAGINAL CULTURE

Vaginal culture may help to diagnose the exact etiology in case of a bacterial or fungal infection. If the microscopic examination for candidal species is negative, vaginal culture for *Candida* species must be done because microscopic examination is not sufficiently sensitive to exclude the diagnosis of *Candida* organisms in symptomatic patients.

In case of clinical suspicion of trichomonal infection, diagnostic test card using NAAT, if available may serve as a reasonable alternative to culture.

CERVICAL CULTURE

In a woman with purulent vaginal discharge, culture of cervical secretions is important for establishing the diagnosis of cervicitis, typically due to *N. gonorrhoeae* or *C. trachomatis*.

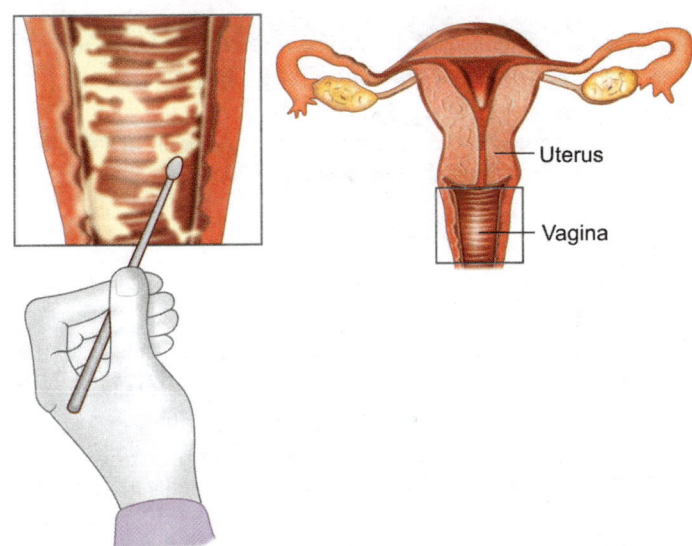

Fig. 26.12: Preparing a wet mount: A sample of vaginal discharge is taken and slide made for microscopic examination.

to reduce the possibility of loss of any trichomonads. Viewing the specimen should not be delayed, since drying could change the result. For example, trichomonads may lose their motility, if the wet smear dries.
- Following the wet mount preparation, the slide must be examined using 10% KOH solution.

KOH PREPARATION

The slide is prepared by placing a drop of vaginal secretion on a slide with a drop of 10–20% KOH and using a coverslip to protect the microscope lens. A coverslip is placed on the slide and air or flame dried before examination is carried out under the microscope. KOH by dissolving the nonfungal elements is useful for detection of candidal hyphae, mycelial tangles, and spores. The test is positive in 50–70% of women with candidal infection. This is particularly useful in diagnosis of candidal vaginitis. Following the examination of the slide, the KOH Whiff test is performed.

KOH WHIFF TEST

Smelling (whiffing) the slide immediately after applying KOH is useful for detecting the fishy (amine) odor of bacterial vaginosis. The odor results from the liberation of amines and organic acids produced from the alkalization of anaerobic bacteria. A positive Whiff test/amine test is suggestive of bacterial vaginosis.

NITRAZINE pH PAPER

Nitrazine pH paper is used to evaluate the pH of vaginal discharge sample, which is collected at the time of per speculum examination. The normal vaginal pH ranges between 3.8 and 4.2. The gynecologist must remember that both blood and cervical mucus are alkaline in nature and their presence may alter the pH of a vaginal sample. The pH

TREATMENT/GYNECOLOGICAL MANAGEMENT

Normal physiological discharge usually requires no treatment. Discharge associated with infections should respond to the specific treatment. If infections like gonorrhea, *Chlamydia*, or trichomoniasis, are suspected, the woman's sexual partner/s must also be tested and treated.

PATIENT EDUCATION

Both the women belonging to premenarchal and the childbearing age groups must be given the following advice:
- Patient must be advised to wipe thoroughly and anteriorly to posteriorly while using toilet paper.
- The importance of wearing loose-fitting, cotton undergarments must be particularly stressed.
- The patient must be advised to avoid using vaginal irritants such as bubble baths and creams. A sitz bath with baking soda may also be helpful.
- The patient must be advised to thoroughly dry up her perineum and avoid unnecessary prolonged exposure to

Abnormalities of the Vagina and Cervix

TABLE 26.8: Treatment summary of various causes of vaginal discharge.

Treatment regimens	Bacterial vaginosis	Vulvovaginal candidiasis	Trichomoniasis
Acute regimens	• Metronidazole (Flagyl), 500 mg orally twice daily for 7 days, forms the first-line treatment or • *Clindamycin phosphate vaginal cream (2%)*: Application of one full applicator (5 g) intravaginally each night for 7 days or • *Metronidazole gel 0.75% (MetroGel vaginal)*: Application of one full applicator (5 g) intravaginally twice daily for 5 days	Topical antifungal agents **(Table 26.4)** or fluconazole 150 mg orally, single dose	Metronidazole, 2 g orally in a single dose
Alternative regimens	Metronidazole, 2 g orally in a single dose or clindamycin (Cleocin), 300 mg orally twice daily for 7 days or metronidazole 375 mg TID, orally for 7 days	Boric acid powder in size-0 gelatin capsules intravaginally once or twice daily for 2 weeks	Metronidazole, 200 mg orally thrice daily for 7 days
Pregnancy	• Metronidazole, 250 mg orally three times daily for 7 days (recommended regimen) or • Clindamycin 300 mg orally twice daily for 7 days • Intravaginal preparations of metronidazole and clindamycin are avoided by some experts during pregnancy	Only topical azole agents such as clotrimazole, miconazole, terconazole, and tioconazole intravaginally for 7–10 days	Metronidazole, 2 g orally in a single dose (usually not recommended in first trimester)
Recurrence	Retreat with an alternative regimen	*For four or more episodes of symptomatic vulvovaginal candidiasis annually*: Initial acute intravaginal regimen for 10–14 days followed immediately by maintenance regimen for at least 6 months (e.g., ketoconazole, 100 mg orally once daily)	Metronidazole, 2 g orally once daily for 3–5 days (note that treatment of sexual partners increases cure rate)

moisture (e.g., wearing a wet bathing suit for prolonged periods of time).

■ THERAPEUTIC OPTIONS

Treatment should be specifically aimed to treat specific bacterial, parasitic, or fungal infection. Treatment of various causes of vaginal discharge has been described in detail previously in the chapter and is summarized in **Table 26.8**.

Alcohol use should be avoided during oral metronidazole therapy and for 24 hours after treatment. Topical antifungal therapy for vaginitis has been described in **Table 26.4**.

COMPLICATIONS

General complications related to vulvovaginitis are as follows:
- Pelvic inflammatory disease
- Intrauterine infections
- Chorioamnionitis
- Postpartum endometritis
- Vaginitis emphysematous
- Preterm labor
- Premature rupture of membranes
- Newborn infections
- Low birth weight babies

■ INFECTION SPECIFIC COMPLICATIONS
Bacterial Vaginosis

- *Pelvic inflammatory disease:* Infection with bacterial vaginosis can cause PID, which can result in complications such as an increased frequency of endometritis, abnormal Papanicolaou (Pap) smears, abdominal pain, uterine bleeding, and uterine and adnexal tenderness. Performance of an invasive gynecological procedure or surgery in a patient with bacterial vaginosis may result in the development of vaginal cuff cellulitis, PID, and endometritis.
- *Pregnancy-related complications:* Bacterial vaginosis during pregnancy can result in complications like premature labor, preterm birth, low-birth weight babies, chorioamnionitis, postpartum endometritis, ectopic pregnancy, and postcesarean section wound infections.
- Bacterial vaginitis in postpartum women can be associated with complications such as endometrial bacterial colonization, plasma-cell endometritis, postpartum fever, and postabortal infection.
- Bacterial vaginosis can also be associated with posthysterectomy vaginal cuff cellulitis.
- Bacterial vaginosis may act as a risk factor for acquisition and transmission of various STDs such as HIV, HSV type 2, gonorrhea, and chlamydial infection.

- Bacterial vaginosis may also serve as a risk factor in development of precancerous cervical lesions.

Chlamydia
- Pelvic infection can often lead to infertility or even absolute sterility.
- Tubal destruction due to chlamydial infection may also result in an increased incidence of tubal pregnancy.
- Chlamydial infection during pregnancy may be associated with an increased incidence of premature births.
- At the time of delivery, chlamydial infection may be transmitted to the fetus resulting in an increased risk of serious eye damage (neonatal conjunctivitis or ophthalmia neonatorum) or pneumonia in the infant. Also, there may be an increased risk of uterine infection in the mother.

Gonorrhea
- In men, infection may extend along the urethra to the prostate, seminal vesicles, and epididymis, resulting in complications such as epididymitis, prostatitis, periurethral abscesses, and chronic urethritis.
- The infection may spread to the periurethral tissues, resulting in formation of abscesses and multiple discharging sinuses (watering-can perineum).
- In women, acute salpingitis may be followed by PID. This may be associated with a high probability of sterility, if not treated adequately.
- Peritoneal spread occasionally occurs and may produce a perihepatic inflammation, resulting in Fitz–Hugh–Curtis syndrome.
- As a result of vertical transmission to the fetus, gonorrhea can cause severe conjunctivitis, also known as ophthalmia neonatorum.
- Disseminated hematogenous gonococcal infection, which rarely occurs, can result in complications such as arthralgia, arthritis, tenosynovitis, and skin lesions.

Genital Herpes
- *Urinary retention:* This may occur due to autonomic neuropathy or due to local reaction around the vulva and urethra because of severe vulval pain. Suprapubic catheterization may be required in these cases.
- *Postherpetic neuralgia:* This may be the cause of chronic vulval pain.

Syphilis
Transplacental passage of treponemal infection at any stage of pregnancy may lead to complications such as polyhydramnios, stillbirths, miscarriage, preterm labor, hydrops, and congenital syphilis.

EVIDENCE-BASED CLINICAL TRIALS

List of references can be scanned through QR code to enable the readers gain deeper insight of the subject by referring to the entire article or its abstract.

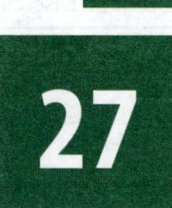

CHAPTER 27

Cervical Intraepithelial Neoplasia (Abnormal Pap Smear)

CASE STUDY

A 38-year-old patient, having two live children, presented to the gynecology clinic for the annual gynecological checkup. She gives a history of having multiple sexual partners in the past. She is presently happily married and in a stable monogamous relationship with her husband. She currently uses oral contraceptive pills for contraception. Though she remembers being treated for genital warts in the past, her previous Pap smear results had been normal. However, this time her Pap smear result is suggestive of high-grade squamous intraepithelial lesion (HSIL).

INTRODUCTION

 Q. Write a short essay on transformation zone.

Cancer of cervix usually is the end stage of the spectrum of disorders progressing from mild through moderate to severe dysplasia and carcinoma in situ (CIS). Cervical intraepithelial neoplasia (CIN) is a premalignant condition of the uterine cervix that arises from the area of metaplasia in the transformation zone at the squamocolumnar junction **(Figs. 27.1A and B)**. Diagnosis of cervical dysplasia/CIN is mainly based on cytological screening (Papanicolaou Test or Pap smear) of the population. CIN refers to squamous cell abnormalities. Glandular cervical neoplasia comprises adenocarcinoma in situ and adenocarcinoma. The peak incidence of occurrence of dysplasias appears to be 10 years earlier than that of frank invasive cancer. CIN is most likely to occur either during menarche or after pregnancy, when metaplasia is most active. Metaplasia becomes less active following menopause, and therefore the risk of developing CIN considerably reduces. If left untreated, most cases of CIN 1 and some cases of CIN 2 may regress spontaneously. The changes like cervical metaplasia, dysplasia, and CIN would be discussed next in this chapter before Pap smear is described.

METAPLASIA

Metaplasia is a pathological change, which refers to the reversible replacement of one type of differentiated cells with another type of mature differentiated cells. As previously described, the squamocolumnar junction represents the transformation zone of the cervix where columnar endocervical epithelium meets the squamous epithelium of ectocervix. The reserve cells lying beneath the columnar epithelium at this junction, sometimes, transform into mature squamous cells. This process is known as metaplasia. However, metaplastic cells are the normal cells without nuclear atypia and do not act as precursors of malignancy. Atypical metaplasia with abnormal nuclear changes acts as a precursor of dysplasia and malignancy. Dysplasia refers to the abnormal maturity of the epithelium. Therefore, proliferative metaplasia without atypical mitotic activity should not be termed as dysplasia. Squamous metaplasia must not be diagnosed as dysplasia or CIN because it does not progress to invasive cancer.

DYSPLASIA

Dysplasia is the process, which refers to an abnormal maturation of cells within the tissue. This process differs from metaplasia in the sense that normal differentiated cells are replaced by abnormal undifferentiated cells, unlike metaplasia in which one type of differentiated epithelial cells are replaced by another type of normal differentiated epithelial cells. Dysplasia is often indicative of an early neoplastic process and is characterized by presence of nuclear changes such as anisocytosis (abnormality in size), poikilocytosis (abnormality in shape), hyperchromatism, and presence of mitotic figures. Dysplasias can be graded as follows:

- *Mild dysplasia or CIN 1:* The undifferentiated cells are confined to the lower one-third of the epithelium. The cells are more differentiated toward the surface. According to Bethesda classification, CIN 1 has been lately described as low-grade squamous intraepithelial lesion (LSIL).

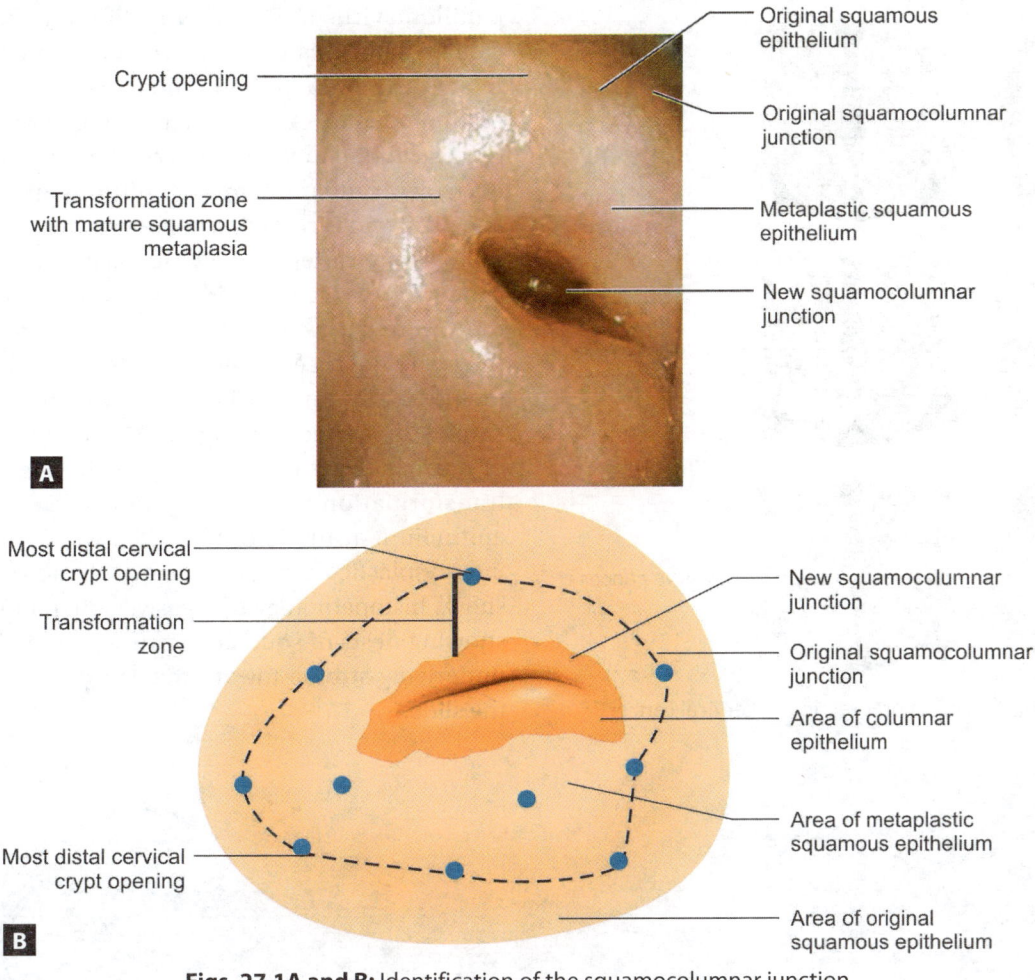

Figs. 27.1A and B: Identification of the squamocolumnar junction.

- *Moderate dysplasia or CIN 2:* Undifferentiated cells occupy the lower 50–75% of the epithelial thickness. The cells show mild-moderate nuclear changes such as moderate nuclear enlargement, hyperchromasia, irregular chromatin, and multiple nucleation.
- *Severe dysplasia and CIS or CIN 3:* In this grade of dysplasia, the entire thickness of epithelium is replaced by abnormal cells. There is no cornification and stratification is lost. The basement membrane, however, remains intact and there is no stromal infiltration.

According to latest Bethesda classification, CIN 2 and CIN 3 lesions are described as HSIL. The presence of HSIL is significant because these lesions have a high-degree potential to progress to invasive cancer that needs to be treated. Sensitivity of Pap smear for detection of HSIL is 70–80% and specificity is 95–98%.

CERVICAL INTRAEPITHELIAL NEOPLASIA OR PREINVASIVE CERVICAL CANCER (STAGE 0)

Histopathological progression of cervical dysplasia is shown in **Figure 27.2**, while the morphological progression of invasive cancer is shown in **Figure 27.3**. The term, CIN can be considered as a precancerous lesion (dysplasia) in which a part or the full thickness of the stratified squamous cervical epithelium is replaced by cells showing varying degrees of dysplasia. CIN represents a spectrum of disease that most commonly affects women during their 40s and 50s. Nearly 90% cases of CIN can be attributed to infection by the human

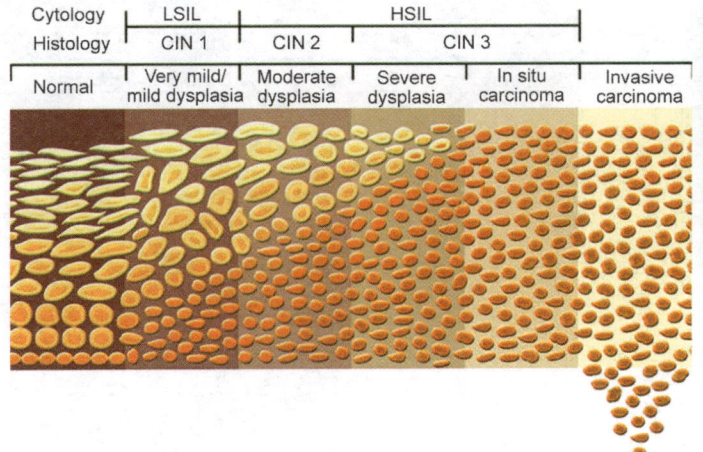

Fig. 27.2: Progression of cervical dysplasia. (CIN: cervical intraepithelial neoplasia; HSIL: high-grade squamous intraepithelial lesion; LSIL: low-grade squamous intraepithelial lesion)

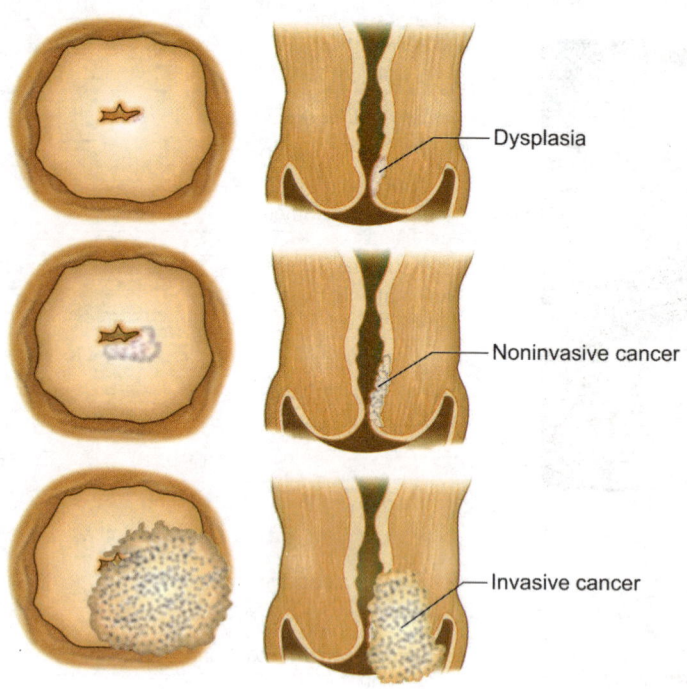

Fig. 27.3: Morphological progression of cervical cancer.

papillomavirus (HPV). CIN is different from the invasive cancer, as in this case the basement membrane remains intact. The intraepithelial neoplasia can be classified as mild, moderate, or severe depending upon the thickness of cervical epithelium involved. Mild degrees of dysplasia may occur with inflammatory conditions like trichomoniasis and HPV and is reversible following treatment; whereas the more severe varieties of dysplasias may progress to invasive cancer in about 10–30% of cases in 5–10 years' time. As the severe degree CIN progresses into an invasive cancer, the neoplastic cells penetrate the underlying basement membrane and invade the stroma with the potential for widespread dissemination. **Figure 27.4A** shows histopathology of normal cervical epithelium, while **Figure 27.4B** shows transformation zone of the normal cervical squamous epithelium at the left hand side, which gets transformed into dysplastic changes at the right hand side. **Figure 27.4C** shows histopathology of invasive squamous cell carcinoma showing nests of squamous cancer, which has invaded the underlying stroma toward the center and left hand side of the slide.

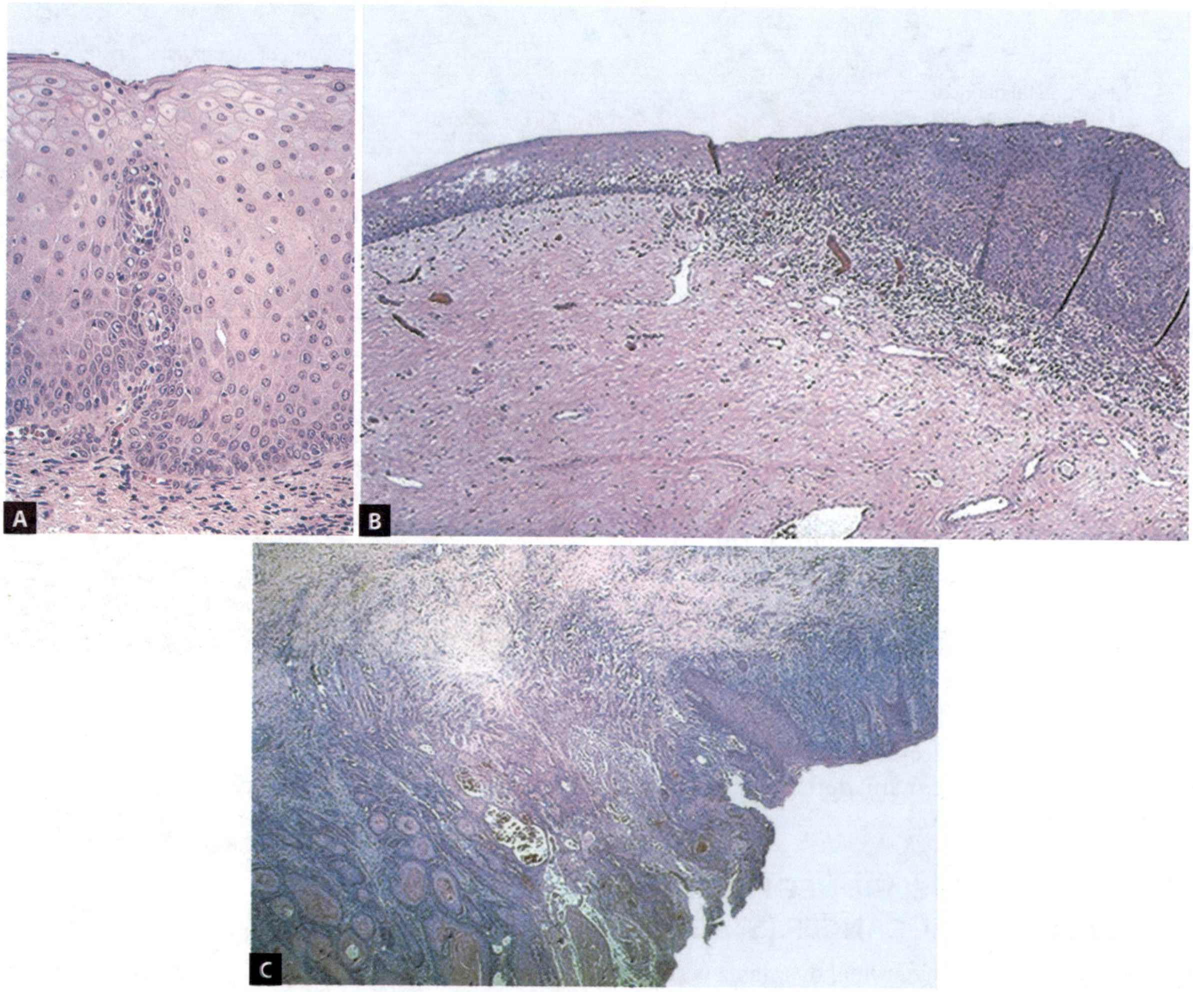

Figs. 27.4A to C: (A) Histopathology of normal cervical epithelium. (B) Transformation of the normal cervical squamous epithelium (at the left) into dysplasia (at the right). (C) Histopathology of invasive squamous cell carcinoma showing nests of squamous cancer, which has invaded the underlying stroma in the center and left.

HISTORY AND CLINICAL PRESENTATION

Precancerous cervical cells usually cause no symptoms and may only be detected by screening.

INFECTION WITH HUMAN PAPILLOMAVIRUS

Infection with HPV is present in 99.7% cases of cervical cancers. HPV can cause self-limited infections as well as persistent infections with recurrent symptoms and repeat infections. The "high risk" types cause cervical cancer. Of these, types 16 and 18 cause 70% of cervical cancers. The "low risk" types cause benign lesions such as genital warts. Types 6 and 11 cause 90% of genital warts.

GENERAL PHYSICAL EXAMINATION

Presence of dysplasia/CIN may be associated with minimal clinical findings on clinical examination.

SPECIFIC SYSTEMIC EXAMINATION

PER SPECULUM EXAMINATION

On inspection, the cervix often appears normal, or there may be cervicitis or erosion, which bleeds on touch.

DIFFERENTIAL DIAGNOSIS

Conditions, which might show resemblance to preinvasive lesions of cervix, are described in **Box 27.1**. Colposcopy aids differentiation. Colposcopic-directed biopsy and histopathological examination serve as the gold standard in arriving at a definitive diagnosis.

MANAGEMENT

> Q. Write a long essay discussing the screening protocol for cervical cancer. Also discuss in detail the management of the case of CIS.
>
> Q. Write a long essay discussing the methods for screening cervical cancer and management of patients whose pap smear is suggestive of high-grade intraepithelial lesions.
>
> Q. Write a short note on screening for cervical cancer.
>
> Q. What is the next step of management in the case study described in the beginning of the chapter?
> In order to confirm the diagnosis of HSIL, colposcopy with biopsy of the suspicious lesions was performed. Following this, loop electrosurgical excisional procedure of the abnormal area was performed. The patient was called for follow-up examination with cytological examination at 6 months and then again at 12 months. Pap smear examination during both these follow-up visits was found to be within normal limits.

BOX 27.1: Differential diagnosis.
- Severe cervicitis, e.g., herpes and syphilis
- Benign ulceration, e.g., trauma
- Foreign body reaction
- Granulomatous cervical conditions
- Granuloma inguinale
- Lymphogranuloma venereum
- Schistosomiasis
- Cervical condylomata

Management of women with CIN aims at preventing the possible progression to invasive cancer at the same time avoiding overtreatment of lesions, which are likely to regress. Management of patients with preinvasive lesions has been described in this chapter, whereas those with invasive lesions have been described in Chapter 28. A Pap smear must be done at the time, when the patient is not actively bleeding. If any locally visible lesion on the cervix is seen, a cervical punch biopsy must be immediately performed. If the Pap smear shows severe dysplasia (HSIL), the next step is to perform a colposcopic-directed biopsy and endocervical curettage. Once the diagnosis of cervical cancer is confirmed on histopathology, staging and grading of the disease are performed. Further management is based on the cancer grade and stage (refer to Chapter 28 for details).

INVESTIGATIONS

The most important investigation, which helps in detection of cervical cancer in its preinvasive stage, is the Pap smear. Pap smear involves cytological analysis of the cells from the squamocolumnar junction, which is an area of rapid cell turnover, squamous metaplasia, and the site of oncogenic transformation. In young women of childbearing age, the squamocolumnar junction is usually readily visible on the ectocervix. With age as the cervical epithelium matures, the squamocolumnar junction may recede within the endocervical canal. As a result, the squamocolumnar junction may be difficult to visualize and to be adequately sampled. The various methods for screening for cervical cancer are summarized in **Flowchart 27.1**.

CYTOLOGIC SCREENING: PAP SMEAR

Since its introduction in the 1940s, cytological screening in form of Pap smear has become the investigation of choice for detection of precancerous lesions of the cervix. The widespread introduction of the Pap test for cervical cancer screening has resulted in significantly reducing the incidence and mortality of cervical cancer in developed countries. Presence of abnormal results on Pap test or symptoms of cervical cancer may mandate further testing in form of colposcopy, colposcopic-directed biopsy, and endocervical

Abnormalities of the Vagina and Cervix

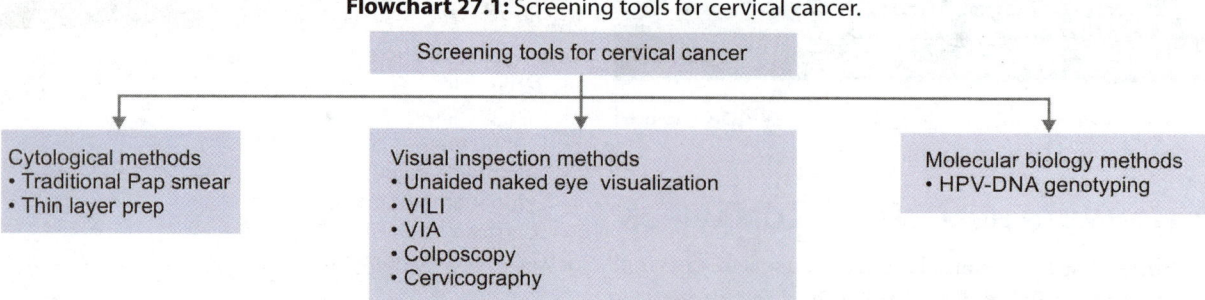

Flowchart 27.1: Screening tools for cervical cancer.

(HPV-DNA: human papillomavirus – deoxyribonucleic acid; VIA: Visual inspection under acetic acid; VILI: Visual inspection under Lugol's iodine)

curettage, which can help in confirming if abnormal cells are dysplastic or cancerous.

PREREQUISITES FOR A SCREENING TEST

The prerequisites for the screening test to be successful are listed in **Box 27.2**.

Since Pap smear is associated with a negative reporting rate of 30%, it is important to repeat Pap smear annually for three consecutive years. If still, the Pap smear continues to remain negative, it should be repeated at 3–5 yearly intervals up to the age of 65 years. After the age of 65 years, Pap smear is not required, because the incidence of CIN drops to 1%.

Prerequisites Before Taking a Pap Smear

- No vaginal douching should be done 48 hours prior to the test.
- Vaginal creams should not be used for 1 week before the test.
- There should be abstinence from sexual intercourse 24 hours prior to the test.

Procedure

- **Figure 27.5** shows the Pap smear kit, while **Figures 27.6A to D** demonstrate the procedure for taking a Pap smear. The patient is made to lie in a dorsal position and adequate light must be used to visualize the cervix and vagina properly.
- A Cusco's speculum must be used to expose the cervix.
- No lubricant should be used on the Cusco's speculum.
- After exposing the cervix, an endocervical brush or a cotton-tipped swab must be placed inside the endocervix and rotated firmly against the canal in order to take an endocervical sample, which is then placed on the glass slide.
- Next the Ayre's spatula must be placed against the cervix with the longer protrusion in the cervical canal.
- The spatula must be rotated clockwise for 360° against the cervix. This would help in scraping the entire transformation zone.
- If it appears that the entire transformation zone has not been adequately sampled, the spatula must be rotated several times.

> **BOX 27.2:** Prerequisites for the screening test.
> - The disease condition for which screening must be done should be an important health problem
> - There should be an accepted treatment option available for the management of disease if diagnosed
> - Services for treatment and diagnosis of the disease should be easily accessible. A suitable method of disease examination must be available
> - There should be a recognizable latent or early symptomatic stage
> - The screening test should be acceptable to the population
> - The natural history of the disease should be adequately understood
> - There should be an agreed policy on whom to treat as patients
> - The screening test should be cost effective in comparison with the expenditure of medical care as a whole

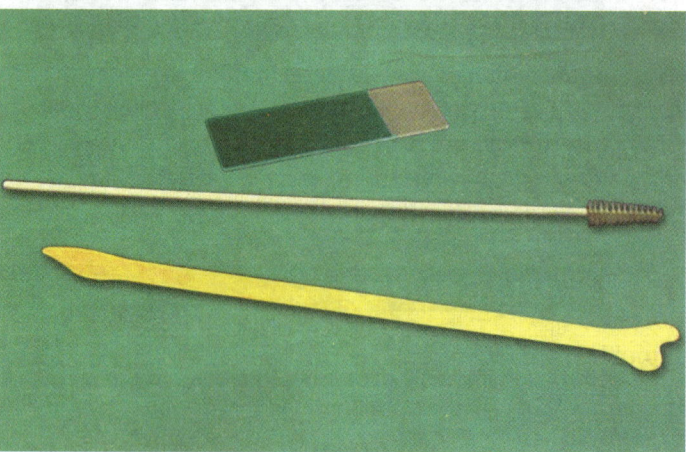

Fig. 27.5: Pap smear kit.

- The sample from the spatula is placed onto the glass slide by rotating the spatula against the slide in a clockwise manner.
- The slide must be immediately fixed with the help of a spray fixative, which is held at a distance of about 9–12 inches.

Qualities of a Good Smear

The smear should be thick enough, but not transparent. Too thin smear may result in formation of artifacts upon drying.

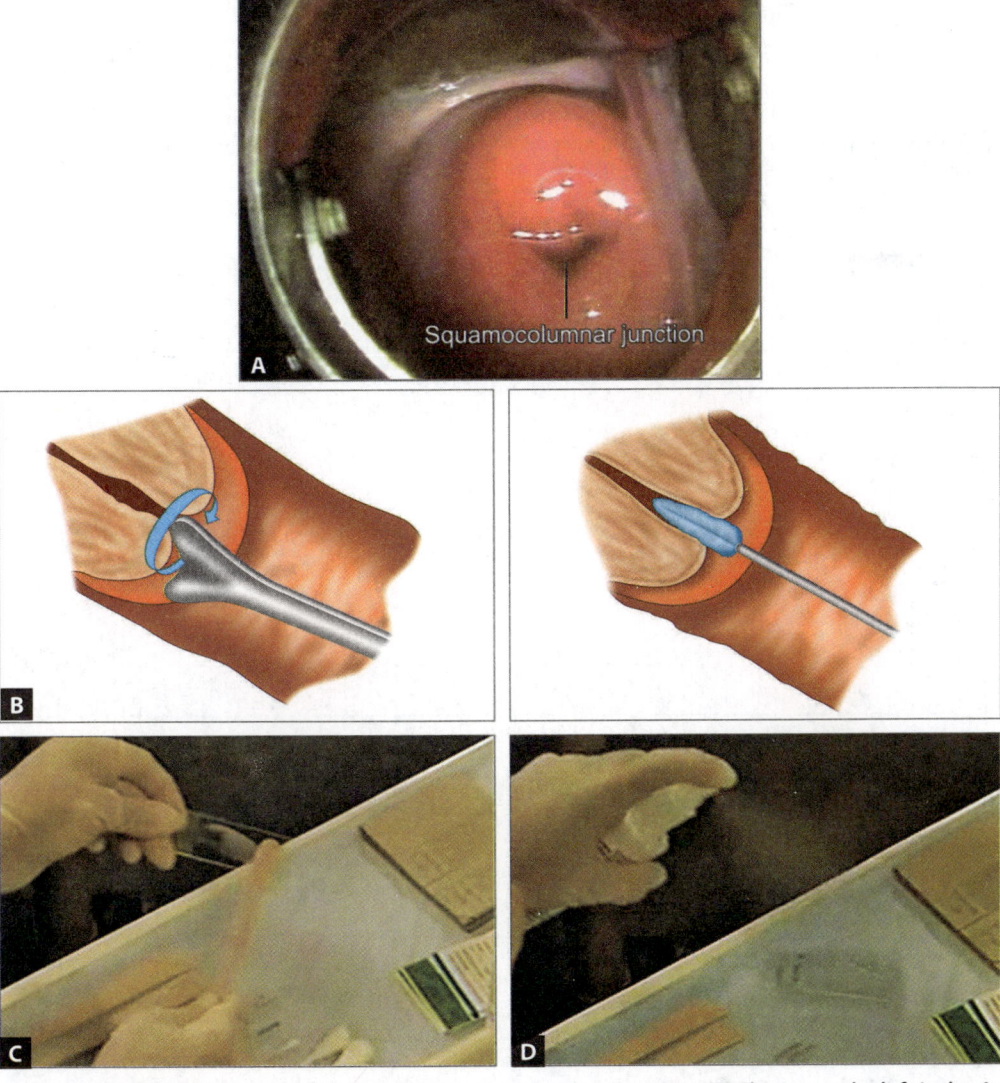

Figs. 27.6A to D: Procedure of taking a Pap smear. (A) Normal squamocolumnar junction; (B) Shown on the left is the Ayre's spatula inserted for taking ectocervical scrapings and on the right is the endocervical brush inserted inside to take endocervical scrapings; (C) Spreading the scrapings on the slide; and (D) Spraying of fixative to fix the slide.

Also, a thin smear might contain too few cells, which might not allow adequate sampling. On the other hand, if the smear is too thick, the Papanicolaou stain will not penetrate.

National Health Service Cancer Screening Programme

National Health Service Cancer Screening Programme (NHSCSP) in the UK helps in identifying individuals who appear healthy but may be at an increased risk of developing cervical cancer in future **(Flowchart 27.2)**. No such national screening program is available in India. Selective private health care centers refer woman above the age of 25 years for regular screening. Women also can get the screening test done as per their own discretion.

In England NHSCSP is available to all the women who are aged 25–64 years. All eligible women who are registered with a GP automatically receive an invitation for cervical screening by mail. Woman's first invitation for routine screening must be sent out 6 months before her 25th birthday, i.e., at the age of 24 and half years. This ensures that the woman would be screened by her 25th birthday. All subsequent invitations for screening must be sent approximately 6 weeks before the woman's test due date. Women, who are between the ages of 25 and 49 years, receive an invitation after every 3 years. On the other hand, women who are aged between 50 and 64 years receive an invitation after every 5 years. Though slightly more costly, 3-yearly cervical screening program is likely to significantly prevent more cancers than 5-yearly screening program in younger women. After 65 years of age, invitation can be sent to women who have had recent abnormal tests. Screening can be performed on request for women who have not had an adequate screening test since the age of 50 years.

Among the women under the age of 25 years, the prevalence of HPV infection is high. As a result,

Abnormalities of the Vagina and Cervix

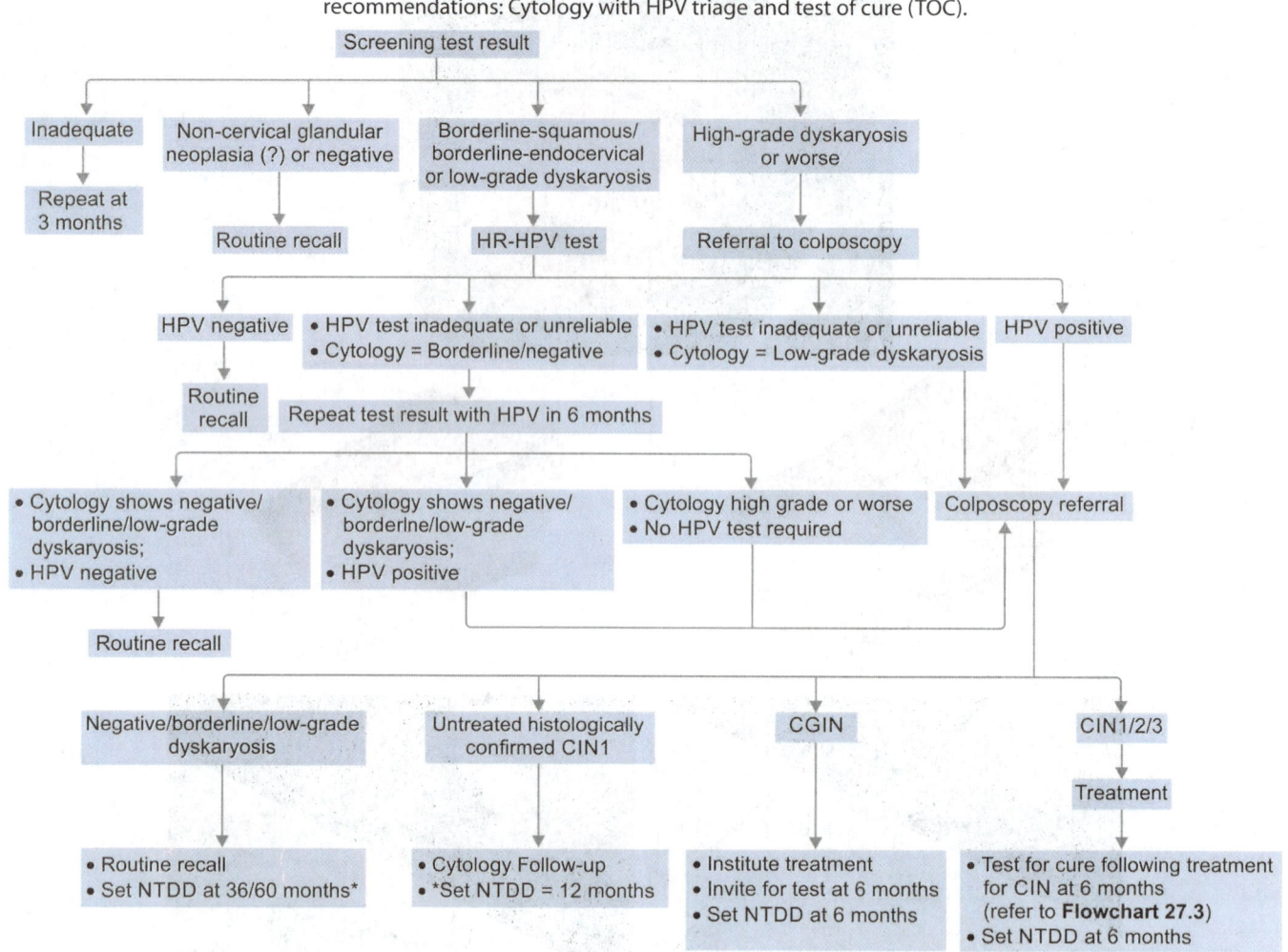

Flowchart 27.2: Screening protocol algorithm and colposcopy management recommendations: Cytology with HPV triage and test of cure (TOC).

(CIN: cervical intraepithelial neoplasia; CGIN: cervical glandular intraepithelial neoplasia; HPV: human papillomavirus; HR-HPV: high-risk human papillomavirus; NTDD: next test due date)
*Women more than 60 years of age who are cytology negative, HPV positive and have a satisfactory and negative colposcopy can be removed from the programme. Women more than 60 years of age who show borderline/low-grade dyskaryosis, HPV positive and have a satisfactory and negative colposcopy should consider large loop excision of the transformation zone (LLETZ) if decline recall at 60 months.

HPV-associated cellular changes are quite common among the sexually active women in this age group. However, majority of low-grade abnormalities related to HPV infection detected in cytology samples taken from women under the age of 25 years are likely to regress spontaneously with time. As a result, the incidence of cervical cancer in this age group is very low. Screening of women under the age of 25 years, therefore, may result in a large number of referrals to colposcopy for further investigation. This may be the cause of increased levels of anxiety for these women.

Additionally, unnecessary treatment may be administered by the colposcopist for abnormalities that are anyway likely to resolve on their own without any further intervention.

Treatment-related complication may result in obstetric complications with future pregnancy, e.g., large loop excision of the transformation zone (LLETZ) may result in preterm labor.

HUMAN PAPILLOMAVIRUS TRIAGE AND TEST OF CURE

Test of cure (TOC) protocol following treatment for CIN 1 is illustrated in **Flowchart 27.3**. Under the high-risk HPV (HR-HPV) triage protocol, women whose cervical samples are reported to be showing borderline changes (of squamous or endocervical type) or low-grade dyskaryosis are subjected to a reflex HR-HPV test. The available evidence shows that HR-HPV testing using Hybrid Capture® 2 assay [Qiagen Gaithersburg, Incorporation, MD, USA (previously Digene Corporation)] technique is a more sensitive screening test than either cytological or colposcopic examination.

Following this test, women who are HPV positive are referred to colposcopy. On the other hand, those who are HR-HPV negative are returned to routine recall. Women whose cervical sample is reported as high-grade dyskaryosis or worse are referred directly for colposcopic examination without being subjected to a HR-HPV test.

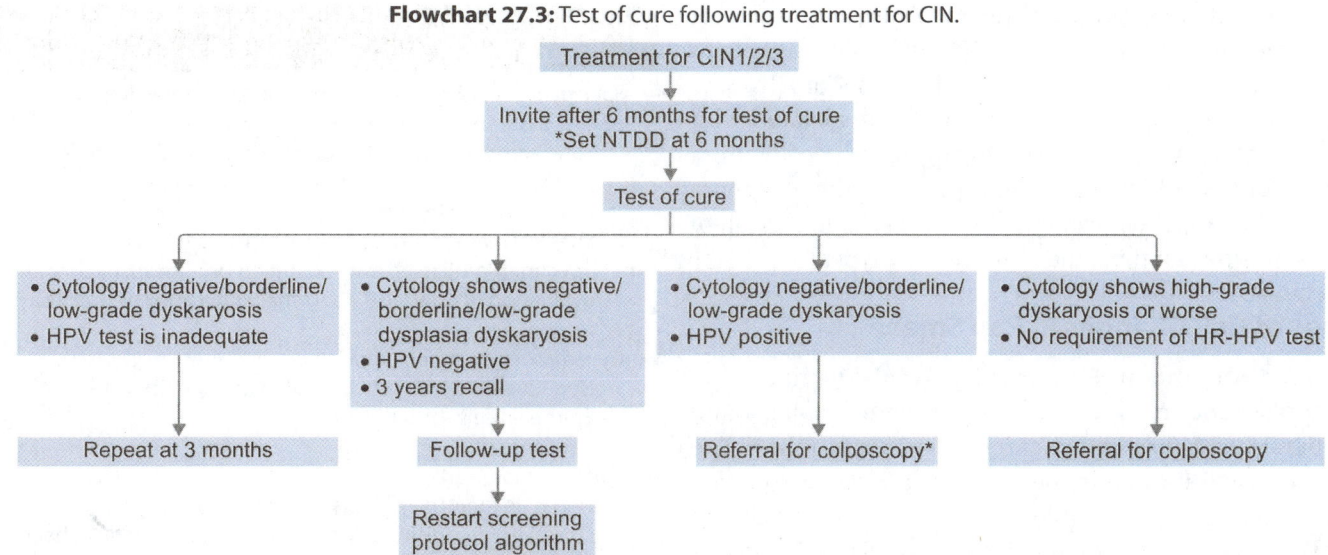

Flowchart 27.3: Test of cure following treatment for CIN.

(CIN: cervical intraepithelial neoplasia; HPV: human papillomavirus; NTDD: next test due date)
*Women who are HR-HPV positive and have borderline/low-grade dyskaryosis or negative cytology are referred back to colposcopy. If colposcopy report is satisfactory or negative, she can be recalled after 3 years.

Introduction of the HPV triage tool has resulted in introducing homogeneity in the referral system of the screening program. This has also helped in reducing the time period of treatment and surveillance from an average of 12 years to 9 months.

Under the HR-HPV "test of cure" protocol, women with all grades of CIN following treatment are invited for screening after 6 months of treatment. During this screening test, women with the findings of borderline change (of squamous or endocervical type), or low-grade dyskaryosis on cytological analysis are subjected to an HR-HPV test. If the HR-HPV test is negative, the woman is recalled for a screening test in 3 years (irrespective of age). She can then be returned to routine recall if the subsequent test result is cytologically negative. Women who are HR-HPV positive are referred back to colposcopy. Women whose cytological analysis reveals high-grade dyskaryosis or worse are referred directly for colposcopic examination without an HR-HPV test.

High-risk HPV as the primary screening test in the cervical cancer screening program is associated with an increased sensitivity and efficacy in comparison with the use of liquid-based cytology (LBC) alone. Also, it helps in increasing the intervals between screening rounds so that the woman may be required to attend the screening tests less frequently. The ARTISTIC trial investigated 24,510 women aged 25–64 years over two screening rounds, approximately 3 years apart (2001–03 and 2004–07) within the NHSCSP in the region of Greater Manchester. The results of this study showed that the primary screening with HR-HPV is likely to detect >90% cases of CIN 2, CIN 3, and invasive cancer. The combination of LBC and additional HR-HPV testing over two screening rounds is likely to be 25% more sensitive than cytology alone for the detection of CIN 3 or CIN 2. It is also 25% more sensitive than LBC in detecting borderline changes. However, in these cases, it is less specific than LBC. The results of the study also showed that the use of HPV testing in a population-based screening program as a primary screening method in combination with the cytology triage served as the most cost-effective method. Primary HR-HPV screening with cytology triage serves as an effective way to classify women > 25 years of age on the basis of their risk for CIN 3+. This is based on the results of the VUSA-screen study (2012) which has shown that HR-HPV positive women with normal cytology are at a lower risk of CIN 3+ in comparison to the HR-HPV positive women with abnormal cytology. On the other hand, negative HR-HPV test offers 50% better protection against the presence of CIN 3 lesions in comparison to negative cytology. HR-HPV, therefore, seems as a feasible alternative to cytological screening. Repeat cytological examination is, however, required after 1 year for HPV-positive women with normal cytology before they can be returned for routine screening. However, routine screening for HPV infection is yet not recommended.

Results of the US Athena study have shown that HPV testing along with separate HPV16 and HPV18 genotype detection serves as an alternative, more sensitive, and efficient strategy for detection of CIN 3+ in comparison to the other screening methods based solely on the cytology. It has also been shown that the reduced specificity of HR-HPV DNA testing can be improved by the addition of HR-HPV genotyping. The POBASCAM (Population Based Screening Study Amsterdam) study has revealed the genotype-specific differences in clearance rates at 6 and 18 months. The lowest clearance rates in women with normal cytology were observed for the genotypes, HPV16, HPV18,

HPV31, and HPV33. Among women who did not clear their HPV infection, persistence of HPV16 infection is likely to be associated with increased detection rates of CIN 3 or greater. Genotyping, therefore, should be associated with an increase in surveillance following referral of women positive for HR-HPV types 16/18. On the other hand, a more conservative approach can be adopted for the follow-up of women positive for the remaining HR-HPV types.

Types of Cell Changes in Pap Smear

According to the WHO, cervical dysplasia has been categorized into mild, moderate, or severe dysplasia and a separate category called carcinoma in situ (CIS). The term "cervical intraepithelial neoplasia" was introduced by Richart (1968). CIN 1 represents mild-to-moderate dysplasia; CIN 2 is an intermediate grade and CIN 3 is severe dysplasia or CIS. However, according to the classification that is the Bethesda System (**Box 27.3**), all cervical epithelial precursor lesions have been divided into two groups: Low-grade squamous intraepithelial lesion (LSIL) and High-grade squamous intraepithelial lesion (HSIL). LSIL corresponds to CIN 1 and HSIL includes CIN 2 and CIN 3. **Figures 27.7A and B** respectively show histopathological changes in case of normal and abnormal Pap smear results. **Figures 27.7C to E** show histopathological changes in case of cervical HPV infection, LSIL, and HSIL, respectively.

Risks Associated with Pap Smear

The risks of cervical cancer screening include the occurrence of false-negative as well as false-positive test results. False-negative test results imply that screening test results may appear to be normal even though cervical cancer is present. This may delay the patient from seeking medical care even if she has symptoms suggestive of cancer. False-positive test results occur when screening test results appear to be abnormal even though no cancer is present. This can cause unnecessary patient anxiety. A false-positive test may be followed by more invasive tests and procedures such as colposcopy, cryotherapy, or loop electrosurgical excision procedure (LEEP), which are associated with their own risks. Also, the long-term effects of these procedures on fertility and pregnancy are not known.

Visual Inspection of Cervix

> **Q.** Write a short essay discussing the methods of visual inspection for screening for cervical cancer.

In areas where facilities for Pap smear screening do not exist, visual inspection with 5% acetic acid (VIA) or visual inspection with Lugol's iodine (VILI) can be done. Application of 5% acetic acid causes dehydration and coagulation of the abnormal areas containing increased

---

BOX 27.3: The Bethesda System (2001) for reporting cervical cytologic diagnoses.

- *Specimen adequacy:* This may be the single most important quality assurance component of the system
  - Satisfactory for evaluation (note presence/absence of endocervical/transformation zone component)
  - Unsatisfactory for evaluation (specify reason)
  - Specimen rejected/not processed (specify reason)
  - Specimen processed and examined but unsatisfactory for evaluation of epithelial abnormality because of specific reason
- *General categorization (optional):*
  - Negative for intraepithelial lesion or malignancy
  - Epithelial cell abnormality
  - Other
- *Interpretation/result:*
  - Negative for intraepithelial lesion or malignancy
  - Observed organisms, such as *Trichomonas, Candida,* bacteria, or cellular changes consistent with herpes simplex virus, are reported
  - Reporting other nonneoplastic findings is optional (i.e., inflammation and atrophy)
- *Epithelial cell abnormalities*
  1. *Squamous cell abnormalities:*
     - Atypical squamous cells (ASC)
     - Atypical squamous cells of undetermined significance (ASCUS)
     - Atypical squamous cells, cannot exclude high-grade squamous intraepithelial lesion
     - Low grade squamous intraepithelial lesion (LSIL), encompassing: human papillomavirus infection/mild dysplasia/cervical intraepithelial neoplasia (CIN 1)
     - High-grade squamous intraepithelial lesion (HSIL), encompassing: Moderate and severe dysplasia, carcinoma in situ (CIS), CIN 2, and CIN 3
     - Squamous cell carcinoma
  2. *Glandular cell abnormalities*:
     - Atypical glandular cells (AGC) (specify endocervical, endometrial, or not otherwise specified)
     - Atypical glandular cells, favor neoplastic (specify endocervical or not otherwise specified)
     - Endocervical adenocarcinoma in situ
     - Adenocarcinoma
- *Others:*
  - List not comprehensive
- Endometrial cells in a woman aged 40 years or older
- Automated review and ancillary testing (include as appropriate)
- Educational notes and suggestions (optional)

---

nuclear material and protein, which turns acetowhite, i.e., opaque and white in appearance (**Figs. 27.8A and B**). The areas of abnormalities can then be biopsied. The dull white plaques with faint borders can be considered as LSIL, while those with sharp borders and thick plaque are suggestive of HSIL. The acetic acid does not affect the mature glycogen producing epithelium. Sometimes instead of acetic acid, Schiller's iodine can be employed. The normal cervical cells contain glycogen, which takes up iodine and turns mahogany brown, while the abnormal area remains unstained (**Figs. 27.9A and B**).

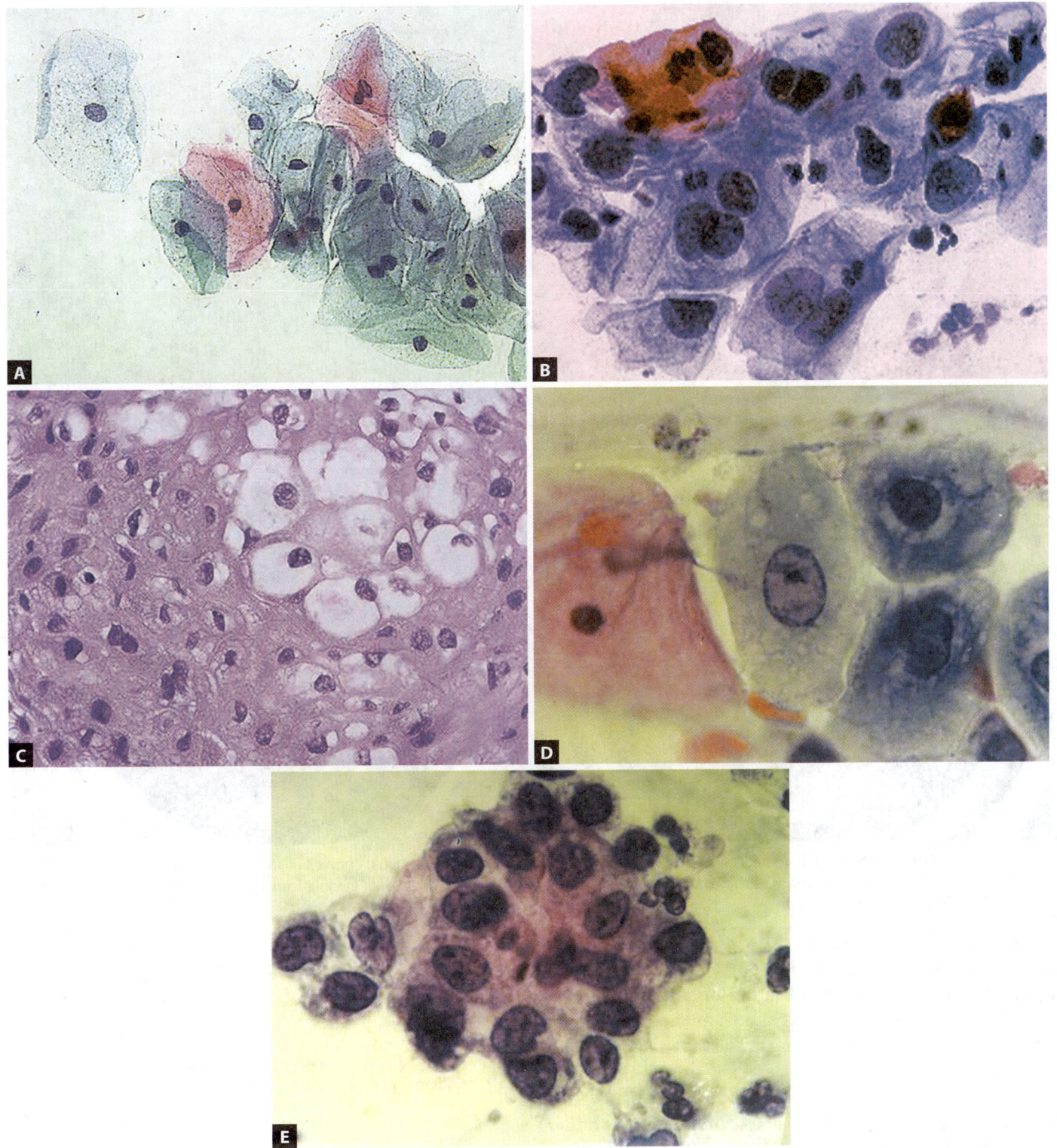

Figs. 27.7A to E: Histopathological appearance. (A) Normal Pap smear result; (B) abnormal Pap smear result; (C) histopathological appearance in case of cervical human papillomavirus infection; (D) histopathological appearance suggestive of low-grade squamous intraepithelial lesion showing hyperchromasia, nuclear irregularities, enlarged pleomorphic nuclei with perinuclear halo; and (E) histopathological appearance suggestive of high-grade squamous intraepithelial lesion showing a marked increase in the nuclear-cytoplasmic ratio, hyperchromasia and irregular nuclear outline.

Liquid-based Cytology in Cervical Screening: A Rapid and Systematic Review

Liquid-based cytology (LBC) is a new way of sampling and preparing cervical cells **(Fig. 27.10)**. While the conventional "Pap smear" involves direct preparation of the slide from the cervical scrape obtained, the procedure of "ThinPrep" involves making a suspension of cells from the sample, which is then used to produce a thin layer of cells on a slide.

606 Abnormalities of the Vagina and Cervix

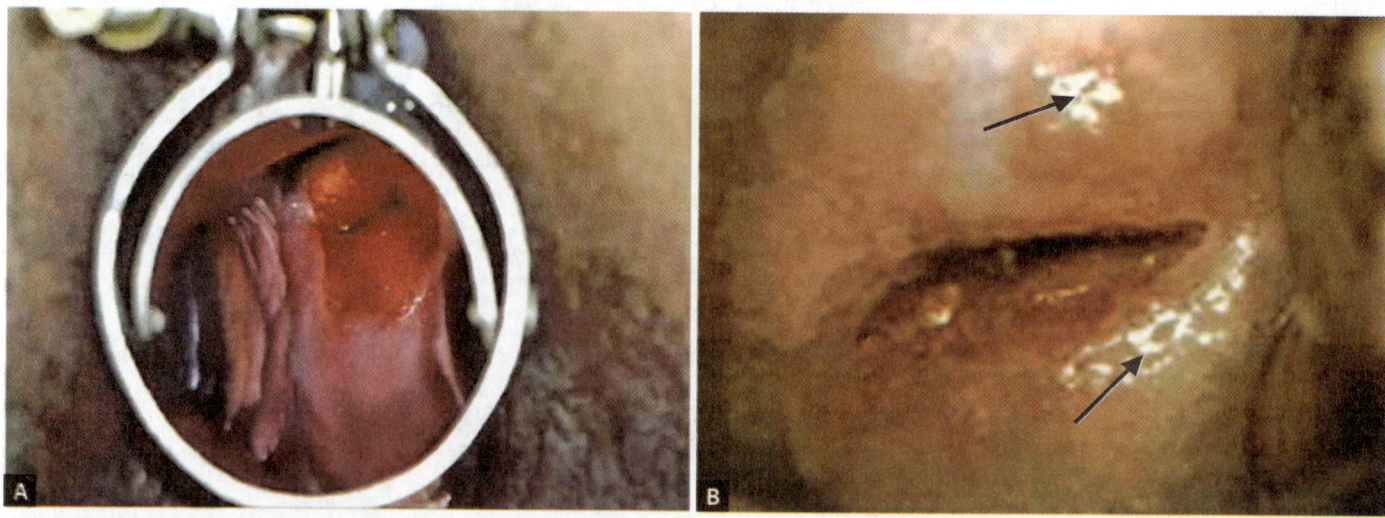

Figs. 27.8A and B: Visual inspection under acetic acid or VIA. (A) Normal cervix after the application of acetic acid; and (B) abnormal cervix following the application of acetic acid (areas of abnormality are indicated by arrows).

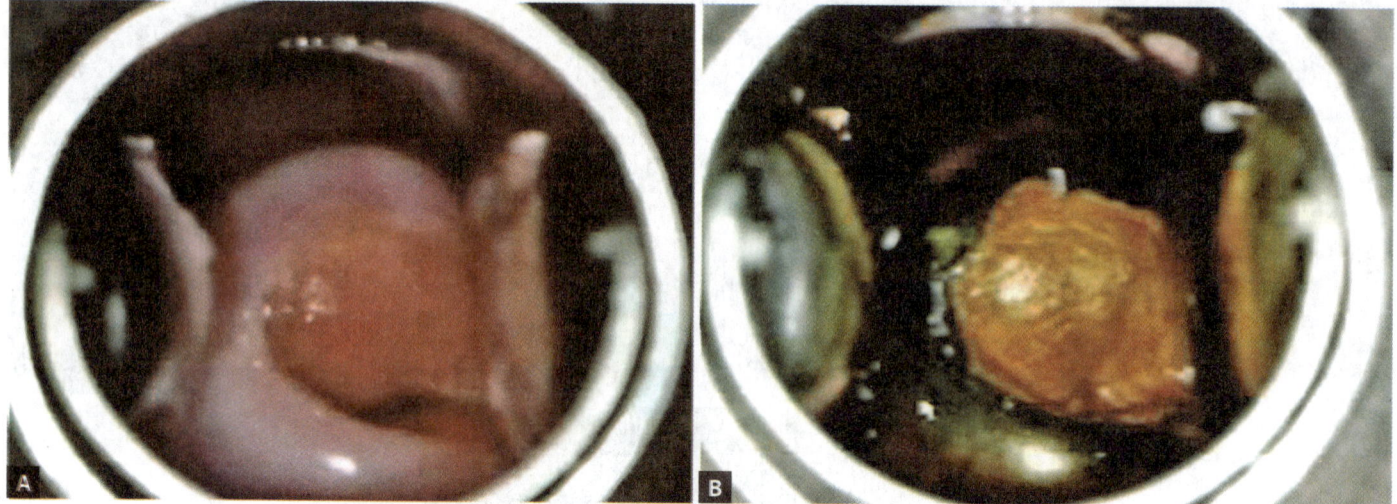

Figs. 27.9A and B: Visual inspection under Lugol's iodine or VILI. (A) Normal cervix before the application of Lugol's iodine; and (B) Normal cervix after the application of Lugol's iodine.

Figures 27.11A and B show the equipment for performing LBC. In this technique, the sample is taken using a plastic spatula, which could either be an endocervical brush or a cervical broom, also known as the Cervex. The figure also shows a vial containing preservative solution into which the endocervical Brush/Cervex is rinsed. Using this technique, the cells collected from the cervix are placed in a preservative fluid, which is then sent to the laboratory rather than being directly spread onto a slide. At the laboratory, the sample is treated to remove unwanted material (blood, mucus, and inflammatory material) and then a thin layer of the cell suspension is placed on the slide for inspection.

Until recently, the Pap smear had remained the principal technology for preventing cervical cancer. However, following a review of the present published literature, liquid-based cytology has now been incorporated within the United Kingdom national screening program. Two systems are presently available, but only one called "the ThinPrep"

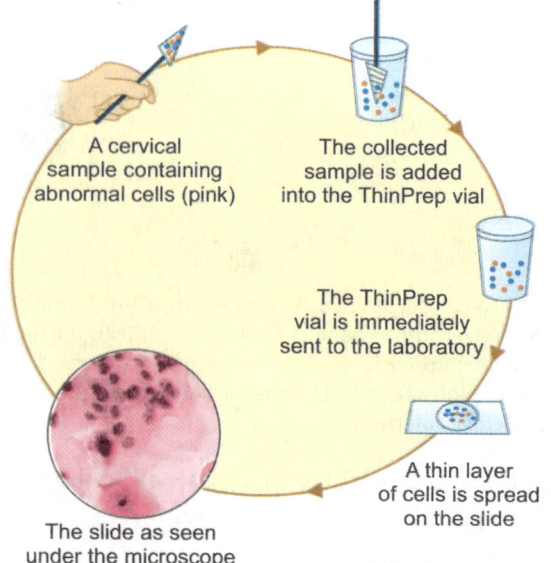

Fig. 27.10: Liquid-based cytology.

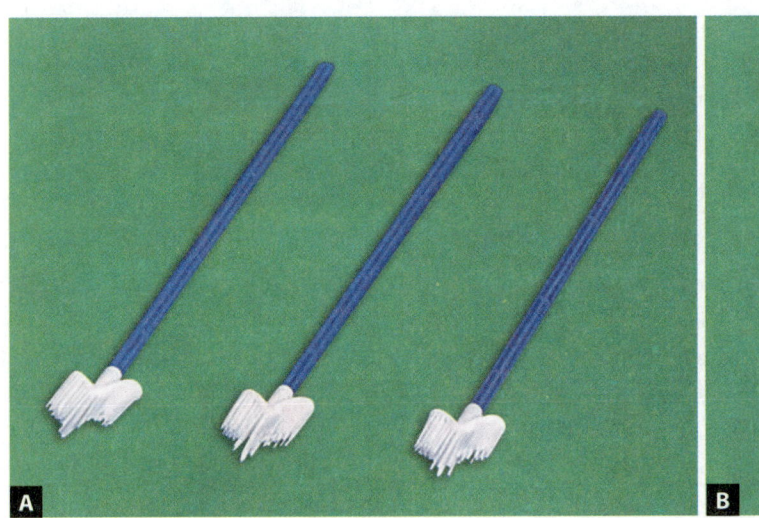
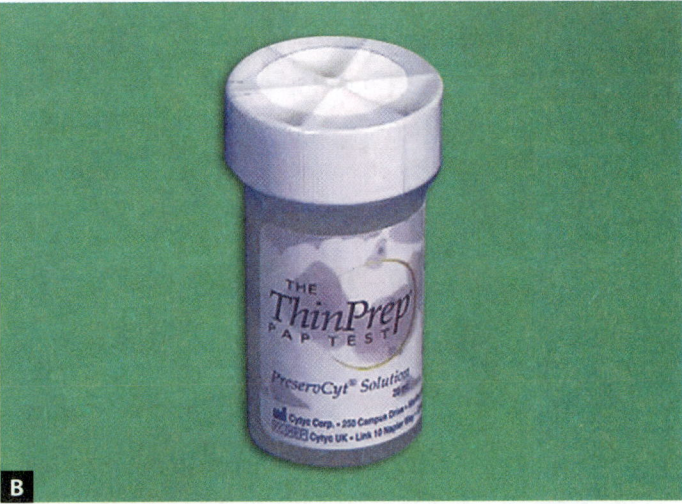

Figs. 27.11A and B: Equipment for liquid-based cytology. (A) Cervex-Brush®; (B) ThinPrep vial.

has been approved by the FDA. There is some evidence that liquid-based cytological methods offer following advantages over traditional smear techniques:

- A reduction in the proportion of inadequate specimens.
- *An improvement in sensitivity rates:* During clinical trials, use of ThinPrep was associated with a reduction in the number of ambiguous interpretations and increased the detection rate of dysplasias by nearly 13%. The use of LBC has mainly helped in reducing the number of inadequate smears from around 9% to around 1%. This has reduced the need to recall women for a repeat smear.
- A possible reduction in specimen interpretation times
- Reduction in the number of false-negative test results by optimizing the collection and preparation of cervical cells.

According to the latest recommendations by the "Screening for cervical cancer: US Preventive Services Task Force" (2012), liquid-based testing has not been shown to significantly improve the accuracy of Pap test in comparison to the conventional cytology testing using a Pap smear.

Colposcopy

If abnormal cells are found in a smear test or LBC, the patient may be referred for a colposcopic examination and/or a colposcopic-directed biopsy. While the Pap smear detects abnormal cells, colposcopy helps in locating the abnormal lesions. A colposcope is like a small microscope with a light and enables the gynecologist to perform a thorough examination of the cervix **(Fig. 27.12)**. **Figures 27.13A and B** show appearance of normal and abnormal blood vessels respectively as observed on colposcopic examination.

Colposcopy is an office-based procedure during which the cervix is examined under illumination and magnification before and after application of dilute acetic acid and Lugol's iodine. The characteristic features of malignancy and premalignancy on colposcopic examination include

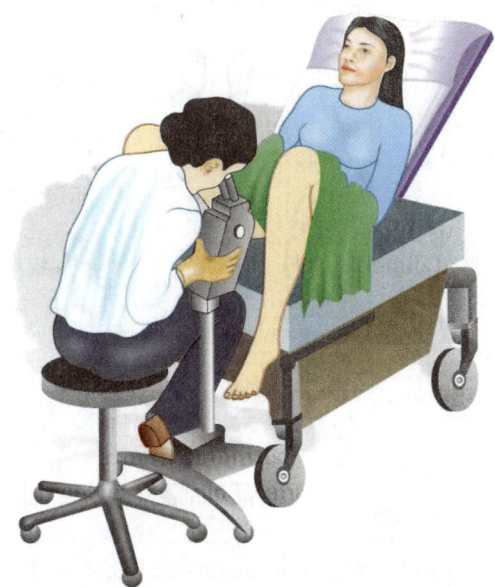

Fig. 27.12: Colposcopic examination.

changes such as acetowhite areas, abnormal vascular patterns, mosaic pattern, punctuation, and failure to uptake iodine stain. Endocervical sampling may accompany colposcopy, particularly in nonpregnant women where the cytology shows AGCs or adenocarcinoma in situ. Satisfactory colposcopy requires visualization of the entire squamocolumnar junction and transformation zone for the presence of any visible lesions. Both a regular white light and a green light are used during colposcopy. The green filter enhances visualization of blood vessels by making them appear darker in contrast to the surrounding epithelium.

The indications for colposcopy are tabulated in **Box 27.4**. The colposcopic examination helps in the following:

- When abnormal cells have been detected on the Pap smear, location and extent of abnormal lesions on the cervix can be assessed with the help of colposcopy.
- Biopsy can be taken from the areas of abnormality.

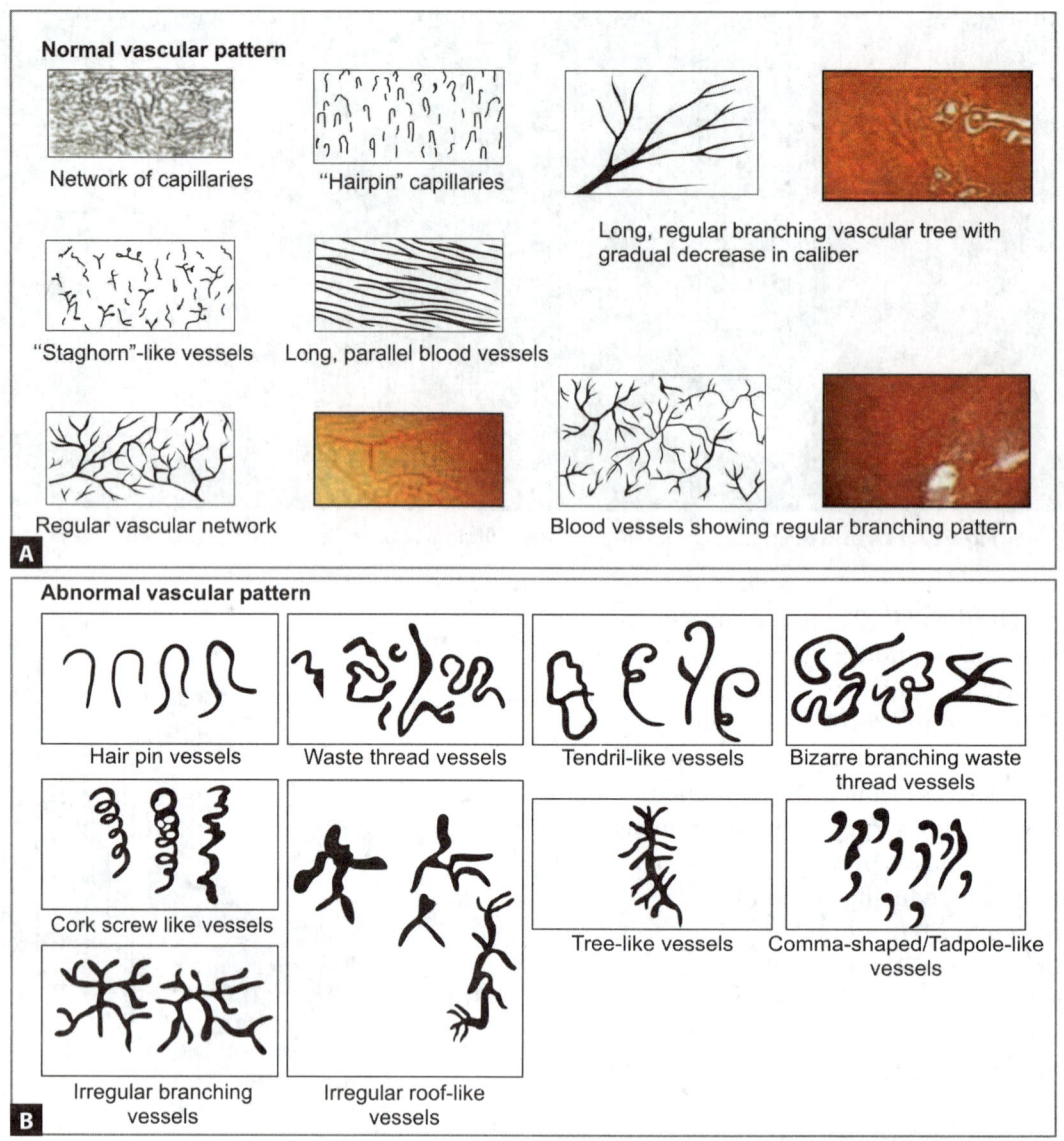

Figs. 27.13A and B: Appearance of blood vessels on colposcopic examination. (A) Normal blood vessels as seen on the surface of cervix; and (B) atypical blood vessel pattern exhibiting bizarre variation in caliber, coarse branching pattern, abnormal proliferation, resulting in nonuniform branching pattern, etc.

- Conservative surgery (e.g., conization) can be performed under colposcopic guidance.
- Colposcopic examination can also be performed during follow-up examination of cases that have undergone conservative therapy.

Procedure

- The patient is placed in the lithotomy position.
- Under all aseptic precautions, a speculum is inserted inside the vagina.
- The colposcope is brought into the position. The perineum, vulva, vagina, and cervix must be examined for presence of lesions using the colposcope's white light and then green light.
- The entire cervix must be viewed both under the low- and high-power magnification. Higher-power magnification helps in visualization of small details and features.

> **BOX 27.4:** Indications for colposcopy.
> - Epithelial cell abnormalities as detected on cervical cytology
> - Presence of high-risk human papillomavirus DNA
> - Suspicious cervical lesions
> - History of in utero diethylstilbestrol exposure
> - Sexual partners of patients with genital tract neoplasia
> - Vulval and vaginal intraepithelial neoplasia
> - Unexplained vaginal bleeding/postcoital bleeding
> - Positive screening test by cervicography/spectroscopy
>
> DNA: deoxyribonucleic acid

- Cervix is visualized after the application of both dilute 5% acetic acid and Lugol's iodine in order to enhance any abnormal epithelial findings. Both acetic acid and Lugol's iodine are applied onto the cervix with the help of a cotton swab and allowed to remain there for at least thirty seconds.

- Under white light, the cervix is visualized for acetowhite changes. The location of the squamocolumnar junction, transformation zone, abnormal and atypical vessels, and areas of acetowhite changes are recorded. On application of Lugol's iodine, the areas of abnormalities such as those with squamous metaplasia, leukoplakia as well as neoplastic tissue do not take up iodine stain and become yellowish in appearance, whereas the normal glycogen containing cervical cells turn deep brown. A scoring system such as "the Reid's Colposcopic Index" **(Table 27.1)** may be used to help the colposcopist in classifying the colposcopic appearance.
- The cervix is reexamined under the green light, which helps in accentuating the margins of the acetowhite areas and in identifying the abnormal blood vessels.

Colposcopic Directed Punch Biopsy (Figs. 27.14A and B)

Following identification of the biopsy site, the cervical punch biopsy forceps are used to obtain the specimen under colposcopic visualization. Specimens are firstly obtained from the most inferior aspect of the cervix to avoid bleeding from the biopsy site and obscuring other biopsy sites. Monsel's paste or silver nitrate can be used to achieve hemostasis after cervical punch biopsy.

The majority of CIN grade I and II lesions regress and aggressive treatment of an adolescent is usually not warranted, because excisional procedures increase the risk of developing cervical stenosis and preterm labor in subsequent pregnancies.

Cervicography

This investigation may be useful when either the procedure of colposcopy or colposcopists are not available for immediate evaluation of the cervix. This procedure involves taking the photograph of the entire cervical os with a 35-mm camera after application of 5% acetic acid. The photographs are then sent to the colposcopist for evaluation in order to select areas for biopsy. Although the sensitivity of colposcopy and cervicography are similar, the specificity of cervicography is much greater than that of colposcopy.

Multimodal Spectroscopy

Multimodal spectroscopy (both reflectance and fluorescence spectroscopies) is the recently discovered technique, which has been found to be useful for early detection of cervical dysplasia. This technology was developed by SpectRx, Inc. Norcross, Georgia, USA. In this technique, light with multiple wavelengths is used for penetrating tissues with different depths. The fluorescence spectrum reveals metabolic changes associated with neoplasia. The reflectance spectrum reveals structural changes associated with neoplasia. This technique is associated with immediate results. This test is an objective one, more accurate than colposcopy and is associated with minimal discomfort. The examination time with this technique is 3–5 minutes versus 20–30 minutes as

TABLE 27.1: Modified Reid's colposcopic index.

Characteristics	Zero point	One point	Two points
Color of acetowhite area	Low-intensity acetowhitening (AW); snow-white, shiny AW; AW beyond the transformation zone	Gray-white AW with shiny surface	Dull, oyster-white or gray AW
Margins and surface configuration of the areas of AW	Lesions with feathered margins; angular jagged lesions; flat lesions with indistinct margins; microcondylomatous or micropapillary surface	Regular lesions with smooth straight outlines	Rolled, peeling edges; internal demarcations (a central area of high-grade change, surrounded by a peripheral area of low-grade change)
Vessels	Fine/uniform vessels, poorly formed patterns of fine punctuations and/ or fine mosaic; presence of vessels beyond the margin of transformation zones; fine vessels with microcondylomatous or micropapillary lesions	Absent vessels	Well-defined coarse punctuation or coarse mosaic pattern; sharply demarcated and randomly and widely placed blood vessels
Iodine staining	Positive iodine uptake showing mahogany brown color Negative uptake of insignificant lesion, i.e., yellow staining by a lesion scoring three points or less on the first three criteria Areas beyond the margin of the transformation zone, conspicuous on colposcopy, evident as iodine-negative areas (such areas are frequently due to parakeratosis)	Partial iodine uptake by a lesion scoring four or more points on the above three categories showing a variegated, speckled appearance	Negative iodine uptake by a significant lesion, i.e., yellow staining by a lesion already scoring four points or more on the first three above-mentioned criteria
Score	0–2: HPV or CIN 1 (low-grade lesions)	3–5: CIN I or CIN II (intermediate-grade lesions)	6–8: CIN II or CIN III (high-grade lesions)

Source: Coppleson M, Dalrymple JC, Atkinson KH. Colposcopic differentiation of abnormalities arising in the transformation zone. Obstet Gynecol Clin North Am. 1993;20(1):83-110.

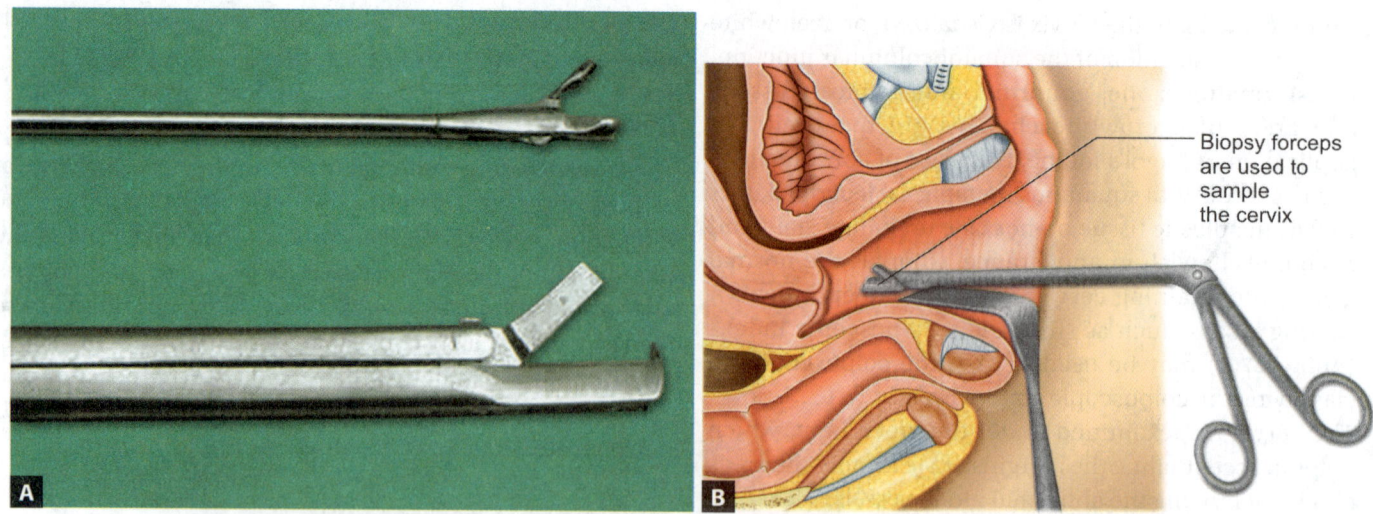

Figs. 27.14A and B: (A) Cervical punch biopsy forceps; and (B) procedure of taking cervical biopsy.

required for colposcopy, thereby resulting in reduced health care costs.

℞ TREATMENT/GYNECOLOGICAL MANAGEMENT

PREVENTION

> Q. Write a long essay on prevention of cervical cancer.
> 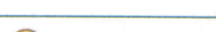 Q. Justify the statement that cervical cancer is a preventable disease.

Cervical cancer is a preventable cancer. There are several levels of prevention which occur:
- *Primordial prevention:* Lifestyle modification and sexual education
- *Primary prevention:* HPV vaccination
- *Secondary prevention:* Screening of preinvasive lesions
- *Tertiary prevention:* Early diagnosis and treatment of preinvasive lesions

Since cervical cancer is a preventable cancer, WHO (2020) has initiated a call for global elimination of cervical cancer. WHO aims to achieve the age-standardized incidence rate (ASIR) <4 per 100,000 women worldwide. The strategy for achieving this target includes the following:
- Achieving full vaccination of 90% girls by the age of 15 years.
- Screening of 70% women using a high-performance test by 45 years of age.
- Treatment of 90% of women identified with cervical disease.

Human Papillomaviruses

Human papillomaviruses are a group of viruses, which contain >100 viruses. Infection with HPV has been considered as one of the most important cause for the development of preinvasive and invasive lesions of the cervix. HPVs infect the stratified squamous epithelium of skin and mucous membranes, where they cause benign lesions, some of which have the potential to progress to invasive cancer. HPV is an epitheliotropic, nonenveloped virus with a proteinaceous coat which encases and protects the viral DNA. The proteinaceous coat is made up of 72 capsomeres composed of major and minor capsid proteins, L1 and L2, respectively. HPV genome (**Fig. 27.15**) is a circular double-stranded DNA, containing 8,000 base-pairs. mRNA is translated into the following proteins: E1, E2, E4, E5, E6, and E7.

While some of these viruses belong to low-risk group and produce wart like, benign growths or papillomas, some types of high-risk HPV have been found to be associated with certain types of cancers, particularly cervical cancer. The presence of the virus may cause morphological abnormalities in the epithelium, including papillomatosis, parakeratosis, and koilocytosis.

Human papillomaviruses are usually transmitted sexually and nearly 40 types of HPV can be sexually transmitted and infect the genital area, including the cervix, vagina, vulva, anus, and penis. Different HPV types and their association with cancer are shown in **Table 27.2**. HPV infections are usually asymptomatic and therefore majority of infections remain unnoticed. Most genital warts are caused by HPV types 6 and 11. Certain high-risk HPV types account for nearly 90% of high-grade intraepithelial lesions and cancer. The IARC (International Agency for Research on Cancer) has described 12 high-risk HPV types (HPV 16, 18, 31, 33, 35, 39, 45, 51, 52, 56, 58, and 59). While infection with low-risk HPV viruses is benign, subclinical, self-limited, and usually regresses spontaneously, persistent cervical infection (infection that lasts for an interval of 6 months or longer) with a high-risk HPV types, especially HPV16 and HPV18, is the most important risk factor for progression to high-grade dysplasia. The HPV types 16 and 18 are most commonly found in association with invasive cancer, CIN 2 and 3 and

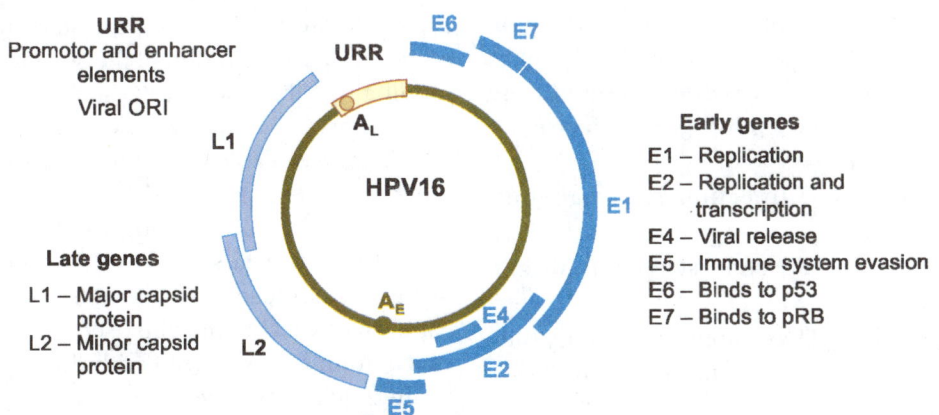

Fig. 27.15: HPV genome.

TABLE 27.2: Human papillomavirus (HPV) types and their association with cancer.

Association with cancer	HPV subtype
High-risk HPV subtypes	HPV types 16, 18, 31, 33, 39, 45, 51, 52, 56, 58, 59, 68, 69, 73, and 82
Probable high risk	HPV types 26, 53, and 66
Intermediate risk	HPV types 30, 31, 33, 39, 51, 52, 58, and 66
Low-risk HPV subtypes	HPV types 6 and 11 (mainly cause genital warts), 40, 42, 43, 44, 54, 61, 70, 72, 81, and CP6108

nearly 47% of women with cancer in all stages. The interval between the acquisition of HPV infection and malignant progression usually takes at least 10 years and is frequently longer. Cervical cancer is, therefore, very uncommon in women under 25 years; the incidence rises progressively for women over 25 years and is highest for women over 40 years.

Human papillomavirus-related cancers occur due to the integration of viral DNA into the cellular DNA and subsequently E6/E7 HPV proteins interact with the cellular tumor suppressor genes, p53, and retinoblastoma genes, thereby prolonging the cell cycle, inhibiting apoptosis and causing malignant transformation and immortalization of cells.

Most of the HPV infections regress on their own. In such cases, there is no cancerous predisposition. However, if the infection persists, it may develop into precancerous or cancerous lesions in future.

Prevention of Human Papillomavirus Infection

Most important way to prevent the occurrence of cervical cancer is to eliminate risk for genital HPV infection by refraining from any genital contact with another individual. For those who want to remain sexually active, a long-term, mutually monogamous relationship with an uninfected partner is the strategy, which is most likely to prevent genital HPV infection. Presently, it is not known whether condoms can provide any protection against HPV infection, because areas not covered by a condom can be infected by HPV.

Human Papillomavirus Vaccination

> Q. With help of a long essay discuss the difference between bivalent and quadrivalent vaccines.

Identification of a viral agent such as HPV as a cause of disease(s) implies that successful prophylactic or therapeutic intervention against the viral agent would be able to prevent the disease(s) it causes. In case of the HPV infection, the vaccine acts as a prophylaxis, for which the HPV-specific neutralizing antibodies (IgA and IgG) are directed against L1/L2 HPV capsid proteins. This helps in preventing the infection of genital mucosa. Vaccines normally have two components:

1. Antigen-specific component to generate immunity specifically against HPV
2. Non-specific component (delivery system), which acts as an adjuvant boosting immune response to specific antigen.

For vaccine preparation, recombinant DNA technology is used for expressing the capsid proteins of HPV, L1 and L2 in the yeast, *Saccharomyces cerevisiae*. These particles self-assemble to form empty shells resembling virus-like particles (VLP). The VLPs have the same outer protein coat as HPV, but no genetic material.

Presently, there are three vaccines available for preventing HPV infection—(1) bivalent Cervarix, (2) quadrivalent Gardasil, and (3) ninevalent Gardasil-9. These are discussed in detail next:

Cervarix®: Cervarix® is a bivalent vaccine that has been developed by GlaxoSmithKline, Middlesex, UK, and gained FDA approval in 2009. This vaccine helps in prevention of high-grade CIN-2/3 and cervical cancer related to HPV types 16 and 18 in girls and women, aged 10–25 years. Besides the HPV types 16 and 18, this vaccine also provides cross-immunity against other high-risk HPV types. It also shows immunogenicity in women, aged 26–55 years. Each dose comprises 20 µg of each, HPV-16 L1 protein and HPV-18 L1 protein. The adjuvant is AS04–monophosphoryl lipid A adsorbed on aluminum hydroxide. This vaccine is

administered via intramuscular route in the deltoid region in three doses, with each dose of 0.5 mL over a 6-month period. The second and third doses are given at 1 month and 6 months after the first dose. The following side effects have been reported with the use of Cervarix:
- *Very common side effects:* Injection site reactions, headache, myalgia, etc.
- *Common side effects:* Gastrointestinal symptoms, rashes, pruritus, itching, etc.
- *Uncommon side effects:* Dizziness, upper respiratory tract infection, induration, paresthesia at the injection site.

Gardasil®-4: Gardasil®-4, a quadrivalent vaccine, developed by Merck & Co., New Jersey, USA, is effective against four strains of HPV (6, 11, 16, and 18). This vaccine has gained approval from the FDA and has been made available in the market since June 2006. Gardasil® has also been approved in the European Union. The vaccine is indicated for women aged 9–26 years and provides protection against high-grade CIN 2/3, cervical cancers, VIN 2/3, and genital warts. Gardasil is also indicated in boys and men between the age of 9 and 26 years for prevention of anal cancer and genital warts. Each dose of Gardasil comprises the following: HPV-6L1 protein (20 µg); HPV-11L1 protein (40 µg); HPV-16L1 protein (40 µg); and HPV-18L1 protein (20 µg). Adjuvant used in this vaccine is AAHS (amorphous aluminum hydroxyphosphate sulfate) Gardasil® is given through a series of three intramuscular injections over a period of 6 months. One dose of 0.5 mL is administered at 0, 2, and 6 months via intramuscular injection in the deltoid or anterolateral thigh. No major adverse effects have been found to be associated with this vaccine, though first day syncope and skin infections (after 2 weeks) have been observed in some patients. Some side effects experienced by the patients include the following:
- *Very common:* Injection site reaction, fever
- *Common:* Bleeding, itching at the site of injection
- *Uncommon:* Urticaria. Bronchospasm, etc.

Gardasil®-9: This is a ninevalent vaccine or nonavaccine, licensed for use since 2014, is not yet available in India. It provides protection against 9 HPV types: 6, 11, 16, 18, 31, 33, 45, 52, and 58. The five additional HPV types included in this vaccine are likely to account for further 15% cases of cervical cancer, thereby resulting in nearly 95% protection. This vaccine is indicated in girls/women between the age of 9 through 45 years and helps provide protection against cervical, vulvar, vaginal, anal, oropharyngeal, other head and neck cancers as well as genital warts. It is also indicated amongst the males between the age of 9 through 45 years and helps provide protection against anal, oropharyngeal, other head and neck cancers, anal precancerous or dysplastic lesions, and genital warts. Gardasil 9 is administered intramuscularly in the dosage of 0.5 mL in the deltoid or anterolateral area of the thigh. For individuals between 9 through 14 years of age, this vaccine can be administered using a two-dose or three-dose schedule. For the two-dose schedule, administration of the second dose should be 6–12 months after the first dose. If the second dose is administered at an interval < 5 months after the first dose, a third dose should be given at least 4 months after the second dose. For the three-dose schedule, Gardasil 9 should be administered at 0, 2 months, and 6 months. For individuals between 15 through 45 years of age, this vaccine is administered using a three-dose schedule at 0, 2 months, and 6 months. Ninevalent vaccine may be used to continue or complete a vaccination series started with other vaccines. If a woman is adequately vaccinated with a bivalent or quadrivalent vaccine, no additional vaccination with a ninevalent vaccine is required.

The high cost of these vaccines has been a cause for concern. Though these vaccines provide protection against the subsequent HPV infection, they do not provide protection against an active infection and cannot be used for treating CIN. HPV infection peaks in early 20s and the cervical cancer occurs in the 40s. Since the vaccines only work if they are administered before HPV infection actually occurs, these vaccines are specifically targeted at girls and women between the ages of 9 and 26 years, before they become sexually active. However, none of these HPV vaccines has been proven to provide complete protection against persistent infection with other HPV types, some of which may cause cervical cancer. Despite this fact, widespread vaccination has the potential to reduce cervical cancer deaths around the world by nearly 70% if all women were to be given this vaccine. There are no major side effects associated with HPV vaccination. Despite receiving HPV vaccination, women who are over the age of 21 years are advised to have a cervical smear test before they are immunized with the vaccine. They would still be required to attend their routine cervical smear test, because there are other types of HPV linked with cervical cancer, which the vaccines are not active against.
- In England as part of the NHS vaccination program, girls and boys who are 12 to 13 years of age are offered routine vaccination with the first dose of first HPV vaccine when they are in the year 8 of school. The second dose is offered 6–24 months following the first dose. Gardasil-4 had been the HPV vaccine previously used in the NHS vaccination program since 2012. However, during the academic year 2021–2022, there has been a switch to Gardasil 9 as the HPV vaccine to be used in the NHS program.
- As per the American Cancer Society, the HPV vaccine is recommended for boys and girls between the age of 9 and 12 years. The vaccine must be administered as soon as possible to the children and young adults, in the age group between 13 through 26 years, who have not been previously vaccinated, or who have not completed their vaccination schedules. As of late 2016, only the ninevalent HPV vaccine is being distributed in the US.
- Screening practices for CIN and cancer should remain unchanged in both vaccinated and unvaccinated women.

Human Papillomavirus Test

Human papillomavirus test is a newer technique, which helps in detecting the presence of HPV infection in the cervix. The HPV test checks directly for genetic material (DNA) of HPV and may be used to determine which women with an ambiguous Pap test result (e.g., ASCUS) are most likely to have underlying precancerous or cancerous changes on their cervix. HPV infection may precede nearly 80% cases of ASCUS and LSIL positive smears in young women. While nearly 80% of such cases are transitory and self-limited and disappear over a year or so, approximately 20% cases may persist and transform to HSIL beyond 30 years of age. Therefore, integration of HPV testing along with cytology screening helps in improving the predictive value of Pap smear and reducing unnecessary colposcopy referrals. Combined HPV testing and Pap smear yields 96% sensitivity as compared to only 60–70% with Pap smear alone. The HPV testing is done either by study of cells in liquid based cytology or endocervical secretion and self-obtained vaginal swab. Though, this test is more sensitive (less likely to produce false negative results), but less specific (more likely to produce false positive results) in comparison to the conventional Pap smear, its role in routine screening is still evolving. Since >99% of invasive cervical cancers worldwide contain HPV, some researchers recommend that HPV testing be done together with routine cervical screening. The routine HPV testing is likely to cause undue alarm to carriers because the prevalence of HPV infection can be as high as 80% among the sexually active population due to high rates of asymptomatic carriers of the infection.

There currently is only one FDA-approved, commercially available test for HPV, the Hybrid Capture, produced by Digene Corporation. The HPV test specifically aims at detecting certain high-risk HPV types, which are known to be associated with cervical cancer. A positive test implies that one of the types of HPV being tested is present and the amount is enough to cause an infection.

Use of Condoms

Though the use of condoms is unlikely to reduce the rates of HPV infection, its use has been found to be useful in preventing potentially precancerous changes in the cervix. Exposure to semen has been found to be associated with an increased risk of precancerous changes, especially CIN 3. Therefore, use of condoms does help in providing some protection.

Nutrition

Fruits, Vegetables, and Antioxidants

Consumption of high amounts of fruits and vegetables (at least five portions) has been found to be associated with a reduced risk of persistent HPV infection. Consumption of high levels of antioxidants, particularly vitamin A, E, and C has also been found to exert a protective role. Higher circulating levels of carotenoids have been found to be associated with a significant decrease in the clearance time of type-specific HPV infection, particularly during the early stages of infection (≤120 days). Another food stuff, which has been observed to exert a protective role in the development of cancer cervix, is folic acid. High levels of folic acid have been found to be inversely related with the risk of developing HPV. Some studies have shown that lower levels of antioxidants coexisting with low levels of folic acid increase the risk of CIN development. Improving folate status in subjects at risk of getting infected or already infected with high-risk HPV may have a beneficial impact in the prevention of cancer. However, presently, the role of various antioxidants and other foodstuffs in cancer prevention is not yet clear as the present evidence regarding the role of folic acid and carotenoids in prevention of cervical carcinoma has largely presented with conflicting results.

TREATMENT OF DYPLASTIC CHANGES

> Q. Write a long essay discussing etiology, pathology, clinical features, diagnosis, and treatment of CIS.
>
> Q. Discuss briefly the diagnosis and treatment of CIS.
>
> Q. Discuss in detail the techniques, advantages, and disadvantages of laser therapy for CIN.

If the smear results are positive, the patient must be followed up with a colposcopy and/or a colposcopic-directed biopsy. In case a preinvasive cervical lesion is detected on colposcopy, the various treatment options, which are available, are as follows:

- *Ablative methods:* Local destructive methods such as cryosurgery, fulguration/electrocoagulation, and laser ablation.
- *Excisional methods:* Excision of the abnormal tissue with cold knife conization, laser conization, LLETZ, LEEP, and needle excision of transformation zone (NETZ).
- *Surgical options:* Surgical options such as therapeutic conization, hysterectomy, or hysterectomy with removal of vaginal cuff if CIS extends to the vaginal vault. HSIL changes have the greatest risk of turning cancerous in the future, thus these need to be definitively treated. The other types of changes may also require further testing, but may not need treatment.

Locally Destructive Methods

Locally destructive/ablative methods are used in the following circumstances:

- There is no evidence of microinvasion or invasive cancer on cytology, colposcopy, endocervical curettage, or biopsy.

- The lesion can be visualized completely and is located on the ectocervix, and there is no involvement of the endocervix.
- The results of colposcopy and biopsy indicate the presence of high-grade cervical dysplasia.

Cryosurgery

Cryosurgery is a locally destructive OPD procedure in which the dysplastic cells are destroyed using freezing agents [CO_2 (–60°C) and nitrous oxide (–80°C)]. The optimal temperature required for effective tissue destruction must be in the range –20°C to –30°C. A cryoprobe is used, usually without any anesthesia or analgesia and causes destruction of the cells by crystallization of intercellular fluid. It uses the "freeze-thaw-freeze" technique in which an ice ball is achieved 5 mm beyond the edge of the probe. The cryoprobe is applied over the area of abnormality for over 9 minutes and destroys the tissue up to the depth of about 4–5 mm. The time required for the procedure is related to the pressure of gas. The higher the pressure of gas, faster is the rate of ice ball formation. Overall, cryosurgery is a relatively safe procedure with fewer complications.

Electrocoagulation

Electrocoagulation is a locally destructive procedure in which the dysplastic cells are destroyed using temperature over 700°C. The procedure is quite painful and is therefore usually performed under general anesthesia. The abnormal tissues are destroyed up to the depth of about 8–10 mm. This procedure can be associated with numerous complications including recurrence of the lesions, bleeding, sepsis, cervical stenosis, and indrawing of the squamocolumnar junction within the cervical canal.

Laser Ablation

Laser ablation is a locally destructive OPD procedure, usually done under local anesthesia, which uses laser energy to destroy the dysplastic cells by boiling, steaming, and exploding the cells. The extensive heat energy liberated causes incineration of the protein and mineral content of the tissues, resulting in a charred appearance at the base of exposed area. The main advantage of this method is that the tissue can be ablated up to the depth of about 7 mm, which is the location of the deepest endocervical gland. Thus, laser ablation can be used in lesions with extensive glandular involvement. The other advantages of laser ablation are that it is associated with minimal bleeding, no infection, minimal postlaser scar formation and does not cause indrawing of the squamocolumnar junction. It is also associated with a rapid post-treatment healing phase.

Excision of the Abnormal Tissue

The advantage of various excisional methods over the locally destructive methods is that the piece of cervical tissue that is removed can be sent for histopathological examination.

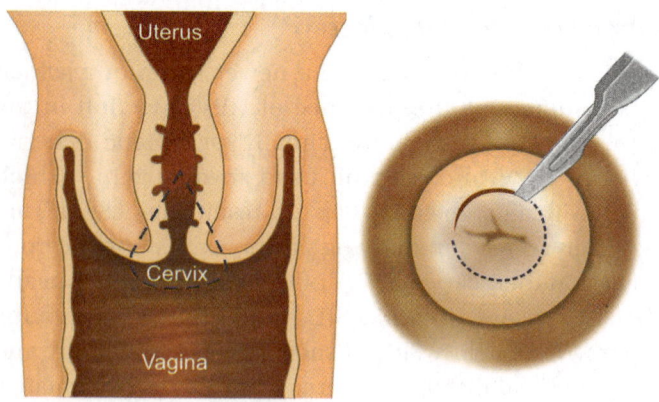

Fig. 27.16: Cone biopsy.

Cone Biopsy

Cone biopsy serves as both a diagnostic and therapeutic procedure. The procedure involves the removal of the entire area of abnormality **(Fig. 27.16)**. It is capable of providing tissue for histopathological examination. The cone biopsy may be performed under general or local anesthesia. This method involves obtaining a wide cone of excision including the entire outer margin of the lesion and the entire endocervical lining. Indications for cone biopsy are as follows:

- The area of the abnormality is large, or its inner margin has receded into the cervical canal.
- The limits of the lesion cannot be visualized by colposcopy.
- The squamocolumnar junction is not completely observable on colposcopy.
- There is discrepancy between the findings of cytology and colposcopy.
- There is a suspicion of microinvasion based on the results of biopsy, colposcopy, or cytology.
- The findings of endocervical curettage are positive for CIN 2 or CIN 3.
- Colposcopist is unable to rule out invasive cancer.

Cold-knife Conization

This procedure is performed with help of a scalpel under anesthesia (either regional or general) and comprises the following steps:

- The patient is placed in dorsal lithotomy position.
- A colposcopic examination may be performed prior to the procedure, and the area of transformation zone may be demarcated using Lugol's iodine or 3–5% acetic acid.
- Under all aseptic precautions, the anterior lip of the cervix may be grasped with help of a single tooth tenaculum.
- A vasoconstrictor solution (vasopressin (0.5 U/mL) or 1:200,000 epinephrine solution) may be injected into the cervix at this time in order to reduce intraoperative blood loss, thereby improving the exposure at the time of surgery.

- A circumferential incision is made just lateral to the outer limit of the transformation zone, usually starting from the posterior side, using a long-handled scalpel with a No. 11 blade **(Fig. 27.17)**. The desired circular incision is made in the region surrounding the endocervical canal using a slight sawing motion, preferably including the entire transformation zone and/or the area of abnormality by inserting the scalpel blade to the desired depth, in the direction slightly toward the endocervical canal. Mayo's scissors can be used to complete and deepen the incision.
- Following excision, the cone bed can be sutured using the modified Sturmdorf type sutures **(Fig. 27.18)**. A rolled gauze pack soaked in ferric subsulfate solution can be placed inside the cervical canal to reduce the amount of bleeding. This pack must be removed by the patient within 12–24 hours.

Laser Excision

This method employs the use of laser energy for obtaining the cone biopsy. In this method, with the help of a colposcope, the margin around the outer limit of the transformation zone may be marked by making a series of dots using carbon dioxide laser **(Fig. 27.19)**. The incision is deepened circumferentially by passing the laser beam progressively across the tissues. The planned outer margin of the cone is circumferentially deepened to the extent depending on the amount of exposure. This is done with a smaller spot size (0.5–1 mm) and a high power density (1,000–1,500 watts/cm^2).

As an alternative technique, the surgeon may plan ablation after marking the outer and inner margins of the planned area of ablation and dividing it into quadrants **(Fig. 27.20)**. Starting from the posterior side, each quadrant is vaporized to a depth of 5–7 mm using a power density of 500–1,000 watts/cm^2.

Large Loop Excision of the Transformation Zone

LLETZ stands for "large loop excision of the transformation zone". In the USA, this procedure is called LEEP—loop electrosurgical excision procedure. This method basically uses low voltage diathermy (30–40 watts) and may be given at the same time as colposcopy. In this procedure, the loop of wire is advanced into the cervix lateral to the lesion until the required depth is reached. The loop is then taken across to the opposite side and a cone of tissue is removed. The area of abnormal cells is removed completely using a loop of wire and electrosurgery **(Fig. 27.21)**. Endocervical curettage is performed following completion of excision. It is an outpatient treatment and is usually performed under local anesthesia. If a large area of tissue needs to be removed, or if the patient is very anxious about the treatment, the surgery may also be performed under general anesthesia.

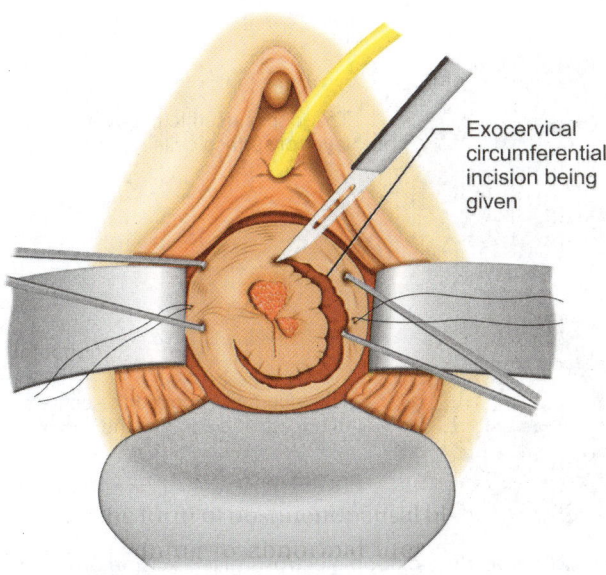

Fig. 27.17: Making a circular incision over the exocervix at the time of cone biopsy.

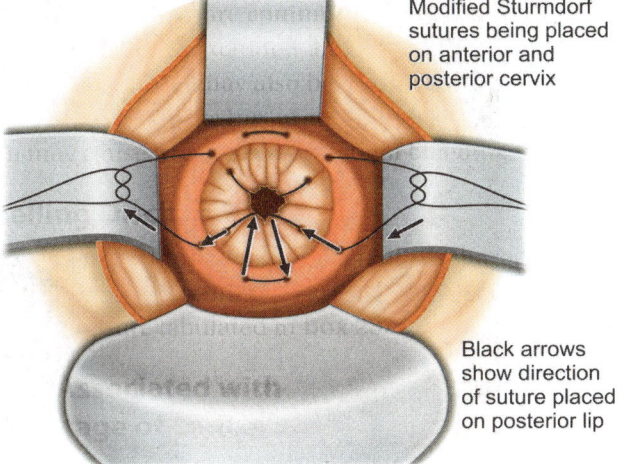
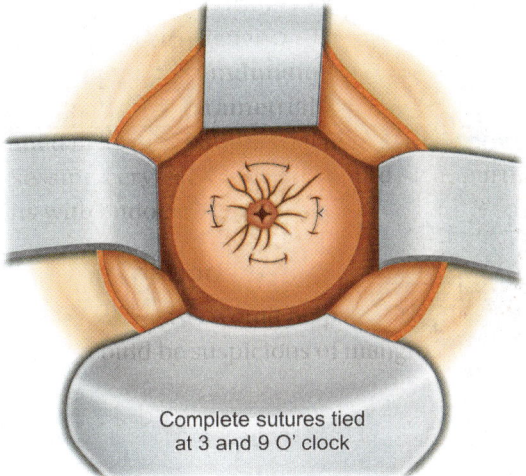

Fig. 27.18: Application of Sturmdorf sutures following cold-knife conization.

616 Abnormalities of the Vagina and Cervix

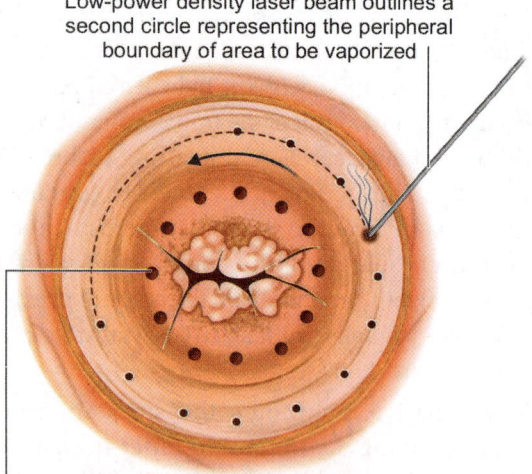

Fig. 27.19: Marking surgical boundaries for laser cervical conization with the help of circle of dots.

Loop Electrosurgical Excision Procedure

In this procedure, a thin wire loop that carries an electric current is used to remove abnormal areas of the cervix **(Figs. 27.22A and B)**. The excised area of the cervix removed is sent to the laboratory for histopathological examination. This electric energy is also used to coagulate the blood vessels on the surface of the cervix. LEEP is even simpler than LLETZ and is applicable anywhere in the lower genital tract whereas LLETZ is applicable only to the cervix.

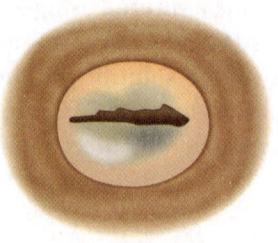
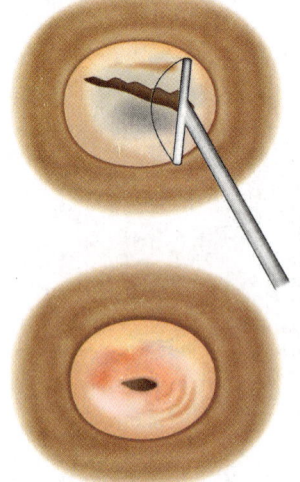

Fig. 27.22A: Procedure of loop electrosurgical excision procedure.

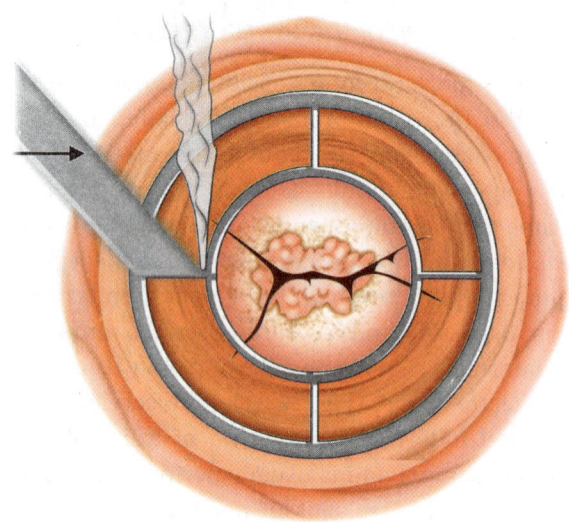

Fig. 27.20: Laser vaporization of the cervix in which the areas planned for vaporization-conization are marked according to quadrants. Each quadrant is vaporized at a time.

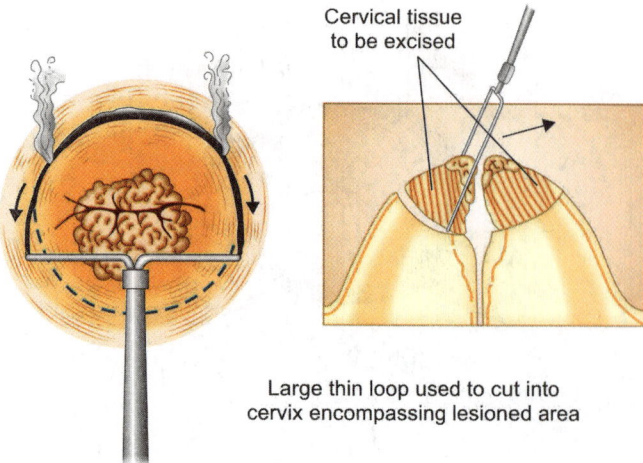

Fig. 27.21: Large loop excision of the transformation zone.

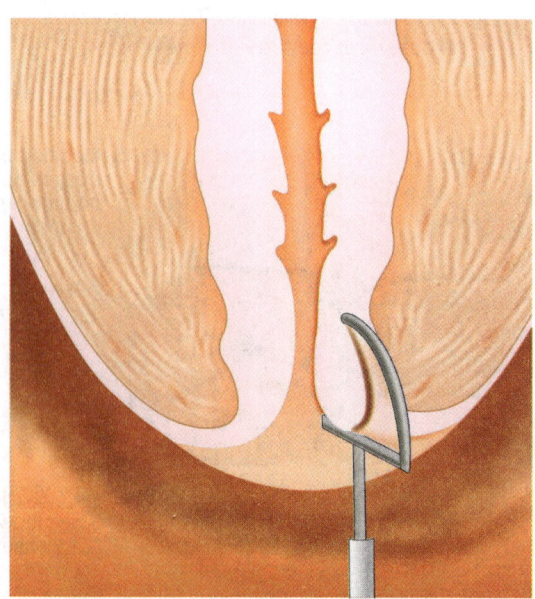

Fig. 27.22B: Procedure of loop electrosurgical excision procedure (magnified view).

Surgical Options

These include therapeutic conization, hysterectomy, or hysterectomy with removal of vaginal cuff.

Therapeutic Conization

The procedure of conization not only provides tissue for histopathological study but can also serve as a therapeutic procedure. Conization includes the entire outer margin of the cervix and endocervical lining, short of internal os. A smaller cone may be desirable in young women as it helps in avoiding complications such as abortion or preterm labor. Complications associated with the procedure include bleeding, sepsis, cervical stenosis, abortion, and preterm labor. Conization may also be done in cases of endocervical dysplasia, when transformation zone cannot be completely visualized or when there is discrepancy in findings between the findings of cytology, colposcopy, and biopsy.

Hysterectomy

Hysterectomy is considered as the treatment of last resort in cases of recurrent high-grade CIN. Hysterectomy may serve as an appropriate option in older and parous women who have attained menopause or those who have completed their families. Hysterectomy can also be performed when it appears that the woman would not be able to comply with the follow-up, recurrence occurs following conservative therapy, if microinvasion exists or if the dysplastic changes are associated with the presence of other pathologies such as fibroids, dysfunctional uterine bleeding (DUB), or uterine prolapse.

Follow-up after Therapy

An abnormal smear must be followed with a repeat smear about 6 months after treatment and then a further smear after about 12 months. Following this, a repeat smear is performed 1 year later in case of CIN 1. In case of CIN 2 or 3, yearly smears are carried out for 9 more years. After that, the frequency is changed to 3 or 5 yearly smears (depending on the patient's age). If the patient has undergone hysterectomy for cervical dysplasia, vault smears are required at 6 months and 1 year after hysterectomy. If these smears are normal, there would be no future requirement for smears.

Treatment of CIN 1

Mild dysplasia (LSIL) is usually due to infection, which should be treated and cytology follow-up done every 3–6 months. Indications for treatment of LSIL are listed in **Box 27.5**.

Expectant Management

Expectant management may be used in patients with biopsy proven CIN 1 with satisfactory colposcopy results. This option must be used only in the patients, who appear compliant

> **BOX 27.5:** Indications for treatment of low-grade squamous intraepithelial lesion (LSIL).
>
> - Persistent LSIL (CIN 1) over 1 year
> - Patient showing poor compliance for follow-up
> - Associated human papillomavirus and human immunodeficiency viral infection

and agree for regular follow-up visits. The patients receiving expectant management must agree for evaluation with Pap smear every at 6 and 12 months. An alternative to Pap testing is HPV DNA testing to be performed at 12 months.

Treatment of CIN 2 and CIN 3

Though the various ablative and excisional procedures can be used as a treatment option for CIN 2 and CIN 3, the preferred treatment option for CIN 2 and CIN 3 is LEEP. Most of the ablative and excisional procedures described previously can be performed on an OPD basis. Since these various therapeutic procedures are associated with a recurrence rate of up to 10%, regular surveillance with cytology or colposcopy is required at 6 months interval. Alternatively, high-risk HPV testing at 6–12 months may be required. Surveillance is continued until two consecutive normal results are obtained. In case any abnormal result is obtained on cytological examination or HPV DNA testing, this must be followed-up by colposcopy.

COMPLICATIONS

PROGRESSION TO INVASIVE CANCER

The main complication of dysplastic cervical changes is progression to cervical cancer if the condition is left untreated.

PROCEDURAL COMPLICATIONS

Complications resulting from cone biopsy are as follows:

Intraoperative and Postoperative Bleeding

Major intraoperative complications rarely occur during cone biopsy. Bleeding may be sometimes heavy and conservative measures (e.g., application of sutures, use of cautery, and application of ferric subsulfate paste) are usually helpful in these cases for controlling hemorrhage. The surgeon may be seldom required to resort to more invasive procedures such as application of a cerclage type stitch, internal iliac artery embolization, or ligation, or hysterectomy in case the bleeding becomes very severe.

Uterine Perforation

Uterine perforation is a rare complication, which is more likely to occur in cases when the uterus is acutely anteflexed or atrophied (postmenopausal women). Extension of the perforation in lateral direction may result in laceration of the uterine artery. In uncommon circumstances, injuries such as broad ligament hematoma or laceration of the bladder and rectum may occur. In these cases, laparoscopy or even laparotomy may be required for management.

Postoperative Bleeding

Bleeding shortly after surgery may be due to inadequate intraoperative hemostasis or a result of vasodilation due to the wearing off of the effect of the vasoconstrictor solution. Delayed hemorrhage may occur 1–2 weeks after surgery and may be due to dissolution of sutures or erosion of a blood vessel during the healing process. This bleeding can be controlled with the help of conservative measures (previously described) or uterine packing. Occasionally, surgical hemostasis under anesthesia may be required.

Infection

Infection occurs rarely if the procedure is performed observing aseptic surgical precautions. Prophylactic antibiotics are usually not required prior to the procedure. However, antibiotics may be prescribed following the procedure if the clinician suspects a risk of infection or in high-risk cases (e.g., history of gonorrhea, pelvic inflammatory disease, etc.). The infection may manifest in many ways, including local cervical inflammation, endometritis, parametritis, salpingitis, pelvic abscess, etc.

Reproductive Effects of Treatment

- Cervical surgery involves removal or destruction of tissue, which may produce many adverse results, thereby affecting the reproductive outcomes. Some of the adverse reproductive outcomes which may occur following the surgical procedures are as follows:
  - *Infertility:* Refer to **Box 27.6** for the likely causes of infertility in these cases.
  - *Second trimester pregnancy loss:* Previous history of cervical conization is associated with an increased risk of second trimester pregnancy loss.

> **BOX 27.6:** Causes of adverse reproductive outcomes in cases of cervical surgery.
>
> - *Alteration of cervical mucus:* Removal of cervical glands may undesirably affect fertility by changing the cervical mucus, which is required for normal sperm migration and sustainability
> - *Premature dilatation of cervix:* Removal or destruction of a large portion of the collagen matrix that forms the cervical stroma may decrease the tensile strength, thereby causing the cervix to dilate prematurely during pregnancy
> - *Increased risk of ascending infection:* Removal of tissue and loss of cervical glands and cervical mucus may theoretically increase the risk of ascending infection
> - *Loss of cervical plasticity:* This may make the membranes more vulnerable to rupture, thereby resulting in preterm premature rupture of membranes
> - *Cervical stenosis:* Scarring from cervical surgery may result in cervical stenosis. This may cause difficulty in cervical dilatation during labor, which may partially or completely obstruct the uterine cavity, interfering with the menstrual flow. In severe cases, hematometra or pyometra can occur. In pregnant women with cervical stenosis, the cervix may fail to dilate normally during labor

- *Preterm premature rupture of membranes:* The risk of preterm premature rupture of membranes may be increased in some women undergoing CIN treatment procedures.
- *Preterm delivery and perinatal mortality:* Preterm premature rupture of membranes associated with various treatment procedures for CIN may result in increased risk for preterm delivery and increased perinatal mortality.
- *Late complications:* Late complications of conization may include complications such as cervical insufficiency and cervical stenosis.

EVIDENCE-BASED CLINICAL TRIALS

List of references can be scanned through QR code to enable the readers gain deeper insight of the subject by referring to the entire article or its abstract.

CHAPTER 28

Cancer Cervix (Postcoital Bleeding)

CASE STUDY

A 62-year-old para 4 woman presented with the complaints of postcoital bleeding since past 2 months. She had been getting regular Papanicolaou (Pap) smear examinations done in the past. The last smear done 1 year back had shown normal pathology. During this visit, a repeat Pap smear was performed which was found to be within normal limits. After ruling out other likely causes of postcoital bleeding in this case, and detecting no significant finding on clinical examination, colposcopic examination was performed. Colposcopy revealed a lesion on the anterior surface of the ectocervix, showing irregular mosaic pattern, surface irregularity, and atypical blood vessel pattern after application of 5% acetic acid. A colposcopic-directed biopsy confirmed the diagnosis of squamous cell carcinoma. Based on clinical staging, the disease was assigned to be stage IA1 (FIGO staging system).

INTRODUCTION

 Q. Discuss the current status of cervical cancer in India and principles of its management.

 Q. Briefly discuss the pathology of cervical cancer.

As per WHO, in the year 2018, an estimated 600,000 women were diagnosed with cervical cancer worldwide. Of these nearly one-fifth cases are contributed by India. Nearly 90% cases of cervical cancer are encountered amongst women belonging to the lower socioeconomic groups.

Cervical cancer can be considered as the fourth most common cancer amongst women. These statistics reflect the global estimates for cervical cancer in the developed countries. In the developing countries, where women do not have access to cervical cancer screening and prevention programs, cervical cancer remains the second most common type of cancer. In India, presently breast cancer has surpassed cervical cancer and has become the most common cancer amongst the women, the second common malignancy being cervical cancer. Cervical cancer can be considered as the most common gynecological malignancy amongst women in India. Cancer of the cervix involves the squamous epithelium of cervix (**Figs. 28.1A and B**), and typically begins at the transformation zone between the ectocervix and endocervix (**Fig. 28.2**). The cervix is the lowermost, narrow, portion of the uterus, which is joined with the upper portion of the vagina. It is anatomically composed of two parts—(1) ectocervix and (2) endocervix. The part of the cervix projecting into the vagina is known as the portio vaginalis or ectocervix, whereas the region of the cervix opening into the uterine cavity is known as the endocervix. The opening of ectocervix inside the vagina is known as the external cervical os, while the opening of the cervix inside the uterine cavity is known as the internal cervical os. The endocervical canal extends between the internal and the external cervical os. The ectocervix is lined by squamous cells, while endocervical cells are mainly of the columnar type. The transformation zone lies at the junction of ectocervix and endocervix. Columnar cells are constantly changing into squamous cells in the transformation zone. Since cells in the transformation zone are constantly changing, this is the most common place for cervical malignancy to develop. Diagrammatic representation of cervical cancer in early stages (stage I and II is shown in **Figure 28.3**).

Mortality due to cervical cancer generally increases with the woman's age, with the highest number of deaths occurring in women in their late seventies. Women who are infected with high-risk human papillomavirus (HPV), genital subtypes are associated with an increased risk of malignant transformation. Widespread use of the Pap smear has dramatically reduced the incidence of cervical cancer in developed countries. As a result, cervical cancer has become relatively uncommon in developed countries having intensive cytologic screening programs. Since, the advent and widespread use of Pap smears, which helps in early detection of preinvasive cervical lesions at an early stage, the incidence of cervical cancer has dramatically decreased in the developed world. However, in many parts of the developing world, cervical cancer continues to cause

Abnormalities of the Vagina and Cervix

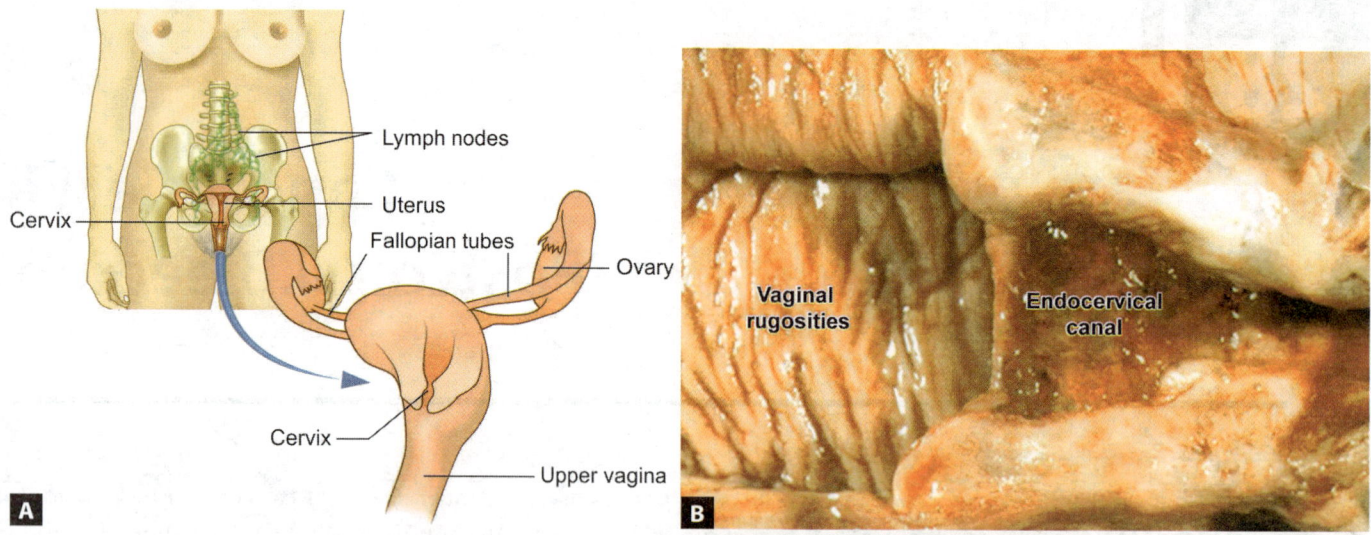

Figs. 28.1A and B: (A) Anatomical location of cervix; (B) Cervical morphology at the region of external cervical os.

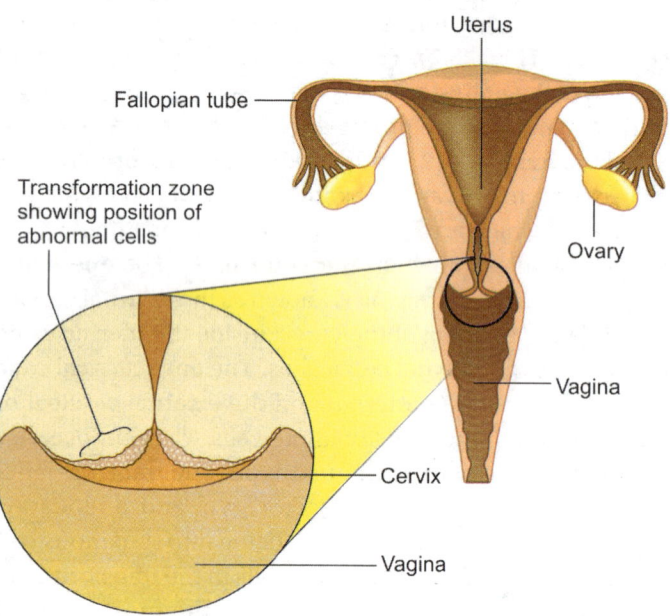

Fig. 28.2: Transformation zone.

significant morbidity and mortality. The various types of malignant tumors in the cervix are enlisted in **Table 28.1**. Out of these, the most common types of cancer in the cervix is squamous cell carcinoma **(Fig. 28.4)**, which is responsible for nearly 80% cases of cancer. Squamous cell carcinoma develops from the cells of ectocervix. **Figures 28.5A and B** show specimen of cervical cancer. The next common type of cancer is adenocarcinoma, which develops from the glandular cells in the endocervical canal.

HISTORY AND CLINICAL PRESENTATION

The factors which are associated with an increased risk of cervical cancer and need to be elicited at the time of taking history include the following.

RISK FACTORS

Q. Enumerate the risk factors and discuss in detail the downstaging and magnitude of cervical cancers in India.

Age

Cancer of the cervix can occur at any age. It is found most often in women older than 40 years, but can occur in younger women. However, it rarely occurs in women younger than 21 years. The average age for occurrence of carcinoma cervix is 47 years. The distribution of cases of cervical cancer is usually bimodal with the peak occurring at two points, first between 35 and 39 years and second between 60 and 64 years of age.

Obstetric History

Women who give birth to babies at young age, particularly the women who have their first delivery before the age of 20 years are at an increased risk. Multiparous women with poor spacing between pregnancies are also at an increased risk.

Sexual History

The factors which are associated with an increased risk of cervical cancer and need to be elicited at the time of taking sexual history include the following:
- Promiscuity or history of having multiple sexual partners.
- History of having a male sexual partner who has had sexual intercourse with more than one person (the more partners the person has, the greater is the risk).
- Young age (<18) at the time of first sexual intercourse
- Having a male sexual partner who has had a sexual partner with cervical cancer. These factors can increase the woman's risk for developing cancer of the cervix,

Cancer Cervix (Postcoital Bleeding)

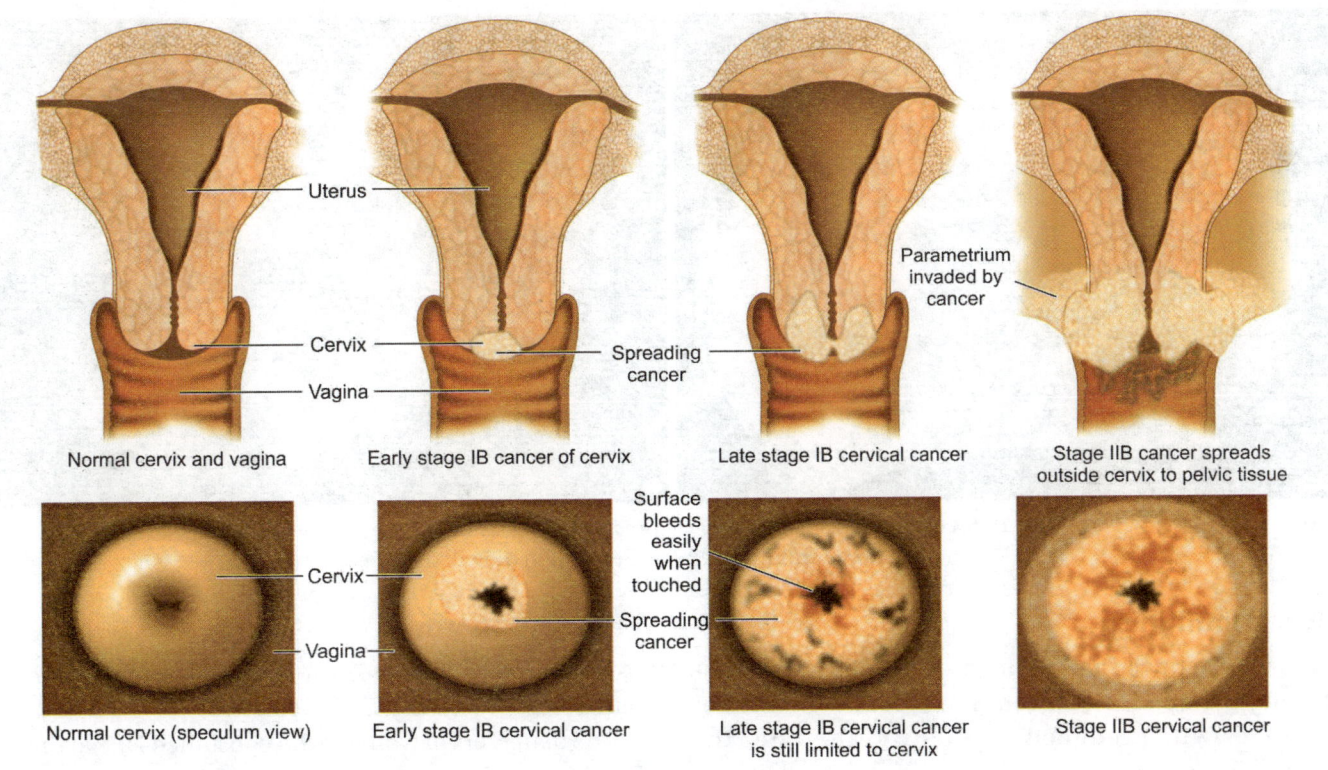

Fig. 28.3: Diagrammatic representation of cervical cancer.

TABLE 28.1: Malignant tumors of the cervix.	
Tumors of the epithelium	**Nonepithelial cell tumors**
Squamous cell carcinoma	Tumors of mesenchymal tissue
• Large cell nonkeratinizing • Large cell keratinizing • Small cell • Verrucous carcinoma	• Endocervical stromal sarcoma • Carcinosarcoma • Adenosarcoma • Leiomyosarcoma • Embryonal rhabdomyosarcoma
Adenocarcinoma	Others
• Common pattern • Adenoma malignum • Mucinous • Papillary • Adenoid cystic • Adenosquamous carcinoma	• Metastatic • Lymphoma • Melanoma • Carcinoid
Endometrioid cancer	
Clear cell	
Stem cell carcinoma	

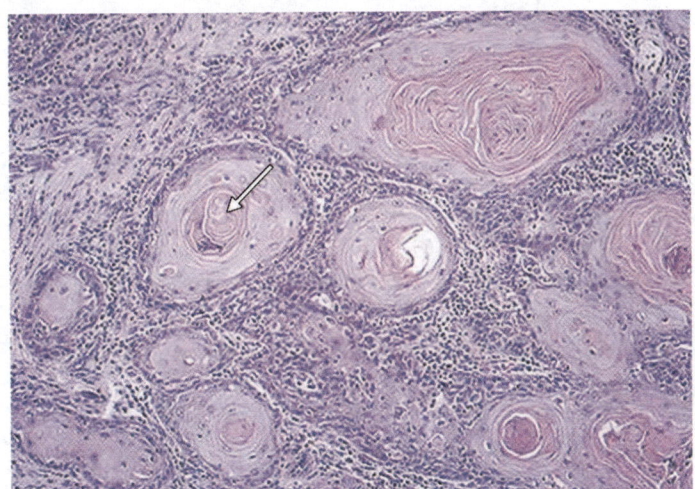

Fig. 28.4: Histopathological appearance of squamous cell carcinoma showing presence of keratin pearls (indicated by arrow).

- *Infection with HPV:* The initiating event in cervical dysplasia and carcinogenesis is infection with HPV. There are 100 different types of HPV, out of which nearly 14 are the high-risk types. Of these, type 16 and 18 are most commonly found in cases of squamous cell carcinoma.

Personal History

- Smoking is associated with an increased risk for development of cancer of cervix.
- Women who do not come for regular health checkups and Pap tests are at an increased risk.

because they increase the chances of acquiring HPV infection, which can lead to dysplasia.
- Women who have had sexually transmitted diseases in the past including the diseases like HIV infection, herpes simplex 2 virus infection, and HPV infection are also at an increased risk of developing cancer of the cervix.

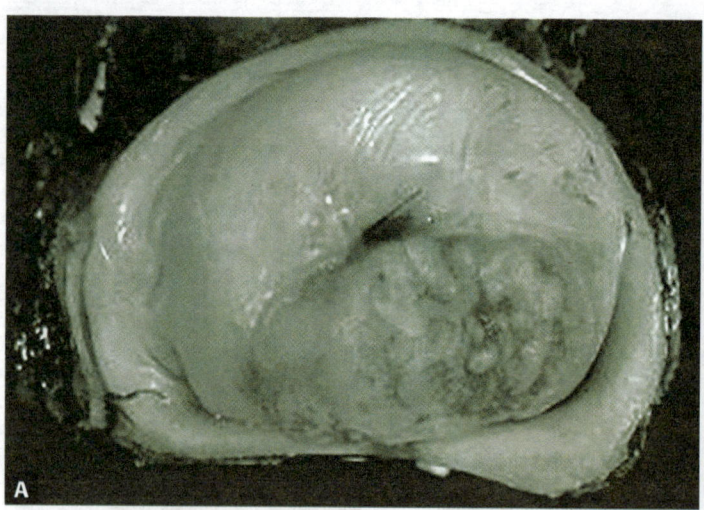 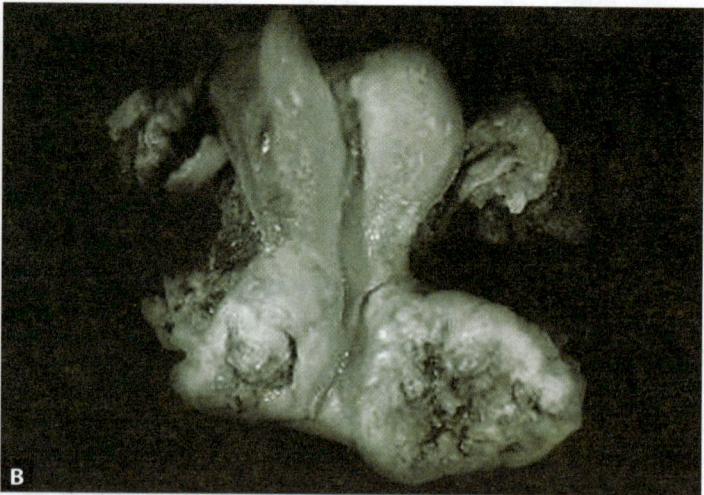

Figs. 28.5A and B: Specimen of cervical cancer. (A) Ulcerative growth of cervix; (B) Hysterectomy specimen showing fungating growth of cervix.

Reduced Immunity

Women with reduced immunity are at an increased risk of developing cervical cancer. Some of the conditions associated with reduced immunity include the following:
- Human immunodeficiency virus infection
- Organ (especially kidney) transplant
- Hodgkin's disease

Previous History of Cancerous Lesions in the Cervix

The woman is at a high risk of developing cancer cervix if she has a previous history of high-grade squamous intraepithelial lesions (HSIL); history of cancer of the cervix, vagina, or vulva, or has not been getting routine Pap tests done in the past. Pap smear is associated with false-negative rate of up to 50%. Therefore, negative Pap smear should not be relied upon in a symptomatic patient.

Previous Vaccination against Cervical Cancer

Two HPV vaccines, quadrivalent Gardasil and bivalent Cervarix have been approved by the US Food and Drug Administration for protection against the HPV subtypes 16 and 18. It is important to take history regarding such vaccination. Since both the vaccines, quadrivalent and bivalent provide protection against only some types of HPV, according to the current guidelines, vaccinated women still require screening with Pap smear.

Socioeconomic Status

Individuals belonging to low socioeconomic classes or low-income groups have been found to be at a high risk of developing cervical cancer. This could be probably due to the fact that poor women may not be able to afford good health care such as having regular Pap tests.

Treatment History

It is important to elicit the history of intake of medicines like diethylstilbestrol (DES), OCPs, etc.

The daughters of women who consumed DES at the time of their pregnancy are at a slightly higher risk of developing cancer of the vagina and cervix. Long-term use of the contraceptive pills for >10 years can slightly increase the woman's risk of developing cervical cancer.

Dietary History

Diets low in fruits and vegetables are linked to an increased risk of cervical and other cancers. Also, women who are overweight are at an increased risk of developing cervical cancer in the future.

Family History

Cervical cancer may run in some families. If the woman's mother or sister had cervical cancer, her chances of getting the disease in future are increased.

CLINICAL PRESENTATION

There may be no symptoms in the early stages of cancer and the woman may be completely asymptomatic. The cervical lesion may be detected at the time of routine Pap smear. The most common symptoms indicative of cervical cancer, which need to be elicited, include the following:

Bleeding

History of abnormal bleeding, spotting, or watery discharge in between periods or after intercourse is an important clinical presentation in cases of carcinoma cervix. In the women of reproductive age group, the presentation could be in the form of postcoital bleeding or intermenstrual bleeding. Various probable causes for intermenstrual bleeding are enlisted in **Box 28.1**. In postmenopausal women, the presentation

BOX 28.1: Causes of intermenstrual bleeding.
- Chronic cervicitis
- Cervical ectopy
- Cervical polyps
- Cervical/vaginal carcinoma
- Varicose veins
- Traumatic ulces

TABLE 28.2: Causes of postcoital bleeding.

Region	Pathology
Vulva	Vulval trauma, vaginitis, and benign or malignant lesions of vulva
Vagina	Senile vaginitis, vaginal tumors
Cervix	Cervical erosions, cervicitis, polyps, decubitus ulcers, and malignancy
Uterus	Senile endometritis, tubercular endometritis, endometrial hyperplasia, polyps, endometrial cancer, AUB, and metropathia hemorrhagica
Fallopian tube	Malignancy
Ovaries	Benign ovarian tumor, granulosa, or theca cell tumors
Systemic diseases	Hypertension, blood dyscrasias
Medicines	Unopposed estrogen, cyclical HRT

(AUB: abnormal uterine bleeding; HRT: hormone replacement therapy)

BOX 28.2: Causes of foul-smelling vaginal discharge.
- Infections (bacterial vaginosis)
- Sepsis
- Infected polyps
- Malignancy

may be in the form of postmenopausal bleeding. To elicit the history pertaining to abnormal uterine bleeding (AUB), kindly refer to Chapter 23. Various causes for postmenopausal bleeding have been described in Chapter 23.

Postcoital bleeding usually indicates a structural lesion of the cervix or vagina. Various causes of postcoital bleeding are enumerated in **Table 28.2**. Infectious etiologies such as *Chlamydia* and gonorrhea are common causes of postcoital bleeding, which must be excluded and treated if required. Uterine or cervical polyps may also be a source of bleeding. Dysplastic or malignant lesion of the cervical or vaginal epithelium may cause irregular or postcoital bleeding.

Foul-smelling Discharge

Often there is also a foul-smelling vaginal discharge and discomfort during intercourse. Various causes of foul-smelling discharge are tabulated in **Box 28.2**.

Symptoms Associated with Advanced Stage of Cancer

In advanced stages of cancer, there may be symptoms like lower abdominal pain, pelvic pain, loss of appetite, weight loss, fatigue, back pain, leg pain, swelling of feet, scanty urination, vesicovaginal or rectovaginal fistula and bone fractures.

GENERAL PHYSICAL EXAMINATION

No specific finding may be detected on the general physical examination. Chronic bleeding may be associated with anemia. Advanced stages of cancer may be associated with cancer cachexia, lymphadenopathy, or pedal edema. Evaluation of supraclavicular, axillary, and inguinofemoral nodes is important to exclude the metastatic disease.

SPECIFIC SYSTEMIC EXAMINATION

PER SPECULUM EXAMINATION

On per speculum examination, cervix must be carefully inspected for presence of any suspicious lesions. Vaginal fornices must also be closely inspected. Squamous cell cancers of the ectocervix may appear as proliferative or cauliflower like, vascular, friable growth, which bleeds on touch; ulcerative lesions or as flat indurated areas. The growth may undergo ulceration and necrosis, which may result in an offensive foul-smelling vaginal discharge. In case of an invasive cancer, the cervix may appear firm and expanded on per speculum examination. This finding, however, needs to be confirmed on digital examination. Detailed description about conducting a pelvic examination has been done in Chapter 22. A per speculum examination may be helpful in detection of abnormal lesions over the cervix. A per speculum examination also enables the gynecologist to simultaneously take the punch biopsy of the suspected lesion. On vaginal examination, both fungating and ulcerative cervical lesions may be identified. Uterus may appear bulky due to occurrence of pyometra in advanced stage when the cervix gets blocked by growth.

RECTAL EXAMINATION

A rectovaginal examination is also essential in cases of suspected cervical malignancy. The rectal examination may reveal thickening and induration of uterosacral ligaments and evaluation of parametrial extension of the disease (identified in form of parametrial nodularity). It is also useful for assessing cervical consistency and size, particularly in patients with endocervical disease.

Breast Examination

Examination of breasts would help in detection of any mass/lump which could be suspicious of malignancy

DIFFERENTIAL DIAGNOSIS

The diagnosis of malignancy is confirmed on biopsy. The biopsy results can help in diagnosing other conditions such as the ulcers of the cervix (tubercular and syphilitic) and polyps (mucus, cervical, and fibroid polyps). In the Indian scenario, one must definitely keep the differential diagnosis of cervical tuberculosis in their minds.

MANAGEMENT

Management of invasive cancer primarily depends on the stage of malignancy, which is essentially based on clinical findings and results of various imaging investigations such as chest radiography, intravenous pyelography (IVP), cystoscopy, proctoscopy, ultrasonography, CT, MRI, and fluorine-18-fluorodeoxyglucose positron emission tomography (FDG-PET). Investigations such as ultrasound examination, both transvaginal sonography and CT examination **(Figs. 28.6 and 28.7)**, are particularly useful in establishing the diagnosis. MRI examination helps in detecting lymph node enlargement of >1 cm in diameter. FDG-PET is positron emission tomography based on the use of radiolabeled compound fluorodeoxyglucose. This investigation is also useful in the determination of lymph node metastasis and has presently become the gold standard investigation. This test is based on the fact that malignant tissue exhibits greater glycolysis in comparison to normal tissues. As a result, FDG accumulates in the malignant tissues resulting in an increased tumor contrast.

Management of cervical cancer changes based on lymph node involvement. Lymph node involvement increases with increasing staging of the disease. Pelvic lymph nodes are involved in 5% cases in stage I, 15% cases in stage II, and 25% in stage III.

INVESTIGATIONS
BIOPSY

Biopsy is usually sufficient for establishing the diagnosis when an obvious tumor growth is present. A punch biopsy forceps can be used for taking biopsy in case of an exophytic growth on the cervix. The biopsy must be preferably taken

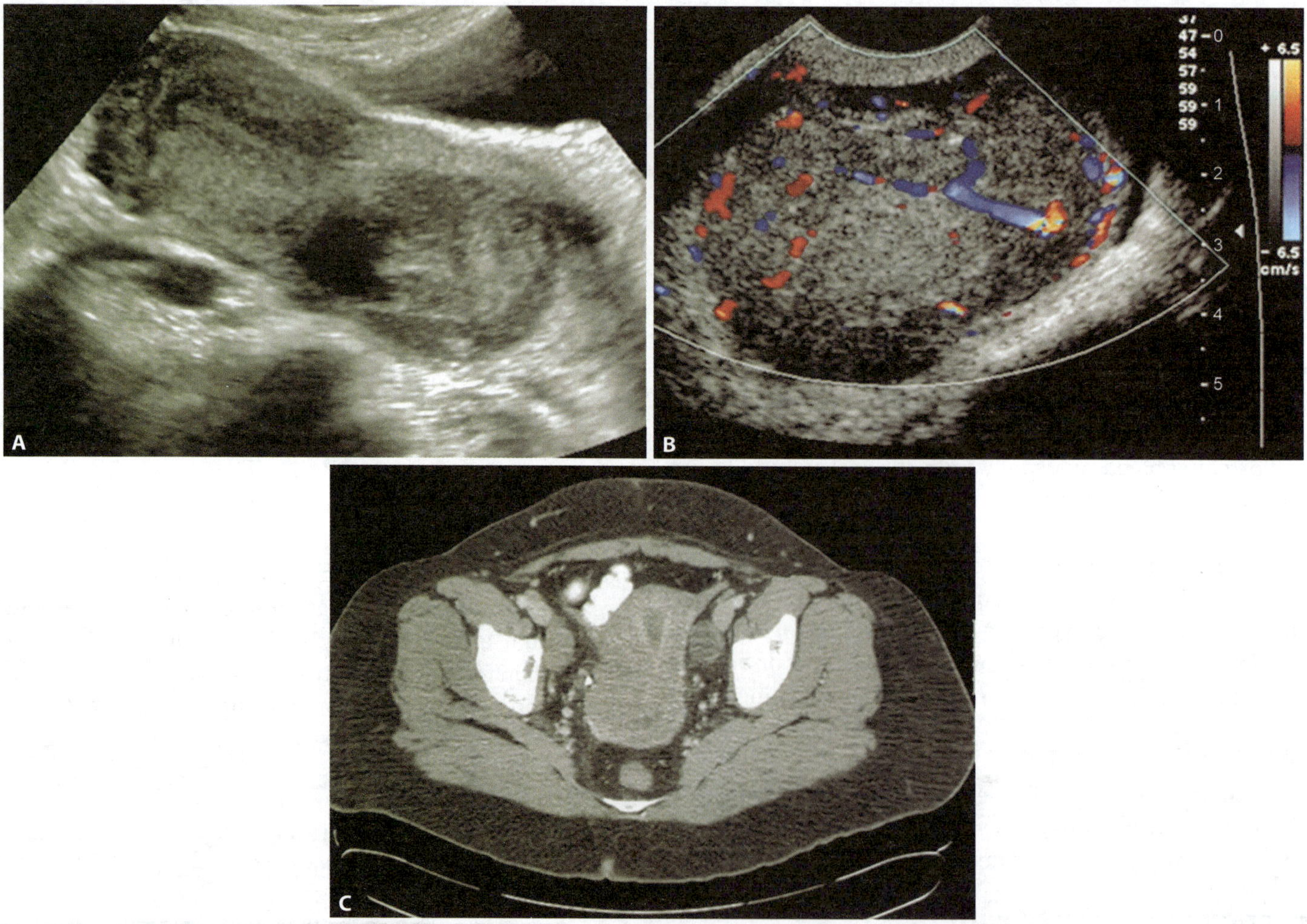

Figs. 28.6A to C: (A) Transabdominal sonography showing solid heterogeneous cervical mass in a 52-year-old postmenopausal patient with the history of abnormal vaginal bleeding. (B) Color Doppler of the same patient showing presence of randomly distributed irregular vessels in the mass arising from the posterior aspect of the cervix. This was highly suggestive of a malignancy; (C) Computed tomography scan of the same patient showing a large lobulated cervical mass with central hypoattenuation.

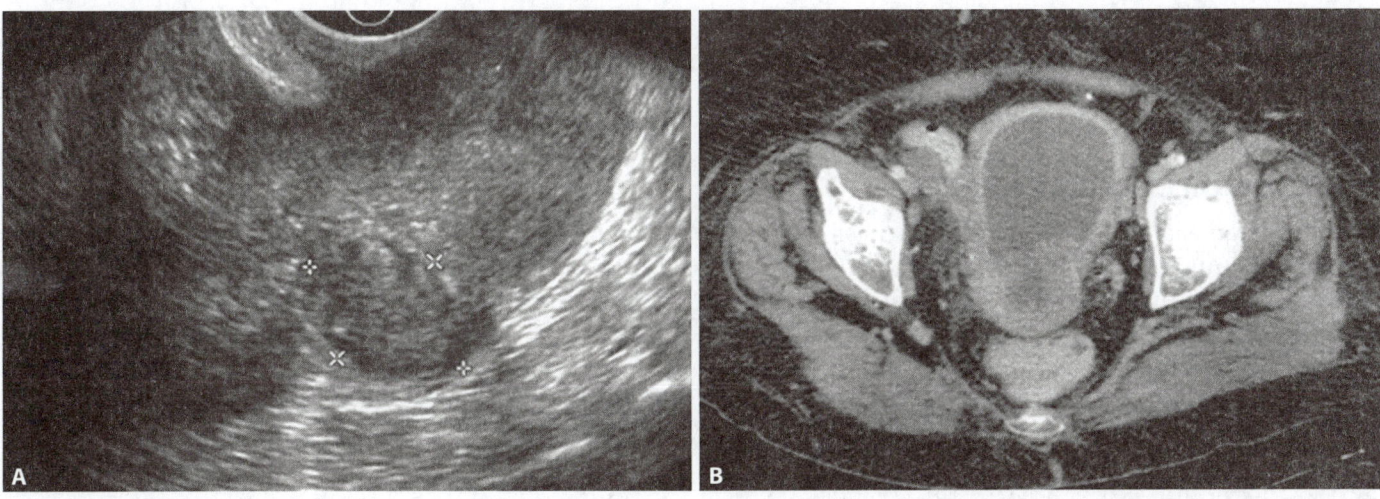

Figs. 28.7A and B: (A) Transvaginal sonography of cervix of a 47-year-old patient with severe suprapubic pain showing presence of a solid cervical mass measuring 3 × 2 × 2.5 cm; (B) CT scan of the same patient showing spread of the cancer.

from the edge of the lesion so that both normal and abnormal tissue can be observed for a better diagnosis. Biopsy must not be taken from the center of the growth because most of the times, it would be necrotic tissue.

COLPOSCOPIC EXAMINATION

If a gross tumor growth is not present, a colposcopic examination with cervical biopsy and endocervical curettage is required to establish the diagnosis. Sometimes diagnosis may not be possible even with colposcopic-directed biopsies, especially in cases of endocervical adenocarcinoma. In these cases, cervical conization may be required. Colposcopic examination is mandatory in cases where early invasive cancer is suspected based on cervical cytology; however, the cervix is normal appearing in these cases. Colposcopic examination has been described in details in Chapter 27. Colposcopic findings suggestive of cervical invasion are abnormal blood vessels, irregular surface contour with loss of surface epithelium, and changes in the color tone. Abnormal-looped vessels, arising from the punctate and mosaic vessels present in cervical intraepithelial neoplasia (CIN), are the most common colposcopic findings, which are suggestive of invasive growth. Colposcopic-directed biopsies may help in detecting frank invasion by the cancerous cells, thereby avoiding the requirement for diagnostic cone biopsy. This enables the clinician to administer treatment without any delay.

In suspected cases of adenocarcinoma, there may be no specific colposcopic appearance. In these cases, endocervical curettage is required as a part of colposcopic examination.

HISTOLOGICAL EXAMINATION

In cases where cervical microinvasion is suspected, cervical conization is required to correctly assess the depth and linear extent of involvement. A significant risk factor predicting

> **BOX 28.3:** Pretreatment investigations in a woman with histologic diagnosis of cervical cancer.
>
> - Physical examination
> - Complete blood count, LFT and KFT
> - Chest radiography
> - Pelvic ultrasound
> - Magnetic resonance imaging
> - Computed tomography scans
> - Laparoscopy
> - Intravenous pyelography or imaging of abdomen with intravenous contrast
> - Barium enema and rectosigmoidoscopy
> - *Cystoscopy:* For visualization of the interior of the urethra and bladder
> - *Proctoscopy:* For visualization of the interior of the rectum
>
> (KFT: kidney function test; LFT: liver function test)

the development of pelvic node metastasis and tumor recurrence is the depth of tumor invasion. Lymph nodes may be positive in 3–8% cases, when the depth of invasion is between 3 and 5 mm. When the depth of invasion is ≤3 mm, metastasis is rarely seen.

PRETREATMENT INVESTIGATIONS

Pretreatment investigations in a woman with histologic diagnosis of cervical cancer are enumerated in **Box 28.3**. These investigations are useful in assessing the spread of metastatic disease. Assessment of renal function is important for staging of cervical cancer. The presence of unilateral or bilateral ureteral obstruction with azotemia often indicates metastatic disease and is associated with poor prognosis.

EXAMINATION UNDER ANESTHESIA

This is an examination of the vagina and cervix after the patient has been administered general anesthesia. This allows the clinician to examine the patient thoroughly without it being uncomfortable for her. The abdomen (especially large bowel, bladder, and rectum) and pelvis are carefully assessed for the spread of metastatic disease. An endometrial biopsy may also be taken to assess the endometrial status.

STAGING OF CERVICAL CANCER

Once the diagnosis of invasive cervical cancer has been established confidently by histological examination, the disease is clinically staged, which involves assessment of the degree of cancer dissemination. The results of bimanual pelvic palpation and cervical inspection and various above-mentioned investigations like colposcopy, endocervical curettage, hysteroscopy, cystoscopy, proctoscopy, IVP, X-ray examination of the lungs and skeleton, cervical conization/biopsy, ultrasonography, CT scan, MRI, PET scanning, etc., help in staging the cervical cancer. When abnormalities are noted on CT, MRI, or PET, radiographic fine needle aspiration can be performed to confirm metastatic disease and individualize treatment planning.

The most commonly used system for staging of cervical cancer is the staging system devised by FIGO, which is based on clinical examination, rather than surgical findings **(Table 28.3 and Fig. 28.8)**. Another staging system in use is the tumor, nodes, metastases (TNM) staging system **(Table 28.3)**, which incorporates lymph node staging unlike the FIGO staging system, which does not incorporate lymph node involvement. The TNM staging system for cervical cancer is analogous to the FIGO stage. Cervical cancer is a clinically staged disease. Though the FIGO staging system does not include any information related to lymph node

TABLE 28.3: TNM and FIGO staging system for cervical cancer.

TNM staging	FIGO Stage	Characteristics
Tx	–	Primary tumor cannot be assessed
T0	–	No evidence of primary tumor
Tis	0	Carcinoma in situ, intraepithelial neoplasia
T1	I	Carcinoma strictly confined to the cervix (extension to the corpus would be disregarded)
T1a	IA	Invasive cancer identified only microscopically, with a maximum depth of invasion ≤ 5 mm*
T1a1	IA1	Measured stromal invasion ≤ 3 mm in depth
T1a2	IA2	Measured stromal invasion > 3 mm and ≤5 mm
T1b	IB	Invasive carcinoma with measured deepest invasion > 5 mm (greater than stage IA), lesion limited to the cervix uteri†
T1b1	IB1	Invasive carcinoma > 5 mm depth of stromal invasion and ≤2 cm in greatest dimension
T1b2	IB2	Invasive carcinoma > 2 cm and ≤4 cm in greatest dimension
T1b3	IB3	Invasive carcinoma > 4 cm in greatest dimension
T2	II	Carcinoma extends beyond the cervix, but not to the pelvic wall; carcinoma involves the vagina but not as far as the lower one-third
T2a	IIA	No obvious parametrial involvement
T2a1	IIA1	Clinically visible lesion ≤ 4.0 cm in the greatest dimension
T2a2	IIA2	Clinically visible lesion > 4.0 cm in the greatest dimension
T2b	IIB	Tumor with parametrial invasion but not up to the pelvic wall
T3	III	Tumor extends to the pelvic wall; on rectal examination, no cancer-free space is found between the tumor and the pelvic wall and/or involves the lower third of the vagina and/or causes hydronephrosis or nonfunctioning kidney
T3a	IIIA	Carcinoma involves the lower third of the vagina, with no extension to the pelvic wall
T3b	IIIB	Tumor extends to the pelvic wall and/or causes hydronephrosis or nonfunctioning kidney
T3c	IIIC	Involvement of pelvic and/or para-aortic lymph nodes (including micrometastasis), irrespective of the tumor size and extent (with r and p notations)‡
T3c1	IIIC1	Pelvic lymph node metastasis only
T3c2	IIIC2	Para-aortic lymph node metastasis
–	IV	Cervical carcinoma has extended beyond the true pelvis or has involved (biopsy proven) bladder mucosa or rectal mucosa. Bullous edema does not qualify as a criterion for stage IV disease
T4	IVA	Spread to the adjacent organs
M1	IVB	Spread to distant organs

Contd...

Contd...

TNM staging	FIGO Stage	Characteristics
Lymph nodes**		
NX	–	Regional lymph nodes cannot be assessed
N0	–	No regional lymph nodes metastasis
N1	–	Regional lymph nodes metastasis

Source: Bhatla N, Berek JS, Cuello Fredes M, Denny LA, Grenman S, Sean T, et al. Revised FIGO staging for carcinoma of the cervix uteri. Int J Gynaecol Obstet. 2019;145(1):129-135. doi: 10.1002/ijgo.12749. (Corrigendum to revised FIGO staging for carcinoma cervix: https://doi.org/10.1002/ijgo.12969) (FIGO: Federation of Gynaecology and Obstetrics; TNM: tumor, node, metastases)
*Imaging (ultrasound, CT, MRI, PET, PET-CT, and MRI-PET) and pathology can be used, when available, to supplement clinical findings with respect to tumor size and extent, in all stages.
†The involvement of vascular/lymphatic spaces does not change the staging. The lateral extent of the lesion is no longer considered. Any patient with positive lymph nodes immediately gets upstaged to stage IIIC.
‡Adding notation of r (imaging) and p (pathology) to indicate the findings that are used to allocate the case to stage IIIC. For example, if imaging indicates pelvic lymph node metastasis, the stage allocation would be stage IIIC1r and if confirmed by pathological findings, it would be stage IIIc1p. The type of imaging modality or pathology technique used should always be documented. When in doubt, the lower staging should be assigned.
**Regional lymph nodes (N), include paracervical, parametrial, hypogastric (obturator), common internal and external iliac, presacral, and sacral group of lymph nodes.

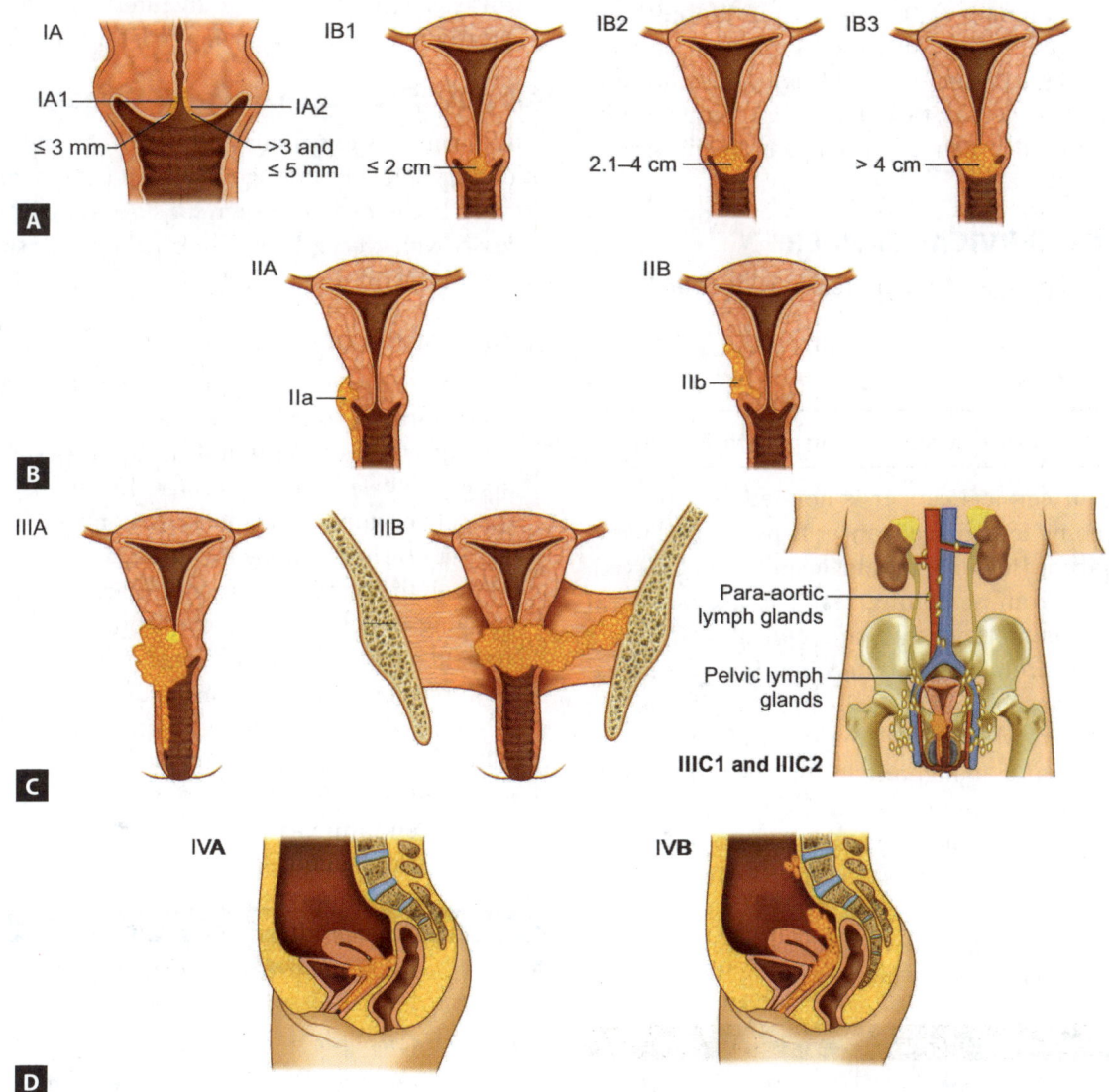

Figs. 28.8A to D: FIGO revised cervical cancer staging: (A) Stage I cancer: Confined to the cervix; (B) Stage II cancer: Cancer spreads beyond the cervix, but not to pelvic wall or to the lower third of vagina; (C) Stage III cancer: Disease spreads to the pelvic side wall or to the lower third of the vagina; (D) Disease has spread beyond the true pelvis to involve either the adjacent organs (bladder/rectum, etc.) or the distant organs (lung/liver, etc.).

involvement, all women with cervical cancer should go through a lymph node evaluation at the time of clinical staging because this information is essential for planning the patient's treatment.

Clinical staging system has been developed by FIGO, based on the belief that cervical cancer is a local disease until late in its course. When there is doubt regarding the allocation of a cancerous lesion to a particular stage, the earlier stage must be selected. As per the new FIGO (2018) staging system, findings of imaging or pathology can be used to decide the exact cancer stage, unlike the staging system (2014), where the clinical staging was largely relied upon.

CANCER GRADING

Cancer grading gives an idea about the degree of malignancy. It is based on the results of the histopathological examination and can be classified as grade 1 (low grade malignancy), grade 2 (moderate grade malignancy), and grade 3 (higher grade malignancy). The more undifferentiated the malignancy, the higher would be its grading. Cervical malignancy is unique because it can be detected at an early preinvasive stage. Nowadays, there has been a trend towards prevention of invasive cancer, which has been already discussed in Chapter 27.

SPREAD OF CERVICAL CANCER

Cancer of cervix spreads through the routes mentioned in **Box 28.4**.

DOWN-STAGING

> **Q. Write a short essay on downstaging of cervical cancer.**

Downstaging for cervical cancer is defined as a process in which screening for cervical cancer is performed using clinical approaches (including visual inspection of cervix). This is distinct from screening test using cytological evaluation. In this method, the paramedical staff with a minimal training would be able to identify any cervical abnormality suggestive of cervical cancer and refer the case early to centers where there are facilities for treatment of premalignant and malignant lesions. Women must also be educated regarding the risk factors, symptoms, and prophylaxis of cervical cancer. This would enable the detection of carcinoma at early stages even in the absence of definite national cancer screening program, especially in developing countries like India where cytological screening may not be possible for every woman.

BOX 28.4: Routes of spread of cancer.
- Direct invasion into the cervical stroma, corpus, vagina, and parametrium
- Lymphatic metastasis
- Blood-borne metastasis
- Intraperitoneal implantation

STAGING

The new staging system for cervical cancer as devised by the FIGO in 2018 is described in **Table 28.3** and **Figures 28.8A to D**. The main differences between the previously used staging system—FIGO 2014 and FIGO 2018—are summarized in **Table 28.4** and are as follows:

Stage IA Disease

In the new staging system, lateral dimension of the lesion was excluded from the stage IA.

Definition of Stage IB Disease

- In the former system, stage IB disease was defined as clinically and macroscopically visible lesions limited to the uterine cervix, having a size greater than stage IA disease.
- In the new staging system, stage IB lesions are defined as invasive lesions limited to the uterine cervix with a size greater than IA, having a depth of invasion >5 mm.

Subclassification of Stage IB Disease

In the former system, tumor size of 4 cm served as the cut-off for classification of sub-stage: Stage IB1 (≤2 cm) and stage IB2 (>2 cm). In the revised system for stage IB disease, substage increases with every 2 cm increase in the tumor size: Stage IB1 (≤2 cm), stage IB2 disease (2.1–4 cm), and stage IB3 (>4 cm).

Incorporation of Nodal Status in Stage III Disease

- A major change in the current staging system is the incorporation of nodal status into stage III disease staging. Cases with lymph node metastasis are now specifically designated as stage IIIC disease, stage IIIC1 for pelvic lymph node metastasis only or stage IIIC2 for para-aortic lymph node metastasis.

Though the primary method of staging remains clinical, imaging as well as results of histopathology can be used to help decide the exact cancer stage. The notations "r" and "p" should be used along with the specific stage (e.g., IIIC1r or IIIC1p) depending on the method used for stage allocation, i.e., imaging or pathology.

In continuation with the new FIGO staging system (2018), a corrigendum was published in 2019, which further made some changes:

TABLE 28.4: Differences between FIGO (2014) and FIGO (2018).

Stages	2014 FIGO system	2018 FIGO system
Stage IB1	Tumor size ≤4 cm	Tumor size ≤2 cm
Stage IB2	Tumor size >4 cm	Tumor size 2.1–4 cm
Stage IB3	N/A	Tumor size >4 cm
Stage IIIC1	N/A	Pelvic lymph node metastasis only
Stage IIIC2	N/A	Para-aortic lymph node metastasis

(FIGO: Federation of Gynecology and Obstetrics)

Cancer Cervix (Postcoital Bleeding)

- Micrometastasis, which was previously not considered is now being considered in stage IIIC
- Presence of lymphovascular space invasion (LVSI) does not change the stage, but must be recorded.
- Extension to the uterine corpus does not change the stage.
- Ovarian involvement does not change the stage.
- Presence of micrometastasis (0.2–2 mm) or isolated tumor (<0.2 mm) does not change the stage but must be recorded.

If one is in doubt, lower stage must be assigned.

℞ TREATMENT/GYNECOLOGICAL MANAGEMENT

Q. Discuss in detail the management of a case of stage I cervical cancer.

Q. Write a long essay discussing the management of stage 1 cervical cancer in a 45-years old woman with postcoital bleeding and dirty vaginal discharge.

Q. Discuss in detail the symptoms, signs, staging, and management of stage IB cervical cancer. How will you prevent it?

Q. What should be the next step of management in the case study mentioned in the beginning of the chapter?
Ans. Since the woman had completed her family, did not want to conserve her uterus and there was no lymphovascular space invasion, a type I extrafascial hysterectomy was performed in this case.

DEFINITIVE TREATMENT FOR INVASIVE CANCER

The treatment of cervical cancer varies with the stage of the disease. As per FIGO (2018) guidelines, early-stage cervical cancer refers to stages IA (IA1 and IA2), IB1, IB2, and IIA1. On the other hand, locally advanced cervical cancer refers to stages IB3, IIA2, and IIB to IV.

- For women with early-stage cervical cancer, modified radical hysterectomy (class II hysterectomy) is recommended over the primary radiation therapy **(Flowcharts 28.1 to 28.3)**.
- For women with locally advanced cancer (stage IB3 to stage IV), chemoradiation is recommended.
- Sometimes, for women with stages IB2, IB3, and IIIA cervical cancer, radical hysterectomy (class III hysterectomy) or modified radical hysterectomy may be employed. Depending on the staging and grading of the cervical cancer, various treatment options are summarized in **Table 28.5** and are described here in details.

EARLY-STAGE CANCER

For women with early stage (IA1, IA2, and IB1) cervical cancer, modified radical hysterectomy (class II hysterectomy) is recommended over the primary radiation therapy. Surgical alternatives to modified radical hysterectomy include the following:

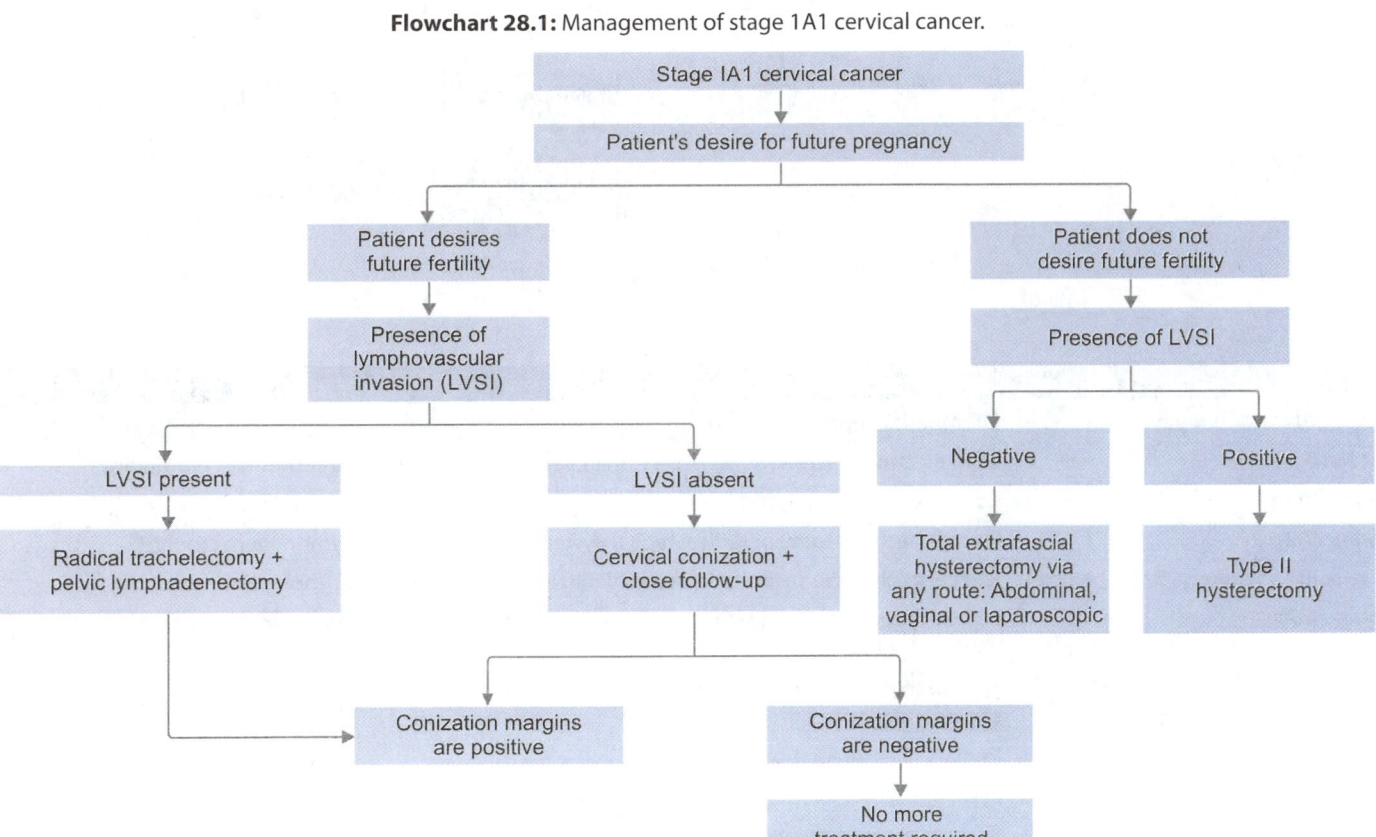

Flowchart 28.1: Management of stage 1A1 cervical cancer.

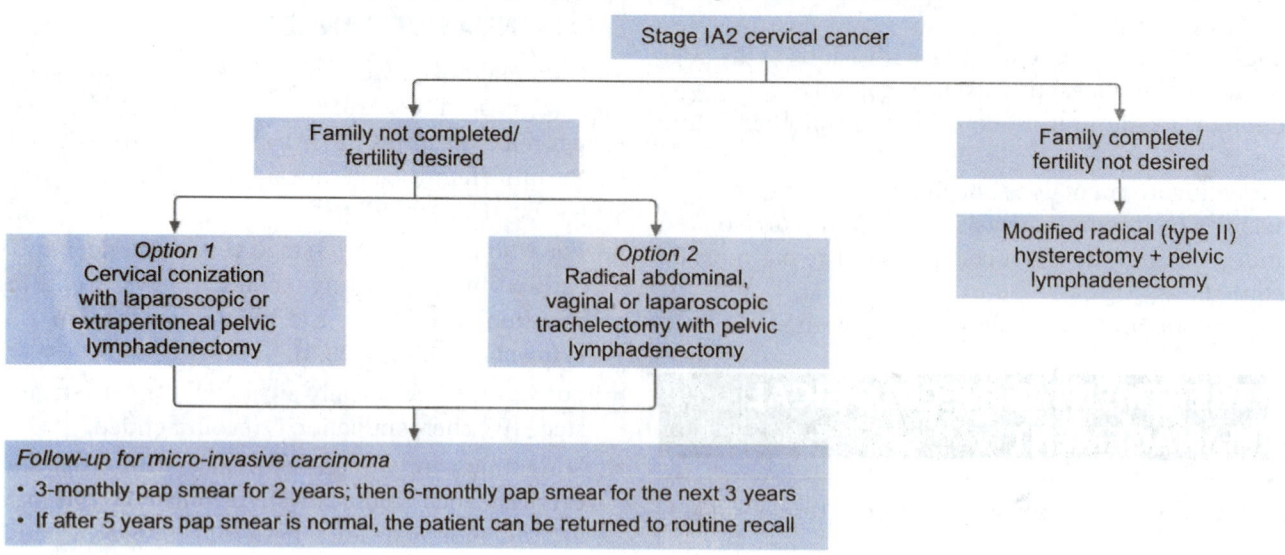

Flowchart 28.2: Management of stage 1A2 cervical cancer.

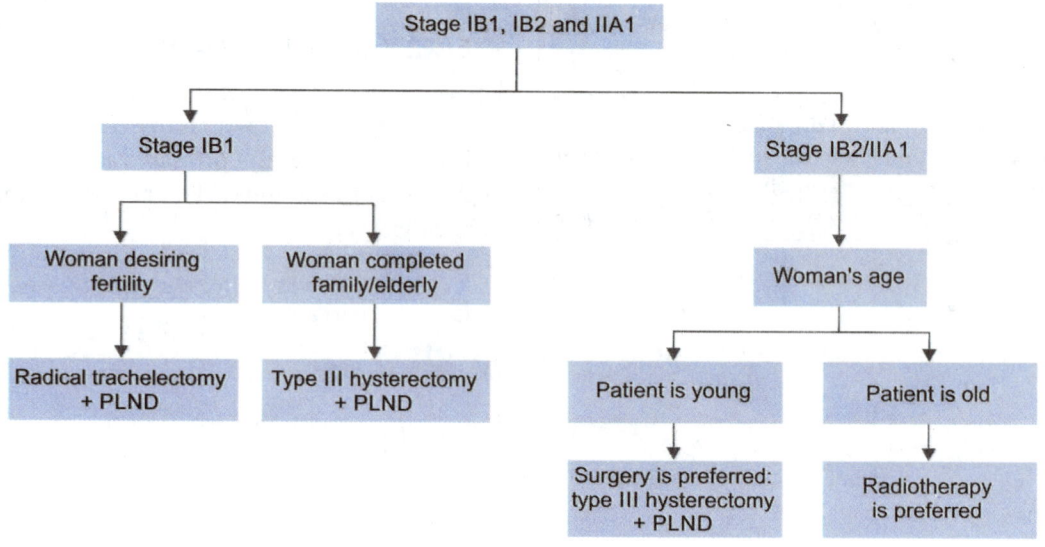

Flowchart 28.3: Management of stage IB1, B2, and IIA1 cervical cancer.

(PLND: Pelvic lymph node dissection)

TABLE 28.5: Summary of treatment of invasive cervical carcinoma.	
Cervical cancer stage	**Therapeutic option**
Stage 0	Loop electrosurgical excision procedure (LEEP), laser therapy, conization, and cryotherapy
Stage IA1	Conization or type I hysterectomy
Stage IA2	Radical trachelectomy or radical type II hysterectomy with pelvic lymphadenectomy
Stage IB1 (invasion > 5 mm, < 2 cm)	Radical trachelectomy or radical type III hysterectomy with pelvic lymphadenectomy
Stage IB2	Radical type III hysterectomy with pelvic and para-aortic lymphadenectomy or primary chemoradiation
Stage IIA1 and IIA2	Radical type III hysterectomy with pelvic and para-aortic lymphadenectomy or primary chemoradiation
Stage IIB, IIIA, and IIIB	Primary chemoradiation
Stage IVA	Primary chemoradiation or primary exenteration
Stage IVB	Primary chemotherapy with or without radiotherapy

- *Cone biopsy or extrafascial hysterectomy:* This can be used for women with microscopic disease with stromal invasion ≤3 mm in depth (stage IA1) who have no evidence of intermediate- or high-risk features.
- *Fertility-sparing surgery:* Fertility-sparing surgery such as radical trachelectomy may be used for women of reproductive age with early-stage disease (lesion size <2 cm and no lymph node metastases) who wish to preserve their fertility.
- *Primary radiation therapy or chemotherapy or chemoradiation therapy:* Chemoradiation or radiation alone or chemotherapy alone may be used for women with poor functional status or medical comorbidities. In this procedure, the whole pelvis is treated to 45 Gy in 25 once-daily fractions of 1.8 Gy.

Though presently there is not enough evidence nevertheless, primary radiotherapy as a standalone procedure does not appear to be an adequate treatment option for early stage cervical cancer in comparison to primary surgery. Radiotherapy must be used as the primary treatment for only those women who are poor candidates for surgery due to the presence of medical comorbidities or poor functional status. Adjuvant radiotherapy may be, however, required for the cases with intermediate risk, defined by the Sedlis criteria **(Box 28.5)**.

Adjuvant chemoradiation rather than adjuvant radiotherapy alone is recommended for women with high-risk factors (Peters' criteria), which include the following:
- Pathologically involved lymph nodes
- Microscopic parametrial invasion
- Positive surgical margins

In these cases, single-agent cisplatin, rather than a combination of cisplatin with 5-fluorouracil (5-FU), must be administered in conjunction with radiotherapy.

Stage IA tumors: As described before, stage IA tumors are mainly diagnosed by microscopic examination. The risk of nodal metastasis in the early invasive tumors (stage IA1) is quite low, only about 0.5%; therefore, the prognosis in these cases is quite good. The 5-year survival rate exceeds 95% with appropriate treatment. The recommended therapy for stage IA1 tumors is described in **Flowchart 28.1**. For effective treatment, there must not be any evidence of lymphovascular space invasion and both endocervical margins and curettage findings must be negative for cancer or dysplasia. If endocervical margins or curettage is positive for dysplasia or malignancy, further treatment is necessary because these findings are predictive of residual disease.

The recommended management in case of stage IA2 cervical cancer is described in **Flowchart 28.2**. The risk of lymph node involvement with stage IA2 disease is as high as 8%, indicating the need for lymphadenectomy, which may be performed via any of the following routes: Vaginal, abdominal, laparoscopic, or robotic. Radical trachelectomy is rapidly emerging as a surgical management option in women with stage IA2 and IB1 disease who desire preservation of uterus and fertility. Criteria for likely candidates are enumerated in **Box 28.6**.

The procedure of trachelectomy involves the removal of whole or at least 80% of the cervix, upper vagina and lymph nodes in the pelvis and cutting Mackenrodt's ligament on either side. A radical trachelectomy can be performed abdominally, vaginally or using laparoscopic or robotic surgery. Patients who are ideal candidates for this procedure have tumors < 2 cm in diameter. This procedure may be accompanied by pelvic lymphadenectomy and cervical cerclage placement. Although complications associated with the procedure are uncommon, women who are able to conceive after surgery are likely to develop preterm labor or late miscarriages. Presently, the experience with this technique is limited. Although early results with this technique look promising, it is uncertain whether the long-term outcome would be similar to that of traditional therapy.

LOCALLY ADVANCED TUMORS (STAGE IB TO IV)

- In locally advanced tumors, chemoradiation has become the mainstay of treatment. Primary surgery is not preferred in women with advanced cervical cancer, because it is unlikely to be curative. Women with advanced cervical cancer may further require

---

BOX 28.5: Sedlis' criteria used to define women at intermediate risk of cancer recurrence following surgery.

- Presence of lymphovascular space invasion (LVSI) plus deep one-third cervical stromal invasion and tumor of any size
- Presence of LVSI plus middle one-third stromal invasion and tumor size ≥2 cm
- Presence of LVSI plus superficial one-third stromal invasion and tumor size ≥5 cm
- No LVSI but deep or middle one-third stromal invasion and tumor size ≥4 cm

---

BOX 28.6: Criteria for choosing likely candidates for radical trachelectomy.

- Stage IA1 with LVSI
- Stage IA2—IB1 (without LVSI)
- Size of the lesion < 2 cm
- No occurrence of metastasis
- Limited endocervical involvement
- Cervical length > 2 cm
- 4–6 weeks following conization
- BMI < 35 kg/m^2
- Desire for future fertility
- No evidence of impaired fertility

(BMI: body mass index; LVSI: lymphovascular space invasion)

adjuvant treatment following surgery, resulting in a high incidence of morbidity. A meta-analysis of RCTs in 2010 has reported the beneficial effects of chemoradiation for women with locally advanced cervical cancer in comparison to radiotherapy alone.

- Chemotherapy is usually administered with either single-agent cisplatin or in combination of cisplatin and FU. External beam radiotherapy (1.8 to 2 Gy for 5 days a week for 5 weeks, i.e., a total of 25 sittings along with a weekly dose of cisplatin, 40 mg/m^2 administered on the first day of the week. Brachytherapy involves administration of 3 weekly applications of 6–8 Gy. Whole of the radiotherapy regimen must be completed over 8 weeks.

  Use of cisplatin may be associated with significant toxicities, including risks of long-standing neuropathy and potentially chronic renal insufficiency. Therefore, in patients with chronic or persistent comorbidities (e.g., patients with chronic renal failure or severe baseline neuropathy), weekly carboplatin treatment is preferred. Gemcitabine also serves as a reasonable substitute to cisplatin.

- In advanced cases of cervical cancer, the most extreme surgery, called pelvic exenteration in which all of the organs of the pelvis, including the bladder and rectum are removed, may sometimes be employed.

- *Surgical management of stages IB3 and IIIA:* Treatment options for stages IB3 and IIA may sometimes include surgical treatment rather than primary chemoradiation. However, surgery alone may be associated with a rate of relapse being at least 30%. Therefore, it may serve as an option in low-risk cases. Surgery, if done in these cases, comprises radical type III hysterectomy along with pelvic and para-aortic lymphadenectomy (**Flowchart 28.3**).

- *Stage IVB:* In patients with disseminated disease, chemotherapy or radiation provides symptom palliation. Palliative radiotherapy is often useful for controlling bleeding, pelvic pain and urinary or partial large bowel obstructions resulting from pelvic disease.

VARIOUS AVAILABLE TREATMENT OPTIONS

> Q. Writing a long essay discussing the role of surgery versus radiotherapy for management of early cervical cancer.

Surgery

Various types of surgical options which can be used in cases of cervical cancer are summarized in **Table 28.6**. Previously, the surgical classification system by Piver-Rutledge (**Table 28.7 and Fig. 28.9**) was used. Nowadays, the Querleu–Morrow classification (**Table 28.8**) system is being commonly used in the clinical practice. As per the updates in this classification system in 2017, the class has been replaced by type and the numbers by letters. Extent of parametrial resection is the key parameter between different types of hysterectomies. This classification system also includes the nerve-sparing hysterectomy. Lymph nodes are dealt with separately.

LYMPHADENECTOMY

Para-aortic lymphadenectomy is performed if the para-aortic nodes are found to be suspicious for metastatic disease at the time of pelvic lymphadenectomy. Four levels of lymphadenectomy are described in **Table 28.9**.

Oophorectomy is usually not necessary in premenopausal women with squamous cell carcinoma of the cervix because ovarian metastases are quite uncommon with squamous cell cancer. However, ovarian metastasis may commonly occur in adenocarcinoma. Therefore, consideration must be given towards the removal of ovaries in these cases.

Recently, it has been shown that patients with parametrial involvement, positive pelvic nodes, or positive surgical margins may benefit from a postoperative adjuvant therapy comprising a combination of cisplatin containing chemotherapy and pelvic radiation.

Surgery versus Radiotherapy

There are advantages to the use of surgery instead of radiotherapy, particularly in younger women in whom

TABLE 28.6: Summary of different surgeries based on the cancer stage.

Cancer stage	Type of surgery	Intent of surgery
Hysterectomy		
Stage IA1	Extrafascial hysterectomy (type A)	Curative for microinvasion
Stage IA1 with LVSI and stage IA2	Modified radical hysterectomy (type B)	Curative for small lesions
Local disease without any obvious metastasis including stage IB1 and IB2, and selected stage IB3–IIA1	Radical hysterectomy (type C1)	Curative for larger lesions
Fertility sparing surgery		
Carcinoma in situ and stage IA1	Simple trachelectomy	Curative for microinvasion (fertility preserved)
Stage IA2–IB1, selective IB2	Radical trachelectomy	Curative for select stage IA2 to IB2 (fertility preserved)

(LVSI: lymphovascular space invasion)

Cancer Cervix (Postcoital Bleeding)

TABLE 28.7: Piver-Rutledge Classification of radical hysterectomy (as adopted by the Gynecological Cancer Group of the European Organization for Research and Treatment of Cancer).

Classification	Description
Type I radical hysterectomy (Simple/extrafascial hysterectomy)	Removal of the uterus and cervix, but not the parametria or more than the upper vaginal margin
Modified radical or type II radical hysterectomy	Removal of the entire uterus, both adnexa, medial half of cardinal and uterosacral ligaments, upper 2–3 cm cuff of the vagina, and pelvic lymphadenectomy. The uterine blood vessels are divided medial to the ureter
Type III radical hysterectomy (Equivalent to the classical Wertheim–Meigs operation)	Removal of the entire uterus, both adnexa, most of the cardinal and uterosacral ligaments, upper one-third of the vagina and pelvic lymphadenectomy. Uterine vessels are ligated lateral to the ureter and ureter is dissected completely to the bladder entry. Uterosacral ligaments are divided at the origin. Cardinal ligaments are divided at the pelvic side wall
Type IV radical hysterectomy (extended radical hysterectomy)	Ureter divided from the pubovesical ligament. Periureteral tissues, superior vesicle artery, and as much as three-fourths of the vagina and paravaginal tissue are excised (in addition to structures removed in type III radical hysterectomy)
Type V radical hysterectomy (partial exenteration)	In addition to the structures removed in type IV hysterectomy, portion of distal ureter and bladder or bowel are also removed

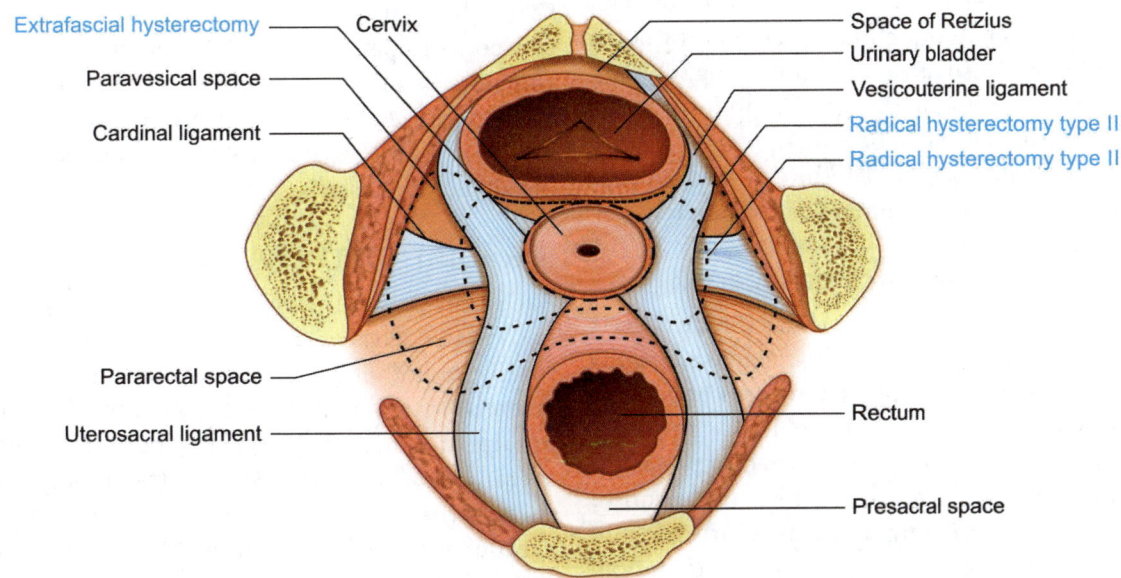

Fig. 28.9: Different types of hysterectomies which can be used in cases of cancer cervix.

TABLE 28.8: Radical hysterectomy: Querleu Morrow classification.

Type of radical hysterectomy	Description
Type A (maximum resection of paracervix)	Extrafascial hysterectomy corresponding to type I radical hysterectomy with a <10 mm vaginal resection
Type B (transection of paracervix at the ureter)	Corresponds to type II radical hysterectomy. Can be of two types: B1 (without additional removal of the lateral paracervical lymph nodes) B2 (with the removal of the lateral paracervical lymph nodes). Also includes > 10 mm vaginal resection
Type C (transection of paracervix at the junction with internal iliac vascular system)	Corresponds to type III radical hysterectomy with the ureter completely mobilized. 15–20 mm of vagina and corresponding paracolpos resected out routinely. It can be of two types: C1 (autonomic nerve preservation) and C2 (without the autonomic nerve preservation)
Type D (laterally extended resection)	Ultraradical procedure mostly indicated at the time of pelvic exenteration, with the entire paracervical resection at the pelvic sidewall including the hypogastric vessels (type D1); type D2 also includes the resection of adjacent fascial musculature

TABLE 28.9: Levels of lymphadenectomy.

Levels	Description
Level 1	External and internal iliac
Level 2	Common iliac (including presacral)
Level 3	Aortic inframesentric
Level 4	Aortic infrarenal

BOX 28.7: Cases where surgery is preferred over radiotherapy.

- Women who are young and in good physical condition with stage IA1, IA2, IB1, IB2, or IIA1
- Presence of associated pathology such as fibroids, tubo-ovarian mass, ovarian tumor, etc.
- Vaginal stenosis
- Müllerian anomaly
- Pregnancy associated with carcinoma cervix

conservation of ovaries is important. Fibrosis and reduced vascularity resulting from radiation therapy can result in chronic bladder and bowel problems, which may be difficult to treat. Moreover, sexual dysfunction can commonly occur following radiation because of vaginal shortening, fibrosis, and atrophy of the epithelium. Surgery is preferred over radiotherapy in the cases listed in **Box 28.7**.

Lesions > 4 cm should not preferably be operated because these patients would require postoperative radiotherapy.

Laparoscopic Surgery in Carcinoma Cervix

Prior to the Laparoscopic Surgery in Carcinoma Cervix (LACC) trial (2018), laparoscopic radical hysterectomy (LRH) was commonly being employed in cases of cervical malignancy and was found to be associated with better short-term outcomes, lower operative complication rates and improved clinical outcomes in comparison to abdominal radical hysterectomy. Disease recurrence and survival rates were found to be similar. As a result, minimum invasive surgery (MIS) was thought to be as adequate and effective as abdominal surgery with respect to surgical and oncological outcomes for surgical management of FIGO stage 1B disease.

The results from phase III LACC trial were presented at the 2018 Society of gynecologic oncology Annual meeting on Woman's Cancer at New Orleans. The LACC trial aimed to compare the standard treatment using laparotomy with MIS via total laparoscopic or total robotic hysterectomy, which was performed using smaller incisions on the abdomen. The open approach was favored, with the women who had undergone laparotomy showing low disease recurrence (7 verses 27), better disease/progression free interval and better overall survival rates. On the other hand, minimally invasive radical hysterectomy was associated with high rates of disease recurrence, poor disease/progression free rates, and poor rates of overall survival. Since no other study was able to find similar outcomes, the results of LACC trial were thought to be attributed due to less radical technique employed with MIS in comparison to open surgery, incorrect manipulation and spread of tumor due to CO_2 insufflation. However, due to the results of this study, laparotomy approach is favored over laparoscopy in cases of both cervical and endometrial cancer. Laparoscopy should be largely limited to tumors <2 cm in size (IB1).

CHEMORADIATION

Chemoradiation helps in covering the benefits of systemic chemotherapy along with the benefits of regional radiation therapy. Use of chemotherapy helps in sensitizing the cells to radiation therapy. Use of chemoradiation has been found to be associated with a significant improvement in progression-free survival as well as the overall survival at 43 months. Chemoradiation is also likely to result in an improved cosmesis and function in comparison to surgical resection with or without adjuvant treatment. Cisplatin-based chemotherapy forms the treatment of choice in patients with advanced-stage cervical cancer. Chemoradiation has been found to be superior to radiation alone because chemotherapy given as a part of concurrent radiation may act systemically and potentially eradicate the distal micrometastasis.

RADIATION THERAPY

Radiation may be used to treat cancer that has spread beyond the pelvis or cancer that has returned. Patients who receive radiotherapy must be closely monitored to assess response to treatment. The tumor may be expected to regress for up to 3 months following radiotherapy. Radiation therapy can be either external (teletherapy) or internal (brachytherapy). Carcinoma of the cervix has two components: (1) central and (2) peripheral. The central component comprises cancerous growth in the cervix, which is best treated by brachytherapy. The peripheral component comprises cancerous growth in the parametrium as well as lymph node metastasis, which is controlled by teletherapy. Two types of radiotherapy, internal and external, are described next in details:

Internal Radiation Therapy

- Internal radiation therapy, also known as brachytherapy, can be administered in the following three ways:
  1. *Intracavitary brachytherapy:* In this method, irradiation using radioactive sources is placed in the body cavity close to the site of the tumor. There is placement of an intrauterine tandem with vaginal ovoids, vaginal cylinders, or vaginal rings which encompass the at-risk paracervical tissues while providing a lower dose distribution.

2. *Interstitial brachytherapy:* In this method, radioactive seeds are implanted directly into the tumor. It is usually used in case of extensive vaginal involvement. The needles are placed with freehanded- or template-based techniques, at times with laparoscopic guidance.
3. *Pulse dosage radiotherapy (PDR) brachytherapy:* PDR uses a single iridium-192 source which is programmed to move through various dwell positions in placed applicators using remote afterloading technology.

Intracavitary brachytherapy involves placing the Selectron tubes inside the patient's vagina. This method helps in delivering radiation directly to the cervix and the surrounding areas. The radioactive balls in the Selectron tube can be withdrawn into the machine when other people come into the patient's room. This helps in keeping the dose of radioactivity to visitors and nurses as low as possible. There are several techniques for administration of brachytherapy: Paris method, Stockholm method, and Manchester method. Of these various methods, the Manchester method is one of the oldest and extensively used systems in the world. This method comprises two insertions. Each insertion lasts for 72 hours with a 1-week interval in between the two insertions. In this method, radiotherapy is administered at two points A and B **(Fig. 28.10)**:

1. **Point A:** This is a fixed point, 2 cm lateral to the uterine axis and 2 cm above the lateral fornix. This point represents the paracervical tissue and the total dosage to this point must not exceed 8,000 rads.
2. **Point B:** This point is 5 cm from the midline at the same level as point A. Point B represents the lateral pelvic wall. Total dose delivered to point B must not exceed 5,000 rads.

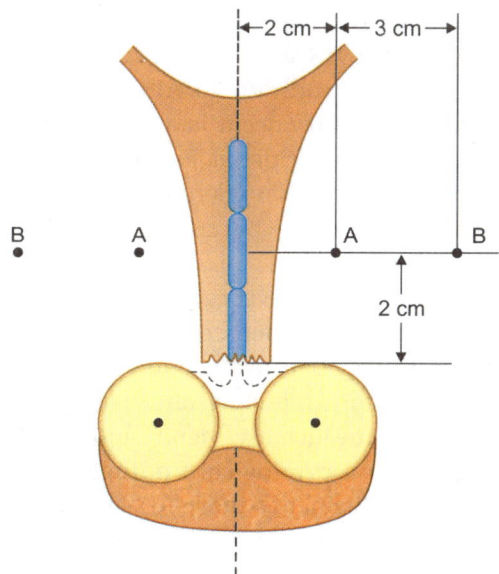

Fig. 28.10: Manchester method for application of brachytherapy.

Based on the current evidence, the National Institute for Health and Care Excellence (NICE, 2006) supports the use of high-dose rate (HDR) brachytherapy for carcinoma of the cervix, provided that the patient has given consent and the arrangements for monitoring the patient are in place.

Prior to the procedure, the patients must receive appropriate counseling and pain management. HDR brachytherapy helps in reducing the radiation hazard to staff and also helps in reducing the length of inpatient treatment.

- For delivering HDR brachytherapy to the cervix, applicators are placed in the cervix and connected to an afterloadings machine which delivers high-dose radiation, usually for a few minutes. The treatment is often repeated several times, a few days apart, on an outpatient basis. While this procedure delivers a high dose of radiation to the cervix and the adjacent areas, tissues, and organs more than a few centimeters away receive a low dose of radiation. Virtually all HDR brachytherapy is given in combination with external-beam radiation therapy.

External Radiation Therapy (Teletherapy)

External radiation therapy involves administration of radiation beams from a large machine onto the body where the cancer is located.

- CT scan is often used for ensuring the accurate targeting of the external radiation beam.
- External radiotherapy is normally administered on an outpatient basis. The treatments are usually given from Monday to Friday, with a period of rest at the weekend.

CHEMOTHERAPY

The most commonly employed chemotherapy regimens use cisplatin, 5-FU, carboplatin, ifosfamide, paclitaxel, cyclophosphamide, etc., and are usually used as a palliative therapy. Chemotherapy is sometimes used in the form of neoadjuvant chemotherapy. This method involves use of chemotherapy before surgery or radiotherapy, to shrink the cancer and to make these treatments more effective.

Pelvic Exenteration

If the cancer recurs in the pelvis after radiation therapy, the gynecologist may need to resort to surgery for removing all pelvic organs. This procedure cures up to 50% of women. This is a major operation that involves removing all of the structures in the pelvic area, including the uterus, cervix, vagina, ovaries, bladder, and rectum. This operation may involve creating two stomas: (1) a colostomy and (2) a urostomy. The operation also involves reconstructing a new vagina.

RECURRENT LESION

In case the disease recurrence occurs after surgery, radiotherapy must be administered for recurrent disease. Vice versa also holds true, i.e., in case recurrence occurs after radiotherapy, surgery (usually exenteration) must be done. Surgery can only be undertaken if the patient is physically fit.

PREGNANT PATIENT WITH CERVICAL CANCER

Pregnancy does not change the course of cervical cancer. The rate of cervical cancer in pregnant patients is similar to that in nonpregnant patients of the same age. In patients with concurrent cervical malignancy and pregnancy, the major dilemma is regarding diagnosis and treatment. Diagnosis usually requires the performance of a cone biopsy, which carries increased risks of hemorrhage and poor perinatal outcome in the first trimester. Conization must not be therefore performed before the second trimester of pregnancy. Also, it must be performed in patients in whom colposcopy findings are consistent with cancer; there is presence of biopsy proven microinvasive cancer or strong cytological evidence of invasive cancer. Following conization, there is no harm in delaying definitive treatment until fetal maturity is achieved in patients with stage IA1 cervical cancer.

Patients with cervical invasion between 3 and 5 mm and evidence of lymphovascular space invasion can be followed up till term and delivered after establishment of pulmonary maturity. They may have cesarean delivery, immediately followed by modified radical hysterectomy and pelvic lymphadenectomy.

Patients having >5 mm cervical invasion, should be treated as having a frankly invasive cancer. The recommended treatment option in these cases is classical cesarean delivery followed by radical hysterectomy and pelvic lymphadenectomy.

Stage III and IV disease must be treated with radiotherapy. If the fetus is viable, it must be delivered by classical cesarean birth and radiation therapy must be started postoperatively. Clinical stage of cervical cancer is the most important prognostic factor during pregnancy.

Most clinicians advocate cesarean delivery in cases with cervical cancer, because of the possibility of the recurrence of the disease at the site of episiotomy. Furthermore, vaginal delivery through a cervix with advanced cervical cancer is associated with an increased risk for hemorrhage, obstructed labor, and infection.

FOLLOW-UP IN CERVICAL CANCER

Following the completion of treatment in cases of cervical cancer, follow-up is essential in cases. Initially, the follow-up can be done every 3-monthly for first 2 years; and 4–6 monthly for next 3 years. In case of normal follow-up at 5 years, the patient can be returned to the screening program as per the national guidelines. At each follow-up visit, the patient must be enquired about any new onset complaints, followed by a complete general physical, per speculum and per abdominal examination. Depending upon the clinical findings, imaging tests (e.g., MRI, CT, or a PET scan) may be ordered.

Effect of the Treatment for Cervical Cancer on Patient's Sexual Life

Removal of ovaries at the time of hysterectomy can result in an early menopause. The symptoms of the menopause can include hot flushes, dryness of skin and vagina, anxiety, and loss of interest in sexual activity. Radiotherapy can cause cervical stenosis and fibrosis, which can result in pain and discomfort at the time of sexual intercourse.

Hormone Replacement Therapy in Women who have Undergone Treatment for Cervical Cancer

Bothersome symptoms such as vasomotor symptoms, vaginal dryness, or dyspareunia can result from treatment-induced menopause. Hormone replacement therapy appears to be a safe treatment option for women with cervical cancer who experience troublesome symptoms following treatment.

ADENOCARCINOMA OF CERVIX

Nearly 80% cases of invasive cancer of cervix are of squamous cell type and arise from the stratified squamous epithelium of the cervix. The second variety of less common type of cancer cervix, known as adenocarcinoma, arises from the mucous membrane of the endocervical canal and accounts for nearly 20% cases of cervical cancer. Increasing number of cases of cervical adenocarcinoma has been reported in the women in their twenties and thirties. Adenocarcinoma in situ (AIS) is believed to be the precursor of invasive adenocarcinoma. In addition to AIS, CIN, or invasive squamous carcinoma may occur in approximately 30–50% cases of cervical adenocarcinoma. Patient with AIS who are treated with conization must undergo close follow-up along with endocervical curettage because conization may miss residual or invasive lesion.

Adenocarcinoma of cervix is associated with poorer prognosis at every stage when compared with squamous cancer. This is mainly because adenocarcinomas tend to grow endophytically and therefore, often remain undetected until the tumor volume increases significantly. Furthermore, the colposcopic and cytological findings for glandular disease are not as distinct as those for squamous lesions. When atypical glandular cells of undetermined significance (AGUS) are diagnosed on Pap smear, the presence or absence of squamous intraepithelial lesion, AIS or adenocarcinoma

Cancer Cervix (Postcoital Bleeding)

TABLE 28.10: Complications due to radical hysterectomy.

Acute complications	Chronic complications
• Blood loss • Fistula formation (ureterovaginal/vesicovaginal fistulas) • Venous thromboembolism/pulmonary embolus • Small bowel obstruction • Febrile morbidity (due to pelvic infection, urinary tract infection, wound infection, pelvic abscess, phlebitis, etc.)	• Bladder dysfunction (especially difficulty in voiding) • Bowel dysfunction • Sexual dysfunction • Lymphocyst formation • Lymphedema • Premature menopause

needs to be confirmed. Adenocarcinoma may be detected on cervical sampling, but less reliably than squamous carcinoma. A definitive diagnosis of cervical adenocarcinoma may require cervical conization for confirmation. Management of cases of cervical adenocarcinoma is same as that of squamous cell carcinoma.

COMPLICATIONS

Therapeutic modalities like surgery, radiotherapy, and chemotherapy can result in numerous complications.

COMPLICATIONS DUE TO SURGERY

Complications which may occur due to radical hysterectomy are tabulated in **Table 28.10**. Other complications which can occur as a result of surgery are as follows.

Premature Menopause

Removal of ovaries in young patients can result in symptoms related to premature menopause.

Urinary Dysfunction

The most frequent complication of radical hysterectomy is urinary dysfunction as a result of partial denervation of the detrusor muscle.

Other Complications

Other complications resulting from surgery may include shortened vagina, ureterovaginal and rectovaginal fistulas, hemorrhage, infection, bowel obstruction, stricture, and fibrosis of the intestine or rectosigmoid colon and bladder.

COMPLICATIONS DUE TO RADIOTHERAPY

During the acute phase of pelvic radiation, the surrounding normal tissues such as the intestines, the bladder and the perineum skin are often affected. As a result, radiotherapy to the pelvic area can cause side effects such as tiredness, diarrhea, and dysuria. These side effects can vary in severity depending on the strength of the radiotherapy dose and the length of treatment. Some of these complications are as follows:

Early Complications

This may include complications such as radiation-induced sickness—nausea/vomiting, radiation induced cystitis, proctitis, abdominal cramps, etc.

- *Cystourethritis:* Inflammation of bladder and urethra can result in complications like dysuria, increased urinary frequency, and nocturia. Antispasmodic medicines are often helpful in providing symptomatic relief. Urine should be examined for possible infection. If urinary tract infection is diagnosed, therapy should be instituted without delay.
- *Gastrointestinal effects:* Gastrointestinal side effects due to radiotherapy include diarrhea, abdominal cramping, rectal discomfort, bleeding, etc. Diarrhea can be either controlled by loperamide (imodium) or diphenoxylate (lomotil). Small, steroid containing enemas are prescribed to alleviate symptoms resulting from proctitis.
- *Sore Skin:* Radiotherapy can result in erythema and desquamation of skin.
- *Tiredness:* Radiotherapy can result in extreme tiredness. Therefore, the patient must be advised to take as much rest as possible.
- *Bowel complaints:* In a small number of cases, the bowel may be permanently affected by the radiotherapy resulting in continued diarrhea. The blood vessels in the bowel can become more fragile after radiotherapy treatment, resulting in hematochezia.

Late Complications

This may include complications such as bowel strictures, intestinal obstruction, radiation-induced rectovaginal or vesicovaginal fistulas, persistent anemia, pyometra, loss of ovarian function, narrowing or shortening of the vaginal orifice resulting in poor sexual quality of life, lymphedema, and lymphocyst formation. Rarely there may be fracture neck of femur or development of second malignancies (e.g., uterine sarcomas).

- *Vaginal stenosis:* Radiotherapy to the pelvis can cause narrowing and shortening of the vaginal orifice, thereby making the sexual intercourse difficult or uncomfortable. This problem can be overcome by prescribing estrogen creams to the patient. Using vaginal dilators or having regular penetrative sex often helps in maintaining the suppleness of the vaginal orifice.
- *Lymphedema:* Lymphedema resulting in the swelling of one or both the legs can commonly occur as a complication of radiotherapy or due to the cancer per se in advanced stages.

SIDE EFFECTS DUE TO CHEMOTHERAPY

Chemotherapy can cause side effects, which may be slightly worse if it is given alongside radiotherapy. Chemotherapy can temporarily reduce the number of normal blood cells, resulting in development of symptoms including increased susceptibility to infection, easy fatigability, anemia, etc. Other side effects, which the chemotherapy drugs can cause, may include oral ulcerations (stomatitis), nausea, vomiting, and alopecia. Nausea and vomiting can be well-controlled with effective antiemetic drugs. Regular use of mouthwashes is important in treating the mouth ulcerations.

SURVIVAL RATES

> Q. What is the prognosis in the cases of cervical cancer.
> Q. What are the prognostic factors in cases of cancer cervix?

5-year survival rate for patients with cervical cancer is shown in **Table 28.11**. Early stage carcinomas are associated with a high 5-year survival rate.

Prognostic Factors

Prognosis depends on the stage of the cancer, followed by the status of the lymph nodes. Outcomes are worse for women where there is involvement of pelvic or para-aortic nodes. Various factors which may affect the prognosis are as follows:

- *Host factors:* Extremes of age (very old or very young age); presence of associated co-morbidities, e.g., diabetes, anemia, etc.
- *Tumor factors:* Tumor stage, size, and grade; extent of lymphovascular space invasion, depth of stromal invasion, histopathological type of tumor, lymph node involvement, etc. Involvement of lymph nodes can be considered as one of the most important prognostic factors because involvement of lymph nodes not only alters the prognosis, it also affects the mode of therapy. Involvement of lymph nodes usually increases with the stage of the disease **(Table 28.12)**.

TABLE 28.11: 5-year survival rate for patients with cervical cancer (nodes negative): 2019 FIGO statistics.

FIGO stage	Five years survival rate
IA1	95.8 (94.4–96.9)
IA2	95 (92.2–96.7)
IB1	91.6 (90.4–92.6)
IB2	83.3 (81.8–84.8)
IB3	76.1 (74.3–77.8)
IIA1	70.3 (65.9–74.3)
IIA2	65.3 (61.6–68.6)
IIIA	40.7 (37.1–44.3)
IIIB	41.4 (39.9–42.9)
IVA	24.1 (21.2–27.1)
IVB	15.4 (13.4–17.6)

Source: Wright JD, Matsuo K, Huang Y, Tergas AI, Hou JY, Khoury-Collado F, et al. Prognostic Performance of the 2018 International Federation of Gynecology and Obstetrics Cervical Cancer Staging Guidelines. Obstet Gynecol. 2019;134(1):49-57. doi:10.1097/AOG.0000000000003311.

TABLE 28.12: Stage-vise lymph node involvement.

Stage	Pelvic lymph node involvement (%)
IA1	0.5
IA2	5
IB	15
IIB	30
IIIB	45
IV	60 and more

EVIDENCE-BASED CLINICAL TRIALS

List of references can be scanned through QR code to enable the readers gain deeper insight of the subject by referring to the entire article or its abstract.

SECTION 6

Uterine, Ovarian, and Tubal Pathology

29. Prolapse Uterus
30. Pelvic Pain
31. Abdominal Lump (Ovarian Cancer)
32. Ectopic Pregnancy
33. Adenomyosis

CHAPTER 29

Prolapse Uterus

CASE STUDY

A 50-year-old G5P5 lady presented with complaints of something descending out of vaginal introitus since past 1 year. According to the patient, the feeling worsens while coughing or standing. On a per speculum examination, a grade II cystocele and a grade I rectocele were noticed. There was no enterocele. Both the cystocele and the rectocele were observed to increase in size when the patient strained. On bimanual examination, uterus was normal-sized, anteverted, and mobile. There has been no history of urinary incontinence. Her previous menstrual history has also been normal. She has completed her family and has five children. All her children were delivered at home by a *dai* (untrained midwife). She works on the farm with her husband. Due to lack of social support, she had to resume her activities immediately following each delivery.

INTRODUCTION

Q. Write a short essay on enterocele.

Uterine prolapse is a descent or herniation of the uterus into or beyond the vagina. It is best considered under the broader heading of "pelvic organ prolapse," which also includes cystocele, urethrocele, enterocele, and rectocele. Anatomically, the vaginal vault has three compartments: an anterior compartment (consisting of the anterior vaginal wall), a middle compartment (cervix), and a posterior compartment (posterior vaginal wall). Weakness of the anterior compartment results in cystocele and urethrocele, whereas that of the middle compartment in the descent of uterine vault and enterocele. The weakness of the posterior compartment results in rectocele. Uterine prolapse involves the middle compartment. Uterine prolapse usually occurs in postmenopausal and multiparous women in whom the pelvic floor muscles and ligaments that support the female genital tract have become slack and atonic. Injury to the pelvic floor muscles during repeated childbirths causing excessive stretching of the pelvic floor muscles and ligaments acts as a major risk factor for causing reduced tone of pelvic floor muscles. Reduced estrogen level following menopause is another important cause for atonicity and reduced elasticity of the muscles of pelvic floor. Uterine prolapse can be classified into four stages based on the Baden–Walker halfway system as described in **Table 29.1**.

Pelvis consists of three compartments: anterior, middle, and posterior (**Fig. 29.1**). The normal female pelvic anatomy is shown in **Figure 29.2**. Descent of the anterior compartment results in cystocele (**Figs. 29.3A to C**) and urethrocele (**Fig. 29.4**), middle compartment in the descent of uterine vault (**Fig. 29.5**) and enterocele (**Fig. 29.6**), and that of the posterior compartment in rectocele (**Figs. 29.7A to C**).

TABLE 29.1: Baden–Walker halfway system for evaluation of pelvic organ prolapse.

Stage	Definition
0	Normal position for each respective site
I	Descent of the uterus to any point in the vagina above the hymen
II	Descent of the uterus up till the hymen
III	Descent of the uterus halfway past the hymen
IV	Total eversion or procidentia

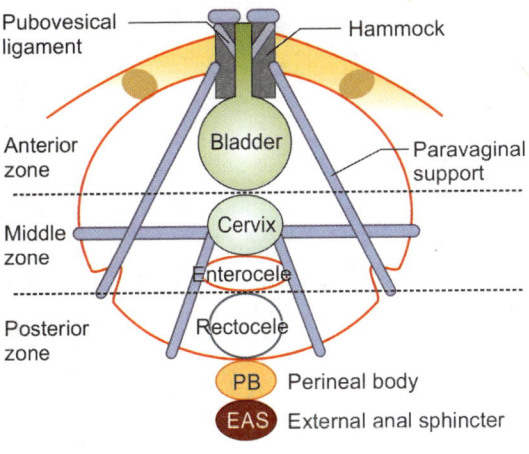

Fig. 29.1: Different pelvic compartments.

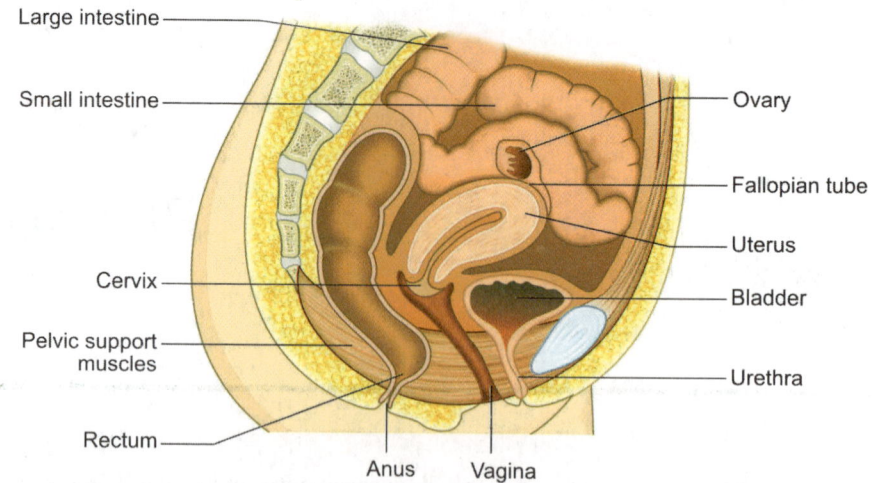

Fig. 29.2: Normal female pelvic anatomy.

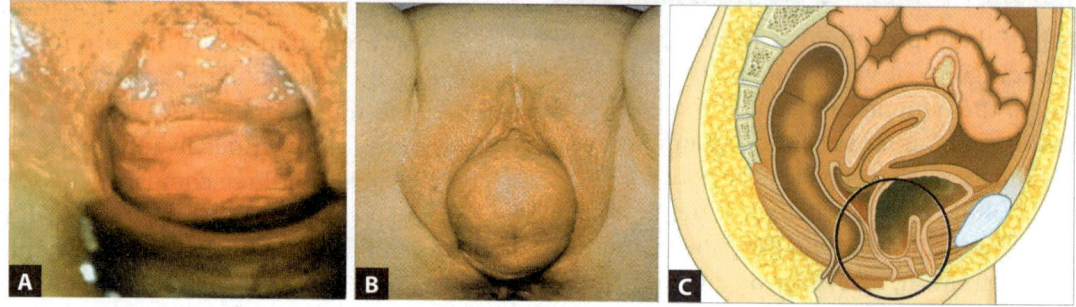

Figs. 29.3A to C: Cystocele. (A) Photograph of grade I cystocele; (B) Photograph of grade III cystocele; (C) Diagrammatic representation of cystocele (demonstrated by the circle).

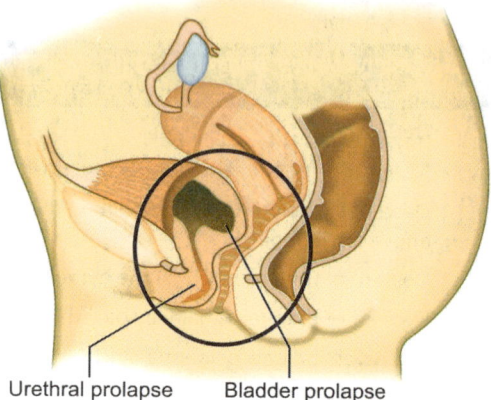

Fig. 29.4: Urethrocele with moderate cystocele.

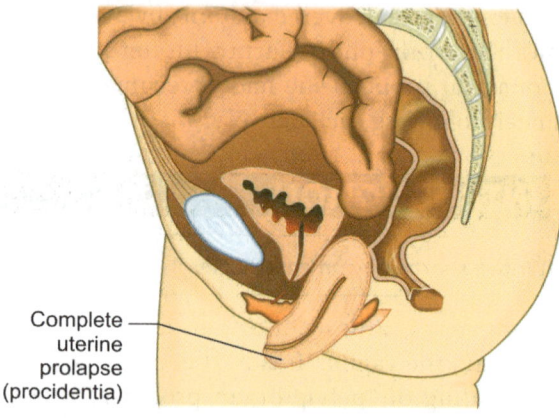

Fig. 29.5: Uterine prolapse.

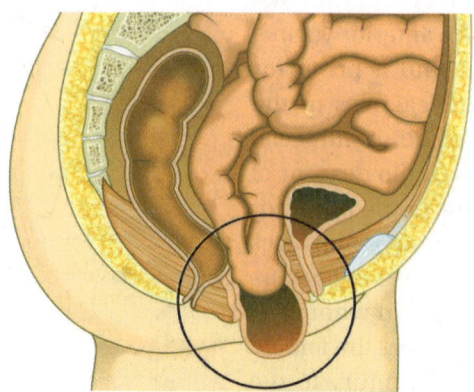

Fig. 29.6: Enterocele.

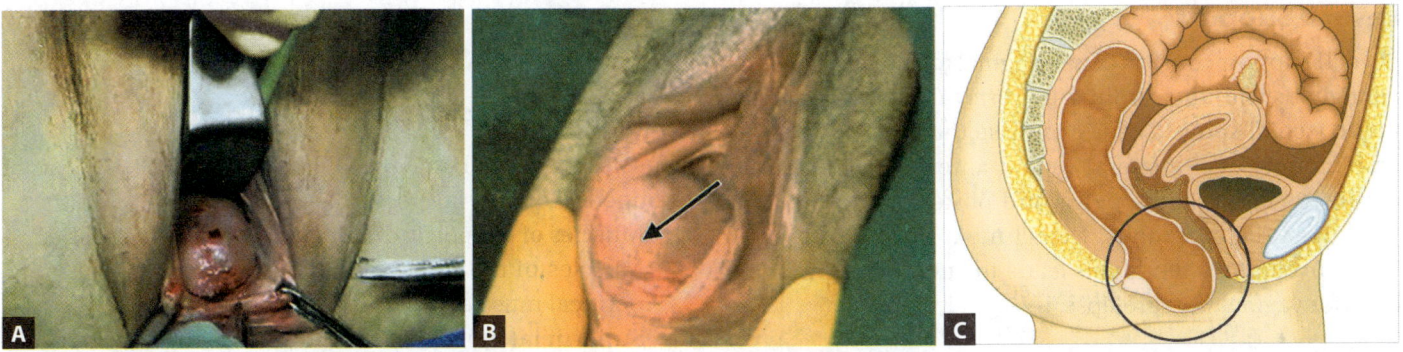

Figs. 29.7A to C: Rectocele. (A and B) Photographic appearance of rectocele; (C) Diagram showing rectocele (demonstrated by the circle).

SUPPORTS OF THE UTERUS

 Q. Briefly discuss the anatomical supports of the uterus.

A basic knowledge of pelvic anatomy and uterine supports is essential for the gynecologist in order to understand the mechanism of prolapse and the methods for correcting it. Thus, the various pelvic supports would be discussed next.

Various support structures of the pelvis are attached to the bony pelvis, which is formed by the pelvic bones (comprising the pubic bone, ilium, and ischium) anteriorly and on either side and posteriorly by sacrum and coccyx. Various pelvic structures including urinary structures (bladder, urethra), genital structures (vagina, cervix, uterus, fallopian tubes, ovaries), and the rectum are present within this "supporting structure." Failure of the pelvic support system allows for descent of one or more of the pelvic organs into the potential space of the vagina, and at its most severe degree, outside the vaginal opening.

Vagina can be divided into proximal (deep), middle, and distal (superficial) thirds. Depending upon the anatomical location of different parts of vagina, three levels of support for vaginal tissues can be defined. Level I support suspends the upper vagina and mainly comprises the cardinal and uterosacral ligaments. Level II support attaches the midvagina along its length to the arcus tendineus fascia of the pelvis. Level III support, on the other hand, results from the fusion of the distal vagina to the adjacent structures and mainly comprises levator ani and perineal muscles. The supports for different parts of vagina have been summarized in **Table 29.2**.

In the supine position, the upper vagina lies almost horizontal and superior to the levator plate. The uterus and vagina have two main support systems. Active support is provided by the levator ani (level III support). On the other hand, passive support is provided by the condensations of the endopelvic fascia (i.e., the uterosacral–cardinal ligament complex, pubocervical fascia, and rectovaginal septum) and their attachments to the pelvis and pelvic sidewalls through the arcus tendineus fascia pelvis (level I and level II support). Contraction of the levator plate creates a flap-valve effect in which the upper vagina is compressed against it during the periods of increased intra-abdominal pressure. When the tone of levator ani muscles decreases, the vagina drops from a horizontal to a semivertical position. This causes widening of the genital hiatus (Gh), thereby predisposing the prolapse of pelvic viscera.

TABLE 29.2: Different levels of support for vaginal tissue.

Different levels of vaginal support	Support elements
Level I (for proximal one-third of vagina)	Cardinal and the uterosacral ligaments
Level II (for middle one-third of vagina)	Paravaginal fascia
Level III (for distal one-third of vagina and the introitus)	Levator ani and perineal muscles

Level I Support

Level I support comprises the attachments of the cardinal (transverse cervical ligaments) and uterosacral ligaments to the cervix and upper vagina (**Fig. 29.8**). Cardinal ligaments fan out laterally and attach to the anterior border of the greater sciatic foramen and ischial spines and the parietal fascia of the obturator internus and piriformis muscles. The cardinal ligaments contain the uterine arteries and provide attachment of uterus to the pelvic side walls. The uterosacral ligaments provide attachment of the cervix to the bony sacrum at the level of S2–S4. Together, this dense visceral connective tissue complex helps in maintaining vaginal length and horizontal axis. It allows the vagina to be supported by the levator plate and positions the cervix just superior to the level of ischial spines. Some other important ligament supports, which help maintain the relationships between the urethra, bladder, vagina, and uterus within the bony pelvis, include the pubourethral ligaments, urethropelvic ligaments, and vesicopelvic ligaments. The pubourethral ligaments provide support to the middle portion of the urethra by anchoring it to the undersurface of the pubic bone. The urethropelvic ligaments are composed of the levator fascia. This ligament provides support to the urethra by helping in its attachment to the tendinous arch. On the other hand, the vesicopelvic ligament provides support to the bladder by facilitating its attachment to the tendinous arch.

Level II Support

Level II support consists of paravaginal attachments that are contiguous with the cardinal–uterosacral ligament complex at the ischial spine. These comprise the connective tissue attachments of the lateral vagina anteriorly to the arcus tendineus fascia of the pelvis and posteriorly to the arcus tendineus rectovaginalis. Detachment of this connective tissue from arcus tendineus leads to lateral or paravaginal anterior vaginal wall prolapse.

Level III Support

Perineal body (Pb) along with superficial and deep perineal muscles of the pelvic floor comprises level III support structures. Together, these structures support the distal one-third of the vagina and introitus. The Pb is not only essential for providing support to the distal vagina but also required for the proper functioning of the anal canal. Damage to level III support structures results in anterior/posterior vaginal wall prolapse, gaping introitus, and perineal descent.

MUSCLES OF THE PELVIC FLOOR

Muscles of the pelvic floor **(Figs. 29.9 and 29.10)** can be grouped into three layers:
1. Muscles of the pelvic diaphragm (levator ani muscle)
2. Muscles of the urogenital diaphragm (deep transverse perineal muscle)
3. Superficial muscles of the pelvic floor (superficial transverse perineal muscle, external anal sphincter, and bulbospongiosus)

Levator Ani Muscle

The levator ani muscle constitutes the pelvic diaphragm and supports the pelvic viscera. It creates a hammock-like structure by extending from the left tendinous arch to the

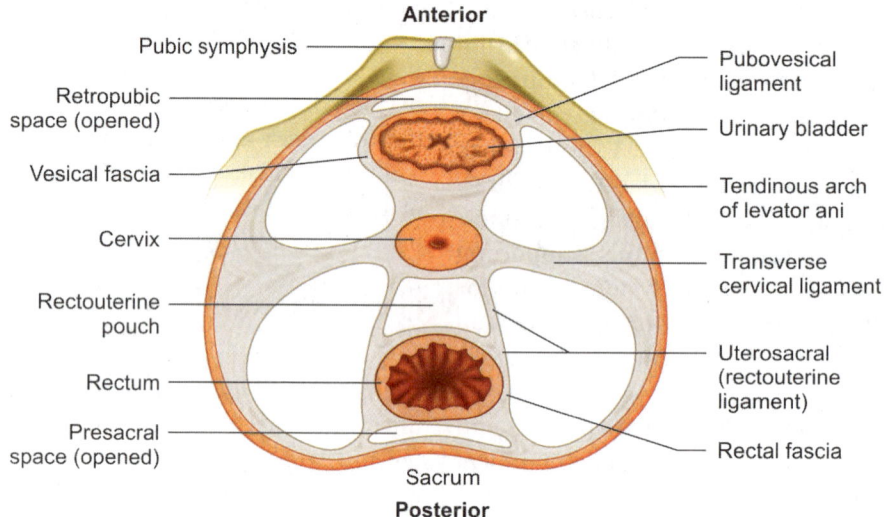

Fig. 29.8: Different ligamentous supports of the uterus.

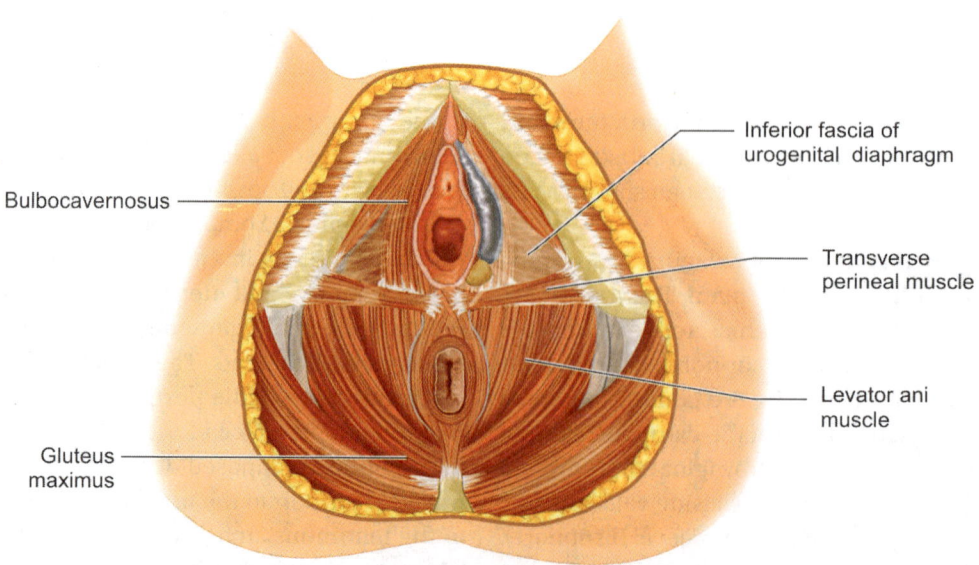

Fig. 29.9: The female perineum.

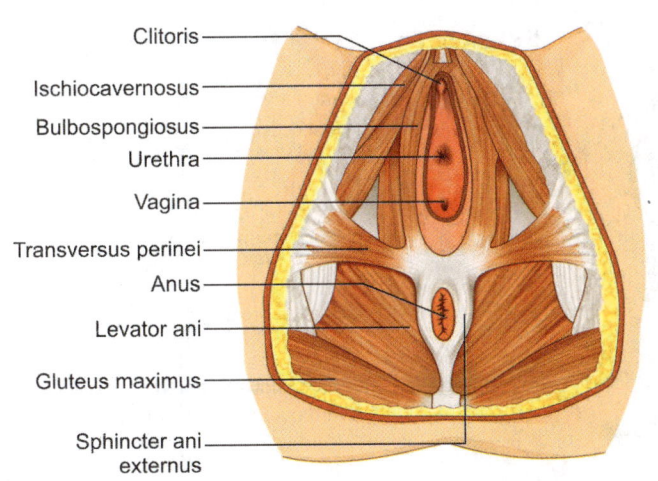

Fig. 29.10: Muscles of the pelvic floor including muscles of the pelvic diaphragm (levator ani muscle), muscles of the urogenital diaphragm (deep transverse perineal muscle), and superficial muscles of the pelvic floor (superficial transverse perineal muscle, external anal sphincter, and bulbospongiosus).

right tendinous arch. The muscle has openings through which the vagina, rectum, and urethra traverse. Contraction of levator muscles tends to pull the rectum and vagina inward, toward the pubic symphysis. This causes narrowing and kinking of both vagina and rectum. The origin of levator ani muscles is fixed on the anterior end because the muscle arises anteriorly either from the bone or from the fascia, which is attached to the bone. As a result, the anterior attachment of the muscle largely remains immobile. On the other hand, levator ani muscles posteriorly get inserted into the anococcygeal raphe or the coccyx, both of which are movable. Thus, the contraction of levator ani muscles tends to pull the posterior attachment toward the pubic symphysis.

The pelvic diaphragm consists of two levator ani muscles, one on each side. Each levator ani muscle consists of three main divisions: pubococcygeus, iliococcygeus, and ischiococcygeus **(Figs. 29.11A and B)**. The pubococcygeus muscle originates from the posterior surface of the pubic bone. It passes backward and lateral to the vagina and rectum to be inserted into the anococcygeal raphe and the coccyx. The inner fibers of this muscle, which come to lie posterior to the rectum, are known as the puborectalis portion of the muscle. These form a sling around the rectum and support it **(Fig. 29.12)**. Some of the inner fibers of puborectalis fuse with the outer vaginal wall as they pass lateral to it. Other fibers decussate between the vagina and the rectum in the region of perineal body. The decussating fibers divide the space between the two levator ani muscles into an anterior portion (hiatus urogenitalis), through which pass the urethra and vagina and a posterior portion (hiatus rectalis), through which passes the rectum. The iliococcygeus is fan-shaped muscle, which arises from a broad origin along white line of pelvic fascia. It passes backward and inward to be inserted into the coccyx. The ischiococcygeus muscle takes its origin from the ischial spine and spreads out posteriorly to be inserted into the front of coccyx. The superior and inferior surfaces of the levator muscles are covered with tough fibrous tissue known as pelvic fascia, which separates the muscles from the cellular tissues of the parametrium above and from the fibrous and fatty tissues of ischiorectal fossa below. This fascia is composed of two components: pelvic component (also known as the endopelvic fascia) and vaginal component (also known as periurethral fascia at the level of the urethra, and the perivesical fascia at the level of the bladder). The "pelvic component" fuses with the "vaginal component" to get inserted into the tendinous arch. Within the two components of the levator fascia are present the various pelvic organs, such as the urethra, bladder, vagina, and uterus, to which it provides support.

Central Tendinous Point of the Perineum or the Perineal Body

The perineal body is a pyramid-shaped fibromuscular structure lying at the midpoint between the vagina and the anus. It lies at the level of the junction between the middle-third and lower one-third of the posterior vaginal wall. Pb assumes importance in providing support to the pelvic organs as it provides attachment to the following eight muscles of the pelvic floor: superficial and deep transverse perineal muscles and levator ani muscles of both the sides, bulbocavernosus anteriorly and external anal sphincter posteriorly **(Fig. 29.13)**.

Deep Transverse Perineal Muscle

Deep transverse perineal muscles run transversely across the pelvic floor and lie within the urogenital diaphragm. They thus lie deep to the superficial transverse perineal muscles and are continuous with the sphincter urethrae muscle anteriorly. They originate from the medial surface of the ischiopubic ramus and get inserted into the midline raphe and the Pb.

Superficial Transverse Perineal Muscle

Superficial transverse perineal muscles arise from the upper and innermost part of the ischial tuberosity and run transversely across the pelvic floor, while lying superficial to the deep transverse perineal muscles. Running medially, they get inserted into the Pb.

Perineal tears occurring at the time of delivery and parturition tend to either divide the decussating fibers of levator ani or cause damage to the Pb. Both these factors can cause the hiatus urogenitalis to become patulous and result in the development of prolapse. Conditions which result in reduced tone of levator muscles tend to increase the dimensions of hiatus urogenitalis, thereby increasing the tendency of pelvic organs to prolapse.

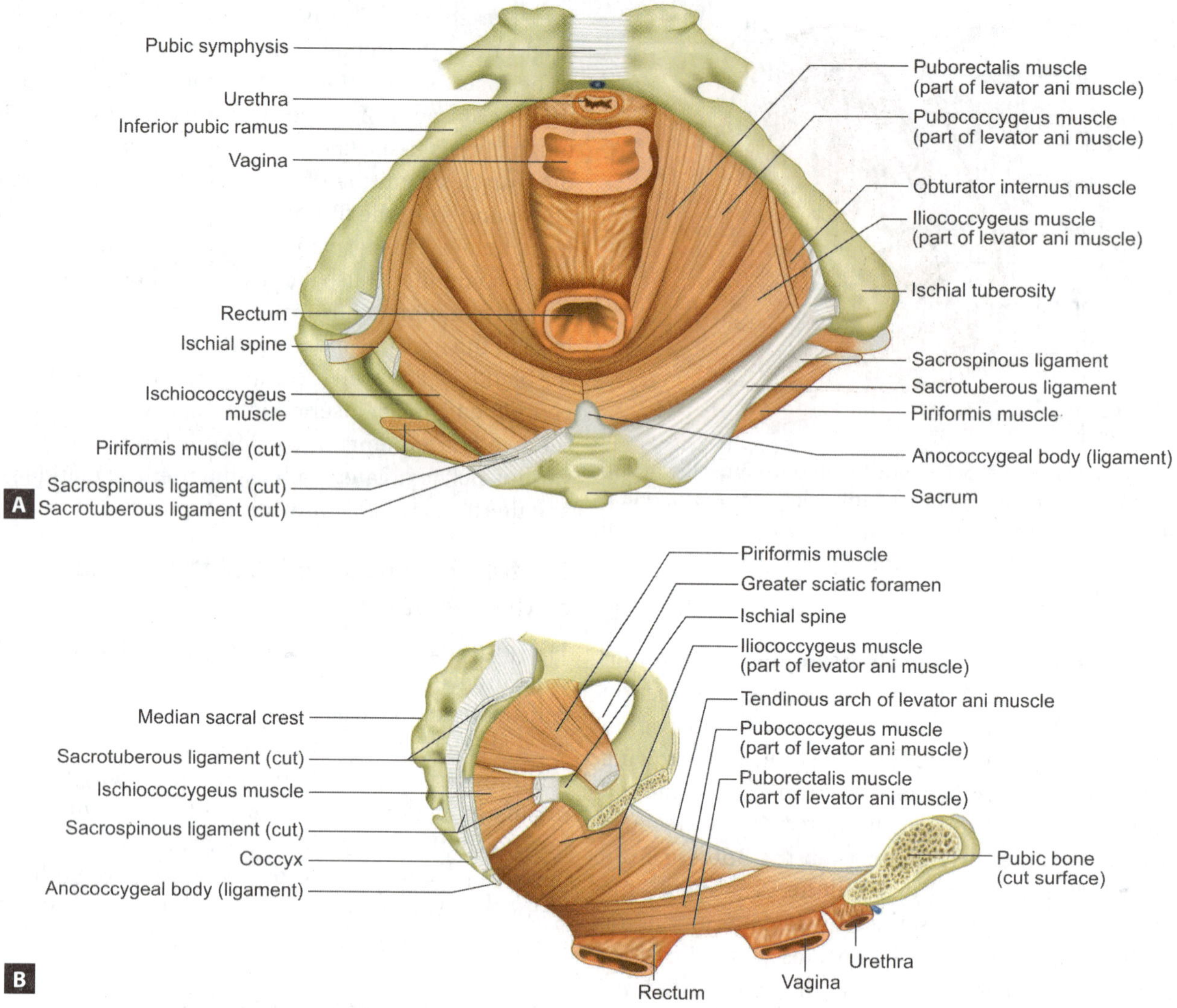

646 Uterine, Ovarian, and Tubal Pathology

Figs. 29.11A and B: Levator ani muscle. (A) Inferior view; (B) Lateral view.

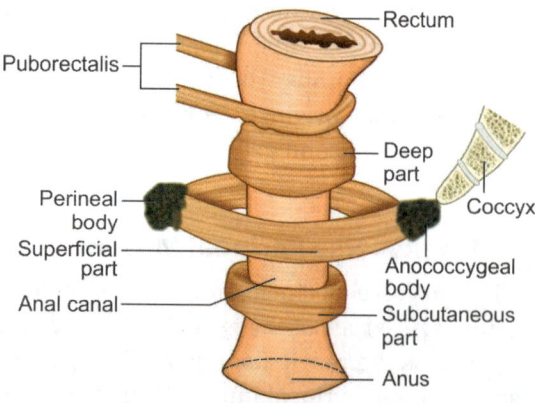

Fig. 29.12: Sling formed by levator ani muscles.

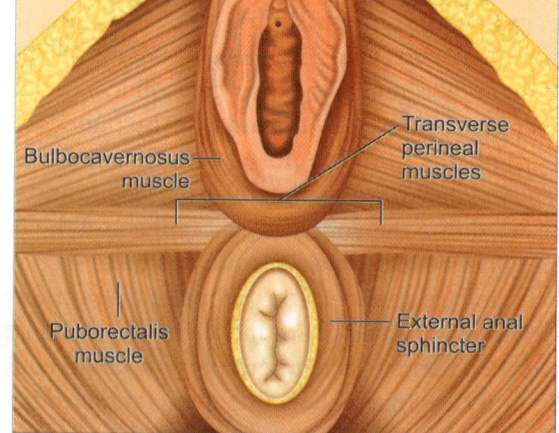

Fig. 29.13: Attachments of perineal body.

HISTORY AND CLINICAL PRESENTATION

RISK FACTORS

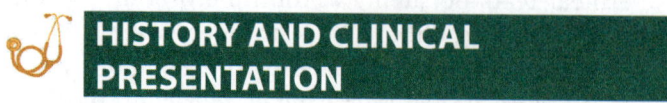

Q. Discuss in detail the causes of uterine prolapse in a woman of childbearing age group.

Risk factors associated with the development of uterine prolapse, which need to be elicited at the time of taking history, are described as follows:

- Obstetrical trauma associated with multiple vaginal deliveries in the past is especially associated with

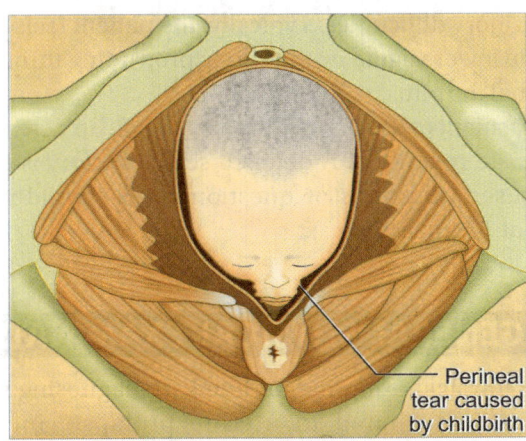

Fig. 29.14: Damage caused by childbirth to the muscles of pelvic floor.

development of prolapse in future **(Fig. 29.14)**. The factors during childbirth which are particularly likely to result in stretching and subsequent weakening of the pelvic support structures, such as the endopelvic fascia, levator muscles, and Pb, are described in the section of obstetric history, which follows later.

- While uterine prolapse is usually more common in multiparous women compared to the nulliparous ones, prolapse may also be sometimes seen in unmarried or nulliparous women. In nulliparous women, prolapse can mainly be attributed to spina occulta and split pelvis, which may result in inherent weakness of the pelvic floor support.
- Decreased estrogen levels (e.g., menopause) resulting in loss of strength and elasticity of pelvic structures. As a result, prolapse is more common in postmenopausal women.
- Increased intra-abdominal pressure (e.g., obesity, chronic lung disease, and asthma)
- History of smoking is particularly important. Not only does smoking act as a risk factor for the surgery but habitual smoking can also have both direct and indirect effects in causing weakness of the pelvic connective tissues. Also, smoking is antiestrogenic in nature.

Medical History

- History of many medical conditions (e.g., obesity, chronic pulmonary disease, smoking, constipation, chronic lung disease, and asthma), which may result in prolapse by causing an increase in intra-abdominal pressure, needs to be asked.
- Abnormalities in connective tissue (collagen), such as Marfan disease and Ehlers–Danlos syndrome, are associated with an increased risk of uterine prolapse.
- In neonates, uterine prolapse is secondary to congenital weakness in the pelvic musculature or defects in innervation.

Obstetric History

Previous obstetric history is particularly important in cases of pelvic prolapse because it may reveal the exact pathology responsible for development of prolapse. Some of the points in the history which need to be asked are as follows:

- *Route of delivery:* Vaginal delivery or delivery by cesarean route plays a crucial role in determining whether the woman may develop vaginal prolapse in future.

  In case of vaginal delivery, the clinician needs to ask whether delivery was taken by untrained midwife, trained midwife, or a doctor? The patient must also be asked about number of previous pregnancies and interval between successive deliveries. Interval between successive pregnancies is especially important because rapid succession of the pregnancies prevents proper puerperal rehabilitation, thereby resulting in a tendency to develop prolapse. In India and many other developing countries, a large number of deliveries are taken by untrained midwives. These untrained midwives tend to adopt certain techniques, which may serve as a risk factor for development of prolapse. Some of these techniques are as follows:

  - Patient is asked to bear down before full dilation of the cervix.
  - Bladder is not emptied before taking the delivery.
  - Untrained midwife usually does not give an episiotomy, which is a surgical incision and prevents perineal muscles from stretching and atonicity. As a result, the second stage of labor may be prolonged, resulting in undue stretching of the pelvic floor muscles.
  - Untrained midwife does not make use of forceps or vacuum in the case of prolonged second stage of labor. Furthermore, ventouse extraction of the fetus before the cervix is fully dilated can also result in overstretching of both the Mackenrodt's ligaments and the uterosacral ligaments and thereby cause prolapse in the long run.
  - Untrained midwife usually uses Crede's method of placental extraction, which involves giving vigorous downward push on the uterus to expel the placenta. This method may weaken the ligaments and muscles, which support the genital tract.
  - Untrained midwife may not stitch the lacerations or tears of the perineum, which occur during the childbirth. Unless sutured immediately, these tears and lacerations may cause widening of the hiatus urogenitalis.
  - Application of fundal pressure by the untrained midwife may also be responsible for prolapse.

- Whether delivery took place at home or hospital? Home delivery may force the woman to resume household activities soon after delivery without taking proper rest or

doing pelvic floor exercises. This may further predispose her to develop prolapse in the long run.
- Whether squatting position was used during delivery? Squatting during delivery may cause excessive stretching of the pelvic floor muscles and ligaments.
- Did the woman use a birthing ball to facilitate the process of normal vaginal delivery? Birthing ball, unlike the squatting position, facilitates fetal descent by causing gentle stretching of the muscles of pelvic floor.
- Woman must be asked about the weight at birth of each baby she has delivered. Delivery of a large-sized baby is likely to stretch the perineal muscles, resulting in patulous introitus and thereby prolapse.

Besides taking history of various risk factors related to prolapse, the gynecologist also needs to take history of different symptoms related to prolapse, as described next.

SYMPTOMS OF PROLAPSE

Symptoms of prolapse are typically exacerbated by prolonged standing or walking and are relieved by lying down. As a result, patients may feel better in the morning, with symptoms worsening throughout the day. Some of these symptoms include:
- Pelvic heaviness or pressure
- *Protrusion of tissue:* The patient often reports of experiencing a "bulge" passing through the vaginal introitus due to which she may experience difficulty while walking and urinating. She may complain of experiencing an annoying protrusion at the vaginal introitus. The patient may complain about a "bearing down sensation" or the feeling that "everything is falling."
- Pelvic pain
- Sexual dysfunction, including dyspareunia, decreased libido, and difficulty achieving orgasm
- *Lower back pain:* There may be feeling of discomfort and aching in the lower back.
- *Constipation:* Rectocele is usually not a cause of constipation, but may be aggravated by it.
- Difficulty in walking
- Urinary symptoms including increased urinary frequency, urgency, and urinary incontinence may be present. Cystocele may be associated with voiding difficulties such as imperfect control of micturition and stress incontinence. If present, these symptoms should be investigated because advanced prolapse may contribute to lower urinary tract dysfunction, including hydronephrosis and obstructive nephropathy.
- Rarely, the prolapsed uterus may become ulcerated (decubitus ulcer), resulting in purulent discharge and bleeding.
- The patient may experience vaginal spotting from ulceration of the protruding cervix or vagina, coital difficulty, lower abdominal discomfort and voiding, and defecatory difficulties. Typically, the patient feels a bulge in the lower vagina or the cervix protruding through the vaginal introitus.

Assessment of quality of life is also helpful in determining appropriate treatment. A detailed sexual history is crucial, and focused questions or questionnaires should include quality-of-life measures.

GENERAL PHYSICAL EXAMINATION

General physical examination helps in diagnosing serious complications related to uterine prolapse, including infection, urinary obstruction, hemorrhage, strangulation with uterine ischemia, urinary outflow obstruction with renal failure, etc.
- If urinary obstruction is present, the patient may exhibit suprapubic tenderness or a tympanitic bladder.
- If infection is present, purulent or blood-stained cervical discharge may be noted.

SPECIFIC SYSTEMIC EXAMINATION

Diagnosis of uterine prolapse is made by performing complete pelvic examination. This must include a rectovaginal examination in order to assess the sphincter tone. The detailed description of pelvic examination has been given in Chapter 22.

PER SPECULUM EXAMINATION

- The vaginal tissue must be evaluated for estrogen status on per speculum examination. Some of the signs of reduced estrogen status include the following:
  - Loss of rugosity of the vaginal wall mucosa
  - Reduced vaginal and cervical secretions
  - Thinning and tearing of the perineal skin
- Examination of the pelvic organ prolapse begins by asking the woman to attempt the Valsalva prior to placing a speculum in the vagina. Patients who are unable to adequately complete a Valsalva maneuver are asked to cough.
- To perform the evaluation of prolapse, a standard Sims' speculum and an anterior vaginal wall retractor are used. The Sims' speculum is placed in the vaginal vault to visually examine the vagina and cervix. The speculum is then replaced into the posterior vaginal wall, allowing visualization of the anterior wall. It is then everted in order to visualize the posterior wall. The point of maximal descent of the anterior, lateral, and apical vaginal walls is noted in relation to the ischial spines and hymen. The level to which the cervix descends on staining can be described as "descends to 2 inches below the introitus," etc. The term "procidentia" should be reserved for patients who have a total uterine prolapse with eversion of the entire vagina.

- Vaginal and cervical mucosa should be carefully examined for atrophy, hypertrophy, and other lesions. Vaginal cytology and biopsy may be required, if any lesions are present.

  Speculum examination helps in answering three questions:

  Whether the level of protrusion comes beyond the hymen, the presenting part of the prolapse (anterior, posterior, or apical), and does the widening of the vaginal hiatus occur with increased intra-abdominal pressure? Answers to these questions help the gynecologists to classify prolapse on the basis of system for quantification of pelvic organ prolapse (POP-Q system).

- In patients with significant degree of uterine prolapse, it is imperative to exclude the potential urinary incontinence. By definition, potential urinary incontinence must be present only when the prolapse is reduced. To test for potential urinary incontinence, the bladder is retrograde filled to maximum capacity (at least 300 mL) with sterile water or saline while replacing and elevating the prolapsed part digitally or with an appropriately fitted pessary. The patient is then asked to cough. If the patient leaks urine, the urinary incontinence is suspected, and the patient must be evaluated by performing a complete urodynamic test.

- In order to check the integrity of the sacral pathways, the bulbocavernous reflex and anal reflex are also evaluated. The presence of both these reflexes suggests normal sacral pathways. The bulbocavernous reflex is elicited by tapping or stroking lateral to the clitoris and observing the contractions of bulbocavernous bilaterally. Innervation of the external anal sphincter is evaluated by stroking lateral to the anus and observing the relative contraction of the anus.

PELVIC EXAMINATION

- Firstly, vaginal examination is carried out in the lithotomy position. The tone of pubococcygeus muscles on each side of the lower vaginal wall must be estimated. For this, two fingers are placed inside the vaginal introitus in such a way that each finger opposes the ipsilateral vaginal wall. The patient is then asked to contract these muscles as if she was attempting to stop the flow of urine during the act of voiding. Any protrusion felt on the vaginal fingers is noted. Following the evaluation of the lateral vaginal support system, the apex (cervix and apical vagina) is assessed. The examination is then repeated with the patient standing and in bearing down position in order to note the maximum descent of prolapse.

  The prolapse can be exaggerated by having the patient strain during the examination or by having her stand or walk prior to examination. The patient is asked to strain as if she was attempting to defecate, or she may also be asked to cough.

- Next, the strength and quality of pelvic floor contraction are assessed by asking the patient to tighten the levator muscles around the examining finger. The diameter of the vaginal introitus and length of Pb must also be assessed.

- A bimanual examination must be performed in order to note the uterine size, mobility, and adnexa. Bimanual examination also helps in ensuring that the pelvic organs are free and not restricted by adhesions or any pathology. Lastly, a rectal examination is performed in order to assess the tone of external sphincter muscles; to note the presence of any palpable pathology, blood on the examining finger, and the rectocele; to differentiate between rectocele and enterocele, strength of the perineum; and to assess the rectovaginal septum. The rectovaginal septum may feel to be unusually thin in between the examining fingers. The examiner needs to differentiate between rectocele and enterocele. For this, the index finger of the clinician's left hand is placed in the rectum with the tip directed upward. Two fingers of the right hand are then placed in the vagina. The patient is asked to strain downward. If a bulge is felt between the examining fingers in the space between the rectum and upper posterior vaginal wall, it is most likely to be an enterocele. On the other hand, if the bulge is felt on the tip of the index finger in the rectum, the bulge is most likely to be a rectocele. The thickness of the perineum can be assessed by feeling the distance between the anal orifice and posterior fourchette, with the finger in the rectum and the thumb pressing against the perineum. Observation of the small bowel peristalsis behind the vaginal wall is definitively indicative of enterocele. In general, bulges at the apical segment of the posterior vaginal wall implicate enterocele, whereas bulges in the posterior wall are most likely to be rectocele. Assessment of both the resting and the contraction tone of pelvic floor muscles must also be done.

Evaluation of the Degree of Prolapse

The Baden–Walker Halfway system as described in **Table 29.1** and **Figures 29.15A to D** is the system which is commonly used for evaluation of pelvic organ prolapse. Another important system which is often used for evaluation of pelvic organ prolapse is the POP-Q system for quantification of pelvic prolapse and is described as follows.

POP-Q System for Quantification of Pelvic Prolapse

> Q. Discuss the POP-Q classification of pelvic prolapse. Discuss the conservative surgeries for genital prolapse.
>
> Q. Describe the latest classification and grading of prolapse. Also discuss management of prolapse in an elderly lady.

In 1966, the International Continence Society defined an organ prolapse (POP-Q system). This system is based on a

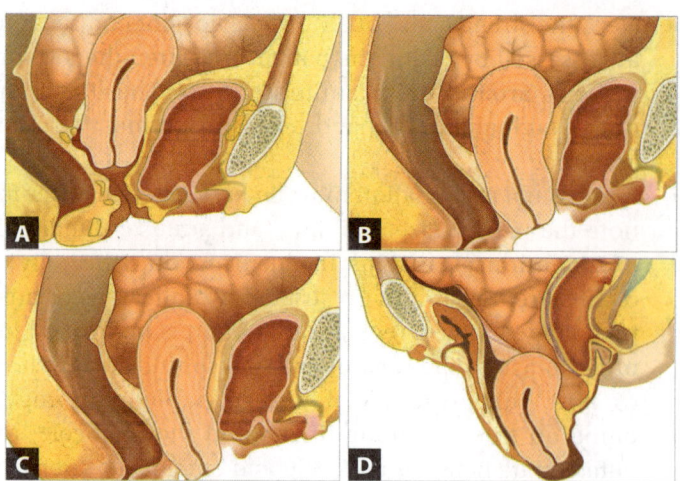

Figs. 29.15A to D: Stages of uterine prolapse. (A) Stage I uterine prolapse; (B) Stage II uterine prolapse; (C) Stage III uterine prolapse; (D) Uterine procidentia.

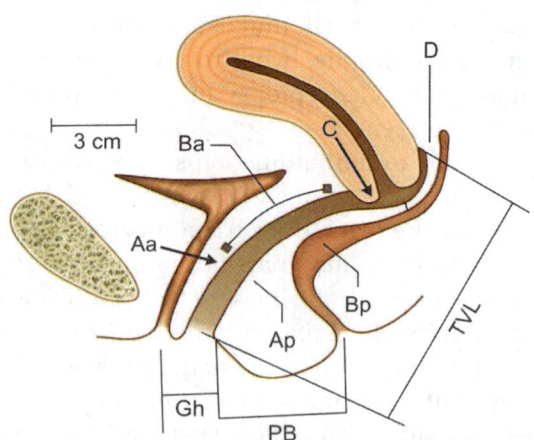

Fig. 29.16: POP-Q system for quantification of pelvic prolapse. (Gh: genital hiatus; PB: perineal body; TVL: total vaginal length)
Source: Bump RC, Mattiasson A, Bø K, Brubaker LP, DeLancey JO, Klarskov P, et al. The standardization of terminology of female pelvic organ prolapse and pelvic floor dysfunction. Am J Obstet Gynecol. 1996;175(1):10-7. doi: 10.1016/s0002-9378(96)70243-0.

series of site-specific measurements of the woman's pelvic organ support system in relation to the hymen in each of the segments. This system is based on the measurement of six points, which are located with the reference to the plane of the hymen: two on the anterior vaginal wall (Aa and Ba), two in the apical vagina (C and D), and two on the posterior vaginal wall (Ap and Bp). All these six points are measured with the patient engaged in maximum protrusion and have been illustrated in **Figure 29.16**.

Anterior vaginal wall points:
- *Point Aa:* This is the point on the anterior vaginal wall in the midline and lies 3 cm above the external urethral meatus, corresponding to the proximal location of the urethrovesical crease. In relation to the hymen, this point's position ranges by definition from −3 (normal support) to +3 cm (maximum prolapse of the point Aa).
- *Point Ba:* This point represents the most distal edge of cervix or vaginal cuff. It is −3 cm in the absence of prolapse. In a woman with total vaginal eversion post hysterectomy, Ba would have a positive value equal to the position of the cuff from the hymen.

Apical vaginal points: The apical points represent the most proximal locations of a normally positioned lower reproductive tract.
- *Point C:* This point represents either the most distal edge of the cervix or the leading edge of the vaginal cuff after total hysterectomy.
- *Point D:* This represents the location of posterior fornix in a woman who still has a cervix. This point is omitted while making measurements, if cervix is absent. It is located at the level of attachment of the uterosacral ligament to the proximal posterior cervix.

Posterior vaginal wall points:
- *Point Ap:* This point is located 3 cm proximal to the hymen on the posterior vaginal wall. Relative to the hymen, the position of this point may range from −3 (normal support) to +3 (maximum prolapse of the point Ap).
- *Point Bp:* This point represents the most distal position of the upper portion of posterior vaginal wall from the vaginal cuff. By definition, this point is at −3 cm in the absence of prolapse. In a woman with total vaginal eversion post hysterectomy, Bp would have a positive value equal to the position of the cuff from the hymen.

Total vaginal length, genital hiatus (Gh), and perineal body (PB): Total vaginal length (TVL) is the greatest depth of vagina (in centimeters) when points C and D are reduced to their fullest position.

In addition to the TVL, remaining measurements include those of the Gh and PB. The Gh is measured from the middle of the external urethral meatus to the midline of the posterior hymenal ring. The PB is measured from the posterior margin of the Gh to the midanal opening.

Assessment of prolapse using the POP-Q system: The POP-Q staging system is shown in **Table 29.3**. While assessing the degree of prolapse using the POP-Q system, the hymenal plane is defined as zero. The anatomical position of these points from the hymen is measured in centimeters. Points above the hymen are described with a negative number, whereas points below the hymen are described using a positive number. It is important to remember that these various measurements can change in accordance with the position of the patient, e.g., whether the patient was standing or in lithotomy position or whether she was asked to strain. Thus, it is important to mention the patient's position at the time of taking measurements.

If the POP-Q examination is performed, firstly the Gh and Pb are measured during the Valsalva maneuver. TVL is the only measurement made while the patient is not engaged in Valsalva maneuver. It is measured by placing the marked

TABLE 29.3: POP-Q staging system for pelvic organ prolapse.

Stage of prolapse	Definition
Stage 0	No prolapse is demonstrated. Points Aa, Ap, Ba, and Bp are all 3 cm above the hymenal ring (value = –3) and either points C or D is at a position above the hymen that is equal to or within 2 cm of TVL. Thus, the quantitation value for point C or D is ≤–(TVL – 2) cm
Stage I	The criteria for stage 0 are not met, but all the points are >1 cm above the level of the hymen (i.e., its quantitation value is ≤–1 cm)
Stage II	The most distal portion of the prolapse protrudes to a point to or above 1 cm above the hymen but no more than 1 cm beyond the hymen (i.e., its quantitation value ≥1 cm but ≤+1 cm)
Stage III	The most distal portion of the prolapse protrudes at least 1 cm below the plane of hymen but protrudes no further than 2 cm less than the TVL (in cm), i.e., its quantitation value is >+1 cm but <+(TVL – 2) cm
Stage IV	Complete eversion of the total length of the lower genital tract is demonstrated. The distal portion of the prolapse protrudes to within 2 cm of the TVL, i.e., its quantitation value is ≥+(TVL– 2) cm

(POP-Q: pelvic organ prolapse quantification; TVL: total vaginal length)

ring forceps at the vaginal apex and noting the distance to the hymen. The apical points C and D are then measured during maximal Valsalva effort. The anterior and posterior vaginal walls are next visualized, and lastly the points Aa, Ba, Ap, and Bp are respectively measured. The urethra is also evaluated during anterior vaginal wall assessment. If the posterior vaginal wall descends, attempts must be made to determine whether rectocele or enterocele is present.

DIFFERENTIAL DIAGNOSIS

Various symptoms related to prolapse could be contributed by several other disorders unrelated to uterine prolapse. For e.g., disorders such as rectal prolapse, presence of vulvar or vaginal cysts/masses, pelvic masses (both adnexal and uterine), or hernia (vaginal or femoral) could produce a sensation of something bulging or protruding through the vaginal introitus. Urinary symptoms such as urinary urgency, frequency, or incontinence could be related to disorders such as incompetence of the urethral sphincters, detrusor overactivity, bladder outlet obstruction, interstitial cystitis, or UTI. Bowel symptoms, such as incontinence of flatus/liquid/solid stools, feeling of incomplete emptying or difficulty in defecation, and urgency to defecate, could be related to disorders such as disruption of anal sphincters or neuropathy, diarrheal disorders, rectal prolapse, inflammatory bowel syndrome, rectal inertia, pelvic floor dyssynergia, hemorrhoids, and anorectal neoplasm. Moreover, sexual symptoms such as dyspareunia, decreased lubrication, reduced sexual sensation, and reduced arousal or orgasm could be related to disorders such as interstitial cystitis, levator ani syndrome, and vulvodynia. Back pain can also result due to lumbar disk herniation or musculoskeletal diseases.

Though the diagnosis of prolapse can be easily established on per speculum and pelvic examinations and it is unlikely to confuse prolapse with any other pathology, congenital elongation of the cervix needs to be ruled out. In cases of congenital elongation of the cervix, the vaginal portion of the cervix is elongated and there is no accompanying vaginal prolapse. As a result, the vaginal fornices are unusually deep. Many a times, decubitus ulceration over the prolapse may resemble an ulcerated cervical fibroid or polyp. A cervical fibroid or polyp can be easily differentiated from cases of uterine prolapse as in case of cervical fibroids, the cervix is high up and in a normal anatomical position.

MANAGEMENT

Q. Write a long essay discussing the management of third-degree prolapse uterus in a para 2 woman aged 30 years.

Q. Discuss the management of nulliparous prolapse in a 25-year-old woman.
Ans. Nulliparous prolapse is likely to be responsible for 1.5–2% cases of genital prolapse in India. The etiology could be related to connective tissue disorders, congenital defects of pelvic floor muscles (e.g., exstrophy of bladder) or congenital defects of spine (e.g., spina bifida occulta). Surgery must aim at providing symptomatic relief, restoration of fertility and reproductive function, and prevention of recurrence. Surgery may involve the use of slings (abdominal or laparoscopic) or transvaginal sacrospinous fixation.

Q. What would be the next step of management in the case study mentioned in the beginning of the chapter?
Ans. In the above-mentioned case study, the prolapse significantly interfered with the patient's day-to-day functioning and prevented her from standing for prolonged periods. Therefore, it needs to be treated. Since the patient was more than 40 years old and did not want to preserve her uterus, a transvaginal hysterectomy was planned. In order to prevent the recurrence of prolapse, surgical treatment for various types of defects must be performed together at the time of surgery. It is very important that the physician carefully inspects the vagina for other prolapses. At the time of hysterectomy in this patient, the following repairs were planned: anterior colporrhaphy, posterior colporrhaphy, and a McCall's culdoplasty. McCall's culdoplasty was performed in this patient in order to obliterate the cul-de-sac and prevent the future development of both vaginal vault prolapse and enterocele.

INVESTIGATIONS

Diagnosis of uterine prolapse is made on pelvic examination. Investigations are directed toward identification of rare but serious complications related to uterine prolapse (infection, urinary obstruction, hemorrhage, strangulation) and for assessing the patient's suitability for anesthesia.

The various laboratory investigations which may be required are as follows:

- *Hemoglobin:* Estimation of hemoglobin levels gives an idea about the patient's anemic status.
- *Urine examination:* Urine analysis is important because it is essential to rule out UTI before undertaking surgery.
- *Blood urea and creatinine levels:* These tests of renal function may be indicated in cases with suspected urinary obstruction.
- Blood sugar
- X-ray chest
- Electrocardiography
- *Urine culture:* It is specifically indicated in cases of suspected UTI.
- *High vaginal swabs:* They are indicated in cases of vaginitis.
- Cervical cultures are indicated for cases complicated by ulceration or purulent discharge.
- Pap smear cytology may be indicated in cases of suspected carcinoma, although this is a rare occurrence.
- *Imaging studies:* A pelvic ultrasound examination may be useful in distinguishing prolapse from other pathologies, especially when other differential diagnoses are suspected on the basis of history and physical examination. Ultrasound also serves as an important investigation modality for diagnosing hydronephrosis and excluding the presence of pelvic masses such as uterine fibroids and adnexal masses.

TREATMENT/GYNECOLOGICAL MANAGEMENT

PREVENTION

Several steps can be taken to prevent the development of uterine prolapse. Some of these steps are as follows:

1. Steps must be taken to minimize obstetrical trauma during vaginal delivery.
2. Second stage of labor must be properly supervised and managed. Earlier it was thought that the routine use of episiotomy in a primigravida would help in preventing undue stretching of the pelvic floor muscles and subsequently prolapse in the long run. However, in the light of present evidence, routine use of episiotomy and its role in preventing prolapse have largely been questioned.
3. Low forceps delivery should be undertaken in cases of delayed second stage of labor.
4. Perineal tear must be immediately and accurately sutured after delivery.
5. Patient must be advised to maintain a reasonable time interval between pregnancies using family planning methods so that too many births at too short intervals are avoided. This helps the pelvic muscles to recover their tone in between pregnancies.
6. Antenatal physiotherapy, postnatal exercises, early postnatal ambulation, and physiotherapy are highly beneficial in preventing prolapse. Adequate rest must be provided to the patient for the first 6 months after delivery, and there must be availability of home help for carrying out heavy domestic duties.
7. Woman should be advised to maintain a healthy body weight. She should be instructed to exercise regularly for 20–30 minutes, three to five times per week. She should be especially advised to do Kegel exercises, which may be done up to four times a day.
8. *Pelvic floor (Kegel) exercises:* Although routine use of Kegel exercises can improve the tone of pelvic floor muscles and stress urinary incontinence, presently there is no high-quality evidence in the form of prospective, double-blinded, randomized trials, which indicates that improvement of pelvic floor muscle tone leads to regression of uterine prolapse. The Kegel floor exercises must be done at least 50–200 times per day, each exercise attempt lasting for about 5–10 seconds.
9. Besides doing regular exercises, the woman must be advised to eat a healthy balanced diet containing appropriate amounts of protein, fat, carbohydrates, and high amounts of dietary fiber (such as whole grain cereals, legumes, and vegetables). A healthy, well-balanced diet can help maintain weight and prevent constipation, which may serve as a predisposing factor for development of prolapse.
10. Patient should be advised to stop smoking. This helps in reducing the risk of developing a chronic cough, which is likely to put extra strain on the pelvic muscles.
11. Prophylactic HRT in menopausal women can avoid or delay the occurrence of prolapse. The use of estrogen replacement therapy, however, has no role in treatment of established cases of uterine prolapse.
12. Woman should be instructed to use correct weightlifting techniques in order to avoid undue straining of the pelvic floor muscles.

NONSURGICAL MANAGEMENT

Expectant management including pelvic floor exercises (Kegel exercises) and pessaries is the current mainstay of nonsurgical management of patients with uterine prolapse. Nonsurgical management must be primarily used in cases with mild degree of uterovaginal prolapse with no or minimal symptoms. Since severe degree of prolapse may interfere with the functioning of urinary tract, such patients should not be managed expectantly.

Pessary Treatment for Prolapse

Pessary is a nonsurgical method for supporting the uterine and vaginal structures. A small pessary may help in maintaining normal uterine position. Pessaries are usually used for attaining temporary relief in cases with symptomatic prolapse. Some indications for using pessaries are enumerated in **Box 29.1**. One of the important indications for using pessary is in young women following childbirth. Immediate surgical treatment must not be advised in a woman suffering from prolapse immediately following childbirth. This is so as the possibility of recurrence of prolapse is high if the surgery is performed within 6 months of delivery. Furthermore, the symptoms of prolapse rapidly improve using conservative measures such as massage and abdominal and perineal exercises. Conservative measures should be advised following delivery for at least 3–4 months.

Presence of infection, such as acute PID and recurrent vaginitis, acts as contraindication for pessary use. The two most common types of pessaries used include ring pessary and donut pessary. Other types are the inflatable ball, cube, and Gellhorn pessaries **(Figs. 29.17A to K)**. The Gellhorn pessary is most often used for patients with significant uterine prolapse and a large introital diameter who have not obtained relief with other pessaries. The Smith–Hodge pessary facilitates retrodisplacement of the uterus and should be used for patients with a well-defined pubic notch and adequate vaginal width. However, the use of pessary requires frequent care and monitoring by a gynecologist.

BOX 29.1: Current indications for the use of pessary.
- Young woman planning a pregnancy in future
- During early pregnancy, immediately after delivery, and during lactation
- Temporary use while clearing infection and decubitus ulcer prior to the actual surgery
- Women unfit for surgery
- Women who do not desire surgery

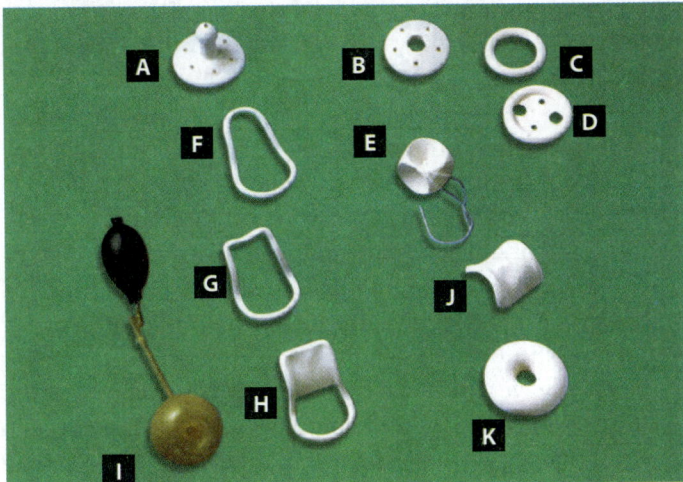

Figs. 29.17A to K: Different types of pessaries used for treatment of uterine prolapse. (A) Gellhorn; (B) Shaatz; (C) Ring; (D) Ring with support; (E) Cube; (F) Smith; (G) Hodge; (H) Hodge with support for cystocele; (I) Inflatoball; (J) Gehrung; (K) Donut.

Pessaries may cause vaginitis, bleeding, ulceration, urinary incontinence, urinary obstruction with retention, fistula formation, and erosion into the bladder or rectum. Most complications result from a retained pessary that had been long forgotten inside the vagina.

Expectant Management

Expectant management involves taking steps to improve conditions which are likely to result in prolapse. This involves treatment of underlying conditions such as chronic cough, obesity, and constipation. Administration of HRT in postmenopausal women helps in improving the tone of the pelvic floor muscles. Postmenopausal women may be administered HRT in the form of conjugated equine estrogens in the dosage of 0.625 mg, 3–4 weeks prior to the surgery. Daily application of estrogen cream may also prove to be useful.

Expectant management also involves regular use of pelvic floor exercises or Kegel exercises. Antibiotic therapy may be indicated for rare cases of prolapse complicated by infection. Steps must also be taken to heal decubitus ulcers prior to surgery. For curing decubitus ulcers, the patient is admitted in the hospital a week prior to the surgery. The prolapsed organs are replaced and packed in position by a tampon or gauze soaked in acriflavine glycerine, which is changed everyday. This action helps in healing the ulcer by restoring circulation to the prolapsed organs. There is usually no need to impregnate the tampon with antibiotics.

SURGERY: DEFINITIVE TREATMENT

Surgery helps in providing relief against symptoms of prolapse and restoring pelvic anatomy, sexual functioning, and human physiologic function (micturition and defecation). Since uterine prolapse is not a life-threatening condition, surgery is indicated only if the patient feels that her condition is severe enough that it warrants correction. Mild prolapse, which is rarely symptomatic, does not require surgical correction. Surgery is usually advised in women over 40 years of age unless it is contraindicated or is hazardous on account of some medical disorders.

Since the surgical treatment for various types of prolapse can be performed together at the time of surgery, it is very important that the physician carefully inspects the vagina for other prolapses. All forms of vaginal relaxation should be treated at the same time as hysterectomy or uterine suspension. It is possible to have vaginal prolapse surgery without the need for hysterectomy or uterine suspension if there is no prolapsed uterus. The main challenge for the pelvic surgeon is to recreate normal pelvic anatomy while restoring normal physiological functioning as far as possible. Experienced gynecologic surgeons can reevaluate the anatomy intraoperatively, noting the

> **BOX 29.2:** Surgical options which can be used in cases of prolapse.
> - Vaginal hysterectomy, posterior culdoplasty, colporrhaphy
> - Vaginal hysterectomy, closure of enterocele sac, total colpectomy, colporrhaphy, colpocleisis
> - Combined vaginal colporrhaphy and abdominal hysterectomy
> - Moschcowitz culdoplasty, sacral colpopexy, and suprapubic urethrocolpopexy
> - Manchester operation
> - Le fort colpocleisis and colporrhaphy
> - Vaginal repair and uterine suspension

strength and consistency of the various support structures (e.g., uterosacral ligaments). If these structures are found to be weak, it may be necessary to use other, stronger reattachment sites, such as the sacrospinous ligament or the presacral fascia, for the correction of the defect. In addition, every possible attempt must be made to prevent the possibility of recurrence of pelvic organ prolapse. For e.g., when performing a retropubic urethropexy for urinary incontinence, a concomitant colpocleisis may avoid the formation of an enterocele in the future. Surgical options which can be used in cases of prolapse are enumerated in **Box 29.2**. The choice of surgery depends on numerous factors:

- Degree of prolapse
- Areas specific for prolapse
- Desire for future pregnancies
- Desire to maintain future sexual function
- Preservation of vaginal function
- Woman's age and general health
- Patient's choice (i.e., surgery or no surgery)
- Medical condition and age
- Severity of symptoms
- Patient's suitability for surgery
- Presence of other pelvic conditions requiring simultaneous treatment, including urinary or fecal incontinence
- Presence or absence of urethral hypermobility
- History of previous pelvic surgery

Although the choice of procedure largely depends on the surgeon's preference and experience, the gynecologist needs to consider numerous factors such as the patient's general health status, degree and type of uterine prolapse, requirement for preservation or restoration of coital function, concomitant intrapelvic disease, and the patient's desire for preservation of menstrual and reproductive function. A careful preoperative evaluation should be carried out in order to identify all concomitant defects associated with uterine prolapse, which should be repaired in order to avoid recurrence of prolapse in future. In a patient with advanced degree of prolapse, additional procedures such as sacrospinous ligament fixation, sacral colpopexy, or colpectomy with colpocleisis may be required to provide adequate support to the vaginal vault.

Preoperative Treatment

Before undertaking the surgical treatment for prolapse, following steps need to be taken:

1. Medical treatment for chronic cough or constipation must be administered.
2. If decubitus ulceration is present over the prolapsed tissue, it first needs to be treated by the application of glycerine acriflavine pack or ring pessaries. Both these strategies help by repositioning the uterus to the normal anatomical position, thereby relieving the kinking of uterine blood vessels, cervical congestion, and ulceration. The surgery must be undertaken only when the decubitus ulceration has regressed.
3. Surgery must be undertaken only when the associated UTI and PID have been aggressively treated.
4. Preoperative estrogen therapy must be given, especially to the elderly postmenopausal patients in whom vaginal epithelium is thin and inflamed.
5. Aseptic vaginal douches should be administered a day before surgery.
6. Full dose of antibiotics (80 mg of gentamycin, 1 g of ampicillin, and 500 mg of metronidazole) must be administered 2 hours before surgery to prevent postoperative pelvic infections.

Principles of Surgery for Pelvic Organ Prolapse

The following principles must be taken into consideration, while undertaking surgery for pelvic organ prolapse:

- At the time of clinical examination, when the patient is made to bear down, the site of primary damage appears first, followed by the sites of secondary damage. The gynecologist must take special note of this site of primary damage. The primary site of damage should be identified first and over-repaired in order to reduce the chances of recurrence.
- Gynecologist must repair all relaxations of the supporting tissues, even if they are minor, in order to prevent recurrence in the future.
- Strength of the various support structures should be evaluated. Even the relatively weak structures can be used, but they must not be used to provide dependable support at the time of reconstruction surgery.
- As far as possible, the surgeon must try to create a normal anatomy. Normal vaginal length should be maintained because a shortened vagina is likely to prolapse again.
- Vagina should be suspended in its normal posterior direction over the levator plate and rectum, pointing into the hollow of the sacrum, toward S3 and S4. The surgeon should avoid suspending the vaginal vault anteriorly to the abdominal wall.
- Cul-de-sac should be closed and rectocele repaired in all cases. A posterior colpoperineorrhaphy should preferably be performed in all cases, where possible.

- Repair of the lower posterior vaginal wall provides some support to the anterior vaginal wall and also lengthens the vagina.
- *Methods for preventing vault prolapse:* Various methods for preventing vaginal prolapse at the time of hysterectomy are enumerated in **Box 29.3**. These various procedures are described as follows.

Culdoplasty

Culdoplasty involves surgical obliteration of the cul-de-sac. The following types are commonly employed in clinical practice:

- *McCall's culdoplasty:* It involves attaching the uterosacral–cardinal ligament complex to the peritoneal surface **(Figs. 29.18A and B)**. The sutures are attached in such a way that when they are tied, the uterosacral–cardinal ligaments are drawn toward the midline. This helps in closing off the cul-de-sac. Additionally, when the sutures are tied, the posterior vaginal apex is drawn up to a higher position, thereby supporting the vaginal vault. The main disadvantage of this type of culdoplasty is a possible increased incidence of kinking or ligating the ureter, because it is so close to the uterosacral ligament. When the uterosacral ligaments are long and strong, the addition of McCall's culdoplasty also helps to reestablish the vaginal length.
- *Moschcowitz culdoplasty:* This process involves the use of circumferential suture for the closure of cul-de-sac **(Fig. 29.19)**.
- *Halban cul-de-sac closure:* The procedure of Halban's culdoplasty is described in **Figures 29.20A to C**. While both the McCall's culdoplasty and the Moschcowitz culdoplasty are performed via the vaginal route. Halban culdoplasty is performed via the abdominal route.

Suspension of Vagina

Suspension of vagina can be done via vaginal route (transvaginal sacrospinous colpopexy) or abdominal route (abdominal sacrocolpopexy). Both these procedures have been discussed in detail later in the text.

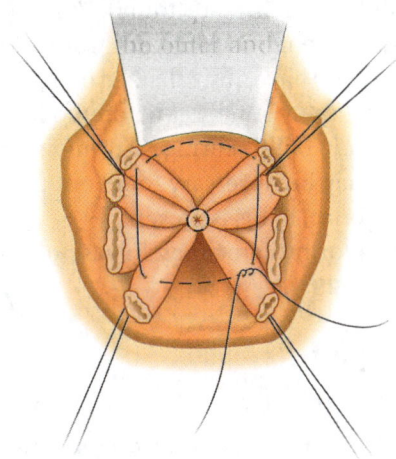

Fig. 29.19: Moschcowitz culdoplasty involving the use of a circumferential suture for closing the cul-de-sac. The first purse-string suture has been placed and tied, closing the peritoneal cavity. The second purse-string suture has been placed 1 cm below the first suture and is yet to be tied.

BOX 29.3: Methods for preventing vaginal prolapse at the time of hysterectomy.

Culdoplasty (obliteration of cul-de-sac):
- McCall's culdoplasty
- Moschcowitz culdoplasty (use of circumferential suture for the closure of cul-de-sac)
- Halban cul-de-sac closure

Suspension of vagina:
- *Vaginal route:* Transvaginal sacrospinous colpopexy
- *Abdominal route:* Abdominal sacrocolpopexy

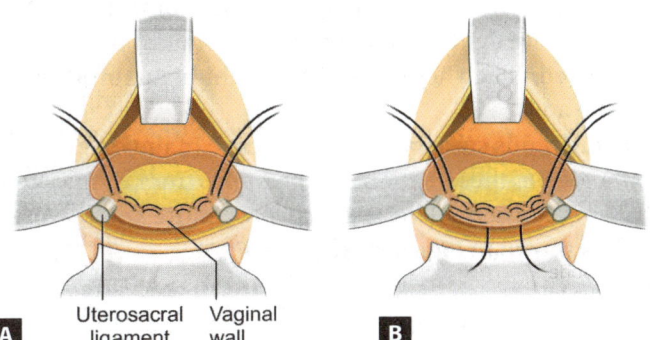

Figs. 29.18A and B: McCall's culdoplasty. (A) Placement of internal sutures; (B) Placement of external suture.

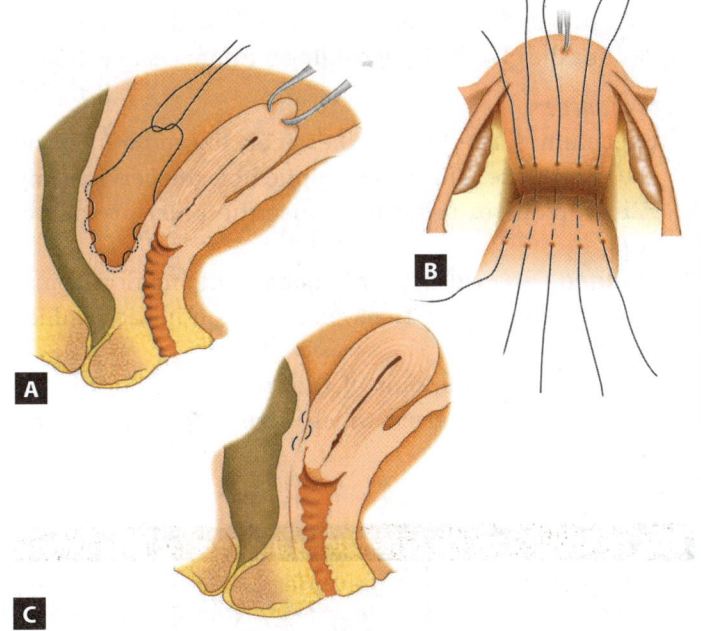

Figs. 29.20A to C: Halban's culdoplasty with uterus in situ. (A) Lateral view showing the attachment of the suture to sigmoid, upper vagina, and lower uterine segment; (B) Superior view of the cul-de-sac; (C) Lateral view of completed closure.

DESCRIPTION OF VARIOUS SURGICAL PROCEDURES

Different types of available surgical options such as hysterectomy, repair of anterior defects, repair of posterior defects, enterocele repair, Manchester repair, and obliterative procedures such as Le Fort colpocleisis would now be described.

Hysterectomy

Surgical removal of uterus or hysterectomy can be done via the vaginal route (vaginal hysterectomy) or through the abdomen (abdominal hysterectomy). Vaginal hysterectomy with pelvic floor repair is suitable for women over the age of 40 years, those who have normal-sized uterus, and those who have completed their families and are no longer interested in retaining their childbearing and menstrual functions. A Kelly stitch may be necessary to relieve the patient of her stress incontinence, if this is present.

Indications for hysterectomy in case of prolapse uterus are listed in **Box 29.4**.

Anterior Repair

Anterior Colporrhaphy

Anterior colporrhaphy operation is one of the most commonly performed surgeries to repair a cystocele and cystourethrocele. This surgery is usually performed under general or regional anesthesia.

Principles of anterior colporrhaphy: It comprises the following steps: excision of a portion of relaxed anterior vaginal wall, mobilization of bladder, pushing the bladder upward after cutting the vesicocervical ligament, and permanently supporting the bladder by tightening the pubocervical fascia.

Steps of surgery:
1. Speculum is inserted into the vagina to expose it during the procedure. Traction is applied on the cervix using Allis forceps in order to expose the anterior vaginal wall.
2. Inverted T-shaped incision is made in the anterior vaginal wall, starting with a transverse incision in the bladder sulcus.
3. Through the midpoint of this transverse incision a vertical incision is given, which extends up to the urethral opening.
4. Vaginal walls are reflected to either side to expose the bladder and vesicovaginal fascia. Bladder is pushed upward, and the vaginal skin is separated from the underlying fascia.
5. Overlying vesicovaginal and pubocervical fascia is plicated with interrupted "0" catgut to correct the vaginal wall laxity and to close the hiatus through which the bladder herniates.
6. Redundant portion of the vaginal mucosa is cut on either side.
7. Cut margins of vagina are apposed together.
8. In women suffering from stress incontinence, a Kelly suture to plicate the bladder neck helps to correct stress incontinence.

Disadvantages: Anterior colporrhaphy is still today the most commonly performed procedure to treat cystoceles, despite several disadvantages. Some of these are as follows:
- It has failure rates in the range of 30–50%.
- It has poor cure rates.
- There is requirement for a repeat procedure.
- Surgery can result in constriction of vagina.
- Constriction and/or shortening of vagina can result in dyspareunia. The surgery is not a true repair; it is just a compensatory procedure, associated with plication of the weakened tissue. Tightening of tissue under the bladder neck can result in voiding dysfunction.

Figures 29.21A to F illustrate the sequence of events in the repair of a midline defect cystocele. The patient has a cystocele due to weakness of the pubocervical fascia in the midline.

Posterior Repair

Posterior Colporrhaphy and Colpoperineorrhaphy

While repairing the rectocele, most surgeons also perform a posterior colporrhaphy. This process involves nonspecific midline plication of the rectovaginal fascia after reducing the rectocele. The lax vaginal tissue over the rectocele is excised. The medial fibers of the levator ani are then pulled together, approximated, and sutured over the top of rectum. This helps in restoring the caliber of the hiatus urogenitalis, and strengthening the Pb. An adequate amount of perineum is also created, which helps in separating the hiatus urogenitalis from the anal canal.

Though this surgery is quite effective in the treatment of the rectocele, these patients often suffer from dyspareunia following surgery. The surgical procedure for rectocele repair is shown in **Figures 29.22A to F**.

Manchester Repair

Manchester repair is performed in those cases where removal of the uterus is not required.

BOX 29.4: Indications for hysterectomy in case of prolapse uterus.
- Removal of a nonfunctioning organ in postmenopausal women
- Uterine or cervical pathology (e.g., large fibroid uterus, endometriosis, pelvic inflammatory disease, endometrial hyperplasia, and carcinoma)
- Bulky uterus
- Patient desires removal of the uterus

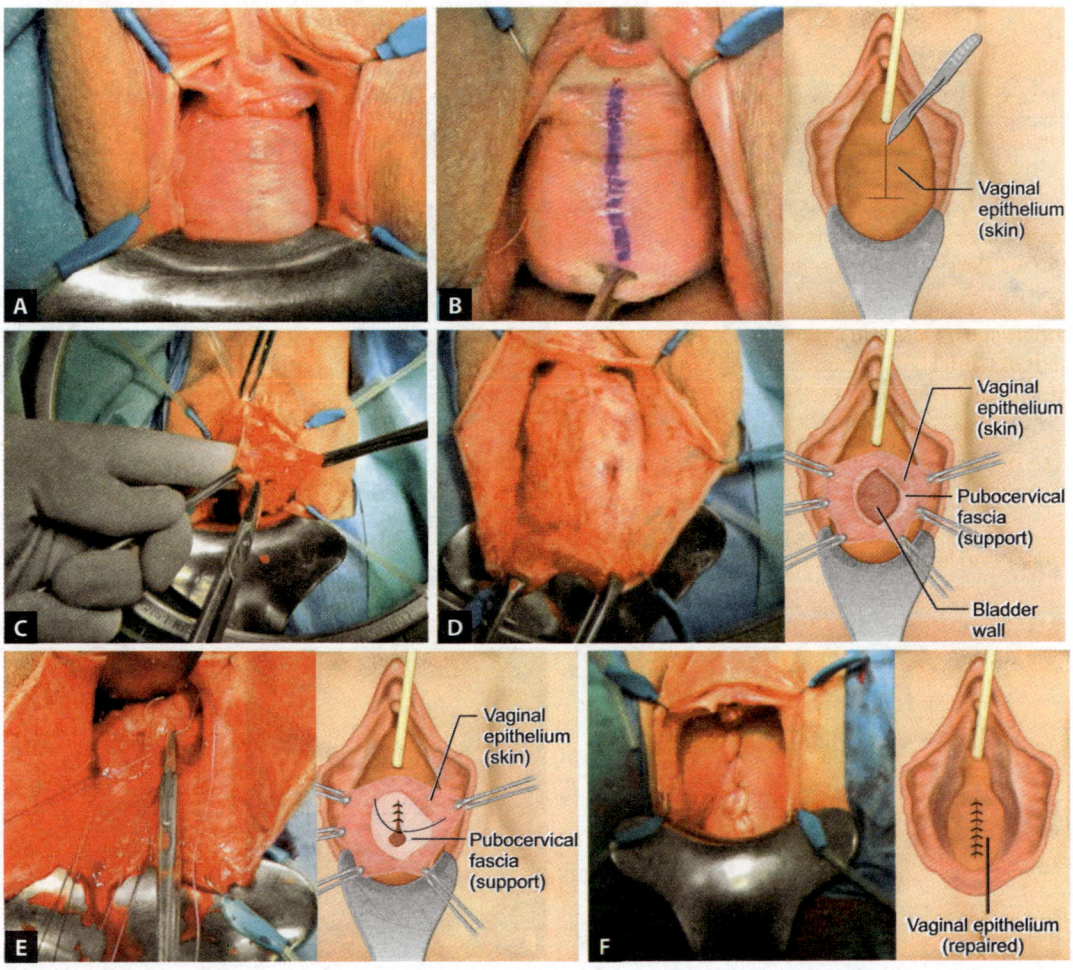

Figs. 29.21A to F: Procedure of cystocele repair. (A) Appearance of cystocele just before giving the incision; (B) Skin incision given over the skin overlying the cystocele; (C) Dissection of the underlying fascia; (D) Dissection of the underlying fascia continued until the midline defect in pubocervical fascia is visualized; (E) The tissue under the bladder plicated and pulled together in the midline, thus reducing the bulge; (F) Closure of the vaginal epithelium.

Indications

Indications of Manchester operation are described as follows:

- Childbearing function is not required.
- Malignancy of the endometrium has been ruled out by performing a dilatation and curettage.
- There is absence of UTI.
- There is presence of a small cystocele with only first- or second-degree prolapse.
- There is absence of an enterocele.
- Symptoms of prolapse are largely due to cervical elongation. The patient requires preservation of the menstrual function.

Procedure

The procedure for Manchester repair (also called Fothergill operation) is described in **Figures 29.23A to M**, and it comprises the following steps:

1. Anterior colporrhaphy is firstly performed.
2. Bladder is dissected from the cervix. A circular incision is given over the cervix.
3. Attachments of Mackenrodt ligaments to the cervix on each side are exposed, clamped, and cut.
4. Vaginal incision is then extended posteriorly around the cervix.
5. Cervix is amputated, and posterior lip of cervix is covered with a flap of mucosa.
6. Base of cardinal ligament is sutured over the anterior surface of cervix.
7. Raw area of the amputated cervix is then covered.
8. Colpoperineorrhaphy is ultimately performed to correct the posterior and perineal defects.

Shirodkar's Modification of Manchester Repair

In Shirodkar's modification of Manchester repair, firstly an anterior colporrhaphy is performed. The cardinal ligaments are exposed, and the pouch of Douglas is opened. The uterosacral ligaments are identified and divided close to the cervix. The amputated uterosacral ligaments are then crossed and stitched in front of cervix. Since in this procedure the cervix is not amputated, the complications related to childbirth can be largely avoided. A high closure of the peritoneum of pouch of Douglas is carried out.

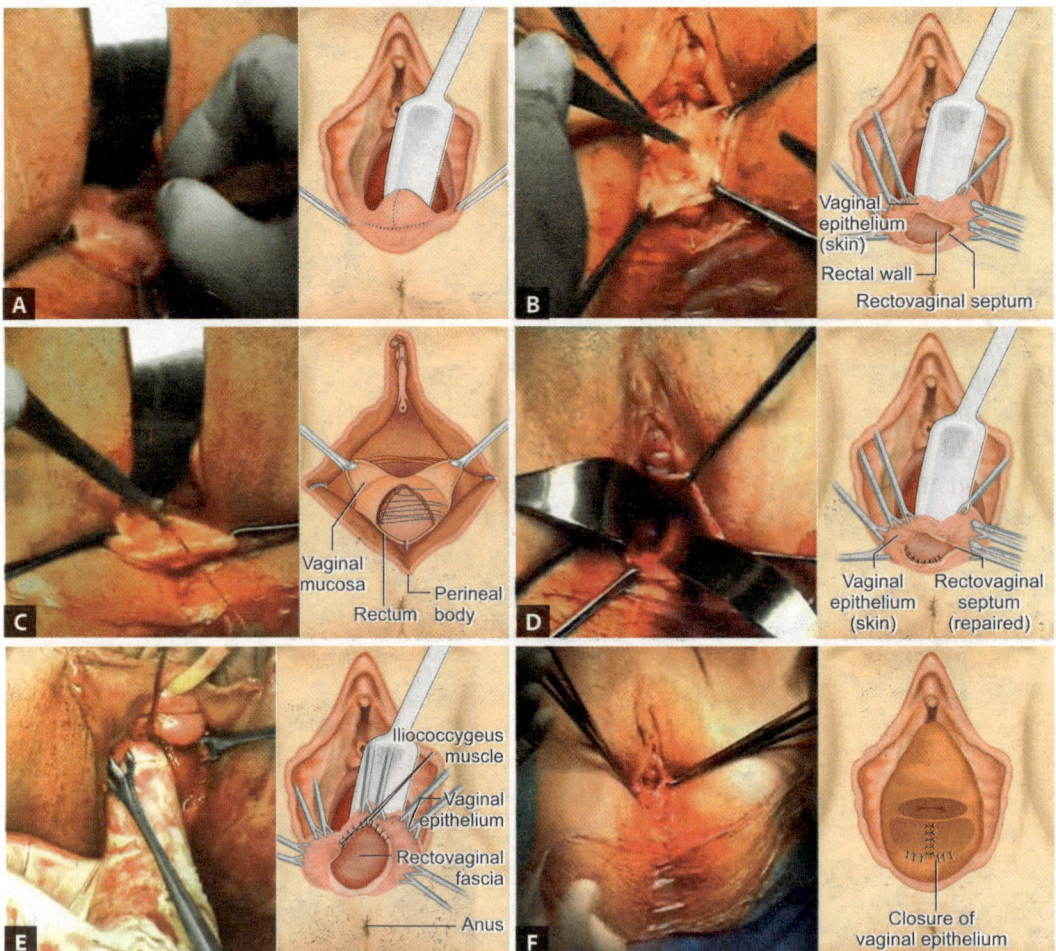

Figs. 29.22A to F: Procedure of posterior colporrhaphy and colpoperineorrhaphy. (A) Rectocele identified and skin incised: a bulge is apparent on the bottom (posterior) floor of the vagina. The dotted line represents the skin incision, performed in this posterior repair procedure; (B) Identification of the fascia break: the defect is readily identified and the rectal wall is found to be protruding through this break in the rectovaginal fascia; (C) The distal defect is repaired; (D) The rectovaginal fascial defect has been repaired; (E) The rectovaginal fascia is reattached to the iliococcygeal muscles bilaterally with permanent sutures; (F) Closure of the vaginal epithelium (skin) completes the operation.

Abdominal Sling Surgery

> **Q.** Discuss briefly about the sling surgery in cases of prolapse.

Sling operations are especially useful in women desirous of retaining their childbearing function, who are suffering from second-degree or third-degree prolapse, or those with nulliparous prolapse. These surgeries aim at buttressing the weakened ligaments (e.g., Mackenrodt and uterosacral ligaments) with the help of synthetic tapes such as nylon and Dacron that are used for forming slings to support the uterus.

- *Principle of sling surgery:* With a fascial strip or prosthetic material (mersilene tape or Dacron), the cervix is fixed to the abdominal wall, sacrum, or pelvis.
- *Commonly performed abdominal sling surgery:* The most commonly performed abdominal sling surgery is abdominal cervicopexy.

Abdominal Cervicopexy

Two musculofascial slings are obtained from the rectus sheath after giving transverse incisions and elevating the fascia from the midline outward and laterally up to the lateral border of rectus abdominis muscle on either side. The uterus is brought into view after opening the peritoneum in the midline. The uterovesical fold of peritoneum is incised, and bladder is mobilized from the front of uterine isthmus. The medial ends of the sling are directed retroperitoneally between the two layers of broad ligament up to the space created in front of the uterine isthmus. The slings are pulled and anchored here with the help of nonabsorbable sutures after ensuring adequate correction of the uterine position. Nowadays, surgeons are commonly using 12 inches long mersilene or nylon tapes instead of the tapes fashioned from the rectus sheath or fascia lata. The use of mersilene tape has a definite advantage over the body tissues because it is an inert material, nonabsorbable, nonirritant having a predictable

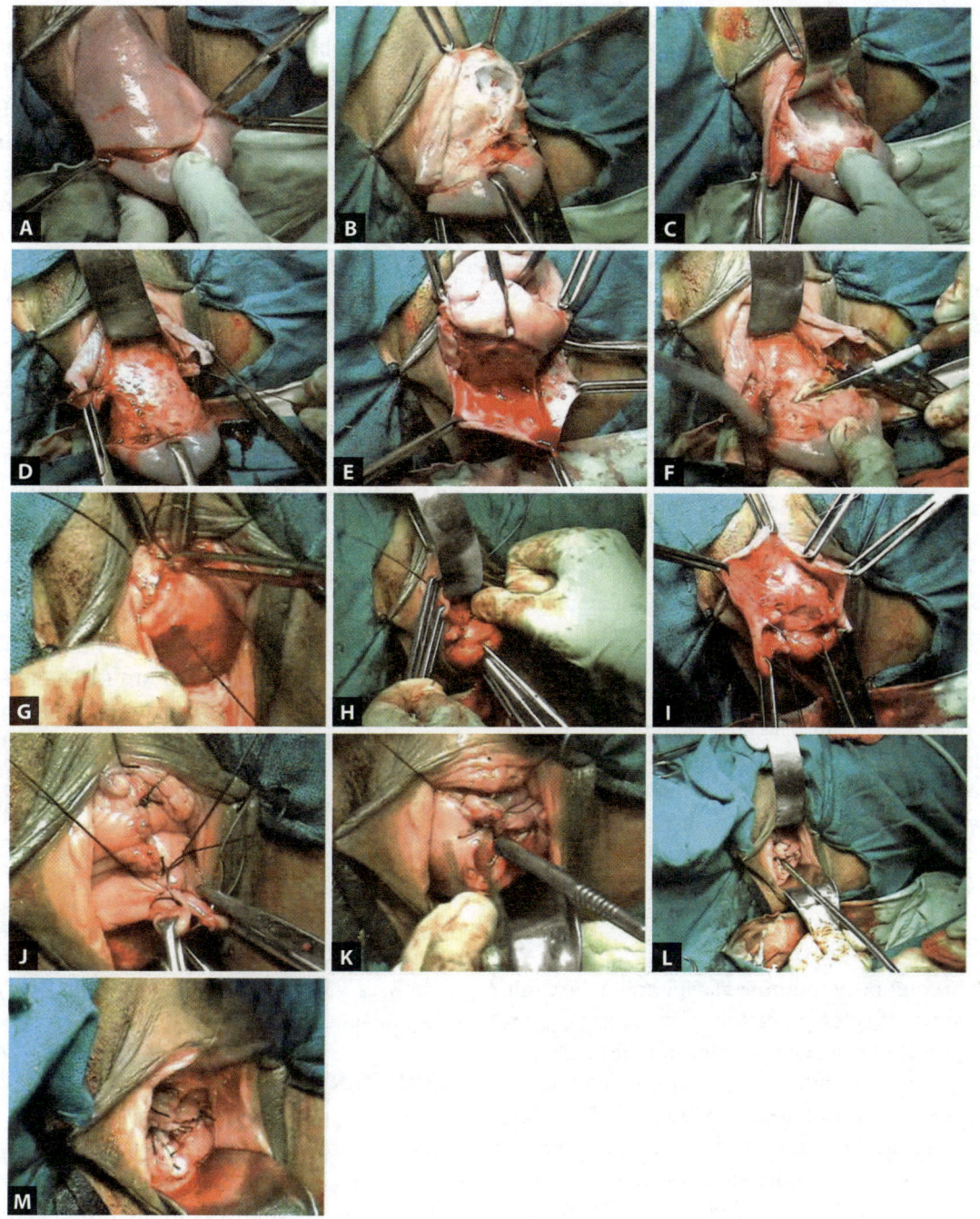

Figs. 29.23A to M: Procedure of Manchester repair. (A) The anterior vaginal wall is separated from bladder; (B and C) Paravesical fascia is dissected out so that bladder is separated from vagina and can be pushed up; (D) The base of cardinal ligament is exposed, clamped, and cut; (E) Posterior vaginal wall is similarly separated from the cervix; (F) The cervix is amputated; (G) Posterior lip of cervix is covered with a flap of mucosa; (H) The base of cardinal ligament is sutured over the anterior surface of cervix; (I) Application of bladder buttressing sutures; (J) Completion of anterior colporrhaphy using interrupted sutures; (K) Formation of anterior lip of cervix; (L) Newly formed cervix at the end of surgery; (M) Appearance of vagina at the end of surgery.

tensile strength. Purandare and Mhatre's modification of this surgery involved attaching the tape posteriorly to the cervix, close to the attachments of the uterosacral ligaments. Some other types of sling surgeries commonly in use are as follows:

- *Khanna's sling surgery:* In this surgery the tape is anchored to the anterior aspect of isthmus and anterior superior iliac spine.
- *Joshi's sling:* Anterior surface of the uterus at the level of internal os is supended to the pectineal ligaments on both sides.
- *Virkud's composite sling operation:* Merseline tape is anchored from the posterior aspect of isthmus to the sacral promontory retroperitoneally on the right side and the anterior abdominal wall/rectus sheath on the left side. Also, the uterosacral ligament is plicated.

- *Soonawala's sling:* Anterior longitudinal ligament on S1 vertebra along right uterosacral ligament is retracted extraperitoneally to S1 vertebra

Vaginal Vault/Uterine Suspension

> Q. Write a long essay discussing the causes and management of vault prolapse.
>
> Q. With the help of a long essay, discuss the diagnosis and management of vault prolapse.
>
> Q. Write a short essay on the surgical management of vault prolapse.

Vault prolapse is a delayed complication of both abdominal and vaginal hysterectomies when the supporting structures, i.e., paravaginal fascia and levator ani muscles, become weak and deficient. It may also result from failure to identify and repair an enterocele during hysterectomy. Uterine suspension procedures involve putting the uterus back into its normal position. Various types of uterine suspensions can be performed either via the abdominal or vaginal route. This may be done by reattaching the pelvic ligaments to the lower part of the uterus to hold it in place (e.g., sacrospinous colpopexy). Another technique uses special materials, which act like sling in order to support the uterus in its proper position (abdominal sacral colpopexy). Recent advances include performing these procedures laparoscopically, thereby considerably reducing postoperative pain and facilitating speedy recovery.

Abdominal Sacral Colpopexy

Abdominal sacral colpopexy comprises suspending the vault to the sacral promontory extraperitoneally using various grafts such as harvested fascia lata, abdominal fascia, dura mater, marlex, prolene, goretex, mersilene, or cadaveric fascia lata **(Figs. 29.24A and B)**. Injury to the ureter, bladder, sigmoid colon, and middle sacral artery should be avoided. Bleeding is the most serious complication of sacral colpopexy due to injury to the presacral venous plexus or the middle sacral artery while operating in the presacral space.

The aim of surgery is to restore the normal pelvic anatomy as far as possible. At the end of the surgery, normal vaginal length should be maintained with its axis directed toward S3–S4 vertebrae. Abdominal sacral colpopexy has the highest cure rate for vault prolapse, probably because of the use of graft tissue with high strength and not relying on the patient's own tissue, which may not be strong enough to hold up the vaginal vault. As a result, sacral colposcopy can also be considered in patients who have had previous failed operations, older patients with poor tissue, or patients with large defects or severe prolapse.

Transvaginal Sacrospinous Ligament Fixation

In this method, the vaginal apex is attached, using permanent sutures, to the sacrospinous ligament. The posterior vaginal wall is opened vertically, following which a window space is created between the vagina and the rectum toward the right sacrospinous ligament. Using Deschamps ligature carrier, a synthetic ligature is used for fixing the vaginal vault to the sacrospinous ligament, 3–5 cm away from the ischial spine **(Figs. 29.25A and B)**. The suture must be placed through the ligament, rather than around it. The two most serious complications from sacrospinous ligament fixation are hemorrhage and nerve injury as a result of damage to the pudendal neurovascular bundle. Thus, the surgeon must try to avoid injuring the pudendal bundle and inferior gluteal vessels as far as possible.

Obliterative Procedures

For patients who cannot undergo long surgical procedures and who are not contemplating sexual activity, obliterative procedures, such as the Le Fort colpocleisis or colpectomy and colpocleisis, are viable options.

Le Fort Colpocleisis

In Le Fort colpocleisis, a patch of anterior and posterior vaginal mucosae is removed. The cut edge of the anterior vaginal wall is sewn to its counterpart on the posterior side. As the approximation is continued on each side, the most dependent portion of the mass is progressively inverted.

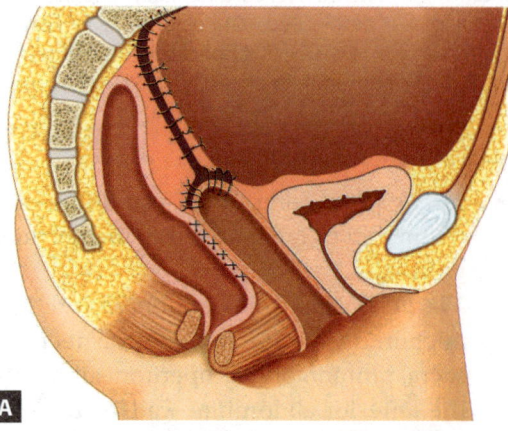
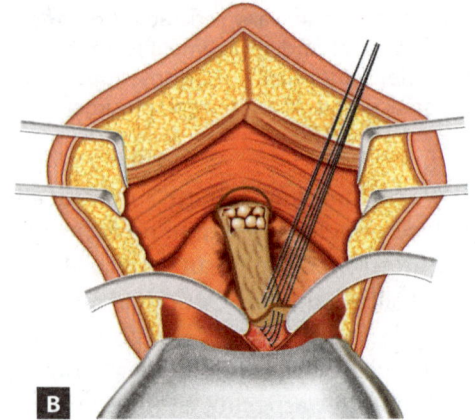

Figs. 29.24A and B: Abdominal sacral colpopexy. (A) Lateral view; (B) Surgery as visualized from the abdominal incision (superior view).

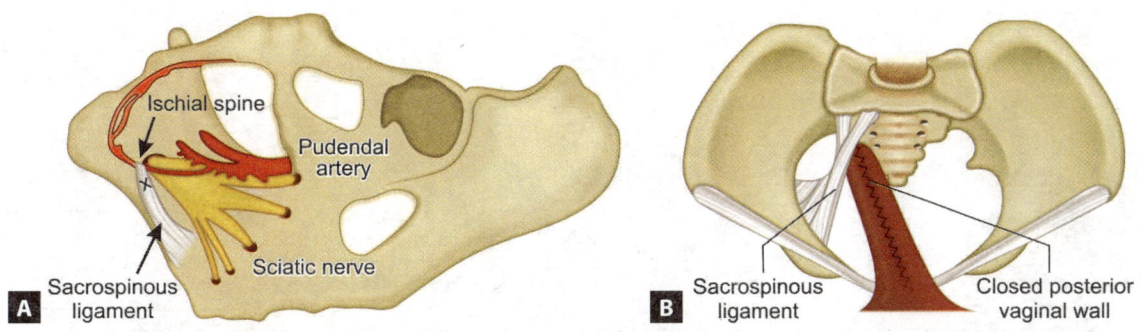

Figs. 29.25A and B: (A) The sacrospinous ligament must be penetrated 3–5 cm medial to the ischial spine at the point marked by "X"; (B) Transvaginal sacrospinous ligament fixation.

A tight perineorrhaphy is also performed to help support the inverted vagina and prevent recurrence of the prolapse. The main problem specific to these obliterative operations is that they limit coital function. Neither does it correct an enterocele because they are both extraperitoneal procedures. Also, there is a 25% incidence of postoperative urinary stress incontinence caused by induced fusion of the anterior and posterior vaginal walls and flattening of the posterior urethrovesical angle. In addition, if the uterus is retained, the patient can later bleed from many causes, including carcinoma.

Indications for Le Fort colpocleisis: Colpocleisis is an excellent operation for the treatment of uterine prolapse or complete vaginal vault prolapse for patients who are:

- Not sexually active
- Have no future plans for sexual activity
- Medically fragile
- Elderly patients who do not require preservation of their sexual functioning

Procedure: It involves excision of rectangular strips of mucosa from the upper portions of anterior and posterior vaginal walls. The exposed submucosal fascia is then closed together. In those frail elderly women who do not wish to be sexually active in the future, colpocleisis acts as a simple, safe, and effective surgical procedure that reliably relieves these women of their symptoms without the potential hazards of vaginal suspension. The procedure is called a total colpocleisis for patients who do not have a uterus and have complete vaginal vault prolapse and a Le Fort colpocleisis for those patients who still have a uterus. Total colpocleisis procedure is often coupled with a tension-free vaginal tape sling procedure for urinary incontinence. The colpocleisis procedure is done through the vagina and essentially closes the vagina on the inside. The patient can no longer engage in sexual intercourse due to the closing up of the vagina. The completed procedure usually leaves the patients with a much-shortened vagina. As a result, the patient becomes incapable of engaging in sexual intercourse. Colpocleisis is an extremely effective operation, which has the advantages listed in **Box 29.5**. The surgical technique of colpocleisis is shown in **Figures 29.26A to E**. The procedure

> **BOX 29.5:** Advantages of colpocleisis.
> - Closes the vagina together
> - Inhibits the patient from future sexual intercourse
> - 90–95% cure rate
> - Can be performed using local anesthesia, epidural or spinal
> - No requirement for general anesthesia
> - Quick procedure, which takes only 45 minutes to perform
> - Minimal pain or complications
> - Can be coupled with tension free vaginal tape sling (incontinence) operation

is associated with disadvantages such as loss of sexual activity and development of stress or urge incontinence. Le Fort's procedure should only be used when there is a good reason to not perform any of the usual procedures for prolapse. This operation is recommended only to patients who are no longer sexually active, nor have plans for future sexual activity. The procedure should never be done before the woman and her partner fully understand that it would result in termination of intravaginal sexual intercourse.

Innovations in Surgery for Uterine Prolapse

> **Q.** Write a long essay critically evaluating the role of mesh in pelvic organ prolapse.

Use of Prosthetic Material for Prolapse Surgery

Synthetic and biological prosthetic material is nowadays commonly being used in cases of pelvic reconstructive surgery, especially in cases where women experience recurrence or in cases of repeat surgery. Anterior colporrhaphy with graft augmentation involves either the use of a prosthetic material to help support the anterior vaginal wall or the placement of a piece of polyglactin 910 mesh into the fold of imbricated bladder wall below the trigone and apical portions of the vaginal vault.

Vaginal or paravaginal repair can also be carried out with graft augmentation. The various types of prosthetic material, which are being used for prolapse surgery, have been listed in **Box 29.6**. The objective of paravaginal defect repair for anterior vaginal wall prolapse is to reattach the detached lateral vaginal wall to its normal place of attachment at the

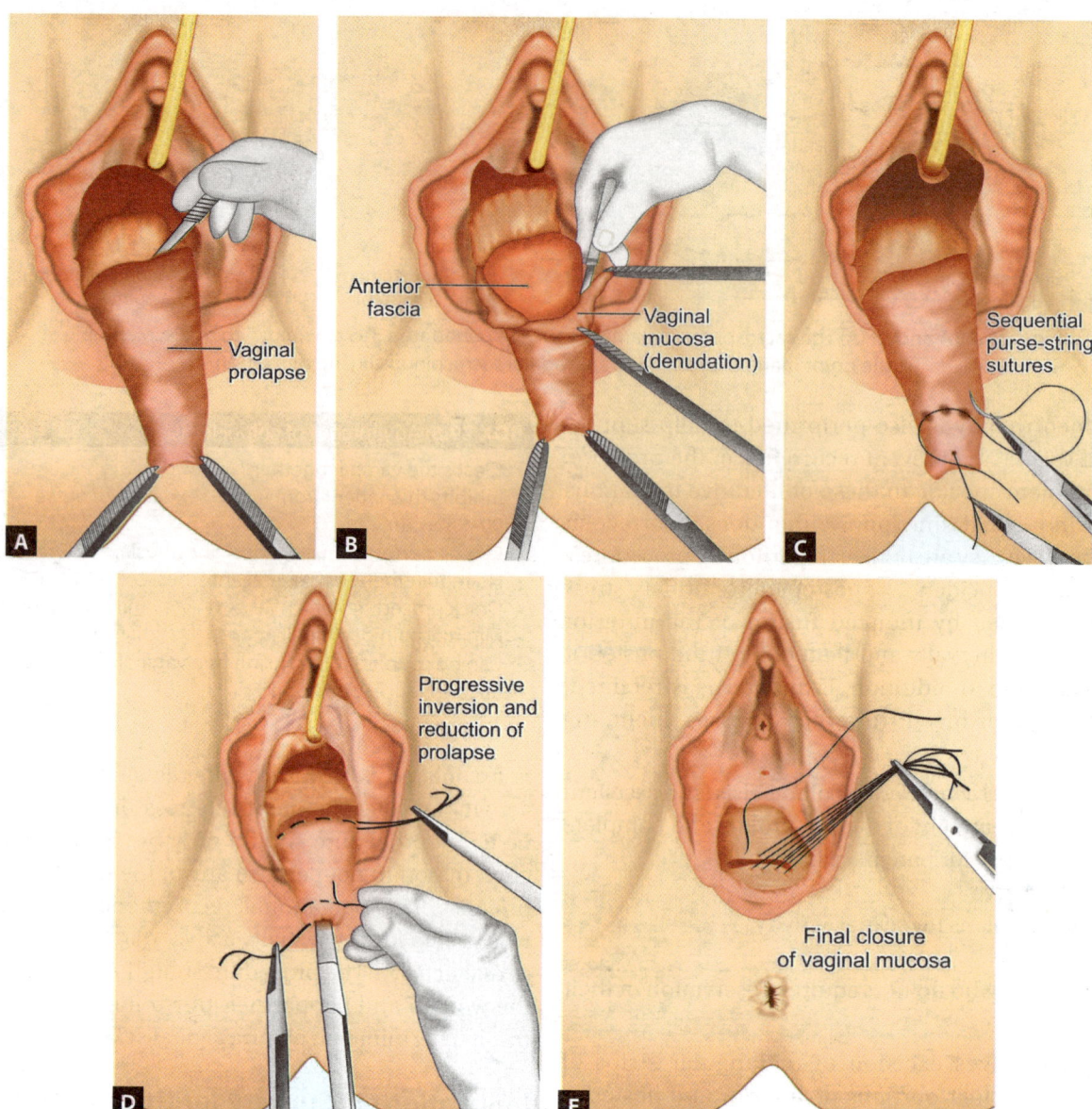

Figs. 29.26A to E: Procedure of colpocleisis. (A) Incision over the mucosa of anterior vaginal wall; (B) Incision and removal of skin. Mucosa is removed from the prolapse to expose the anterior fascia (pubocervical fascia) and posterior fascia (rectovaginal fascia); (C) Suturing. The mucosa has been removed, and the underlying strong tissues (pubocervical and rectovaginal fascia) are identified. The tissue is sewn together in a circular fashion (like the drawstrings on a purse); (D) Reducing the prolapse. The most protruding portion of the vagina is inverted (pushed in upon itself), and the last suture placed is tied. The suture holds the rest of the vagina from coming back out or prolapsing; (E) Final closure of vaginal mucosa. After multiple circular sutures are placed and the prolapse is progressively reduced, the prolapse is completely reduced back into the patient's vagina and pelvis. The skin edges from the original incision are then closed using sutures.

BOX 29.6: Various types of prosthetic material being used for prolapse surgery.

Synthetic materials:
- Nonabsorbable (Marlex, Prolene)
- Absorbable polyglactin (Vicryl)

Biological materials:
- Autologous material (rectus fascia, fascia lata)
- Xenografts (porcine dermis or porcine small intestine submucosa)

New systems:
- Polypropylene tapes
- Apogee and perigee

---

level of the white line or "arcus tendineus fasciae pelvis," which is done using a vaginal or retropubic approach.

Transobturator tension-free vaginal mesh techniques can also be used for management of anterior vaginal wall prolapse. These techniques facilitate a tension-free placement of an allograft, xenograft, or polypropylene mesh implant without trimming of the vagina or suturing of the mesh to the vagina. The involved "systems" allow selective application of anterior, posterior, or total vaginal implants. Therefore, the requirement for hysterectomy is potentially eliminated. The mesh implants have arms that are delivered with trocars or special devices through anatomical landmarks via the obturator membrane or the ischiorectal fossa. Some of the currently available commercial kits have been listed in **Table 29.4**. **Figure 29.27** shows perigee system for transobturator cystocele repair. The graft is depicted in the center and has the dimensions of 5 × 10 cm. The graft has four arms that come out laterally and are attached to the pelvic sidewalls with the help of needles. The pink needles are superior needles, which are used for attaching the bladder neck arms. The grey needles are inferior needles, which are used for attaching the apical arms of the graft to the arcus tendineus. **Figures 29.28A and B** show that the graft has been placed in position under the bladder. It provides an entire new floor of support for the bladder from side to side. The skin of vagina is closed over the graft. The growth in tissue occurs rapidly, causing the graft to get incorporated and soon become a part of the patient's anatomy. High rate of anatomical cure due to the use of tension-free vaginal tape has been demonstrated in the uncontrolled short-term case studies. These techniques are still awaiting safety and efficacy studies. Nevertheless, they are still increasingly being used in clinical practice. Before undertaking the procedure, the patients must be counseled regarding the serious adverse results of transvaginal mesh repair including pain, dyspareunia, etc.

Laparoscopic Surgery for Prolapse

Nowadays, laparoscopic procedures are commonly being performed for the cases of prolapse. Some of these are described next:

- Cervicopexy or sling operations with or without laparoscopic paravaginal repair or vaginal repair
- Vaginal hysterectomy/laparoscopic vaginal hysterectomy/laparoscopic hysterectomy/total laparoscopic hysterectomy along with colposuspension
- Vaginal hysterectomy/laparoscopic vaginal hysterectomy/laparoscopic hysterectomy/total laparoscopic hysterectomy along with laparoscopic pelvic reconstruction
- Rectocele repair and levatorplasty
- Enterocele repair with suturing of uterosacral ligaments
- Anterior or posterior colpopexy

All types of sling operations can be performed by laparoscopy. Associated vaginal or paravaginal defects can also be repaired via laparoscopic route. Vaginal anterior and posterior colporrhaphy can be done either before or after laparoscopy. Laparoscopic vault suspension culdoscopy

TABLE 29.4: Commercial transvaginal mesh kits available.

Company	Device	Implant material
American Medical Systems Inc., Minnetonka, MN	Apogee/Perigee®	Intepro polypropylene InteXen® porcine dermis
Gynecare/Ethicon, Johnson and Johnson, Somerville, NJ	Anterior Prolift®	Gynemesh-PS® polypropylene
CR Bard Inc., Murray Hill, NJ	Avaulta Plus®	Polypropylene + porcine collagen

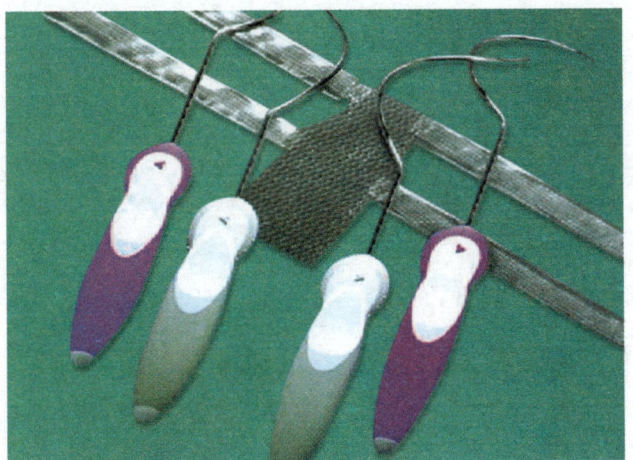

Fig. 29.27: Perigee system for transobturator cystocele repair.

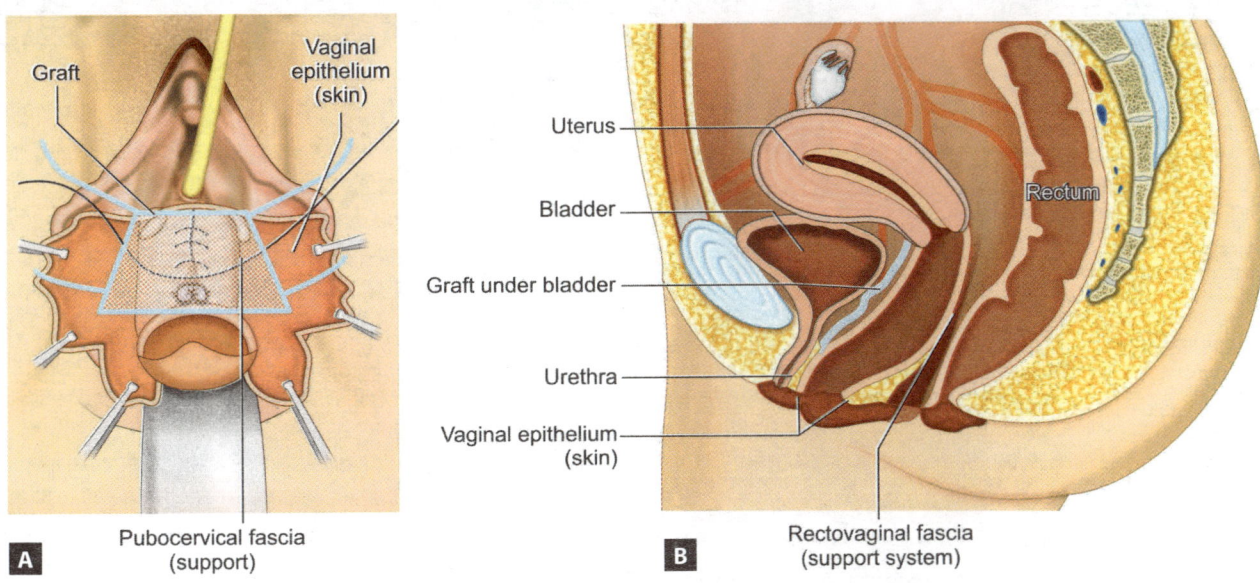

Figs. 29.28A and B: Graft has been placed in position under the bladder. (A) Front view; (B) Side view.

can be performed along with vaginal hysterectomy, laparoscopic-assisted vaginal hysterectomy, laparoscopic hysterectomy, and total laparoscopic hysterectomy. This helps in correcting mild laxity and prevents vault prolapse. Advantages of laparoscopic surgery for prolapse include small incision, better view, minimal packing, minimal bowel and tissue handling, short recovery period, less pain, and insignificant scar tissue formation.

COMPLICATIONS

Uterine prolapse, if not corrected, can interfere with bowel, bladder, and sexual functions and result in the development of the following complications:

- Ulceration
- Infection/urosepsis (including due to pessary use)
- Urinary incontinence
- Constipation
- Fistula
- Postrenal failure
- Decubitus ulceration.

EVIDENCE-BASED CLINICAL TRIALS

List of references can be scanned through QR code to enable the readers gain deeper insight of the subject by referring to the entire article or its abstract.

CHAPTER 30

Pelvic Pain

CASE STUDY

A 25-year-old nulliparous patient presented with complaints of chronic pelvic pain (CPP) for last 2 years. The pain is mainly present in the lower back and abdomen and typically exacerbates at the time of menstrual periods. During this time, the pain becomes severe enough to interfere with the quality of life for last two years, when she got married. The patient gives history of experiencing mild-to-moderate pain at the time of sexual intercourse. The patient also gives history of experiencing primary infertility for last two years, when she got married. On bimanual pelvic examination, localized areas of tenderness were felt in the pelvic region. However, no nodularity or thickness of uterosacral ligaments, cul-de-sac or rectovaginal septum was felt.

INTRODUCTION

The International Association for the Study of Pain has defined pain as an unpleasant sensory and emotional experience associated with actual or potential damage to the tissues. This implies that pain is associated with both a sensory and an emotional component. American Congress of Obstetrics and Gynecology has defined CPP as cyclic or noncyclic pain, emanating from the pelvic area, which has been present for 6 months or more. The pain often localizes to the pelvis, infraumbilical part of anterior abdominal wall, lumbosacral area of the back or buttocks and often leads to functional disability. It may also be present in the perineal region and produce discomfort in the anus, rectum, coccyx and sacrum. It is often associated with symptoms such as premenstrual pain, dysmenorrhea, dyspareunia, exercise related pain, or cramping, with or without menstrual exacerbation of sufficient severity to cause functional disability or require medical care. The pain may be a steady or it may come and go. It can feel like a dull ache, or it can be sharp and may be generalized or localized. The pain may be mild, or it may be severe enough to negatively affect health-related quality of life.

Chronic pelvic pain is not a disease, but a symptom, which rarely reflects a single pathologic process. Different neurophysiological mechanisms may be involved in the pathophysiology of CPP. Patient's history is crucial and is generally of utmost importance for reaching a correct diagnosis. CPP is common in women of the reproductive and older age groups and causes disability and distress. In many cases no obvious cause for the pain can be found even after conducting numerous investigations including laparoscopy. Since the pathophysiology of CPP is not well understood, its treatment is often unsatisfactory and limited to symptom relief.

■ IDENTIFYING THE CAUSE OF PELVIC PAIN

The most important question for the patient and the clinician is to identify the cause of pain. In general the three most common sources of pain include:

Pain of Somatic Origin

This type of pain arises from skin, muscles and bone tissue and is commonly described by the patients as throbbing, stabbing or burning type of pain.

Pain of Visceral Origin

This type of pain arises from internal organs and tends to be diffuse and more generalized.

Pain of Neuropathic Origin

The pain of neuropathic origin arises from damaged nerve fibers and may be described as numbness, pins and needles, and may produce electric current like sensations.

The main contributing factors in women with CPP are identified by history and physical examination in most cases. Many disorders of the reproductive tract, urological organs, gastrointestinal (GI), musculoskeletal and psychoneurological systems may be associated with CPP. The various gynecological and nongynecological causes for CPP have been enumerated in **Table 30.1** and are described in the section of differential diagnosis of this chapter.

Since CPP can be caused due to numerous pathologies and pathology in one organ can commonly lead to dysfunction in the other, women with CPP may have more than one cause for pain and other overlapping symptoms.

TABLE 30.1: Causes of chronic pelvic pain.

Gynecological causes	Gastrointestinal causes
• Endometriosis, chocolate cyst of ovary • Ovarian adhesions, polycystic ovarian disease • Chronic pelvic inflammatory disease, pelvic and tubal adhesions • Pelvic tuberculosis • Uterine fibroids and adenomyosis • Benign or malignant ovarian tumors • Premenstrual syndrome	• Irritable bowel syndrome • Chronic intermittent bowel obstruction • Diverticulitis, colitis, appendicitis • Carcinoma rectum
Renal causes	**Musculoskeletal disease**
• Ureteric or bladder stones • Urinary tract infection, interstitial cystitis, radiation cystitis • Bladder malignancy	• Abdominal wall myofascial pain • Degenerative joint disease including muscle strains and pain • Disk herniation, rupture or spondylosis
Psychiatric/neurological cause	**Miscellaneous causes**
• Abdominal epilepsy, abdominal migraines • Depression, sleep disturbances, somatization • Nerve entrapment, neurologic dysfunction	• Familial Mediterranean fever • Herpes zoster • Porphyria

Thus a comprehensive evaluation of multiple organ systems and psychological state is essential for complete treatment. Most important causes for CPP include endometriosis, symptomatic leiomyomas, interstitial cystitis and irritable bowel syndrome (IBS). Diagnosis and treatment of pain in relation to endometriosis would be discussed in this chapter. Evaluation and management of pain secondary to that of leiomyomas has been discussed in Chapter 24. The most common symptoms related to endometriosis are dysmenorrhea, dyspareunia and low back pain which worsen during menses.

ENDOMETRIOSIS

> Q. Write a short essay on endometriosis.
> Q. Write a short essay discussing the chocolate cysts.

Endometriosis is one of the most common causes of CPP in women belonging to the reproductive age groups and may be associated with infertility in nearly 30–40% cases. Endometriosis is characterized by occurrence of endometrial stroma and glands outside the uterus in the pelvic cavity, including all the reproductive organs as well as on the bladder, bowel, intestines, colon, appendix and rectum **(Fig. 30.1)**. Endometrial lesions have been identified in virtually all tissues and organs of the female body with the exception of the spleen. In normal women, endometrial glands and stroma are largely limited to the uterus. The ectopic endometrial tissue, both the glands and the stroma, are capable of responding to cyclical hormonal stimulation and has the tendency to invade the normal surrounding tissues. Endometriosis is a disease, which is largely encountered in the women belonging

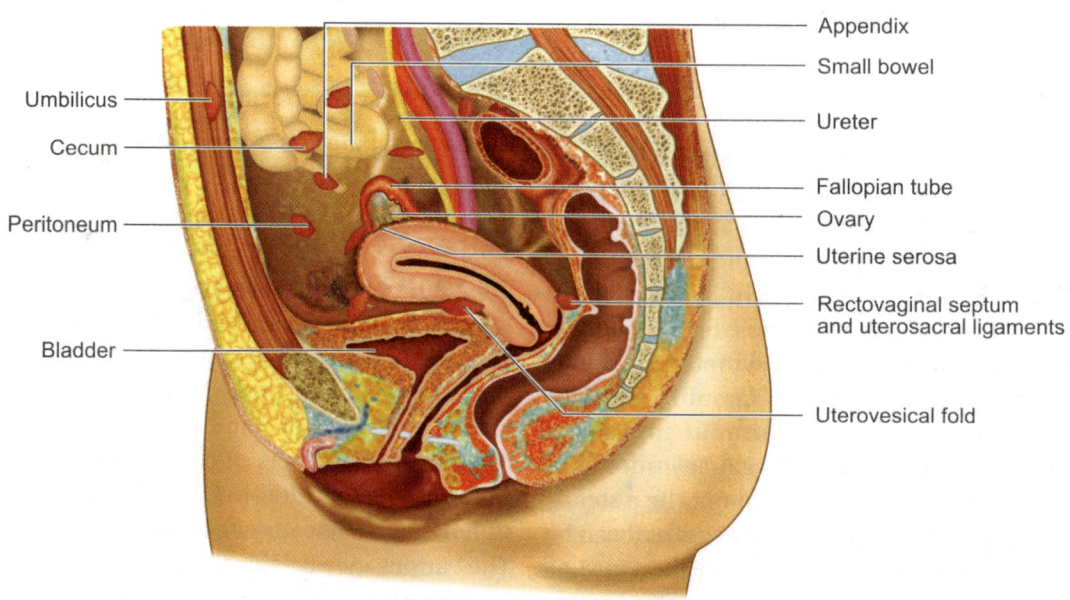

Fig. 30.1: Common sites of endometriotic lesions.

to the reproductive age group. It is a leading cause of disability in women of reproductive age, responsible for causing dysmenorrhea, pelvic pain and subfertility. The common sites for the occurrence of endometriosis include the ovaries, the pouch of Douglas, uterosacral ligaments and serosal surface of the uterus, bladder, sigmoid colon, appendix, cecum, uterine scars, etc. The ovary is the most common site for endometriosis. Lesions can vary in size from spots to large endometriomas. The classic lesion is a chocolate cyst of the ovary that contains old blood that has undergone hemolysis. On gross microscopic examination, the tunica albuginea appears to be thickened. Red vascular lesions may be well marked on the under surface of the ovary. Once intracystic pressure inside the chocolate cyst rises, the cyst perforates, spilling its contents within the peritoneal cavity. This can cause severe abdominal pain typically associated with endometriosis exacerbations. The inflammatory response may result in the development of adhesions which may further increase the disease related morbidity.

Endometriotic lesions can also involve the uterine serosa and the anterior surface of the bladder. Involvement of uterine serosa and formation of dense adhesions can lead to fixed retroversion of the uterus. Posteriorly, the disease may cause obliteration of the cul-de-sac and form dense adhesions between the posterior vaginal wall or cervix and the anterior rectum. This can be responsible for producing severe dyspareunia, dyschezia and alteration of bowel habits. Deep endometriotic nodules can also cause infiltration of the uterosacral ligaments and rectovaginal septum. Through contiguous spread, endometriosis may invade the rectovaginal septum and the anterior rectal wall. It may also involve the upper rectum and sigmoid colon, resulting in cyclical rectal bleeding (hematochezia). The ileum, appendix and cecum may also be involved, resulting in intestinal obstruction.

In the beginning, the endometriotic lesions appear as red colored, papular vesicles. With the passage of time, these lesions progressively change their appearance from dark red to bluish-black appearance. Scarring in the surrounding tissues may give it a puckered appearance. Old inactive lesions of endometriosis may appear as powder burnt areas.

Malignant Transformation of Endometriomas

While majority of endometriomas are benign, they may sometimes serve as precursors to epithelial ovarian cancers, most commonly endometrioid adenocarcinoma or clear cell carcinoma. The clotted blood in the endometriomas is likely to be rich in ferrous/ferric ions, which could be the cause of oxidative stress predisposing the woman to develop carcinoma. Due to the apparent link between endometriosis and certain types of ovarian cancers, endometriosis nowadays is considered to be a premalignant condition for type 1 tumors.

Pathogenesis of Endometriosis

> Q. Enumerate the theories behind the origin of endometriosis.
>
> Q. Write a long essay on the mechanism of origin of extrauterine endometriosis. Also discuss its signs, symptoms and management.
>
> Q. Discuss in detail the etiopathology of endometriosis.
>
> Q. Write a short essay discussing the immunological aspects of endometriosis.

The pathogenesis of endometriosis is yet not clear. Retrograde menstrual flux is considered as an essential element in the pathogenesis of endometriosis. However, it is yet not clear why endometriosis develops only in a limited number of women, despite the fact that retrograde menstruation is seen in almost all women. Endometriosis is an estrogen-dependent disease, characterized by the regression of lesions following treatment with drugs that block estradiol synthesis. Endometriosis is considered to be a complex, multifactorial disease, involving interplay between several factors. Some likely pathogenetic mechanisms for endometriosis are described here.

Retrograde Menstruation

The most widely accepted theory for pathogenesis of endometriosis involves retrograde menstruation (**Fig. 30.2**). According to this theory, reflux of degenerated menstrual endometrium through the Fallopian tubes occurs during menstrual cycles. This tissue subsequently gets implanted on the pelvic peritoneum and the surrounding structures and starts growing. These refluxed cells implant in the pelvis, bleed in response to cyclic hormonal stimulation and increase in size along with progression of symptoms at the time of menses. Although retrograde menstruation seems to be the most likely cause involved in the pathogenesis of endometriosis, this theory does not explain the full spectrum of the disease. For example, this theory is unable to explain the presence of endometrial implants at remote sites such as the lung, pleura, endocardium, etc.

Theory of Coelomic Metaplasia

According to this theory, peritoneal epithelium can be "transformed" into endometrial tissue under the influence of some unknown stimulus. The possible stimulus could be the chronic inflammation or chemical irritation from refluxed menstrual blood. Coelomic metaplasia is also believed to explain the occurrence of endometriosis in women who have undergone total hysterectomy and are not taking estrogen replacement.

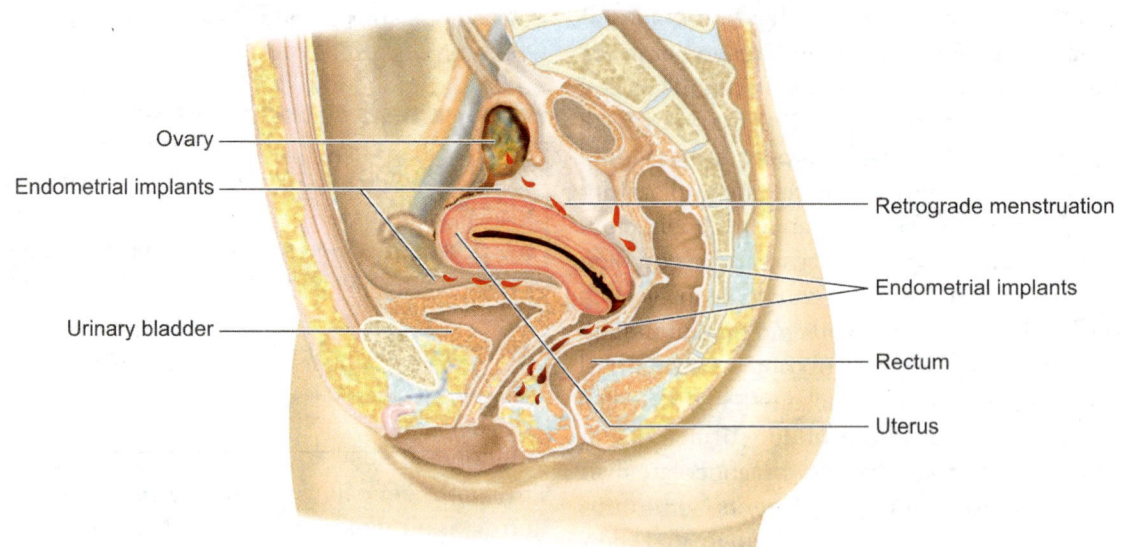

Fig. 30.2: Basic anatomy of retrograde menstruation.

Metastatic Theory of Lymphatic and Vascular Spread

Metastatic deposition of endometrial tissues at ectopic sites via lymphatic and vascular route has been postulated as another theory responsible for the pathogenesis of endometriosis. This pathway may explain the occurrence of endometriosis at distant, noncontiguous sites such as lung, pleura, etc. Ovarian endometriosis is also believed to be caused by lymphatic spread, although superficial ovarian endometriosis may also be due to implantation via retrograde menstruation.

Immunological Defects

Immunological defects such as impaired activity of T cells and natural killer cells are believed to increase the susceptibility of a woman to endometriosis. Humoral antibodies to endometrial tissue have also been found in sera of women with endometriosis. The peritoneal fluid in women with endometriosis may show the presence of macrophages and natural killer cells.

Genetic Factors

Familial tendency for endometriosis may be found in as many as 15–20% individuals with endometriosis.

Induction Theory

The induction theory proposes that some hormonal or biologic factor(s) may induce the differentiation of undifferentiated cells into endometrial tissue. These substances could be either exogenous agents or released directly from the endometrium. Although many factors have been recognized, their tendency to cause endometriosis is limited only to some women, but not to all.

Müllerian Rests

The "Müllerian rests" present in the ovary and pelvis are of paramesonephric origin and respond to ovarian hormone production resulting in development of the endometriotic lesions. This theory can also explain the presence of deep infiltrating lesions in the absence of superficial endometriosis. The validity of this theory is further strengthened by the fact that endometriosis is often observed in adolescent girls with Müllerian anomalies and outflow obstruction.

Hormonal Dependence

Estrogen has been established as having a causative role in the development of endometriosis. Besides ovary, other peripheral tissues can also create estrogens through aromatization of ovarian and adrenal androgens. Endometriotic implants have been shown to express the enzymes such as aromatase and 17β-hydroxysteroid dehydrogenase type 1, which are respectively responsible for conversion of androstenedione to estrone and estrone to estradiol. Moreover, the endometrial implants are deficient in 17β-hydroxysteroid dehydrogenase type 2, which inactivates estrogen.

Angioneogenesis

Angioneogenesis and vascular endothelial growth factor (VEGF) secretion is likely to play an important role in persistent and recurrent disease. Therefore antiangiogenetic drugs are likely to become novel adjuvant treatment modalities in future for the management of endometriosis.

HISTORY AND CLINICAL PRESENTATION

Taking proper history and conducting appropriate physical examination in a woman can help in narrowing the differential diagnosis and guide further tests and investigations. The most important part of history is taking a detailed history regarding pain. The following characteristics related to pain need to be enquired:

- *The exact area of pain localization:* The pain may be localized to the pelvis, lower back, perineal region or the lower abdomen.
- *The severity and duration of pain:* The clinician needs to assess whether the pain is acute or chronic in nature and whether it is mild or severe in intensity. A significant number of women with endometriosis remain asymptomatic. The clinician must remember that the degree of visible endometriosis may have no correlation with the degree of pain or other symptoms. However, the pain may correlate with the depth of tissue infiltration caused by the endometriotic lesion. Though the endometriotic lesions commonly cause CPP, at times, there may be acute exacerbations of pelvic pain caused by chemical peritonitis due to leakage of old blood from an endometriotic cyst.
- The aggravating or relieving factors for pain must be enquired.
- Timing during the day when the pain occurs or increases in intensity.
- *Correlation of pain with menstrual cycles:* Chronic pelvic pain due to endometriosis is commonly associated with dysmenorrhea and low back pain that worsens during menses. The diagnosis of endometriosis should be considered especially if a patient develops dysmenorrhea after years of pain-free menstrual cycles. Secondary dysmenorrhea has been observed to occur twice as commonly in women with endometriosis in comparison to controls. Pain due to endometriosis typically commences prior to menses.
- *Details related to the menstrual cycle:* The details related to menstrual cycle (e.g., cycle length, duration of menstrual flow, etc.) also need to be elicited because increased exposure to menstruation (i.e., shorter cycle length, longer duration of flow and nulliparity), acts as a risk factor for the development of endometriosis.
  - The patient needs to be asked if the pain follows any cyclic pattern and whether it remains same all the time or varies at different times of the day. Cyclic pain is the pain that accompanies bleeding at the time of menstruation. Cyclical pain associated with hormonal changes taking place during the menstrual cycle is likely to result from endometriosis or adenomyosis, while a nonhormonal pattern of pain may be more indicative of a musculoskeletal pathology or other conditions such as adhesions, IBS, or interstitial cystitis. However, the clinician should be careful before reaching any conclusion because pain caused by IBS and interstitial cystitis may also sometimes fluctuate based on hormone levels.
- The effect the pain has on the patient's quality of life needs to be assessed.
- Relation of pain to bowel movements or urination needs to be asked.
- The clinician needs to take history regarding any correlation between the symptoms of pain and the sexual intercourse. Relation of pain with deep penetration during intercourse or dyspareunia needs to be asked. Deep dyspareunia may result due to scarring of the uterosacral ligaments, nodularity of the rectovaginal septum, obliteration of cul-de-sac and/or uterine retroversion. All these reasons are also responsible for producing lower backache. These symptoms may get exaggerated during menses. A woman presenting with a combination of dysmenorrhea, CPP and dyspareunia is most likely to be suffering from endometriosis.
- Other questions which need to be asked at the time of taking history include:
  - The patient's age
  - Any previous history of sexually transmitted disease (STD) or pelvic inflammatory disease (PID)
  - Symptoms indicative of malignancy such as unexplained weight loss, hematochezia, perimenopausal irregular bleeding, postmenopausal vaginal bleeding, or postcoital bleeding, should prompt an investigation to rule out malignancy.

OBSTETRIC HISTORY

Injury to the ilioinguinal nerve or hypogastric nerves during Pfannenstiel incision for cesarean section delivery may be the cause of lower abdominal pain. In a nulliparous woman with infertility, pain may be due to endometriosis, pelvic adhesions or PID. History of using oral contraceptive pills (OCPs) or any other methods of birth control need to be asked.

SURGICAL HISTORY

Prior history of abdominal surgery increases the woman's risk for developing pelvic adhesions, especially if infection, bleeding or large areas of denuded peritoneal surfaces were involved. Certain disorders may persist and therefore information regarding prior surgeries for endometriosis, adhesive surgery or malignancy must be sought.

PSYCHOSOCIAL HISTORY

It is important to investigate all contributing factors related to the pain including psychological, social and environmental causes.

PREVIOUS TREATMENT HISTORY

The patient needs to be asked if she has ever undergone an assessment or treatment for pain in the past. The patient needs to be asked if she has been taking any medicines or if she has ever suffered from psychiatric disorders like depression or anxiety.

CLINICAL PRESENTATION

> **Q. Write a long essay discussing the clinical features of pelvic endometriosis.**

Patients with endometriomas may present with variable symptoms, such as pelvic pain, back pain, dysmenorrhea, or dyspareunia, or they may present with infertility or a pelvic mass. Endometriosis may be present in about 35–50% patients with infertility. Endometriosis may present in form of a unilateral or bilateral adnexal mass (may be due to presence of an endometrioma). A ruptured endometrioma may present with an acute abdomen, low-grade fever, and an elevated white blood cell count. The most important objective during the evaluation of an adnexal mass is to rule out malignancy. Suspicion of malignancy is great in cases of postmenopausal women with an ovarian cyst that is complex in appearance.

GENERAL PHYSICAL EXAMINATION

Initial examination begins with the assessment of the woman's general appearance including the woman's facial expression, pallor, degree of agitation and vital signs. Altered vital signs such as elevated temperature, hypotension and tachycardia could be indicative of presence of underlying intra-abdominal pathology. Constant low-grade fever is commonly present in inflammatory conditions such as diverticulitis and appendicitis. Higher temperature may be associated with conditions such as advanced stages of PID, pyelonephritis or advanced peritonitis.

Evaluation of the patient's pulse and blood pressure may help in assessment of hypovolemia. Reduced blood pressure (hypotension) and tachycardia may indicate the underlying hypovolemia. If hypovolemia is present, an intravenous access must be established prior to completion of the examination.

EVALUATION OF THE PATIENT'S POSTURE

Evaluation of the patient's posture may point toward underlying musculoskeletal pathology. Patient's posture should be evaluated in three directions: (1) anterior, (2) posterior and (3) lateral. The back must be examined posteriorly for the presence of structural deformities such as scoliosis, kyphosis, lordosis, etc., and symmetry of the shoulders, gluteal folds and knee creases also needs to be assessed. Asymmetry may be indicative of underlying musculoskeletal disease. The clinician must also evaluate the mobility of spine by asking the patient to bend in forward and sideways direction at the waist. Limitation in forward flexion may be indicative of underlying orthopedic or musculoskeletal disease. The clinician can assess the abnormal tilting of the pelvic bones by simultaneously placing the medial side of his/her open palm on each side of patient's pelvis between the anterior superior iliac spine and posterior superior iliac spine. In normal individuals, the anterior superior iliac spine lies about 1 cm below the level of posterior superior iliac spine. Distances greater than this may be suggestive of abnormal tilt and could be associated with osteoarthritis and other orthopedic problems.

SPECIFIC SYSTEMIC EXAMINATION

ABDOMINAL EXAMINATION

Both abdominal and pelvic examinations must proceed slowly and gently because both the abdominal and pelvic components of the examination may be painful. The abdominal examination can help to identify areas of tenderness and the presence of masses or other anatomical findings which may help in reaching the accurate diagnosis. The method of performing abdominal examination has been described in details in Chapter 22. The abdomen must be inspected for the presence of previous surgical scar marks. Presence of previous surgical scars increases the possibility of postoperative adhesions, which could be an important cause of pelvic pain. Anterior abdominal wall must also be inspected for the signs of hernia. Hernias involving the anterior abdominal wall or pelvic floor may be associated with CPP. Palpation of the abdomen must systematically explore each abdominal quadrant and begin away from the area of indicated pain. Superficial palpation of the anterior abdominal wall by the clinician may reveal sites of tenderness or knotty muscles which may reflect nerve entrapment or myofascial pain syndromes. Deep palpation of the lower abdomen may identify pathology originating from the pelvic viscera. Palpation of the outer pelvis, back and abdomen may reveal trigger points that may indicate a myofascial component to the pain.

Following inspection and palpation, auscultation must be done. Presence of high-pitched bowel sounds is characteristic of bowel obstruction.

However, a lack of findings during the abdominal or pelvic examination does not rule out intra-abdominal pathology because many patients with a normal abdominal and pelvic examination may subsequently show pathologic findings on laparoscopic examination. Carnett's sign can be performed to distinguish whether the pain is due to an intra-abdominal pathology or pathology in the anterior abdominal wall.

Carnett's Sign for Patients with Pelvic Pain (Fig. 30.3)

The test is performed with the patient lying supine on the table. While the clinician places a finger on the painful,

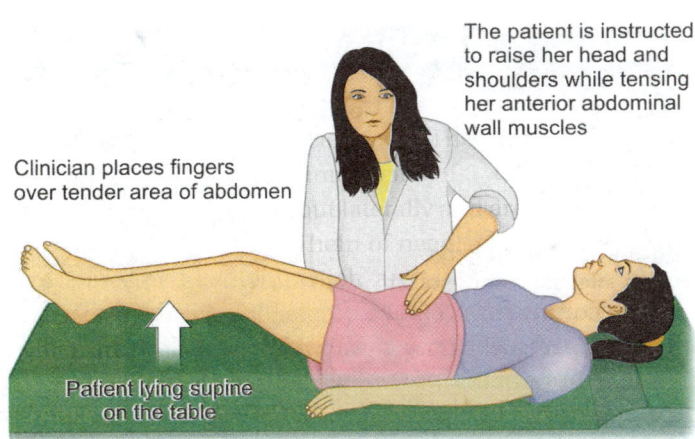

Fig. 30.3: Performing Carnett's sign for patients with pelvic pain.

tender area of the patient's abdomen, the patient is instructed to raise her head and shoulders while tensing the anterior abdominal wall muscles. A positive test occurs when the pain increases during this maneuver and is typical of anterior abdominal wall pathology and indicates myofascial cause of the pain. On the other hand, tenderness originating from inside the abdominal cavity usually decreases with this maneuver. In addition, Valsalva maneuver during head and shoulder elevation may display diastasis of the rectus abdominis muscle or hernias. Diastasis recti can be differentiated from the case of ventral hernias. With diastasis, the borders of rectus abdominis muscle can be palpated bilaterally along the entire length of the protrusion.

PELVIC EXAMINATION

Detailed description of the method for conducting the pelvic examination has been described in Chapter 22. The pelvic examination should commence with inspection of the external genitalia.

Per Speculum Examination

- Vagina and vulva must be inspected for presence of generalized changes and any local lesions. Findings of purulent vaginal discharge or cervicitis may be indicative of PID.
- Presence of bluish-black puckered spots, which are tender to touch may be noted on per speculum examination. This feature of endometriosis is pathognomonic of endometriosis. Bleeding through the vagina could be due to pregnancy-related complications, benign or malignant reproductive tract neoplasia or acute vaginal trauma. Cervical motion tenderness is commonly associated with peritoneal irritation and may be seen with PID, appendicitis and diverticulitis.

Bimanual Pelvic Examination

Tenderness upon pelvic examination is best detected at the time of menses when the endometrial implants are likely to be the largest and most tender. Since the pelvic examination must be performed slowly and gently, it should begin with a single-digit of one-hand. A moistened cotton swab should be used to elicit point tenderness in the vulva and vagina. Following the single-digit examination, a bimanual examination should be performed. During the pelvic examination, it is important to determine whether any manipulations reproduce the pain especially upon the palpation of the uterus or rectum. The bimanual examination may reveal the following findings:

- Nodularity and thickening of the uterosacral ligaments and the cul-de-sac may be present in cases of moderate to severe endometriosis. Women with minimal or mild endometriosis may have focal tenderness of the uterosacral ligaments or cul-de-sac without palpable nodules.
- Pain with deep palpation of the vaginal fornices may be observed with endometritis and cervical motion tenderness may be noted with PID.
- The uterus may be fixed in retroversion, owing to adhesions. Besides endometriosis, immobility of the uterus could be related to pelvic inflammatory disease, malignancy or adhesive disease from prior surgeries. Evaluation of adnexa may reveal masses or tenderness.
- A bluish nodule may be seen in the vagina due to infiltration from the posterior vaginal wall.
- Myofascial tenderness involving the puborectalis and coccygeus muscles may be noted by firmly sweeping the index finger across these muscles.
- Tenderness of urethra and bladder are potential indicators of urethral diverticulum or interstitial cystitis respectively. The patient should be checked for point tenderness along the bladder or other musculoskeletal structures.
- The size of the uterus must be assessed on pelvic examination. While an irregularly enlarged uterus is indicative of leiomyomas, a regularly enlarged uterus with softening could indicate adenomyosis or pregnancy.
- Adnexal tenderness with or without enlargement may indicate ovarian endometriosis. On the other hand, failure to reproduce localized tenderness during the pelvic examination may point towards a nongynecologic disorder. A tender adnexal mass may be suggestive of ectopic pregnancy, tuboovarian abscess, or ovarian cyst with torsion, hemorrhage or rupture.

Finally a rectovaginal examination must be performed. This should include the palpation of rectovaginal septum. A rectal examination may show rectal or posterior uterine masses, presence of nodules in the uterosacral ligaments, cul-de-sac or rectovaginal septum and/or pelvic floor point tenderness. The rectovaginal nodule suggestive of deep infiltrating endometriosis (DIE) may be easily palpated on rectovaginal examination, especially during menstruation when it becomes tender and more prominent. Nodularity of the rectovaginal septum could also be due to neoplasia. Palpation of hard stools or hemorrhoids on rectovaginal examination may indicate GI disorders.

DIFFERENTIAL DIAGNOSIS

> Q. Discuss in brief the differential diagnosis of CPP.

The etiology of CPP in women is poorly understood. Although a specific diagnosis is not found in the majority of cases, the four most commonly diagnosed pathologies include endometriosis, adhesions, IBS and interstitial cystitis. The various causes for CPP are listed in **Table 30.1**. Various points in the history, clinical examination and results of laboratory investigations can point toward the specific cause of pelvic pain **(Table 30.2)**.

MANAGEMENT

The discovery of exact pelvic pathology or cause of pain helps the clinician in instituting therapy appropriate to the etiology. The management plan for a patient suffering from CPP is described in **Flowchart 30.1**. The treatment needs to be individualized and must be decided after taking various parameters into consideration. Some of these include patient's age, requirement for preserving future reproductive function, main presenting complains for which the patient sought treatment (for example, pain or infertility), severity of symptoms, extent of disease and patient's attitude toward her problem.

Warning signs of malignancy include unexplained weight loss, hematochezia, perimenopausal, postmenopausal or postcoital bleeding.

INVESTIGATIONS

> Q. Write a long essay discussing the investigations and management of endometriosis in a 30-year-old woman.

Since CPP can be caused due to numerous pathologies and pathology in one organ can commonly lead to dysfunction in the other, women with chronic pain may have more than one cause of pain and overlapping symptoms. Thus, a comprehensive evaluation of multiple organ symptoms and psychological state is essential for complete treatment. The main issue in evaluating patient with CPP is distinguishing between gynecologic and nongynecologic causes of the pain. This would enable the gynecologist to institute the most appropriate course of further investigations and management. A definite diagnosis and the cause of the pain cannot always be elicited clinically. If the gynecological cause of pain cannot be established with surety, the gynecologist can make use of the hormonal suppression test to distinguish between the gynecological and nongynecological causes of pain. The hormonal suppression test is a functional study that provides a practical means of making this distinction and uses progestogens to create a hypoestrogenic environment. If the pain emanates from a gynecologic source or is exacerbated by normal menstrual physiology, the symptoms should improve significantly with hormone suppression.

Negative investigations at least assure the woman that no serious condition prevails and also help in eliminating

TABLE 30.2: Significance of selected findings on history, physical examination and diagnostic investigations.

Finding	Possible significance
History	
Hematochezia	Gastrointestinal malignancy/bleeding
History of pelvic surgery, pelvic infections, or use of an intrauterine device	Adhesions
Nonhormonal pain fluctuation	Adhesions, interstitial cystitis, irritable bowel syndrome, musculoskeletal causes
Pain fluctuates with menstrual cycle	Adenomyosis or endometriosis
Perimenopausal or postmenopausal irregular vaginal bleeding	Endometrial cancer
Postcoital bleeding	Cervical cancer or cervicitis (e.g., chlamydia or gonorrhea)
Unexplained weight loss	Systemic illness or malignancy
Physical examination	
Lack of uterus mobility on bimanual examination	Endometriosis, pelvic adhesions
Nodularity or masses on abdominal, bimanual pelvic and/or rectal examination	Adenomyosis, endometriosis, hernias, malignancy, tumors
Pain on palpation of outer back and outer pelvis	Abdominal/pelvic wall source of pain, trigger points
Point tenderness of vagina, vulva, or bladder	Adhesions, endometriosis, nerve entrapment, trigger points, vulvar vestibulitis
Positive Carnett's sign	Myofascial or abdominal wall cause of pain
Diagnostic studies	
Abnormal urine analysis or urine culture	Bladder malignancy, infection
Elevated leukocyte count, increased level of C-reactive protein	Infection, systemic illness, or malignancy (elevated/decreased white blood cell count or anemia)
Elevated erythrocyte sedimentation rate	Infection, malignancy, systemic illness
Positive culture tests for gonorrhea or *Chlamydia*	Pelvic inflammatory disease
Transvaginal ultrasound abnormalities	Adenomyosis, endometriosis/endometriomas, malignancy

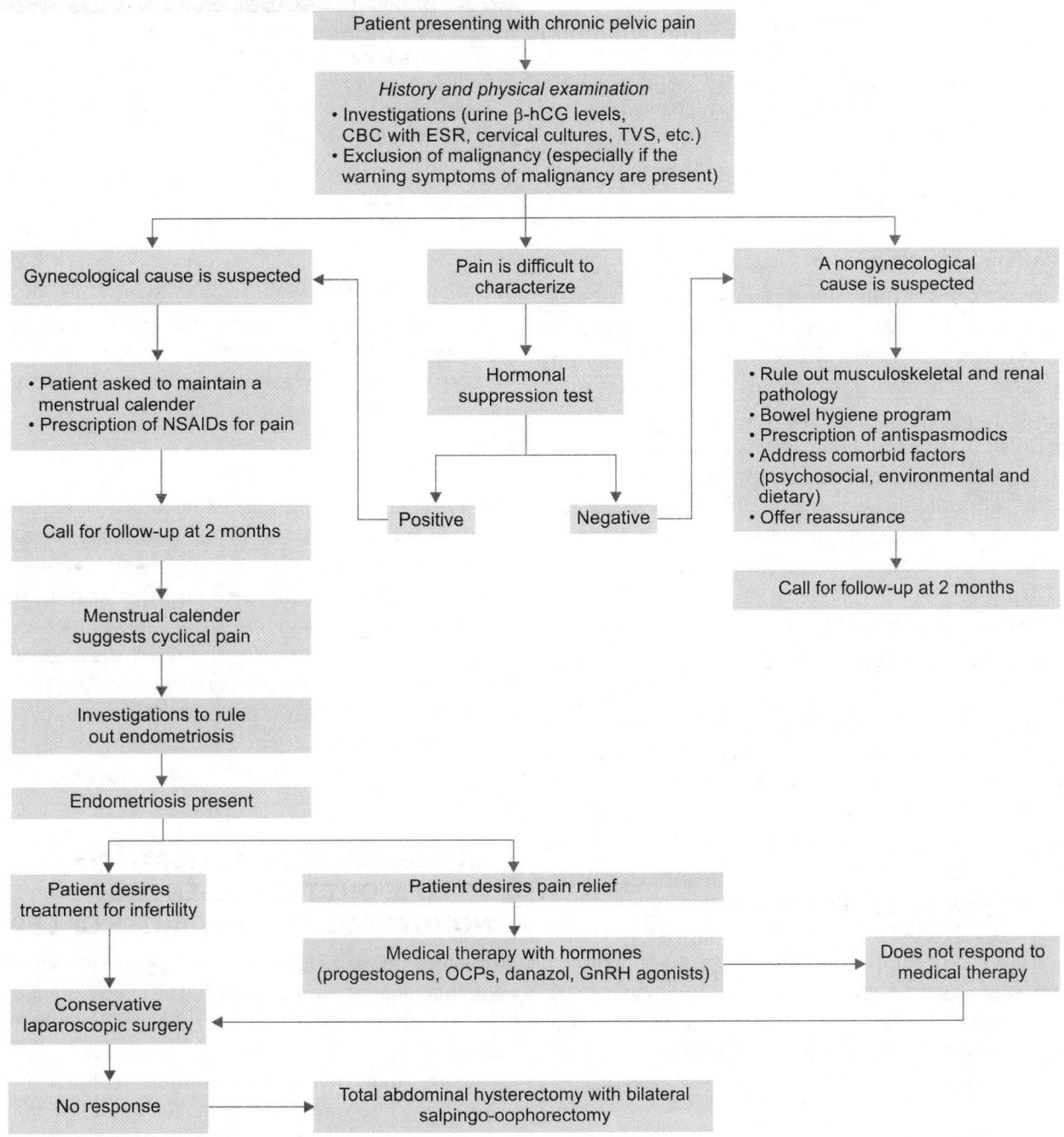

Flowchart 30.1: Algorithm for the management of chronic pelvic pain in women.

(CBC: complete blood count; ESR: erythrocyte sedimentation rate; GnRH: gonadotropin-releasing hormone; hCG: human chorionic gonadotropin; NSAIDs: nonsteroidal anti-inflammatory drugs; OCPs: oral contraceptive pills; TVS: transvaginal ultrasound)

the cancer phobia. Other investigations which may facilitate diagnosis are described here.

Urine β-hCG Levels

Determination of urine β hCG levels is important to rule out pregnancy related complications.

Complete Blood Count

Elevated leukocyte count points toward infection, whereas reduced hemoglobin level suggests anemia, which could be the result of chronic or acute blood loss.

Urine Analysis/Urine Culture

Urine analysis helps in excluding out the presence of possible urolithiasis, cystitis and urinary tract infection.

Cervical Cultures

Vaginal swabs may help in detecting infection such as gonorrhea and Chlamydia.

Serum Cancer Antigen 125 Test

Cancer antigen 125 (CA 125) levels may be increased to values >35 IU/mL in nearly 80% cases of endometriosis.

Serial measurement of CA 125 have a low sensitivity in detecting endometriosis, but the progressively decreasing serum CA 125 level is a useful prognostic indicator of treatment outcome. However, normal post-treatment values do not mean that endometriosis is absent. Increased CA 125 levels may be associated with numerous other conditions such as tuberculosis, PID, malignant epithelial ovarian tumors, chronic liver disease, etc.

> **BOX 30.1:** Appearance of lesions of endometriosis
> - Brown/black (powder-burn/gunmetal lesions)
> - Clear (atypical) nodules
> - Peritoneal windows
> - Classic blue-black blisters
> - Flame-like blisters
> - White plaques
> - Macroscopically normal peritoneum may have microscopic endometrial glands

IMAGING STUDIES

Ultrasound examination (both transabdominal and transvaginal) is the most commonly used investigation which may help in revealing the pelvic pathology responsible for producing pain. Imaging investigations such as computed tomography (CT) and magnetic resonance imaging (MRI) may be helpful in some cases. Though these diagnostic modalities help in identifying the individual lesions, these modalities are not helpful in assessing the extent of endometriosis. Doppler ultrasound may be used for diagnosis of pelvic congestion.

Transvaginal Sonography

Ultrasound examination, especially TVS forms the diagnostic modality of choice in most cases of CPP due to gynecological causes. Transvaginal sonography is a useful method for identifying the classic chocolate cyst of the ovary and typically shows a cyst containing low-level homogenous internal echoes consistent with old blood. The cyst wall may be thickened and irregular. There may be multiple cysts in different phases of ovulation. TVS serves as a useful method for both identifying and ruling out deep rectal endometriosis and/or an ovarian endometrioma. The following ultrasound characteristics are helpful in diagnosing an ovarian endometrioma in premenopausal women: Unilocular mass with ground glass echogenicity, one to four compartments (locules), and no papillary structures with detectable blood flow.

CT/MRI Examination

In cases, where sonographic findings are equivocal or non-diagnostic, CT examination must be widely used to reach the correct diagnosis. MRI is too costly imaging modality and therefore cannot be recommended as an investigation for routine use. However, MRI examination may be helpful in detecting rectovaginal endometriosis and cul-de-sac obliteration in >90% of cases where ultrasound examination proved to be nonconclusive.

ENDOSCOPY

Endoscopic investigations such as cystoscopy, laparoscopy, sigmoidoscopy and colonoscopy may also be employed depending upon the symptoms of each individual patient.

In patients with CPP and urinary symptoms, cystoscopy is typically advised. If GI symptoms are dominant, flexible sigmoidoscopy or colonoscopy may be warranted. For many women with a likely gynecological cause for their CPP, laparoscopy may be performed.

Diagnostic Laparoscopy

Diagnostic laparoscopy, backed by biopsy remains the gold standard for diagnosis of pelvic pathology. Laparoscopy detects small nodules of endometriosis which may remain undetected clinically. Laparoscopy can also detect pelvic adhesions and small inflammatory pelvic masses. Varied appearance of the lesions of endometrosis as observed on laparoscopic examination is described in **Box 30.1**. Biopsy of the suspected lesions is preferable over visual inspection. Therapeutic treatment such as adhesiolysis and cauterization of endometriotic lesions can be applied in the same sitting.

RADIOLOGICAL INVESTIGATIONS TO RULE OUT THE PRESENCE OF NONGYNECOLOGICAL CAUSES OF CPP

Radiological studies may be required in case of nongynecological causes of CPP. These investigations must be ordered in accordance with the patient's history and examination.

Some such investigations include barium studies (especially if GI pathology is suspected), radiography of joints (if musculoskeletal pathology is suspected) and intravenous pyelography (in case of renal pathology). In patients with bowel symptoms, barium enema may indicate internal or external obstructive lesions, malignancy and diverticular disease or irritable bowel disease.

℞ TREATMENT/GYNECOLOGICAL MANAGEMENT

 Q. Write a long essay discussing the medical management of endometriosis.

 Q. Discuss in detail the management of a 30-years old lady presenting with primary infertility and grade 4 endometriosis.

> Q. Discuss the pathogenesis and management of endometriosis in a 40-years old lady who has completed her family.
>
> Q. Write a short essay on surgical treatment of endometriosis.
>
> Q. What is the next step of management in the case study mentioned in the beginning of the chapter?
>
> Ans. In this patient, the history points toward the likelihood of endometriosis as the likely diagnosis. However, since the main complaint of the patient is infertility rather than chronic pelvic pain, she must undergo a thorough basic evaluation for other causes of infertility before diagnostic laparoscopy is undertaken.

In many women with CPP, treatment begins with identification of a source of pain and treatment is dictated by the diagnosis. However, in other cases, pathology may be identified and treatment is directed toward dominant symptoms. Treatment should be directed at the underlying cause of pelvic pain. The patient should be given a menstrual calendar to document the correlation of pain with the menstrual cycle. She should be advised to return after 2 months to review her symptoms and the calendar. Such record of pain also guides the gynecologist regarding the severity of pain and to decide whether the pain is sufficiently severe and truly disrupts the patient's quality of life to justify proceeding with more invasive diagnostic modalities or surgery.

If a nongynecological cause of pelvic pain is suspected, the patient should be instructed to follow a course of proper bowel hygiene for at least 2 months. If her symptoms get alleviated, she should continue this program for 6 more months. However, if the menstrual calendar suggests a gynecologic etiology (e.g., endometriosis) for pelvic pain, exploratory laparoscopy can be considered. At the time of laparoscopy, the following procedures can be undertaken: destruction of endometrial implants, uterosacral transection, lysis of adhesions and evacuation of endometriomas. These simple laparoscopic procedures may help in relieving symptoms in the majority of appropriately selected patients.

Management of patients with endometriosis may be expectant, medical, or surgical and is usually based on the presenting complaints and the disease staging. Each modality of treatment is associated with its own specific advantages and disadvantages which are described in **Table 30.3**.

One of the main criteria, which help the gynecologist to decide whether to consider medical or surgical management, is whether the patient's main complaint is infertility or pelvic pain. The algorithm for treatment of endometriosis is described in **Flowchart 30.2**. While medical therapy has a role in the symptomatic management of endometriosis, it has no role in the management of endometriosis-associated infertility. In fact, hormonal therapy may rather enhance infertility.

Before starting empirical treatment, other causes of pelvic pain should be ruled out, as far as possible. Initial treatment comprises of using analgesic drugs, especially NSAIDs or COCPs. Use of levonorgestrel-releasing intrauterine system (LNG-IUS) or continuous progestogens can be considered if estrogenic preparations are contraindicated or give rise to side effects. These therapies can be used for long term if effective and well tolerated. Patients in whom the initial therapies (NSAIDs, OCPs, and progestins) do not prove to be successful can be considered for GnRH agonists. The use of GnRH agonists is preferred over androgenic agents such as danazol and gestrinone because the latter drugs can cause unacceptable androgenic side-effects. Initially, a trial of GnRH agonists is tried for 2–3 months. This can be further continued for 6 months if the patient experiences relief from pain. This is likely to be more cost-effective than initial laparoscopy with local ablation in case of clinically suspected endometriosis given that the incidence of long-term symptom recurrence is similar for both the strategies.

Majority of medical therapies act by suppression of the ovaries and induction of amenorrhea. This merely inactivates and does not remove the local disease. Symptoms, therefore, may recur following the cessation of therapy in a high proportion of patients. Since both medical and surgical treatments are associated with a high risk of recurrence following the interruption of therapy, medical treatment may be required to be instituted on an intermittent basis in the long term. These treatment strategies are described here.

STAGING OF ENDOMETRIOSIS

> Q. Write a long essay discussing the staging of endometriosis.

Before initiating treatment for endometriosis, it is important to classify the disease as minimal, mild, moderate or severe **(Table 30.4 and Figs. 30.4A to D)**. The American Fertility

TABLE 30.3: Advantages and disadvantages associated with different treatment modalities.		
Treatment	**Advantages**	**Disadvantages**
Surgical therapy	*Beneficial for infertility:* • Possibly better long-term results • Definitive diagnosis and treatment • Associated with a much lower rate of recurrence	• Expensive • Invasive
Medical therapy	It is associated with reduced initial cost and is effective for providing relief from pain.	Adverse effects are commonly present; it is unlikely to improve fertility and is associated with a high recurrence rate

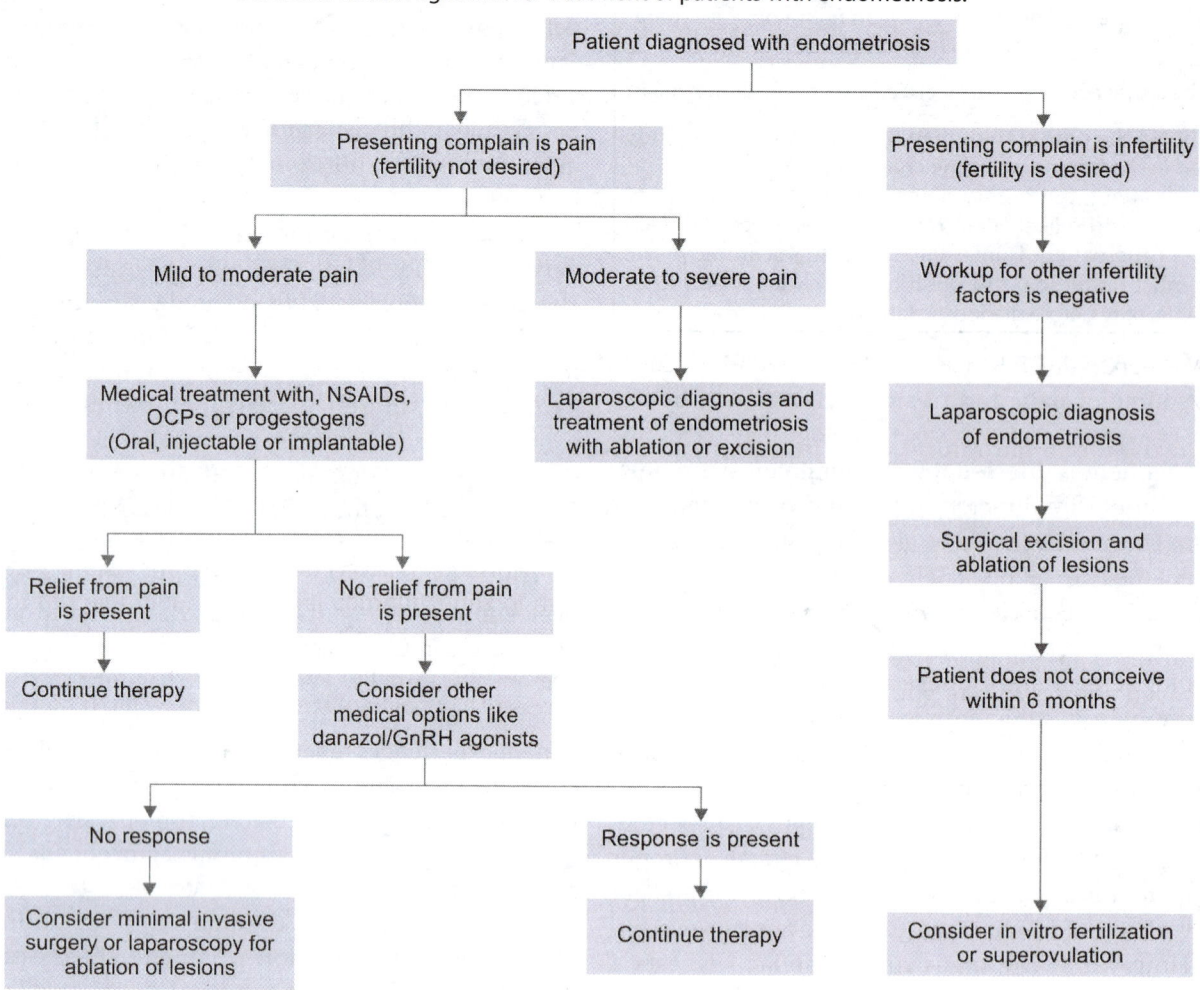

Flowchart 30.2: Algorithm for treatment of patients with endometriosis.

(GnRH: gonadotropin-releasing hormone; NSAIDs: nonsteroidal anti-inflammatory drugs; OCPs: oral contraceptive pills)

TABLE 30.4: Stage of endometriosis in accordance to the points assigned.

Stage of endometriosis	Points
Stage I (minimal)	1–5
Stage II (mild)	6–15
Stage III (moderate)	16–40
Stage IV (severe)	>40

Society's revised staging for endometriosis is currently the most widely used staging system. In this scoring system, point scores are assigned based on the number of lesions, their bilaterality, size of the lesions, depth of endometrial implants, presence and extent of adnexal adhesions and degree of obliteration of the pouch of Douglas **(Table 30.5)**. It, however, does not take into account the complaints such as infertility or pelvic pain. This classification is a fairly accurate method of recording laparoscopic findings and can help standardize the patient's findings and documenting the patient's baseline condition and subsequent progress. Staging is based on location, diameter and depth of lesions and density of adhesions. Stages range from minimal to severe disease. Despite this standardization, the correlation between stage and extent of disease remains controversial.

TREATMENT FOR ENDOMETRIOSIS-ASSOCIATED PAIN

Analgesics

Pain is a cardinal symptom of endometriosis. Studies have demonstrated elevated prostaglandin levels in peritoneal fluid and endometriotic tissue in women with endometriosis. As a result, NSAIDs are widely used analgesics in clinical practice.

Before prescribing NSAIDs to the patient, clinicians must discuss the role of NSAIDs in provision of pain relief along with its side-effects profile, including risk of gastric ulceration and cardiovascular disease. In conclusion, the effectiveness of NSAIDs (naproxen) in treating endometriosis-associated dysmenorrhoea is not well-established owing to a lack of studies.

Pelvic Pain

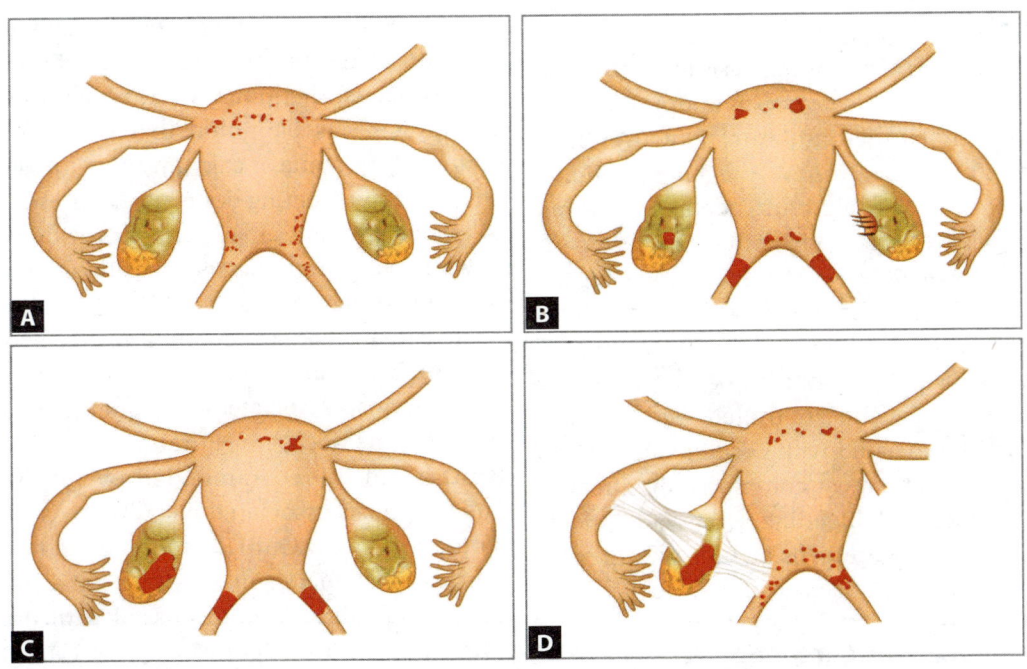

Figs. 30.4A to D: Staging system of endometriosis as devised by the American Society of Reproductive Medicine: (A) Stage I: minimal; (B) Stage II: mild; (C) Stage III: moderate and (D) Stage IV: severe.

TABLE 30.5: Revised American Fertility Society classification of endometriosis (1996).

Peritoneum			
Endometriosis	<1 cm	1–3 cm	>3 cm
Superficial	1	2	4
Deep	2	4	6
Ovary			
Right superficial	1	2	4
Right deep	4	16	20
Left superficial	1	2	4
Left deep	4	16	20
Posterior cul-de-sac obliteration			
Partial		Complete	
4		40	
Ovary			
Adhesions	<1/3 enclosure	1/3 to 2/3 enclosure	>2/3 enclosure
Right filmy	1	2	4
Right dense	4	8	16
Left filmy	1	2	4
Left dense	4	8	16
Tube			
Right filmy	1	2	4
Right dense	4*	8*	16
Left filmy	1	2	4
Left dense	4*	8*	16

*If the fimbriated end of the Fallopian tube is completely enclosed, the point assignment is changed to 16.
Source: Revised American Society for Reproductive Medicine classification of endometriosis: 1996. Fertil Steril. 1997;67:817-21. doi: 10.1016/s0015-0282(97)81391-x

Hormonal Therapies

Endometriosis is considered predominantly an estrogen-dependent disease. Thus, hormonal suppression might be an attractive medical approach to treat the disease and its symptoms. Currently, hormonal contraceptives, progestogens, antiprogestogens, GnRH agonists, and aromatase inhibitors are in clinical use. The guideline development group (GDG) recommends that clinicians must take patient preferences, side-effects, efficacy, costs, and availability into consideration when choosing hormonal treatment for endometriosis-associated pain. Presently, there is no significant evidence supporting the efficacy of a particular treatment strategy over the others. Management plans must be individualized, taking into consideration various parameters, described previously. Woman should be able to make an informed choice based on a good understanding of the disease process and its effect on her body.

Hormonal Contraceptives

A systematic review by Vercellini et al., 2003 has shown that use of low-dose cyclic OCPs is effective in reducing pain symptoms in patients with endometriosis. Continuous rather than the cyclic use of OCPs is likely to be more effective for pain control. Clinicians may consider the use of a vaginal contraceptive ring or a transdermal (estrogen/progestin) patch to reduce endometriosis-associated dysmenorrhea, dyspareunia, and CPP. Due to their good safety profile, combined OCPs are useful for long-term use.

Progestogens and Antiprogestogens

Continuous administration of progestogens is likely to cause inhibition of ovulation. They also exert an antiproliferative effect on the endometriotic implants, causing their decidualization and eventual atrophy. A recent systematic Cochrane review by Brown et al., (2012) determined that there was no evidence to suggest a benefit of progestogens over other treatments. However, continuous progestogens serve as an effective therapy for the alleviation of painful symptoms associated with endometriosis. Nevertheless, progestogens must be used with caution due to the scarcity of data and absence of placebo-controlled studies. Also, progestogens may be associated with certain side effects, which can limit its use. The most common side effect of progestogens is breakthrough bleeding. Other side effects reported with the use of progestogens include weight gain, breast tenderness, bloating, headache, nausea, etc.

Levonorgestrel-releasing Intrauterine System

Levonorgestrel-releasing intrauterine system does not suppress ovulation but acts locally on the endometrium. Due to its locally mediated action, LNG-IUS is likely to serve useful for the management of endometriosis-associated pain. Three studies (Petta et al., 2005; Gomes et al., 2007; and Ferreira et al., 2010) have investigated the potential of LNG-IUS for management of endometriosis-associated symptoms. These studies have concluded that LNG-IUS is effective for the management of endometriosis-associated pain as well for the maintenance of pain control following surgical treatment.

Gonadotropin-releasing Hormone Agonist

Gonadotropin-releasing hormone analogs [e.g., leuprolide (lupron), goserelin (zoladex)] produce a hypogonadotropic-hypogonadic state by inhibiting the secretion of gonadotropins by causing the downregulation of pituitary gland. Initial administration of GnRH agonists stimulates the pituitary resulting in the release of FSH and LH. However, chronic administration of GnRH agonists leads to the down regulation of pituitary GnRH receptors, causing the suppression of hypothalamic-pituitary-ovarian axis, thereby resulting in anovulation. Currently, goserelin and leuprolide acetate are the most commonly used GnRH agonists. The efficacy of GnRH agonists is comparable to danazol in relieving pain. However, these drugs mainly help in suppressing pain and may show no improvement in infertility. The results from the Cochrane review by Brown et al. (2010) suggest that GnRH agonist (GnRHa) is more effective than placebo but inferior to the LNG-IUS or oral danazol in providing relief from the endometriosis-associated pain. The most common side effects associated with the long-term use of GnRH agonists include the hypoestrogenic side effects, especially reduction of the bone density. This can be prevented through addition of either oral or transdermal estrogens in combination with various progestogens, or tibolone (add-back therapy) to GnRHa therapy if it is used for more than 6 months. However, use of progestogens alone or calcium supplements is unlikely to be effective in preventing bone loss. Antiresorptive agents such as bisphosphonates may help in providing bone protection in women in whom the add-back therapy is contraindicated or is not tolerated.

It can be concluded that GnRH agonists, with and without add-back therapy, are effective in the relief of endometriosis associated pain, but there is limited evidence regarding its dosage or duration of treatment. No specific GnRHa can be recommended over another in relieving endometriosis associated pain. There is evidence of severe side effects with GnRHa (e.g., reduced bone density, hot flushes, insomnia, vaginal dryness, reduced libido, headache, etc.) which should be discussed with the woman before prescribing GnRH agonists to her. Careful consideration must be given before prescribing GnRH agonists to the young women and adolescents, because these women may not have reached maximum bone density.

Androgenic Agents

Danazol: Danazol, a synthetic androgen, is the derivative of ethinyl testosterone, which has been shown to be highly effective in relieving the symptoms of endometriosis by inhibiting pituitary gonadotropins (FSH and LH). This may result in the development of a relative hypoestrogenic state. Danazol probably provides pain relief by producing endometrial atrophy. A Cochrane review by Farquhar et al., 2007 has shown that Danazol in the dosage of 400–600 mg daily is effective in treating the symptoms and signs of endometriosis. However, its use is limited by the occurrence of androgenic side effects **(Table 30.6)**. Recent studies indicate that vaginal danazol may be better tolerated. According to the European Society of Human Reproduction and Embryology (ESHRE) recommendations (2013), danazol should not be used if any other medical therapy is available, due to occurrence of severe side effects (acne, greasy skin, deepening of voice, hirsutism, vaginal spotting, weight gain, muscle cramps, etc.). Atherogenic effects on the lipid profile have also been reported. However, neither danazol nor gestrinone cause any adverse effect on the bone density. Therefore,

TABLE 30.6: Adverse effects caused by danazol.

Cause of side effect	Side effect caused
Estrogen deficiency	Headache, flushing, sweating, atrophic vaginitis and breast atrophy
Androgenic effect	Acne, edema, hirsutism, deepening of the voice and weight gain

these serve as beneficial alternatives to GnRH analogues in women who are susceptible to bone loss or those in whom estrogenic addback preparations are contraindicated.

Gestrinone: It is a 19-norsteroid derivative having antiestrogenic, antiprogestogenic, antigonadotrophic, and androgenic properties. It has a long half-life and is therefore administered twice weekly orally in a dose of 1.25–2.5 mg. The consumption of this drug induces amenorrhea in 50–100% of women with endometriosis. Resumption of menses occurs after cessation of treatment. Though the use of gestrinone can cause androgenic side effects, these are less intense in comparison to danazol. Gestrinone has been found to be as effective as GnRH agonists for providing relief from pelvic pain associated with endometriosis for up to 6 months after cessation of therapy.

Aromatase Inhibitors

The most common third-generation aromatase inhibitors, letrozole and anastrozole, are reversible inhibitors of the enzyme aromatase, which compete with androgens for aromatase-binding sites. Even though the evidence for increased expression of aromatase P450 in endometriotic tissue still remains controversial; aromatase inhibitors have been studied for treatment of pain in women with endometriosis. Two systematic reviews evaluating the potential of aromatase inhibitors for the treatment of endometriosis-associated pain (Ferrero et al., 2011; Nawathe et al., 2008) have concluded that future studies are required to assess if aromatase inhibitors would be useful in long term for improvement of pain symptoms in comparison to the conventional therapy.

Use of these agents is likely to result in hypoestrogenic side effects, such as vaginal dryness, hot flushes, and reduced bone mineral density.

Adjuvant Therapy

This includes the use of tricyclic antidepressants such as amitriptyline and antiepileptics such as gabapentin for the management of chronic pain of endometriosis in patients who are resistant to the conventional therapies.

Surgical Treatment

Surgical treatment involving elimination of endometriotic lesions (through excision, diathermy, or ablation/evaporation), division of adhesions (for restoring pelvic anatomy), and interruption of nerve pathways for alleviation of pain has long been used for the management of endometriosis-associated pain. Surgical treatment of endometriomas must preferably be via laparoscopic cystectomy.

Laparotomy and laparoscopy are equally effective in the treatment of endometriosis-associated pain. Operative laparoscopy (excision/ablation) is more effective for the treatment of pelvic pain associated with all stages of endometriosis, compared to diagnostic laparoscopy only.

Laparoscopic surgery is usually associated with less pain, shorter duration of hospital stay, quicker recovery, and better cosmesis, in comparison to laparotomy. Therefore, laparoscopic surgery is usually preferred to open surgery.

If the clinician having relevant experience with laparoscopy is not available, the patient should be referred to a centre of expertise because operative laparoscopy for advanced disease may be associated with a significant risk. When the lesions of endometriosis are identified at the time of diagnostic laparoscopy, clinicians are recommended to surgically treat these for reducing endometriosis-associated pain. While laparoscopic surgery is effective for the treatment of pain secondary to endometriosis, long-term recurrence of pain can occur in nearly 50% individuals.

Ablation versus Excision of Endometriosis

Clinicians may consider using either ablation or excision of peritoneal endometriosis for reducing endometriosis-associated pain because both the procedures have been found to be equally effective.

Laparoscopic Uterosacral Nerve Ablation versus Presacral Neurectomy

The minimally invasive procedure, laparoscopic uterosacral nerve ablation (LUNA), has not been found to be useful for alleviation of pain related to endometriosis. Presacral neurectomy (PSN), on the other hand, has been found to be beneficial for treatment of endometriosis-associated midline pain as an adjunct to conservative laparoscopic surgery. However, PSN is a procedure requiring high degree of skill. Moreover, it may be associated with an increased risk of adverse effects such as bleeding, constipation, urinary urgency, etc.

Hysterectomy for Endometriosis-associated Pain

Hysterectomy with removal of the ovaries and all visible endometriosis lesions can be considered as a treatment option in women who are not desirous of future childbearing and have failed to respond to more conservative treatments. Prior to the surgery, women should be informed that hysterectomy might not necessarily cure the symptoms or the disease because disease excision may be incomplete.

Prevention of Adhesions following Endometriosis Surgery

There are a number of barrier, fluid, and pharmacological agents, which have been used for prevention of adhesions at the time of gynecological surgery. Some such agents include oxidized regenerated cellulose (Interceed®), polytetrafluoroethylene surgical membrane (Gore-Tex®), fibrin sheet, sodium hyaluronate, carboxymethylcellulose combination (Seprafilm®), polyethylene oxide and carboxymethylcellulose gel (Oxiplex/AP®), icodextrin 4% (Adept®), hyaluronic acid products and polyethylene glycol hydrogel (SprayGel®), etc. Studies have shown that the use of oxidized regenerated cellulose helps in preventing adhesion formation during operative laparoscopy for endometriosis. On the other hand, use of icodextrin after operative laparoscopy for endometriosis is not likely to prevent adhesion formation. Therefore, its use is not recommended.

TREATMENT OF ENDOMETRIOSIS-ASSOCIATED INFERTILITY

Causes of Infertility in Endometriosis

 Q. Discuss briefly the role of endometriosis in infertility.

The possible mechanisms for infertility in patients with endometriosis are described in **Box 30.2**.

Endometrial Fertility Index

Adamoson (2010) introduced the endometrial fertility index (EFI), which acts as a measure of probable prognosis in the patients with endometriosis regarding the chances of spontaneous conception in 3 years without assistance.

The variables used for calculating EFI is the least function (LF) score, which is calculated by adding the scores of fallopian tube, fimbra and ovary on both the sides determined intraoperatively following the surgical intervention **(Table 30.7)**. For calculating the total LF score, the lowest score for the left side is added to the score on right side **(Fig. 30.5)**.

Management in Mild/Moderate Cases

In case of minimal/mild lesions of endometriosis diagnosed at the time of laparoscopic examination, excision or ablation of the implants should be performed, followed by timed intercourse with or without controlled ovarian hyperstimulation (COH) for 3–6 months. If the patient fails to conceive, intrauterine insemination (IUI) after 2–3 cycles of COH may be followed by in vitro fertilization (IVF).

Management in Moderate/Severe Cases

For moderate-to-severe disease, surgical excision of the lesions followed by treatment by IUI or IVF is recommended. Resection of endometriomas has not been shown to improve fertility potential and must be only performed for gynecological indications, such as pelvic pain. As previously described, medical therapy delays pregnancy and has no role in improving the fertility potential. However, medicines like GnRH-agonists can be used in ovulation induction protocols. IVF should be the first-line treatment option in the presence of peritubal adhesions. In patients with poor ovarian reserve, donor oocytes may be employed for IVF.

BOX 30.2: Mechanisms for infertility in endometriosis.
- Deformity of pelvic organs
- Alteration of peritoneal environment
- Increase in macrophages
- Reduced sperm motility
- Phagocytosis of spermatozoa
- Interference with oocyte pickup

TABLE 30.7: Description of terms of least function terms.

Structure	Score	Dysfunction	Description
Tube	3	Mild	Slight injury to serosa of the fallopian tube
	2	Moderate	Moderate injury to serosa or muscularis of the fallopian tube; moderate limitation in mobility
	1	Severe	Fallopian tube fibrosis or mild/moderate salpingitis isthmica nodosa; severe limitation in mobility
	0	Nonfunctional	Complete tubal obstruction, extensive fibrosis or salpingitis isthmica nodosa
Fimbria	3	Mild	Slight injury to fimbria with minimal scarring
	2	Moderate	Moderate injury to fimbria, with moderate scarring, moderate loss of fimbrial architecture and minimal intrafimbrial fibrosis
	1	Severe	Severe injury to fimbria, with severe scarring, severe loss of fimbrial architecture and moderate intrafimbrial fibrosis
	0	Nonfunctional	Severe injury to fimbria, with extensive scarring, complete loss of fimbrial architecture, complete tubal occlusion or hydrosalpinx
Ovary	3	Mild	Normal or almost normal ovarian size; minimal or mild injury to ovarian serosa
	2	Moderate	Ovarian size reduced by one-third or more; moderate injury to ovarian surface
	1	Severe	Ovarian size reduced by two-thirds or more; severe injury to ovarian surface
	0	Nonfunctional	Ovary absent or completely encased in adhesions

Source: Adamson GD, Pasta DJ. Endometriosis fertility index: the new, validated endometriosis staging system. Fertil Steril. 2010;94(5):1609-15. doi: 10.1016/j.fertnstert.2009.09.035. PMID: 19931076.

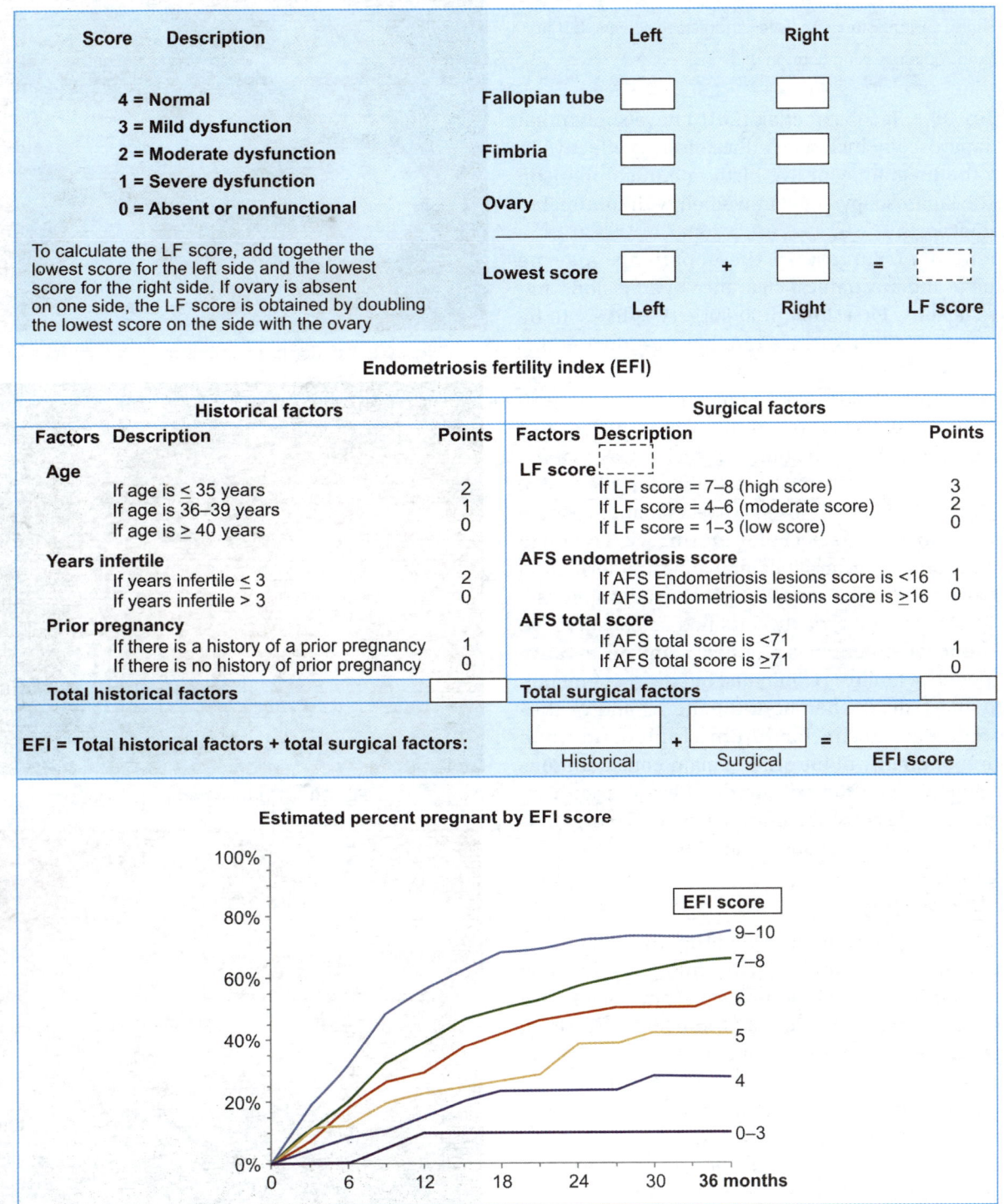

Fig. 30.5: Endometrial fertility index (EFI) surgery form.
(AFS: American Fertility Society)

Treatment Options

Hormonal Therapies

Use of hormonal treatment (e.g., danazol, GnRH analogues, OCPs, etc.) for suppression of ovarian function is unlikely to improve fertility in cases of minimal to mild endometriosis.

Surgical Treatment

If the medical therapy does not prove to be successful, the gynecologist may have to resort to surgical treatment. Surgical treatment is the preferred approach for treatment of infertile patients with advanced endometriosis. Some indications for surgery in cases of endometriosis are

BOX 30.3: Indications of surgery in endometriosis.
- Endometriomas >4 cm in size
- Severe dyspareunia/dysmenorrhea
- Failure of long suppression with GnRH agonists to achieve fertility

(GnRH: gonadotropin releasing hormone)

listed in **Box 30.3**. Jacobson et al. (2010) have shown that operative laparoscopy including adhesiolysis is effective in increasing the pregnancy or live birth rate in comparison to diagnostic laparoscopy alone in women with minimal to mild endometriosis.

The benefit of surgery in these patients may be entirely due to the mechanical clearance of adhesions and obstructive lesions. First attempt at surgery is likely to be associated with highest success rate because during this time, the surgical planes are best defined. During the repeated attempts, the surgical planes may not be well defined due to the formation of adhesions. In case of infertility, the surgery must be timed in such a way that the couple gets an opportunity to stay together for atleast 4–6 months following surgery. In case it appears that the couple may not be able to stay together following surgery, it is best to postpone the surgery because bilateral adhesion formation may occur again within 4–6 months following adhesiolysis.

Surgical care can be broadly classified as conservative when reproductive potential is retained, semiconservative when reproductive ability is eliminated but ovarian function is retained and radical when both the uterus and ovaries are removed. Age, desire for future childbearing and deterioration of quality of life are the main considerations when deciding on the extent of surgery. Besides removing the endometriotic lesions, the minimal invasive surgery is also useful in restoration of patient's fertility.

Laparoscopic Surgery

Laparoscopy can help in establishing the diagnosis of endometriosis by identifying the following lesions: endometriotic nodules or lesions having blue-black or a powder-burned appearance **(Figs. 30.6 and 30.7)**. However, the lesions can be red, white, or nonpigmented. Peritoneal defects and adhesions are also indicative of endometriosis. Laparoscopy can also detect presence of blood **(Fig. 30.8)** or endometriotic deposits in cul-de-sac and its obliteration.

Besides diagnosis of endometriotic lesions at various locations, laparoscopy can also help in treating the patient. Powder-burn lesions over the uterine surface may be amenable to laser obliteration **(Figs. 30.9 and 30.10A and B)**. Some of the endometrial lesions are cystic or nodular and can be excised. Laparoscopic surgery can also be used for excision of adhesions **(Figs. 30.11A and B)**. With the advent of robot-assisted laparoscopy, a laparoscopic approach is even more widely accessible. Similar outcomes have been demonstrated by robotic-assisted laparoscopy in comparison to traditional laparoscopy for the management of endometriosis.

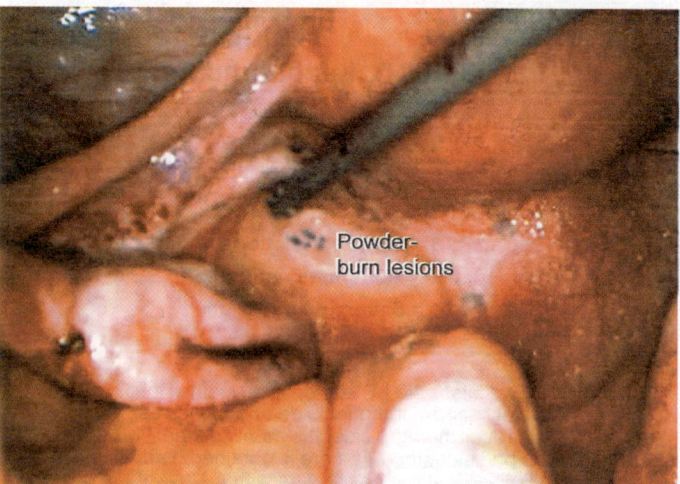

Fig. 30.6: Powder-burn lesions over endometrial surface.

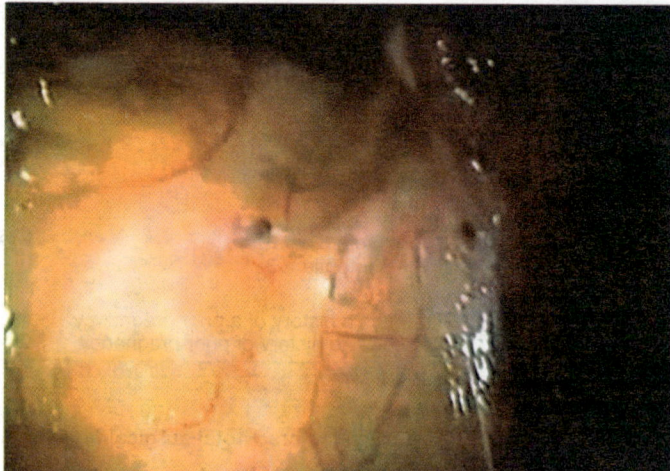

Fig. 30.7: Nodular endometrial lesions.

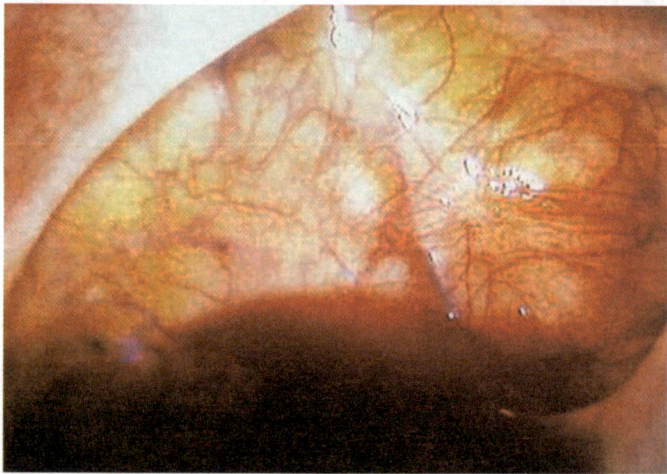

Fig. 30.8: Presence of blood in cul-de-sac.

Until recently, surgery in infertile patients with limited disease was thought to be no better than expectant management. However, according to the recent evidence, laparoscopic surgery has been found to significantly improve the fertility rates among infertile women with minimal or mild endometriosis. Infertile patients with documented endometriosis can also benefit from the same reproductive techniques such as superovulation, in vitro fertilization, etc.

The usefulness of conservative surgery for pain relief is unclear, but it appears that immediate postoperative efficacy is at least as high as that with medical treatment and long-term outcomes may be considerably higher. Since laparoscopy is much more expensive in comparison to the medical treatment, some physicians advocate that the overall costs can be reduced by making aggressive use of empiric medical treatment before surgery is considered. Definitive surgery, which includes hysterectomy and oophorectomy, is reserved for use in women with intractable pain who no longer desire pregnancy. Women who have undergone oophorectomy must be treated with estrogen replacement therapy in order to prevent the side effects related to premature menopause. When the diagnosis of endometriosis is made at laparoscopy, surgical ablation of the lesions is frequently performed.

Surgical treatment improves pregnancy rates and is the preferred initial treatment for infertility caused by endometriosis. Surgery also appears to provide better long-term pain relief than medical treatment. Bilateral oophorectomy and hysterectomy are treatment options for patients with intractable pain, if childbearing is no longer desired.

Conservative Surgery

The aim of conservative surgery is to destroy visible endometriotic implants and lyse peritubal and periovarian adhesions that are a source of pain and may interfere with

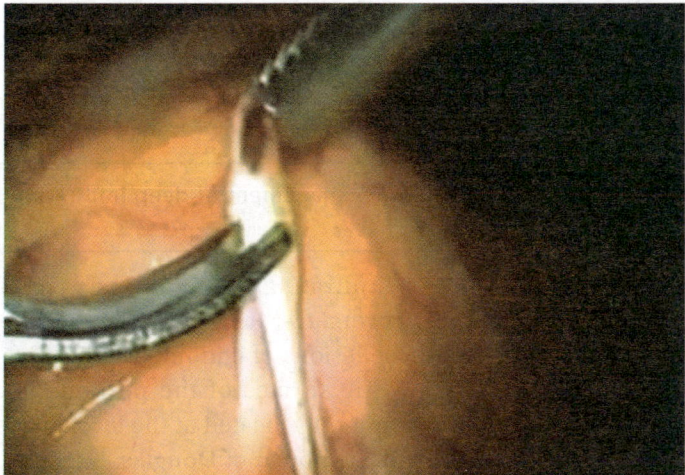

Fig. 30.9: Laparoscopic excision of nodular endometrial lesions overlying the round ligament.

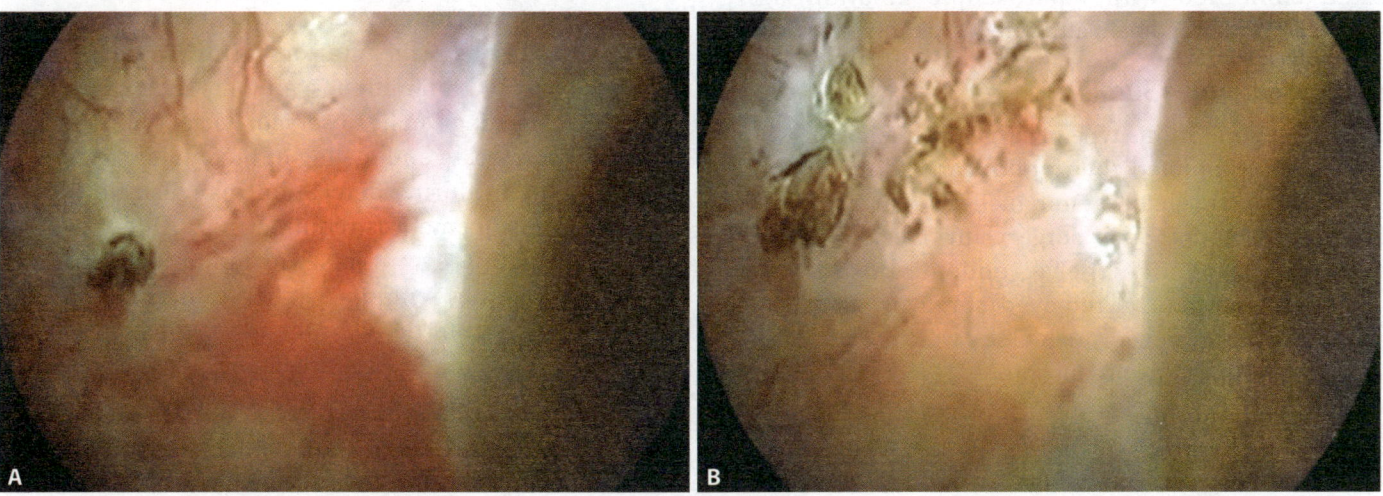

Figs. 30.10A and B: Appearance of the uterine surface after the ablation of endometriotic lesions.

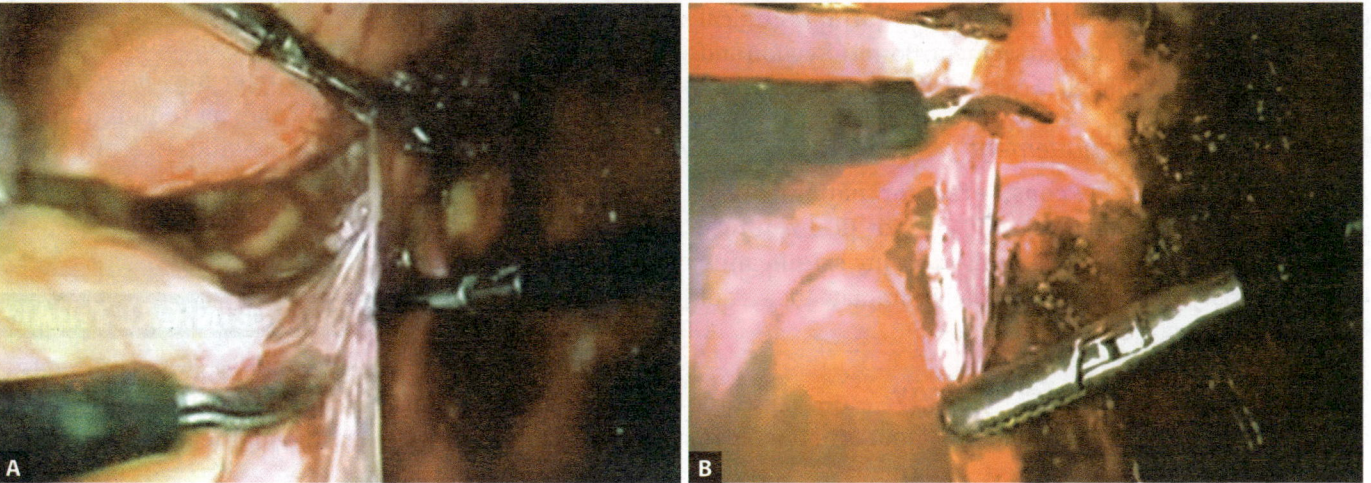

Figs. 30.11A and B: Laparoscopic excision of endometrial adhesions.

ovum transport. The laparoscopic approach is the widely used method for conservative treatment of endometriosis. Ablation can be performed with laser or electrodiathermy. Ovarian endometriomas can be treated by drainage or cystectomy. Tubal flushing with oil-soluble media has been shown to improve pregnancy rates in women with endometriosis-associated infertility.

Presacral neurectomy may be used to relieve severe dysmenorrhea. The nerve bundles are transected at the level of the third sacral vertebra and the distal ends are ligated. Some authors advocate prophylactic ligation of the middle sacral artery and vein in order to prevent potential vascular injury. Constipation is a long-term adverse effect of this procedure.

Nodularity of the uterosacral ligaments may contribute to dyspareunia and low back pain. The transmission of neural pathways is via the Lee-Frankenhäuser plexus. Laparoscopic uterine nerve ablation (LUNA) is performed to interrupt the pain fibers. Potential complications of this procedure include uterine prolapse and pelvic denervation. A systematic review of trials of LUNA found no advantage in terms of pain relief when compared to placebo. However, when combined with laparoscopic ablation, LUNA significantly reduced pain attributed to endometriosis.

Semiconservative Surgery

The indication for this type of surgery is mainly in women who have completed their childbearing, are too young to undergo surgical menopause and are debilitated by the symptoms. Such surgery involves hysterectomy and cytoreduction of pelvic endometriosis. Ovarian endometriosis can be removed surgically because the remaining functioning ovarian tissue which is left behind is sufficient for hormone production.

Radical Surgery

This involves total hysterectomy with bilateral oophorectomy and cytoreduction of visible endometriosis. Adhesiolysis is performed to restore mobility and normal intrapelvic organ relationships. Ureteric obstruction may warrant surgical release or excision of a damaged segment. Bowel resection and anastamosis may be required in cases of intestinal obstruction.

Definitive Surgical Management

Oophorectomy may be considered for patients who have completed childbearing and do not desire future pregnancy. Though bilateral oophorectomy significantly reduces the risk, it does not completely eliminate the risk of endometrioma recurrence.

Assisted Reproductive Technology

If the patient does not conceive after 6 months of operative laparoscopy or in cases of severe endometriosis lesions, assisted reproductive techniques (in vitro fertilization and superovulation) can be considered. IVF protocol for endometriosis comprises long suppression of hypothalmo-pituitary-ovarian axis using two doses of GnRH agonists. For further details related to such techniques, kindly refer to Chapter 34.

DEEP INFILTRATING ENDOMETRIOSIS OF PELVIS

> Q. Discuss in detail the management of deep infiltrating endometriosis.

The definition of deep infiltrating endometriosis (DIE) presently remains controversial. Most clinicians believe that DIE comprise of those lesions of endometriosis which penetrate >5 mm below the surface of the peritoneum. These lesions are most commonly located at the level of the uterosacral ligaments and the pouch of Douglas. However, these lesions may often extend along the rectovaginal (RV) septum, thereby infiltrating and extending backward into the rectum and sigmoid colon resulting in the obliteration of the cul-de-sac. DIE may be associated with severe pelvic pain, severe dysmenorrhea and/or severe dyspareunia. In the presence of rectal infiltration, symptoms such as dyschezia and rectal bleeding can be observed. Rectal symptoms, e.g., urgency to defecate and feeling of incomplete evacuation and rectal pain during defecation may also be present. Adequate management is required to provide relief from such debilitating symptoms. Hormone-based medical treatment provides temporary relief. Hence, laparoscopic excision can be considered as the most suitable treatment option for DIE. Surgery comprising of radical resection of DIE lesions without hysterectomy and oophorectomy is now considered as an appropriate treatment option. Bimanual examination and investigations such as transvaginal ultrasonography (TVUS) and transrectal ultrasonography (TRUS), prior to the surgery help in mapping the disease. Mobilization of the anterior vaginal wall and resection of the lesion en bloc with the vaginal wall is recommended. Repair of bowel, bladder, and ureter may be required in case of injury. Rectal excision may be required in cases of bowel occlusion and rectal bleeding. Use of LNG-IUS is recommended for patients with incomplete resection experiencing the recurrence of symptoms.

EVIDENCE-BASED CLINICAL TRIALS

 List of references can be scanned through QR code to enable the readers gain deeper insight of the subject by referring to the entire article or its abstract.

CHAPTER 31

Abdominal Lump (Ovarian Cancer)

CASE STUDY

A 60-year-old, para 3 woman presented to the gynecology OPD with the complaints of a lump in the abdomen, which has been increasing in size since past 6 months. There also has been anorexia, bloating sensation, vague pain in the left iliac fossa, fatigue, weakness, and increased frequency of micturition since last 1 month. Patient has experienced severe weight loss of nearly 10 kg over past 6 months. There was no significant personal history or family history of cancers. The woman has been menopausal since last 10 years and never had any gynecological problems in the past. On per abdominal examination, a small mass of the size of a lemon was palpable in the left iliac fossa. The mass appeared fixed with restricted mobility. The abdomen was soft and nontender with no evidence of ascites. Vaginal examination revealed the presence of a solid, nodular, irregular-shaped, and fixed mass of size of a lemon arising from left ovary. An ultrasound examination revealed an ovarian mass of size 6 cm having mixed echogenicity, thick wall, and papillary projections. CA 125 levels were performed which were found to be elevated (>35 IU/L).

BOX 31.1: Causes for an abdominal lump.

Pelvic masses:
- Adenomyosis
- Endometrial hyperplasia and cancer
- Bladder cancer
- Ovarian masses (benign and malignant)
- Ectopic pregnancy
- Uterine fibroids (especially pedunculated subserous fibroids)

Extrapelvic masses:
- Distended bladder (hypogastric region)
- Cholecystitis (right hypochondriac region)
- Colon cancer (iliac, hypogastric, and umbilical regions)
- Bowel obstruction (iliac, hypogastric and umbilical regions)
- Diverticulitis (iliac, hypogastric and umbilical regions)
- Gallbladder tumor (right hypochondriac region)
- Hydronephrosis (lumbar regions)
- Cancer of the kidneys (lumbar regions)

INTRODUCTION

There can be various causes for presence of an abdominal lump in a patient presenting to the gynecological OPD. Some of these causes are listed in **Box 31.1**.

EXTRAPELVIC MASSES

Of the various causes for the presence of abdominal mass listed in **Box 31.1**, cancer ovary as the cause for the presence of abdominal mass would be primarily discussed in this chapter. It is important for the gynecologist to detect the presence of ovarian malignancy at an early stage because detection of malignancy at an early stage is associated with a far better prognosis. If the malignancy is diagnosed at stage I, there is an almost 90% survival rate at 5 years; but if diagnosed at an advanced stage, as are most cases, the 5-year survival rate is <30%. Furthermore, ovarian malignancy often remains undetected due to its nonspecific presentation.

OVARIAN MASSES

Q. Write a short note on epidemiology of ovarian tumors.

Ovarian cysts are the most common ovarian masses encountered among women belonging to the reproductive age group. Ovarian cysts can be either neoplastic or non-neoplastic in nature (**Figs. 31.1A and B**). Ovarian neoplasms (tumors) can be benign or malignant in nature. Most ovarian tumors (80–85%) are benign and occur in the women between 20 and 44 years.

Non-neoplastic cysts of ovary are extremely common and can occur at any age (early reproductive age until perimenopause). These cysts are also known as functional cysts and include follicular cysts, corpus luteum cysts, and theca lutein cysts.

Functional Cysts

These cysts develop due to accumulation of fluid in unruptured Graafian follicles or follicles that have ruptured and sealed. These cysts may be multiple and are usually

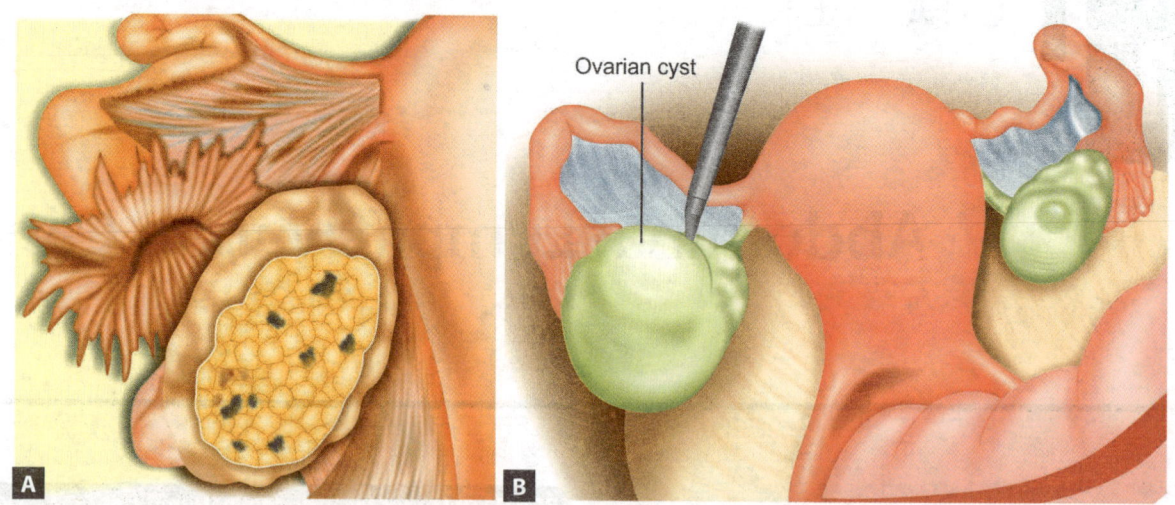

Figs. 31.1A and B: (A) Cancerous mass in right ovary; (B) A cyst arising from right ovary.

small in size (1.1–1.5 cm). However, sometimes they can grow up to 3–4 cm in size. Spontaneous rupture of these cysts can cause pelvic pain and bleeding.

All the functional cysts of the ovary are benign and usually do not cause any symptoms or require surgical management. Follicular cyst is the most common functional cyst of the ovary, which rarely becomes >7–8 cm in size. Corpus luteum cysts are less common than follicular cysts. Luteal cysts tend to have thicker walls in comparison to the follicular cysts. Corpus luteum cysts may sometimes rupture, resulting in the development of hemoperitoneum, and requiring surgical treatment. Theca lutein cysts are the least common of the functional ovarian cysts. They may be associated with molar gestation, diabetes, Rh isoimmunization, or ovulation induction by use of clomiphene citrate, human chorionic gonadotropin (hCG), human menopausal gonadotropin, or gonadotropin-releasing hormone analogs. Theca lutein cysts may be quite large (up to 30 cm), are multicystic and regress spontaneously.

Most follicular ovarian masses resolve spontaneously in 4–8 weeks. Persistence of an ovarian lesion for >6–12 weeks is an important sign indicating the presence of neoplastic ovarian masses.

TYPES OF OVARIAN NEOPLASTIC GROWTH

 Q. Write a short note on histogenesis of ovarian tumors and its significance.

Neoplastic growths of the ovary can be either benign or malignant in nature. Histological classification of neoplastic ovarian growths is shown in **Box 31.2**.

Human ovarian tumors are divided into three major categories, which are named according to their histological patterns and directions of differentiation—(1) epithelial tumors; (2) sex cord stromal tumors; and (3) germ cell tumors. Most ovarian cancers (approximately 95%) are of epithelial type, which originate from the coelomic epithelium or mesothelium of the ovary.

Epithelial Tumors

 Q. Write a short note on Brenner's tumor.

Epithelial tumors are of the following histopathological types:
- Serous tumors which are similar to the epithelium of fallopian tube (most common subtype).
- Mucinous tumors which are similar to the endocervical mucosa.
- Endometrial tumors which are similar to the endometrium.
- Clear cell (mesonephroid) tumors
- Brenner tumors which contain cells similar to the transitional epithelium of the bladder. The WHO classification of different types of the epithelial tumors has been detailed in **Box 31.2**.

  Most malignant ovarian cancers are derived from the surface epithelium of the ovary, with 90–95% of malignant tumors being epithelial cell carcinomas. Metastatic ovarian cancer arising from nonovarian primary cancer may account for further 5% of the cases.
- Serous and mucinous cystadenocarcinomas are the most common types of invasive epithelial ovarian cancers (EOCs) accounting for nearly 65–70% of cases. Nonepithelial ovarian cancer (e.g., germ cell tumors such as ovarian teratomas and sarcomas) is much less common. Germ cell tumors usually affect younger women and tend to behave very differently from other types of ovarian cancer. As mentioned in **Box 31.2**, ovarian tumors could be either benign, malignant, or have a borderline potential. Benign growths are noncancerous whereas malignant growths are cancerous.

BOX 31.2: Histological classification of neoplastic ovarian growths.

I. *Surface epithelial tumors* (70%)
- *Serous tumors* (70%):
  - Benign 25%:
    - Cystadenoma and papillary cystadenoma
    - Surface papilloma
    - Adenofibroma and cystadenofibroma
  - Of borderline malignancy (carcinomas of low malignant potential):
    - Cystadenoma and papillary cystadenoma
    - Surface papilloma
    - Adenofibroma and cystadenofibroma
  - Malignant:
    - Adenocarcinoma, papillary adenocarcinoma, and papillary cystadenocarcinoma
    - Surface papillary carcinoma
    - Malignant adenofibroma and cystadenofibroma
- *Mucinous tumors* (20%)
  - Benign:
    - Cystadenoma
    - Adenofibroma and cystadenofibroma
  - Of borderline malignancy (carcinomas of low malignant potential):
    - Cystadenoma
    - Adenofibroma and cystadenofibroma
  - Malignant:
    - Adenocarcinoma and cystadenocarcinoma
    - Malignant adenofibroma and cystadenofibroma
- *Endometrioid tumors* (2%):
  - Benign
    - Adenoma and cystadenoma
    - Adenofibroma and cystadenofibroma
  - Of borderline malignancy (carcinomas of low malignant potential):
    - Adenoma and cystadenoma
    - Adenofibroma and cystadenofibroma
  - Malignant:
    - Carcinoma
      - Adenocarcinoma
      - Adenoacanthoma
      - Malignant adenofibroma and cystadenofibroma
    - Endometrioid stromal sarcomas
    - Mesodermal (Müllerian) mixed tumors, homologous and heterologous
- *Clear cell (mesonephroid) tumors* (1%):
  - Benign
  - Of borderline malignancy (carcinomas of low malignant potential)
  - Malignant: Carcinoma and adenocarcinoma
- *Brenner tumors* (1%):
  - Benign
  - Of borderline malignancy (proliferating)
  - Malignant
- *Mixed epithelial tumors:*
  - Benign
  - Of borderline malignancy
  - Malignant
- *Undifferentiated Carcinoma*
- *Unclassified Epithelial Tumors*

II. *Sex cord stromal tumors* (5–10%)
- *Granulosa-stromal cell tumors:*
  - Granulosa cell tumor
  - Tumors in the thecoma-fibroma group
    - Thecoma
    - Fibroma
    - Unclassified
- *Androblastomas, Sertoli–Leydig cell tumors:*
  - Well-differentiated:
    - Tubular androblastoma and Sertoli cell tumor (tubular adenoma of Pick)
    - Tubular androblastoma with lipid storage and Sertoli cell tumor with lipid storage (folliculome lipidique of Lecene)
    - Sertoli-Leydig cell tumor (tubular adenoma with Leydig cells)
    - Leydig cell tumor and hilus cell tumor
  - Of intermediate differentiation
  - Poorly differentiated (sarcomatoid)
  - With heterologous elements
- *Gynandroblastoma*
- *Unclassified*

III. *Germ cell tumors* (15–20%)
- Dysgerminoma (most common malignant germ cell tumor)
- Endodermal sinus tumor
- Embryonal carcinoma
- Polyembryoma
- Choriocarcinoma
- Teratomas (most common benign germ cell tumor)
  - Immature
  - Mature
    - Solid
    - Cystic
      - Dermoid cyst (mature cystic teratoma)
      - Dermoid cyst with malignant transformation
  - Monodermal and highly specialized:
    - Struma ovarii
    - Carcinoid
    - Struma ovarii and carcinoid
    - Others
- Mixed Forms

IV. *Lipid (lipoid) cell tumors*

V. *Gonadoblastoma*
- Pure
- Mixed with dysgerminoma or other form of germ cell tumor

VI. *Soft tissue tumors not specific to ovary*

VII. *Unclassified tumors*

VIII. *Secondary (metastatic) tumors*

IX. *Tumor-like conditions*
- Pregnancy luteoma
- Hyperplasia of ovarian stroma and hyperthecosis
- Massive edema
- Solitary follicle cyst and corpus luteum cyst
- Multiple follicle cysts (polycystic ovaries)
- Multiple luteinized follicle cysts and/or corpora lutea
- Endometriosis
- Surface-epithelial inclusion cysts (germinal inclusion cysts)
- Simple cysts
- Inflammatory lesions
- Paraovarian cysts

Serous Tumors

Serous cystadenomas and cystadenocarcinomas are amongst the most common cystic ovarian neoplasms accounting for nearly 50% of all the ovarian neoplasms. Out of these, 60–70% are benign, whereas 20–25% are malignant. These tumors are characterized by the presence of papillary excrescences both on the surface and within the loculi. In case of carcinoma, the papillary excrescences are coarse and friable and may spread to the peritoneal surface. The benign tumors may contain straw-colored fluid, while this fluid may be blood stained in case of malignant tumors.

Mucinous Tumors

> **Q.** Write a short note mucinous cystadenoma of ovary.

Mucinous tumors are multiloculated which commonly contain loculi filled with mucinous contents. If the tumor ruptures, it may result in the formation of pseudomyxoma peritonei.

Borderline Ovarian Tumors

> **Q.** Write a short note on the epidemiology of borderline tumors.

The borderline ovarian tumors are a group of tumors with low malignant potential lying in between the benign and malignant tumors. These tumors usually occur at an earlier age (i.e., 30–50 years) in comparison to the invasive ovarian malignancy which occurs in older women between the age of 50 and 70 years. While borderline tumors remain confined to the ovary for a long period of time, they can also metastasize. Nearly 20–25% of borderline malignant tumors may spread beyond the ovary. The criteria for the diagnosis of borderline tumors are as follows:
- *Clinical criteria:* Age, CA-125 levels and the healthcare center at which the tumor was diagnosed.
- *Ultrasound criteria:* Size (diameter) of the lesion, presence of solid areas, epithelial proliferation with papillary formation and pseudostratification, "microcystic pattern" comprising of papillary projections, solid component(s) and/or septa. These tumors are typically associated with the absence of true stromal invasion (i.e., without any tissue destruction).

Histological features of borderline ovarian tumors include: multilayering of the epithelium, budding of epithelium, presence of mitotic activity and nuclear atypia, and absence of stromal invasion.

Treatment is same as that of ovarian cancer and comprises staging laparotomy and total abdominal hysterectomy (TAH) and bilateral salpingo-oophorectomy (BSO) with omentectomy. Lymphadenectomy can be omitted in the primary surgery. Appendectomy may be required in malignant borderline tumors. Fertility preserving surgery can be considered in younger women. However, this is likely to be associated with a higher rate of recurrence (20–25% vs. 5% after radical surgery). Furthermore, laparoscopic surgery is likely to be associated with a higher recurrence rate. Postsurgery follow-up becomes essential in cases of borderline tumors because these tumors are likely to have a high recurrence rate. While stage 1 tumors may be associated with a recurrence rate of 1%, stage 2 tumors may have a recurrence rate as high as 40%. While postsurgery follow-up is important in these cases, no therapy, either chemotherapy or radiotherapy has been found to be useful presently.

Despite the similarity between the borderline tumors and ovarian cancer, there appear to be distinct differences between the two—fertility drugs can cause borderline ovarian tumors but not ovarian cancer. Use of OCPs/salpingectomy is protective for ovarian cancer, but not borderline tumors. Mutations such as p53 and HER2 are dangerous for ovarian cancer, but beneficial in cases of borderline tumors.

Sex Cord Stromal Cell Tumors

All ovarian tumors in this category are derived from the sex cord and stromal components of the developing gonad. During the normal course of development, the embryonic sex cords develop into the sertoli cells in the testis and granulosa cells in the ovary. On the other hand, the stroma or mesenchyme develops into the Leydig cells of the testis and the theca and corpus lutein cells of the ovary. As a result, the sex cord stromal tumors in the ovary may contain one or more of different types of cells—granulosa cells, theca cells, lutein cells, Sertoli cells, Leydig cells, and fibroblasts, in varying combinations. The most common tumors in this category are the fibromas, which are composed entirely of fibroblasts. Next in frequency is the granulosa cell tumor, generally an estrogenic neoplasm, followed by thecomas.

Fibromas

These tumors are relatively common (4% of all ovarian tumors) and are unilateral in 90% cases. These are solid, spherical, encapsulated, grayish-white, well-differentiated lesions. These tumors are composed of well-differentiated fibroblasts. As the name suggests, the fibroma has a firm consistency and is composed of a network of spindle-shaped cells. Ovarian fibromas > 6 cm in size may be associated with ascites and right-sided hydrothorax in nearly 40% cases. This is also known as Meigs' syndrome. Meigs' syndrome may also be associated with other solid ovarian tumors such as granulosa cell tumors and Brenner tumors.

Granulosa Cell Tumors

Granulosa cell tumors are the most common type of sex-cord stromal tumors. These tumors can be of two types:

(1) adult type (95%) and (2) juvenile types (5%). While the adult type can occur in any age group, juvenile type usually occurs during childhood and adolescence. The tumor marker in these cases is inhibin. FOXL2 mutation may be present in the adult type. These tumors can occur at any age and are composed of cells which are identical to the granulosa cells of the Graafian follicle. Functionally, active granulosa cell tumors are responsible for producing estrogen. This can cause precocious sexual development in young girls. In adult women, this can cause endometrial hyperplasia, fibrocystic disease of the breast, abnormal uterine bleeding (AUB), amenorrhea, endometrial carcinoma, etc. In postmenopausal women, this tumor can cause postmenopausal bleeding. The histopathological examination may show the presence of Call-Exner bodies which can be considered as primitive follicles comprising of granulosa cells arranged haphazardly around a space containing eosinophilic fluid (**Fig. 31.2**). The anaplastic type of granulosa cell tumor is associated with nearly 65% chances of malignancy.

Granulosa cell tumors are low potential malignant tumors. If diagnosed in the early stage, surgery is the primary modality of treatment. Extent of surgery depends upon the patient's age and disease stage. There is strong evidence that feminizing tumors of the ovary are associated with carcinoma endometrium. Therefore, endometrial biopsy is required if conservative surgery is planned because there is 25–50% risk of endometrial hyperplasia and a 5% risk of endometrial cancer. Chemotherapy and radiotherapy may be useful for metastatic or recurrent disease. These tumors are associated with a good prognosis and a 10 years survival rate of 90%. Bleomycin, etoposide, and cisplatin (BEP) regimen may be useful in adult granulosa cell tumor. Other medications which have proved to be useful include paclitaxel and carboplatin or taxanes and bevacizumab.

Germ Cell Tumors

 Q. Write a short note on germ cell tumors.

Germ cell tumors arise from totipotent germ cells. Germ cell tumors tend to affect only one ovary, and most are curable even if they are diagnosed at an advanced stage. Of the various germ cell tumors, endodermal sinus tumor is likely to be most virulent. Different types of germ cell tumors are enumerated in **Flowchart 31.1** and are described below in details:

Teratomas

 Q. Write a short essay on dermoid cyst of ovary.

Ovarian teratomas are a complex group of tumors that are subdivided into three major categories: (1) immature, (2) mature, and (3) monodermal and highly specialized. The

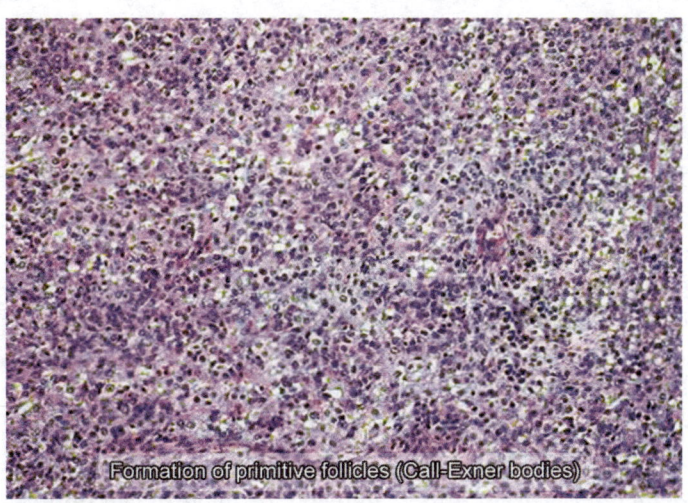

Fig. 31.2: Histopathological pattern of granulosa cell tumor.

Flowchart 31.1: Different types of germ cell tumors.

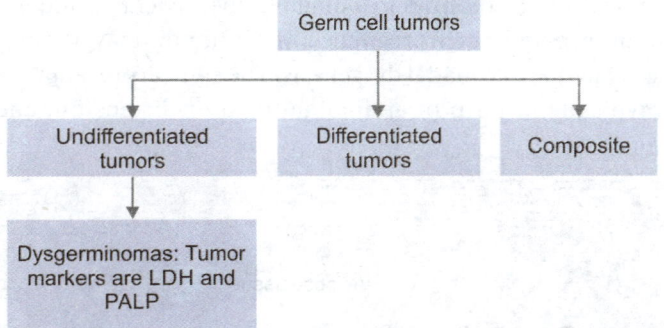

(LDH: lactate dehydrogenase; PALP: placental alkaline phosphatase)

majority of germ cell tumors are benign cystic teratomas, also known as dermoids.

Immature Teratomas

Immature teratomas primarily contain immature tissues, most commonly of neuroectodermal origin. However, they may sometimes also contain varying quantities of mature tissue as well. Immature teratomas are essentially malignant.

Mature Teratomas

Unlike the immature teratomas, the mature teratomas are exclusively composed of mature tissues (**Figs. 31.3 and 31.4A and B**). Mature teratomas could be either solid or cystic (dermoid cysts). In most cases, the tumor contains elements derived from all three germ layers. The dermoid cysts are benign ovarian masses, which may appear as masses having various sonographic appearances ranging from anechoic to echogenic due to variety of internal contents. The solid areas may be due to the presence of hair follicles in combination with the calcified elements within dermoid. These materials are responsible for producing echogenicity within the cyst. These cysts may contain hair, which because of its high echodensity may produce a typical acoustic shadow. Other types of tissues which may be present include teeth, bone, cartilage, thyroid tissues, bronchial tissues, and sebaceous material. Though dermoid cysts are usually benign in nature, epidermoid carcinoma may occur in approximately 2% of cases.

Monodermal Tumors

The best known monodermal and highly differentiated teratoma of the ovary is the struma ovarii, which is also known as the thyroid tumor of the ovary and is composed entirely of the thyroid tissue. Another common monodermal tumor of the ovary is carcinoid tumor.

Dysgerminoma

These germ cell tumors are the female homologue of the testicular seminoma. They constitute 1–2% of all malignant ovarian tumors and 50% of all germ cell tumors. Dysgerminomas are usually malignant and commonly affect both the ovaries. Nearly 10–15% cases are bilateral. This tumor is more common in women in their twenties and is a common neoplasm in pregnancy. These tumors may be rarely associated with gonadal dysgenesis. The clinical presentation is typically in form of abdominal pain or distension, and palpable mass per abdomen. The tumor has a typical elastic, rubbery consistency and has a firm smooth capsule. The cut surface of the tumor is yellowish-grayish with areas of degeneration and hemorrhage. Though the tumor does not secrete any hormones, it can secrete tumor markers such as lactate dehydrogenase, placental alkaline phosphatase, and β-hCG. Ultrasound shows presence of a solid tumor, divided into different lobules having irregular internal echogenicity, with smooth lobulated contours and well-defined borders. Doppler examination reveals masses with high vascularity. Surgery is the mainstay option for management option in all the stages. Staging laparotomy is done to assess the tumor stage. Most tumors are stage 1 at the time of diagnosis. KIT mutations, which may be present in nearly one-third cases, are associated with an advanced stage at the time of presentation. Chemotherapy comprises IV bleomycin, etoposide and cisplatin. VAC (vincristine, actinomycin, and cyclophosphamide), and VBP (vinblastine, bleomycin, and cisplatin) regimens can also be used.

In a woman desiring fertility, conservative surgery may be done. In case of a pregnant woman with dysgerminoma, surgery can be done in the second trimester, whereas chemotherapy is preferred in the third trimester. Surgery is usually sufficient for stage IA disease, whereas chemotherapy must be used for rest of the stages (IB to IV). Recurrence rate of these tumors is low and 5-years survival rate in stage I is 95%.

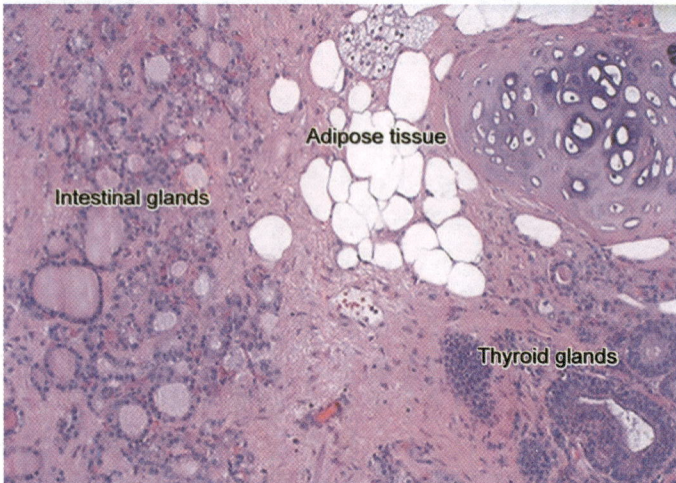

Fig. 31.3: Histological picture of a mature teratoma showing adipose tissue and intestinal glands at the right and thyroid tissue on the left.

Yolk Sac Tumors

One of the most highly malignant forms of primitive germ cell tumor is the endodermal sinus tumor or yolk sac tumor, which summarizes yolk sac development. This tumor characteristically contains papillary units termed as Schiller–Duval bodies. These are composed of papillary projections surrounding the central blood vessels protruding into a network of spaces lined by primitive neoplastic cells. Yolk sac tumors characteristically produce α-fetoprotein, which can be detected in the patient's serum.

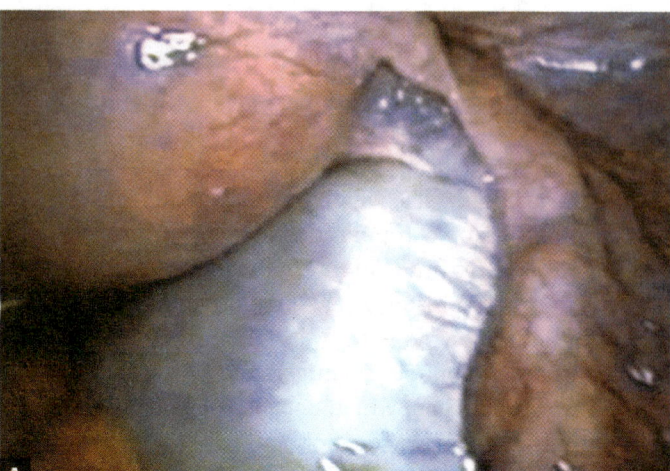
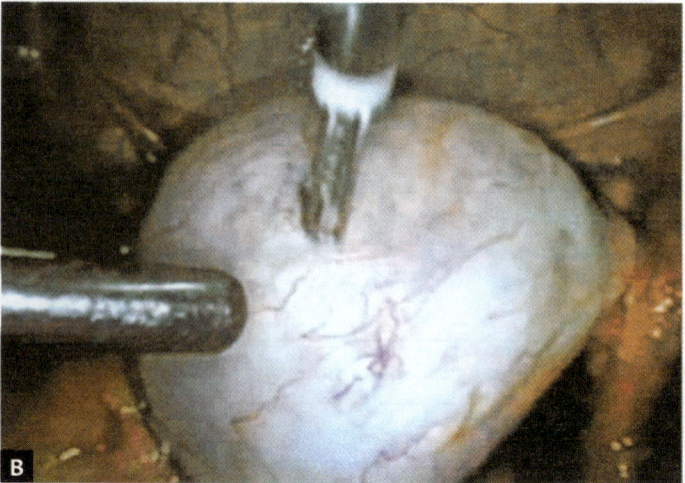

Figs. 31.4A and B: Laparoscopic appearance showing a teratoma arising from the ovary.

OVARIAN CANCER

Ovarian cancer is the fourth most common cause of cancer-related deaths in women and is the seventh most common cancer diagnosed. An estimated 200,000 cases and 125,000 deaths due to ovarian cancer occur worldwide annually. Its incidence is highest among the high-resource countries with the incidence being 9.3 per 100,000 women. Ovarian cancer has accounted for 4% all new cancer cases in women in the year 2017. This cancer assumes importance because it is usually diagnosed in the advanced stage and is likely to be asymptomatic in the early stage. Advanced stage is associated with a poor prognosis, a 5-year survival rate of 46%. Early diagnosis is likely to improve the survival rates by 94%.

This type of cancer develops most often in women aged 50–70 years. Nearly 80% of the cancers are epithelial cell cancers which originate from the surface epithelium of the ovaries.

Other types of ovarian cancers include germ cell tumors, sex cord stromal cell tumors, and metastatic cancers. Primary peritoneal cancer and primary fallopian tube cancer are rare malignancies but share many similarities with ovarian cancer. Also, clinical management of these three types of cancers is similar. Therefore, peritoneal, ovarian, and fallopian tube cancers are considered as a single entity and they follow a common staging system. The cancer terminology has also changed. The term, "cancer ovaries, fallopian tube, and peritoneum" is used rather than the term "cancer ovaries". Ovarian cancers are classified as type 1 and type 2 tumors **(Table 31.1)**. Based on the histologic, genetic, and molecular evidence, it can be presumed that 80% of tumors that had been classified as originating in the ovaries or peritoneum may have developed in the fallopian tubes in reality. This could be related to the pattern of spread of ovarian malignancy.

Pattern of Spread of Ovarian Malignancy

The most common pattern of spread of EOC is through the exfoliation of the cancer cells that implant along the surfaces of the peritoneal cavity. Exfoliation of the cancer cells that implant along the surfaces of the peritoneal cavity tends to follow the circulatory path of the peritoneal fluid. As a result, metastases are typically seen on the posterior cul-de-sac, paracolic gutters, right hemidiaphragm, liver capsule, and peritoneal surfaces of the intestine, their mesenteries and the omentum. Though the lumen of the intestines is rarely invaded by the malignant cells, progressive agglutination of the bowel loops often takes place, resulting in functional intestinal obstruction. This condition is known as carcinomatous ileus.

Other less common modes of spread of ovarian cancer include lymphatic and hematogenous spread **(Figs. 31.5A and B)**. Lymphatic spread can lead to the involvement of pelvic and para-aortic group of lymph nodes. Lymphatic spread above the diaphragm can result in the involvement of supraclavicular lymph nodes. Hematogenous spread can occur to organs like lungs and liver.

TABLE 31.1: Difference between type I and type II.

Feature	Type I tumors	Type II tumors
Origin	Ovarian origin	Fallopian tube origin
Description	Less aggressive tumors	More aggressive tumors
Types	Endometrioid, mucinous, clear cell, borderline and low-grade serous tumors, low-grade adenocarcinomas, not otherwise specified (NOS)	Conventional high grade serous carcinoma, undifferentiated carcinoma, malignant mixed mesodermal tumors (carcinosarcomas), and high-grade adenocarcinomas
Progression	These tumors show gradual spectrum of changes (benign–borderline–low-grade carcinoma)	Highly aggressive tumors showing rapid progression
Disease at the time of diagnosis	The tumor is usually indolent and confined to the ovary	Extraovarian disease is likely to be present
p53 mutation	Absent	P53 mutation is likely to be present in 80% cases.
Prognosis	Good	Poor

HISTORY AND CLINICAL PRESENTATION

RISK FACTORS FOR OVARIAN CANCER

The causes responsible for development of ovarian cancer are not yet completely understood. Some factors are known to increase a woman's chance of developing ovarian cancer—these need to be elicited at the time of taking history **(Table 31.2)** and are described below:

Age

Ovarian cancer is more common in the women belonging to the age group between 50 and 70 years, with the peak incidence of the disease occurring at the age of 62 years. The risk of developing ovarian cancer is very low in young women and increases as women get older. 30% of epithelial ovarian tumors in postmenopausal women and 7% in premenopausal women are likely to be malignant.

Personal history of cancer: Women who have previously had cancer of the breast, uterus, colon, or rectum are at a higher risk of developing ovarian cancer in future.

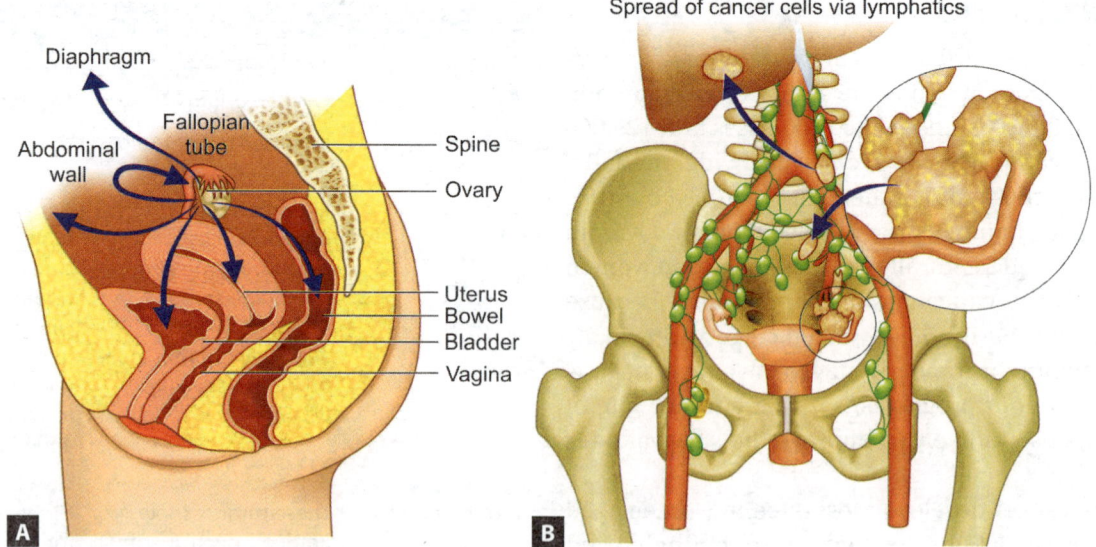

Figs. 31.5A and B: Spread of ovarian cancer. (A) Spread of ovarian cancer via transcoelomic implantation; (B) Spread of ovarian cancer via lymphatics.

TABLE 31.2: Women at high risk for developing ovarian cancer.

Incessant ovulation	Genetic factors	Family history
• Infertility (not the fertility inducing drugs or ART) • Endometriosis • PID • PCOS • Obesity • Increasing age (EOC) • HRT after menopause	5–10% ovarian cancers are associated with the following genetic factors: • Germline mutation of BRCA-1 gene (15–45% risk) • Germline mutation of BRCA-2 gene (13–23% risk) • Lynch syndrome: 9–12% cases • Mutations of the tumor suppressor p53 protein	• Autosomal dominant inheritance pattern • Lifetime risk: 1.5% • One first-degree relative having ovarian cancer with age < 50 years: risk is 30–45% • One first-degree relative and other second degree relative having ovarian cancer with age < 50 years: risk increases by 2–10 folds. • Survivors of breast cancer are also associated with an increased risk of ovarian cancer

(ART: assisted-reproductive technology; EOC: epithelial ovarian cancer; HRT: hormone replacement therapy; PCOS: polycystic ovarian syndrome; PID: pelvic inflammatory disease)

Lifestyle Factors

- *Body mass index:* Having an increased body mass index (overweight or obese) is associated with an increased risk of developing ovarian cancer. However, future research is required to significantly prove this fact.
- *Diet:* Eating a diet, high in animal fats and low in fresh fruit and vegetables, may increase the woman's risk of developing ovarian cancer.

Family History

It is important to take the family history of cancers such as ovarian cancer, breast cancer, endometrial cancer, colorectal cancer, etc.

Family history of ovarian cancer can be considered as one of the most important risk factors for the development of ovarian cancer. Women who have a first-degree relative (mother, daughter, or sister) with ovarian cancer are at an increased risk of developing the disease. This risk is even higher in women who have two or more first-degree relatives with ovarian cancer. Besides detecting the occurrence of ovarian cancer in an isolated relative, the presence of "familial breast ovarian cancer syndrome" also needs to be detected. Nearly 5–10% cases of ovarian cancers may be caused by an inherited genetic defect. Therefore, prophylactic oophorectomy may be considered in some women who are at an increased risk of developing ovarian cancer.

Hereditary ovarian cancer syndrome: Women with hereditary ovarian cancer syndromes have a lifetime probability of 25–50% for developing ovarian cancer in future. This is in contrast to the lifetime probability of 1–1.5% for developing ovarian cancer in a 35-years-old woman having a family history of ovarian cancer in one isolated relative. In case of familial ovarian cancer syndrome, ovarian cancer may occur in a first- or second-degree family members (both maternal and paternal lineage) at an early age (under 50 years) or it may occur in multiple members (i.e., two to four generations). Some of the hereditary ovarian syndromes include:

- *The Lynch II syndrome:* Cancers of the colon, breast, endometrium, and ovary with hereditary nonpolyposis colorectal cancer
- *Breast-ovarian cancer syndrome:* Usually, occurs in association with a BRCA1 or BRCA2 mutation. The

absolute lifetime risk for development of ovarian cancer is 15–45% with BRCA1 gene mutation, whereas it is 13–23% with BRCA2 mutation. Hereditary ovarian cancers, particularly those caused by mutations in the BRAC1 gene occur approximately 10 years earlier in comparison to those with nonhereditary tumors. Mutations in the BRCA1 or BRCA2 genes are inherited in an autosomal dominant pattern. Therefore, a complete pedigree analysis must be carefully evaluated in all patients with EOC.

Menstrual and Obstetric History

- *Increased menstrual span:* Patients with a history of early menarche and late menopause are associated with an increased risk for ovarian cancer as well as endometrial cancer.
- Women with a history of nulliparity or low parity are at an increased risk for development of ovarian cancer. On the other hand, women who have had children in the past or had breastfed their babies are at a reduced risk. Multiparity acts as a protective factor in the development of ovarian cancers. Since parity is inversely related to the risk of ovarian cancer, having at least one child is protective for the disease, with a risk reduction of 0.3–0.4. Breastfeeding the children may also act as a protective factor against development of cancer. Various reproductive and endocrine factors, which need to be elicited at the time of taking history and could be associated with an increased or decreased risk of ovarian cancer, are respectively tabulated in **Table 31.1** and **Box. 31.3**.
- Women with endometriosis are at an increased risk of developing ovarian cancer.
- *Infertility and fertility treatments:* Presently, it is not clear if the risk of ovarian cancer is increased by taking treatment with ovulation inducing drugs for infertility, or undergoing HRT. More research would be required in future to find out whether the risk of ovarian cancer is increased by these above-mentioned factors.
- *Menopausal HRT:* Some studies have shown that women who take unopposed estrogen in the form of HRT for 10 or more years may be at an increased risk of developing ovarian cancer. However, when HRT is stopped, the risk of ovarian cancer gradually reduces to the level similar to the women who have not taken HRT. HRT must not be administered in cases of women with endometrioid cancers or sex cord ovarian tumors who have undergone treatment. It can be administered in cases of germ cell tumors and other epithelial ovarian malignancies (e.g., serous cell tumors). Risk is more with estrogen only therapy. The clinician must weigh the potential benefits of therapy with its risks before prescribing HRT. Women prescribed such therapy should come for a regular follow-up. HRT should be preferably administered

> **BOX 31.3:** Factors reducing the risk of ovarian cancer.
>
> *Physiological prophylaxis:*
> Events like pregnancy, childbirth and lactation provide protection against ovarian cancer
>
> *Chemoprophylaxis:*
> - 5-years use of oral contraceptives results in 50% reduction in the risk of ovarian cancer (type 1) for 30 years after stopping the pills
> - Use of ibuprofen also associated with a reduced risk of ovarian cancer (type 1)
> - Drugs like tamoxifen, hydroxyretinoic acid, and acetaminophen may have a role in the prevent of ovarian cancer: No definite evidence available
>
> *Surgical prophylaxis:*
> - Bilateral tubal ligation is likely to reduce the risk of ovarian cancer (type 2) by 20–45%
> - Salpingectomy reduces the risk of ovarian cancer by 42%
> - Oophorectomy in women at high risk is also found to be protective

2 years following the completion of treatment since the chances of tumor recurrence are highest in the first 2 years following the completion of therapy.

- *Oral contraceptive pills:* Women taking the contraceptive pill are at a reduced risk of developing ovarian cancer. Women who use OCPs for 5 or more years are likely to experience approximately 50% reduction in the likelihood of development of ovarian cancer.
- *History of menstrual cycles:* It is important to take the history regarding menstrual cycles in the woman because most ovarian tumors, even bilateral ones, do not affect the menstrual cycles. The only tumors causing menorrhagia are granulosa cell tumors and theca cell tumors because both these types of ovarian tumors are associated with increased estrogen secretion. On the other hand, masculinizing tumors may cause amenorrhea and virilization. Postmenopausal bleeding may occur in cases of benign Brenner tumors and feminizing tumors of the ovary.

Environmental Factors

- *Cigarette smoking:* Present or past history of smoking is likely to be associated with an increased risk of mucinous ovarian cancers, but not other types of EOC.
- *Genital use of talcum powder:* Genital use of talc has been thought to be associated with an increased risk of ovarian cancer because talc is structurally similar to asbestos, which is a known carcinogen. Moreover, talcum powder is sometimes contaminated with asbestos. However, the relationship between EOCs and the genital use of talcum powder (talc) presently remains controversial.

CLINICAL PRESENTATION

The clinical presentation in case of an epithelial ovarian carcinoma may be either acute or subacute **(Table 31.3)**. Women who present in an acute fashion are typically

TABLE 31.3: Clinical presentation in case of epithelial ovarian cancer.	
Acute presentation	**Subacute presentation**
• *Pleural effusion:* Shortness of breath • *Bowel obstruction:* Severe nausea and vomiting • Venous thromboembolism	• *Adnexal mass:* Discovered on a routine pelvic examination or an imaging study performed for another indication • *Pelvic and abdominal symptoms:* Bloating, urinary urgency or frequency, difficulty in eating or early satiety, pelvic or abdominal pain

those with advanced disease who present with a condition requiring urgent assessment and management (e.g., pleural effusion and bowel obstruction). The type or severity of symptoms usually does not correspond to the disease stage or severity. The pathophysiology of abdominal symptoms in women with disease confined to the ovary or pelvis is not well-understood. In women with advanced disease, abdominal symptoms may be due to the presence of ascites and omental or bowel metastases.

Symptoms

Most women with early-stage cancer of the ovary do not have any symptoms for a long time. This is an important cause for late diagnosis of ovarian cancer. A few symptoms which do develop are quite nonspecific and may be indicative of other gastrointestinal pathologies. Some of the symptoms which could be suggestive of ovarian cancer and need to be elicited while taking the history include the following:

- *Abdominal bloating/distension:* Quite often ovarian malignancy may present as a large intra-abdominal mass and ascites. Both these could be responsible for producing abdominal distension and bloating.
- Pelvic or abdominal pain or dyspareunia
- Loss of appetite or early satiety
- Pressure symptoms such as increased urinary urgency and frequency could result due to an ovarian tumor placed in the uterovesical pouch. On the other hand, a tumor impacted in the pouch of Douglas (POD) may cause constipation.
- Nausea, vague indigestion, constipation, or diarrhea
- Feeling of tiredness, unexplained loss of weight, anemia, and cachexia
- Rapidly increasing abdominal swelling and dyspnea due to development of ascites
- *Pain:* Normally, the benign ovarian tumors cause no abdominal pain and are comfortably placed in the abdominal cavity which is distensible. Large intra-abdominal tumors, on the other hand, may cause abdominal discomfort and difficulty in walking. Acute abdominal pain may develop if the ovarian tumor undergoes torsion, rupture, or hemorrhage. If the tumor undergoes torsion, the woman may develop acute abdominal pain, vomiting and at times low-grade fever.
- Rarely, there may be abnormal vaginal bleeding (postmenopausal bleeding or menorrhagia). Presence of estrogen secreting granulosa cell tumors may produce menometrorrhagia and episodes of abnormal uterine bleeding. However, women with postmenopausal bleeding should be assessed for uterine pathology before proceeding with an evaluation for ovarian cancer. In case of AUB and/or presence of an adnexal/uterine mass, endometrial sampling should be performed preoperatively because in this case, the most likely diagnosis is endometrial cancer rather than ovarian cancer.
- *Rectal bleeding:* This may be sometimes present in some women with EOC. However, it is unlikely that this would be present as the only presenting symptom and deserves further evaluation for an EOC only if other clinical features suggestive of an ovarian malignancy are present (e.g., adnexal mass, hereditary ovarian cancer syndrome, etc.)
- Presence of ascites, omental metastases, or bowel metastases in the late stages of the disease may produce symptoms such as abdominal distension, bloating, constipation, nausea, and early satiety.
- *Presence of lump in the abdomen:* This could be related to the presence of ovarian malignancy per se or development of omental cake due to infiltration of the omentum by malignant cells.
- *Paraneoplastic syndrome:* Rarely, women with EOC may present with a paraneoplastic syndrome, which may be associated with symptoms such as cerebellar degeneration, polyneuritis, dermatomyositis, hemolytic anemia, disseminated intravascular coagulation, acanthosis, and nephrotic syndrome.

Features suggestive of Malignancy

> **Q. Discuss briefly the features suggestive of malignant ovarian growth?**

Some features suggestive of malignancy on history and clinical examination are enlisted below:

- *Rapidity of growth:* A rapidly growing tumor is highly suggestive of malignancy, while a slow growing tumor is more likely to be benign. A tumor which has been rapidly increasing in size over the past 6 months is suggestive of malignancy.
- *Consistency of the mass:* The growth which appears to be solid, nodular, and irregularly shaped on vaginal examination is more likely to be malignant. On the other hand, growths which are smooth, cystic, and have regular margins are more likely to be benign.
- *Fixation of the tumor:* Malignant tumors are more likely to be adherent to the underlying structures and have a restricted mobility in comparison to the benign masses which are not adherent to the underlying structures and have a greater mobility.

- *Presence of ascites:* Presence of free fluid in the abdominal cavity is usually indicative of peritoneal metastasis or at least the fact that the tumor has perforated the ovarian capsule. However, in this case no ascitic fluid was present on per abdominal examination.
- *Cancer cachexia:* Cachexia, associated with severe degrees of weight loss, muscle wasting, weakness, and fatigue typically occurs with malignant growths. A benign tumor is usually not painful unless there is an underlying complication. A malignant tumor, on the other hand, is associated with pain in the abdomen.

GENERAL PHYSICAL EXAMINATION

Findings on general physical examination such as anemia, unexplained weight loss, unilateral nonpitting edema of the leg, pleural effusion, and hepatic enlargement are suggestive of advanced stage of the malignant disease. The lymph nodes must be palpated because they (especially the supraclavicular nodes) could often be enlarged in presence of malignancy.

SPECIFIC SYSTEMIC EXAMINATION

ABDOMINAL EXAMINATION

Abdominal Examination of the Swelling

The typical ovarian cyst results in an abdominal swelling which is detected on inspection. The method of examination of an intra-abdominal swelling has been detailed in Chapter 22. The movement of abdominal wall over the swelling can be observed when the patient takes a deep inspiration. On abdominal palpation, the upper and lateral limits of the tumor can be defined. However, in most of the cases it is impossible to identify the lower pole of the tumor except in case of a small cyst with a long pedicle. The surface of the ovarian tumor is smooth although it may be slightly bossed with multilocular cysts. Small cysts are generally movable from side to side, but large, especially the malignant ones may be fixed. The consistency of the cystic tumor is tense and cystic and a fluid thrill can be elicited. All patients with a possible ovarian cyst should be examined carefully for the presence of ascites because the presence of the ascites is a strong indicator that the tumor is malignant. In some cases, even benign tumors may be associated with ascites, e.g., Meigs syndrome associated with fibroma, Brenner tumor, and occasionally granulosa cell tumor.

Ascites

Abdominal distension due to ascites is a common feature associated with malignant ovarian growth. In most of the cases, ascites can be differentiated from large ovarian growths on abdominal examination (Chapter 22). With a large ovarian cyst, the percussion note over the tumor is dull, whereas both the flanks are resonant. In cases of ascites, the note is dull over the flanks, while the abdomen in the midline is resonant. The physical signs of shifting dullness and fluid thrill may be obtained. A sample of ascitic fluid must be taken to look for malignant cells.

PELVIC EXAMINATION

Detailed description of pelvic examination has been done in Chapter 22. Pelvic examination helps in assessment of the adnexa for presence of any lumps or mass. The most important sign of an ovarian tumor is presence of pelvic mass on physical examination. Presence of a solid, irregular, fixed pelvic mass is highly suggestive of an ovarian malignancy. In addition, if there is presence of an upper abdominal mass or ascites, the diagnosis of ovarian cancer is almost certain. As a general rule, under normal circumstances ovaries must become nonpalpable in women who are at least 1 year past menopause. Presence of any palpable pelvic mass in these patients should arouse the suspicion of malignancy. The method of conducting pelvic examination has been described in details in Chapter 22. The physical signs on bimanual examination vary according to the size of the ovarian tumor. With small tumors, the uterus can be palpated without difficulty and the ovarian mass be outlined bimanually. A large ovarian cyst usually displaces uterus to the opposite side and it may get difficult to outline the uterus with larger sized cysts. Even with a large cyst, the lower pole of the tumor should be palpable through one of the fornices. The lower pole of the ovary appears firm and rounded in appearance with a characteristic feel and fluctuations can usually be obtained between the finger placed in the vagina and external hand. The ovarian mass needs to be differentiated from uterine mass on bimanual examination. The cardinal sign which helps in distinguishing a mobile ovarian tumor from a uterine tumor is that when the ovarian tumor is raised up by the abdominal hand, the cervix remains stationary to the vaginal fingers. However, in case of a mass of uterine origin, rising up of tumor by abdominal hand results in simultaneous movement of the vaginal fornices. In all cases, the POD should be examined carefully for presence of any nodules. The vaginal examination may reveal fixed nodules in the POD. A common site for metastasis is the POD and these deposits are often palpable on vaginal examination. Presence of hard nodules in the POD is a strong indicator of malignancy.

BREAST AND CHEST EXAMINATION

Both the breasts should be examined for the presence of any lump or nodule. This is especially important due to the familial association of breast cancer with ovarian cancer. A chest examination should be carried out to particularly rule out pleural effusion.

DIFFERENTIAL DIAGNOSIS

Different types of ovarian tumors have been described earlier in the text. Various other common causes of abdominal lump which need to be excluded before establishing the correct diagnosis of an ovarian tumor are enumerated in **Box 31.1** at the beginning of the chapter. Some other likely diagnoses include the following:

- *Gastrointestinal pathology:* Since the cases of ovarian cancer mainly present with gastrointestinal symptoms, it is important to rule out any underlying gastrointestinal pathology in these cases. In the Indian scenario, abdominal tuberculosis could be an important cause of gastrointestinal symptoms such as abdominal distension, bloating, early satiety, etc. Therefore, it becomes important to rule this out.
- *Myomas:* Myomas, especially pedunculated uterine leiomyomas can commonly result in an abdominal lump. The myoma can be differentiated from ovarian cyst based on clinical examination. A myoma is usually hard and firm, whereas a typical ovarian cyst has a cystic consistency.
- *Extraovarian primary cancers:* It is also important to exclude extraovarian primary cancers such as those of gastrointestinal tract (e.g., gastric cancer with Krukenberg ovarian metastases) and breast cancer which could metastasize to the ovaries. Secondary ovarian malignancies comprise 5–10% of the total cases. These tumors are likely to be typically bilateral and solid.
- *Synchronous tumors:* It is also important to exclude synchronous primary cancers of the ovary and endometrium which may be present simultaneously at the same time. Synchronous primary cancers of the ovary and endometrium may be present in about 10% of women with ovarian cancer and 5% of women with endometrial cancer. Treatment in these cases must be a combination of treatment for each case according to the cancer stage.

MANAGEMENT

Q. Classify ovarian tumors and describe the staging of ovarian malignancies. Also discuss the management of immature teratomas.

Q. Enumerate the causes for presence of a lower abdominal mass in a 40-years old woman. With help of a long note discuss the management of a malignant ovarian tumor.

Q. Discuss in detail the management of a 45-year-old woman with advanced epithelial ovarian cancer.

Q. Discuss the management of epithelial ovarian tumor with help of a long essay.

Q. Write a long essay discussing the diagnosis and management of benign ovarian tumors.

Q. Write a long essay on the management of stage 2 epithelial ovarian carcinoma.

Q. Write a long essay on diagnosis and also outline the management of malignant ovarian tumors.

Q. What would be the most appropriate management in the case study described in the beginning of the chapter?
Ans. In the above-mentioned case study, after taking into consideration the patient's age and findings of ultrasound examination, the suspicion of malignancy must be definitely ruled out by the clinician. The best modality of diagnosis in patient with suspected ovarian cancer is surgical staging on exploratory laparotomy.

Evaluation of Adnexal Lesion

The most important step of management in these cases comprises classifying the adnexal mass as benign or malignant. An ovarian mass observed on ultrasound examination does not require further imaging characterization if it is obviously malignant, e.g., presence of concurrent omental implants, other evidence of peritoneal disseminated disease, lymphadenopathy, pleural effusion, hydronephrosis, etc. Also, simple unilocular cysts < 5–6 cm in size, with no solid components in a premenopausal woman, are likely to be benign and do not require further imaging. Simple cysts that are larger may warrant additional imaging during the future follow-up visit to document whether these cysts have undergone resolution. This is particularly important because such cysts can undergo torsion and may need to be removed surgically if they persist. On the other hand, lesions found in postmenopausal women and those that have solid components on ultrasound examination require further evaluation, usually within 6 weeks.

- *Management in premenopausal women:* In case of premenopausal women, if the adnexal mass does not show any feature of malignancy (i.e., the mass is freely mobile, cystic in consistency, and of regular contour) a period of observation of no more than 2 months can be allowed during which hormonal suppression with OCPs can be used. A benign mass would regress, while a malignant mass would be persistent and would mandate surgical removal. Management in case of simple cysts has been described in **Flowchart 31.2**.
- *Management in postmenopausal women:* It takes 3–5 years after the menopause for the ovaries to atrophy. As previously mentioned, in postmenopausal women ovaries must not be palpable. There is no such thing as physiologic enlargement of the postmenopausal ovary. Since there are no follicles or corpus luteum in postmenopausal ovary, no such cysts can arise. Therefore, palpable ovary in postmenopausal women must be considered as a significant finding. Management algorithm in case of a postmenopausal woman with an ovarian cyst is described in the **Flowchart 31.3**.

Evaluation in Cases of Suspected Malignancy

Management for ovarian cancer initially includes taking history, conducting physical examination, and evaluation

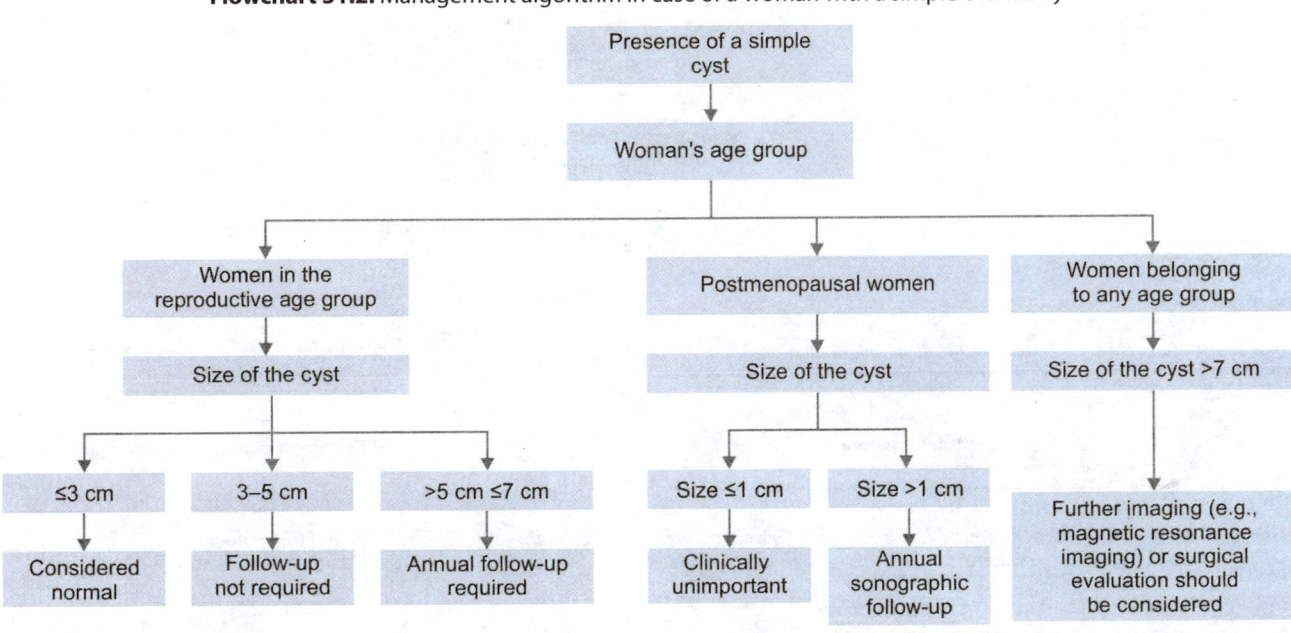

Flowchart 31.2: Management algorithm in case of a woman with a simple ovarian cyst.

of serum CA 125 levels in combination with imaging (ultrasound, MRI, and CT). Neither imaging results nor CA 125 levels alone are sufficiently accurate in diagnosing ovarian cancer. The diagnosis and management of ovarian carcinoma require surgical exploration. The staging of ovarian cancer is done on exploratory laparotomy. Surgical staging is particularly important because subsequent treatment and prognosis are determined by the disease stage. Patients with advanced stage disease must go through debulking or cytoreductive surgery to remove as much of the tumor and its metastasis as possible, provided that the patient is medically fit for a major surgery. Surgery is almost always performed in all women with suspected ovarian cancer, even when advanced. Aims of performing a surgical procedure are listed in the **Box 31.4**.

Primary surgical cytoreduction (usually without any chemotherapy) forms the preferred management plan for patients with stage I and II ovarian cancer. Primary surgical cytoreduction followed by systemic chemotherapy is the preferred initial management for women with stage III or IV EOC.

However, there are some exceptions to the diagnosis via a surgical procedure, which are listed in **Box 31.5**. Such patients must be treated with neoadjuvant chemotherapy. Initial evaluation in these patients must be carried out with the help of imaging and either paracentesis, thoracentesis, or image-guided biopsy from a peritoneal implant prior to treatment. The FIGO system (2014), used for cancer staging is summarized in **Table 31.4**.

New Staging System for Cancer Ovaries, Fallopian Tubes, and Peritoneum Devised by FIGO in 2014

As per the new staging system devised by FIGO in 2014, carcinoma, ovaries, fallopian tube, and peritoneum are considered as a single entity. Other changes done in the staging system are as follows:

- *Stage I:* Apart from ovaries, fallopian tube has also been added. Also, stage IC has been further subclassified as stage IC1, IC2, and IC3 based on whether the tumor capsule ruptured prior to or during the surgery or there is a presence of malignant cells in the ascitic fluid or peritoneal washing.
- *Stage II:* Apart from ovaries, fallopian tubes and peritoneum have also been included. Previously included stage IIC has been removed.
- *Stage III:* Involvement of retroperitoneal lymph nodes has been included. Stage IIIA1 has been further classified into subgroups based on the details regarding the size of enlarged retroperitoneal lymph nodes.
- *Tumor, node, and metastasis (TNM) classification:* Also, there has been the addition of TNM classification to the FIGO staging.

INVESTIGATIONS

BLOOD TESTS

The following blood tests help in assessing the patient's fitness for anesthesia:

- Full blood count
- Kidney function tests (including blood urea and serum creatinine)
- Liver function tests (including total proteins and albumin levels)
- Serum electrolytes
- Blood sugar levels.

Flowchart 31.3: Management algorithm in case of a postmenopausal woman with an ovarian cyst.

```
Presence of ovarian cyst (≥1 cm)
in postmenopausal women
            ↓
Measurement of CA-125 levels along
with transvaginal-sonography
            ↓
    Calculation of RMI I
    ↓                    ↓
RMI < 200 (low risk      RMI ≥ 200 (increased risk
of malignancy):          of malignancy)
Management by general
gynaecologist
    ↓                    ↓
Features of the cyst    CT scan (abdomen/pelvis)
                         ↓
                    Referral to gynaecological
                    oncology for MDT review
                    ↓              ↓
                High-risk of    Low-risk of
                malignancy      malignancy
                    ↓              ↓
                Laparotomy:     Laparotomy: Pelvic
                Full staging    clearance
                procedure by    (TAH + BSO +
                a trained       omentectomy +
                gynaecological  peritoneal cytology)
                oncologist in   by a trained
                a cancer centre gynaecologist in a
                                general gynaecology
                                or cancer ward
```

Features of the cyst branches:

- **Asymptomatic, simple cyst <5 cm, unilocular, unilateral**
  - *Conservative management:* Re-assessment in 4–6 months with CA-125 levels and TVS
  - Discharge from follow-up after 1 year if the cyst remains unchanged or reduces in size
    - Resolution → Discharge
    - Persistent/unchanged → Repeat assessment in another 4–6 months
    - Change in features → Consider intervention
  - Individualise treatment after discussion with the woman

- **Symptomatic, non-simple, size ≥ 5 cm, multilocular, bilateral**
  - *Consider surgery:* Salpingo-oophorectomy (usually bilateral): laparoscopic route can be adopted
  - Surgery to be preceded with preoperative counselling that a full staging laparotomy may be required if there is an evidence of malignancy on laparoscopy
  - Removal of surgical specimen (without intraperitoneal spillage) in a laparoscopic retrieval bag via umbilical port

(BSO: bilateral salpingo-oophorectomy; CT: computed tomography; MDT: multidisciplinary team; RMI: risk of malignancy index; TAH: total abdominal hysterectomy; TVS: transvaginal scanning)

BOX 31.4: Aims of performing a surgical procedure.

- Obtaining the tissue for biopsy to help confirm the diagnosis
- Assessing the extent of disease (i.e., surgical staging)
- Attempting optimal cytoreduction (which may be essential for successful treatment especially in advanced cases)

BOX 31.5: Women who are poor candidates for aggressive initial surgical cytoreduction.

- Patients with a complex ovarian cyst in whom an extraovarian primary tumor has not been excluded
- Imaging findings suggestive of an extensive disease (liver or pulmonary metastases, disease in the porta hepatis, massive ascites, etc.)
- Women with a poor performance status (e.g., elderly patients or those having medical comorbidities)

TUMOR MARKERS

CA 125 Levels

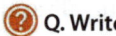 **Q. Write a short essay on CA 125.**

CA 125 is a surface glycoprotein found on the surface of ovarian cancer cells and on some normal tissues. A high CA 125 level could be a sign of cancer or other conditions. The CA 125 test should not be used as a standalone test to diagnose ovarian cancer because it is associated with a sensitivity of 50–60%. Therefore, this test is not very reliable.

TABLE 31.4: Staging of carcinoma ovaries, fallopian tube, and peritoneum based on TNM and FIGO staging.

TNM categories	FIGO stage	Stage
*Primary tumor*		
TX		Primary tumor cannot be assessed
T0		No evidence of primary tumor
T1	I	Tumor limited to ovaries (one or both) of fallopian tube(s)
T1a	IA	Tumor limited to one ovary or fallopian tube; capsule intact, no tumor on ovarian surface. No malignant cells in ascites or peritoneal washings
T1b	IB	Tumor limited to both ovaries and fallopian tubes; capsules intact, no tumor on ovarian surface. No malignant cells in ascites or peritoneal washings
T1c	IC	Tumor limited to one or both ovaries with any of the following: capsule ruptured, tumor on ovarian surface, malignant cells in ascites or peritoneal washings
T1c1	IC1	Surgical spill
T1c2	IC2	Capsule ruptured before surgery or presence of the tumor cells on ovarian or fallopian tube surface
T1c3	IC3	Malignant cells in the ascites or peritoneal washings
T2	II	Tumor involves one or both ovaries or fallopian tube with pelvic extension (below pelvic brim) or primary peritoneal cancer
T2a	IIA	Extension and/or implants on uterus and/or tube(s) and/or ovaries
T2b	IIB	Extension to and/or implants on other pelvic tissues
T3	III	Tumor involves one or both ovaries or fallopian tubes, or primary peritoneal cancer, with cytologically or histologically confirmed spread to the peritoneum outside the pelvis and/or metastasis to the retroperitoneal lymph nodes
	IIIA1	Positive retroperitoneal lymph nodes only (cytologically or histologically proven)
	IIIA1 (i)	Metastasis up to 10 mm in greatest dimension
	IIIA1 (ii)	Metastasis > 10 mm in greatest dimension
T3a	IIIA2	Microscopic extrapelvic (above the pelvic brim) peritoneal involvement with or without positive retroperitoneal lymph nodes
T3b	IIIB	Macroscopic peritoneal metastasis beyond the pelvis up to 2 cm in greatest dimension, with or without metastasis to the retroperitoneal lymph nodes
T3c	IIIC	Macroscopic peritoneal metastasis beyond the pelvis more than 2 cm in greatest dimension, with or without metastasis to the retroperitoneal lymph nodes (includes extension of tumor to capsule of liver and spleen without parenchymal involvement of either organ)
T4	IV	Growth involving one or both the ovaries with distant metastasis. If pleural effusion is present, there must be a positive cytological test result to allot a case to stage IV; parenchymal liver metastasis also equals stage IV.
*Regional lymph nodes (N)*		
TNM categories	**FIGO stages**	
NX		Regional lymph nodes cannot be assessed
N0		No regional lymph node metastasis
N1	IIIC	Regional lymph node metastasis
*Distant metastasis (M)*		
TNM categories	**FIGO stages**	
M0		No distant metastasis
M1	IV	Distant metastasis (excludes peritoneal metastasis)

(FIGO: International Federation of Gynecology and Obstetrics; TNM: tumor, node and metastasis)

However, it is associated with a specificity of 90%. This test is approved by the Food and Drug Administration for monitoring a woman's response to ovarian cancer treatment and for detecting its return after treatment. Values of CA 125 > 35 IU/mL are found in over 80% of cases with nonmucinous EOCs. Estimation of CA 125 levels is not reliable because it can also be raised in presence of benign conditions such as endometriosis, tuberculosis, leiomyomas, liver or kidney disease, and pelvic inflammatory disease. The cut-off value of CA-125 in premenopausal women is considered as 200 IU/mL, whereas in postmenopausal women, it is considered as 35 IU/L.

HEA-4 (Human epididymis protein 4)

This is a new useful biomarker in cases of ovarian cancer having a sensitivity of 73% and specificity of 95%. As previously mentioned, CA-125 levels are used as a prognostic marker. Using a combination of both C-125 and HEA-4 as a prognostic marker is likely to be associated with a sensitivity of 94–95%.

CA19-9

This marker is likely to be raised in cases of mucinous carcinomas, torsion of dermoid cysts, etc.

IMAGING STUDIES: ULTRASOUND

Ultrasonography (both transabdominal and transvaginal) is accurate in differentiating tumors of the ovary from other types of tumors of the pelvis, in >90% of the patients (**Figs. 31.6 to 31.11**). Discrimination between benign and malignant lesions of the ovary can be made on the basis of ultrasonic patterns.

At the time of evaluation an adnexal mass using ultrasound, it is important to assess the risk of malignancy of that mass. This is usually done using IOTA (International ovarian tumor analysis) simple rules, which is stepwise evaluation of the adnexal mass by ultrasound.

Iota Simple Rules

This comprises the following steps:
- *Step 1*: Assessing the origin of mass, whether ovarian or extraovarian.

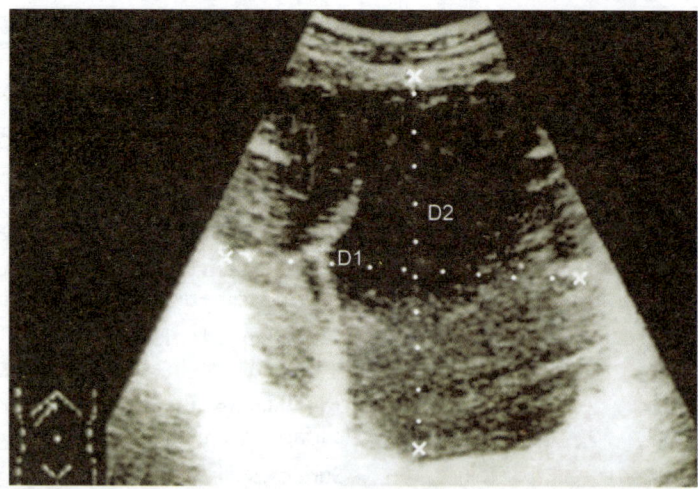

Fig. 31.7: Transabdominal sonography showing presence of a large thin-walled cyst of right ovarian origin with multiple septa and numerous internal echoes.

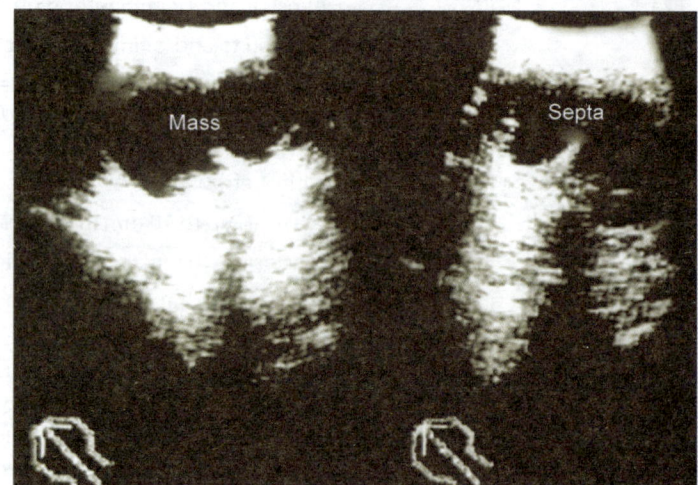

Fig. 31.8: Transvaginal sonography showing presence of a single cystic mass with septa arising from left adnexa.

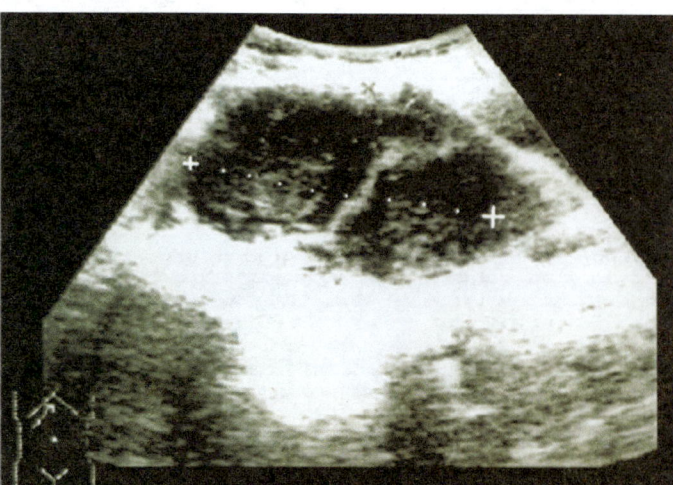

Fig. 31.6: Transabdominal sonography showing a multiloculated mass with presence of cystic areas along with a few brightly echogenic areas. Differential diagnosis of mucinous cystadenoma and dermoid cyst were established.

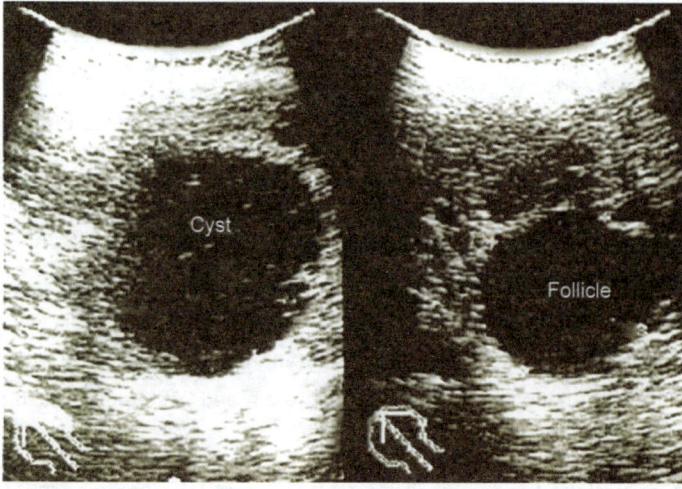

Fig. 31.9: Transvaginal sonography revealing the presence of an ovarian cyst (with multiple internal echoes) on the right side. On the left side, the ovary is normal with the presence of a dominant follicle.

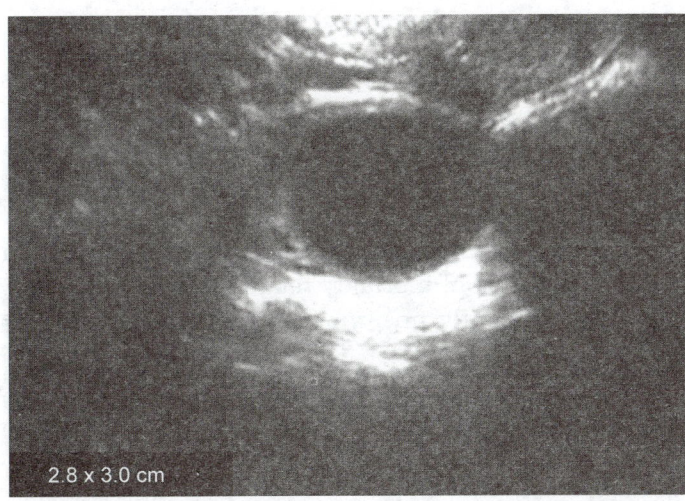

Fig. 31.10: Transvaginal sonography showing presence of a small, smooth-walled cystic mass suggestive of a functional cyst.

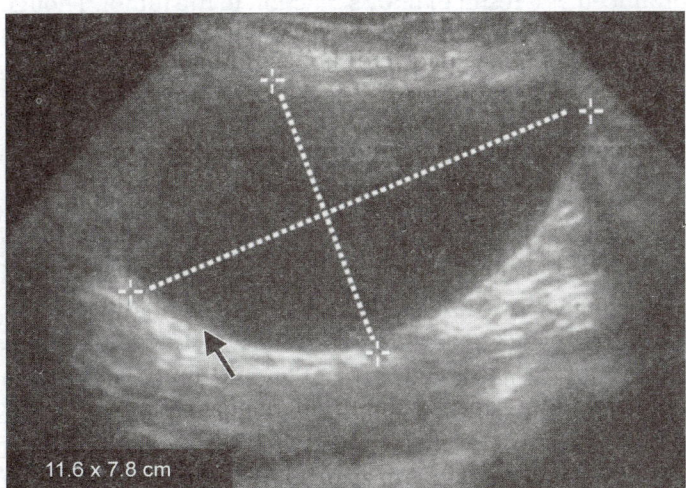

Fig. 31.11: Transabdominal sonography showing presence of a large cyst of size 12 cm × 8 cm in a patient aged 52 years.

- *Step 2:* In case of the mass of ovarian origin, it needs to be categorized as benign, intermediate, or malignant.
- *Step 3:* Categorization of the patient as high risk or low risk:
  - *Low-risk:* Premenopausal women without any additional risk factors
  - *High-risk:* Postmenopausal or premenopausal women with additional risk factors

IOTA group has also described ultrasound "rules" (**Table 31.5**), which helps in classifying the masses as benign, malignant, or uncertain. These rules are likely to be associated with a sensitivity of 80–90%.

Doppler flow studies of the ovarian artery may also help in differentiating between benign and malignant growths. Normally, a high resistance pattern (resistive index > 0.70) is indicative of a benign growth. In malignant tumors due to increased blood supply, the resistance index is usually low (<0.4) and there is a high peak velocity. The scoring system

TABLE 31.5: IOTA Group ultrasound "rules" for classification of masses as benign or malignant.

Characteristics	B-rules (benign)	M-rules (malignant)
Consistency: Cystic/solid	Unilocular cysts	Irregular solid Tumor
Presence of solid components	The largest solid component <7 mm	The largest solid component ≥7 mm
Ascites	Absent	Present
Presence of acoustic shadowing	Present	Absent
Papillary structures	Less than four papillary structures	Four or more papillary structures
Surface: Smooth/irregular	Smooth	Irregular
Tumor diameter	Largest diameter < 100 mm	Largest diameter ≥ 100 mm
Blood flow	No blood flow	Very strong blood flow

TABLE 31.6: Doppler blood flow in the adnexal mass scoring system.

Findings on Doppler blood flow analysis	Score
No blood flow	1
Minimal blood flow	2
Moderate blood flow	3
High blood flow	4

for evaluation of Doppler blood flow in the adnexal mass is described in **Table 31.6**. A blood flow score of >3 along with vascularity of the papilla present in the solid area in the central part of the mass is indicative of malignancy.

Other signs suggestive of malignancy include presence of irregular solid parts within the mass, indefinite margins, papillary projections extending from inner wall of the cyst, presence of ascites, hydronephrosis, pleural effusion, matted bowel loops, omental implants, other evidence of peritoneal disseminated disease, and lymphadenopathy. Size of tumor may also give clues regarding the nature of the mass. Larger tumors, usually >8 cm in size have been thought to be associated with higher risk of malignancy in comparison to the smaller ones.

RISK OF MALIGNANCY INDEX (RMI-4)

In case, the mass appears to be uncertain following the application of IOTA rules, the RMI or risk of malignancy index must be used for evaluating the mass. The most recent RMI in use is RMI-IV (**Box 31.6**). Previously used indices RMI-1 to RMI-3 (**Table 31.7**) are different from RMI-4 in aspect of not including size of the tumor as one of the parameters. RMI 4 is calculated as a product of ultrasound score (U) × menopausal score (M) × CA 125 × tumor size. RMI-4 is likely

> **BOX 31.6:** Risk of malignancy index 4.
>
> *Definition:* Combination of four presurgical features:
> 1. Serum CA-125 (CA-125)
> 2. Menopausal status (M)
> 3. Ultrasound score (U)
> 4. Tumor size
>
> *Calculation:*
> RMI = U × M × CA-125 × S
>
> *Note:* U = ultrasound score. The ultrasound result is scored 1 point for each of the following characteristics: multilocular cysts, solid areas, metastases, ascites, and bilateral lesions.
> U = 1 (for an ultrasound score of 0), U = 1 (for an ultrasound score of 1), U = 4 (for an ultrasound score of 2–5). The menopausal status is scored as 1 = premenopausal and 3 = postmenopausal; serum CA-125 is measured in IU/mL and can vary from 0 to 100 or even 1,000 of units
> S = Tumor size in cm [A tumor size (single greatest diameter) < 7 cm, yields S = 1 and size ≥ 7 cm yields S = 2]
> A score > 450 for RMI-4 is suggestive of malignancy

TABLE 31.7: Scoring system for various RMI indices (1 to 4).

Score parameter	RMI-1	RMI-2	RMI-3	RMI-4
Premenopausal	1	1	1	1
Postmenopausal	3	4	3	4
Ultrasound feature: None	0	1	1	1
Ultrasound feature: 1	1	1	1	1
Ultrasound feature: 2–5	3	4	3	4
CA-125				
Tumor size <7 cm				1
Tumor size ≥ 7 cm				2
Score calculation	U × M × CA-125	U × M × CA-125	U × M × CA-125	U × M × CA-125 × S
Significant score	>250	>200	>200	>450

to be associated with a sensitivity of 91% and a specificity of 80%. If the RMI is high (RMI-1 ≥ 250 or RMI-4 ≥ 450), the women must be referred to a gynecological oncologist for management in the cancer center. Here, the woman must be preferably managed by a multidisciplinary team. In case, the RMI is low (RMI-1 < 250 or RMI-4 < 450), the woman must be managed by a general gynecologist.

RISK OF OVARIAN MALIGNANCY ALGORITHM

Both the indices, RMI and risk of ovarian malignancy algorithm (ROMA) are used for categorization of women into high-risk and low-risk groups. Parameters taken into consideration in this index include:
- Measurement of CA-125 and HEA-4 levels
- Woman's premenopausal or postmenopausal status

RISK OF OVARIAN CANCER ALGORITHM (ROCA)

This model, developed by UK Collaborative Trial of Ovarian Cancer Screening (UKCTOCS) is used for screening of women > 50 years of age. This involves serial measurement of CA 125 levels and TVS.

None of the screening modalities have been proven to reduce the risk of mortality related to ovarian cancer. Therefore, presently no proper screening modality for ovarian cancer is available.

OVASURE TEST

This test, based on proteomic analysis measures the level of six protein markers in the woman's blood sample to calculate her probability of developing an ovarian cancer. Some of these protein markers are produced by a tumor and rest are produced as a result of body's reaction to the tumor. Though this test is coming up in a big way, there is presently limited evidence regarding its efficacy.

OTHER IMAGING MODALITIES

CT and/ or MRI

Sonographic diagnosis of a malignant tumor necessitates further evaluation (e.g., CT or MRI). If these investigations also suggest ovarian cancer, then the best approach is laparotomy for staging and treatment. Of these various modalities, CT scan (**Fig. 31.12**) is preferred and helps in evaluation of the following: peritoneal involvement, upper abdominal involvement, and lymph nodal involvement. MRI scans help in accurate characterization of ovarian tumors (**Fig. 31.13**) and are also particularly helpful for examining metastatic spread of the cancer to the brain and spinal cord.

Barium Enema

This is a test to see whether the cancer has invaded the colon or rectum. Nowadays, barium enema has been largely replaced by colonoscopy in order to assess the colonic invasion.

Positron Emission Tomography

In this test, radioactive glucose is given to detect malignancy. Since the cancerous tissues utilize glucose at a higher rate than normal tissues, the radioactivity tends to get concentrated in the area of malignancy. A scanner can spot the radioactive deposits. In some instances, this test has proved useful in estimating the spread of ovarian cancer. However, the test is expensive and is therefore not routinely done.

BIOPSY

There is no place for routine FNAC or tru-cut biopsy of the tumor. If ascites is present, ascitic fluid can be aspirated

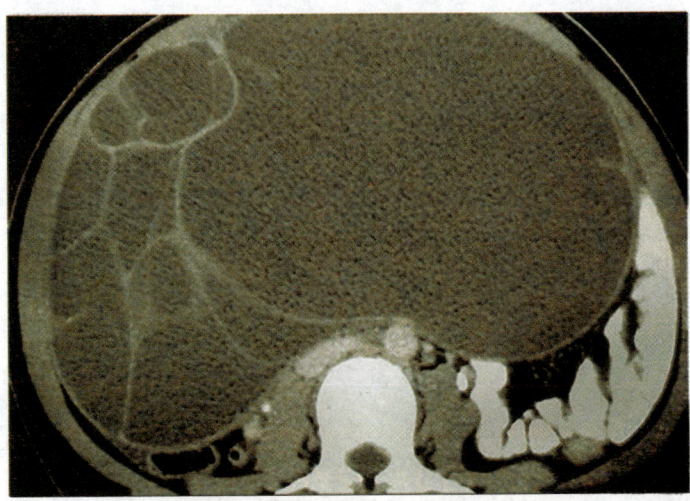

Fig. 31.12: Computed tomography scan showing a well-circumscribed mass arising from the left ovary having septations with a homogeneous higher-than-water attenuation. Diagnosis of mucinous cystadenoma was made.

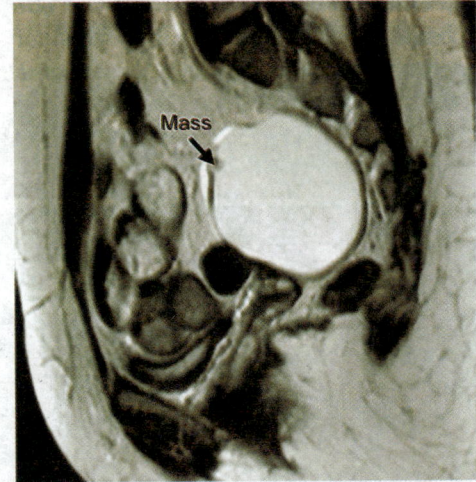

Fig. 31.13: T1-weighted image on magnetic resonance imaging showing a benign serous cystadenoma. The mass is smooth walled, having homogenous consistency with no internal septae or lobulations.

for cytology. However, this test is not confirmative because malignancy cannot be ruled out if even if the test is negative. FNAC, percutaneous biopsy, or diagnostic paracentesis has a role in ruling out a primary peritoneal malignancy, if there is diffuse carcinomatosis without presence of an obvious ovarian mass. This would help the clinician in planning for neoadjuvant chemotherapy.

PREOPERATIVE EVALUATION

Once the ovarian malignancy has been diagnosed or suspected, a preoperative evaluation must be done in order to evaluate the extent of malignancy prior to undertaking surgery. The preoperative evaluation helps in excluding other primary cancers (e.g., gastrointestinal malignancy), which could be metastatic to the ovary. The preoperative evaluation in case of ovarian malignancy comprises the following investigations:

- *Chest X-Ray:* This procedure may be done to determine whether ovarian cancer has metastasized to the lungs. Chest X-rays can help in the detection of pleural effusion.
- *Colonoscopy and barium enema:* Colonoscopy/barium enema must be performed to exclude involvement of the colon by cancerous growth. Upper gastrointestinal series or gastroscopy may also be performed if symptoms indicate gastric involvement.
- *Intravenous pyelography:* IV pyelography is done in order to assess the urinary tract for invasion by the cancerous mass. Presence of hydronephrosis could be due to obstruction of the urinary tract by malignant growth.
- *Cervical Cytology:* Although Pap test has low sensitivity for detection of ovarian malignancy; this test may help in ruling out the presence of uterine or endocervical cancer causing metastatic involvement of the ovaries.

EXPLORATORY LAPAROTOMY

Sometimes cancer of the ovary cannot be diagnosed before an exploratory laparotomy is carried out. The staging of ovarian cancer is done at the time of exploratory laparotomy **(Figs. 31.14A to H)**. Surgical staging helps in estimating the spread of cancer. Staging of the ovarian cancer is particularly important because subsequent treatment depends upon the stage of the disease. Once a stage has been assigned, it does not change, even if the cancer later spreads to other areas of the body or comes back following surgery.

Pre-requisites: A gynecological oncologist must be available. ICU facilities as well as the facilities for frozen section must be present. There must be an easy access to blood and blood products. Patient consent must be taken for surgical staging/blood transfusion/colostomy/intraperitoneal (IP) chemotherapy, etc.

Steps: Besides estimating the stage of cancer spread, exploratory laparotomy also helps in removing most of the cancerous tissue larger than about 0.5 inch and helps in taking out the tissue samples. These tissue samples help the clinician in deciding stage of the tumor. The steps of surgical staging are described below:
- A midline or a paramedian abdominal incision is given in order to allow adequate access to the upper abdominal cavity especially in cases where there is a possibility of malignancy.
- At the time of surgery, the ovarian tumor must be removed intact and a frozen histological section should be obtained.
- Any intra-abdominal free fluid or that presents in the POD must be submitted for cytological analysis.
- If no free fluid is present, peritoneal washings should be performed by instilling and recovering 50–100 mL of

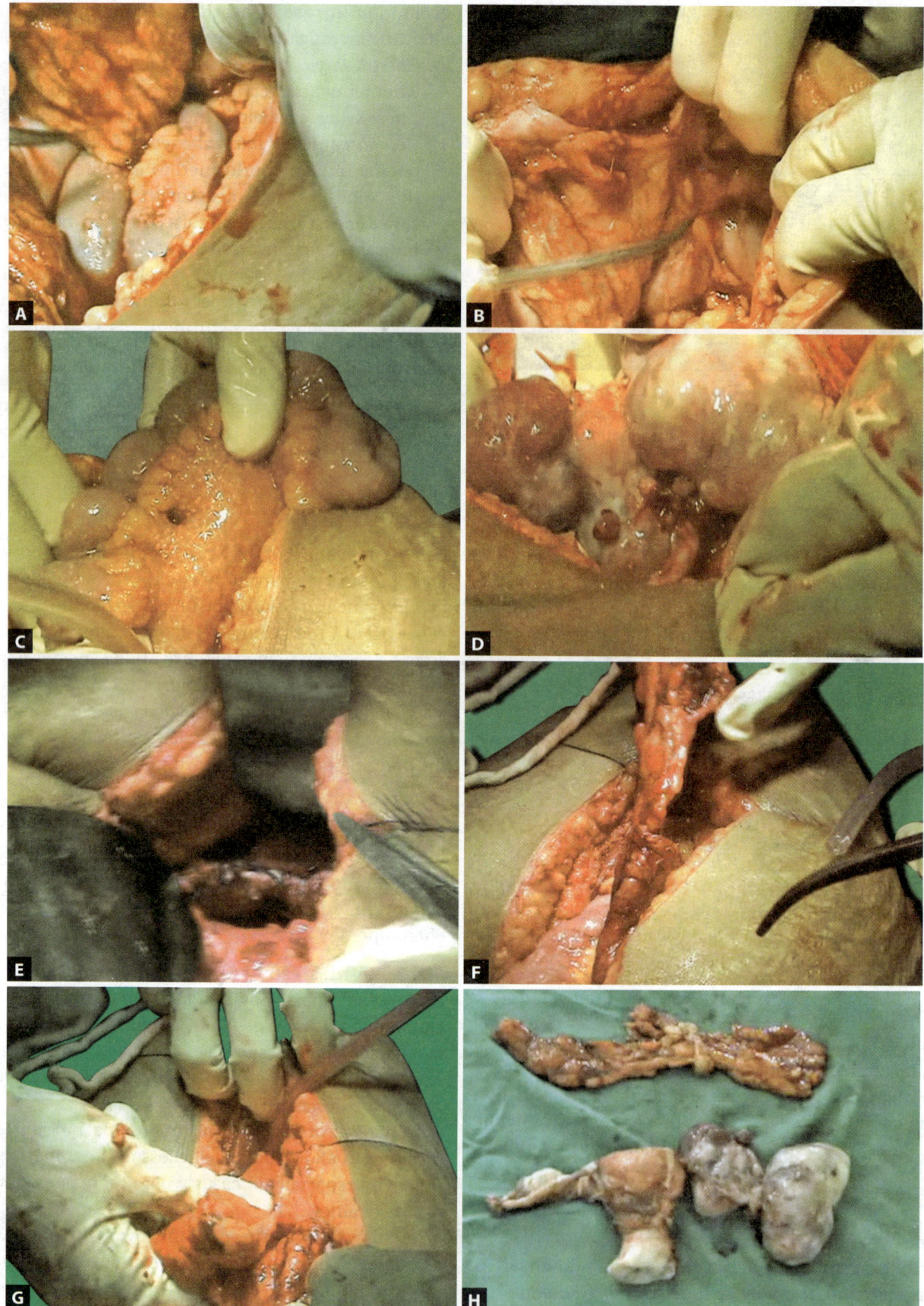

Figs. 31.14A to H: Exploratory laparotomy performed in a 52-year-old patient. (A) Peritoneal surface of uterus studded with cancer deposits; (B) omental surface showing deposits; (C) Mesentery studded with cancer deposits; (D) Polypoidal cancerous growth arising from the left ovary; (E) Vaginal vault closed with continuous sutures following hysterectomy; (F and G) Infracolic omentectomy; (H) Specimen of uterus, ovaries, and omentum which had been removed during surgery.

saline from the pelvic cul-de-sac, each paracolic gutter and beneath each hemidiaphragm.
- A systematic exploration of all intra-abdominal surfaces and viscera must be performed. The gynecologist must proceed in a clockwise fashion from the cecum, moving cephalad along the paracolic gutter and the ascending colon to the right kidney, the liver, and gall bladder, the right hemidiaphragm, transverse colon and then down to the left gutter, and descending colon and the rectosigmoid.
- Biopsy must be taken from any suspicious areas and peritoneal adhesions. If there is no evidence of the disease but the disease is nevertheless suspected, multiple IP biopsies must be performed.
- The diaphragm must be sampled.
- Ovarian tumor must be resected out. Frozen section of the tumor must be obtained and sent immediately for histopathological analysis. In case of positive histological evidence of malignancy, TAH along with (TAH + BSO) must be performed.
- Infracolic omentectomy, which involves resection of omentum from the transverse colon needs to be performed.
- Exploration of retroperitoneal spaces to evaluate the pelvic and para-aortic lymph nodes also needs to be done.

The FIGO cancer is subsequently done based on the findings of clinical examination and/or surgical exploration. If the cancer comes back after initial treatment, this is known as recurrent cancer.

ROLE OF LAPAROSCOPY

Laparoscopic surgery is not commonly employed in cases of ovarian cancer due to risk of recurrence postoperatively. Also, insufflation at the time of laparoscopy is likely to promote the cancer spread, causing a limited tumor to convert into a widespread tumor. Minimal invasive surgery can be best employed under the following circumstances:
- Early stage cancer or borderline tumor
- In advanced staged cancer, only for debulking or for insertion of IP catheters.
- Taking biopsies in case planning HIPEC.

GRADING

Grading of ovarian cancer is done by evaluating the histopathological appearance of cells on the basis of microscopic examination. The tumor grading gives an idea about the degree of malignancy and how quickly the cancer is likely to progress. There are three cancer grades: (1) grade I (low grade); (2) grade II (moderate grade), and (3) grade III (high grade).

1. *Low-grade cancer:* The cancer cells are well-differentiated and look very much like the normal cells of the ovary. They usually grow slowly and are less likely to spread.
2. *Moderate-grade cancer:* The cancer cells are less well-differentiated and appear more abnormal in comparison to the low grade cells.
3. *High-grade cancer:* The cells look very abnormal and may show a high grade of anaplasia. These cancers are highly malignant, which tend to grow very quickly and are highly likely to spread.

REPORTING THE DIAGNOSIS OF EOC

This must include the following:
- *Site of origin:* Whether ovary/fallopian tube or peritoneum. This assumes importance because the primary peritoneal tumors are likely to have the worst prognosis. In cases of primary peritoneal malignancy, the ovary may be normal looking and tumor-free.
- *Disease stage*
- *Disease grade*

TREATMENT/GYNECOLOGICAL MANAGEMENT

PREVENTION

Screening for Ovarian Cancer

> Q. Discuss in detail the screening for ovarian malignancy.
>
> Q. Write a short note discussing risk reduction in familial gynecological cancer.

Presently, research studies are being carried out to assess whether ovarian cancers can be detected at an early stage so that they can be treated more effectively. Some of the tests which are being considered in various research trials include estimation of CA 125 levels or performing a transvaginal ultrasound. It is important to identify an appropriate screening test, which can detect ovarian cancer in its early stages because survival rates from ovarian cancer are related to the stage at diagnosis. 5-year survival rates of over 90% have been reported for the minority of women with stage I disease. Since presently, it is not known whether these screening tests could help in detection of ovarian cancers at an earlier stage, or help reduced the cancer-related mortality, currently there exists no national screening program for ovarian cancer.

Screening not recommended: Screening for ovarian cancers is not recommended for women with average risk, who does not have a personal or family history of ovarian cancer or personal history of breast cancer.

Screening is recommended: Screening for ovarian cancer is recommended in high-risk women. This is inclusive of the following:
- Women having a strong family history of ovarian cancer or breast cancer in one or more first-degree relatives.

- Women with BRCA mutation or lynch syndrome
- Women with a previous history of breast cancer.

In high-risk women, screening must begin from the age of 30-35 years or 10 years prior to the age when the youngest family member was affected.

DEFINITIVE THERAPY

The treatment of a patient with ovarian cancer must be planned by a multidisciplinary team comprising of a gynecological oncologist, a clinical or medical oncologist, radiologist, pathologist, a gynecological oncology nurse specialist, dietician, physiotherapist, occupational therapist, and clinical psychologist, or counselor. The issues which need to be discussed with the patient before undertaking therapy include: the type and extent of the treatment the patient would receive, the advantages and disadvantages of the treatment, any other treatment options that may be available, and any significant risks or side effects of the treatment.

Stage IA (Grade I Disease)

Primary treatment for stage I EOC is surgical, i.e., a TAH and a BSO and surgical staging. The uterus and contralateral ovary can be preserved in woman with stage IA, grade I disease who desire to preserve their fertility. However, such women must be periodically monitored with routine pelvic examinations and determination of serum CA 125 levels.

Stage IA and IB (Grade II and III) and Stage IC

Treatment options in this case include additional chemotherapy or radiotherapy besides surgery as described above. Chemotherapy is the more commonly used option and comprises either single agent or multiagent chemotherapy. The most commonly used single agent chemotherapy in the past was melphalan which was administered orally on a "pulse" basis for 5 consecutive days, every 28 days. Radiotherapy could be administered either in the form of IP radiocolloids (P 32) or whole abdominal radiation.

According to the current treatment recommendations, the treatment must be in form of either cisplatin or carboplatin or combination therapy of either of these drugs with paclitaxel for three to four cycles.

FERTILITY PRESERVING SURGERY

Fertility preservation (unilateral salpingo-oophorectomy on the affected side) can be considered as an option for women with stage IA and 1B grade 1 EOC in young women desiring pregnancy. It can also be considered for stage 1A and 1B invasive carcinoma, grade 2 (in whom chemotherapy had been given previously). Some prerequisites before considering fertility preserving surgery are as follows:
- Mass is 10 cm or smaller as viewed on the sonogram.
- Mass has a distinct border, but no solid areas.
- No associated ascites is observed.
- Serum CA-125 levels are within normal limits (<35U/mL).
- She has no family history of ovarian cancer.
- She is willing for regular follow-ups.

Even if conservative surgery is being planned, complete surgical staging should be performed. The staging should include collection of peritoneal washings, omentectomy, appendectomy, and lymph node biopsies. A thorough abdominal exploration and biopsy of any abnormal areas must be performed. Endometrial biopsy should also be performed to exclude endometrial cancer. At the time of surgery, the contralateral ovary is not usually biopsied, if it appears to be normal. Cryopreservation of the oocyte/ovarian tissue must be considered in these cases. Young women with a well-differentiated lesion of one ovary, who have undergone conservative surgery, must go through hysterectomy and removal of the remaining ovary upon completion of their families, or by the age of 35 years.

Stage II, III, and IV

Debulking surgery or cytoreductive surgery is performed in these cases. This involves an initial exploratory procedure with the removal of as much disease as possible (both tumor and the associated metastatic disease).

CYTOREDUCTIVE SURGERY

Cytoreductive surgery (Box 31.7) includes abdominal hysterectomy and BSO, complete omentectomy and resection of metastatic lesions from the peritoneal surface. The gynecologist must take the biopsies or remove some of the lymph nodes in the abdomen and pelvis. They may also have to remove the omentum, appendix, and part of the peritoneum. Resection of rectosigmoid colon should be attempted in women with bulky abdominal disease in case maximal cytoreduction appears to be a likely option. Bowel surgery is of little value in case of grossly unresectable disease, except for relieving gastrointestinal obstruction. Gastrointestinal surgery can add significant morbidity to surgical treatment. In case, the patient has ascites, ascitic fluid must be collected, and sent for cytological examination. In case of absence of ascites, peritoneal washings must be collected after instillation of normal saline in the paracolic gutters. Extent of surgery can be standard, radical, or ultraradical (Flowchart 31.4) depending upon the stage of the cancer

At the time of surgery, exploratory laparotomy is carried out in a systematic manner, in which the status of various organs such as pelvic organs, small and large intestine, mesentery, appendix, stomach, liver, gallbladder, spleen, omentum, diaphragm, the entire peritoneum, and retroperitoneal structures such as the kidneys, pancreas, and lymph nodes, are assessed. The affected adnexa should be removed intact and a frozen section must be obtained to confirm the diagnosis. Biopsies must be taken from all suspicious areas. If suspicious areas cannot be obviously seen, multiple random biopsies are taken from peritoneal surfaces, including the POD, bladder peritoneum, paracolic gutters, and bowel mesentery, to help detect micrometastases. The diaphragm should be biopsied or scraped for cytology. Any adhesions or peritoneal surface irregularities should also be sampled.

The omentum is resected rather than biopsied. Resection of the omental cake must be performed even when optimal cytoreduction is not possible in order to reduce the tumor bulk and postoperative ascites formation. Pelvic and para-aortic node sampling is performed to exclude the possibility of microscopic stage III disease. Suspicious nodes are removed. Lymph nodes are randomly sampled in case there are no suspicious nodes. Para-aortic nodes, especially those above the inferior mesenteric artery, are involved more commonly than pelvic nodes. Appendectomy is performed as part of the routine staging procedure.

Cytoreduction can be a complicated surgery and should ideally be done by a specialist gynecological oncologist. The goal of cytoreductive surgery is resection of the primary tumor and all the metastatic disease. If this is not possible, the goal must be to reduce the tumor burden by resection of the tumor to an "optimal status". Potential benefits of aggressive primary surgical management (cytoreduction) in women with EOC are listed in **Box 31.8**.

Optimal Cytoreduction

The Gynecologic Oncology Group (2004) has defined optimal cytoreduction as leaving residual disease having <1 cm maximum tumor diameter. The volume of residual disease remaining after cytoreductive surgery shows an inverse correlation with the survival rates. Therefore, in cases where it is technically feasible, all visible tumor tissue must be resected at the time of initial surgery. Cytoreduction must preferably be performed by gynecologic oncologists experienced in this surgery so as to achieve optimal cytoreduction. Certain areas in the abdomen may not be easily accessible or may be unresectable, e.g., large tumor plaques on the diaphragm or liver, tumor involving the mesentery, etc. In these cases, other therapeutic options like CO_2 laser, ultrasonic aspirator, argon beam coagulator, or loop electrosurgical excision may be used.

If the initial surgical attempt at cytoreduction was not an optimal one, then chemotherapy followed by secondary

> **BOX 31.7:** The procedure of cytoreductive surgery.
>
> *Preoperative preparation:*
> - Nutritional assessment
> - Assessment of intercurrent medical diseases, which should be under optimum control (e.g., good glycemic control in women with diabetes)
> - *Preoperative laboratory tests:*
>   – A complete blood count
>   – Liver and renal function tests
>   – Serum electrolytes and glucose
>   – Coagulation tests
>   – Baseline CA 125 levels
>   – Chest radiograph
>   – Electrocardiogram
>   – Computed tomography of the abdomen
>   – Liver imaging helps to determine whether metastatic disease, if present, is confined to surface implants or whether a partial hepatic resection of parenchymal disease may be required
>
> *Surgery:*
> - Abdominal hysterectomy and bilateral salpingo-oophorectomy
> - Complete omentectomy
> - Collection of ascitic fluid (if present) or collection of peritoneal washings (after instillation of normal saline in the paracolic gutters)
> - Resection of metastatic lesions from the peritoneal surface
> - Biopsy of the lymph nodes in the abdomen and pelvis
> - Random biopsies are taken from peritoneal surfaces, including the pouch of Douglas bladder peritoneum, paracolic gutters, and bowel mesentery
> - Diaphragm should be biopsied or scraped for cytology
> - Any adhesions or peritoneal surface irregularities must be biopsied
> - Pelvic and para-aortic node sampling
> - Appendectomy
>
> *Postoperative preparation:*
> Maintenance of fluid electrolyte balance

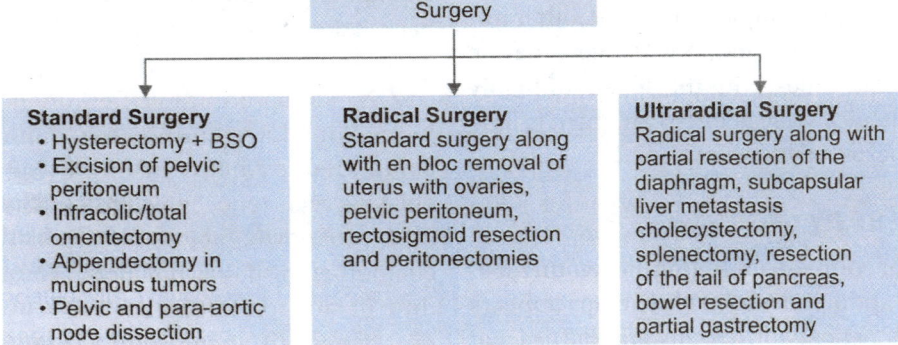

Flowchart 31.4: Extent of surgery based on the cancer stage.

(BSO: bilateral salpingo-oophorectomy)

BOX 31.8: Potential benefits of cytoreduction in women with epithelial ovarian cancer.

- Removal of bulky disease helps in rapidly improving the disease-related symptoms (e.g., abdominal pain, increased abdominal girth, dyspnea, early satiety, etc.
- Removal of tumor bulk may help improve host immune competence by reducing the production of immunosuppressive cytokines [e.g., interleukin-10, vascular endothelial growth factor(VEGF)], which are normally produced by the tumor tissue
- Cytoreductive surgery is also believed to increase chemosensitivity due to resection of areas with poor blood supply and necrosis. Cytoreduction enables the residual disease to become well-perfused and therefore mitotically active, thereby maximizing the effect of chemotherapeutic agents.
- Improvement of the patient's quality of life and nutritional status by achieving the following:
  - Reduction in the volume of ascites
  - Restoration of adequate intestinal function, resulting in an improvement in the overall nutritional status of the patient
  - Improving the patient's ability to withstand subsequent chemotherapy
  - Removal of cancer invading bowel, lessens sepsis
  - Removal of a large tumor reduces pain

BOX 31.9: Indications for chemotherapy.

- Early stage ovarian (stage IB or IC) cancer (after surgery in order to reduce the chance of the cancer recurrence): Adjuvant chemotherapy
- Moderate or high-grade ovarian cancer (after surgery)
- Neoadjuvant chemotherapy before surgery in advanced stage ovarian cancer
- Stage IV cancer with distant metastasis

surgical cytoreduction may be beneficial, but survival is not as high as that achieved with optimal cytoreduction at the time of primary surgery.

A second attempt at cytoreduction after chemotherapy for suboptimally debulked disease is usually not as successful as an aggressive initial surgical debulking. However, if the initial surgical attempt at cytoreduction was not a maximal surgical effort, then chemotherapy followed by secondary surgical cytoreduction might be beneficial. The two modalities used in the postoperative treatment of newly diagnosed advanced stage EOC are IV chemotherapy alone or a combination of IV and IP chemotherapy. A choice between these options is dependent on the amount of disease remaining after surgery. Combination IV/IP treatment is reserved for women with optimally cytoreduced EOC. On the other hand, patients with suboptimal cytoreduction (having >1 cm of residual disease following surgery) are treated with IV chemotherapy instead of IP because the IP administered chemotherapy drugs have limited penetration into larger tumors. For patients with no clinical evidence of disease and negative tumor markers at the completion of chemotherapy, a reassessment laparotomy or "second-look" surgery may be performed. In the present times, with the advent of highly sensitive imaging modalities such as PET-scan, there is little role of second-look laparoscopy.

RADIATION THERAPY

Radiation therapy is not commonly used for the treatment of ovarian cancer. Whole abdominal radiation therapy appears to be a useful option for patients with metastatic disease that is microscopic or completely resected. The current evidence suggests that the whole abdominal radiation is inappropriate for the patients with macroscopic residual disease. Radiotherapy may be rarely used to treat an area of cancer that has come back after surgery and chemotherapy, when other treatment options are no longer appropriate. It can also be used as palliative therapy in order to reduce bleeding or symptoms of pain and discomfort. It has been successfully used in the treatment of recurrent germ cell tumors which are very radiosensitive. Radioactive isotopes of gold (Au 198) or phosphorus (P 32) have been used intraperitoneally in combination with external radiotherapy.

CHEMOTHERAPY

Q. Write a short note on role of chemotherapy in ovarian malignancies.

Q. Write a short essay discussing about chemotherapy in epithelial ovarian cancer.

Various indications for chemotherapy are enumerated in **Box 31.9**. Chemotherapy is often recommended after surgery for women with moderate or high-grade ovarian cancer or those with stage IB or IC cancer. Generally, six sessions of chemotherapy are given, over 5–6 months. In advanced-stage ovarian cancer, chemotherapy is sometimes given before surgery (neoadjuvant chemotherapy), to shrink any residual tumor. Women who are given neoadjuvant chemotherapy are given three cycles of chemotherapy before the surgery, followed by three further cycles after the surgery. In case of stage IV cancer with distant metastasis, chemotherapy is the main treatment modality, which is used. In women with early-stage ovarian cancer, chemotherapy is given after surgery to reduce the chance of the cancer recurrence. Though chemotherapy cannot guarantee that the cancer will not come back, it does help in reducing the risk of disease recurrence.

International Collaboration on Ovarian Neoplasms (ICON) study, a multicenter, open randomized trial has helped in determining that platinum-based adjuvant chemotherapy helps in improving overall survival and delaying recurrence in women with early-stage EOC having poor prognostic factors or in patients receiving adjuvant chemotherapy if they had not been completely staged at the time of surgery. European Organisation for Research and Treatment of Cancer (EORTC), Adjuvant ChemoTherapy in Ovarian Neoplasm (ACTION) collaborators from a randomized phase III trial have also shown similar findings. The benefit of adjuvant chemotherapy appeared to be limited to patients with nonoptimal staging, i.e., patients with more risk of unappreciated residual disease.

A systematic review and meta-analysis by Winter Roach has demonstrated that chemotherapy is likely to confer significant benefit both in terms of overall and disease-free survival. Platinum-based chemotherapy should be offered to reduce risk of recurrence except in women where adequate surgical staging has revealed a well-differentiated disease confined to one or both ovaries with intact capsule. Presently, for patients with high-risk early-stage disease and for advanced-stage ovarian cancer, the recommended treatment is chemotherapy comprising of platinum-taxane combination for six cycles. Platinum-based therapy is likely to be more effective than the nonplatinum-based chemotherapy. Moreover, the use of combination therapy is likely to improve the survival rates in comparison to the use of platinum alone.

Types of Chemotherapy

Intraperitoneal chemotherapy: Chemotherapy can be instilled directly into the abdomen and pelvis through a thin tube. The drugs destroy the cancer cells in the abdomen and pelvis. Use of IP chemotherapy is likely to extend the overall survival by 12–17 months in women with advanced ovarian cancer who have been completely cytoreduced. Presently, the role of IP chemotherapy remains unclear and it is not widely used probably due to its high rate of toxicity. According to the results of a new study, OV21/PETROC trial, a randomized phase II trial, presented at the 2016 American Society of Clinical Oncology (ASCO) Annual Meeting, a combination of IP (carboplatin based) and IV chemotherapy is likely to be more effective than IV chemotherapy alone in women with optimally resected advanced ovarian cancer following neoadjuvant chemotherapy. This therapy is not only well tolerated, it also helps in reducing the progressive disease rate by nearly 19% at 9 months. Combination of IP cisplatin and IP paclitaxel in ovarian cancer (as devised by GOG 172) comprises the following regimen: IV paclitaxel 35mg/m^2 over 24 hours on day 1, followed by IP cisplatin 100 mg/m^2 in 1,000 mL of normal saline on day 2. Finally, IP paclitaxel must be administered in the dosage of 60 mg/m^2 on day 8. This entire regimen must be repeated once in 3 weeks for 6 cycles.

Systemic chemotherapy: Systemic chemotherapy may be either taken in orally or injected intravenously. The drugs enter the bloodstream and destroy or control cancer throughout the body. IV chemotherapy is given as a session of treatment, usually over several hours. This is followed by a rest period of a few weeks, which allows the patient's body to recover from any side effects of the treatment. Together, the treatment and the rest periods are known as a cycle of chemotherapy. Most women are given six cycles of chemotherapy.

Intravenous chemotherapy: Presently, platinum- and taxane-based combination therapy has been recommended as the first-line treatment for EOC. For patients with advanced EOC, IV carboplatin [dosed by AUC (area under the curve) = 6 (range 5–7.5)] is administered with IV paclitaxel (175 mg/m^2 over 3 hours) repeated every 3 weeks for six cycles. Phase III studies have demonstrated that carboplatin produces response rates and survival outcomes similar to cisplatin. Moreover, the use of carboplatin is associated with reduced toxicity in comparison with cisplatin. The recent trend is, therefore, to replace cisplatin with carboplatin. Since the renal and gastrointestinal toxicities of carboplatin are modest compared to those with cisplatin, the patients being treated with carboplatin do not require prehydration as that required by cisplatin. The following regimens can be used:

- Docetaxel (75 mg/m^2) and carboplatin (AUC = 5) IV every 3 weeks for six cycles. Due to the potential risk of neutropenia, the use of prophylactic growth factors during therapy is also recommended.
- Cisplatin (75 mg/m^2) plus paclitaxel (135 mg/m^2 over 24 hours) every 3 weeks for six cycles. Dose-dense treatment comprises carboplatin (AUC = 6 on day 1) and weekly paclitaxel (80 mg/m^2 days 1, 8 and 15) every 3 weeks for six cycles.

There is currently no role for the addition of a third chemotherapeutic agent in addition to carboplatin and paclitaxel. A randomized, phase 3 trial conducted by the GOG (2001) has shown that the combination of IV paclitaxel with IP cisplatin in comparison with IV paclitaxel plus cisplatin alone is likely to improve survival in patients with optimally debulked stage III ovarian cancer.

Alternative regimens include the following:

- *Incorporation of angiogenesis inhibitors (bevacizumab):* Presently, there has been increased interest toward the incorporation of angiogenesis inhibitors (bevacizumab) and other VEGF targeting agents into the first-line treatment for patients with EOCs. This medication is being used not only as the primary modality of treatment, but also for maintenance, consolidation and in cases of recurrence. Bevacizumab is humanized monoclonal antibody which binds with VEGF, thereby preventing it from binding to its receptor. This blocks growth and maintenance of blood vessels feeding the cancer cells. The Gynecologic Cancer Inter Group (GCIG) ICON 7 (International Collaborative Ovarian Neoplasm) trial, a multicentric RCT and the complementary GOG-0218 (ClinicalTrials.gov number, NCT00262847) have indicated that incorporation of bevacizumab to platinum and taxane-based chemotherapy improves progression-free survival but not the overall survival rates or the quality of life in patients with stage IV disease and those with residual disease following surgery. Therefore, the use of angiogenesis inhibitors along with chemotherapy in the first-line setting for treatment of EOC is presently not recommended by most clinicians. It is administered in the dosage of 15 mg/kg body weight every 3 weekly for 6 cycles. Women with EOCs who are treated with bevacizumab may be associated with complications such as new or worsening hypertension, proteinuria, thrombotic events, bleeding, altered wound healing, and gastrointestinal perforation. As a result, monitoring with investigations such as hemogram, LFT, and KFT must be done when administering this drug. Early detection of these complications, especially gastrointestinal perforation might help in reducing the morbidity and mortality associated with the use of bevacizumab.

- *Novel angiogenesis-inhibiting agents:* There have been several ongoing clinical trials evaluating other antiangiogenic agents for treatment of women with EOC. Some of these agents are enumerated in **Table 31.8**.

NEOADJUVANT CHEMOTHERAPY PROTOCOL

This involves administration of systemic chemotherapy prior to definite surgery in cases of enhanced (stage 3) EOC. This involves administration of three to four cycles of chemotherapy prior to debulking surgery. Another six cycles of chemotherapy are administered following the surgery.

Primary surgery versus interval debulking surgery following neoadjuvant chemotherapy in advanced-stage disease: Two multicentric randomized trials, European Organisation for Research and Treatment of Cancer (EORTC) and chemotherapy or upfront surgery (CHORUS) have investigated whether the strategy of performing primary surgery followed by chemotherapy or that of performing interval debulking surgery after neoadjuvant chemotherapy (three to four cycles of chemotherapy administered prior to surgery) is likely to result in better survival rates and a more complete cytoreductive surgery. The results of these trials have shown that the patients undergoing primary cytoreductive surgery followed by chemotherapy are likely to have similar outcomes in terms of survival to the patients, with advanced ovarian cancer, or those with poor performance status or those with large tumor burden, undergoing interval debulking surgery following neoadjuvant chemotherapy. Interval debulking is associated with reduced morbidity and lesser number of major resections. Patients with no residual disease following cytoreductive surgery and those who respond to platinum-based chemotherapy (platinum-sensitive) are likely to have a better survival rate. Results from the EORTC trial have also shown that the patients with stage IIIC and less extensive metastatic tumors are likely to have higher survival rates with primary surgery, in comparison to those with stage IV disease and large metastatic tumors.

Benefits: Neoadjuvant chemotherapy is likely to be associated with the following advantages:
- No survival benefits
- Reduced surgical morbidity
- Allows optimal debulking
- Reduced postoperative complications
- Chances of tumor assessment for platinum sensitivity.

TREATMENT OF RECURRENT DISEASE

The management in case of relapsed or recurrent ovarian cancer is decided based upon the platinum-free interval (PFI). This can be defined as the extent of time that has passed between the completion of platinum-based treatment and the recognition of the disease relapse. Based on the amount of PFI, patients can be classified as follows:
- *Patients with a PFI of 6 months or longer:* Such patients are considered to have "platinum-sensitive" **(Table 31.9)**

TABLE 31.8: Novel angiogenesis inhibiting agents.

Angiogenesis inhibiting agents	Description
Aflibercept (VEGF-Trap)	A fusion protein which binds to both VEGF receptors, VEGFR1 and VEGFR2
AMG386	An angiopoietin antagonist (peptide-Fc fusion protein) which prevents angiopoietin-1 and angiopoietin-2 from binding to their tyrosine kinase receptors
Nintedanib (BIBF 1120)	An oral angiokinase inhibitor which aims at VEGFR-1, -2, and -3, PDGFR-alpha/beta, FGFR-1, -2, and -3, members of the sarcoma viral oncogene homolog (Src) family, and fms-like tyrosine kinase 3
Pazopanib	A novel antiangiogenic agent which specifically targets VEGFR-1, -2, and -3, PDGFR-alfa/beta, FGFR-1 and -3, and c-kit
Cediranib (AZD 2171)	A novel antiangiogenic agent which specifically targets VEGFR-1, -2, and -3, PDGFR-alfa/beta, FGFR-1, and c-kit

(FGFR: fibroblast growth factor receptors; PDGFR: platelet-derived growth factor receptors; VEGFR: vascular endothelial growth factor receptors)

TABLE 31.9: Response of the tumor to therapy with platinum.

Response to platinum	Description
Platinum-sensitive tumor	No occurrence of tumor up to 12 months of chemotherapy (disease free interval of 12 months)
Platinum-resistant	Reoccurrence of tumor within 6 months of completion of chemotherapy (disease free interval of <6 months)
Platinum-refractory	Tumor recurrence occurs within 4 weeks of administration of chemotherapy
Partial-sensitivity	Tumor recurrence occurs with 6–12 months of completion of chemotherapy

disease. A combination of cisplatin and taxol is the drug of choice in these cases.

- *Patients with a PFI of <6 months:* Such patients are considered to have "platinum-resistant" disease. For the patients who experience disease recurrence, chemotherapy is the mainstay of treatment. Surgery is reserved only for selective cases. Patients with "platinum-sensitive" disease have a high probability of responding again to platinum-based treatment at the time of relapse.

For women with recurrent "platinum-resistant" disease, second-line chemotherapy comprising of combinations different to carboplatin, with or without the addition of taxol, are usually indicated. Sequential single agent chemotherapy with pegylated liposomal doxorubicin, which is not associated with significant side effects (e.g., hair loss, myelosuppression, etc.), is usually used in 4-weekly cycles. Single agent regimens are usually adopted due to their ease of administration and low toxicity. Other chemotherapeutic agents without cross-resistance, which can be used in these cases, include gemcitabine, anthracyclines, topoisomerase inhibitors (etoposide and topotecan) and others (e.g., tamoxifen).

Second-line chemotherapy regimens are associated with a much lower response rate in comparison to the first-line chemotherapeutic regimens.

Role of Surgery for Recurrent Disease

Surgery can be employed for recurrent disease in the following cases:
- Progression free interval of at least 12 months
- Optimum resection appears possible
- Response to first-line therapy was good
- Good performance status
- Locally recurrent EOC.

HYPERTHERMIC INTRAPERITONEAL CHEMOTHERAPY

Hyperthermic intraperitoneal chemotherapy (HIPEC) is administered intraoperatively and serves as a treatment option for advanced surface spread of cancer within the abdomen. This therapy involves peroperative IP infusion of cisplatin in the dosage of 70 mg/m^2 in 1 L of saline solution heated to 40–42°C. This fluid is allowed to remain inside for about 1–1.5 hours, following which it is removed. Systemic chemotherapy is administered after 2–4 weeks. Prophylactic antibiotics are administered for a week. Liquid diet can be given to the patient after 3 days of therapy.

Advantages

Hyperthermic intraperitoneal chemotherapy is associated with the advantages listed in **Box 31.10**.

> **BOX 31.10:** Advantages of hyperthermic intraperitoneal chemotherapy (HIPEC).
>
> - Direct delivery of cytotoxic drug to cancer cells
> - Improved absorption of the drug by the cancer cells due to heated solution
> - High peritoneal concentration of the drug
> - Lesions 2–3 mm or smaller are likely to be exposed to high drug concentrations
> - Systemic toxicity is much less
> - Avascular tumors are likely to be associated with high drug concentrations

FOLLOW-UP AFTER TREATMENT FOR OVARIAN CANCER

Presently, there is no optimal follow-up protocol for cases of ovarian cancer. Follow-up protocol depends upon parameters such as disease staging, type and extent of surgery, and the patient's performance status. Generally, the follow-up is done every monthly for 3 months, 6-monthly for a year and yearly for the lifetime. Each follow-up visit must involve taking a detailed history and clinical examination. PVR (prevaginal rectal) examination must be done to assess the anal canal for oresence of any nodular masses in the rectum. Follow-up also involves vault smear and regular tests to check the level of CA-125 in the patient's blood. PET-CT is useful investigation to help deduct any recurrence. Often, the CA-125 level will begin to rise before any clinical symptoms suggestive of cancer recurrence develop. In the MRC OV05/EORTC 55955 collaborative trial, it was shown that institution of early treatment on the basis of increased CA-125 concentrations is not likely to be associated with a survival benefit in comparison with delayed treatment on the basis of clinical recurrence. Therefore, the value of routine measurement of CA-125 in the follow-up of patients with ovarian cancer who attain a complete response after first-line treatment presently remains unclear.

Therefore, presently, the measurement of CA-125 levels has limited role in deciding the management of cancer recurrence. As a result, presently the treatment for cancer recurrence is delayed until she starts showing symptoms, or the results of an examination or scan make it clear that the cancer has come back. Different types of tumor markers **(Table 31.10)**, based on the histological pattern of the tumor, are being tried under research settings. If the cancer comes back, treatment is usually given with chemotherapy. Many different types of chemotherapy can be used for women in this situation. The same chemotherapy drugs that were given initially can be used or different ones may be tried. Occasionally, it may be possible to remove tumors using surgery. Radiotherapy may be used to treat particular areas or to relieve symptoms.

TABLE 31.10: Different types of tumor markers being tried to detect cancer recurrence.

Epithelial tumors	Germ cell tumors	Stromal tumors
• CA 125 antigen • BRCA-1 and BRCA-2 • Carcinoembryonic antigen • Galactosyltransferase • Tissue polypeptide antigen	• Alpha-fetoprotein • Human chorionic gonadotropin	• Inhibin

BOX 31.11: Factors affecting the prognosis of ovarian cancer.

- The stage of the cancer
- The type and size of the tumor
- The patient's age and general health
- Whether the cancer has been diagnosed for the first time or there has been cancer recurrence

COMPLICATIONS

- *Poor prognosis:* Cancer of the ovaries has the worst prognosis in comparison to any other type of gynecologic cancer. As a result, it is the fifth most common cause of cancer deaths in women. Some factors, which may affect prognosis in cases of ovarian cancer, are listed in **Box 31.11**.

- *Metastasis:* The ovarian cancer is one of the most aggressive types of cancers, which can spread directly to the surrounding tissues, through the lymphatic system to other parts of the pelvis and abdomen and through the bloodstream to the distant body organs, mainly the liver and lungs.

- Ascites and/or pleural effusion and/or peritonitis

- *Side effects related to chemotherapy:* These include anorexia, bone marrow damage, constipation, diarrhea, hair loss, increased risk of infection, etc.

- *Premature menopause:* TAH with BSO for ovarian cancer in a patient who has yet not attained menopause is likely to result in premature menopause, resulting in symptoms such as hot flushes, dry skin, reduced sexual desire, and dryness of the vagina, which can make sexual intercourse uncomfortable. Such women should be prescribed HRT following treatment for ovarian cancer. This could help in reducing some of the problems caused by premature menopause.

EVIDENCE-BASED CLINICAL TRIALS

List of references can be scanned through QR code to enable the readers gain deeper insight of the subject by referring to the entire article or its abstract.

CHAPTER 32

Ectopic Pregnancy

CASE STUDY

A 24-year-old nulliparous woman, married since last 1 year, presented with 3 months' amenorrhea to the A&E department with vaginal bleeding and severe abdominal pain particularly confined to the left iliac fossa since past few hours. She had done a home pregnancy test, which was positive. Vaginal examination revealed cervical motion tenderness and a normal-sized uterus. An ultrasound examination and urine human chorionic gonadotropin (hCG) levels were ordered. Urine hCG levels were found to be raised and TVS examination revealed an adnexal mass (about 1 cm in size) and an empty uterus.

INTRODUCTION

> Q. Write a long note discussing the etiology and pathology of ectopic pregnancy.
>
> Q. Discuss in detail he etiopathogenesis of tubal ectopic pregnancy.

Ectopic means "out of place." In an ectopic pregnancy, the fertilized ovum gets implanted outside the uterus as a result of which the pregnancy occurs outside the uterine cavity **(Fig. 32.1)**. It usually occurs as a result of delay or prevention in passage of the blastocyst to the uterine cavity, resulting in its premature implantation in the extrauterine tissues.

Most commonly, i.e., in nearly 95% of cases, the fertilized ovum gets implanted inside the fallopian tube. The ovum buries into the tube and induces a decidual reaction in the cells of the endosalpinx. However, this reaction is feeble. Also, there occurs invasion of the trophoblastic cells into the wall of the fallopian tube. As a result, there is a high risk of choriodecidual hemorrhage and erosion or rupture of the tube wall.

Since the uterus itself is under the influence of the hormones of corpus luteum and trophoblast, there occurs generalized enlargement, increased vascularity, tissue hypertrophy, and decidual reaction in the endometrium.

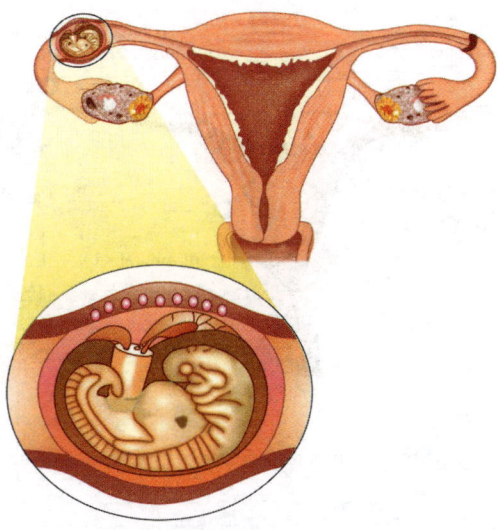

Fig. 32.1: Ectopic pregnancy.

TABLE 32.1: Average incidence for site of implantation of ectopic pregnancy at various locations.

Extrauterine location	Incidence of occurrence
Fallopian tube	95–96%
• Ampulla (middle portion of tube): 70% • Isthmus (part of the tube closer to the uterus): 12% • Infundibulum/fimbria (distal portion of tube): 11% • Cornual/interstitial (within the uterine muscles): 2%	
Ovarian	<3%
Cervical	<1%
Abdominal • Primary • Secondary [intraperitoneal or extraperitoneal (broad ligament)]	0.9–1.4%
Cesarean scar	<1%
Intramural	<1%
Heterotopic (combination of ectopic and intrauterine pregnancies)	1–3%

Other extrauterine locations where an ectopic pregnancy can get implanted include the ovary, abdomen, or cervix. Average incidence for occurrence of pregnancy at various locations is enumerated in **Table 32.1** and is also shown in

Figure 32.2. The incidence of ectopic pregnancy ranges from 1 in 25 to 1 in 250, with the average being 1 in 100. Assisted reproductive techniques (ARTs) may be associated with >5% cases of ectopic pregnancy.

The extrauterine locations do not have sufficient space or nurturing tissues to support a growing pregnancy. Since none of these areas have been equipped by nature to support a growing pregnancy, with the continuing growth of the fetus, the gestational sac and the organ containing it burst open **(Figs. 32.3A to D)**. This can result in severe bleeding, sometimes even endangering the woman's life. A classical ectopic pregnancy normally does not develop into a live birth. Although spontaneous resolution of ectopic pregnancy can sometimes occur, patients are at risk of tubal rupture and catastrophic hemorrhage. Ectopic pregnancy is estimated to occur in 2% of all pregnancies. It remains a major cause of maternal morbidity and mortality when misdiagnosed or left untreated.

COURSE OF ECTOPIC PREGNANCY

On an average, the isthmic pregnancy may survive for 6–8 weeks, ampullary pregnancy for 8–12 weeks, and interstitial pregnancy for about 4 months. The ectopic pregnancy is likely to have the following outcomes:

- *Tubal abortion:* The pregnancy gets aborted/expelled out through the tubal fimbria. It may either get completely absorbed or there may be complete or incomplete abortion. If the internal bleeding continues to occur, the condition may become symptomatic. Severe intra-abdominal bleeding may require immediate surgical intervention. No further treatment may be required in cases with minimal bleeding. While tubal abortion is more common in ampullary pregnancies, rupture is most likely in isthmic pregnancies.
- *Tubal mole:* The embryo dies due to faulty environment and gets converted into a carneous mole.
- *Tubal rupture:* The fallopian tube may rupture due to its thin lumen at the isthmus and ampulla. The lumen is incapable of distension due to burrowing in and erosion

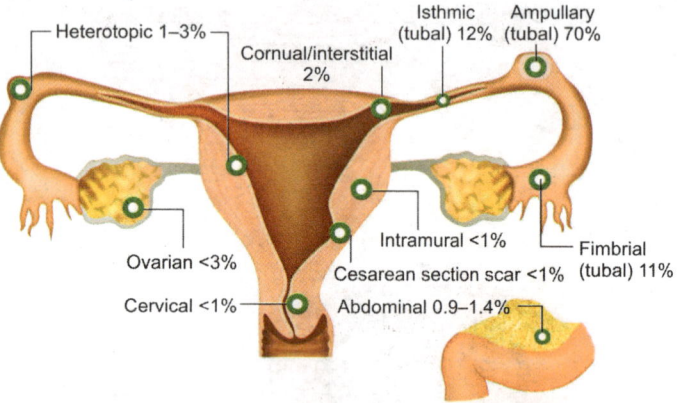

Fig. 32.2: Common sites for occurrence of ectopic pregnancy.

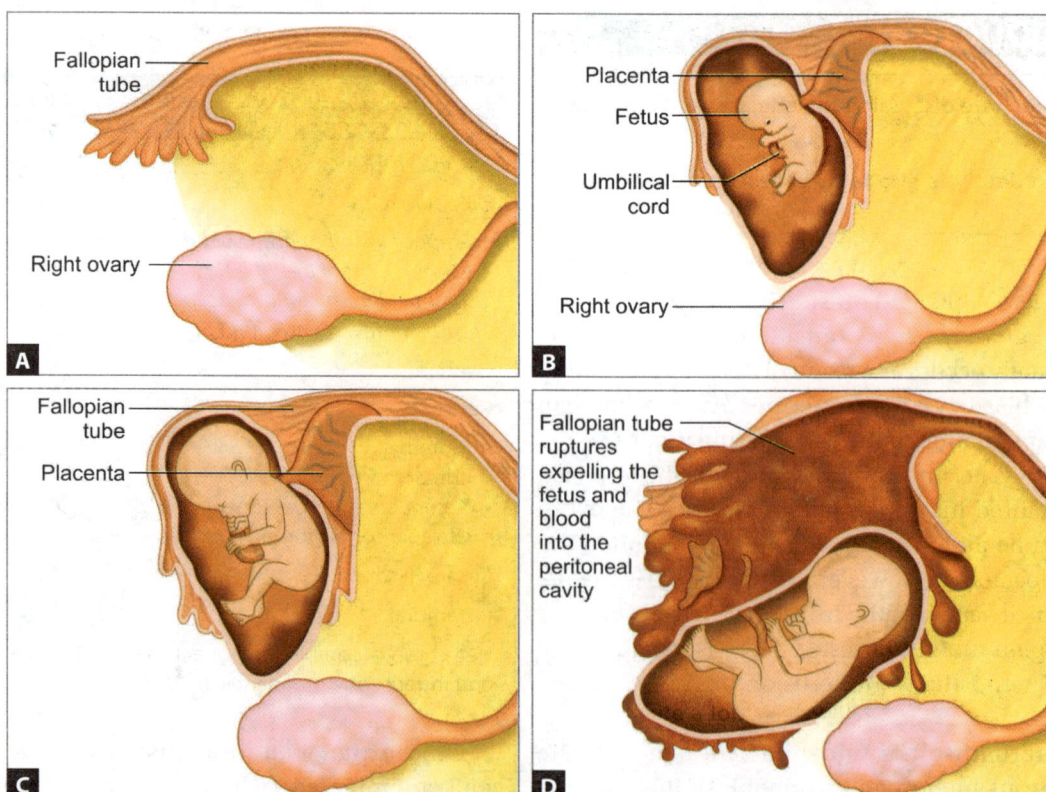

Figs. 32.3A to D: Course of ectopic pregnancy with the increasing gestational age. (A) Condition of tube before pregnancy; (B) Condition at 8 weeks' ectopic pregnancy; (C) Condition at 12 weeks' ectopic pregnancy; (D) Ultimate condition: ruptured ectopic pregnancy.

> **BOX 32.1:** Factors associated with an increased risk of rupture.
> - History of never having used any contraception
> - History of tubal damage, infertility, induction of ovulation, etc.
> - High level of human chorionic gonadotropin (at least 10,000 IU/L)

by the blastocyst. Factors which are associated with an increased risk of rupture in suspected cases of ectopic pregnancy are listed in **Box 32.1**.

Tubal rupture is usually intraperitoneal and may result in severe bleeding and partial or complete extrusion of chorionic villi, resulting in hemodynamic instability and shock-like features. Rarely, the rupture may be extraperitoneal. If the rupture occurs in the broad ligament, this may result in the development of a broad ligament hematoma. Tubal rupture may cause intense hemorrhage, which can prove to be fatal if emergency laparotomy is not performed. Salpingectomy is the most commonly used surgical approach when the tube has ruptured. Ruptured ectopic pregnancy is the most important cause of maternal mortality in the first trimester. Therefore, it is important to identify and manage tubal pregnancy well before it ruptures.

- *Chronic ectopic adnexal mass:* The products of conception are partially extruded out through the fimbriae or partial rupture. After a slight or moderate bleeding, the hemorrhage may get arrested and result in the formation of an adnexal mass involving the tube and ovaries.
- *Fetal survival to term*: This usually does not occur as the fetus is commonly unable to develop beyond 6 weeks of gestation.
- *Spontaneous resolution:* In some cases, the ectopic pregnancy may just regress spontaneously on its own. Such patients can be safely managed expectantly, without requiring any surgical or medical intervention. It is difficult to predict which patients will experience uncomplicated spontaneous resolution. Women who are hemodynamically stable and have an initial hCG concentration of <2,000 IU/L, which may be found to be declining, appear to be the likely candidates who may experience uncomplicated spontaneous resolution.

HISTORY AND CLINICAL PRESENTATION

RISK FACTORS

The risk factors/etiological factors for ectopic pregnancy are listed below and described in detail. These need to be elicited at the time of taking history:

- *Idiopathic:* One-third of ectopic pregnancies occur in women with no known risk factors.
- *Prior history of an ectopic pregnancy:* This can be considered as the most important risk factor for the occurrence of ectopic pregnancy. The risk of future ectopic pregnancy is about 15% after the first ectopic pregnancy, and 25% after the second.
- *History of pelvic infections, including infections such as PID, STD, salpingitis, and tuberculosis:* Infection in the pelvis is an important risk factor for ectopic pregnancy and increases the risk by 6–10 times. Pelvic infections may be caused by sexually transmitted organisms, such as chlamydia or gonorrhea, with chlamydial being the most common cause. However, nonsexually transmitted bacteria (e.g., tuberculosis) can also cause pelvic infection and increase the risk of an ectopic pregnancy. Infection causes ectopic pregnancy by damaging the tubal ciliary epithelium or obstructing the fallopian tubes, causing delay in transport of the fertilized ovum along the fallopian tube. Additionally, infection-related scarring and partial blockage of the fallopian tubes are likely to further prevent the movement of fertilized ovum into the uterine cavity.
- *Tubal surgery:* Prior surgeries to the fallopian tubes, including tubal reconstructive surgery, tubal sterilization, reversal of tubal sterilization, etc. Risk of ectopic pregnancy with failure of tubal sterilization is based on the technique used and the patient's age, with the risk being 65% with the failure of bipolar cauterization, 29% with the failure of silicon rubber band, 43% with failure of interval salpingectomy, and 20% with the failure of postpartum salpingectomy. Risk of ectopic pregnancy with reversal of sterilization methods is based on the method used at the time of sterilization, site of tubal occlusion, and residual tubal length. While reanastomosis of cauterized tube is associated with 15% risk, reversal of Pomeroy's method is associated with <3% risk of ectopic pregnancy. On the other hand, tubal reconstructive surgery may be associated with four to five times increased risk of ectopic pregnancy.
- *Endometriosis and pelvic scar tissue (pelvic adhesions):* This can further narrow the fallopian tubes and disrupt the transportation of egg, thereby increasing the chances of an ectopic pregnancy.
- Fibroid tumor of the uterus
- *Failure of IUCDs and progesterone-only hormonal contraception:* Pregnancy occurring even after the use of contraception is more likely to be ectopic in nature. Risk of ectopic pregnancy associated with failure of various methods of contraception is as follows:
  - *CuT*: 4%
  - *Progestasert*: 17%
  - *Minipills*: 4–10%
  - *Norplant*: 30%

The use of progesterone-only hormonal contraceptive devices is likely to cause altered tubal mobility, resulting in the development of ectopic pregnancy. The use of an IUCD per se does not increase the risk of ectopic pregnancy. However, a normal pregnancy is unlikely with an IUD in place, so if a woman becomes pregnant while using an IUCD, it is more likely to be ectopic.

- *Congenital abnormalities of tubes:* These may include abnormalities such as tubal hypoplasia/tortuosity, congenital diverticula, accessory ostia, tubal stenosis, tubal elongation, and intramural polyps.
- *Smoking:* It is a risk factor in about one-third of ectopic pregnancies and may contribute to decreased tubal motility by causing damage to the ciliated cells in the fallopian tubes.
- *Assisted reproductive techniques:* Infertility problems and the use of ovulation induction drugs and techniques for assisted conception such as ovulation induction (especially using gonadotropins), IVF-embryo transfer (ET), and gamete intrafallopian transfer (GIFT) (4–7% risk for ectopic pregnancy) are likely to increase the risk for ectopic pregnancy. ART may also increase the risk of heterotopic pregnancy by as high as 1%.
- Patients who have had several induced abortions
- Having multiple sexual partners also increases the risk of an ectopic pregnancy.

CLINICAL PRESENTATION

Ectopic pregnancy can be difficult to diagnose in the beginning because symptoms are often very similar to those of a normal early pregnancy. These can include missed periods, breast tenderness, nausea, vomiting, or frequent urination. In cases of acute ectopic pregnancy, patients can present with a wide spectrum of clinical presentation from asymptomatic appearance at one end of the spectrum to the patient in shock with acute abdomen at the other end of the spectrum. Patients may often experience symptoms such as nausea, vomiting, fainting attack, and syncope due to reflex vasomotor disturbances.

The typical triad on history for ectopic pregnancy includes bleeding, abdominal pain, and a positive pregnancy test result. The classical symptoms of ectopic pregnancy, which can occur in both ruptured and unruptured cases, are listed in **Box 32.2**. Of these, pain is the most consistent feature, present in nearly 95% patients. Pain may be variable in nature. Amenorrhea is another symptom which is often encountered. Nearly 60–80% patients may present with delayed periods or slight spotting at the time of expected menses. Vaginal bleeding is likely to be scanty and dark brown in color.

BOX 32.2: The classical triad of symptoms in cases of acute ectopic pregnancy.
- Abdominal pain
- Amenorrhea
- Vaginal bleeding

However, while these symptoms are typical for an acute ectopic pregnancy, they do not imply that an ectopic pregnancy is necessarily present and could also represent other conditions. In fact, these symptoms may also be associated with a threatened abortion in nonectopic pregnancies. The symptoms of an ectopic pregnancy typically occur 6–8 weeks after the last normal menstrual period, but they may occur later, if the ectopic pregnancy is not located in the fallopian tube.

When bleeding occurs, the clinical presentation can be suggestive of miscarriage. Many women with ectopic pregnancy may show no signs and symptoms. As a result, almost half of the cases are not diagnosed at the time of the first prenatal visit. Pain may be felt in the pelvis, abdomen, lower back, or sometimes may even be referred to the patient's shoulder or neck, especially in cases of hematoperitoneum. Most women describe the pain as sharp and stabbing in nature. It may be confined to one side of the pelvis and may come and go or vary in intensity. Acute blood loss in some cases may result in the development of dizziness or fainting and hypotension. Malaise, weakness, dizziness, and a sense of passing out on standing can represent serious internal bleeding, and mandates immediate laparotomy. Leakage of blood from the fallopian tube may cause irritation of the diaphragm, resulting in shoulder pain. Moreover, pooling of blood in pouch of Douglas (POD) may cause an urge to defecate.

On the other hand, diagnosis of chronic ectopic pregnancy is made on clinical suspicion. The patient usually presents with a history of having an attack of acute pain in abdomen from which she has recovered. She may present with a period of amenorrhea, vaginal bleeding, dull pain in the abdomen, and bowel and bladder complaints such as dysuria, increased frequency or retention of urine, and rectal tenesmus.

GENERAL PHYSICAL EXAMINATION

Though the physical examination may be completely unremarkable in a woman with a small, unruptured ectopic gestation, following signs are usually observed on general physical examination in cases of unruptured ectopic gestation:

- Normal signs of early pregnancy (e.g., uterine softening and breast changes)
- Abdominal pain and tenderness
  On the other hand, a patient with ruptured ectopic pregnancy in shock may appear restless, in extreme agony, may look blanched, pale, and may be sweating with cold clammy skin.
- Extreme abdominal pain and tenderness
- Evidence of hemodynamic instability (hypotension, tachycardia, collapse, signs and symptoms of shock)

- *Hypotension*: Low blood pressure could be related to significant amount of intraperitoneal bleeding. In severe cases, even shock may be present.
- Signs of peritoneal irritation (abdominal rigidity and guarding)

SPECIFIC SYSTEMIC EXAMINATION

ABDOMINAL EXAMINATION

Significant abdominal tenderness suggests ruptured ectopic pregnancy, especially in a patient with hypotension who presents with rigidity, guarding, and rebound tenderness. Abdomen is tense, and there may be shifting dullness, especially if free fluid is present in the peritoneal cavity.

The signs of unruptured ectopic pregnancy on examination include lower abdominal tenderness with or without rebound and pelvic tenderness, usually much worse on the affected side.

PELVIC EXAMINATION

The following findings may be observed on vaginal examination:
- Vaginal bleeding may be observed on per speculum examination. Many a times, there may be minimal bleeding.
- Uterine or cervical motion tenderness on vaginal examination may suggest peritoneal inflammation.
- Uterus may be soft, bulky, and deviated to opposite side.
- Uterine size does not correspond to the period of gestation.
- Adnexal mass may be palpated in the fornix (with or without tenderness).
- POD may appear full, and uterus may appear as if it is floating in water.

The presence of a normal or slightly enlarged uterus and a palpable adnexal mass on vaginal examination and symptoms such as vaginal bleeding and pelvic pain with manipulation of the cervix significantly increase the likelihood of an ectopic pregnancy. Clinical examinations are not diagnostic because up to 30% of patients with ectopic pregnancies may have no vaginal bleeding, 90% may have a palpable adnexal mass, and up to 10% have negative pelvic examinations. The overall likelihood of ectopic pregnancy is nearly 39% in a patient with abdominal pain and vaginal bleeding but no other risk factors. The probability of ectopic pregnancy increases to 54% if the patient has other risk factors (e.g., history of tubal surgery, ectopic pregnancy, or PID, or an IUCD in situ at the time of conception). Gynecologists should therefore remember that no combination of physical examination findings can reliably exclude ectopic pregnancy. Abdominal rigidity, involuntary guarding, and severe tenderness as well as evidence of hypovolemic shock, such as orthostatic blood pressure changes and tachycardia, should alert the clinician to a surgical emergency; this may occur in up to 20% of cases.

TABLE 32.2: Differential diagnoses of ectopic pregnancy.

Obstetric causes	Gynecological causes	Nongynecological causes
• Threatened or incomplete miscarriage • Molar gestation • Septic abortion • Early pregnancy with pelvic tumors	• Ovarian/adnexal torsion • PID • Ruptured or hemorrhagic corpus luteum • Salpingitis • Degenerating fibroids/torsion of pedunculated fibroids • Abnormal uterine bleeding • Endometriosis • Tubo-ovarian abscess	• Appendicitis • Cholecystitis • Diverticulitis • Splenic rupture • Urinary calculi/renal colic • Urinary tract infection • Gastroenteritis • Intraperitoneal hemorrhage • Perforated peptic ulcer

(PID: pelvic inflammatory disease)

DIFFERENTIAL DIAGNOSIS

The possible differential diagnoses in cases of ectopic pregnancy are listed in **Table 32.2**.

MANAGEMENT

Q. What is the most likely diagnosis in the case study mentioned in the beginning of the chapter? What would be the best treatment option in this case?
Ans. The patient is young and desires future pregnancy. Since the patient is hemodynamically stable and no cardiac activity was observed on ultrasound examination, the two most commonly used treatment modalities, which can be considered in this case, include medical and surgical options (laparoscopic salpingostomy).

Nowadays most cases of early unruptured tubal ectopic pregnancy can be successfully treated either with minimally invasive surgery or with medical management using methotrexate (MTX). Various treatment options used nowadays in cases of ectopic pregnancy are summarized in **Table 32.3**. Whenever the tubal ectopic pregnancy is diagnosed or suspected, the patient should be admitted immediately to the hospital. If the patient is in a state of shock, it needs to be treated first. Transfusion with blood, plasma, or substitutes needs to be arranged as soon as possible. If the patient is in shock, resuscitation and surgery at the same time can be lifesaving. Immediate laparotomy and clamping of the bleeding vessels may be the only way of saving the life of a moribund patient. Management plan for a patient with suspected ectopic pregnancy has been summarized in **Flowchart 32.1**. Presently, laparoscopic surgery has become the standard surgical approach for

TABLE 32.3: Various treatment options used nowadays in cases of ectopic pregnancy.		
Expectant management	**Medical management**	**Surgical management**
Awaiting spontaneous resolution of tubal ectopic pregnancy (tubal abortion): • Monitoring of β-hCG levels • Monitoring the patient for signs of shock/rupture	*Systemic therapy:* • Methotrexate *SAM therapy:* Local (ultrasound or laparoscopic salpingocentesis): • Methotrexate • Potassium chloride • Hyperosmolar glucose • Mifepristone • Prostaglandins (PG $F_{2\alpha}$) • Actinomycin D	*Radical management:* Salpingectomy (laparoscopic/laparotomy) *Conservative management:* • Salpingostomy • Salpingotomy • Segmental resection • Milking or fimbrial expression

(hCG: human chorionic gonadotropin; PG $F_{2\alpha}$: prostaglandin $F_{2\alpha}$; SAM: surgically administered medical)

management of ectopic pregnancy. Most cases of ectopic pregnancies, even in the presence of hemoperitoneum, heterotopic pregnancy, or interstitial pregnancy, may be treated by a laparoscopic procedure. However, the type of surgical approach adopted depends on the surgeon's preference and expertise in laparoscopy. The use of single-port laparoscopy [also referred to as laparoendoscopic single-site surgery (LESS)] for ectopic pregnancy is also being employed at some places.

INVESTIGATIONS

Diagnosis of acute ectopic pregnancy is mainly made based on the findings of clinical examination. The following investigations must be done in the suspected cases of ectopic pregnancy.

BLOOD GROUP TYPING (ABO AND RH TYPE)

Blood typing (ABO and Rh) and antibody screen should be done in all pregnant patients with bleeding to identify Rh-negative pregnant patients in whom bleeding would be associated with an increased risk of Rh isoimmunization. Such patients require to be injected with 50 μg of anti-D immune globulins (RhoGAM) to prevent the occurrence of hemolytic disease of the newborn. Blood must be typed and crossed in order to ensure availability of blood products in case of excessive blood loss. Hemoglobin or hematocrit levels must be measured serially in order to quantify blood loss.

COMPLETE BLOOD COUNT

Estimation of hemoglobin and/or hematocrit must be done in these patients for evaluation of maternal anemia. In cases of tubal rupture with severe intra-abdominal bleeding, measurement of platelet count and/or coagulation tests is also indicated. If administration of MTX is considered in cases of unruptured ectopic gestation, a CBC must be done as a part of the pretreatment laboratory evaluation.

URINE OR SERUM BETA HUMAN CHORIONIC GONADOTROPIN LEVELS

In the emergency department, pregnancy is diagnosed by determining the levels of β-hCG in the urine or serum. This hormone may be detected in the urine and blood as early as 1 week before an expected menstrual period. While urine testing may detect levels up to 20–50 IU/L, serum testing may detect levels as low as 5 IU/L. In most cases of suspected ectopic pregnancy, screening is initially done with urine pregnancy test. Determination of serum β-hCG levels is a time-consuming procedure and may not be a practical option at the time of emergency. However, if pregnancy is strongly suspected, even when the urine pregnancy test has a negative result, serum testing becomes necessary. Single serum β-hCG levels are of little value in predicting ectopic pregnancy. The quantitative level of β-hCG found in ectopic pregnancy varies. In a normal pregnancy, the β-hCG levels double every 48–72 hours until they reach 10,000–20,000 mIU/mL. Normal intrauterine pregnancies are associated with a doubling time of 1.4–2.1 days. Diagnosis of biochemical pregnancy is made in women. According to the ACOG recommendations (2018), an increase in serum hCG of <53% in 48 hours confirms an abnormal pregnancy. The increase in hCG concentration is at a much slower rate in most, but not all, cases of ectopic and nonviable intrauterine pregnancies. A falling, slow-rising, or plateauing hCG concentration is most consistent with a failed pregnancy (e.g., anembryonic pregnancy, tubal abortion, spontaneously resolving ectopic pregnancy, and complete or incomplete abortion).

A single serum measurement of the β-hCG concentration, however, cannot definitely identify the presence of an intrauterine gestational sac. Although women with an ectopic pregnancy tend to have lower β-hCG levels than those with an intrauterine pregnancy (IUP), there is considerable overlap. Therefore, serial β-hCG measurement is often used for women with first-trimester bleeding or pain, or both. However, similar to a single measurement, serial measurement of β-hCG levels also cannot confirm the intrauterine location of the

Flowchart 32.1: Management of patients with suspected diagnosis of ectopic pregnancy.

(β-hCG: beta human chorionic gonadotropin; EP: ectopic pregnancy; IUP: intrauterine pregnancy)

gestational sac. In a patient with a subnormal increase in β-hCG concentration, nonviability is assumed, and more invasive investigations must be used for differentiating between miscarriage and ectopic pregnancy. Though the falling β-hCG levels confirm nonviability, at the same time they do not rule out ectopic pregnancy. The lack of an IUP when the β-hCG level is above the discriminatory zone represents an ectopic pregnancy or a recent abortion.

Discriminatory Zone of Beta Human Chorionic Gonadotropin

The discriminatory zone of β-hCG is the level above which a normal IUP is reliably visualized in nearly 100% cases. Ectopic pregnancy is suspected if TAS does not show an intrauterine gestational sac and the patient's β-hCG level is >6,500 mIU/mL (6,500 IU/L) or if TVS does not show an intrauterine gestational sac and the patient's β-hCG level is 1,500 mIU/mL (1,500 IU/L) or greater.

A negative ultrasound examination at hCG levels below the discriminatory zone is suggestive of an early viable IUP or an ectopic pregnancy or nonviable IUP. Such cases where the location of gestational sac (whether intrauterine or extrauterine) cannot be identified on ultrasound examination are termed as "pregnancy of unknown location."

Serum Human Chorionic Gonadotropin Levels Above the Discriminatory Zone

Visualization of an intrauterine gestational sac at serum hCG levels above the discriminatory zone almost always excludes the presence of an ectopic pregnancy. However, there may be some exceptions to this rule such as heterotopic pregnancy, or the pregnancy in a rudimentary uterine horn or cornual pregnancy.

Diagnosis of an extrauterine pregnancy is almost certain if there is an absence of an intrauterine gestational sac and presence of a complex adnexal mass at hCG concentrations above the discriminatory zone. The presence of embryonic cardiac activity or a definite yolk sac in this adnexal mass is a certain evidence of an ectopic gestation. In these cases, treatment of ectopic pregnancy should be started.

The diagnosis is less certain if there is an absence of a complex adnexal mass or an intrauterine gestational sac on ultrasound examination with serum hCG levels > 1,500 IU/L. The absence of intrauterine gestational sac in the presence of serum β-hCG levels above the discriminatory zone may sometimes be indicative of a multiple gestation, since there is no proven discriminatory level for multiple gestations. Therefore, in these cases, TVS examination and serum β-hCG concentration must be repeated again after 2 days. If an IUP is still not observed on TVS, then the pregnancy is abnormal. In these cases, serial follow-up with serum β-hCG levels is required:

- If the serum hCG concentration is observed to be increasing or has plateaued, treatment for ectopic pregnancy can be instituted.
- If the serum hCG concentration is observed to be decreasing, this is most consistent with a failed pregnancy (e.g., miscarriage, blighted ovum, and tubal abortion). The rate of fall is slower with an ectopic pregnancy than with a complete abortion. Weekly hCG concentrations should be monitored in these cases until the serum hCG levels become undetectable.

Serum Human Chorionic Gonadotropin Levels Below the Discriminatory Zone

In case serum β-hCG levels are below the discriminatory zone, evaluation of serum hCG levels must be repeated after 3 days in order to observe the trend. As previously mentioned, in normal viable intrauterine gestation, serum hCG concentration usually doubles every 1.4–2 days until 6–7 weeks of gestation. A normally rising hCG concentration should be evaluated with TVS examination when serum hCG levels reach the discriminatory zone. At that time, an IUP or an ectopic pregnancy can be diagnosed. If the hCG concentration does not double over 72 hours, then the pregnancy is most likely abnormal (an ectopic gestation or IUP that is destined to abort). The clinician can be reasonably certain that a normal IUP is not present in these cases. A falling hCG concentration is also most consistent with a failed pregnancy.

IMAGING STUDIES

Ultrasonography, especially TVS or endovaginal ultrasonography, should be the initial investigation of choice for symptomatic women in their first trimester. TVS can be performed either in the outpatient clinic or emergency department to diagnose IUP. TVS has been reported to have sensitivity of 90%, specificity of 99.8%, with positive and negative predictive values of 93% and 99.8% respectively. TVS can detect intrauterine gestational sac at 4-5 weeks of gestation and at β-hCG levels as low as 1,500 IU/L. On the other hand, TAS can detect intrauterine gestational sac at 5-6 weeks of gestation and at β-hCG levels of 1,800 IU/L.

Signs of an Intrauterine Pregnancy on Transvaginal Sonography

The presence of a gestational sac with a sonolucent center (>5 mm in diameter) is indicative of an IUP. Gestational sac is surrounded by a thick, concentric, echogenic ring located within the endometrium and contains a fetal pole, yolk sac, or both. A normal gestational sac, an ovoid collection of fluid adjacent to the endometrial stripe, can be visualized by means of the transvaginal probe at a gestational age of about 5 weeks. It can often be seen when it is 2 or 3 mm in diameter and should be consistently seen at 5 mm. Since a pseudogestational sac is often associated with an ectopic pregnancy, the presence of a sac alone cannot confirm IUP. The earliest embryonic landmark, the yolk sac, appears when the sac is 8 mm or more in diameter, usually during the fifth week of gestation. Cardiac activity can be seen with endovaginal scanning when the embryo reaches 4–5 mm in diameter, at a gestational age of 6–6.5 weeks.

Probably Abnormal Intrauterine Pregnancy

The IUP visualized on TVS is probably abnormal if the gestational sac is larger than 10 mm in diameter without a fetal pole or with a definite fetal pole but without cardiac activity. In these cases, the gestational sac frequently has an irregular or crenated border.

Definite Ectopic Pregnancy

Signs of a definite ectopic pregnancy on TVS examination are as follows:

- *Thick, bright echogenic, ring-like structure, which is located outside the uterus, having a gestational sac containing an obvious fetal pole, yolk sac, or both:* This usually appears as an intact, well-defined tubal ring (Doughnut's or Bagel's sign, **Fig. 32.4**). Though this finding confirms the diagnosis of ectopic pregnancy, it may not always be present. Another sign specific to ectopic pregnancy is the blob sign. This is seen as a small conglomerate mass next to the ovary, with no evidence of any gestational sac or embryo.
- *Empty uterus (Fig. 32.5) or the presence of a pseudogestational sac:* A trilaminar endometrial pattern is seen in the uterus in cases of ectopic pregnancy. The presence of pseudogestational sac and decidual cyst on TVS is also an indicator of ectopic pregnancy. Pseudogestational sac is typically formed due to endometrial changes and fluid collection in the endometrial cavity occurring with implantation of extrauterine pregnancy because all pregnancies induce an endometrial decidual reaction. Sloughing of decidua can create an intracavity fluid collection, known as the pseudosac. Difference between the gestational sac associated with IUP and pseudogestational sac associated with ectopic pregnancy is described in **Table 32.4**. Decidual cyst, another feature of ectopic pregnancy, can be identified as an anechoic area within the endometrium, but remote from the canal. It is often present at the endometrium–myometrium border.
- Empty uterus on TVS images in patients with a serum β-hCG level greater than the discriminatory cutoff value is considered to be an ectopic pregnancy until proven otherwise. An empty uterus may also represent a recent abortion. However, in that case, serum β-hCG levels would not be greater than the discriminatory cutoff value.
- Presence of an adnexal sac with fetal pole and cardiac activity is the most specific sign of ectopic pregnancy. Another useful guide while looking for ectopic pregnancy is the presence of corpus luteum, which may be observed in ipsilateral ovary in 85% cases.
- Cystic or solid adnexal or tubal masses (including the tubal ring sign, representing a tubal gestational sac)

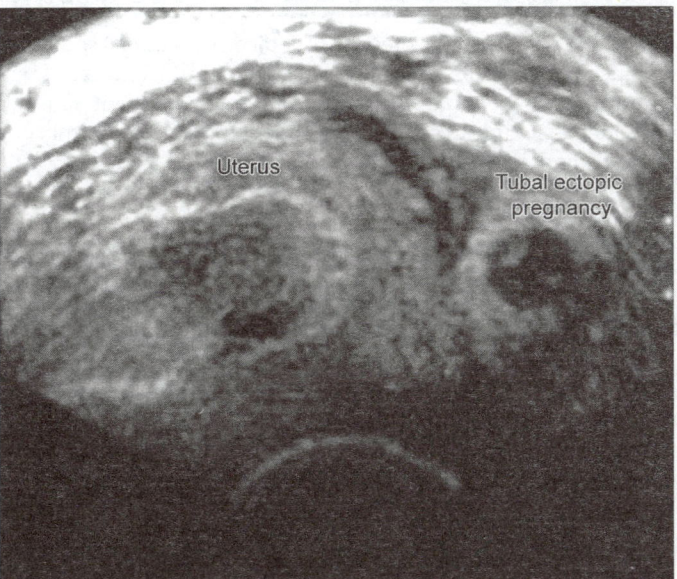

Fig. 32.5: Ectopic pregnancy in left tube showing an empty uterus with or without the presence of free fluid in the pouch of Douglas and a complex tubal adnexal mass.

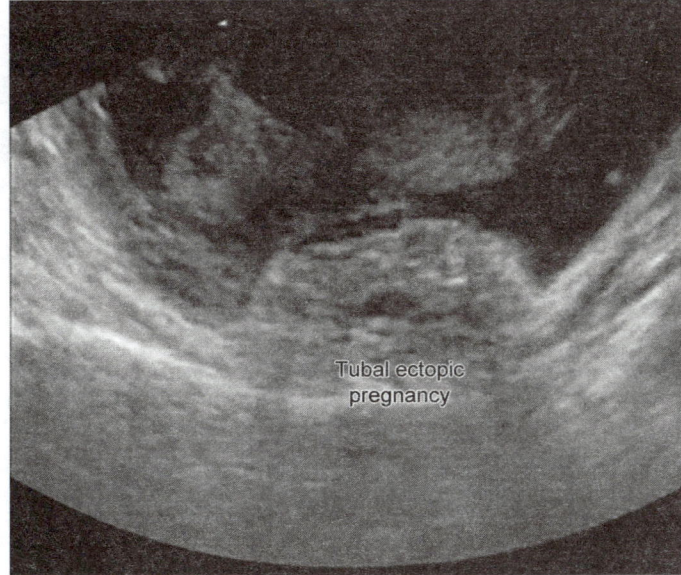

Fig. 32.4: Ultrasound examination showing the Bagel's sign, which can be defined as the thickened fallopian tube due to the presence of gestational sac inside it. In this picture, there is a thick, bright echogenic, ring-like structure, which is located outside the uterus, having a gestational sac containing an obvious fetal pole and yolk sac. This usually gives the appearance of an intact, well-defined tubal ring (Doughnut's or Bagel's sign).

TABLE 32.4: Difference between the gestational sac and pseudogestational sac.

Parameter	Early gestational sac associated with intrauterine pregnancy	Pseudogestational sac associated with ectopic pregnancy
Location of sac	Eccentrically placed	Centrally placed
Placement	It is placed below the midcavity line echo and is buried into the endometrium	It is placed along the midcavity line between the endometrial layers
Shape	Usually round	Ovoid
Borders	Double ring sign (this is a sign specific of gestational sac)	Single layer
Doppler color flow	High blood flow	Avascular

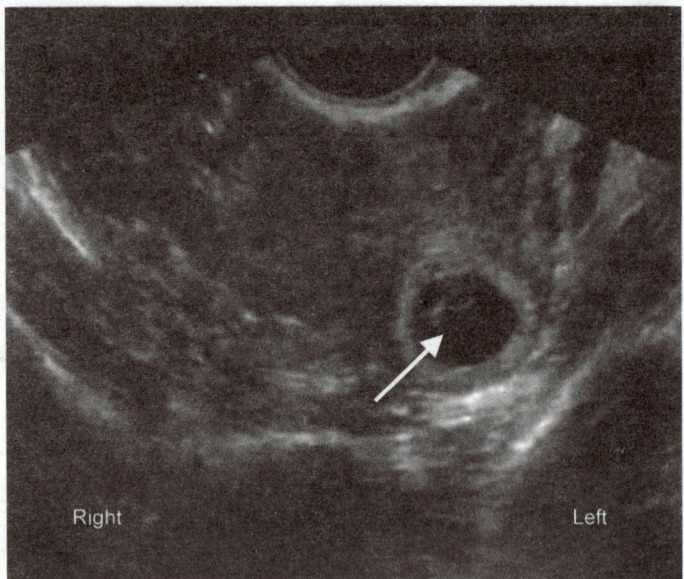

Fig. 32.6: Cornual ectopic pregnancy (indicated by arrow) shows the presence of a gestational sac in the left horn of the bicornuate uterus. A gestational sac with a sonolucent center can be identified. It is surrounded by a thick, concentric, echogenic ring located within one of the horns of bicornuate uterus and contains a fetal pole.

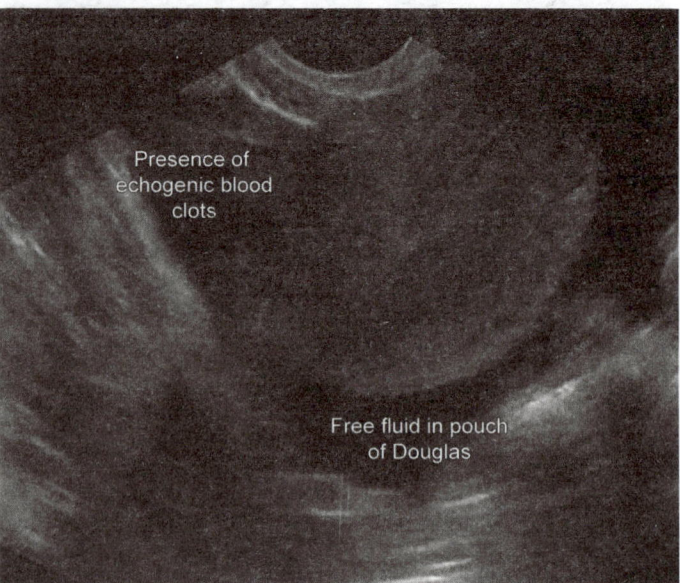

Fig. 32.8: Free fluid in the pouch of Douglas, which is suggestive of a tubal ectopic pregnancy.

TABLE 32.5: The criteria for TVS diagnosis of ectopic pregnancy.

Stage	TVS finding
Type 1A	Well-defined tubal ring displaying fetal heart
Type 1B	Well-defined tubal ring displaying no fetal heart
Type 2	Ill-defined tubal mass
Type 3	Free pelvic fluid, empty uterus, displaying no adnexal mass

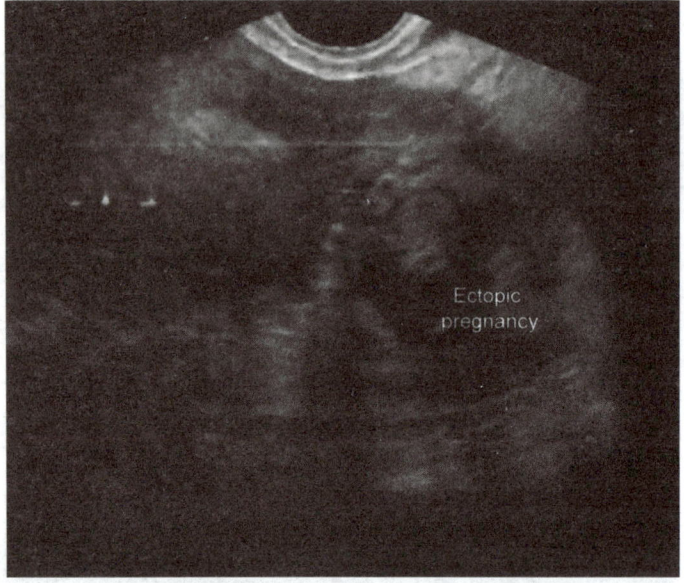

Fig. 32.7: Left-sided ectopic pregnancy.

(Figs. 32.6 and 32.7) and severe adnexal tenderness with probe palpation are also suggestive of ectopic pregnancy.
- Hematosalpinx (presence of free fluid or blood in the fallopian tubes) and echogenic or sonolucent cul-de-sac fluid
- *Ruptured ectopic pregnancy*: In case of a ruptured ectopic pregnancy, the ultrasonographic findings include the presence of free fluid or clotted blood in the cul-de-sac (**Fig. 32.8**) or intraperitoneal gutters (Morison's pouch).

The criteria for TVS diagnosis of ectopic pregnancy, given by Rottem et al. (1991), are described in **Table 32.5**.

If a low-risk patient's ultrasonography is negative for IUP, she is hemodynamically stable, and has a β-hCG level < 1,500 mIU/mL, the physician should take another β-hCG measurement after 48 hours. Patients with nondiagnostic TVS results and a β-hCG level of 1,500 mIU/mL or greater are at an increased risk for ectopic pregnancy and may require a surgical consultation and must remain under vigilance. Serial measurement of β-hCG and progesterone concentrations may also be useful when the diagnosis remains unclear.

OTHER TESTS

Serum Progesterone Levels

Serum progesterone levels have been used by some in assessment of an ectopic pregnancy. While a value of 25 ng/mL is associated with normal pregnancies in 98% of cases, a value of <5 ng/mL identifies a nonviable pregnancy without regards to the location of pregnancy. Most women with an ectopic pregnancy would show serum progesterone levels somewhere in between these two values, limiting the clinical usefulness of progesterone in diagnosing an ectopic pregnancy. Therefore, serum progesterone levels < 15 ng/mL could be indicative of ectopic pregnancy. Measurement of the serum concentration of progesterone has been investigated as a potentially useful adjunct to serum β-hCG measurement, since progesterone levels are stable and independent of gestational age in the first trimester. Rapid progesterone analysis can identify two important subgroups of patients in the emergency department with symptomatic first-trimester bleeding or pain, or both: stable patients with progesterone levels above 22 ng/mL, who have a high (but not certain) likelihood of viable IUP, and patients with levels of 5 ng/mL or less, who almost certainly have a nonviable pregnancy. Invasive diagnostic testing (e.g., D&C) could be offered to the latter, as could treatment with MTX, without fear of interrupting a potentially viable IUP. Serum progesterone levels can detect pregnancy failure and identify patients at risk for ectopic pregnancy, but they are not diagnostic of ectopic pregnancy. Sensitivity for diagnosis of ectopic pregnancy is very low (15%); therefore, 85% of patients with ectopic pregnancy will have normal serum progesterone levels. Therefore, serum progesterone levels are not routinely measured because the results of this test merely confirm the provisional diagnosis, which had already been established, by hCG measurements and TVS.

Other Hormonal Levels

Recently, levels of some newer hormones are being measured as indicators of ectopic pregnancy. These include placenta protein 14 (PP-14), which is reduced in cases of ectopic pregnancy. Levels of pregnancy-associated plasma protein A (PAPP-A), PAPP-C (Schwangerschaft protein 1) appear to have low value in detection of cases of ectopic pregnancy. On the other hand, levels of cancer antigen 125 (CA-125), maternal serum creatine kinase, and serum alpha-fetoprotein (AFP) are elevated in cases of ectopic pregnancy.

Color Flow Doppler Examination

Blood flow in the arteries of the fallopian tube, which contains an ectopic pregnancy, is approximately 20–45% higher in comparison to the opposite tube. As a result, the Doppler waveforms in the tube containing an ectopic pregnancy show low impedance flow. Color Doppler may also demonstrate a "ring of fire" appearance due to an increased blood flow in the tubal mass **(Figs. 32.9A and B)**. However, investigations such as TVS and serum hCG measurements are usually sufficient for establishing the diagnosis in the usual clinical practice, and routine Doppler ultrasound examination is not normally required.

Magnetic Resonance Imaging

Though magnetic resonance imaging can be used for diagnosing ectopic pregnancy, it is not usually used due to high costs involved.

■ DIAGNOSTIC PROCEDURES

Laparoscopic Examination

Diagnostic laparoscopic examination can be considered as the gold standard investigation for diagnosis of ectopic pregnancy **(Figs. 32.10 and 32.11)**. However, it must be done only if the patient is hemodynamically stable. If the diagnosis of ectopic pregnancy is confirmed on laparoscopy, definitive treatment (salpingectomy or salpingostomy) may be carried out during the same sitting. Medical treatment must not be carried out in these cases because it is associated with an additional risk and does not show any proven benefit.

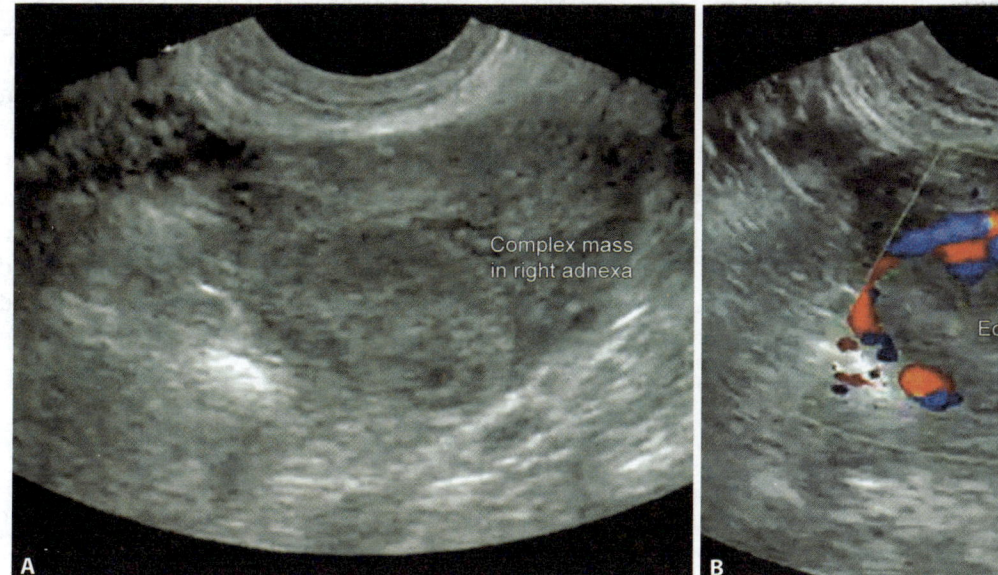

Figs. 32.9A and B: (A) Complex right echogenic adnexal mass in this figure represents hematosalpinx (presence of free fluid or blood in the fallopian tubes); (B) Doppler ultrasound in the same case showing a "ring of fire" appearance due to increased vascularity of the surrounding fallopian tube.

724 Uterine, Ovarian, and Tubal Pathology

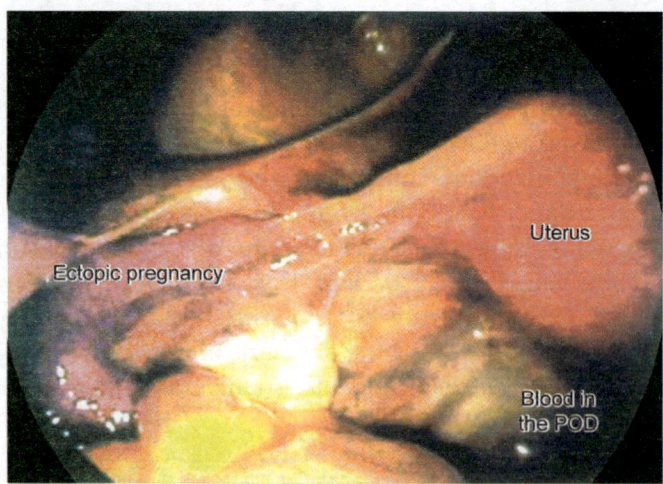

Fig. 32.10: Unruptured ectopic pregnancy in the ampulla of the right tube. (POD: pouch of Douglas)

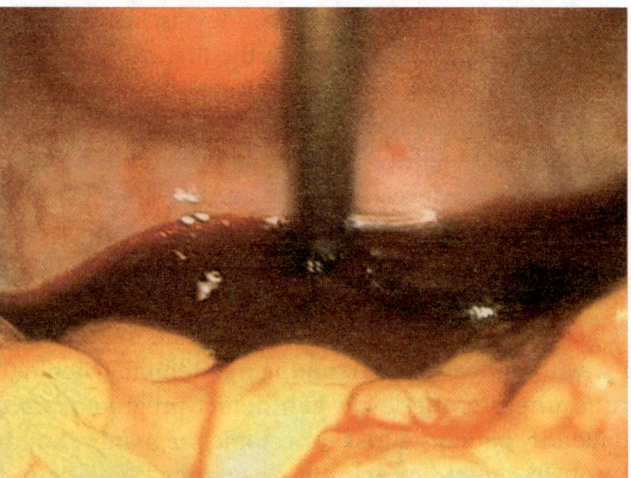

Fig. 32.12: Presence of clotted blood in the pouch of Douglas.

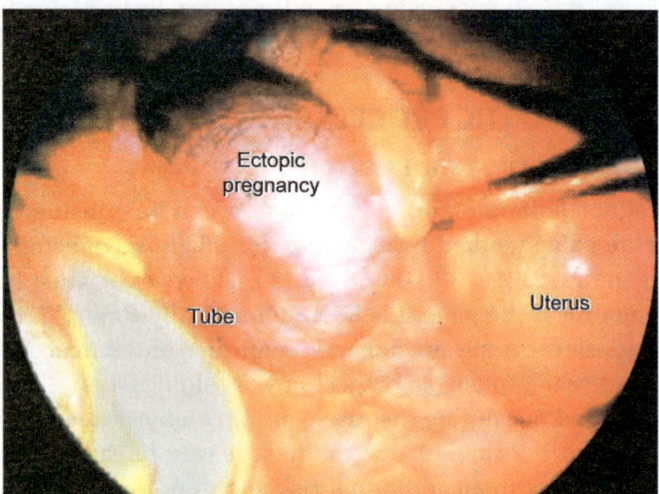

Fig. 32.11: Unruptured tubal ectopic pregnancy on the right side.

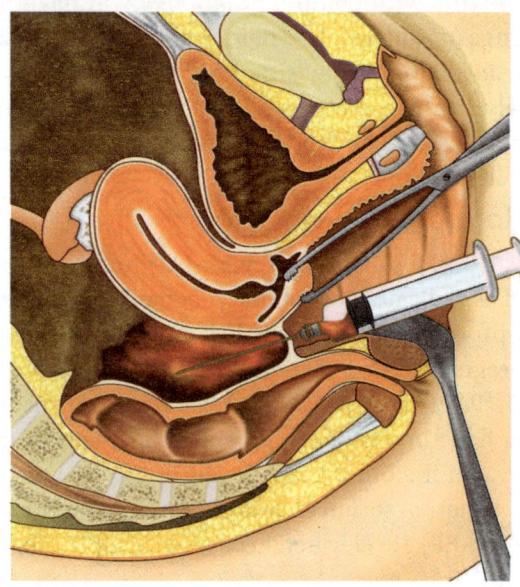

Fig. 32.13: Procedure of culdocentesis. The process of culdocentesis showing extraction of blood from pouch of Douglas.

Culdocentesis

Culdocentesis can be defined as the aspiration of fluid from the POD. An investigation commonly done in the past, it is rarely done nowadays due to the availability of high-quality ultrasound scan. This procedure used to be performed using a 16–18-gauge lumbar puncture needle, inserted via the posterior fornix into the POD. The tap was considered as positive if 0.5 mL or more of nonclotting blood was aspirated out. The presence of nonclotted blood in the POD (**Figs. 32.12 and 32.13**) is diagnostic of chronic hemorrhage in the abdomen, which may be due to a ruptured ectopic pregnancy or as a result of some other cause of hemorrhage, e.g., a ruptured ovarian cyst. Therefore, a positive culdocentesis test for blood may not always be diagnostic for ectopic gestation. Nowadays, this test has been largely replaced by ultrasound examination.

Dilatation and Curettage

Dilatation and curettage is recommended in suspected cases of incomplete abortion versus ectopic pregnancy. The curettings obtained on D&C must be sent for histopathological examination (HPE). Identification of decidua without chorionic villi is suggestive of ectopic pregnancy, whereas the presence of chorionic villi suggests incomplete abortion. Arias-Stella reaction on HPE is suggestive, but not diagnostic, of ectopic pregnancy. Arias-Stella reaction refers to atypical endometrial changes characterized by hypertrophy and vacuolization of glandular epithelial cells, associated with marked nuclear pleomorphism, enlargement, and hyperchromasia.

DIAGNOSTIC CRITERIA FOR NONTUBAL ECTOPIC PREGNANCY

Diagnostic criteria for various types of nontubal ectopic pregnancy are summarized in **Boxes 32.3 to 32.9**.

> Q. With the help of a short essay, describe heterotopic pregnancy.

BOX 32.3: Diagnostic criteria for a cervical pregnancy.

- *Definition*: Ectopic pregnancy, which is implanted in the uterine endocervix
- *Incidence*: 1 in 9,000 pregnant women
- *Risk factors*:
  – Previous induced abortion
  – Previous cesarean delivery
  – Asherman's syndrome
  – IVF
  – DES exposure
  – Leiomyomas
- *Ultrasound criteria*:
  – Empty uterus
  – Barrel-shaped cervix
  – Presence of the gestational sac below the level of the internal cervical os
  – Absence of the "sliding sign" (helps in differentiating cervical ectopic pregnancy from an aborting intrauterine pregnancy; upon application of gentle pressure on the cervix with the help of a probe, the implanted ectopic pregnancy does not appear to slide against the probe, whereas gestational sac of an abortus would slide)
  – Presence of peritrophoblastic blood flow around the gestational sac using color Doppler
- *Clinical criteria (Paulman and McEllin)*:
  – Uterine bleeding, no cramping following amenorrhea
  – Cervix distended, thin walled, soft in consistency
  – Enlarged uterine fundus may be felt
  – Internal os is closed
  – External os is partially open
- *Histopathological criteria (Rubin's)*:
  – Cervical glands present opposite to placenta
  – Placental attachment to the cervix must be below the entrance of uterine vessels
  – Fetal elements are absent from corpus uteri
- *Biochemical investigations*: Single, raised serum β-hCG levels

(β-hCG: beta human chorionic gonadotrophin; DES: diethylstilbestrol; IVF: in vitro fertilization)

BOX 32.4: Diagnostic criteria for a cesarean scar pregnancy.

- *Definition*: Pregnancy in which implantation of the gestational sac occurs within the scar of a previous cesarean surgery
- *Ultrasound criteria*:
  – Empty uterine cavity
  – Anterior location of gestational sac at the level of the internal os
  – Gestational sac is embedded at the site of the previous lower uterine segment cesarean section scar
  – Thin or absent layer of myometrium between the gestational sac and the bladder
  – Evidence of prominent trophoblastic/placental circulation on Doppler examination
  – Endocervical canal is empty
- *Magnetic resonance imaging*: It can be used as a second-line investigation, if the diagnosis is equivocal on TVS
- *Biochemical investigations*: No biochemical investigation is routinely required

(TVS: transvaginal sonography)

BOX 32.5: Diagnostic criteria for an interstitial pregnancy.

- *Definition*: Pregnancy where the gestational sac develops in the uterine part of the fallopian tube. It constitutes only 5% of all tubal ectopic pregnancies and is associated with a high rate of complications, especially late rupture
- *Ultrasound criteria*:
  – Empty uterine cavity
  – Products of conception/gestational sac laterally located in the interstitial (intramural) part of the tube
  – Less than 5 mm of myometrium surrounding the gestational sac in all imaging planes
  – Presence of the "interstitial line sign" (an echogenic line extending from the gestational sac to the endometrial echo complex)
  – Sonographic findings in two dimensions can be further confirmed using three-dimensional ultrasound
- *Magnetic resonance imaging*: It can be used as a second-line investigation, if the diagnosis is equivocal on TVS
- *Biochemical investigations*: A single serum beta human chorionic gonadotrophin (β-hCG) or in some cases repeat serum β-hCG levels in 48 hours may be helpful in deciding further management

(TVS: transvaginal sonography)

BOX 32.6: Diagnostic criteria for cornual pregnancy.

- *Definition*: Pregnancy, which develops in the cavity of a rudimentary horn in the unicornuate uterus or cornua of a bicornuate or septate uterus
- *Ultrasound criteria*:
  - Only a single interstitial portion of fallopian tube is visualized in the main uterine body
  - Gestational sac is mobile and separate from the uterus and completely surrounded by myometrium
  - Vascular pedicle adjoining the gestational sac to the unicornuate uterus
- *Biochemical investigations*: A single serum beta human chorionic gonadotrophin (β-hCG) or in some cases repeat serum β-hCG levels in 48 hours may be helpful in deciding further management

BOX 32.7: Diagnostic criteria for an ovarian pregnancy.

- *Definition*: A rare form of nontubal ectopic pregnancy where the gestational sac is present in the ovary. The most important risk factor for the development of ovarian pregnancy is the use of IUCD
- *Ultrasound criteria*: No specific agreed criteria for ultrasound diagnosis of ovarian ectopic pregnancy. Some of the likely features include:
  - Empty uterine cavity
  - Wide echogenic ring with an internal anechoic area on the ovary. A yolk sac or embryo is visualized less commonly
  - Not possible to separate the gestational sac from the ovary on gentle palpation (negative sliding organ sign)
  - Corpus luteum can be identified separately from the suspected ovarian pregnancy
  - Color Doppler may help in the detection of a fetal heart pulsation within the ovary
  - Complex echogenic adnexal mass with free fluid in the pouch of Douglas could be representative of a ruptured ovarian ectopic pregnancy
- *Spiegelberg criteria (on laparotomy)*:
  - Ipsilateral tube is intact and separate from the sac
  - Sac occupies position of the ovaries
  - Sac is connected to the uterus via ovarian ligament
  - Ovarian tissue is found on its wall on histopathological study
- *Biochemical investigations*: A single serum beta human chorionic gonadotrophin (β-hCG) or in some cases repeat serum β-hCG levels in 48 hours may be helpful in deciding further management

(IUCD: intrauterine contraceptive device)

BOX 32.8: Diagnostic criteria for an abdominal pregnancy.

- *Definition*: Form of an ectopic pregnancy where the embryo grows and develops outside the uterine cavity in the abdomen. Also, the other female internal genitalia such as fallopian tube, ovary, or broad ligaments are not involved. Abdominal pregnancy can be of two types: primary and secondary. Primary abdominal pregnancy occurs when the conceptus first implants inside the abdomen. Secondary abdominal pregnancy occurs when the conceptus escapes out of a rent from the primary sites and implants in the abdomen. Implantation site could be intraperitoneal or extraperitoneal (in the broad ligament). Secondary abdominal pregnancy could have the following fate:
  - *Death of ovum*: Complete absorption
  - *Placental separation*: Massive intraperitoneal hemorrhage
  - *Infection*: Fistulous communication with intestines, bladder, vagina, or umbilicus
  - *Death of the fetus*: Occurs in majority of cases and may be associated with mummification or adipocere formation or calcification to lithopedion
  - *Continuation till term*: Very rare and may be associated with fetal malformation
- *Ultrasound criteria*:
  - Absence of an intrauterine gestational sac
  - Absence of both an evidently dilated tube and a complex adnexal mass
  - Gestational cavity surrounded by loops of bowel, with peritoneum separating the two
  - With the application of pressure of the transvaginal probe toward the posterior cul-de-sac, the gestational sac appears to be widely mobile
- *Magnetic resonance imaging*:
  - Serves as a useful diagnostic adjunct for diagnosis in advanced cases
  - Identification of placental implantation over vital structures, such as major blood vessels or bowel
  - Help in planning the surgical approach
- *Studdiford criteria (primary abdominal pregnancy—on laparotomy)*:
  - Both tubes and ovaries are normal
  - Absence of uteroperitoneal fistula
  - Pregnancy related exclusively to the peritoneal surface and young enough to rule out the possibility of secondary implantation
- *Biochemical investigations*: A single serum beta human chorionic gonadotrophin (β-hCG) or in some cases repeat serum β-hCG levels in 48 hours may be helpful in deciding further management

> **BOX 32.9:** Diagnostic criteria for heterotopic pregnancy.
>
> - *Definition:* Rare complication of pregnancy in which both extrauterine or ectopic pregnancy and intrauterine pregnancy occur simultaneously
> - *Clinical criteria:* Heterotopic pregnancy should be suspected with the presence of risk factors such as:
>   – Woman presenting after assisted reproductive technologies
>   – Woman with an intrauterine pregnancy complaining of persistent pelvic pain
>   – Persistently raised beta human chorionic gonadotrophin (β-hCG) level following miscarriage or termination of pregnancy
> - *Ultrasound criteria:* Presence of an intrauterine pregnancy with a coexisting ectopic pregnancy
> - *Biochemical investigations:* A single serum β-hCG or in some cases repeat serum β-hCG levels in 48 hours may be helpful in deciding further management

 ## TREATMENT/OBSTETRIC MANAGEMENT

> Q. Write a short note on modern management of ectopic pregnancy.
>
> Q. With the help of a long essay, discuss the diagnosis and management of unruptured tubal ectopic pregnancy.
>
> Q. Discuss in detail the diagnosis and management of unruptured tubal ectopic pregnancy.
>
> Q. Write a long essay discussing the recent trends in the management of ectopic pregnancy.
>
> Q. Write a long essay discussing the medical management of ectopic pregnancy.
>
> Q. Discuss in detail the diagnosis and management of unruptured tubal ectopic pregnancy.
>
> Q. Write a long essay discussing the recent trends in the management of ectopic pregnancy.

Various treatment options for ectopic pregnancy include expectant, medical, and surgical management (**Flowchart 32.2**). Before deciding the treatment option in a woman with ectopic pregnancy, she and her partner must be fully involved in deciding the relevant management. They must be provided with the written information regarding the various treatment options, and carefully explained about the advantages and disadvantages associated with each approach. Before deciding the appropriate surgical management, the opposite tube and ovary must definitely be examined. The procedure must then be performed after taking into consideration the patient's age, future reproductive capacity, and the nature of lesion. Decisions regarding management should be based on the following inclusion criteria:

- *Patient's hemodynamic stability*: Treatment of an ectopic pregnancy varies, depending on how medically stable the woman is. Surgery is the only treatment option which must be used in hemodynamically unstable patients.
- Size of ectopic pregnancy
- Location of the pregnancy

The various treatment options for ectopic pregnancy are described below in detail.

■ EXPECTANT MANAGEMENT

> Q. Write a short essay, discussing the conservative management of unruptured tubal ectopic pregnancy.
>
> Q. Write a short note on nonsurgical management of ectopic pregnancy.

Expectant management of ectopic pregnancy is based on the assumption that a certain proportion of all ectopic pregnancies will regress spontaneously and be slowly absorbed. Such pregnancies will not progress to tubal rupture. This may be a possibility in cases where the hCG levels appear to be falling and the woman appears clinically well. If the initial hCG level is <200 mIU/mL, nearly 70% of the patients may experience spontaneous resolution, whereas 30% may require laparoscopic salpingostomy. The criteria for expectant management of ectopic pregnancy are described in **Box 32.10**. During spontaneous resolution, β-hCG levels may take 4–67 days (mean 20 days) to return to nonpregnant levels. The percentage fall in serum hCG levels by day 7 is a better indicator than the percentage fall by day 2. An important warning which obstetricians need to remember is that tubal pregnancies are known to rupture even when the serum hCG levels are low.

At the time of expectant management, the patient must be hospitalized with strict monitoring of clinical symptoms. Her hemoglobin levels must be estimated daily. The β-hCG levels must be measured at every 48-hour interval for three measurements to confirm that it continues to decline, and then at weekly intervals until it becomes undetectable or <10 IU/L. TVS must be done twice weekly. Expectant treatment should be abandoned if a patient experiences significant increase in abdominal pain, serum hCG starts to increase or fails to decrease, or the patient shows signs of tubal rupture. Some contraindications for expectant management are mentioned in **Box 32.11**.

■ MEDICAL MANAGEMENT (METHOTREXATE)

> Q. Write a long essay discussing the medical management of ectopic pregnancy.
>
> Q. Write a short note on medical management of ectopic pregnancy.

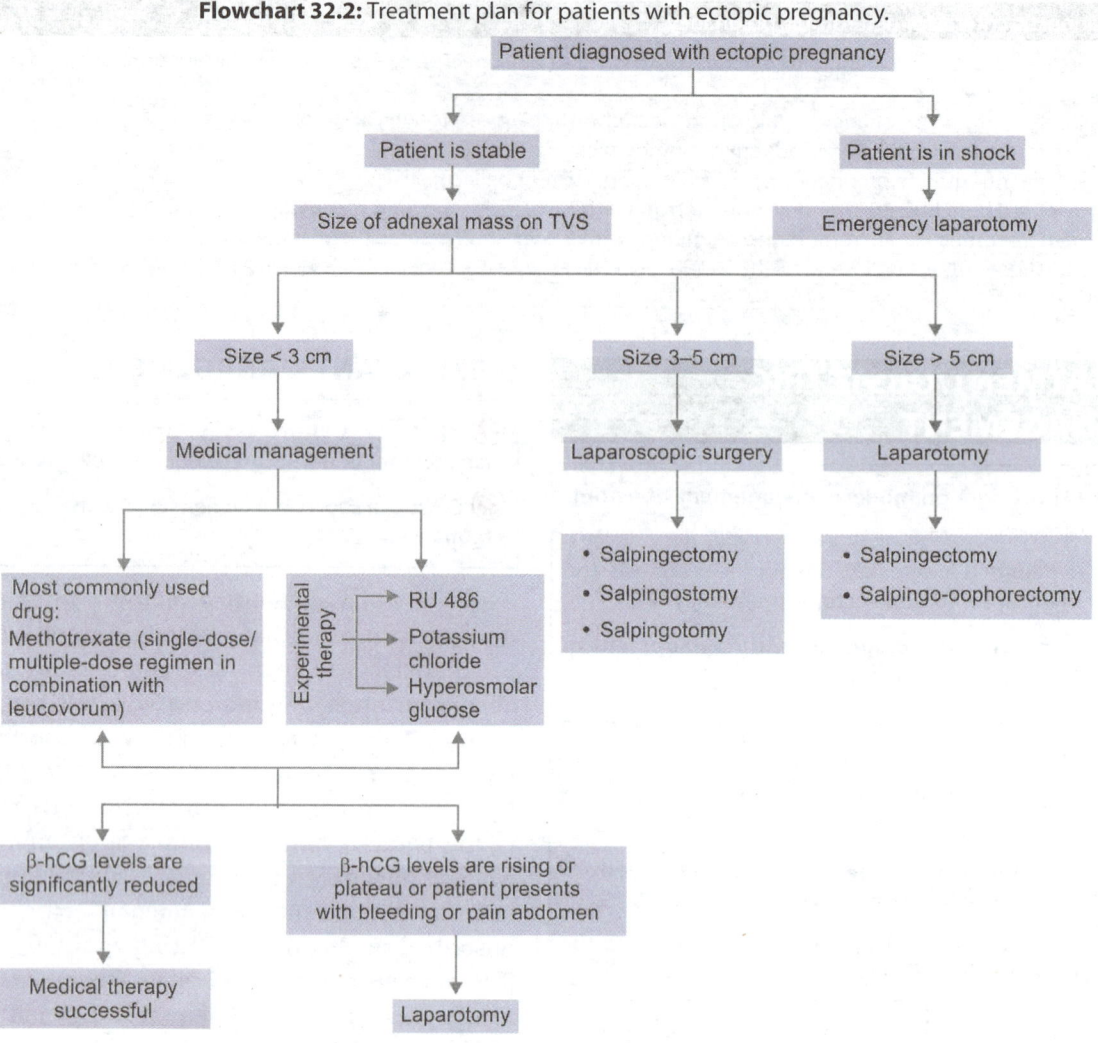

Flowchart 32.2: Treatment plan for patients with ectopic pregnancy.

(β-hCG: beta human chorionic gonadotrophin; TVS: transvaginal sonography)

BOX 32.10: Criteria for expectant management of ectopic pregnancy.

- Patient is hemodynamically stable
- Tubal ectopic pregnancy only (no other type of ectopic pregnancy)
- Serum human chorionic gonadotropin (hCG) levels ≤ 200 mIU/mL and are declining
- Size of ectopic pregnancy is <3.5 cm without heartbeat
- Hemoperitoneum is <50 mL
- No signs of rupture or acute bleeding on TVS
- The patient has been made aware of the risks involved; she accepts the risks and is able to comply with follow-up

(TVS: transvaginal sonography)

BOX 32.11: Contraindications for expectant management of ectopic pregnancy.

- Patient is hemodynamically unstable
- Presence of signs of impending or ongoing rupture of ectopic mass
- Serum hCG levels ≥ 200 mIU/mL, are increasing, or are not declining
- Noncompliant patient, who is unwilling or unable to follow-up with monitoring
- Patient does not have timely access to a medical institution

While surgery remains the main modality of treatment worldwide, medical management is sometimes employed in a stable patient with a medically treatable ectopic pregnancy or in the presence of other medical conditions which would make the risk of surgery unacceptable. An early ectopic pregnancy can sometimes be treated with an injection of MTX, which stops the growth of the embryo. With the advancement in science and technology over the years, modification and refinements of the protocols for medical therapy of ectopic pregnancy have now allowed for single-dose outpatient therapy. While MTX presently remains the most effective and commonly used drug in medical therapy for treatment of an ectopic pregnancy, other protocols, using drugs such as potassium chloride, hyperosmolar glucose, RU 486, and prostaglandins, have also been used. These drugs may be administered orally, systemically, and locally into the ectopic pregnancy under direct vision. However, these therapies are largely experimental at present since there is limited experience in using them, and the efficacy of such treatment modalities over standard MTX protocol has not been established. Administration of medical treatment is likely to be associated with minimal hospitalization, usually outdoor treatment, and quick recovery. Medical treatment may be associated with success rates as high as 90%, with proper case selection. Besides being useful in cases of tubal ectopic pregnancy, MTX therapy also helps in an early resolution of placental tissues in case of abdominal pregnancy. Before administration of MTX, the prerequisites mentioned in **Box 32.12** must be fulfilled.

Methotrexate is a folic acid antagonist, which acts by inactivating the enzyme dihydrofolate reductase, thereby inhibiting the synthesis of pyrimidines, which interferes with deoxyribonucleic acid (DNA) synthesis in actively dividing cells, including trophoblasts. When administered to properly selected patients, it has been found to be associated with a success rate of up to 94%. Side effects of MTX therapy include bone marrow suppression, elevated liver enzymes, rash, alopecia, stomatitis, nausea, and diarrhea. The time to resolution of the ectopic pregnancy is usually between 3 and 7 weeks following MTX therapy. MTX can be administered systemically (IV, IM, or orally) or via direct local injection into the ectopic pregnancy sac. Though the local injection of MTX can be given either via transvaginal or laparoscopic route, this route is commonly not used. MTX is most commonly administered via the IM route.

One of the best predictors of success of medical therapy is the initial serum β-hCG levels. Success rates of >90% can be achieved with single-dose MTX when hCG levels are <5,000 mIU/mL. Success rates with single- dose MTX have been observed to progressively decrease as serum hCG levels increase. The overall success rate (approximately 90%) with multiple-dose MTX therapy has been found to be similar to that associated with single-dose MTX therapy. However, presently the single-dose approach is more commonly used in comparison to the multidose regimen because it is less expensive, involves less intensive monitoring, and does not require folinic acid rescue. Absolute and relative contraindications to MTX therapy have been described in **Box 32.13**.

Protocol for Single-dose Methotrexate

The protocol for single-dose MTX is described in **Box 32.14**. Patients treated with MTX should be followed closely. On discharge from oncology unit, the women should be advised that she may experience some pain in the abdomen as the pregnancy resolves. Mild abdominal pain could be due to tubal abortion or tubal distention because of hematoma formation. Severe abdominal pain, however, can be a sign of actual or impending tubal rupture, warranting immediate attention.

> **BOX 32.12:** Prerequisites for starting medical treatment of ectopic pregnancy.
>
> - Patient is hemodynamically stable and does not have pelvic pain
> - Patient desires future fertility
> - Patient appears to be reliable and compliant, who will return for posttreatment follow-up care
> - Ectopic pregnancy smaller than 4 cm in diameter and no fetal heart activity on TVS or smaller than 3.5 cm with the presence of cardiac activity and absence of any free fluid in the pouch of Douglas
> - There is no evidence of tubal rupture
> - Serum hCG is below 5,000 IU/L, with minimal symptoms
> - Availability of facilities for follow-up care following the use of methotrexate
> - Patient agrees to use reliable contraception for 3–4 months post-treatment
> - Patient has no underlying severe medical condition or disorder
> - Investigations such as CBC, LFT, and KFT need to be done prior to administration of methotrexate to ensure that there is no underlying abnormality suggestive of hepatic, renal, or bone marrow impairment
> - Patient does not have any known contraindications to methotrexate
> - Patient is not currently taking nonsteroidal anti-inflammatory drugs, diuretics, penicillin, and tetracycline group of drugs
> - Patient does not have a coexisting intrauterine pregnancy
> - Patient is not breastfeeding

(CBC: complete blood count; hCG: human chorionic gonadotropin; KFT: kidney function test; LFT: liver function test)

> **BOX 32.13:** Contraindications to methotrexate therapy.
>
> *Absolute contraindications*
> - Patient is hemodynamically unstable
> - Presence of signs of impending ectopic mass rupture (i.e., severe or persistent abdominal pain or >300 mL of free peritoneal fluid outside the pelvic cavity)
> - Pregnancy and lactation
> - Hepatic, renal, or hematologic dysfunction, e.g., liver disease with a transaminase level two times greater than normal and renal disease with a creatinine level > 1.5 mg/dL (133 µmol/L)
> - Overt or laboratory evidence of immunodeficiency with a white blood cell count < 1,500/mm^3 (1.5 × 10^9/L)
> - Active pulmonary disease
> - Peptic ulcer disease
> - Alcoholism, alcoholic liver disease, or other chronic liver disease
> - Active pulmonary disease
> - Preexisting blood dyscrasias, such as bone marrow hypoplasia, leukopenia, thrombocytopenia [platelet count < 100,000/mm^3 (100 × 10^9/L), or significant anemia
> - Known sensitivity to methotrexate
> - Coexistent viable intrauterine pregnancy
> - Patient is unwilling to be compliant with post-therapeutic monitoring, or there is lack of timely access to a medical institution
>
> *Relative contraindications*
> - Large ectopic size (≥3.5 cm)
> - Presence of embryonic cardiac activity
> - High human chorionic gonadotropin (hCG) concentration (>5,000 mIU/mL)
> - Presence of fetal cardiac activity
> - Presence of fluid in the peritoneal cavity
> - *Other relative contraindications requiring further research*: Sonographic evidence of a yolk sac, isthmic location of ectopic mass rather than ampullary, high pretreatment levels of folic acid, etc.

> **BOX 32.14:** Protocol for single-dose methotrexate.
>
> *Pretreatment investigations*:
> - CBC
> - Blood group typing (ABO and Rh) and antibody testing
> - Liver function and kidney function tests
> - Measurement of serum β-hCG levels
> - TVS
>
> *Pretreatment prerequisites*:
> - Written informed consent must be obtained from the patient and her partner
> - Woman's weight and height must be obtained, and her BSA must be calculated
>
> *Day 0 (day of treatment)*:
> - Methotrexate needs to be injected in the dosage of 50 mg/m² of BSA IM injection
> - BSA is calculated using the following formula:
>   BSA = Square root [(height in cm × weight in kg)/3,600]
> - RhoGAM (50 IU) is administered intramuscularly if the patient is Rh negative
> - Advise patients not to take vitamins with folic acid until complete resolution of the ectopic pregnancy occurs
> - Folinic acid supplements to be discontinued
> - They should also refrain from strenuous exercises, alcohol consumption, and intercourse for the same period
>
> *Day 4*: Measurement of the β-hCG levels must be performed, and serve as the baseline level against which subsequent levels are measured
>
> *Day 7*:
> - Serum β-hCG levels are measured on day 7
>   - If the decline in serum hCG levels on day 7 is >15% since day 4 or >25% in comparison to the measurement of day 1, weekly hCG levels must be obtained until they have reached the negative level
>   - If the difference in serum hCG levels is <15% on day 7, repeat the dose of methotrexate and begin new day 1
>   - If fetal cardiac activity is present on day 7, repeat the dose of methotrexate and begin new day 1
>   - If even after 3–4 doses of methotrexate, β-hCG levels are not decreasing or fetal cardiac activity persists, surgical intervention may be required
> - If the weekly levels plateau or increase, a second course of methotrexate may be administered
> - Second dose of methotrexate may also be required if decline in β-hCG levels is <25% on day 7
> - If no drop has occurred by day 14, surgical therapy is indicated
> - If the patient develops increasing abdominal pain after methotrexate therapy, repeat a TVS to evaluate for possible rupture
> - Aspartate transaminase levels, CBC, and TVS also need to be done
>
> *Weekly*:
> - Measure serum β-hCG concentrations, until levels become <15 IU/L
> - Perform TVS
>
> *Anytime*: Perform laparoscopy if the patient has severe abdominal pain, acute abdomen, or if the ultrasound examination reveals blood in the abdomen
>
> (β-hCG: beta human chorionic gonadotropin; BSA: body surface area; CBC: complete blood count; TVS: transvaginal sonography)

Protocol for Multidose Methotrexate Regimen

Multidose regime of MTX may be considered for women with cervical or cornual ectopic pregnancies, after discussion with gynecology consultant (**Box 32.15**). In this regimen, MTX is administered in the dose of 1 mg/kg body weight via IM route every other day alternately along with leucovorin in the dose of 0.1 mg/kg body weight. Leucovorin (also called folinic acid, N5-formyl-tetrahydrofolate or citrovorum factor) is given to bypass the metabolic block caused by MTX, thereby rescuing normal cells from toxicity. Follow-up with liver function test (LFT), complete blood count (CBC), kidney function test (KFT), and serum β-hCG levels is required at baseline, day 4, and day 7 until the serum β-hCG levels decrease. On day 4, β-hCG levels may be the same or increased because syncytiotrophoblasts are not affected by MTX, whereas cytotrophoblasts are affected. Therefore, β-hCG measurement of day 7 is likely to be more specific. Weekly follow-up must be with serum β-hCG levels until serum β-hCG is no longer detected.

Irrespective of the type of regime being followed, some precautions, which need to be taken at the time of MTX administration, are listed in **Box 32.16**. Failure of medical therapy requires surgical treatment.

The use of MTX can be associated with other side effects such as gastritis, stomatitis, enteritis, conjunctivitis, bone marrow suppression, and hepatotoxicity. Therefore, patient monitoring with the help of investigations such as CBC, KFT, and LFT becomes essential.

Single-dose versus Multiple-dose Regimen

Treatment with MTX has not been found to be associated with impaired future fertility, adverse pregnancy outcome, or an increased risk for recurrent ectopic pregnancy.

> **BOX 32.15:** Methotrexate multidose regime.
>
> *MTX regime*
> - MTX to be administered IM or IV in the dose of 1 mg/kg IM, on alternate days (day 1, day 3, day 5, and day 7) for total of four doses
> - Leucovorin calcium must be administered orally in the dosage of 0.1 mg/kg body weight IM on alternate days (30 hours after previous MTX injection)—day 2, day 4, day 6, and day 8
> - hCG levels are initially drawn on day 1, day 3, day 5, and day 7
> - Consider alternate-day injection until the decline in β-hCG levels is 15% or more in 48 hours or four doses of MTX have been given
> - If the decline in serum hCG levels is >15% from the previous measurement, treatment is stopped, and surveillance phase begun
> - Surveillance phase consists of weekly hCG measurements until the levels become <5 IU/L or undetectable
> - If the decline in hCG levels is <15% from the previous level, the patient is given an additional dose of MTX 1 mg/kg IM followed by oral leucovorin 0.1 mg/kg the next day
>
> (hCG: human chorionic gonadotropin; MTX: methotrexate)

> **BOX 32.16:** Precautions to be taken at the time of methotrexate administration.
>
> - If treatment is on an outpatient basis, facilities for rapid transportation to a tertiary care center must be in place
> - Vaginal intercourse and new conception must be avoided until serum human chorionic gonadotropin (hCG) levels become undetectable
> - Pelvic examination must be avoided following methotrexate therapy due to theoretical risk (5–10%) of tubal rupture
> - Due to the theoretical risk of tubal rupture, the patient must be advised to report immediately in case of vaginal bleeding, abdominal pain, dizziness, syncope, etc.
> - Exposure to the sun must be avoided to reduce the risk of methotrexate dermatitis
> - Intake of foods and multivitamins containing folic acid must be best avoided
> - Use of nonsteroidal anti-inflammatory drugs must be preferably avoided due to the risk of development of complications such as bone marrow suppression, aplastic anemia, and gastrointestinal toxicity

A single-dose regimen is usually preferred over a multiple-dose regimen. Multiple-dosage regimen, however, may be used in cases of interstitial pregnancy.

Pain Following Treatment

Patients receiving MTX may experience mild abdominal pain of short duration after receiving the medication. This can commonly occur due to tubal abortion or tubal distention as a result of hematoma formation and is known as separation pain or resolution pain. This pain can usually be controlled with acetaminophen. The use of nonsteroidal anti-inflammatory drugs is best avoided because of the potential risk of clinically significant drug interaction with MTX in some patients taking both the drugs.

At times, the pain may be of severe intensity. In these cases, it is important to assess the patient's hemodynamic stability. Women with severe pain who are hemodynamically stable often do not require any surgical intervention. A patient with severe pain may be further evaluated with TVS. Findings suggestive of hemoperitoneum raise clinical suspicion of tubal rupture. Women with severe pain should be closely observed for hemodynamic changes, which may accompany a tubal rupture. Falling hCG levels do not preclude the possibility of tubal rupture. If tubal rupture is suspected, immediate surgery is required.

Combination Therapy of Methotrexate with Mifepristone

Treatment of ectopic pregnancy using a combination of MTX with mifepristone is presently being tried in the research settings. However, the use of mifepristone is not yet approved for treatment of ectopic pregnancy in the United States.

Surgically Administered Medical Treatment

The aim of surgically administered medical (SAM) treatment is to cause trophoblastic destruction without any systemic side effects. In this method, trophotoxic substances are injected into the ectopic pregnancy sac or into the affected tube under the guidance of laparoscope or TAS or TVS with or without falloposcopic control. Various trophotoxic substances which can be used include MTX, potassium chloride, mifepristone, prostaglandin F2α (PGF2α), hyperosmolar glucose solution, actinomycin D, etc. Local administration of MTX is associated with following advantages: increased tissue concentration of MTX at local site is associated with reduced systemic side effects, reduced rates of hospitalization, and greater preservation of fertility. Follow-up in these cases involves measurement of serum β-hCG levels twice weekly till levels decrease to <10 IU/L. TVS must be done on a weekly basis for 4–6 weeks and then on a monthly basis. Hysterosalpingography must be done after 6 months for checking tubal patency.

■ SURGICAL TREATMENT

The option of surgical treatment must be considered if an adnexal mass suggestive of ectopic pregnancy can be observed on TVS examination or there are clear signs demonstrating the presence of an ectopic pregnancy on ultrasound examination. If no abnormality is imaged on ultrasound examination, there is a high probability that an ectopic pregnancy would not be visualized at the time of surgery. Surgical treatment in the form of conservative surgery (tube-sparing approach), open surgery (laparotomy), or minimal invasive surgery (laparoscopy) are the commonly used treatment options. The procedures which can be performed at the time of both laparotomy and laparoscopy include salpingectomy or salpingotomy. In a hemodynamically stable patient, a laparoscopic approach is preferable to laparotomy. Moreover, in a stable woman with a reasonable probability of future normal tubal function in the affected tube, salpingostomy is preferred over salpingectomy. Main disadvantage associated with laparoscopic salpingostomy is that it is associated with a higher rate of persistent trophoblastic tissue in comparison to open salpingostomy. If the woman does not conceive in the first 12–18 months following surgical therapy for ectopic pregnancy, or her contralateral tube is damaged or absent, the clinician must resort to the option of IVF. Some indications for surgical therapy are described in **Box 32.17**.

Surgical treatment is associated with reduced requirement of time for resolution of the ectopic pregnancy and avoidance of the requirement for prolonged monitoring.

Some prerequisites which must be taken into consideration before starting surgical therapy include the following:

- Treatment needs to be explained to the woman and her partner, and written informed consent must be obtained.

> **BOX 32.17:** Indications for surgical therapy.
>
> - Candidate not suitable for medical therapy (not willing to comply with post-treatment medical therapy follow-up or contraindications to the use of methotrexate)
> - Failed medical therapy
> - Heterotopic pregnancy with a viable intrauterine pregnancy
> - Patient is hemodynamically unstable and requires immediate treatment
> - Impending or ongoing rupture of the ectopic mass
> - Absence of timely access to a medical institution for managing tubal rupture
> - Patient desires permanent method of contraception

- Patient's blood sample needs to be typed and cross-matched (ABO and Rh), and blood needs to be arranged. Anti-D immunoglobulins need to be administered to women who are Rhesus negative.

The following steps need to be taken in women who are hemodynamically unstable:
1. Immediate resuscitation
2. Securing immediate IV access by inserting large-bore venous cannula
3. Sending blood for full blood count and cross-matching and arranging at least four units of blood
4. Informing the theater staff, anesthetist, and on-call gynecology consultant
5. Foley's catheter must be inserted prior to starting the procedure.

The urgency of the situation must be stressed to all concerned. The surgery must not be delayed and should be performed even before blood and fluid losses have been completely replaced.

Type of Surgical Approach

Surgical therapy may be either in the form of open laparotomy or via the laparoscopic route. Nowadays, the trend is toward using a conservative approach for surgery. Numerous factors need to be considered before deciding the type of surgical approach to be used. Some of these factors include history of multiple prior surgeries, pelvic adhesions, skill of the surgeon and surgical staff, availability of the equipment, condition of the patient, and size and location of ectopic pregnancy. As previously described, a laparoscopic approach to the surgical management of tubal pregnancy must be used in hemodynamically stable patients. On the other hand, management of tubal pregnancy in the presence of hemodynamic instability should be by laparotomy. There is no role for medical management in the treatment of tubal pregnancy or suspected tubal pregnancy when a patient is showing signs of hypovolemic shock.

Conservative Surgery

Conservative surgery aims at preserving the tube and can be done via laparoscopic route or microsurgical laparotomy.

The choice of technique in these cases depends upon the location and size of gestational sac, condition of tubes, and accessibility to the gestational sac. Indications for conservative surgery include the following: the patient desires fertility, and contralateral tube is damaged or was previously removed. Various conservative surgeries could include the following:

- *Linear salpingostomy*: This is usually indicated in cases of unruptured ectopic pregnancy < 2 cm in the ampullary region. In this method, a linear incision is given on the antimesenteric border over the site of ectopic pregnancy. If the procedure is done via laparotomy, the products of conception can be removed by fingers. In case the procedure is being done by laparoscopy, the products of conception can be removed by gentle suction and irrigation. In either case, the incision site is kept open and allowed to heal by secondary intention.
- *Linear salpingotomy*: Procedure is similar to linear salpingostomy, except that the incision is not left open, rather closed in two layers with 7-0 interrupted vicryl sutures.
- *Segmental resection and anastomosis*: This procedure may be indicated in unruptured isthmic pregnancy. End-to-end anastomosis may be done immediately or later.
- *Milking or fimbrial expression*: This procedure may be ideal in cases of distal ampullary or infundibular pregnancy. Milking of pregnancy through abdominal ostium (transfimbrial extraction) had been advocated in the past if the hemorrhage was easy to control and pregnancy was fimbrial. However, the risk of recurrent/persistent ectopic pregnancy in these cases is likely to be twice as high. There is also likely to be a risk of rupture and bleeding in the long run. Therefore, this procedure is no longer recommended.

Follow-up after conservative surgery comprises measurement of weekly serum β-hCG levels till it comes out negative. In case β-hCG titers increase, MTX therapy can be administered.

Laparoscopic Surgery

Benefits of Laparoscopic Management of Tubal Pregnancy

Laparoscopy can be used for diagnosis, evaluation, and treatment of cases of ectopic pregnancy. Laparoscopy can simultaneously be used for the diagnosis and management of other causes of infertility (e.g., peritubular adhesions can be released, and endometriotic lesions can be treated). Laparoscopic management is associated with considerably reduced postoperative morbidity, duration of hospital stay, complication rate, and time duration of return to normal activity level. Most cases of ruptured as well as unruptured tubal pregnancy can be treated laparoscopically.

Laparoscopic management is a useful method for reducing hospital stay, complications, and return to normal activity. The main advantages of laparoscopic surgery are enumerated in **Box 32.18**.

Complications due to Laparoscopic Management of Ectopic Pregnancy

In experienced hands there is no specific complication directly related to laparoscopic procedure, but if the surgeon is not trained enough in laparoscopy then the chance of the complications as described in **Box 32.19** is there. However, in experienced hands, the chances of these complications are extremely rare. Altogether, laparoscopic procedure has a much lower complication rate in comparison to the conventional surgery.

Laparotomy

There are times when laparotomy is favored over the laparoscopic approach. Some of these indications are described in **Box 32.20**.

Laparotomy is usually preferred in cases of hemodynamic instability or when ectopic pregnancy is cervical, interstitial, abdominal, etc. It is also preferred in patients having large hematoma due to large ruptured ectopic pregnancy or in case of presence of >1,500 cc hemoperitoneum. A patient with cardiac diseases and chronic obstructive pulmonary disease should not be considered a good candidate for laparoscopic management. Laparoscopic management of ectopic pregnancy may also be more difficult in patients who have had previous lower abdominal surgery or those who may also be at an increased risk for complications with general anesthesia combined with pneumoperitoneum, e.g., the elderly patients.

The surgical procedure performed during laparotomy is usually salpingectomy, which is described later in the text.

Laparotomy Versus Laparoscopy

Laparoscopy is usually reserved for patients who are hemodynamically stable. Ruptured ectopic pregnancy may not necessarily require a laparotomy if the patient is stable. However, in the presence of large clots, laparotomy must be considered.

Reproductive outcome: It is likely to be similar with both laparotomy and laparoscopy, with identical rates of IUP.

Surgical Procedures during Laparotomy or Laparoscopy

Salpingectomy

Salpingectomy involves removal of ectopic pregnancy along with the fallopian tube of affected side.

Regardless of the route of approach (whether laparotomy and laparoscopy), salpingectomy is indicated in the situations enumerated in **Box 32.21**. The clinician has the option for choosing between partial and total salpingectomy. The choice for partial versus total salpingectomy is based on the patient's age and her desire to conceive in future. Partial salpingectomy is usually done in those cases who might opt for tubal reanastomosis at a future date.

Total salpingectomy is usually performed in those cases where IVF appears to be the likely treatment option.

BOX 32.18: Advantages of laparoscopic surgery.
- Reduced postoperative pain
- Faster recovery
- Short hospital stay
- Lower rate of postoperative complications such as wound infection
- Cost-effectiveness
- Reduced postoperative analgesic requirement
- Reduced adhesion formation

BOX 32.19: Complications due to laparoscopic surgery.
- Missed diagnosis
- Bleeding
- Incomplete removal of ectopic pregnancy
- Visceral Injury
- Leakage of purulent exudates
- Intra-abdominal abscess
- Hernia

BOX 32.20: Indications for laparotomy.
- Patient is hemodynamically unstable
- Cervical, interstitial, or abdominal ectopic pregnancy
- Patients having large hematoma due to large ruptured ectopic pregnancy
- Presence of >1,500 cc hemoperitoneum
- Patients with underlying cardiac diseases and chronic obstructive pulmonary disease
- History of abdominal surgery in the past
- Patients at increased risk of complications with general anesthesia

BOX 32.21: Indications for salpingectomy.
- Tube is severely damaged
- There is uncontrolled bleeding
- There is a recurrent ectopic pregnancy in the same tube
- There is a large tubal pregnancy of size > 5 cm
- Ectopic pregnancy has ruptured
- Woman has completed her family, and future fertility is not desired
- Ectopic pregnancy has resulted due to sterilization failure
- Ectopic pregnancy has occurred in a previously reconstructed tube
- Patient requests sterilization
- Hemorrhage continues to occur even after salpingotomy
- Cases of chronic tubal pregnancy

Procedure of salpingectomy: It involves the following steps:
1. If done via the laparoscopic route, laparoscopic scissors and diathermy or endoloops are used.
2. Loop using No. 1 catgut is passed over the ectopic pregnancy, following which the stitch is tightened, and then the tubal pregnancy is cut distal to the loop stitch.
3. Tubo-ovarian artery is also clamped, cut, and ligated, while preserving the utero-ovarian artery and ligament.
4. Mesosalpinx must be continued to be clamped, cut, and ligated until the tube is free and can be removed.
5. Following the excision and removal of tube, the pedicles are ligated using a 2-0 or 3-0 synthetic absorbable suture.
6. If using laparoscopy, the excised tissue is removed piecemeal or using a tissue removal bag.

Partial Salpingectomy

Partial salpingectomy may be sometimes performed instead of complete salpingectomy if the pregnancy is in the midportion of the tube, none of the indications for salpingectomy are present, and the patient appears to be a candidate for tubal reanastomosis in future. In these cases, a clamp is placed through an avascular area in the mesosalpinx under the ectopic pregnancy. This creates spaces through which two free ties are placed, which are tied around the tube on each side of the ectopic pregnancy. The isolated portion of the tube containing the ectopic pregnancy is then cut and removed.

Follow-up: All patients who have not had the entire ectopic pregnancy removed by salpingectomy need to have their weekly hCG levels observed until these levels return to nonpregnant values. If during this time span the hCG level either plateaus or rises, the patient must be treated with MTX. Patients should be advised to use some form of effective contraception until their hCG levels have returned to nonpregnant levels.

Salpingotomy

Tube-sparing salpingostomy or salpingotomy is a procedure in which the gestational sac is removed, without the removal of tube, through a 1 cm long incision on the tubal wall. This surgery is preferred over salpingectomy because not only is salpingotomy less invasive but it is also associated with comparable rates of subsequent fertility and ectopic pregnancy. Laparoscopic salpingotomy should especially be considered as the primary modality of treatment if the woman has contralateral tube disease and desires future fertility.

When salpingotomy is used for the management of tubal pregnancy, follow-up protocols (weekly serum β-hCG levels) are necessary for the identification and treatment of women with persistent trophoblastic disease. Persistent trophoblast is detected by the failure of serum hCG levels to fall as expected after the initial treatment.

Procedure: After infiltrating the mesosalpinx with vasopressin [20 IU in 50 mL normal saline (NS)], 1–2 cm longitudinal incision is made on the antimesenteric side of the tube. The incision can be made using carbon monoxide or argon laser. Laparoscopic scissors can be used for extending the incision. Bleeding points can be ablated using bipolar diathermy. A syringe filled with saline is inserted deep into the incision, and the fluid is injected forcefully in such a way so as to dislodge the ectopic pregnancy and clots. The contents of ectopic pregnancy and clots are then aspirated out. Following this, the bed of the ectopic pregnancy must be irrigated well. In case some trophoblastic tissue remains, prior injection of vasopressin may lead to anoxia and death of the trophoblasts, preventing postoperative growth. Bleeding may be controlled by applying pressure with blunt tissue forceps for 5 minutes.

Postoperative follow-up: Regular follow-up must be done following surgery in order to ensure that the patient's hCG levels have returned to zero. This may take several weeks. Elevated hCG levels could mean that some ectopic trophoblastic tissue, which was missed at the time of removal, is still remaining inside. This tissue may have to be removed using MTX or additional surgery.
- Patient must be instructed to visit the clinician after 1 week for removal of sutures.
- Patient must be counseled that she may experience mild bleeding or pain during the first postoperative week. In case of mild pain, she can use simple analgesic drugs available over the counter. In case of pain or bleeding of severe intensity, she must be instructed to report to the clinician immediately.

Salpingostomy/Salpingotomy Versus Salpingectomy

The choice between salpingostomy or salpingectomy for the treatment of ectopic pregnancy presently remains controversial. Both the procedures are associated with similar rates of operative morbidity.

All tubal ectopic pregnancies can be treated by partial or total salpingectomy. The main disadvantage of salpingostomy/salpingotomy is the potential risk of persistent or recurrent ectopic pregnancy. Salpingostomy/salpingotomy is therefore performed in women who are hemodynamically stable, and who want to conserve their fertility. Also, in these cases, the tubal ectopic pregnancy should be unruptured, have a size < 5 cm, and the site of ectopic pregnancy must be easily accessible. This procedure may also be indicated when contralateral tube is absent or damaged. To decide between salpingostomy/salpingotomy and salpingectomy, Chapron et al. (1993) have devised a scoring system **(Table 32.6)** based on the patient's gynecological history and appearance of pelvic organs. The main rationale behind the scoring system is to help decide the risk of recurrent ectopic pregnancy. Conservative surgery is indicated with a score of 1–4. More radical treatment is required with a score of 5 or more, otherwise there may be a high risk of recurrence.

Some situations where salpingectomy, instead of salpingostomy/salpingostomy, is preferred are listed in **Box 32.22**.

TABLE 32.6: Scoring system by Chapron et al. (1993) to decide between salpingostomy/salpingotomy and salpingectomy.

Fertility-reducing factor	Score
Antecedent one ectopic pregnancy	2
Antecedent each further ectopic pregnancy	1
Antecedent adhesiolysis	1
Antecedent tubal microsurgery	2
Antecedent salpingitis	1
Solitary tube	2
Homolateral adhesions	1
Contralateral adhesions	1

Source: Chapron C, Pouly JL, Wattiez A, Mage G, Canis M, Bouquet J, et al. Laparoscopic management of tubal ectopic pregnancy. Eur J Obstet Gynecol Reprod Biol. 1993;49(1-2):73-9.

BOX 32.22: Indications for performing salpingectomy instead of salpingostomy.

- Uncontrolled bleeding from the implantation site
- Recurrent ectopic pregnancy in the same tube
- Severely damaged tube
- Large tubal pregnancy (i.e., >5 cm)
- Women who have completed their childbearing
- Women who may be treated with IVF in future

Laparoscopic Surgery

Laparoscopic Salpingectomy

Laparoscopic salpingectomy **(Figs. 32.14A to C)** involves the use of bipolar cautery for desiccation of tube. The rest of the procedure is same as that performed during laparotomy.

Tube-sparing Salpingotomy

The procedure of laparoscopic salpingotomy **(Figs. 32.15A to G)** is same as that described with laparotomy before.

Medical Versus Surgical Treatment

Systemic treatment with MTX has been found to be as effective as laparoscopic salpingostomy. At the same time, medical treatment is more cost-effective in comparison to the surgical treatment.

Prospects of Future Conception

Some women who have had ectopic pregnancies in past may have difficulty becoming pregnant in future. This difficulty is more common in women who also had fertility problems before developing ectopic pregnancy. The likelihood of a repeat ectopic pregnancy increases with each subsequent ectopic pregnancy. If the patient has had one ectopic pregnancy, there is an approximately 15% chance of developing another one in future. This risk increases to as high as 32% in women who have had two consecutive ectopic pregnancies in the past. Approximately 30% of women treated for ectopic pregnancy are expected to have future difficulty in

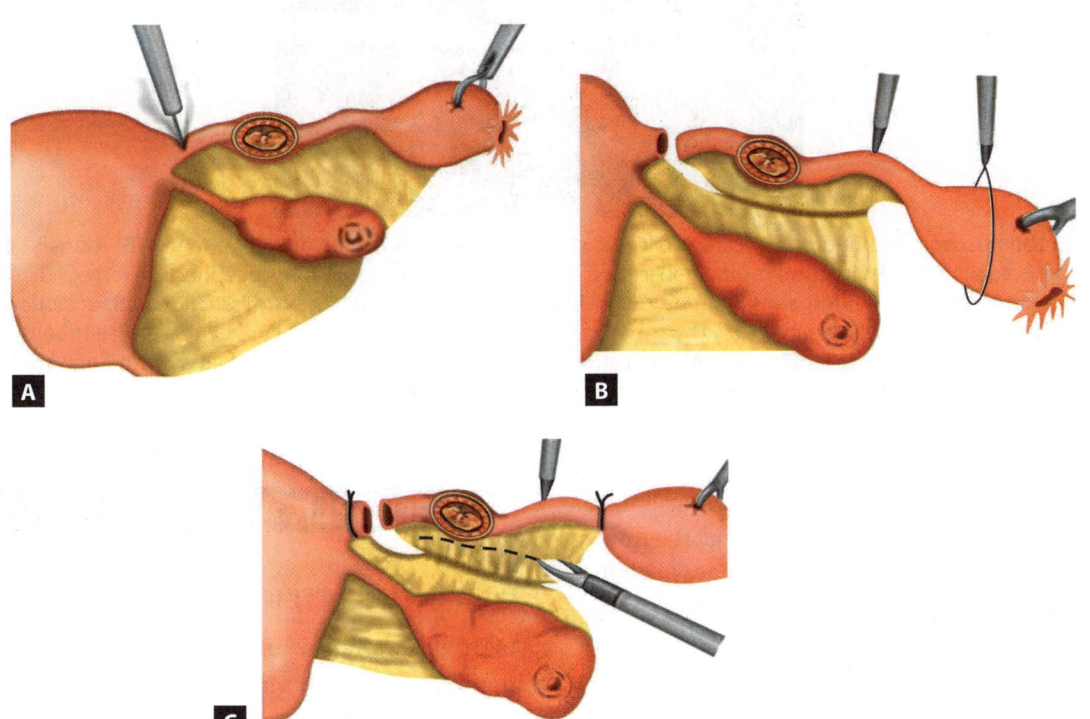

Figs. 32.14A to C: Procedure of laparoscopic salpingectomy. (A) Bipolar cautery is used to desiccate the tube at its insertion into the uterus; (B) Pretied surgical loop is placed over the fallopian tube with the help of grasping forceps; (C) Fallopian tube is resected and then removed.

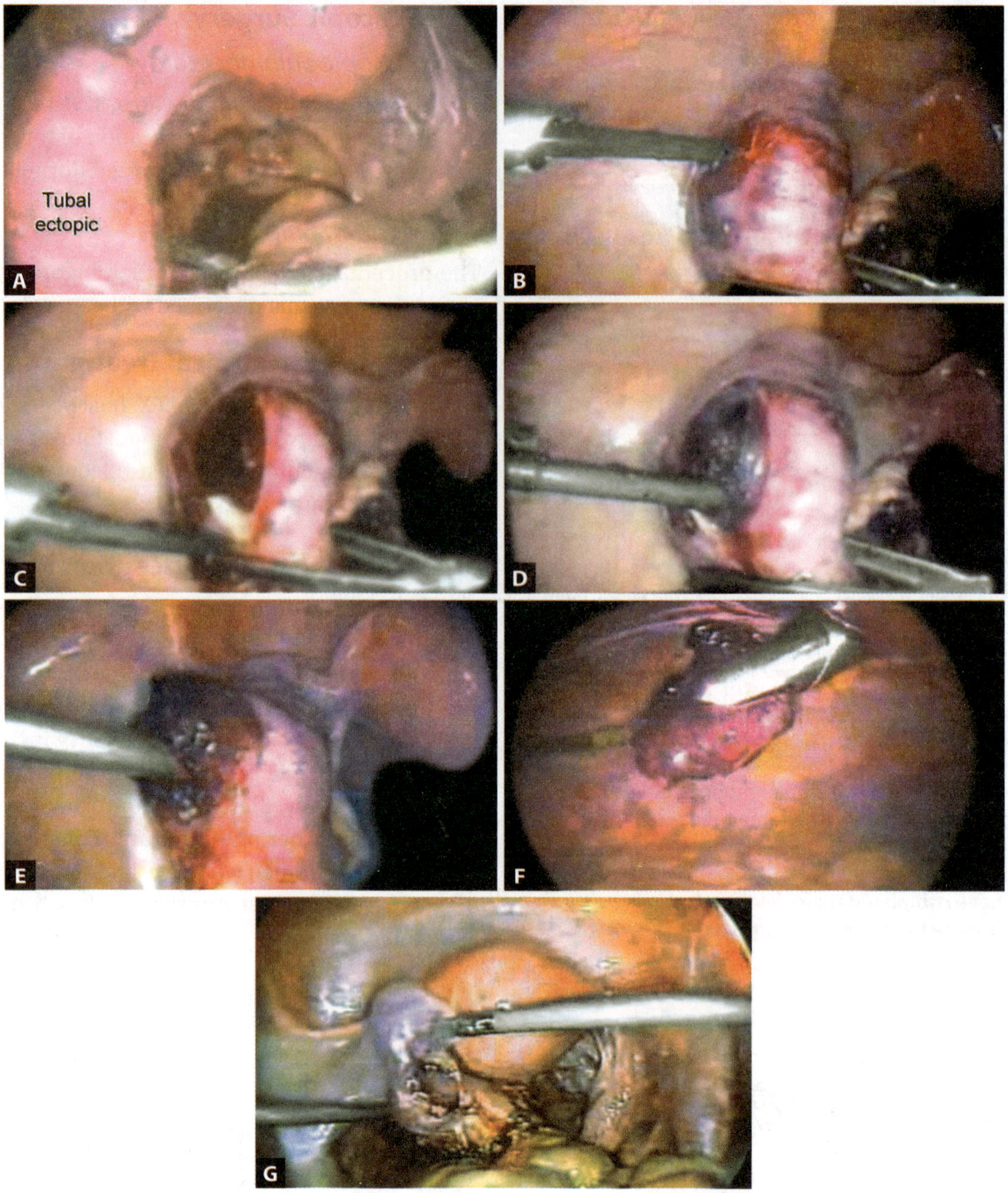

Figs. 32.15A to G: Laparoscopic salpingotomy. (A) Laparoscopic view showing the tubal ectopic pregnancy; (B) A small 1 cm linear incision given over the tubal ectopic; (C) The salpingotomy incision is then enlarged; (D) The products of conception are removed from the tube using a combination of hydrodissection with irrigating solution under high pressure and gentle blunt dissection with a suction irrigator; (E) The contents of the tube being completely removed; (F) The tubal contents are removed out of pelvic cavity; (G) The tube is carefully irrigated and inspected underwater for hemostasis. Bleeding points can be controlled by pressure or coagulated with light application of bipolar coagulation. The salpingotomy incision is left unstitched once bleeding has been controlled.

conceiving. The overall future conception rate in this case can be expected to vary between 70% and 85%. Moreover, results of the Demeter randomized trial (2013) show that the mode of treatment (medical, surgical, or conservative) does not appear to influence future fertility in cases with ectopic pregnancy.

TREATMENT OF NONTUBAL ECTOPIC PREGNANCY

Management options in cases of nontubal ectopic pregnancy are summarized in **Table 32.7**.

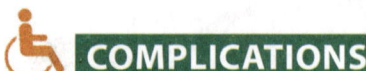

COMPLICATIONS

LIFE-THREATENING HEMORRHAGE

As the pregnancy in tubal location grows and starts increasing in size, it may cause the fallopian tube to rupture. Hemorrhage due to tubal rupture and intra-abdominal bleeding is an important cause for mortality and morbidity in these cases.

TABLE 32.7: Management options of various types of ectopic pregnancy based on their location.

Cervical pregnancy	Cesarean scar pregnancy	Interstitial pregnancy	Ovarian pregnancy	Heterotopic pregnancy	Abdominal pregnancy
• Medical management with methotrexate can be considered • Surgical methods may be associated with a high failure rate • Surgical management may be used in women suffering from life-threatening bleeding	• Counseling the woman that such pregnancies may be associated with severe maternal morbidity and mortality • Medical and surgical interventions with or without additional hemostatic measures should be considered in women with first-trimester pregnancy • Although the present evidence is insufficient, the current literature favors surgical approach in comparison to the medical approach • There are some studies exploring the role of uterine artery embolization or uterine artery chemoembolization prior to the use of suction curettage in these patients. Though these procedures are likely to reduce the blood loss in comparison to the use of systemic methotrexate, presently there is no definite evidence proving this	• Nonsurgical management is an acceptable option in stable patients • Expectant management is only suitable for women with low or significantly falling beta human chorionic gonadotropin (β-hCG) levels in whom the addition of methotrexate is unlikely to improve the outcome • Management in these cases involves excision of the rudimentary horn via laparoscopy or laparotomy • A pharmacological approach using methotrexate has been shown to be effective, although there is insufficient evidence available regarding its use	• In case laparoscopy is required for diagnostic purposes, surgical treatment is preferred • In case surgery is associated with high risk, systemic methotrexate therapy can be used • Methotrexate therapy is also useful in the presence of persistently raised β-hCG levels or residual trophoblast disease	• If the intrauterine pregnancy is nonviable or if the woman does not wish to continue with the pregnancy, methotrexate therapy should be considered • In case of clinically stable women, local injection of potassium chloride or hyperosmolar glucose with aspiration of the sac contents can be considered • Surgical removal of the ectopic pregnancy is the method of choice for all women, whether hemodynamically stable or not • Expectant management should be used in cases where the ultrasound findings point toward a nonviable pregnancy	• Early abdominal pregnancy must be removed via laparoscopic route • Alternatively, systemic methotrexate with ultrasound-guided feticide can be used • Laparotomy must be used in cases of advanced abdominal pregnancy

RUPTURE OF ECTOPIC PREGNANCY

Rupture of ectopic pregnancy is a medical emergency responsible for significant maternal mortality and morbidity. It may be associated with features of shock and warrants immediate resuscitation of the patient and an emergency laparotomy to resect out the ruptured tube and control the intraperitoneal hemorrhage. Antishock treatment comprises the following:

- IV line should be established, and crystalloids should be started.
- Blood sample should be collected for blood-grouping, cross-matching, bleeding time, and clotting time.
- Foley's catheterization must be done.
- Colloids must be used for volume replacement.

Emergency laparotomy involves the following:

- It is based on the principle of quick in and quick out.
- It involves rapid exploration of the abdominal cavity.
- Salpingectomy is the definitive surgery. Resected sample of the tube must be sent for HPE.
- Blood transfusion may be required to revive the patient.
- Autotransfusion may be done in cases where donated blood is either not available or not acceptable to the patient.

PERSISTENT ECTOPIC PREGNANCY

Persistent ectopic pregnancy is the complication of salpingotomy/salpingostomy when the residual trophoblastic tissue continues to survive due to incomplete evacuation of the ectopic pregnancy. Diagnosis is usually made when serum β-hCG levels continue to be raised postoperatively. If untreated, this is likely to result in life-threatening hemorrhage. Risk factors for development of persistent ectopic pregnancy are as follows:

- Early ectopic pregnancy (<6 weeks' amenorrhea)
- Small-sized ectopic pregnancy (<2 cm in size)
- High serum β-hCG levels preoperatively (>3,000 IU/L), and postoperative day-1 titer is <50% of the preoperative level.
- Implantation medial to the salpingostomy site

Management comprises surgical intervention in the form of total or partial salpingectomy if medical therapy was administered previously. In case surgical management was done previously, medical management can be tried in cases of persistent ectopic pregnancy.

FUTURE FERTILITY OUTCOME

> Q. Discuss, with the help of a short essay, fertility outcome following ectopic pregnancy.

Women with initial ectopic pregnancy are likely to have lower chances of future conception in comparison to the women who had a miscarriage. This is probably due to the fact that the same underlying pathology, i.e., tubal damage (with the most likely risk factor being PID) is likely to be responsible for both infertility and ectopic pregnancy.

Also, these women are likely to have an increased risk of repeat ectopic pregnancy in their future pregnancies, with the risk being 15% after the first ectopic pregnancy, and 25% after the second. With the shift in management strategies adopting tubal conservative approach, chances of fertility have improved, but the risk of recurrence has increased.

EVIDENCE-BASED CLINICAL TRIALS

List of references can be scanned through QR code to enable the readers gain deeper insight of the subject by referring to the entire article or its abstract.

CHAPTER 33

Adenomyosis

CASE STUDY

A 45-year-old para 2 woman who has completed her family has presented with a history of heavy menstrual bleeding since last 4 days. She has been experiencing this problem over the past 4 years. Besides being associated with heavy bleeding, her periods are also occurring frequently, every 10–15 days. She also complains of severe abdominal pain during her periods. Her pain has not responded to treatment with NSAIDs or hormonal preparations. There is no history of dyschezia or dyspareunia.

INTRODUCTION

 Q. Write a short note on adenomyosis.

Adenomyosis is a condition in which there is a growth of endometrial cells inside the uterine myometrium (usually >2.5 mm beneath the basal endometrium) **(Figs. 33.1A to C)**. It is associated with myometrial hypertrophy and the lesions may be diffuse (present throughout the myometrium) or focal (localized lesions) or present as adenomyomas. Adenomyoma is a form of

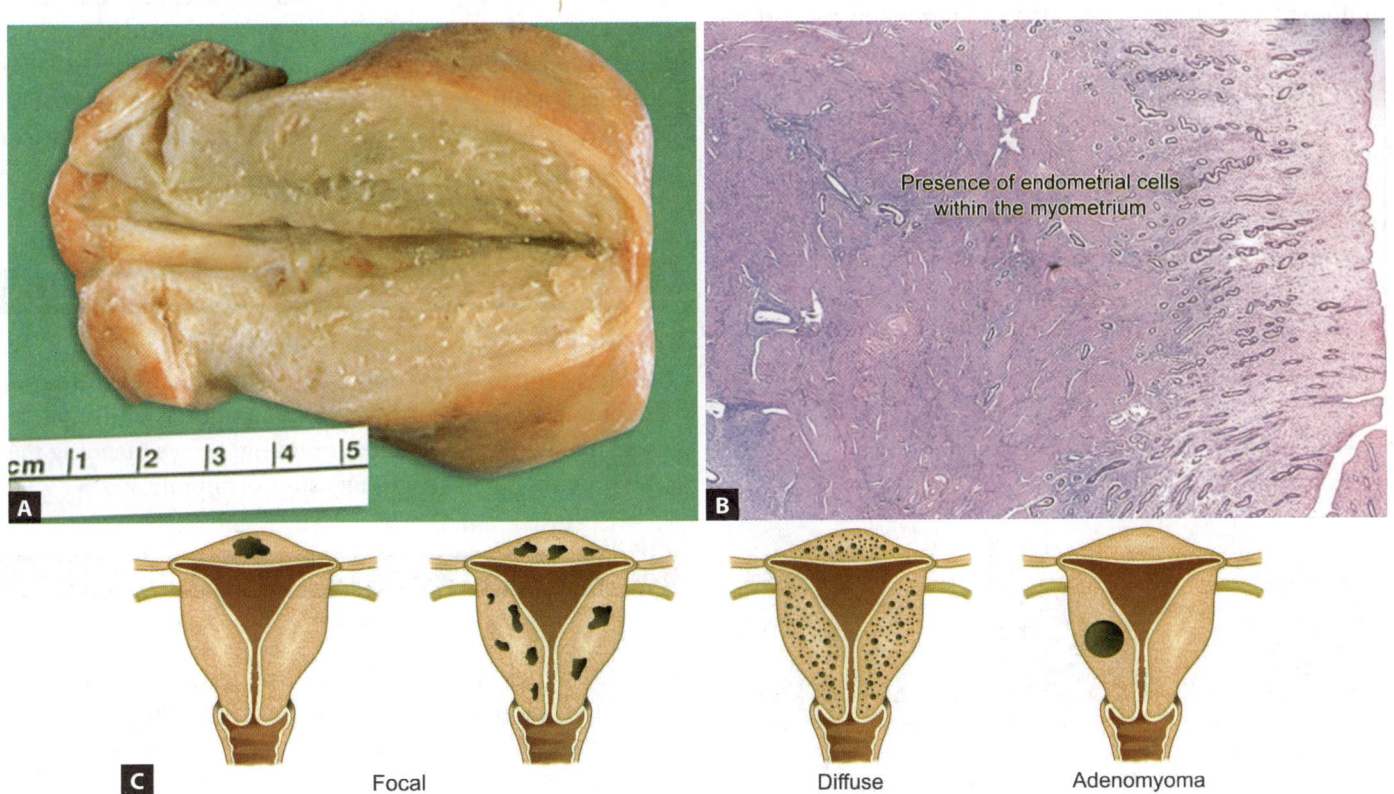

Figs. 33.1A to C: Adenomyosis (A) Cut specimen of the uterus; (B) Histopathological appearance of adenomyosis; (C) Different lesions of adenomyosis.

circumscribed nodular aggregate of tissues composed of benign endometrial glands surrounded by endometrial stromal component, which is bordered by leiomyomatous smooth muscle. Microscopically, there are ectopic, non-neoplastic endometrial glands and stroma, surrounded by hypertrophic and hyperplastic myometrium.

The majority of cases of adenomyosis are diagnosed following histological examination of hysterectomy specimens, with a prevalence varying between 5% and 70%. The prevalence in general population, however, remains unclear.

The majority of cases are reported among women in the age groups of 40–50 years and there is a positive association with parity. No association has been observed with age at menarche, menopausal status, or age at hysterectomy or its indication.

ASSOCIATED PATHOLOGY

Nearly 80% of women with adenomyomas may also have other lesions, most common being the leiomyomas. Other lesions which may frequently occur in these cases include endometrial polyps, endometrial hyperplasia (with or without atypia), adenocarcinoma, and pelvic endometriosis. Presence of adenomyosis, however, has no adverse effect on cancer survival.

ETIOLOGY

Abnormal ingrowth and invagination of the basal endometrium into the subendometrial myometrium at the endometrial-myometrial interface is likely to result in the development of adenomyosis **(Figs. 33.2A to C)**. Though the exact cause of adenomyosis remains unknown, various factors, such as hormonal, genetic and immunological, are likely to play a role in the pathogenesis of adenomyosis. Some likely causes are as follows:

- *Uterine trauma:* Various causes of uterine trauma that may break the barrier between the endometrium and myometrium include surgical procedures such as cesarean section, tubal ligation, and pregnancy termination. Pregnancy is another factor which can break this barrier.

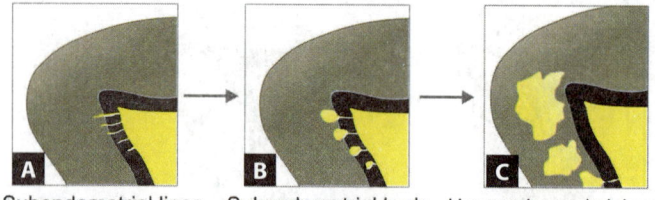

Figs. 33.2A to C: Growth of ectopic endometrial glands and stroma into the myometrium resulting in various ultrasound findings. (A) Subendometrial lines; (B) Buds; (C) Expansion to hyperechogenic islands in the myometrium.

- *Estrogen dominance:* Conditions associated with the localized production of excessive estrogens may predispose the woman to develop adenomyosis.
- *Abnormal level of various cytokines:* Increased levels of interleukin 18 (IL-18) receptor mRNA (messenger RNA) and the ratio of IL-18 binding protein to IL-18, and dysregulation of leukemia inhibitory factor.

HISTORY AND CLINICAL PRESENTATION

HISTORY

If detailed history had not been taken during the time of gynecological check-up, it must be taken now, at the time of admission. The details, which need to be elicited at the time of taking history, are described in Chapter 22.

CLINICAL PRESENTATION

Nearly 35% of women with adenomyosis uteri are asymptomatic.

Commonly occurring symptoms include menorrhagia (unresponsive to hormonal therapy or uterine curettage) and progressively increasing dysmenorrhea. Menorrhagia can occur in nearly 40–50% cases, dysmenorrhea in 10–30% cases, and metrorrhagia in 10–12% cases. Menorrhagia may be due to dysfunctional contractility of the myometrium, endometrial hyperplasia, and anovulation. Other rare symptoms may include pelvic pain, backache, dyspareunia, dyschezia, and subfertility. These symptoms are more likely to be associated with endometriosis. Also, pain rather than bleeding is a more prominent symptom with endometriosis. Older women tend to be more symptomatic in comparison to younger women.

GENERAL PHYSICAL EXAMINATION

This involves assessment of patient's vital signs, similar to that done during the time of gynecological examination (Chapter 22). General physical examination is unlikely to be associated with any significant finding. Heavy bleeding may sometimes result in signs suggestive of anemia.

SPECIFIC SYSTEMIC EXAMINATION

PELVIC EXAMINATION

- Uterus may become diffuse and enlarged in cases of diffuse adenomyosis. Uterus may be enlarged to about 12–14 weeks in size and may be globular, nontender to touch, soft, and boggy. Uterine size of <14 weeks is indicative of adenomyosis. Irregular, firm uterus, >14 weeks in size is more suggestive of uterine fibroids

- In cases of adenomyosis, uterus is uniformly distended, whereas in the cases of fibroid, uterus is irregularly distended.
- In cases of adenomyosis the uterus is mobile/non-tender, whereas in cases of endometriosis it is fixed and tender due to the presence of adhesions.
- Adenomyosis is associated with uterine fibroids in about 6–20% cases.

TABLE 33.1: Features of adenomyosis on ultrasound and MRI.

Imaging feature	Ultrasound description	MRI description
Direct features	• Tiny myometrial cysts • Hyperechoic nodules or striations • Poor definition of the endometrial-myometrial interface	• Tiny myometrial cysts • Myometrial foci of high signal intensity on T1-weighted images
Indirect features	• Diffuse myometrial heterogeneity associated thin hypoechoic linear striations within a heterogeneous myometrium • Diffuse asymmetric or symmetric widening of the myometrial walls	• Junctional zone thickening • Abnormal myometrial signal intensity • Large, regular, asymmetric uterus without leiomyomas

DIFFERENTIAL DIAGNOSIS

Before making the diagnosis of adenomyosis, the following conditions need to be ruled out:

- *Endometriosis:* Congestive dysmenorrhea is likely to be associated with two main differential diagnoses: adenomyosis or endometriosis. Endometriosis is commonly associated with symptoms such as dyschezia or dyspareunia, whereas adenomyosis is not.
- *Leiomyomas:* Adenomyosis is most commonly confused with leiomyomas. Transvaginal ultrasonography is an effective, noninvasive, and relatively inexpensive procedure for establishing the diagnosis of adenomyoma, preoperatively. In case of inconclusive findings on TVS, one can resort to MR examination.
- *Endometrial polyp:* Presence of endometrial polyp can be confirmed through TVS.
- *Endometrial hyperplasia/cancer:* Endometrial biopsy helps in the diagnosis of endometrial hyperplasia/cancer. This diagnosis is more likely in younger perimenopausal women with abnormal uterine bleeding having presence of comorbidities such as hypertension, diabetes, and obesity with a history of anovulation.

MANAGEMENT

Q. Discuss the management plan in context of the case study described in the beginning of the chapter.

Different surgical and medical modalities of treatment have been used for the management of cases of adenomyosis uteri. Medical management can be considered as the first-line treatment option for providing symptomatic relief. This would be discussed further in the text.

INVESTIGATIONS

Presently, there is lack of a reliable, noninvasive diagnostic test for diagnosing adenomyosis. No serum markers for the diagnosis of adenomyosis are currently available. Some investigations, which are commonly performed, include the following:

ULTRASOUND EXAMINATION

Transvaginal sonography is better than transabdominal sonography in demonstrating the subtle features suggestive of adenomyosis uteri. Ultrasound may show heterogeneous myometrium with irregular cystic spaces giving salt and pepper appearance of the myometrium. The endometrium-myometrium junction is typically distorted. Some features suggestive of adenomyosis on TVS and MRI are enlisted in **Table 33.1**. **Figure 33.3** shows morphological Uterus Sonographic Assessment (MUSA) criteria for diagnosis of adenomyosis as described by Van den Bosch et al. (2015).

Presently, there is no consensus regarding whether one or some of these criteria should be used for making the diagnosis of adenomyosis. Most authorities presently use three or more of these criteria for making the diagnosis of adenomyosis. A recent meta-analysis has indicated that ultrasound features such as presence of myometrial cysts, linear myometrial striations, poor delineation or distortion of the endomyometrial junction, and a heterogeneous myometrium are associated with an increased probability of the presence of disease **(Fig. 33.4)**. Preferential thickening of the posterior wall is another important feature of adenomyosis.

In the normal woman, the myometrium has three distinct sonographic layers of which the middle layer is the most echogenic and the inner layer is hypoechoic relative to the middle and outer layers. This hypoechogenicity is responsible for producing the subendometrial or myometrial halo. The presence of adenomyosis uteri can cause alterations in the sonographic appearance of these zones. Studies regarding the accuracy of TVS for detection of adenomyosis have reported the rates of sensitivity varying between 53 and 89% and specificity varying between 50 and 99%. Three-dimensional ultrasonography is likely to offer higher accuracy in determining uterine volume and pathology.

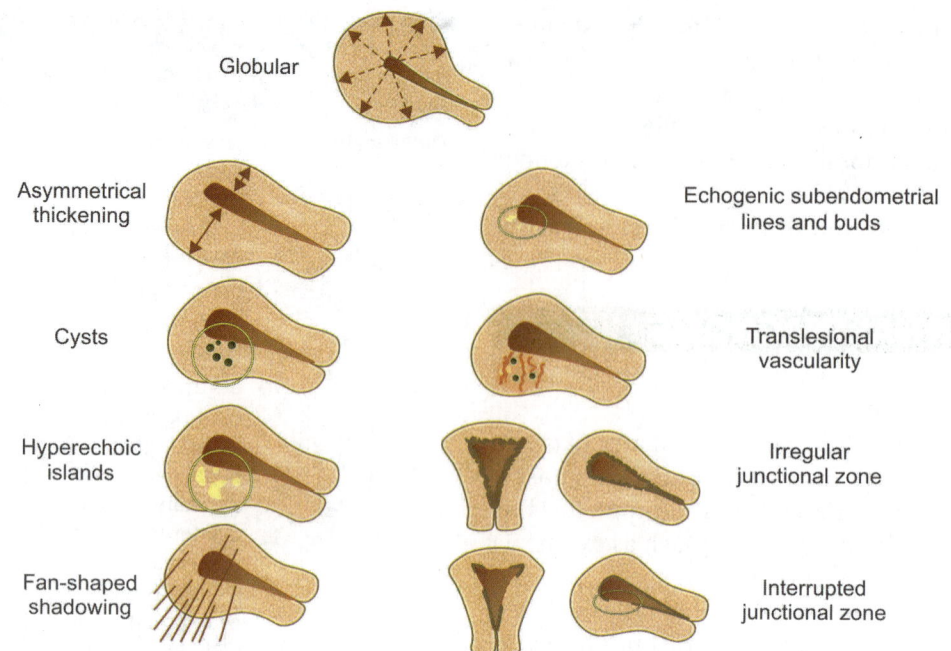

Fig. 33.3: Morphological Uterus Sonographic Assessment (MUSA) criteria for diagnosis of adenomyosis.
Source: Van den Bosch et al (2015)

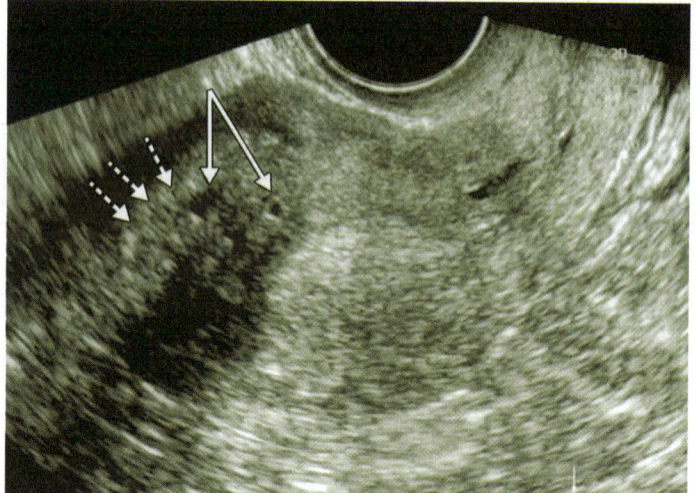

Fig. 33.4: Ultrasound showing mottled texture of the myometrium and presence of hypoechoic areas within the hyperechoic area in the fundal region which is suggestive of adenomyosis.

Fig. 33.5: Sagittal T1-weighted MR image showing diffuse, even thickening of the junctional zone (as depicted by arrows) which is consistent with the diagnosis of diffuse adenomyosis.

MAGNETIC RESONANCE IMAGING

This is superior to ultrasound for the diagnosis of adenomyosis. There has been growing evidence to support the use of MRI in the diagnosis of adenomyosis uteri. MRI may be considered when findings on TVS appear to be inconclusive. Main indication of doing MRI is while planning a conservative surgery in order to delineate the exact extent of the adenomyoma. However, its high cost and limited availability may impede its routine use. The presence of heterotopic endometrial glands and stroma in the myometrium appear as bright foci within the myometrium on T1-weighted MR images (**Fig. 33.5**). Adjacent smooth muscle hyperplasia may present as areas of reduced signal intensity on MRI. On MRI examination, there is considerable variation in the thickness of junctional zone, ranging from 2 to 8 mm. The appearance of diffuse or focal widening of the junctional zone on MRI is suggestive of adenomyosis uteri. Several studies which have compared the accuracy of TVS and MRI have found both these techniques to have comparable sensitivities and specificities. Nevertheless, MRI is less observer-dependent. MRI has proved to be superior to TVS in the presence of associated leiomyomas or additional pathologies. MRI is more useful in distinguishing adenomyosis from fibroids in an enlarged uterus.

- *CT scan:* There is no role of CT scan for diagnosis of adenomyosis.

- *Cancer antigen 125 (CA-125):* Level of CA-125 in the peripheral blood may be raised.
- *Other investigations:* These may include investigations such as hemoglobin (to rule out anemia) and pap smear (to rule out cervical carcinoma).
- *Histopathological examination:* The final diagnosis is established by histopathological examination of the hysterectomy specimen.

TREATMENT/OBSTETRIC MANAGEMENT

> Q. Write a long essay discussing the management and treatment of adenomyosis

MEDICAL THERAPY

Several hormonal and nonhormonal medications such as nonsteroidal anti-inflammatory drugs, mefenamic and tranexamic acid, combined oral contraceptive pills, danazol, gonadotropin-releasing hormone (GnRH) agonists, and Mirena® intrauterine contraceptive device (IUCD) are being used in an off-label manner to provide symptomatic management in the cases of adenomyosis, without the involvement of surgery.

Newer drugs such as aromatase inhibitors are also being investigated for their use in cases of adenomyosis. Presently, there is limited evidence regarding the use of medical, non-hormonal therapy for the treatment of cases of adenomyosis. These treatment strategies are likely to result in a variable and unpredictable degree of symptomatic relief, which is usually limited to the duration of treatment. Present evidence also indicates that temporary reversion of adenomyosis and symptomatic improvement can be observed by using medical suppressive hormonal therapy (e.g., oral contraceptive pills, high-dose progestins, selective estrogen receptor modulators, selective progesterone receptor modulators, the levonorgestrel releasing intrauterine device, aromatase inhibitors, danazol, GnRH analogs, etc.). Reduction in the size of adenomyoma foci is likely to be caused by drugs such as danazol, GnRH analogs, aromatase inhibitors and levonorgestrel-releasing intrauterine system (LNG-IUS). Presently, the most preferred treatment option is combined oral contraceptive pills in combination with NSAIDs. LNG-IUS would serve as the best long-term treatment option. In refractory cases, eventually surgery is required.

- *Nonsteroidal anti-inflammatory drugs:* These drugs help in reducing pain by decreasing the formation of prostaglandin precursors by causing nonselective reversible inhibition of COX-1 (cyclooxygenase 1) and COX-2 (cyclooxygenase 2). This helps in preventing the conversion of arachidonic acid into prostaglandins. Though the use of NSAIDs may be associated with reduced pain and bleeding, it may result in side effects such as gastrointestinal bleeding.

  Selective COX-2 specific inhibitors, such as celecoxib or etoricoxib are also being increasingly used to provide relief from pain and bleeding. Presently, there is limited evidence to show any improved efficacy of selective COX-2 inhibitors over NSAIDs in treatment of congestive dysmenorrhea associated with adenomyosis.

- *Combined oral contraceptive pills:* Use of low-dose, continuous combined oral contraceptives with withdrawal bleeding after every 4–6 months may be effective in relieving menorrhagia and dysmenorrhea associated with adenomyosis. Oral contraceptive pills act by causing the suppression of following: hypothalamic and pituitary gonadotropin production, ovarian folliculogenesis and ovarian steroid production. However, there is no specific randomized study related to this therapy in cases with adenomyosis.

- *Progesterone-only pills:* Progesterone only pills are likely to cause a significant reduction in pain and bleeding by causing endometrial decidualization and atrophy. They are also likely to cause alleviation of local hyperestrogenism. However, their use may be ineffective in about one-third of the patients. Its use may frequently result in metrorrhagia in varying severity. Also, their role in diminishing uterine volume presently remains doubtful.

- *Gonadotropin-releasing hormone analogs:* These drugs are likely to cause reduction in secretion of gonadotropins, thereby resulting in ovarian quiescence and induction of a pseudomenopausal hypoestrogenic state. Administration of GnRH analogs is likely to be useful for the treatment of adenomyosis uteri by reducing uterine volume and providing symptomatic relief. However, these benefits are rapidly reversed following the cessation of treatment. Moreover, they are also likely to cause skeletal and general side-effects. There could be a role for long-term use of GnRH therapy in association with add-back therapy as described with uterine fibroids and endometriosis (Chapters 24: HMB due to Leiomyomas and 30: Pelvic Pain)

- *Danazol:* This drug acts on androgen receptors as an androgen agonist. It also has antiestrogen and antigonadotropic actions. The use of danazol has largely become outdated due to its androgenic side-effects. Danazol-loaded intrauterine device has been used as a noninvasive method for the treatment of infertile women with adenomyosis uteri. This method is likely to result in pregnancy following the discontinuation of treatment. Moreover, it is associated with preservation of both menstrual and ovulatory functions and a significant decrease in dysmenorrhea.

- *Levonorgestrel-releasing intrauterine system:* LNG-IUS has been tried as the treatment option of moderate or severe dysmenorrhea and/or menorrhagia associated with adenomyosis. It acts by causing decidualization of endometrial lining, downregulation of estrogen receptors on adenomyotic foci and reduction in the production of prostaglandins. Its use is likely to result in the size of adenomyotic foci, significant reduction in menstrual bleeding, and reduced uterine volume and pain symptoms. However, it may be associated with side effects such as irregular bleeding and amenorrhea. There is some evidence that the presence of deep lesions of adenomyosis is associated with the failure of endometrial ablation. In these situations, LNG-IUS has also been successfully used for the treatment of adenomyosis-associated menorrhagia, especially when inserted immediately after endometrial ablation.

A prospective randomized control trial by Ozdegirmenci et al. (2011) has shown that use of LNG-IUS is likely to result in significant improvement in level of hemoglobin in patients with adenomyosis-associated menorrhagia, which is comparable to that attained with hysterectomy. Although both the treatment modalities are likely to result in an improvement in health-related quality of life, LNG-IUS seems to have superior effects on psychological and social life. It is likely to serve a promising alternative therapy to hysterectomy.

- *Aromatase inhibitors:* These drugs act by inhibiting the enzyme aromatase, which is involved in the conversion of androstenedione and testosterone to estrone and estradiol respectively. These drugs help in reducing the volume of adenomyoma and pelvic pain. However, these drugs may result in side effects such as hot flushes and nausea. Aromatase inhibitors are likely to have an efficacy similar to GnRH agonist in reducing the volume of adenomyoma and improving symptoms.
- *Newer drugs:* Some newer drugs which have been tried in cases of adenomyosis include selective estrogen receptor modulators (SERM), dienogest, and ulipristal acetate. Dienogest is an oral progestin that has been investigated extensively in the treatment of adenomyosis. The long-term use of dinogest is likely to be well-tolerated and effective in patients with symptomatic adenomyosis. The most common adverse effects associated with dineogest include metrorrhagia (96.9%) and hot flushes (7.7%). Recently therapeutic agents like selective progesterone receptor modulators (SPRMs) such as ulipristal acetate and selective estrogen receptor modulators (SERMs), such as clomiphene, tamoxifen, toremifene, raloxifene, ospemifene, lasofoxifene, etc., are being increasingly used in cases of adenomyosis. However, there is still requirement of well deigned randomized trials for evaluating the efficacy of SERMs and SPRMs in cases of adenomyosis. Some studies have shown that ulipristal acetate is likely to be a good alternative treatment option for women with adenomyosis who want to preserve their fertility. Ulipristal had been previously used in the cases of fibroids. However, its use has been found to be associated with hepatitis, which can progress to acute liver failure in some cases, even requiring liver transplantation. As a result the European medical Board has now suspended the use of ulipristal acetate except in cases where it is used as a contraceptive agent because it is require in very low doses for this indication.

SURGICAL MANAGEMENT

Hysterectomy

Total hysterectomy with or without bilateral salpingo-oophorectomy is the treatment of choice in elderly patients who are past their childbearing age or those who have completed their childbearing. Decision to perform a hysterectomy is usually based on the presence of other pathologies such as leiomyomas or failure of medical or conservative management in cases of menorrhagia. Most preferred route of hysterectomy is vaginal hysterectomy because it is associated with reduced duration of hospital stay, lower cost and fewer complications.

Conservative surgery may be performed in the younger patients.

Conservative Surgery

Conservative surgery involving preservation of uterus may involve partial or complete resection of the uterine myomas. These surgeries are likely to be associated with the risk of recurrence as well as an increased risk for scar rupture in future pregnancies. Moreover, there is paucity of adequate evidence regarding the efficacy of these procedures. The type of surgery is based on the kind of adenomyosis:

- *Focal adenomyosis:* In case of focal adenomyosis, surgery comprises adenomyomectomy.
- *Diffuse adenomyosis:* In case of diffuse adenomyosis, surgical procedures comprise Osada's procedure and wedge resection.

Osada Procedure

Osada surgery is a fertility preserving surgery in cases with diffuse adenomyosis involving multiple flap reconstruction of the uterine wall following wide excision of adenomyosis. The uterus is opened by flaps so that the entire uterus is opened. Following this, the adenomyomas are resected from each quadrant, taking care to leave at least 1 cm residual myometrium. Once the resection is complete, the uterus is repaired by suturing it using triple-flap method. This surgery is likely to result in a significant reduction in pain as well as bleeding postsurgery in women who desire to conceive in future. This surgery also enables the woman to carry on their pregnancy till term without the risk of uterine rupture.

Other Conservative Procedures

Uterine Artery Embolization

Uterine artery embolization (UAE) is presently developing as an effective and safe method for the treatment of adenomyosis. UAE, by causing reduction of the uterine blood flow by blocking the uterine artery, has been shown to reduce the symptoms associated with adenomyosis uteri and to improve the quality of life. In the latest meta-analysis by de Bruijn et al. (2017), short-term improvement was achieved in about 90% patients whereas long-term improvement was achieved in about 75% patients with pure adenomyosis. UAE can be considered as a recognized treatment option for women with adenomyosis having concurrent fibroids. However, there is still a lack of randomized clinical trials showing favorable clinical outcomes related to the use of UAE. In this regard, there is a multicentric, randomized, non-blinded QUESTA trial, ongoing in Netherland. The trial started in November 2015 and the primary outcomes were expected by 2020. The outcomes were yet not out by the time of publication of this book. The main factor determining whether UAE can replace hysterectomy in treatment of adenomyosis is its ability to preserve fertility. However, the chances of a subsequent successful pregnancy following the procedure are presently unclear. Further randomized trials are required in this aspect.

For details related to UAE, kindly refer to Chapter 24: HMB due to Leiomyomas.

Endomyometrial Ablation

Endometrial ablation or resection can be considered as an option for women with superficial adenomyosis, presenting with the complaints of menorrhagia. However, the option of endometrial ablation cannot be used in women desiring future pregnancy. Moreover, this procedure is likely to be associated with an increased failure rate in patients with deep adenomyosis.

Magnetic Resonance-guided Focused Ultrasound

Magnetic resonance-guided focused ultrasound (MRgFUS) has also been tried as a noninvasive option for the treatment of adenomyosis. However, further studies are required in future for assessment of the overall safety and long-term effectiveness of MRgFUS for the treatment of adenomyosis.

COMPLICATIONS

- Adenomyosis can be associated with considerable morbidity due to the presence of debilitating symptoms such as menorrhagia, dysmenorrhea, chronic pelvic pain, etc.
- Coexistence of pelvic abnormalities such as uterine fibroids, endometrial hyperplasia, and endometrial adenocarcinoma.
- *Effect on fertility:* Adenomyosis is not thought to be a direct cause of infertility. However, it may interfere with the implantation of embryo in the endometrium. It is also likely to be associated with an increased risk of first trimester miscarriages. In case adenomyosis is present in association with a known cause of infertility (e.g., endometriosis, etc.), the outcome is worse in comparison with the outcome in absence of adenomyosis.

EVIDENCE-BASED CLINICAL TRIALS

 List of references can be scanned through QR code to enable the readers gain deeper insight of the subject by referring to the entire article or its abstract.

SECTION 7

Abnormalities in Conception

34. Infertility
35. Amenorrhea

CHAPTER 34

Infertility

CASE STUDY

A 28-year-old woman married since last 5 years presented to the gynecology OPD along with her husband with a complaint of infertility. The couple has been practicing regular sexual intercourse since last 2 years. On general physical examination, there was no significant finding except that the patient's BMI was 27. There were no signs of hyperandrogenism (hirsutism), galactorrhea, or thyroid dysfunction. The woman's menstrual history revealed that she has been having irregular menstrual cycles since last 3 years. The cycle duration ranges within 30–35 days. The cycles last for approximately 4–5 days. However, the woman has been observing a progressive decrease in the amount of menstrual blood flow over the past few months. The couple had previously visited an infertility specialist 6 months back who had ordered a semen analysis. The result of this investigation was within normal limits.

INTRODUCTION

> Q. With the help of a long essay, define primary infertility. Discuss various diagnostic modalities and therapeutic options in infertility.

Infertility is defined as the inability to conceive even after trying with unprotected intercourse for a period of 1 year for couples in which the woman is under 35 years and 6 months of trying for couples in which the woman is over 35 years of age. Investigations may be started earlier in a woman with irregular menstrual cycles or in the presence of known risk factors for infertility, such as endometriosis, history of PID, and reproductive tract malformations, or having a male partner with known or suspected poor semen quality.

Fertility is defined as the capacity to reproduce or the state of being fertile. Fecundability is the probability of achieving a pregnancy each month, which is approximately 20–25%. Taking an average fecundability of 20% per cycle, the cumulative pregnancy rate over 3 months of exposure is 57%, over 6 months is 72%, over 1 year is 85%, and over 2 years is 93%. On the other hand, fecundity can be defined as the ability to achieve a live birth within 1 menstrual cycle. The factors which are likely to influence fecundability include the woman's age at time of planning pregnancy and the frequency of sexual intercourse. With regular unprotected sexual intercourse, 94% of fertile women aged 35 years or younger are likely to conceive after 3 years of trying.

Infertility commonly results due to the disease of the reproductive system, in either a male or a female, which inhibits the ability to conceive and deliver a child. Approximately 6.1 million people in the United States, or roughly 10–15% of the individuals belonging to the reproductive age group, are affected by infertility. Approximately one in six couples is affected by infertility and there are a number of factors **(Table 34.1)**, both male and female, that can cause the condition. In fact, in nearly 35% of cases the cause is attributed to the male, in 50% the cause can be attributed to female (35% due to tubal and pelvic pathology and 15% due to ovulatory dysfunction), 5% of cases can be attributed to unusual causes, and in remaining 10% of cases the causes are unknown. Though both male and female factors are responsible for producing infertility, female factor infertility would primarily be discussed in this chapter. Amongst the female causes of infertility, both ovulatory dysfunction and tubal pathology are responsible for approximately 40% cases each of infertility. Nearly 10% cases are due to an unexplained pathology, whereas the remainder 10% cases are due to relatively uncommon/unusual problems such as uterine pathology **(Fig. 34.1)**.

TABLE 34.1: Causes of infertility (both male and female factors).

Causes of infertility	Percentage of cases
Male causes	35%
Female causes:	50%
• Tubal and pelvic pathologies	35%
• Ovulatory dysfunction	15%
Unusual causes	5%
Unexplained causes	10%

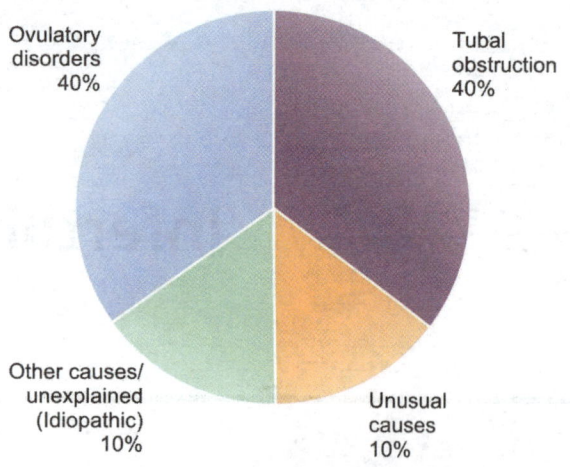

Fig. 34.1: Female causes of infertility.

Since nearly 40–50% cases of infertility are likely to be due to combined causes, the evaluation for infertility must focus on the couple as a whole and not on one or the other partner. Both the partners must be encouraged to attend the clinic at the time of each appointment.

HISTORY AND CLINICAL PRESENTATION

Infertility is a problem that may involve both male and female partners; therefore, the initial assessment must involve both the partners. The initial evaluation must include a detailed reproductive history and at least two semen analyses at a laboratory that is qualified to perform the testing. The consultation is grossly incomplete if only the woman is evaluated. Anxiety is very common in couples desiring pregnancy, and many couples may seek consultation only after a few months of unprotected intercourse. Diagnostic testing must not be performed if the couple has not attempted to conceive for at least 1 year, unless the woman is 35 years old or older, or there is a history of male factor infertility, endometriosis, tubal factor, exposure to diethylstilbestrol (DES), PID, or pelvic surgery. In many cases, attempts at alleviation of anxiety through reassurance and briefly explaining the physiology of reproduction are usually enough to lessen the couple's anxiety.

HISTORY FROM THE FEMALE PARTNER

During the consultation, the following history should be taken from the woman.

History of Presenting Complaints

- *Type of infertility:* A detailed medical history regarding the type of infertility (primary or secondary), its duration, and if any treatment for this had been sought in the past. Primary infertility implies that the woman had never been able to conceive in the past. Secondary infertility implies that the woman had conceived in the past (irrespective of the outcome of pregnancy, whether she progressed till term or had a miscarriage) but is presently not being able to conceive.
- *Patient's age:* It is important to know the woman's age because increasing age of women (>35 years) is associated with reduced fertility. The present evidence indicates that age-related decline in female fertility is largely due to progressive follicular depletion and a high rate of abnormalities (particularly aneuploidy) in the aging oocytes. The available evidence also indicates a decrease in the pregnancy rate and an increase in the time to conception with an increase in the age of the male partner. However, since this decline is rarely observed before the age of 45–50 years, male factors contribute very little toward the overall age-related decline in fertility.
- *Duration of infertility:* Duration of the couple's attempts for becoming pregnant, whether or not they have ever had children or a positive pregnancy test together with same or a different partner in the past, needs to be asked. Number and outcome of any previous pregnancies including ectopic pregnancy and/or miscarriages also need to be determined.
- *Thyroid dysfunction or galactorrhea:* Symptoms suggestive of thyroid disease, pelvic or abdominal pain, and galactorrhea must be asked. Thyroid dysfunction is commonly associated with menstrual abnormalities and reduced fertility. Galactorrhea or milk secretion from the breasts is often a manifestation of pineal gland tumor and may be associated with amenorrhea.
- *Previous history of Pap smears:* Previous history of abnormal Pap smears or undergoing treatment for cervical intraepithelial neoplasia could be responsible for producing cervical stenosis.
- *History of vaginal or cervical discharge:* This must be enquired. The infections could be at times responsible for producing infertility, e.g., infection with *Chlamydia* can cause PID and tubal blockage, resulting in subsequent infertility.

Sexual History

Sexual history must be taken in detail in order to enquire about the frequency of sexual intercourse, use of lubricants (e.g., K-Y gel) that could be spermicidal, use of vaginal douches after intercourse, and history of any sexual dysfunction. History of sexual dysfunction such as an absence of orgasm or painful intercourse (dyspareunia) must be enquired. History related to the frequency of intercourse and presence of deep dyspareunia (suggestive of endometriosis) also needs to be enquired. The use of any form of contraception including natural methods, medical methods, and surgical form of contraception (e.g., vasectomy and tubal ligation) needs to be asked. Overall pattern of sexual activity during the period of time the couple has been trying to conceive, specifically in relation to ovulation, needs to be asked. The patient should also be asked if she had ever used ovulation-predictor kits or has been prescribed ovulation-promoting medications such as clomiphene citrate (CC).

The patient should be explained about the period of fertility. The optimal chances for pregnancy occur if the patient has intercourse in the 6 days before ovulation, with day 6 being the actual day of ovulation. Sometimes, simply advising the patients to adjust the timing of their intercourse can result in a significantly increased chance for pregnancy.

Patient's Lifestyle

A detailed history regarding the patient's lifestyle, consumption of alcohol and tobacco, use of recreational drugs of abuse (amount and frequency), occupation, and physical activities must be asked.

Menstrual History

The age of attaining menarche and puberty must be asked. The woman should be questioned in detail about her menstrual history and asked about the frequency, cycle length, patterns since menarche, and history of dysmenorrhea. Regular menstrual cycles are usually ovulatory in nature, while irregular cycles may be anovulatory in nature. A history of weight changes, hirsutism, frontal balding, and acne should also be addressed. History of progressively worsening dysmenorrhea, newly developed dyspareunia, and physical findings of focal tenderness or nodularity of cul-de-sac point toward endometriosis. Irregular or infrequent menstrual cycles are usually indicative of ovulatory dysfunction.

Obstetric History

The patient should be enquired about details regarding previous pregnancies (including miscarriages or medical terminations of pregnancy and previous history of live births), dead babies, or stillborn children. She should also be asked if she has ever undergone evaluation regarding infertility issues and any medical or surgical management that had been instituted. The patient should be asked about outcome of each of the previous pregnancies, interval between successive pregnancies, and the presence of any other complications associated with any pregnancy. If the patient has ever experienced pregnancy losses, she should be asked about the duration of pregnancy at the time of miscarriage; hCG levels, if they were done; ultrasonographic data, if available; and the presence or absence of fetal heartbeat as documented on the ultrasound report. History of previous pregnancy is particularly important because couples who have conceived before usually have a better prognosis in comparison to those who have never conceived. A history of past obstetric hemorrhage suggesting postpartum pituitary necrosis (i.e., Sheehan syndrome) must be asked.

Past History

A previous history of pelvic infection, endometriosis, fibroids, cervical dysplasia, septic abortion, ruptured appendix, ectopic pregnancy, and gynecological surgery, e.g., abdominal myomectomy, adnexal surgery, and surgery of cervix, fallopian tube, pelvis, and abdomen, raises the suspicion for tubal or peritoneal disease. Past or current episodes of sexually transmitted diseases or PIDs must also be enquired. The patient must be asked if she is currently receiving any medical treatment, the reason for treatment, and if she has any history of allergies. She must be asked if she had been using intrauterine copper devices or any other form of contraception in the past.

Family History

Family history of birth defects, mental retardation, early menopause, or reproductive failure needs to be taken.

HISTORY FROM THE MALE PARTNER

- Determination of the period of infertility at the time of taking history is most important. The history should include several points specific to the patient's sexual functioning including history of impotence, erectile dysfunction, premature ejaculation, change in libido, etc. The history should include several points specific to the patient's sexual functioning such as the precise nature of dysfunction, for e.g., whether the problem is in attaining or sustaining an erection, or whether there is difficulty with penetration due to insufficient rigidity. The presence or absence of nocturnal and morning erections and their quality must be asked. The patient must be enquired if he is taking any treatment, both pharmacologic and nonpharmacologic, for treatment of his problem. Complaints of reduced libido may also be associated with depression, loss of interest in daily activities, a decline in erectile function, fatigue, etc. Thus, history related to these symptoms must also be elicited. Additionally, the time period since which these complaints have been present must be enquired from the patient.
- History related to the frequency of intercourse or use of any lubricants which may be toxic to sperms must be enquired.
- History of pain during both time of ejaculation and erection must be enquired. The time of pain onset, its localization to any specific organ, and the quality of pain must also be asked.
- History of testicular trauma, previous sexual relationships, history of any previous pregnancy, and the existence of offspring from previous partners must also be asked. History of undergoing previous treatment for infertility including semen analysis must also be asked.

- Any complaints specific to the genitourinary structures, such as complaints of a dull ache or fullness in the scrotum or nonradiating pain on one side, dysuria, and dyspareunia, must also be asked.
- History of exposure to environmental toxins, such as excessive heat, radiation, and chemicals such as heavy metals, glycol ethers, or other organic solvents needs to be asked.

Medical History

- History of treatment for malignancy (especially chemotherapy or radiotherapy), regardless of site, should be documented.
- History of medical disorders such as diabetes, chronic obstructive pulmonary disease, renal insufficiency, hemochromatosis, and hepatic insufficiency, which may contribute to male subfertility, must be asked.
- History of systemic illness, particularly a febrile illness, and any recent weight gain or loss in last 6 months must be asked.

Surgical History

History of any surgery related to genitourinary organs such as orchidopexy, repair of inguinal hernia, epispadias or hypospadias repair, prostate surgery, bladder reconstructions, and bladder or testicular surgeries needs to be asked. The patient should be asked specifically if there is a history of a vasectomy.

Treatment History

The dose and duration of the use of certain prescription drugs which can affect sperm count, motility, and morphology must be documented. Some of the drugs which can commonly affect semen parameters by reducing spermatogenesis include calcium channel blockers, spironolactone, chemotherapy drugs, anabolic steroids, etc. The patient must also be asked about the ingestion of herbal drugs or drugs belonging to other alternative systems of medicine and other over-the-counter medications. Many times the patient may not disclose this history unless specifically enquired. Any of these substances may be responsible for affecting spermatogenesis.

Social History

Cigarette smoking, excessive alcohol consumption, and consistent marijuana use are all known to be gonadotoxins. A careful history of the use of these agents and other illicit drugs must be part of the complete male infertility evaluation. Cigarette smoking has been thought to cause changes in sperm morphology, production, and motility while chronic alcohol use may contribute to infertility by causing erectile dysfunction and hypogonadism. Simply eliminating these agents can improve semen parameters in the absence of other physical findings.

Patients should be asked about recreational activities, as some activities, such as long-distance cycling, may put pressure on the perineal area and result in possible impairment of erectile function. Certain occupations which result in exposure of male genital organs to high temperatures such as men working in blast furnaces may be the reason behind the patient's infertility.

Family History

It is important to elicit family history of birth defects or reproductive failure. The family history must include a discussion regarding the presence of testicular or other genitourinary malignancies specifically related to prostate or bladder in other family members. The patient should be queried regarding siblings or extended family members who may have had similar fertility problems. It is especially important to ask about the family history of cystic fibrosis because this genetic disease could be responsible for producing infertility by causing congenital absence of vas deferens. According to the ACOG recommendations, screening for cystic fibrosis should be made available to all the couples seeking preconceptional care and not just to those with a personal or family history of cystic fibrosis. The screening should be specifically offered to couples belonging to racial or ethnic groups with a high risk for cystic fibrosis (e.g., Caucasians, particularly those of Ashkenazi Jewish descent).

GENERAL PHYSICAL EXAMINATION

General physical examination requires routine measurement of the patient's vital signs including pulse rate, blood pressure, and temperature. Other important aspects of general physical examination include measurement of the following parameters:

- *BMI:* Measurement of the patient's height and weight to calculate the BMI. Calculation of BMI is important because extremely low or extremely high BMI may be associated with reduced fertility. Moreover, abdominal obesity may be associated with insulin resistance.
- *Thyroid examination:* Note for thyroid enlargement, nodule, or tenderness.
- *Eye examination:* It must be performed in order to establish the presence of exophthalmos, which may be associated with hyperthyroidism.
- *Stigmata of Turner's syndrome:* The presence of epicanthus, low-set ears and hairline, and webbed neck can be associated with chromosomal abnormalities.
- *Breast examination:* It must be performed in order to evaluate breast development and assess the breasts for the presence of abnormal masses or secretions, especially galactorrhea. This opportunity must be taken by the gynecologist to educate patients about breast

self-examination during the early days of their menstrual cycles.

- *Signs of androgen excess*: Signs of androgen excess such as hirsutism, acne, deepening of the voice, and hypertrichosis must be looked for. Androgen deficiency during early gestation may result in development of ambiguous genitalia. Reduced androgen exposure in childhood may present as delayed pubertal development, while in adulthood as reduced sexual function, infertility, and ultimately, loss of secondary sexual characteristics.
- *Examination of extremities:* The extremities must be examined in order to rule out malformations, such as shortness of the fourth finger or cubitus valgus, which can be associated with chromosomal abnormalities and other congenital defects.
- *Examination of the skin:* The skin must be examined for the presence of acne, hypertrichosis, and hirsutism.
- *Examination of the secondary sexual characteristics:* Failure of development of secondary sexual characteristics must always prompt a workup for hypopituitarism. Loss of axillary and pubic hair and atrophy of the external genitalia should lead the physician to suspect hypopituitarism in a previously menstruating young woman who develops amenorrhea. Tanner stages of development of breasts and pubic hair have been described in Chapter 35.

SPECIFIC SYSTEMIC EXAMINATION

ABDOMINAL EXAMINATION OF FEMALE PARTNER

The abdominal examination should be done to detect the presence of abnormal masses in the abdomen. Masses felt in the hypogastrium could be arising from the pelvic region.

PELVIC EXAMINATION OF FEMALE PARTNER

Per Speculum Examination

A thorough gynecologic examination has already been described in Chapter 22. The distribution of hair pattern on the external genitalia should be particularly noted. The inspection of the vaginal mucosa may indicate a deficiency of estrogens or the presence of infection. Cervical stenosis can be diagnosed during a speculum examination. Complete cervical stenosis is confirmed by the inability to pass a 1–2 mm probe into the uterine cavity.

Bimanual Examination

Bimanual examination should be performed to establish the direction of the cervix and the size and position of the uterus.

The gynecologist should look for the presence of any mass, tenderness, or nodularity in adnexa or cul-de-sac. Various pelvic pathologies such as fibroids, adnexal masses, tenderness or pelvic nodules indicative of infection, or endometriosis can be detected on bimanual examination. Many uterine defects related to infertility such as the absence of vagina and uterus, and presence of vaginal septum can be detected during the pelvic examination. Tenderness or masses in the adnexae or posterior cul-de-sac (pouch of Douglas) are suggestive of chronic PID or endometriosis. Palpable tender nodules in the posterior cul-de-sac, uterosacral ligaments, or rectovaginal septum are additional signs of endometriosis.

EXAMINATION OF MALE PARTNER

The patient should be examined for age-appropriate development of male secondary sex characteristics, gynecomastia, or hirsutism. The structures of male external genitalia which must be evaluated include the penis, scrotum, testes, epididymis, spermatic cord, and vas deferens. The clinician must examine the external genitalia for the presence of following abnormalities:

- Scrotum must be carefully and thoroughly palpated, and the presence of all scrotal structures should be confirmed, along with their size and consistency.
- Presence of congenital abnormalities of the genital tract, e.g., hypospadias, cryptorchidism (undescended testes), and absence of the vas deferens (unilateral or bilateral), must be assessed.
- Testicular size, presence of tenderness on palpation of testicle, and presence of any associated mass must be assessed. If any mass is palpated, it must be verified whether it is arising from the testicles or is separate from it.
- Urethra must be assessed for the presence of any stenosis, diverticulum, etc.
- *Presence of an inguinal hernia or varicocele:* A varicocele can be exaggerated during physical examination by asking the patient to perform the Valsalva maneuver while standing. The varicocele normally disappears when the patient lies down. A long-standing varicocele may result in testicular atrophy. If the varicocele is large, it may be visible during inspection, resulting in "bag of worms" appearance.
- Complete physical examination should also include a digital rectal examination.

DIFFERENTIAL DIAGNOSIS

The process of human reproduction begins with the deposition of spermatozoa, during sexual intercourse, into the vagina. The spermatozoa migrate through the cervix and uterine cavity to the fallopian tubes where they meet the egg, and fertilization takes place. The embryo then travels back down the fallopian tube and enters the uterine cavity where implantation takes place. As a result, female factor infertility can result from various causes including cervical, uterine, ovarian, or tubal factors.

754 Abnormalities in Conception

CAUSES OF MALE INFERTILITY

> **Q.** Write a short essay discussing the etiopathology of male infertility.

Some of the likely causes of male infertility are tabulated in **Table 34.2**.

CAUSES OF FEMALE INFERTILITY

Cervical Factor Infertility

The uterine cervix plays an important role in capturing, nurturing, and then transporting and capacitating the sperms after intercourse. The cervix ultimately releases the mature sperms into uterus and fallopian tube. Cervical factors account for 5–10% cases of infertility. Cervical factor infertility can most commonly result due to abnormalities of the mucus–sperm interaction and narrowing of the cervical canal due to cervical stenosis. Both these causes of cervical infertility would now be discussed.

Mucus–Sperm Interaction

In normal women, at the beginning of the menstrual cycle, cervical mucus is scanty, viscous, and very cellular. This mucus does not allow the sperms to pass into the uterine cavity. Mucus secretion from the cervix increases during the midfollicular phase and reaches its maximum approximately 24–48 hours before ovulation. Just prior to ovulation, the mucus becomes thin, watery, alkaline, stretchable,

TABLE 34.2: Causes of male infertility.	
Cause	**Prevalence**

• Hypothalamic pituitary disease (secondary hypogonadism):
– *Congenital disorders:* Kallmann syndrome, Laurence–Moon–Biedl syndrome, Prader–Willi syndrome, lower oculocerebral syndrome, familial cerebellar ataxia, etc.
– *Acquired diseases:*
  - *Tumors:* Pituitary macroadenomas (macroprolactinomas and nonfunctioning adenomas)
  - *Infiltrative diseases:* Sarcoidosis, histiocytosis, tuberculosis, fungal infections, transfusion siderosis, hemochromatosis, etc.
  - *Vascular lesions:* Pituitary infarction and carotid aneurysm
  - *Hormonal:* Hyperprolactinemia, estrogen excess, glucocorticoid excess, and androgen excess
  - *Drugs:* Opioid-like or other central nervous system-activating drugs, including many psychotropic drugs, GnRH analogs (agonists and antagonists), etc.
  - *Systemic illness:* Any serious systemic illness or chronic nutritional deficiency
	1–2%

• Testicular disease:
– *Congenital or developmental disorders of the testes:* These include Klinefelter's syndrome, Y chromosome microdeletions, cryptorchidism, varicoceles, and other less common disorders
  - Klinefelter's syndrome
  - Autosomal and X chromosome defects
  - Y chromosome and related defects
  - *Defective androgen receptor or synthesis:* Men with congenital androgen insensitivity due to androgen receptor or postreceptor abnormalities and those with 5-alpha-reductase deficiency are nearly always infertile
  - Disorders of the estrogen receptor or estrogen synthesis
  - Inactivating mutation in FSH receptor gene
  - Myotonic dystrophy
– *Acquired disorders of the testes:*
  - *Drugs:* Cyclophosphamide, chlorambucil, antiandrogens (flutamide, cyproterone, spironolactone), ketoconazole, cimetidine, etc.
  - Radiation
  - *Environmental factors:* Environmental toxins such as lead, cadmium, and mercury, exposure of testes to high temperature (e.g., workers in blast furnace)
  - Antisperm antibodies
  - *Systemic disorders:* Chronic renal insufficiency, cirrhosis, or malnutrition
	30–40%

• Post-testicular defects (disorders of sperm transport): – *Abnormalities of the epididymis:* Absence, dysfunction, or obstruction of the epididymis – *Abnormalities of the vas:* Bilateral obstruction, ligation, or altered peristalsis of the vas deferens results in infertility, infection (gonorrhea, *Chlamydia*, tuberculosis) resulting in the development of obstruction – *Defective ejaculation:* Spinal cord disease or trauma, sympathectomy or autonomic disease (e.g., diabetes mellitus), erectile dysfunction, mechanical obstruction (condoms and diaphragm use), premature ejaculation, infrequency of intercourse, etc.	10–20%
• *Idiopathic:* Failure to conceive with an apparently normal female partner despite having repeatedly normal semen analyses	40–50%

(FSH: follicle stimulating hormone)

acellular, and elastic in appearance due to increase in the concentration of salt and water in the mucus under the influence of estrogen. In this type of cervical mucus pattern, multiple microchannels are formed so that the spermatozoa can travel through the mucus into the uterine cavity, and the mucus also acts as a filter for abnormal spermatozoa and cellular debris present in the semen. Furthermore, during this phase, the mucus assumes a fern-like pattern (**Fig. 34.2**) when allowed to dry on a slide under the microscope. Following ovulation, under the effect of progesterone, the cervical mucus changes its character. During this stage, the mucus becomes opaque, viscid, and may become hostile, resistant, and impenetrable to sperms.

Cervical Stenosis

Cervical stenosis can cause infertility by blocking the passage of sperm from the cervix to the intrauterine cavity. It can be congenital or acquired in etiology, resulting from surgical procedures, infections, hypoestrogenism, and radiation therapy.

Uterine Factor Infertility

Uterus is the ultimate destination for the fertilized egg and the site for embryo implantation and fetal growth. Therefore, uterine factors may be associated with primary infertility or recurrent pregnancy wastage and premature delivery. Uterine factors may affect either the endometrium or the myometrium and are responsible for nearly 2–5% cases of infertility. They can be congenital or acquired and would be discussed below.

Congenital Defects

Abnormalities in the development of Müllerian ducts may result in a spectrum of congenital/Müllerian duct abnormalities, varying from total absence of the uterus and vagina (Mayer–Rokitansky–Küster–Hauser syndrome) to minor defects such as arcuate uterus and vaginal septa (transverse or longitudinal). The classification of Müllerian anomalies by the American Fertility Society (AFS, 1988) has been described in Chapter 13. The relationship between Müllerian anomalies and infertility is not entirely clear except when there is absolute absence of the uterus, cervix, or vagina.

Acquired Causes

> **Q. Write a short essay on intrauterine adhesions.**

- *Drug-induced uterine malformations:* The drug DES, used for treating patients with a history of recurrent miscarriages during 1950s, was found to be responsible for producing numerous defects such as malformations of the uterine cervix, irregularities of the endometrial cavity (e.g., T-shaped uterus), malfunction of the fallopian tubes, menstrual irregularities, and development of clear cell carcinoma of the vagina.
- *Asherman's syndrome:* Development of adhesions or synechiae within the endometrial cavity may result in its partial or total obliteration. This could be due to Asherman's syndrome, which may develop following a vigorous dilatation and curettage procedure (Chapter 13). Development of adhesions or synechiae within the endometrial cavity may result in its partial or total obliteration.
- *Endometritis:* Endometritis or inflammation of the uterine cavity due to infections such as tuberculosis could be associated with an increased risk of infertility.
- *Leiomyomas:* The impact of fibroids on fertility presently remains controversial and has been a subject of extensive debate. Uterine fibroids have been covered in detail in Chapter 24. As a sole factor, fibroids probably account for only 2–3% of infertility cases.

Leiomyomas are more common in nulliparous or relatively infertile women, but it is not known whether infertility causes myomas or vice versa or whether both the conditions have a common cause. The general view is that the uterus, which is deprived of pregnancy, consoles itself with myomas. This has been aptly summed up by the saying, "Fibroids are rewards of virtue, babies the fruit of sin." Postponement of pregnancy results in uninterrupted estrogenic stimulation of the uterus, which can act as a predisposing factor for development of myoma. The presence of myomas may then discourage the development of pregnancy. However, mere presence of myomas in an infertile patient should not be considered as a cause of her infertility. Firstly, she should be investigated for all the common causes of infertility (including the tubal, ovarian, male factors, etc.). Only after all the other common causes

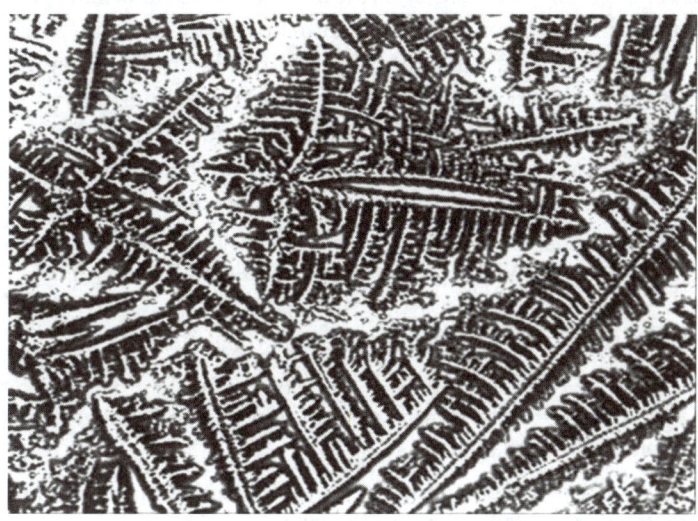

Fig. 34.2: Ferning pattern of the cervical mucus.

of infertility in a woman have been ruled out, the presence of myomas may be considered as a cause for infertility in a woman. The extent to which the presence of myomas can influence fertility in a woman depends upon the position of fibroids inside the uterus, the number of fibroids, and their size.

Myomas can cause infertility through the following mechanisms:

- *Distortion of the endometrial cavity:* Presence of submucous myomas may distort the endometrial cavity, thereby interfering with normal implantation. Thus, submucous myomas are most likely to affect the woman's fertility, followed by interstitial myomas and lastly the subserosal myomas. Subserosal myomas are located farthest from the endometrial cavity; as a result, they are associated with minimum effect on fertility. Removal of fibroids that distort the uterine cavity may be indicated in infertile women, where no other factors have been identified, and in women about to undergo IVF. Besides causing distortion of the uterine cavity, myomas may also cause dysfunctional uterine contractions, which may interfere with sperm migration, ovum transport, or nidation. Furthermore, the growth of myoma is dependent on estrogen production. Thus, uterine myomas in a woman are often associated with anovulation, which may play a role in producing infertility. Also, AUB and dyspareunia associated with uterine myomas can cause infertility to some extent.
- *Anatomical location of the fibroid:* The anatomical location of myoma inside the uterus can affect fertility. For e.g., the presence of large submucous fibroids in the vicinity of cervix may result in displacement of cervix, which can prevent normal deposition of sperms at the cervical os, or a submucosal myoma impinging on the intramural portion of the fallopian tube can interfere with the proper transportation of ovum.
- *Inflammation:* Biological factors such as infiltration of inflammatory cells (macrophages) and production of inflammatory mediators [cytokines, monocyte chemoattractant protein-1 (MCP-1), prostaglandin F2-α, etc.] due to the presence of fibroids may be responsible for producing infertility.
- *Indirect evidence:* Since there is very limited direct evidence in the form of prospective randomized controlled trials regarding the role of myoma in producing infertility, we have to depend on indirect evidence. The indirect evidence is mainly available in two forms. The first one is studying the effect of fibroids based on the outcomes of ARTs [IVF, GIFT, etc.]. The second is assessing the outcome of fertility following removal of myomas. Various studies have indicated pregnancy rates of 44–62% following myomectomy.

Ovarian Factor Infertility

> Q. Describe in detail the physiology of ovulation. How will you manage a case of dysovulatory infertility?
>
> Q. Describe in detail the ovarian factors involved in infertility and their management.

Oogenesis occurs in the ovary from the first trimester of embryonic life and is completed by 28–30 weeks of gestation. By then, approximately 6–7 million oogonia are present. This can be considered as the maximal oogonial content of the gonad. They are arrested at the prophase stage of the first meiosis division. Subsequently, the number of oocytes irretrievably decreases until the menopause is attained because of a continuous process of atresia. At birth, the pool of oocytes is reduced to approximately 2 million. By menarche, approximately 500,000 oocytes are present. These oocytes are used throughout the reproductive years until menopause.

The ovulatory process begins after the maturation of hypothalamus–pituitary–ovarian axis, and there occurs production of gonadotropins, such as FSH and LH, under the regulation of GnRH. Though a cohort of follicles gets recruited every month, only a single oocyte ultimately gets selected, develops to the preovulatory stage, and is known as the dominant follicle. LH surge occurring during the midpoint of the menstrual cycle triggers the ovulatory process and stimulates the formation of the corpus luteum. Following ovulation, the luteal phase begins under the influence of progesterone secreted by corpus luteum. Furthermore, ovulation induces the resumption of meiosis by the oocyte, which had been arrested at the prophase stage.

Causes of Ovulatory Dysfunction

Ovulatory dysfunction results in an alteration in the frequency and duration of the menstrual cycle. Anovulation or failure to ovulate is one of the most common causes for infertility. An absence of ovulation can also be associated with primary or secondary amenorrhea, or oligomenorrhea. Amenorrhea as a cause of infertility has been discussed in detail in Chapter 35. Rise in the prevalence of infertility with increase in the woman's age could be related to reduction in the ovarian reservoir. PCOS, a common endocrine disorder in women, frequently results in infertility by causing ovulatory dysfunction. Classification of various ovulatory disorders as devised by the WHO is described in **Table 34.3**.

Polycystic Ovarian Syndrome

> Q. Discuss the importance of lifestyle changes in the etiology and management of PCOS.
>
> Q. Discuss in detail the etiology of hyperandrogenism and metabolism of androgens in a female.

Infertility

TABLE 34.3: The WHO classification of ovulatory disorders.

WHO class	Pathology	Causes	Incidence	Treatment strategy
WHO Class 1: Hypogonadotropic hypogonadal anovulation (FSH < 2 IU/L)	Low or low-normal levels of serum FSH and low serum estradiol concentrations	Excessive exercise or low body weight	5–10% of women	• Lifestyle modification • Human menopausal gonadotropin (hMG) (FSH and LH preparations)
WHO Class 2: Normogonadotropic, normoestrogenic anovulation	Normal levels of gonadotropins and estrogens. However, FSH secretion during the follicular phase of the cycle is subnormal	Women with PCOS	Most common, accounting for 70–85% of cases	• Weight modulation • Aromatase inhibitors • Clomiphene citrate or other selective estrogen receptor modulators • Metformin or other insulin-sensitizing agents • Gonadotropin therapy • Laparoscopic ovarian diathermy • Assisted reproductive technology
WHO class 3: Hypergonadotropic hypoestrogenic anovulation (FSH > 8 U/L)	High-to-normal levels of gonadotropins and low levels of estrogen	Women with primary gonadal failure (previously called premature ovarian failure) or gonadal dysgenesis	Accounts for 10–30% cases	Gonadotropin therapy and IVF with donor oocytes
Hyperprolactinemic anovulation	Inhibition of gonadotropin and estrogen secretion due to hyperprolactinemia; gonadotropin concentrations in this condition are usually normal or decreased			Bromocriptine or other dopamine agonist (only in cases of hyperprolactinemia and anovulation)

(FSH: follicle stimulating hormone; LH: luteinizing hormone; PCOS: polycystic ovarian syndrome)

> **Q.** Write a long note on the diagnostic procedures and treatment in a case of PCOS.
>
> **Q.** Write a long note discussing the diagnostic criteria, etiopathogenesis, and recent advancements in the treatment of PCOS.
>
> **Q.** Write a long essay discussing the pathogenesis of PCOS. Also discuss the diagnosis and management of infertility caused by PCOS.
>
> **Q.** Write a short essay on pathogenesis of PCOS.
>
> **Q.** Write a short essay on PCOS.

Polycystic ovarian syndrome is the most common cause of hyperandrogenic chronic anovulation. The pathophysiology of PCOS is described in **Flowchart 34.1**. According to the American Society of Reproductive Medicine (ASRM) and the European Society of Human Reproduction and Embryology (ESHRE) joint consensus meeting in November 2003, the diagnosis of PCOS should be made, when two of the following three criteria are met (Rotterdam's criteria):

1. *Infrequent or absent ovulation:* Irregular cycles are defined as cycles lasting for >35 days or <21 days or <8 cycles/year, which may continue for >3 years post menarche and may occur until the perimenopause.

2. *Clinical or biochemical features of hyperandrogenism:* Biochemical hyperandrogenism is associated with the following parameters: free androgen index (FAI) or calculated bioavailable testosterone or calculated free testosterone levels.

   FAI = 100 × [total testosterone/sex hormone-binding globulin (SHBG)]

   Levels of androstenedione or dehydroepiandrosterone sulfate (DHEAS) should be considered if total or free testosterone levels are not elevated. However, these provide limited additional information regarding the diagnosis of PCOS.

   Clinical symptoms of hyperandrogenism include acne, alopecia, and hirsutism in adults. In adolescents, the symptoms include acne or hirsutism.

3. *Ultrasound features of PCOS:* Previous ultrasound criteria included the presence of multiple small cysts of the size 0.5–1 mm, (usually >10 in number) along the periphery of the ovary, giving rise to the "necklace appearance" on the ultrasound. Hyperplasia of the stroma results in an increase in the ovarian volume to >8 mL or 9 cm^3.

Besides these, other important features of PCOS include the following:

- Increased LH levels, LH:FSH ratio

758 Abnormalities in Conception

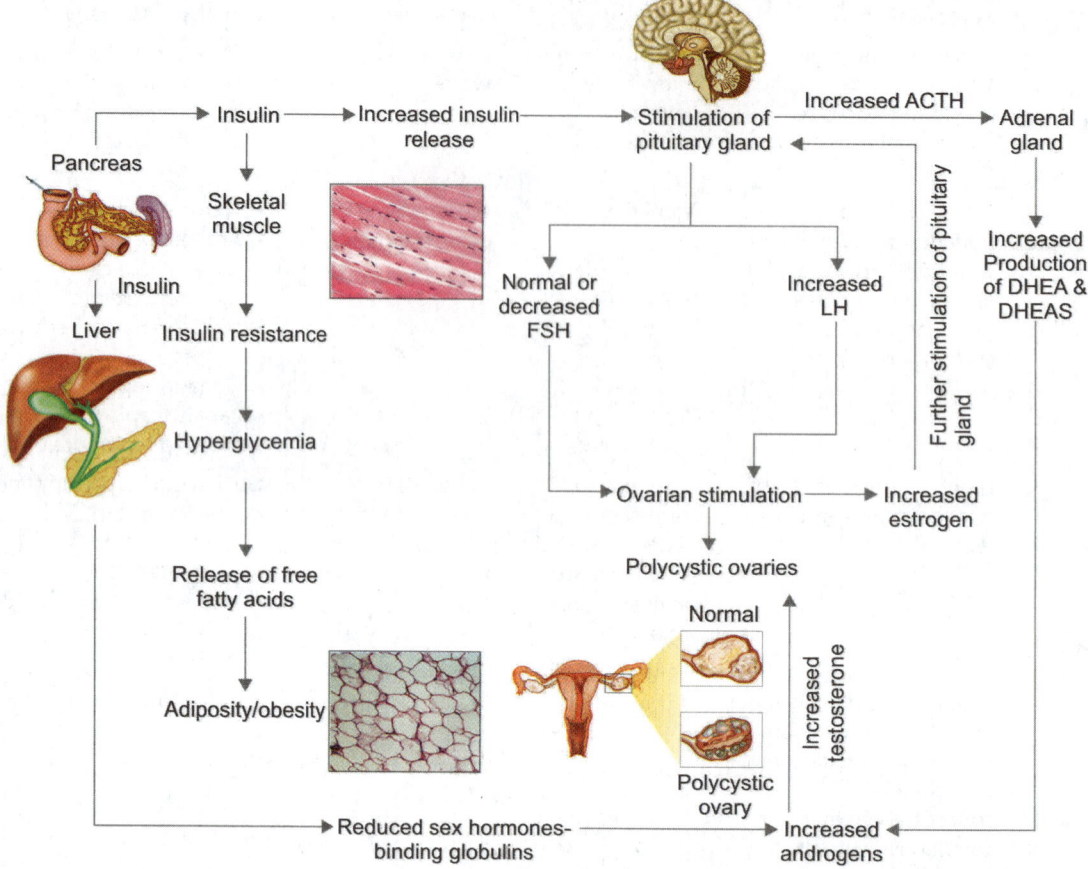

Flowchart 34.1: Pathophysiology of PCOS.

(ACTH: adrenocorticotropic hormone; DHEA: dehydroepiandrosterone; DHEAS: dehydroepiandrosterone sulfate; FSH: follicle stimulating hormone; LH: luteinizing hormone; PCOS: polycystic ovarian syndrome)

- Insulin resistance
- Obesity.

The revised version of these guidelines was published by the ESHRE/ASRM in 2018. In these guidelines the Rotterdam's criteria have been endorsed with a few changes:

- *Diagnosis of PCOS amongst adolescents:* Both hyperandrogenism and ovulatory dysfunction are required for making the diagnosis of PCOS in young girls within 8 years of menarche. In these patients, ultrasound is not recommended.
- *Ultrasound criteria:* They are strengthened in view of advancements in the scanning technology. New ultrasound criteria for the diagnosis of PCOS include the presence of ≥20 follicles per ovary and/or an ovarian volume ≥ 10 ml. The evaluation must be done using endovaginal ultrasound transducers with a frequency bandwidth of 8 MHz, and the clinician must ensure that no corpora lutea, cysts, or dominant follicles are present. In case of transabdominal ultrasound reporting, focus should be toward measuring the ovarian volume with a threshold of ≥10 mL. Old ultrasound criteria have been described previously.
- *Anti-Müllerian hormone (AMH) levels:* Measurement of AMH levels is yet not considered adequate for the diagnosis.

The diagnostic criteria for PCOS developed by the National Institute for Health are as follows:

- Clinical evidence of hyperandrogenism (e.g., hirsutism and acne) and/or hyperandrogenemia (e.g., elevated total or free testosterone levels). PCOS is associated with mild-to-moderate hyperandrogenism and/or hyperandrogenemia. On the other hand, signs of markedly elevated androgen levels, such as clitoromegaly, temporal balding, and deepening of the voice, are suggestive of an androgen-producing tumor.
- Oligoovulation (i.e., cycle duration >35 days or <8 cycles per year)
- Exclusion of related disorders (e.g., hyperprolactinemia, thyroid dysfunction, androgen-secreting tumors, and 21-hydroxylase-deficient nonclassical congenital adrenal hyperplasia)

Grossly, the ovaries of most women with PCOS are bilaterally enlarged and globular and have a thickened capsule **(Fig. 34.3)**. Due to the presence of a smooth glistening capsule, the ovaries often have an "oyster shell" appearance.

The tunica albuginea is often thickened diffusely, and many cysts 3–7 mm in diameter are present in the periphery on cut section **(Fig. 34.4)**. Corpora lutea are rarely present due to the absence of ovulation. The clinical

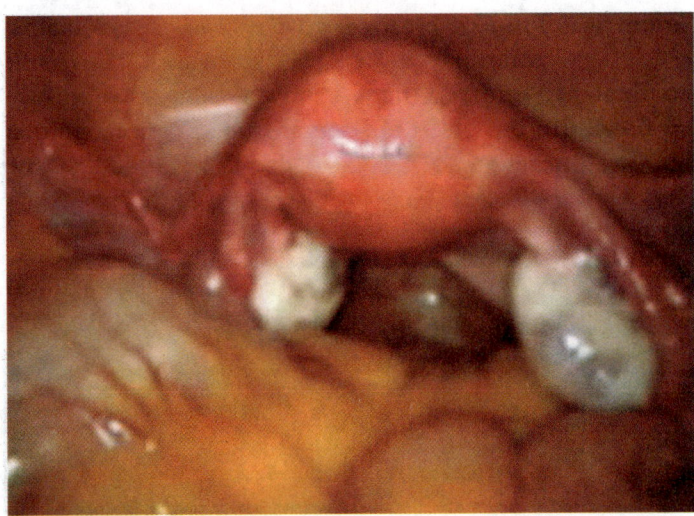

Fig. 34.3: Bilateral polycystic ovaries as observed on laparoscopic examination.

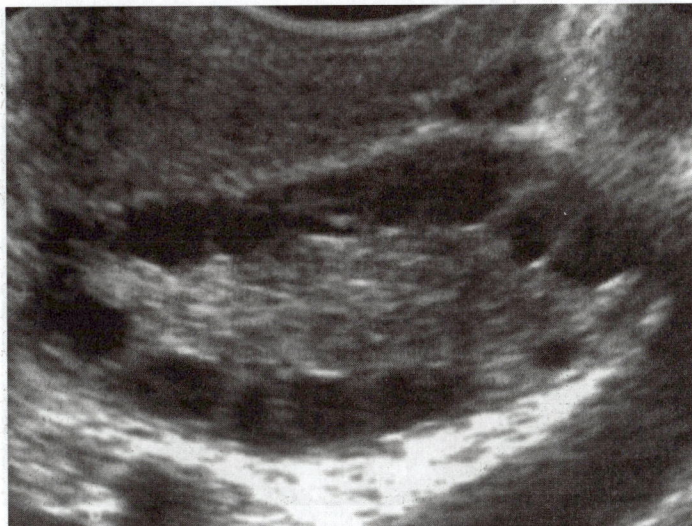

Fig. 34.4: TVS showing a row of intermediate-sized subcapsular follicles present peripherally in both the ovaries, suggestive of PCOS.

syndrome accompanying this pathologic finding is typically characterized by massive obesity, severe hirsutism due to excessive ovarian production of androgens, glucose intolerance with insulin resistance, and hyperuricemia.

Women with PCOS invariably are well estrogenized, with normal breast development and abundant cervical mucus on examination. Patients with PCOS often have excess unopposed circulating estrogen, increasing their risk of developing endometrial cancer. The insulin resistance associated with PCOS increases a patient's risk of diabetes mellitus by two-to-fivefold. Therefore, testing for glucose intolerance should be considered. The diagnosis of PCOS is primarily clinical, although laboratory studies may be needed to rule out other causes of hyperandrogenism. The following laboratory investigations must be done:

- *Androgen levels:* Increased levels of androgens such as testosterone, epiandrostenedione, and dehydro-epiandrosterone may point towards the underlying pathology. Significantly elevated testosterone levels (>200 ng/mL) or DHEAS levels (>700 mg/mL) indicate a possible androgen-secreting tumor (ovarian or adrenal). On the other hand, slightly raised testosterone (>80 ng/mL, <200 ng/mL) or DHEAS levels (>300 ng/mL, <700 mg/mL) are associated with PCOS.
- Raised serum concentrations of LH with normal FSH levels often result in an increased LH:FSH ratio of >2.
- Increased levels of 17-alpha hydroxyprogesterone (>800 ng/dL)
- Increased fasting insulin levels (>10 mIU/L), and increased fasting glucose/insulin ratio > 4.5 (normal 2.4–4.5).

Two important biochemical features associated with PCOS include insulin resistance to a standard glucose challenge and compensatory hyperinsulinemia and obesity. Weight loss in patients with PCOS helps in reducing the levels of insulin and androgens. The androgen is converted to estrogen, primarily estrone, in the periphery. Estrogen feedbacks on the central nervous system hypothalamic–pituitary unit to induce inappropriate gonadotropin secretion with an increased LH:FSH ratio. It stimulates GnRH synthesis and secretion in the hypothalamus, causing preferential LH release by the pituitary gland. Selective inhibition of FSH secretion by increased ovarian inhibin levels may also occur in PCOS. The increased LH secretion stimulates theca cells in the ovary to produce excessive androgen. The androgen also inhibits production of SHBGs, resulting in increased free androgen levels, thereby predisposing affected women to hirsutism. The absence of follicular maturation in the ovaries is related to the reduced estradiol production by the ovaries apparently resulting from combination of inadequate FSH stimulation and inhibition by the increased concentrations of intraovarian androgens. The low levels of SHBG probably facilitate tissue uptake of free androgen, leading to increased peripheral formation of estrogen and perpetuating the acyclic chronic anovulation. The androgenic basis for the inappropriate estrogen feedback is partly shifted to the ovaries. The increased estrogens (and perhaps androgens) may also stimulate fat cell proliferation, leading to obesity. The current data suggest that there is no defect in the hypothalamic–pituitary axis in PCOS but rather that peripheral alterations result in abnormal gonadotropin secretion.

Tubal Factors

Q. Write a long essay discussing the causes of infertility in females. How will you manage a case of tubal block.

Q. Evaluate the tubal factors in infertility, and outline the management of tubal block in a 25-year-old nulliparous woman.

Q. Write a short essay discussing the diagnosis of tubal factors in infertility.

The fallopian tubes play an important role in reproduction. After ovulation, the fimbriae pick up oocyte from the peritoneal fluid, which has accumulated in the cul-de-sac. The epithelial cilia in the tubal epithelium then transport the oocyte up to the ampulla. The capacitated spermatozoa are transported from the cervix through the endometrial cavity into the ampulla of fallopian tube, where fertilization ultimately occurs. Fallopian tube abnormalities or tubal damage or obstruction may result in either infertility or abnormal implantation or ectopic pregnancy.

Causes of Tubal Obstruction

Pelvic inflammatory disease: PID is typically associated with gonorrheal and chlamydial infections. Formation of peritoneal adhesions secondary to PID can compromise the motility of fallopian tubes. Furthermore, obstruction of the distal end of the fallopian tubes results in accumulation of the normally secreted tubal fluid, creating distention of the tube. This subsequently causes damage to the epithelial cilia and may result in development of hydrosalpinx **(Figs. 34.5 and 34.6)**.

Other Causes of Tubal Obstruction

> Q. Write a short essay discussing the implications of reproductive tract infections in infertility and their management.
>
> Q. Write a short essay discussing the microorganisms involved in female infertility.

Tubal obstruction can commonly result due to formation of scar tissue and adhesions due to infections (especially *Chlamydia* and gonorrhea), endometriosis, pelvic tuberculosis, and salpingitis isthmica nodosa (i.e., diverticulosis of the fallopian tube) or abdominal or gynecological surgery. Tubal obstruction prevents the ovum from entering or traveling down the fallopian tube and meeting the sperm. Damage to the ciliary epithelial of the fallopian tube as a result of infection can result in the development of abnormal implantation or an ectopic pregnancy. Ectopic pregnancy has been discussed in detail in Chapter 32.

Peritoneal Factors

The uterus, ovaries, and fallopian tubes are all present in the same space within the peritoneal cavity. The released ovum from the ovary often gets extruded into the peritoneal cavity into the cul-de-sac from where it is picked up by the fimbriae. Anatomical defects or physiologic dysfunctions of the peritoneal cavity, including infection, adhesions, and adnexal masses, may cause infertility.

Peritoneal Defects

Endometriosis: It is an enigmatic disease characterized by the growth of endometrial tissue outside the uterus, which

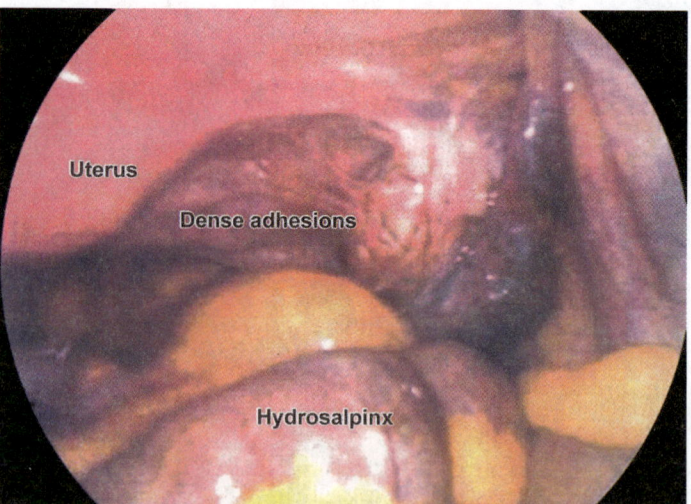

Fig. 34.5: Laparoscopic appearance of hydrosalpinx arising from left tube.

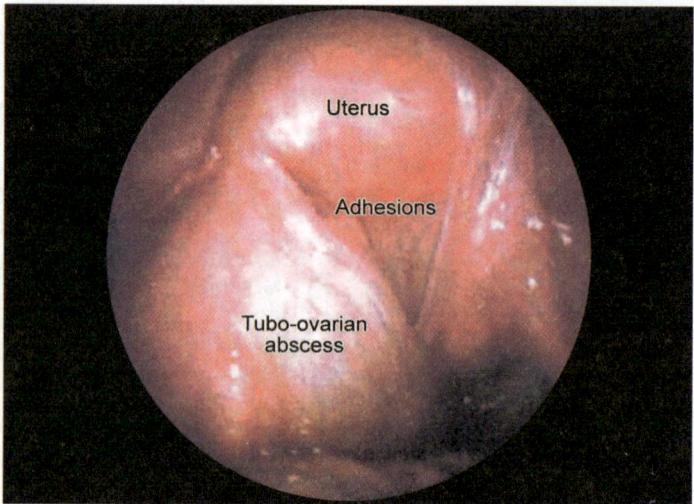

Fig. 34.6: Laparoscopic findings showing the presence of a tubo-ovarian mass.

may affect a woman's fertility. For detailed management of endometriosis, kindly refer to Chapter 30.

Endometriotic lesions vary from microscopic to macroscopic size. Classic endometriosis appears as bluish-black pigments, (i.e., "powder-burn lesions") that affect the peritoneal surfaces of the bladder, ovary, fallopian tubes, cul-de-sac, and bowel. Nonclassic endometriosis may appear as red-, tan-, or white-colored lesions and vesicles. Medical treatment of minimal or mild endometriosis has not been shown to increase the pregnancy rates. Moderate-to-severe endometriosis should be treated surgically. Different mechanisms through which endometriosis results in infertility are described in **Table 34.4**.

■ FACTORS AFFECTING BOTH SEXES

Environmental and Occupational Factors

Excessive radiation may damage the germinal cells. It has yet not been proven whether exposure to heavy metals,

TABLE 34.4: Different mechanisms through which endometriosis results in infertility.	
Type of endometriosis	**Cause for infertility**
Severe endometriosis	• Damage to the fallopian tubes due to the presence of adhesions • Damage to the ovaries due to the presence of endometriomas
Minimal and mild endometriosis	• Increased peritoneal macrophages that increase phagocytosis of the sperms, reduced sperm binding to the zona pellucida, proliferation of peritoneal lymphocytes, increased production of cytokinin and immunoglobulins, and defective activity of natural killer cells • Ovulatory disorders such as luteal phase deficiency, oligo-ovulation, and luteinized unruptured follicle syndrome

such as lead, excessive heat, microwave radiation, and ultrasonography, may be responsible for inducing infertility.

Toxic Effects Related to Tobacco, Marijuana, and Other Drugs

Smoking has been associated with infertility in both males and females. Various chemical substances in tobacco such as nicotine and polycyclic aromatic hydrocarbons have been observed to block spermatogenesis and decrease testicular size. In women, various chemicals present in the tobacco smoke are thought to affect the transportation of sperm and ova across the fallopian tube by altering the cervical mucus and cilial epithelium, respectively.

Marijuana and its metabolite, delta-9-tetrahydro-cannabinol, inhibit the secretion of LH and FSH in women, thereby inducing ovulatory and luteal phase dysfunction. Also, marijuana use affects male fertility by reducing the sperm count and quality of the sperm. The use of heroin, cocaine, and crack cocaine may produce similar effects. Chronic alcoholism in women may induce ovulatory dysfunction, thereby producing infertility. Alcohol use by males interferes with the synthesis of testosterone and may reduce sperm concentration. Alcoholism may also inhibit sexual response and cause impotence.

Exercise

Exercise should be encouraged as part of normal activity. However, compulsive exercise is deleterious, especially for long-distance runners, athletes, dancers, etc. In these women, excessive exercise could also result in amenorrhea. In males, excessive exercise has been associated with oligospermia.

Inadequate Diet Associated with Extreme Weight Loss or Gain

Both excessive weight gain and loss may have an impact on the woman's fertility. Although weight loss associated with anorexia nervosa or bulimia induces hypothalamic amenorrhea, obesity may be associated with anovulation and oligomenorrhea. In men, obesity has been associated with decreased sperm quality.

MANAGEMENT

Q. What minimum investigations must be offered in the case study mentioned in the beginning of the chapter?
Ans. Since the causes of infertility can be multifactorial, a systematic approach is typically used and involves testing for male, ovulatory, uterotubal, and peritoneal factors. Since the evaluation for male factor infertility has already been done in the form of semen analysis, the next step should be toward evaluation of ovulatory factors. These must include tests such as serum progesterone level, serum basal FSH level, and CC challenge test (CCCT).

Q. What advice must be given in this case?
Ans. Couples concerned about their fertility should be informed that about 84% of couples in the general population will conceive within 1 year if they do not use contraception and have regular sexual intercourse. Of those who do not conceive in the first year, about half will do so in the second year (cumulative pregnancy rate of 92%). Regular sexual intercourse after every 2–3 days is likely to maximize the overall chances of natural conception, as spermatozoa survive in the female reproductive tract for up to 7 days after insemination. In this case, the sexual history revealed that the couple had reasonable knowledge regarding the female reproductive cycle and had been having regular unprotected sexual intercourse. The main abnormality detected on the general physical examination was an increased BMI. Also, the menstrual cycles were irregular. Both these things raised suspicion toward the likely ovulatory dysfunction in this patient. Keeping in mind the diagnosis of anovulatory cycles, the woman was advised the following investigations: pelvic ultrasound examination, serum progesterone levels 1 week before the expected time of menses, serum LH:FSH ratio, fasting insulin levels, and serum testosterone levels. In view of the raised BMI, the woman was advised lifestyle changes in order to reduce her weight. She was advised to indulge in brisk walking for 30 minutes every day. She was also referred to the nutrition specialist to help her devise a proper dietary plan in order to bring her weight under control.

Evaluation of the couple is the starting point for treatment of infertility as it may suggest specific causes and appropriate treatment modalities. Patient evaluation should begin by taking detailed history from both the partners. Sometimes simple reassurance and explanation about the physiology of menstrual cycle and importance of having regular intercourse is sufficient in achieving pregnancy. Although the history and physical examination is able to provide important information, specific diagnostic tests are also required to evaluate infertility. Once the cause of infertility has been identified, treatment must be aimed at correcting the underlying etiologies. Besides instituting corrective measures, the couple must be counseled to observe certain changes in lifestyle such as ceasing smoking, reducing excessive caffeine and alcohol consumption, and maintaining appropriate frequency of sexual intercourse (every 1–2 days around the anticipated time of ovulation).

INVESTIGATIONS

Evaluation of infertile couples should be organized and thorough. Diagnostic tests should start from the simplest tests (e.g., semen analysis and pelvic ultrasonography) onto the more complex and invasive ones (e.g., laparoscopy). Also, the evaluation of fertility must first begin with tests for the assessment of male fertility. Semen analysis is the most commonly performed test of male infertility, which yields tremendous amount of information as to the potential causes of male infertility. The tests which are useful for the initial evaluation of an infertile couple are listed in **Box 34.1**.

■ SCREENING TESTS

There are some general screening tests which need to be done, if not done previously for all women presenting for an infertility workup.

Pap Smear

Pap smear is recommended for all sexually active women belonging to the reproductive age group. Tests such as ABO blood group typing, Rh typing, and antibody screening (in Rh-negative women) are also recommended if not done previously.

Screening for Cystic Fibrosis

The American Congress of Obstetricians and Gynecologists and American College of Medical Genetics recommend that screening for cystic fibrosis should be offered to all individuals with a family history of cystic fibrosis, reproductive partners of individuals with cystic fibrosis, and couples planning a pregnancy wherein one or both the partners are Caucasians or Ashkenazi jews. This test must also be available to all patients on request.

Immunity for Rubella

All women attempting pregnancy with undocumented previous rubella infection or vaccination should be tested for immunity. If found to be seronegative, they must be vaccinated. The CDC recommends that women need not avoid pregnancy for >1 month after vaccination. It also recommends that women without a history of any previous infection or evidence of immunity or vaccination against varicella must receive two doses of vaccine and avoid pregnancy for 1 month after each dose.

Screening for Sexually Transmitted Diseases

Screening for sexually transmitted infections is recommended for all women at moderate-to-high risk for infection. Current recommendations from the CDC include screening for the following diseases:

- Screening of all pregnant women for Chlamydia and gonorrhea (using nucleic acid-based tests)
- Screening for syphilis using rapid plasma reagin (RPR) test
- Screening for hepatitis B using hepatitis B surface antigen (HBsAg)
- Voluntary screening for HIV type 1 virus at the time of first prenatal visit

■ EVALUATION OF THE MALE PARTNER

> Q. Write a short essay discussing the treatment of abnormal semen analysis in an infertile couple.
>
> Q. Write a long essay regarding evaluation of the male partner in case of an infertile couple.
>
> Q. Describe the diagnosis and management of male infertility with the help of a long essay.
>
> Q. Discuss in detail the anatomy of a normal sperm and parameters of normal semen analysis.

Semen Analysis

A comprehensive semen analysis must be performed in a certified andrology laboratory. The male patient should be instructed well in advance that they must provide a semen sample after a period of abstinence of 2–5 days. This sample is collected through masturbation, and must be collected into a container, which is nontoxic to the sperms. The semen is usually not collected from condom samples because it may contain a spermicidal agent. The patient is discouraged

---

BOX 34.1: Workup of an infertile couple.

Minimal investigations (required in most couples):
- Semen analysis to assess male factors
- Menstrual history, assessment of LH surge in urine prior to ovulation, and/or luteal phase progesterone level to assess ovulatory function and endometrial receptivity
- Hysterosalpingography to assess tubal patency and uterine cavity
- Day 3 serum FSH and estradiol levels to assess ovarian reserve

Additional tests required in select couples:
- Pelvic ultrasound to assess for uterine myomas and ovarian cysts
- Laparoscopy to diagnose endometriosis or other pelvic pathology

Additional tests for assessment of ovarian reserve in women >35 years of age: Clomiphene citrate challenge test, ultrasound for early follicular antral follicle count, day 3 serum inhibin B level, or anti-Müllerian hormone measurement
- Assessment of thyroid function

(FSH: follicle stimulating hormone; LH: luteinizing hormone)

from attempting to collect a sample through intercourse as coitus interruptus is not a reliable means for sample collection. Ideally, the specimen must be collected at the same andrology laboratory, which would conduct the test. If the sample is collected at home, it should be transported to the laboratory within 30 minutes to ensure the accuracy of the results. The primary values that are evaluated at the time of semen analysis include the volume of the ejaculate, sperm motility, total sperm concentration, and sperm morphology, motility, and viability. The odds of male infertility increase with the number of major semen parameters (sperm concentration, mobility, and morphology) in the subfertile range. The probability is 2–3 times higher in the presence of one abnormal parameter, 5–7 times higher in the presence of two abnormal parameters, and nearly 16 times higher in the presence of all three abnormal parameters. Spermatogenesis takes approximately 72 days. Therefore, the sperm analysis must be repeated after 3 months if any of the parameters appear abnormal or as soon as possible in case of gross sperm deficiency.

Normal parameters for semen analysis are described by the WHO (2010) in **Table 34.5**. The fifth edition has been mainly criticized for suggesting the reference ranges of semen parameters as the mainstay factor in the evaluation of male infertility. In 2021, the WHO published the sixth edition **(Table 34.6)**, a revised reference criteria for semen analysis, which included the data of previous fifth edition along with the addition of new data of fertile men whose partners conceived within 12 months, collected during the time extending between 2010 and 2020. The newly added data also included two countries in southeast Asia, which were underrepresented in the previous edition, along with two countries from Asia, one from Africa, which lacked representation in the previous edition. The sixth edition addresses the drawbacks of the fifth edition and has abandoned the reference values and emphasizes that multiple criteria must be applied for establishing the diagnosis of male infertility. With the growing awareness that chromosomal abnormalities and gene mutations could be responsible for a wide spectrum of male infertility, genetic and genomic testing have been given more attention in this sixth edition. This edition aims at assisting fertility/infertility diagnosis, assessment of male reproductive health, guiding the choice of ART procedure, monitoring the response to treatment, measuring the efficacy of male contraception, updating the semen analysis procedures, and eliminating the outdated tests (such as human cervical mucus). The sixth edition also highlights the importance of sperm DNA fragmentation (SDF) and genetic evaluation in the context of male infertility. SDF assay has been introduced for an extended assessment of semen, which can be requested in certain clinical scenarios.

Interpretation of Semen Analysis

Abnormal semen analysis results can be attributed to various unknown reasons such as short period of sexual abstinence and poor sexual stimulus. Therefore, it is important to repeat the semen analysis at least 1 month later before reaching a diagnosis. The terminology associated with abnormal results of semen analysis is described in **Table 34.7**. To establish the diagnosis of azoospermia, the semen specimen must be centrifuged at high speed (3,000 g for 15 minutes), following which the pellet must be examined under high magnification (400×). The absence of sperms must be documented on at least two separate occasions.

A low semen volume (<1.5 mL) in association with azoospermia or severe oligozoospermia is suggestive of genital tract obstruction, which is commonly due to two causes. These include either congenital absence of the vas deferens or obstruction of ejaculatory ducts. Low semen pH is indicative of congenital absence of vas deferens.

TABLE 34.5: Parameters for semen analysis: lower reference limits (95% CI) in fertile men (WHO, 5th Edition, 2010).

Parameter	Normal range
Volume	1.5 mL (1.4–1.7 mL)
Sperm concentration	15 (12–16) million/mL or greater
Total sperm number	39 (33–46) million spermatozoa per ejaculate or more
Motility	32% forward progression, 40% total motility (progressive + nonprogressive motility)
Morphology	Normal sperms (>4%) using "strict" Tygerberg method
Vitality	58 (55–63)% or more live

Source: Cooper TG, Noonan E, von Eckardstein S, Auger J, Baker HW, Behre HM, et al. World Health Organization reference values for human semen characteristics. Hum Reprod Update. 2010;16(3):231-45.

TABLE 34.6: Normal parameters for semen analysis (WHO, 6th Edition, 2021).

Parameter	Normal range
Volume	1.3–1.5 mL (1.4 mL)
Liquefaction time	Within 60 minutes
Viscosity	<3 (scale 0–4)
pH level	pH level 7.2–7.8
Total sperm number	39 million (35–40 million) spermatozoa per ejaculate or more
Motility	Total motility should be 42% (40–43), progressive motility should be 30% (29–31), nonprogressive motility should be 1%
Morphology	Normal sperms (>4%)
Vitality	54 (50–56)
Round cells	Fewer than 5 million cells/mL
Sperm agglutination	<2 (scale of 0–3)

TABLE 34.7: Terminology associated with abnormal results of semen analysis.

Terminology	Interpretation	Causes
Normozoospermia	Normal ejaculate as defined by the WHO reference values	
Hypospermia	Decrease in semen volume to <2 mL per ejaculation	
Hyperspermia	Increase in semen volume to >8 mL per ejaculation	
Aspermia	No ejaculate	
Azoospermia	Absence of sperms in the semen	Congenital absence or bilateral obstruction of the vas deferens or ejaculatory ducts
Oligozoospermia	Concentration of sperms fewer than 20 million sperms/mL	Ejaculatory dysfunction such as retrograde ejaculation, genetic conditions, or hormonal disturbances
Asthenozoospermia	Sperm motility of <50%	Extreme temperatures
Teratospermia	An increased number of sperms with abnormal morphology at the head, neck, or tail level	
Teratozoospermia	Sperm morphology less than the WHO reference	
Oligoasthenoteratozoospermia	*Disturbance of all three variables*: (1) Motility, (2) morphology, and (3) sperm concentration	
Cryptozoospermia	Few spermatozoa recovered after centrifugation	

In the presence of normal pH of seminal fluid, transrectal ultrasound (TRU) examination must be performed. In case TRU shows dilated seminal vesicles, this is indicative of ejaculatory duct obstruction.

White blood cells are normally not present in the seminal fluid. Increased white blood cells in the seminal fluid ejaculate are an indicator of genital infection/inflammation. Leukocytes in the seminal fluid may release reactive oxygen species, which may be related with poor quality of semen. Though presently, there is no evidence-based cutoff limit for the diagnosis of possible infection, clinically accepted cutoff value is considered as 1 million leukocytes/mL of ejaculate. When the round cell count exceeds 5 million cells/mL, additional tests must be performed to differentiate leukocytes from immature sperms and identify those men having true leukocytospermia (>1 million leukocytes/mL). These individuals may require additional evaluation for genital tract infections or inflammation.

Determination of Serum Testosterone Levels

Serum testosterone levels, particularly that of total testosterone, free testosterone, LH, and FSH, must be measured if hypogonadism is suspected as a cause for infertility. Morning values are preferred to afternoon blood samples because testosterone is secreted in the morning. Hypogonadism is the only cause of male infertility that can successfully be treated with hormone therapy.

Karyotyping

Routine karyotyping is usually not required. It may be performed in the following circumstances:
- Karyotyping the male partner in the presence of severe oligospermia
- Karyotyping the women in case of very early premature menopause (prior to the age of 40 years)
- Karyotyping both partners in case of recurrent pregnancy losses.

Detailed description of other tests for male infertility besides semen analysis is beyond the scope of this chapter.

EVALUATION OF THE FEMALE PARTNER

> Q. Write a long essay on evaluation and management of secondary infertility in a female patient.
>
> Q. Write a long essay regarding the evaluation of a female partner who presents with primary infertility.

A complete evaluation of the female reproductive tract must involve cervical, uterine, endometrial, tubal, peritoneal, and ovarian factors. Since thyroid disease and hyperprolactinemia can cause menstrual abnormalities and infertility, serum thyroid TSH and prolactin levels must be checked first before instituting further investigations.

Evaluation of Cervical Factor

> Q. Write a short note regarding cervical factors in infertility.

Postcoital Test (Sims or Huhner Test)

> Q. Write a short essay on postcoital test.

Postcoital test aims at identifying the cervical factor infertility by testing the characteristics of cervical mucus. The couple is advised to have intercourse in the early hours of morning and present to the clinic as soon as possible in the morning. Ideally, the male partner must have abstained from ejaculation at least 48 hours prior to the test. The mucus, which is aspirated from the cervical canal, is spread over the glass slide and then examined under the microscope. This test involves both a gross and microscopic examination to grade the cervical mucus. Normally, there are 10–50 motile sperms per high power field. The presence of <10 sperms is considered abnormal and requires the performance of a proper semen analysis. However, many researchers consider the presence of a single motile sperm in most fields as a "positive" or normal test result. Normally, the sperms show progressive mobility. The presence of a jerky or rotatory mobility could be due to the presence of antisperm antibodies. A smear must be taken from the posterior fornix, which serves as a control. Physical properties of cervical mucus such as volume, pH, viscosity (length to which the cervical mucus can be stretched), and fern test are also studied. The most common cause for a "negative" postcoital test is improper timing. While of historical interest, this test is no longer routinely performed in the standard infertility workup because it has been found to be associated with poor predictive value. Furthermore, infertility due to cervical factors can be easily overcome by performing intrauterine inseminations (IUIs).

Tests for Uterine Factor

The commonly used investigations include hysterosalpingogram (HSG), pelvic ultrasonography, and endometrial biopsy.

Operative procedures such as laparoscopy and hysteroscopy are often necessary for confirmation of the final diagnosis.

Screening Tests for Chlamydia trachomatis

Before undergoing uterine instrumentation, women should be offered screening for *Chlamydia trachomatis* using an appropriately sensitive technique. In case the results for the test of *Chlamydia trachomatis* are positive, women and their sexual partners should be referred for appropriate management with antibiotic treatment and contact tracing. Prophylactic antibiotics may be considered before uterine instrumentation if screening has not been carried out.

Hysterosalpingogram

The HSG is the most frequently used diagnostic tool for evaluation of the endometrial cavity as well as the tubal pathology **(Fig. 34.7)**. If performed meticulously under fluoroscopic guidance, HSG helps in providing accurate information about the endocervical canal, endometrial cavity, cornual ostium, patency of the fallopian tubes **(Fig. 34.8)**, and status of the fimbriae. Tubal patency is indicated by spillage of dye into the endometrial cavity. HSG is able to accurately define the shape and size of the

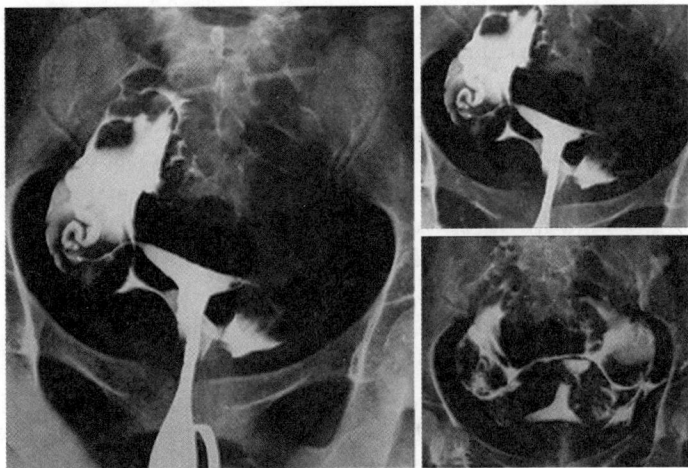

Fig. 34.7: Normal hysterosalpingogram showing bilateral spillage of dye.

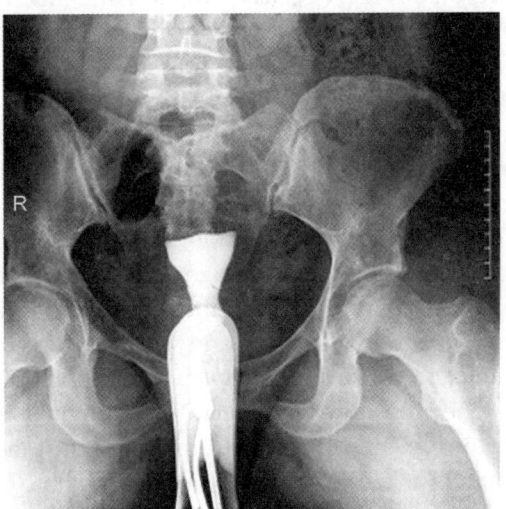

Fig. 34.8: Hysterosalpingogram showing bilateral cornual block.

uterine cavity. It can help diagnose uterine developmental anomalies (e.g., unicornuate uterus, septate uterus, bicornuate uterus, and uterus didelphys), submucous myomas, adnexal masses, intrauterine adhesions, and endometrial polyps. Furthermore, the HSG also provides indirect evidence regarding the presence of pelvic adhesions and uterine, ovarian, or adnexal masses. Normal uterine cavity is symmetrical and triangular in shape. It is widest at the level of cornual orifices near the fundus. HSG is best performed during the 2–5-day interval period immediately following end of menses.

Timing: The HSG should be performed postmenstrually during the early follicular phase, usually after the end of menstrual bleeding and before the occurrence of ovulation. At this time, the endometrium is thin, and the HSG can help delineate the minor defects. Additionally, performance of HSG before the occurrence of ovulation eliminates the possibility of accidental irradiation to the fetus in case of an undiagnosed pregnancy.

Procedure: It involves the following steps:
1. Patient is made to lie on the examination table either in lithotomy position, with her feet held up with stirrups, or in dorsal position with her knees bent.
2. Posterior vaginal wall is retracted using a Sims speculum, and the anterior lip of cervix is held with a tenaculum.
3. Procedure is performed after taking strict aseptic precautions. The cervix is cleansed with a povidone-iodine solution (betadine).
4. After cleaning the cervix, a catheter is inserted through the cervix inside the uterine cavity.
5. Speculum and tenaculum are removed, and the patient is carefully situated underneath the fluoroscopy device.
6. Contrast material is inserted through the catheter into the uterine cavity, fallopian tubes, and peritoneal cavity, and fluoroscopic images are taken. Initially, oil-based dye, lipoidal, was used as the contrast media. However now, water-soluble contrast material is generally being preferred as it helps in preventing the development of possible complications such as oil embolism.
7. X-ray pictures are taken as the uterine cavity begins to fill. Following this, additional contrast material is injected inside the uterine cavity so that the tubes fill up and the dye begins to spill into the abdominal cavity. More X-ray pictures are taken as the spillage of dye occurs. The X-ray images can help in determining whether the fallopian tubes are patent or blocked and whether the blockage is located at the proximal or distal end of the fallopian tube.
8. When the procedure is complete, the catheter is removed.

Since the injection of dye can sometimes cause cramping, the woman is asked to remain lying on the table for a few minutes following the completion of the procedure in order to let her recover from this cramping. Normal HSG findings with bilateral spillage have been previously discussed in Chapter 13. HSG in the patient whose ultrasound had revealed the presence of bilateral masses suggestive of hydrosalpinx is shown in **Figures 34.9A and B**.

Indications: Women who are not known to have comorbid disorders (such as PID, previous ectopic pregnancy, or endometriosis) should be offered HSG as a screening test for tubal occlusion. HSG serves a reliable, noninvasive, cost-effective test for ruling out tubal occlusion. Where appropriate expertise is available, hysterosalpingo-contrast sonography (HyCoSy) can be considered as an appropriate cost-effective alternative to HSG for women who are not known to have any comorbidities. Women who are thought to have comorbidities should be offered laparoscopy with dye instillation so that tubal and other pelvic pathologies can be assessed at the same time.

In comparison to laparoscopy, HSG is less invasive, does not require general anesthesia, and is able to reveal the internal structure of the uterus and tubes. Also, it is associated with a much lower rate of complications, such as injury to the bowel or blood vessels. Though HSG has only a moderate sensitivity, it has a very high specificity in detection of tubal pathology. This implies that when HSG reveals obstruction, there is a high degree of probability that this is a false-positive result, and the tube is probably patent. On the other hand, when the HSG demonstrates patency, it is highly unlikely that the tube would be actually occluded. Also, HSG may also not prove to be useful for diagnosis of peritubal adhesions or endometriosis.

Hysterosalpingogram is usually not associated with any infectious complications. However, routine prophylactic treatment with doxycycline 100 mg twice a day for 5 days, beginning 1–2 days before HSG, is usually justified because of the potential drastic consequences of a postprocedural infection. Antibiotic prophylaxis is especially indicated when the tubal disease is highly suspected or HSG reveals distal tubal obstruction because in these cases the risk for acute salpingitis is increased, and treatment can prevent clinical infection.

Saline Infusion Sonography

Saline infusion sonography (SIS) provides a simple and inexpensive method for evaluating the uterine cavity and assessing tubal patency. Detailed description of the procedure has been done in Chapter 24. The procedure is well tolerated by patients and can be performed in the OPD. In comparison to HSG, SIS helps in eliminating the risks

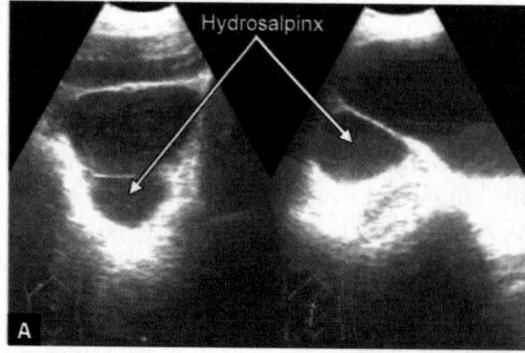 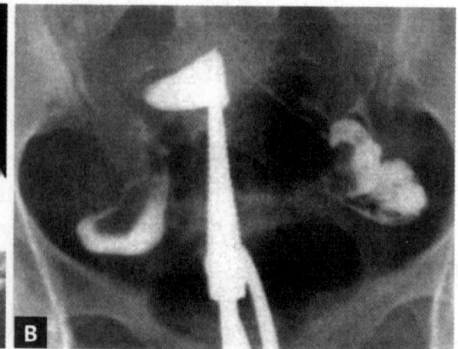

Figs. 34.9A and B: (A) Transabdominal sonography revealing the presence of bilateral mass with multiple internal echoes suggestive of hydrosalpinx; (B) Hysterosalpingogram in the same patient showing the presence of mass bilaterally.

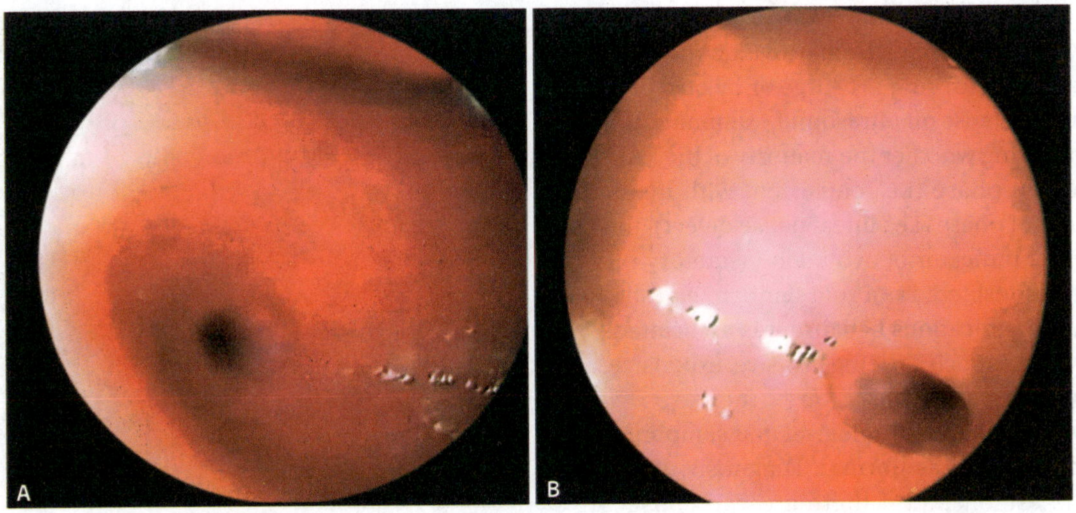

Figs. 34.10A and B: Hysteroscopic evaluation of tubal ostium. (A) Right sided; (B) Left sided.

associated with the use of dye and radiation required by HSG. SIS helps in diagnosing intracavitary uterine abnormalities and tubal patency. SIS should be performed during days 6–12 of the menstrual cycle prior to the occurrence of ovulation. Thin uterine endometrium during this phase allows better detection of intrauterine lesions. In addition, this ensures that an undiagnosed pregnancy is not disrupted.

While SIS can confirm tubal patency, it does not provide information about the contour of the tubes. Thus, if a patient has a history of endometriosis or other tubal disease, laparoscopy is preferred.

Ultrasonography

Pelvic ultrasonography (both transabdominal and transvaginal) has become an important tool in the evaluation and monitoring of infertile patients, especially during ovulation induction. It has become an important part of the routine gynecologic evaluation because it allows precise evaluation of the uterus, endometrial cavity, and adnexa (especially the ovaries). Pelvic sonograms also help in the early detection of uterine fibroids, endometrial polyps, ovarian cysts, adnexal masses, and endometriomas. Ultrasonography can help in diagnosing conditions such as ectopic pregnancy, polycystic ovaries, and persistent corpus luteum cysts. In the diagnostic evaluation of the infertile couple, ultrasound examination of the endometrium has no proven value. Although ultrasound examination cannot be used to evaluate endometrial receptivity, it does help in the identification of important uterine pathology in infertile women (e.g., presence of congenital malformations, septate uterus, and bicornuate uterus).

Hysteroscopy

Hysteroscopy is a method for direct visualization of the endometrial cavity, which is commonly performed as an OPD procedure using local anesthesia (i.e., paracervical block). Hysteroscopy is a definitive method used for both the diagnosis and the treatment of intrauterine pathology, which is likely to have an effect on the fertility. While performing hysteroscopy, solutions such as hyskon (previously used) and glycine and sorbitol (used nowadays) are used for intrauterine instillation. Hysteroscopic examination helps in evaluation of tubal ostia **(Figs. 34.10A and B)**. Hysteroscopic examination helps in both the diagnosis and the treatment of endometrial pathology. Hysteroscopic surgery can also be used for treatment of intrauterine pathologies such as uterine synechiae, endometrial polyps, submucous myomas, removal of foreign bodies (e.g., intrauterine devices), and lysis of intrauterine adhesions produced by Asherman's syndrome. In patients undergoing hysteroscopy, performing laparoscopy simultaneously helps in avoiding the requirement for HSG.

Endometrial Biopsy

> **Q. Write a long essay describing the physiology of luteal phase and the management of luteal phase defects.**

The endometrial lining constantly changes in response to the various hormones secreted during different phases of the menstrual cycle. Detailed description of the procedure of endometrial biopsy has been done in Chapter 23. A diagnosis of luteal phase dysfunction is made on the basis of the lack of correlation between the findings on endometrial biopsy and day of the menstrual cycle. During the follicular phase of the menstrual cycle, the endometrium exhibits a proliferative pattern. The growth is stimulated by rising levels of estrogen derived from the dominant ovarian follicle. Progesterone secreted by the corpus luteum causes secretory transformation of the endometrium. The endometrium in anovulatory women is always in the follicular phase. Unopposed estrogen stimulation can cause endometrial proliferation, resulting in endometrial hyperplasia.

Pathologists date the endometrium by estimating the number of days that have passed since ovulation. Ovulation can be detected by measuring LH surge or by observing the signs of follicular collapse on ultrasound examination.

Besides evaluating whether the maturity of the secretory endometrium is in phase (i.e., consistent with menstrual cycle date) or out of phase (i.e., luteal phase defect), this test is also an indirect indicator of ovulation (secretory phase). However, it is not considered as a gold standard investigation for either of these indications because it is associated with several disadvantages such as being invasive, expensive, and uncomfortable.

Agreement between the histological and sampling dates by 2 days is considered as normal. Diagnosis of a luteal phase defect is established if there are two consecutive endometrial biopsy specimens showing histology >2 days out of phase with the actual biopsy date. This is however not diagnostic of luteal phase defect because nearly 50% of normal fertile women may have a 2-day lag in the maturation of endometrium. The delayed endometrial maturation is thought to be caused due to deficiency in the production of progesterone by the corpus luteum. However, up to 50% of normal fertile women may have a 2-day lag in endometrial maturation on a single biopsy. Endometrial biopsy was once considered as the basic element in the evaluation of infertility for establishing the diagnosis of luteal phase. However, this is no longer the situation because endometrial dating cannot guide the clinical management of women with reproductive failure and/or infertility due to the above-described factors. Therefore, presently this investigation has no place in the diagnostic evaluation of infertility.

Tubal and Peritoneal Factors

The two most frequent tests used for diagnosis of tubal pathology are laparoscopy and HSG. HSG has been previously described. Therefore, only laparoscopy would be described here. Noninvasive or minimally invasive investigation, which may serve as an alternative to HSG for testing tubal patency, includes *Chlamydia* antibody testing and/or HyCoSy. More invasive tests such as laparoscopy with chromotubation and fluoroscopic/hysteroscopic selective tubal cannulation may be required to confirm the diagnosis of suspected tubal pathology. An endoscopic procedure known as falloposcopy is sometimes used for delineating fallopian tube pathology.

Laparoscopy

The laparoscope is one of the greatest developments in gynecologic instrumentation.

The laparoscope was first used to visualize the pelvic cavity. Gynecological laparoscopy is used for diagnosis as well as treatment of pelvic pathology. During laparoscopic examination, a laparoscope is used for visualizing the pelvic area, uterine surface, anterior and posterior cul-de-sac,

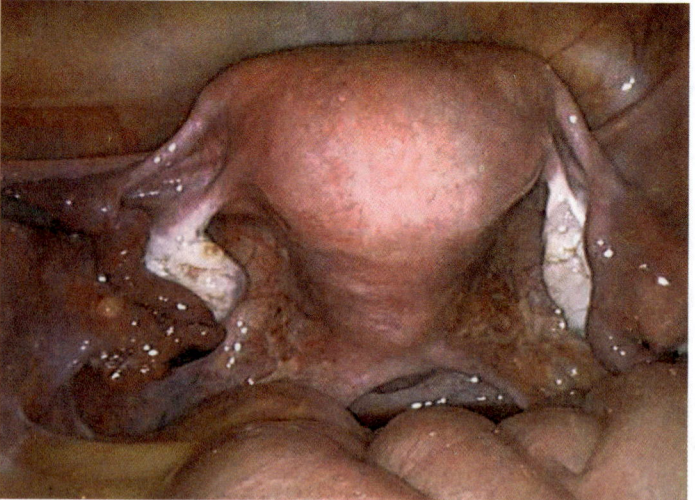

Fig. 34.11: Normal laparoscopic view of the pelvis.

fallopian tubes, and ovaries **(Fig. 34.11)**. Gynecological laparoscopy is commonly used for diagnosing and treating endometriosis, PID, ectopic pregnancy, and removal of adhesions and scar tissue. Laparoscopy can be used for monitoring the effects of ovulation induction medicines on the ovaries, and taking biopsies from ovarian cysts. Diagnostic laparoscopy may be performed under deep sedation and local anesthesia, while operative laparoscopy typically requires general anesthesia. Injection of a dye solution through the cannula inserted inside the cervix permits evaluation of tubal patency (chromotubation) **(Figs. 34.12A to C)**. Indigo carmine dye is usually preferred over the dye methylene blue due to the possible risk of acute methemoglobinemia. Laparoscopy is an invasive and expensive procedure. Moreover, findings at laparoscopy usually do not change the initial management of the infertile couple when the initial investigations performed for evaluation of infertility were either normal or there was severe male factor infertility.

Laparoscopy is contraindicated in patients with probable bowel obstruction, bowel distention, cardiopulmonary disease, or shock due to internal bleeding. It is associated with the risk of complications such as bowel perforation, uterine and pelvic vessel injury, and bladder trauma. Therefore, the procedure must preferably be performed by a skilled and experienced surgeon. Currently, laparoscopy has become the gold standard method for detection of tubal patency. In suspected cases of endometriosis or pelvic adhesions, diagnostic laparoscopy and chromotubation are preferred. Ablation of implants and lysis of adhesions can also be performed at the time of laparoscopy.

Falloposcopy

Falloposcopy is defined as transvaginal microendoscopy of the fallopian tubes and enables the gynecologist to directly visualize the entire lumen of the fallopian tube.

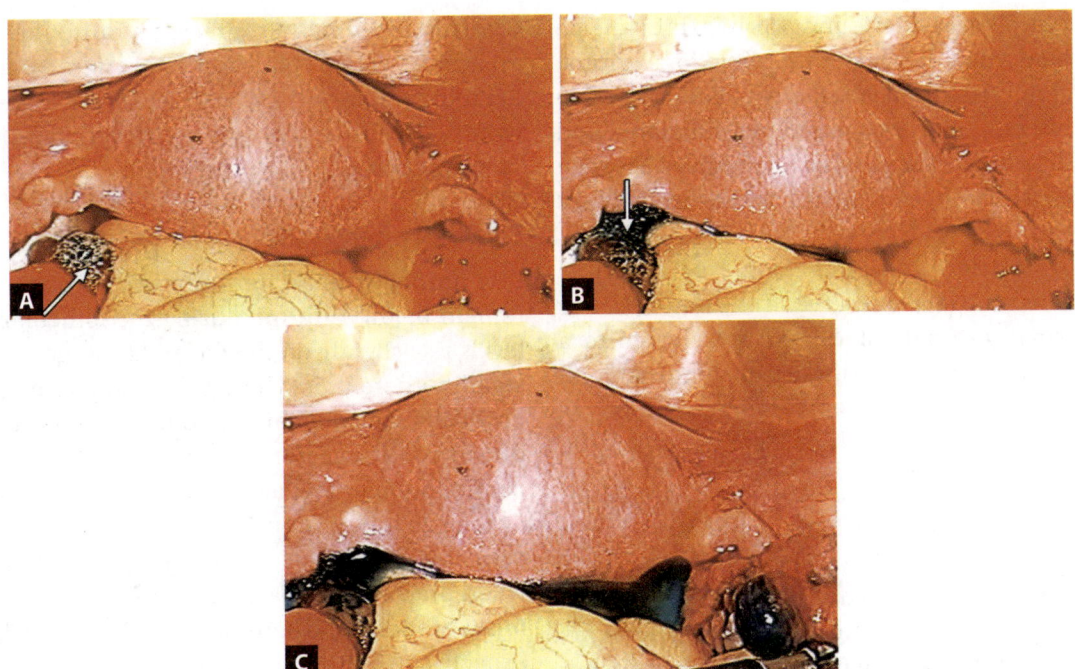

Figs. 34.12A to C: Laparoscopic test for tubal patency. (A) Slight spillage of dye from right-sided tube (indicated by the arrow); (B) Spillage of dye more pronounced on the right side (indicated by the arrow); (C) Bilateral spillage of dye on both the sides.

Chlamydia Antibodies

Chlamydia trachomatis IgG antibody testing is a simple, inexpensive, noninvasive test with some evidence supporting its use as a method for predicting the presence of tubal disease. Studies suggest that antibodies to *Chlamydia* are more predictive of infertility than an abnormal HSG or a history of previous use of a copper intrauterine device.

Hysterosalpingo-Contrast Sonography

In this method, echogenic contrast media is injected transcervically, following which ultrasound is used for visualizing the uterus, tubes, and adnexa. It is a safe, well-tolerated, quick, and easy method for obtaining information related to tubal status, the uterine cavity, ovaries, and the myometrium.

Ovarian Factors

 Q. Discuss in detail the tests for ovulation.

Checking the Ovarian Reserve

Diminished ovarian reserve can refer to a reduction in quality or quantity of oocytes, or a reduction in reproductive potential. Since many patients nowadays are presenting for diagnostic evaluation later in their lifespans, identification of diminished ovarian reserve is becoming increasingly important. The level of ovarian reserve and the age of the female partner are the most important prognostic factors in the fertility workup. The level of ovarian reserve is supposed to decrease with age. Checking for ovarian reserve is specifically indicated in patients aged 35 years or older.

Other circumstances where testing for ovarian reserve may also be required include the following:
- Unexplained infertility
- Family history of early menopause
- History of some ovarian surgery in the past (e.g., ovarian cystectomy or drilling, unilateral oophorectomy, chemotherapy, or radiation therapy)
- Poor response to exogeneous gonadotropin secretion.

Presently, there is no ideal test for assessing ovarian reserve. Though a number of screening tests are being used, none of the tests have been found to be extremely accurate in predicting the fertility potential. For women over 35 years of age and younger women having risk factors for premature ovarian failure, the test commonly used for testing ovarian reserve is determination of day 3 FSH level. Other tests which are being used include the CC challenge test (CCCT), antral follicle count (AFC), and levels of AMH.

CCCT: This test involves oral administration of 100 mg CC on days 5 through 9 of the menstrual cycle, followed by measurement of estradiol and FSH levels on day 3 and measurement of FSH levels on day 10. Women with good ovarian reserve usually produce sufficient amount of estradiol from small follicles early in the menstrual cycle, thereby maintaining FSH at a low level. In contrast, women with a reduced pool of follicles and oocytes are unable to produce sufficient amount of ovarian hormones, which is unable to inhibit the pituitary secretion of FSH, causing the FSH levels to rise early in the cycle.

Day 3 FSH concentration: A day 3 FSH concentration < 10 mIU/mL is suggestive of adequate ovarian reserve, whereas

FSH levels varying between 10 and 15 mIU/mL can be considered as borderline. The upper threshold for a normal FSH concentration varies from laboratory to laboratory due to the use of different FSH assay reference standards and various methodologies for assay. In general, values between 10 and 25 mIU/mL have been reported as the threshold for normal FSH levels.

An elevated FSH level on either day 3 or day 10 is suggestive of reduced ovarian reserve. If the day 3 FSH or CCCT is abnormal, the patient should be referred to a reproductive endocrinologist to discuss further treatment options such as aggressive ovulation induction, IVF, or use of donor oocytes.

AFC: The number of antral follicles (defined as follicles measuring 2–10 mm in diameter) can be measured with the help of ultrasound examination. In a normal woman, the number of antral follicles in the ovary is proportional to the number of primordial follicles remaining. Therefore, as the number of primordial follicles decrease, the number of visible small antral follicles also decline. On TVS, a low AFC ranging from 4 to 10 antral follicles between days 2 and 4 of a regular menstrual cycle is suggestive of poor ovarian reserve. Although AFC is a good predictor of ovarian reserve and response, it is less predictive of oocyte quality, the ability to conceive with IVF, and pregnancy outcome. Low AFC has, however, high specificity for predicting poor response to ovarian stimulation and treatment failure.

AMH: Since AMH is usually derived from the granulosa cells of the small (<8 mm) preantral and early antral follicles, its levels are independent of gonadotropins and exhibit very little variation within and between the cycles. As a result, serum AMH levels can be measured on any day of the cycle. AMH levels reflect the size of the primordial follicle pool. Therefore, in a normal adult woman, levels of this hormone progressively reduce with the gradual decline in the pool of primordial follicle with age. AMH levels are almost undetectable at the time of menopause. Low AMH values (0.2–0.7 ng/mL) have high sensitivity and specificity for predicting poor response to stimulation protocols, but not for predicting pregnancy. On the other hand, AHM level >5 ng/mL is indicative of hyper-responders, thereby suggesting that such patients can go for ovarian hyperstimulation syndrome (OHSS). Measurement of AMH helps identify reduced ovarian follicle pool in some patients (e.g., those receiving chemotherapy or radiotherapy for cancer).

Inhibin B levels: Inhibin is secreted by the granulosa cells of smaller antral follicles. However, its concentration is likely to increase in response to exogenous GnRH stimulation. Therefore, levels of inhibin B are usually not regarded as a reliable measure of ovarian reserve.

Ovarian volume: Progressive follicular depletion is associated with a reduction in ovarian volume. Therefore, ovarian volume (L × W × 0.52) shows a good correlation with the number of oocytes retrieved, but poorly with the pregnancy rates.

Serum Progesterone Levels

In a normal woman, serum progesterone levels generally remain below 1 ng/mL during the follicular phase. These levels rise slightly on the day of LH surge (1–2 ng/mL) and steadily thereafter. The levels of this hormone peak 7–8 days following ovulation and decline again. Measurement of serum progesterone levels is the simplest, most common, objective, and reliable test of ovulatory function as long as it is appropriately timed. A serum progesterone concentration of <3 ng/mL implies anovulation, except when drawn immediately after ovulation or just before the onset of menses, when the lower levels might be naturally expected.

Ideally, the serum progesterone levels should be measured approximately 1 week before the expected menses when the serum concentration is at or near its peak. As previously believed, day 21 value is not the best time to measure serum progesterone concentration. The exact time for measurement varies with the overall length of menstrual cycle, aiming for approximately 1 week before the expected menses. If the serum progesterone concentration is <3 ng/mL, the patient must be evaluated for causes of anovulation. Minimum investigations required in these cases include determination of serum levels of prolactin, TSH, FSH, and assessment for PCOS. Presently, there is no consensus on minimum serum progesterone concentration, which defines normal luteal function and documents ovulation. A midluteal serum progesterone level > 10 ng/mL is commonly considered as a standard. A properly timed serum progesterone concentration can be considered as the simplest and most reliable method when the clinician's aim is to confirm ovulatory function in a woman with regular monthly menses.

Ovulation Prediction Kit

An over-the-counter urinary ovulation prediction kit helps in detecting midcycle LH surge in the urine. Therefore, this test is highly effective for calculating the timing of the LH surge that consistently indicates ovulation. LH surge is a brief event and typically lasts between 48 and 50 hours from start to finish. This test is usually positive on a single day and occasionally on 2 consecutive days. To detect the LH surge, testing is done daily, beginning 2–3 days before the day of expected LH surge based on the overall cycle length. Ovulation usually occurs 14–26 hours after detection of LH surge (and indicative color change in the kit) and almost always within 48 hours. Therefore, the interval of greatest fertility includes the day LH surge is detected and the following 2 days.

For accurate prediction of ovulation in couples requiring IUI, LH monitoring appears to be the most appropriate choice. In a few patients where this method fails, serial TVS examination can be used to provide the necessary information.

Ultrasound

Serial ultrasonographic examination can be performed to confirm follicular rupture or ovulation. Ultrasound examination is also helpful in diagnosing PCOS **(Fig. 34.4)**.

Basal Body Temperature

Basal body temperature (BBT) charts can be used for predicting ovulation. In this method, the woman is asked to measure her oral temperature with an oral glass or mercury thermometer, the first thing when she wakes up in the morning or after at least 3 hours of uninterrupted sleep. She should measure her temperature throughout the entire duration of her menstrual cycle for at least three menstrual cycles. The temperatures are then plotted on a graph paper.

Basal body temperature varies between 97.0°F and 98.0°F during the follicular phase of the cycle and rises by 0.4–0.8°F over the average preovulatory temperature during the luteal phase. The thermogenic shift in BBT occurs when serum progesterone levels rise above 5 ng/mL, usually occurring for up to 4 days following ovulation. In a normal ovulating woman, there occurs a rise in body temperature by 0.5–1.0°C immediately following ovulation under the thermogenic effect of progesterone **(Fig. 34.13)**. This increase in temperature remains sustained throughout the luteal phase. The temperature again falls to baseline just before or after the onset of menses. This biphasic pattern is evident in ovulatory women. Besides providing an evidence for ovulation, BBT recording can also help in determining the approximate time of ovulation. BBT recording can also reveal an abnormally long follicular phase or a short luteal phase. Treatment of these may help in improving fertility. Though an easy, noninvasive, and cost-effective procedure, taking the temperature daily can become cumbersome. BBT serves as a useful method for couples who are reluctant or unable to pursue more formal and costly evaluations.

TREATMENT/OBSTETRIC MANAGEMENT

INITIAL MANAGEMENT

A treatment plan should be generated based on the diagnosis established through the findings of laboratory investigations, clinical history and examination, duration of infertility, and the woman's age. General principles for management of infertile couple are described in **Box 34.2**.

TREATMENT OF MALE INFERTILITY

> Q. Discuss in detail the advances done in the management of infertility due to male factors.
>
> Q. Define azoospermia. Discuss in detail its causes and management.
>
> Q. Write a long essay on antisperm antibodies.
>
> Q. Discuss briefly management of oligospermia in cases of infertility.
>
> Q. Write a short essay on oligospermia.

The treatment of male factor infertility has been described in **Flowchart 34.2**. In most cases of male factor infertility due to oligospermia, IUI is the treatment of choice if >2 million sperms are recovered after the sperm wash. Men with hypogonadotropic hypogonadism should be offered treatment with gonadotropin drugs because these are effective in improving fertility. Patients with ejaculatory sexual dysfunction may benefit from a prescription for phosphodiesterase type 5 inhibitors, e.g., sildenafil.

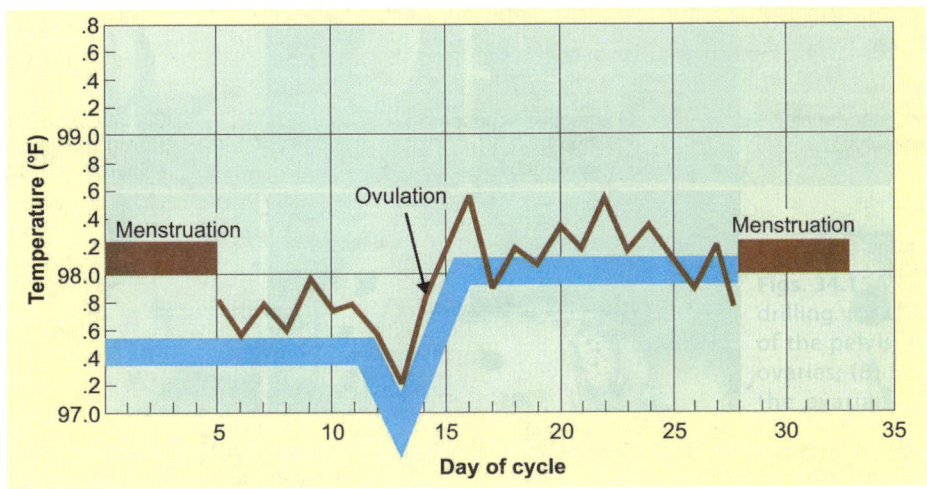

Fig. 34.13: Basal body temperature method.

The use of drugs such as antiestrogens, gonadotropins, androgens, bromocriptine, or kinin-enhancing drugs is not recommended. These have not been shown to be effective in improving male factor infertility. Men with leukocytes in their semen should not be offered antibiotic treatment unless the presence of infection has been confirmed because there is no evidence that the use of antibiotics improves pregnancy rates.

Where appropriate expertise is available, men with obstructive azoospermia should be offered surgical correction of epididymal blockage because it is likely to restore patency of the duct and improve fertility. Other options which can be considered as an alternative to surgery include surgical sperm recovery and IVF. Though men with varicoceles are commonly offered surgery as a form of fertility treatment, this has not been observed to improve the pregnancy rates.

TREATMENT OF CERVICAL FACTORS

Chronic cervicitis may be treated with antibiotics. The easiest and most successful treatment option for infertility related to cervical factors is artificial IUI in conjunction with ovulation-inducing agents. Low-dose estrogen therapy may provide some benefit in cases with reduced secretion of cervical mucus. In case of unsuccessful attempts at IUI, IVF must be used as the next option.

Artificial Intrauterine Insemination

Artificial insemination can be performed by depositing the sperms at the level of internal cervical os (cervical insemination) or inside the endometrial cavity (IUI). Since cervical insemination is associated with low success rates in comparison with IUI, the latter is more commonly used. IUI may be performed either during a natural cycle (unstimulated IUI) or following ovulation induction

> **BOX 34.2:** General principles for management of infertile couple.
> - Involvement of both the partners in evaluation and management of infertility
> - Lifestyle modifications to enhance fertility
> - Couple should be advised to quit smoking and reduce exposure to environmental toxins
> - Woman should be asked to abstain from alcohol, reduce excessive intake of caffeine, and maintain BMI <23 kg/m^2
> - Providing emotional support and taking into consideration the couple's emotional, financial, and social requirements
> - *Counseling the couple regarding the fertile period:* The patient should be explained that normal sperm retains its ability to survive in the female reproductive tract for about 3–5 days, while the oocyte remains viable for about 12–24 hours following ovulation. Therefore, for conception to occur, intercourse must occur while the ovum is still alive, with the highest estimated conception rates associated with intercourse 2 days before ovulation. However, timed intercourse is less likely to result in fertility and is supposed to further increase the patient's anxiety. Therefore, for most couples, the gynecologist must recommend the couple to have intercourse every 2–3 days. This strategy helps in avoiding unnecessary stress and at the same time ensures high fertility rate
> - Evaluation and management of infertility as per the established guidelines
> - *Identification of the likely cause of infertility:*
>   – *Reversible cause:* Medical or surgical therapy to correct the etiology
>   – *Irreversible cause:* Treatment modalities such as assisted reproductive technology, gamete donation, adoption, and gestational carrier

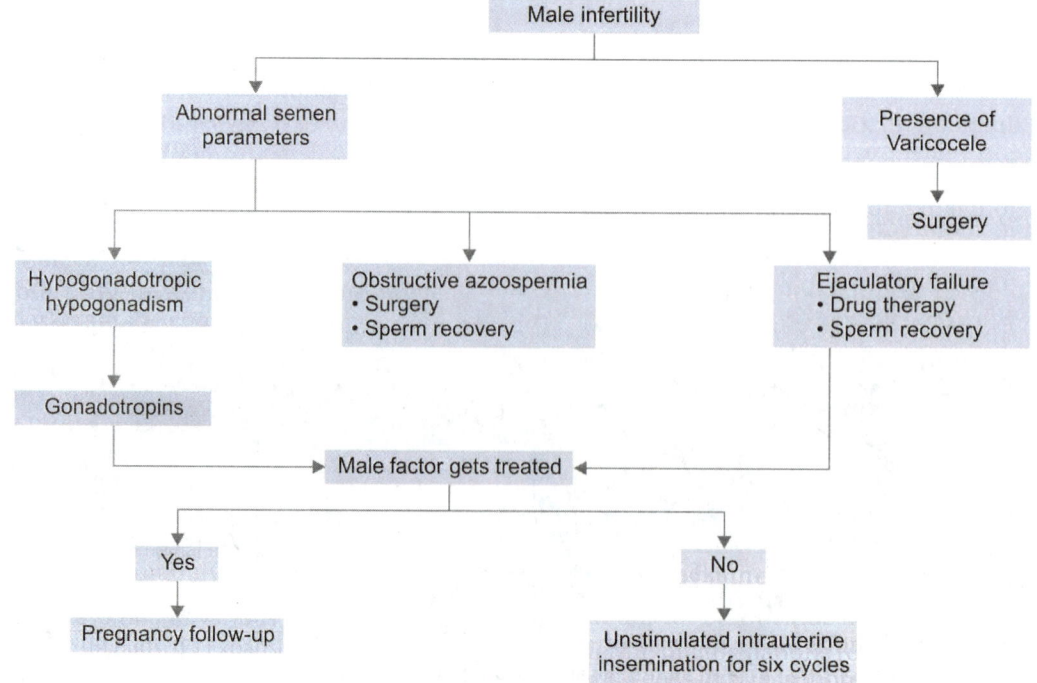

Flowchart 34.2: Treatment of male infertility.

with CC or gonadotropins (stimulated IUI). The average pregnancy rate achieved after a natural cycle IUI is 8%. This rate increases by 5–10% in the stimulated cycles. Of all the successful pregnancies achieved by IUI, 85% are achieved within the first four cycles of IUIs. Artificial insemination can be of two types: (1) homologous and (2) heterologous. While homologous insemination refers to the use of sperm from the patient's partner, heterologous insemination refers to the use of frozen donor sperms that have been quarantined for at least 6 months.

Indications for IUI
Important indications for IUI are enumerated in **Box 34.3**.

Procedure
The procedure is performed 30–34 hours after the spontaneous LH surge or 36 hours after the administration of 10,000 U of hCG.
1. Timing for the procedure is very crucial while dealing with IUI because sperms should be injected at the precise time when ovulation has occurred or is about to occur.
2. *Sperm preparation:* At the time of expected ovulation, a fresh semen sample is collected from the male partner and processed in the lab by washing in a culture medium or using a density gradient column. After sperm preparation, the spermatozoa are enhanced in motility and become activated and ready to fertilize an oocyte.
3. *IUI:* The prepared semen sample is delivered inside the endometrial cavity using an IUI catheter.
4. Following the injection of the sperms, the patient must remain in the recumbent position for at least 10–15 minutes.

TREATMENT OF UTERINE FACTORS
Surgical Intervention
Surgical treatment involves lysis of uterine septae and uterine synechiae, surgical treatment of uterine anomalies (e.g., bicornuate uterus). Uterine synechiae and septae are corrected using operative hysteroscopy. This surgery is performed during the early follicular phase. Once the synechiae/septae have been resected, an intrauterine balloon is left for 7 days inside the uterine cavity to prevent the recurrence of adhesions. Endometrial polyps may also be removed through operative hysteroscopy associated with a dilatation and curettage, if required. Treatment of fibroids may be required if they are associated with abnormal uterine bleeding or if they are thought to be the cause of infertility. Three modalities which are commonly used for treatment of myomas, i.e., medical treatment, surgical treatment (conventional laparotomy, operative laparoscopy, and operative hysteroscopy), and embolization are described in Chapter 24. Women having an irreparable uterine defect may require a gestational carrier (surrogate mother). Treatment of infertility in women with luteal phase defect is best dealt with the help of ovulation-inducing agents rather than with progesterone.

TREATMENT OF TUBAL FACTORS OF INFERTILITY
The treatment of tubal factor infertility has undergone tremendous changes, especially during the last few decades with the widespread use of tubal microsurgery and ARTs.

Microsurgery
Tubal obstruction due to elective sterilization is usually repaired using microsurgical technique **(Figs. 34.14A to F)**. Before undertaking microsurgery, it is important to determine the type of tubal ligation technique that had been employed in that particular case. This knowledge helps the clinician in predicting the success rate for surgery. For example, tubal cauterization results in the destruction of a large amount of tissue; so tubal reanastomosis, if performed in the remnant part of fallopian tube, may not prove to be successful.

Before undertaking reanastomosis, the lengths of proximal and distal fragments of the fallopian tubes from the point of tubal ligation need to be determined. In order to achieve a successful reanastomosis, the final tube length should measure at least 4.5 cm. If fimbriectomy had been performed previously, no treatment option is available other than IVF. The best candidates for tubal reanastomosis are patients who had undergone tubal ligation by the method of Falope ring, Filshie clip, or Pomeroy's technique. The pregnancy rate following a tubal reanastomosis performed by surgeons skilled in microsurgery varies from 70% to 80%. However, the procedure is also associated with an ectopic pregnancy rate varying between 7% and 10%.

Laparoscopy
Nowadays, laparoscopic surgical approach is widely being used for the treatment of multiple tuboperitoneal pathologies, using techniques such as electrocautery, endocoagulation, lasers, and ultrasonography.

Laparoscopy for lysis of adhesions may be indicated in patients with severe pelvic adhesions that compromise the bowel, ovaries, and tubes along with the obliteration of the cul-de-sac. Lysis of adhesions should be meticulous, using hydrodissection and fine instruments. Blunt dissection

---

BOX 34.3: Indications for intrauterine insemination.
- Unexplained infertility
- Cervical factor infertility
- Failure to conceive after ovulation induction treatment
- Immunological causes (antisperm antibodies)
- Couples with minimal-to-mild endometriosis
- Mild–moderate male factor infertility and other causes of male infertility such as ejaculatory failure and retrograde ejaculation

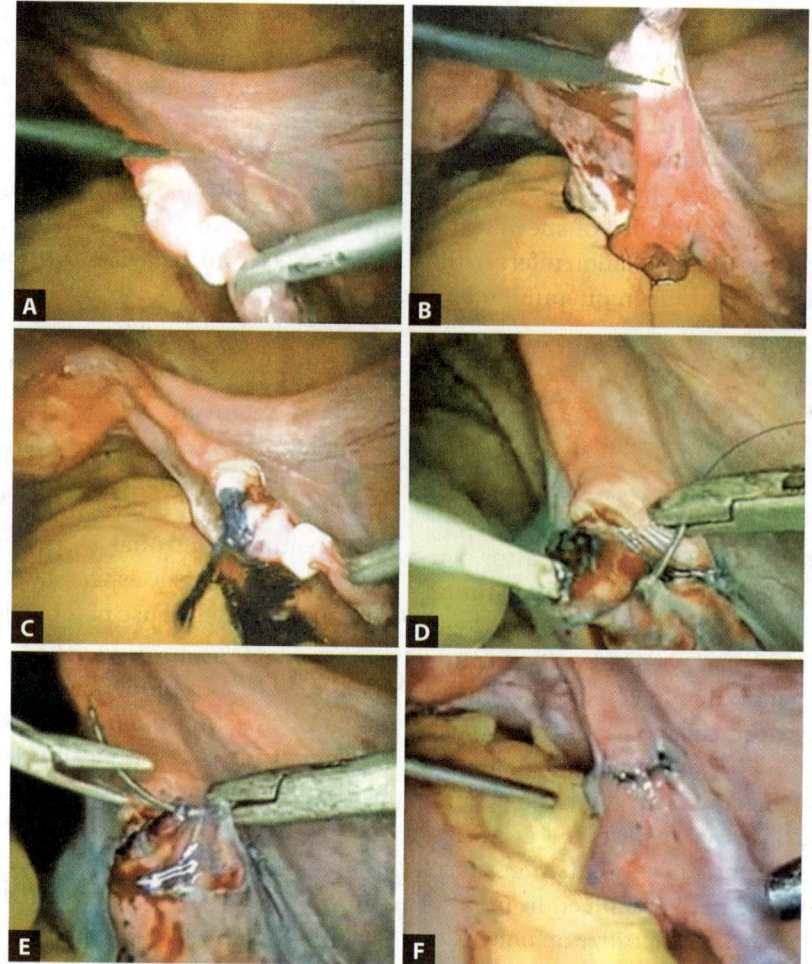

Figs. 34.14A to F: Steps of tubotubal anastomosis. (A) Grasping the portion of the tube in which tubal ligation had been performed; (B) Transecting the blocked portion of the tube; (C) Chromopertubation performed to check the patency of the proximal segment; (D) Stitching the cut segments; (E) Stitching the cut at the ends of the tube; (F) Appearance of tube following the completion of recanalization procedure.

should be avoided. Constant irrigation with Ringer's lactate solution and heparin prevents fibrin formation.

Meticulous hemostasis must be maintained at all times. Fimbrial phimosis and periadnexal disease can also be treated by fimbrioplasty using laparoscopy.

Treatment of hydrosalpinx (distal tubal obstruction) with salpingostomy can be performed through microsurgery or operative laparoscopy. The success of either procedure is related to the diameter of the hydrosalpinx and damage to the ciliated epithelium. If the ciliated epithelium has been destroyed, the outcome of the procedure is poor. In these cases, it is better to perform a salpingectomy in preparation for future IVF. Treatment of tubal factor infertility has been described in **Flowchart 34.3**. Various surgical procedures for improving tubal patency are listed in **Table 34.8**. Since reconstructive surgery for proximal tubal occlusion is not always successful, IVF appears to be the preferable option. IVF is a proven method of treatment of tubal factor infertility and has the following advantages and disadvantages **(Table 34.9)** in comparison with tubal reconstruction.

TREATMENT OF OVARIAN FACTORS

> Q. A 25-year-old nulliparous woman has presented with oligomenorrhea and infertility. Discuss in detail the investigations and management to be done in this case.
>
> Q. Write a long essay discussing the diagnosis, problem, and management of anovulation.

In case of patients with ovulatory dysfunction, the most appropriate treatment option is to begin with ovulation-inducing drugs. The treatment can be begun immediately before other potential causes of infertility have been investigated. Women with ovulatory disorders due to hyperprolactinemia should be offered treatment with dopamine agonists such as bromocriptine. In cases where anovulation is the only obstacle to be overcome, most couples would conceive promptly on using ovulation induction agents. In these cases, the various ovulation induction agents which can be used include CC, letrozole, human menopausal gonadotropin (hMG), hCG, recombinant FSH, and recombinant LH.

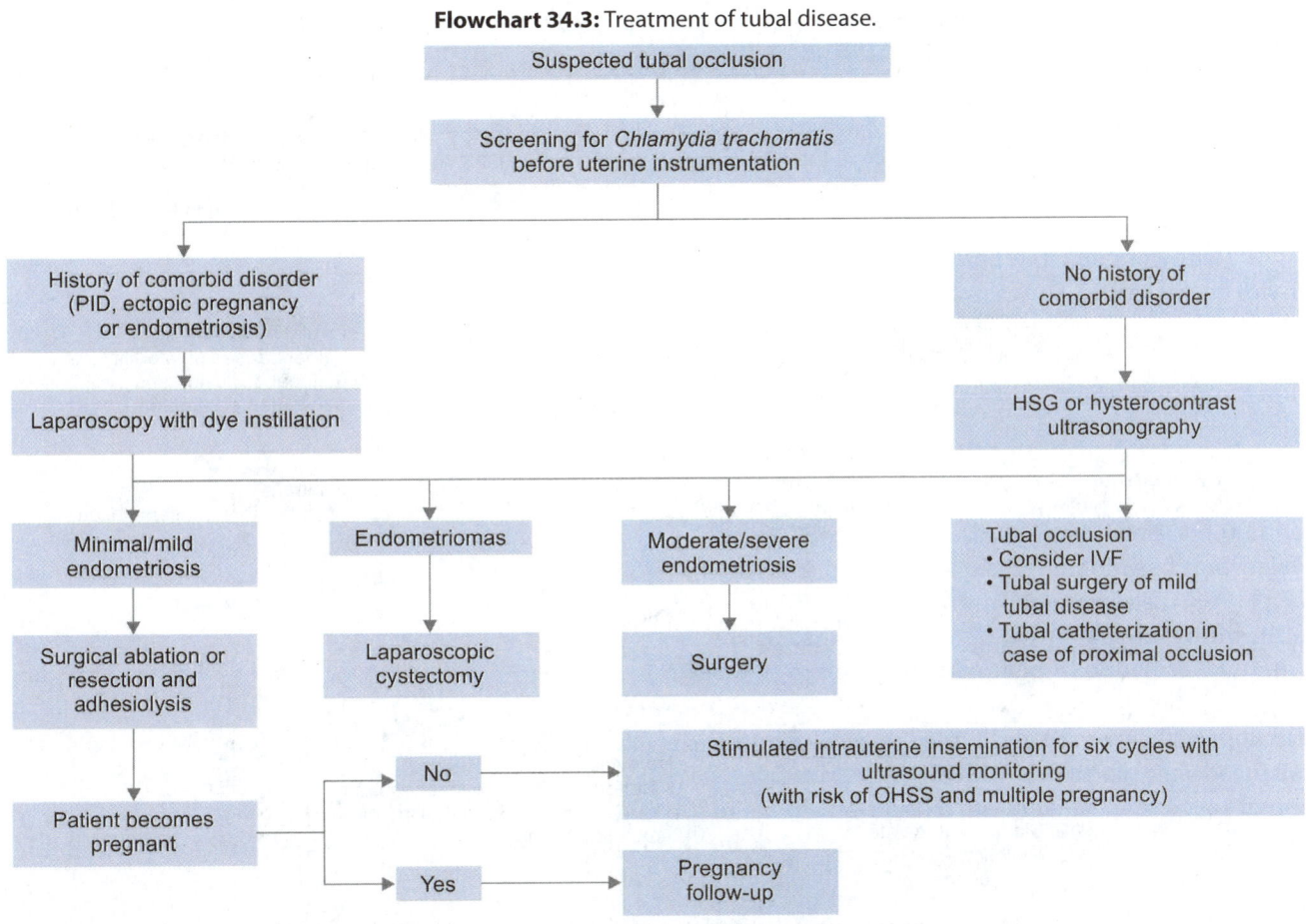

Flowchart 34.3: Treatment of tubal disease.

(HSG: hysterosalpingogram; OHSS: ovarian hyperstimulation syndrome)

TABLE 34.8: Surgical procedures for improving tubal patency.	
Type of tubal pathology	Surgical procedure
Distal obstruction	• *Fimbrioplasty:* The lysis of fimbrial adhesions or dilatation of fimbrial strictures • *Neosalpingostomy:* Creation of a new tubal opening in a distally occluded tube
Proximal obstruction	• Hysteroscopic or fluoroscopic tubal catheterization • Tubocornual anastomosis by laparotomy

TABLE 34.9: Characteristic features of IVF as a treatment option for tubal factor infertility.	
Advantages	Disadvantages
• Good success rate per cycle (about 30%) • Less invasive than tubal surgery • Can help overcome other factors of subfertility, if present (e.g., male factor, cervical factor, and reduced ovarian reserve) • Site and extent of tubal damage are not vital for the end result	• High cost per cycle and possible requirement for multiple cycles • Necessity for IVF each time a pregnancy is desired • Frequent injections of ovulation-inducing agents and monitoring is essential • High risk of complications such as multiple gestation, ovarian hyperstimulation syndrome, and slightly higher absolute risk of some adverse perinatal outcomes

Treatment of infertility due to ovarian factors has been described in **Flowchart 34.4**.

Clomiphene Citrate

> Q. Write a short essay on clomiphene citrate.

Clomiphene citrate is a nonsteroidal selective estrogen receptor modulator (SERM) with both estrogen antagonist and agonist effects. It is largely believed to exert its antiestrogen effect by competing with estrogen receptors at the level of hypothalamus, pituitary, and ovaries. By blocking the estrogen receptors within the hypothalamus, CC alleviates the negative feedback effect exerted by endogenous estrogens. As a result, the GnRH release gets normalized. Therefore, the secretion of FSH and LH is able to reestablish the normal process of ovulation and is capable of normalizing follicular recruitment, selection,

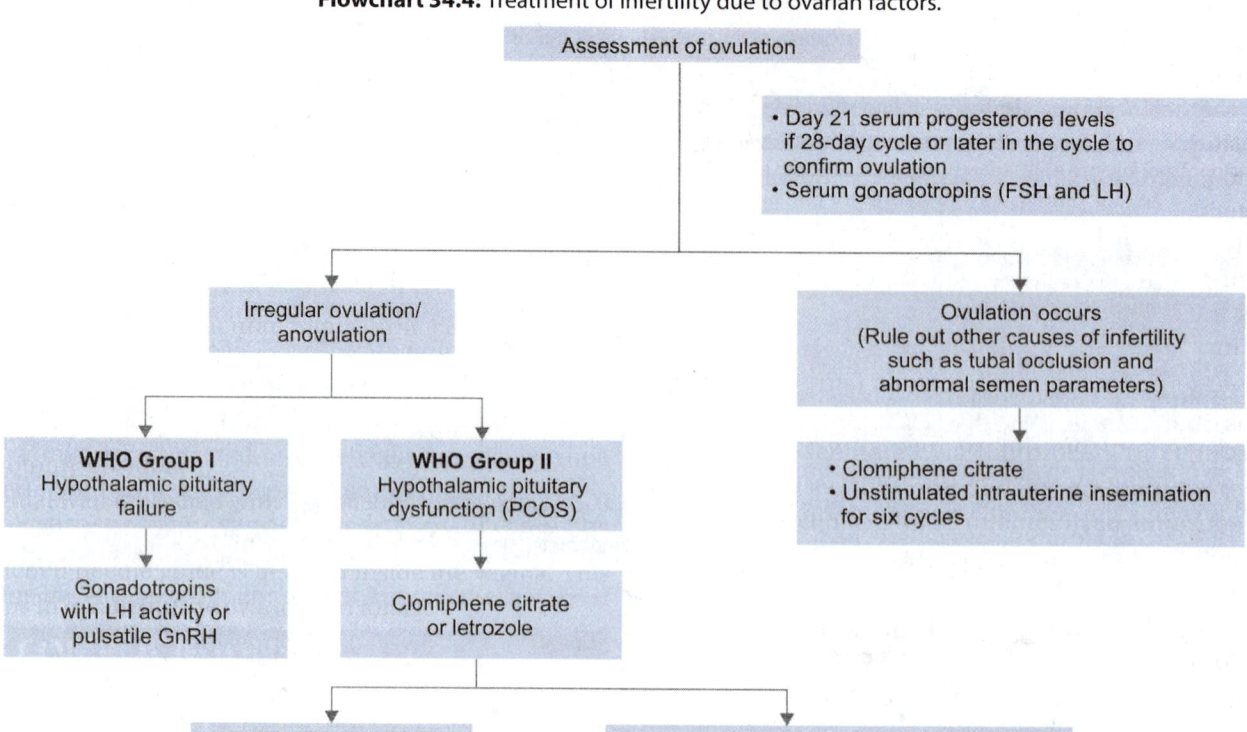

Flowchart 34.4: Treatment of infertility due to ovarian factors.

(hMG: human menopausal gonadotropin; FSH: follicle stimulating hormone; rFSH: recombinant FSH; uFSH: urinary FSH; LH: luteinizing hormone; PCOS: polycystic ovarian syndrome)

and development. CC can also be prescribed to women with unexplained fertility problems.

The standard dose of CC is 50 mg PO once a day for 5 days, starting on the day 3–5 of the menstrual cycle or after progestin-induced bleeding. Response to CC is monitored using pelvic ultrasonography, starting on day 12 of the menstrual cycle. The follicle should develop to a diameter of 23–24 mm before a spontaneous LH surge occurs.

However, women who are being prescribed CC should be informed that this drug may be associated with the risk of multiple pregnancies. Women undergoing treatment with CC should be offered ultrasound monitoring during at least the first cycle of treatment to ensure that they receive a dose that minimizes the risk of multiple pregnancy. Another important adverse effect associated with the use of this drug is the thickening of the cervical mucus under the antiestrogenic effect of CC. This may create an iatrogenic cervical factor, which may be responsible for producing infertility in a patient who has otherwise ovulated. Other adverse effects which may be rarely associated with CC include hot flashes, scotomas, dryness of the vagina, headache, and ovarian hyperstimulation. The use of CC is contraindicated in cases of ovarian cyst, pregnancy, and liver disease. Its use is also controversial in patients with a history of breast cancer. Anovulatory women with PCOS, having a BMI of >25 who have not responded to CC alone, should be offered metformin in combination with CC. Women who are prescribed metformin should be informed about the side effects, such as nausea, vomiting, and other gastrointestinal disturbances, associated with its use. Clomiphene resistance is defined where there is no conception even after three cycles of ovulation induction with CC. On the other hand, clomiphene failure is defined when there is no conception even after six cycles of ovulation induction with CC.

Letrozole

Aromatase inhibitors such as letrozole are commonly used nowadays for induction of ovulation. More about letrozole has been described later in the text.

Human Menopausal Gonadotropins

Human menopausal gonadotropin and its derivatives are indicated for ovulation induction in patients with primary amenorrhea and/or infertility, who did not respond to ovulation induction with CC. hMG (Menopur®) contains 75 U of FSH and 75 U of LH per mL, although the concentration may vary in the range of 60–90 U for FSH and for LH in the range of 60–120 U. The new generations of available gonadotropins are produced by genetically engineered mammalian cells, i.e., Chinese hamster ovary cells.

Multiple adverse effects and complications that may occur following the use of the gonadotropins include multiple pregnancy, ectopic pregnancy, miscarriages, ovarian torsion, and rupture and OHSS. Due to the risk of various side effects, especially OHSS, the administration of hMG and its derivatives should be directly supervised by a reproductive endocrinologist under ultrasound guidance and daily determinations of estradiol, FSH, and LH levels. Cutoff of follicular size and endometrial thickness for marking the follicular and endometrial maturity is 17 mm and 7 mm, respectively.

In case the above therapies do not work, some modified regimens can be employed:

- *High-dose extended CC regimen:* Dosage of CC can be increased to a maximum of 200–250 mg/day in case there is no response to a standard dose. This regimen of clomiphene may be employed for women who cannot receive exogenous gonadotropins.
- *Ovulation trigger:* Despite clomiphene-induced follicular development, sometimes absent or inadequate midcycle surge of LH may result in the failure of ovulation. In this situation, single-dose IM injection of exogenous hCG (5,000–10,000 IU) can be used for triggering ovulation when the ovarian follicles have attained maturity (size of leading follicle 18–20 mm on TVS). The clinician must note that premature administration of hCG acts like a premature LH surge and may result in follicular atresia. Ovulation occurs approximately 36–44 hours after the hCG injection.

Administration of hCG may sometimes be associated with the risk of OHSS. In case of a presence of up to two follicles having the size of 17 mm, hCG can be administered. The risk of OHSS increases with the presence of multiple intermediate cycles. In case OHSS is suspected, it is preferable to administer decapeptide or gonadotropins (e.g., leuprolide) over hCG. Though there is an initial flare response with the administration of gonadotropins, this is later followed by a sustained release of FSH and LH, thereby reducing the chances of OHSS.

Gonadotropin-Releasing Hormone

Synthetic GnRH (e.g., gonadorelin) has a chemical composition similar to native GnRH and is indicated for patients with hypothalamic dysfunction, especially those who do not respond to CC. This drug is administered in a pulsatile fashion every 60–120 minutes, intravenously or subcutaneously, using a delivery pump in the starting dose of 5 µg/pulse intravenously or 5–25 µg subcutaneously. The administration of GnRH should be extended throughout the luteal phase, or this should be supplemented with the administration of exogenous hCG. Intensive monitoring of folliculogenesis is not required in these patients due to low risk of ovarian hyperstimulation.

Laparoscopic Ovarian Drilling

Being an invasive procedure, laparoscopic ovarian drilling (LOD) must be done as a last resort when the medical methods fail to achieve pregnancy. The procedure must be done carefully because it can reduce the ovarian component. This can also interfere with ovarian function by hampering the blood flow.

TREATMENT OF POLYCYSTIC OVARIAN SYNDROME

Algorithm for treatment of patients with PCOS is described in **Flowchart 34.5**. Some commonly used treatment options for PCOS include ovulation-inducing medicines such as letrozole, CC, insulin-sensitizing agents (such as Glucophage and metformin), dietary changes (low glycemic diet), and surgery (ovarian drilling). The primary first-line treatment strategy for PCOS is weight loss with the help of lifestyle modifications such as diet and exercise. Modest weight loss helps in lowering the androgen levels, improving hirsutism, normalizing menstrual cycles, resuming ovulation, and reducing insulin resistance. However, it may take months before these results become apparent. Besides facilitating fertility, the aims of treatment in women with PCOS are to control hirsutism, prevent endometrial hyperplasia from unopposed acyclic estrogen secretion, and prevent the long-term consequences of insulin resistance. The treatment must be individualized according to the needs and desires of each patient. The use of OCPs or cyclic progestational agents can help maintain a normal endometrium and also reduce the increased risk of endometrial hyperplasia and carcinoma.

For the woman with PCOS who wants to conceive, previously CC was used as the first-line therapy for ovulation induction because of its high success rate and relative simplicity and inexpensiveness. However, CC has a longer half-life due to which some women may experience an increased risk of complications such as multiple gestation and OHSS. Also, some women may not ovulate with CC. Therefore, in the present times, letrozole has been recommended as the first-line therapy for ovulation induction in women with PCOS. Other possible therapeutic approaches for ovulation induction include the use of insulin-sensitizing agents, gonadotropins (perhaps preceded by GnRH analogs), FSH alone, pulsatile GnRH, etc. Algorithm for treatment of patients with PCOS suffering from hirsutism is described in **Flowchart 34.6**.

Clomiphene Citrate

Clomiphene citrate has been described previously in the text.

Gonadotropins

Women with PCOS having BMI within normal range, who have not responded to CC, can be treated with

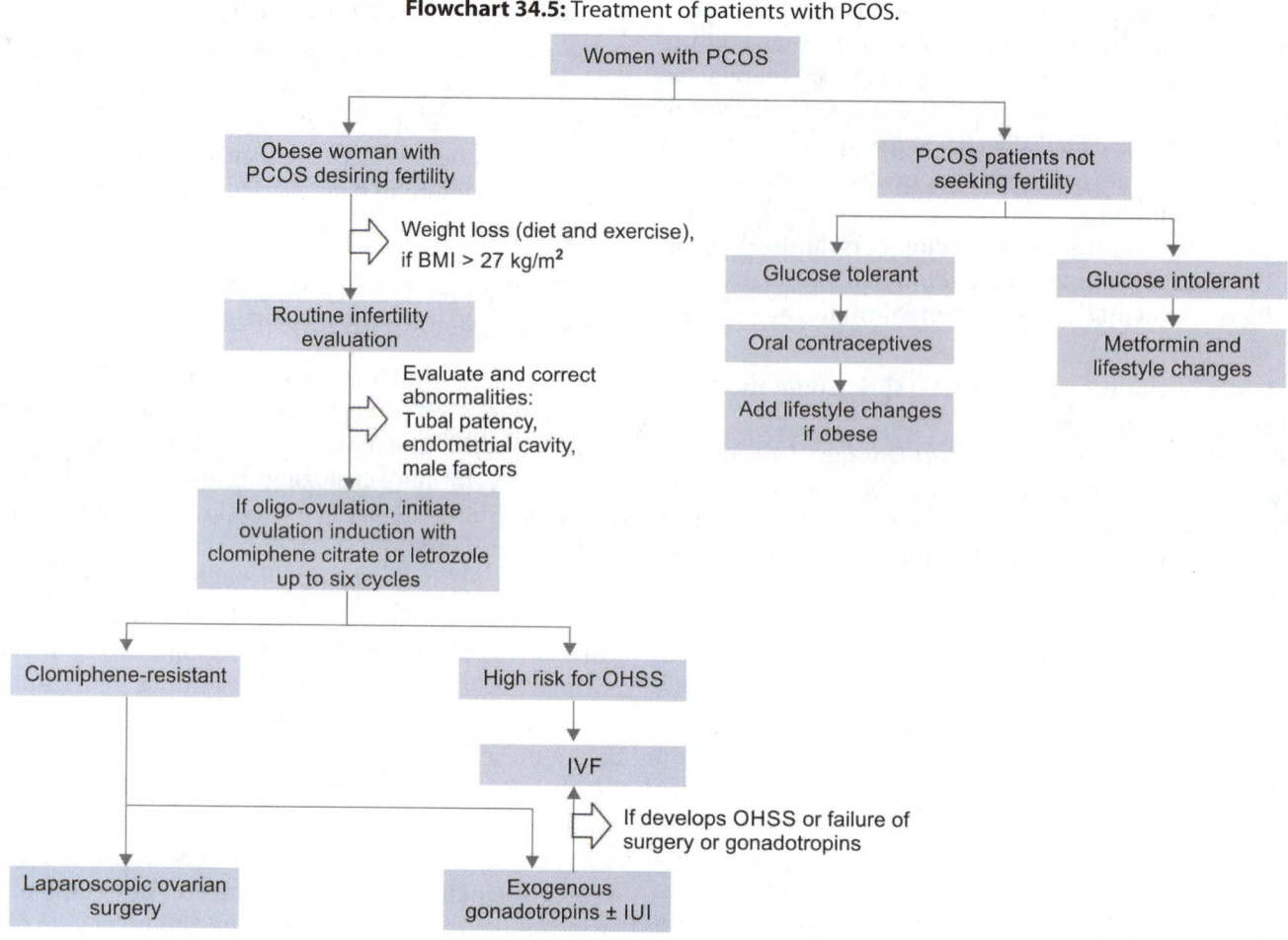

Flowchart 34.5: Treatment of patients with PCOS.

(IUI: intrauterine insemination; OHSS: ovarian hyperstimulation syndrome; PCOS: polycystic ovarian syndrome)

gonadotropins. hMG, urinary FSH, and recombinant FSH are equally effective in achieving pregnancy.

Laparoscopic Ovarian Drilling

Women with PCOS who have not responded to CC should be offered LOD because it is as effective as gonadotropin treatment and is not associated with an increased risk of multiple pregnancy. This procedure involves creation of approximately 4–20 holes, having a size of 3 mm diameter and 3 mm depth to be made in each ovary, preferably on the antimesenteric side **(Figs. 34.15A to D)**. Women who are unable to conceive naturally following the previously mentioned therapeutic options often respond to ARTs, including IVF.

Tamoxifen

Tamoxifen citrate is a SERM, which is extensively used for the secondary chemoprevention of hormone-responsive breast cancer. It is now also being used for ovulation induction in PCOS. Tamoxifen has lower antiestrogenic effects on the endometrium and cervix in comparison to clomiphene.

Aromatase Inhibitors

Aromatase inhibitors, such as letrozole and anastrozole, inhibit the action of the enzyme aromatase, which is responsible for the process of aromatization (conversion of androgens into estrogens). As a result, estrogen levels are dramatically reduced, releasing the hypothalamic–pituitary axis from its negative feedback. As per the new ESHRE guidelines (2018), letrozole, a third-generation aromatase inhibitor, is considered as the first-line pharmacological therapy for PCOS patients who want to conceive. Nowadays, letrozole is preferred over anastrozole for ovulation induction because letrozole has been more extensively studied and appears to be more effective. Also, it is preferred over CC because of the reasons mentioned in **Box 34.4**.

Dosage: Letrozole is administered in the dosage of 2.5 mg/day starting on day 2 or 3 for a 5-day period, following a spontaneous menses or progestin-induced bleed. This dosage can be increased to 5 mg/day, in case there is no response to 2.5 mg dose, with a maximal dose of 7.5 mg/day. In case of no response to the maximal dose, sequential dose escalation using a step-up or the step-stair protocol of letrozole can be tried; it comprises the following dosage:

- *Day 1:* 2.5 mg (one 2.5 mg tablet)
- *Day 2:* 5 mg (two 2.5 mg tablets)
- *Day 3:* 7.5 mg (three 2.5 mg tablets)
- *Day 4:* 10 mg (four 2.5 mg tablets)
- *Day 5:* 12.5 mg (five 2.5 mg tablets)

Started on days 3–7 of the menstrual cycle

Flowchart 34.6: Management of hirsutism.

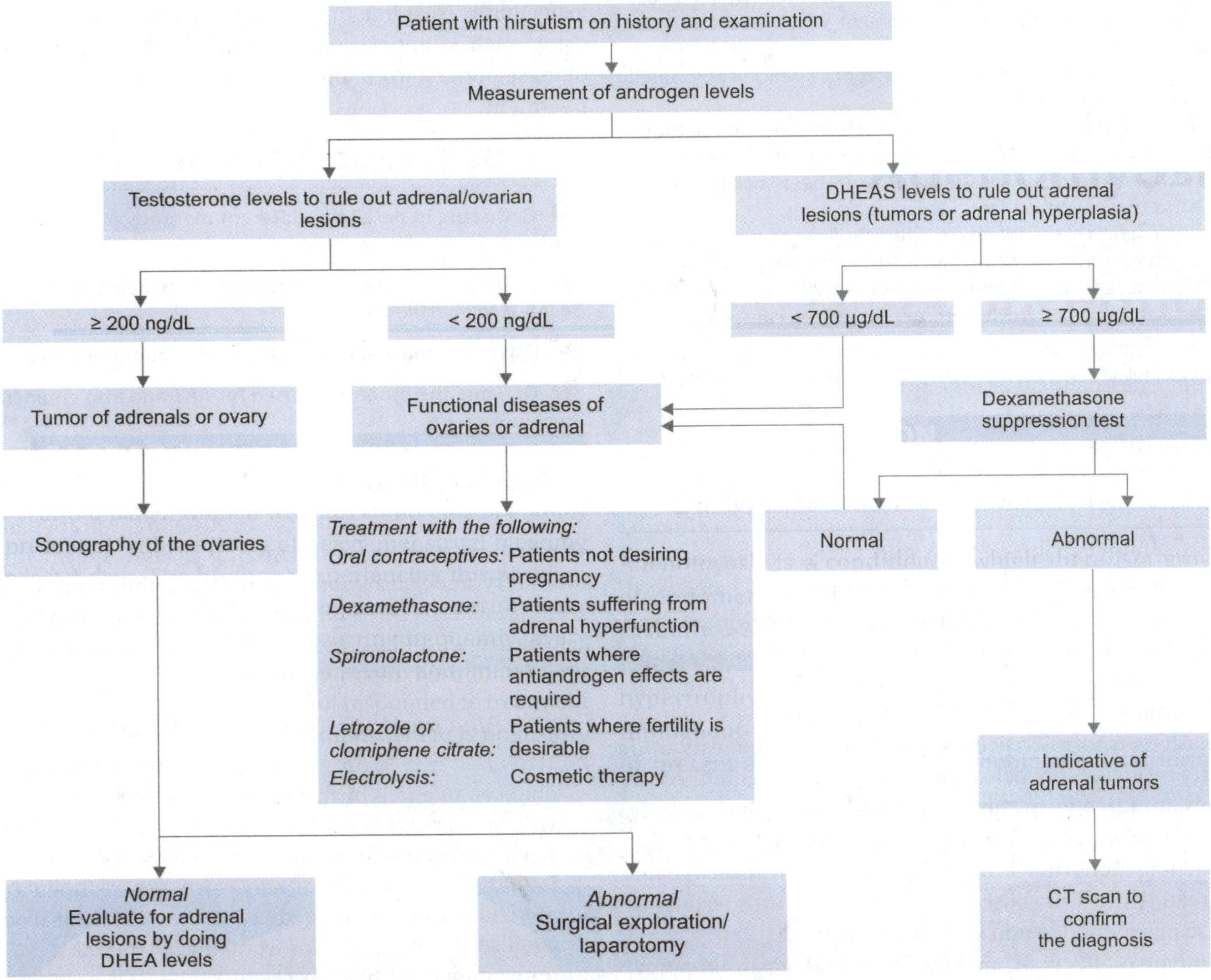

```
Patient with hirsutism on history and examination
                        │
                        ▼
            Measurement of androgen levels
                   /              \
                  /                \
Testosterone levels to rule          DHEAS levels to rule out adrenal
out adrenal/ovarian lesions          lesions (tumors or adrenal hyperplasia)
      /        \                          /              \
 ≥ 200 ng/dL   < 200 ng/dL            < 700 μg/dL      ≥ 700 μg/dL
     │              │                      │                │
 Tumor of      Functional diseases of                  Dexamethasone
 adrenals      ovaries or adrenal                      suppression test
 or ovary                                                /        \
     │                                                Normal    Abnormal
 Sonography                                                        │
 of the ovaries                                              Indicative of
                                                             adrenal tumors
                                                                   │
                                                             CT scan to
                                                             confirm
                                                             the diagnosis
```

Treatment with the following:
- **Oral contraceptives:** Patients not desiring pregnancy
- **Dexamethasone:** Patients suffering from adrenal hyperfunction
- **Spironolactone:** Patients where antiandrogen effects are required
- **Letrozole or clomiphene citrate:** Patients where fertility is desirable
- **Electrolysis:** Cosmetic therapy

Normal — Evaluate for adrenal lesions by doing DHEA levels

Abnormal — Surgical exploration/laparotomy

(DHEA: dehydroepiandrosterone; DHEAS: dehydroepiandrosterone sulfate)

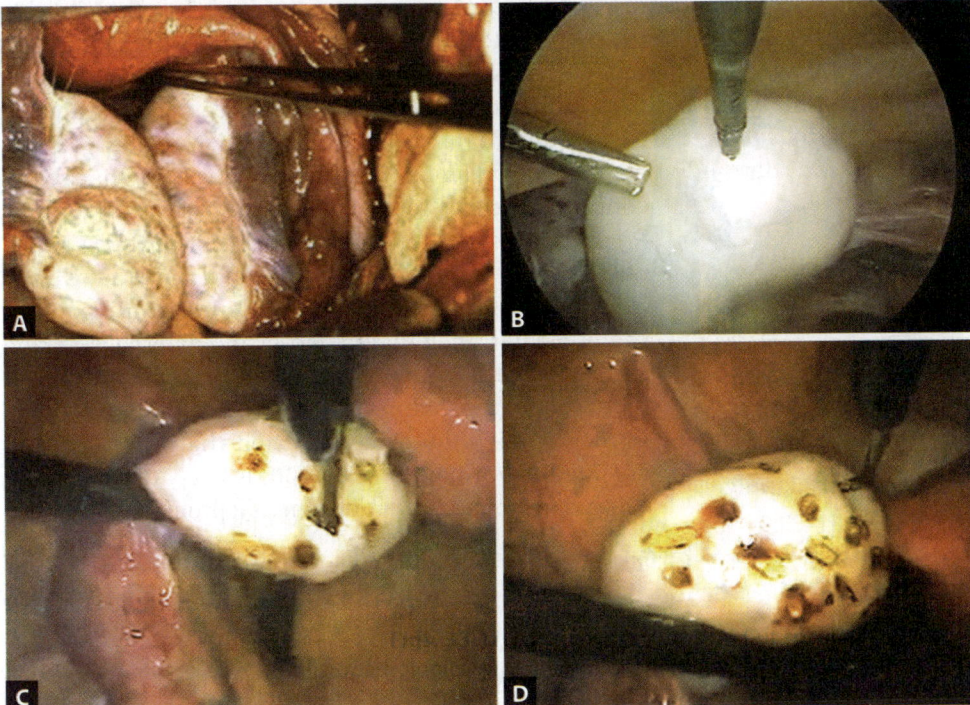

Figs. 34.15A to D: Laparoscopic ovarian drilling. (A) Laparoscopic visualization of the pelvis in an effort to locate the ovaries; (B) Lifting the ovaries out of the ovarian fossa and placing them over the cervicouterine junction; (C) The procedure of laparoscopic ovarian drilling using electrocauterization; (D) Appearance of the ovary following the procedure.

BOX 34.4: Advantages of letrozole over CC.

- High rate of monofollicular development, which reduces the risk of multiple pregnancies
- Shorter half-life (48 hours vs. 2 weeks for CC), which is associated with a lower risk of OHSS
- No direct antiestrogenic adverse effects on the endometrium, due to the absence of peripheral estrogen receptor blockade and the shorter half-life. This is likely to be associated with a reduced risk of miscarriage
- Lower serum estradiol levels, which is likely to be a probable advantage for women with endometriosis undergoing IVF
- Outcomes of live birth rates in oligoovulatory women with PCOS are likely to be better with letrozole (as per the latest data)

(CC: clomiphene citrate; IVF: in vitro fertilization; OHSS: ovarian hyperstimulation syndrome; PCOS: polycystic ovarian syndrome)

Metformin

> Q. Discuss briefly the use of metformin in gynecology.

Patients with PCOS, having a BMI >25 are often resistant to treatment with CC alone. These patients commonly have other problems, such as hyperinsulinism and hyperandrogenism, associated with acanthosis nigricans. This group is amenable to metformin treatment in combination with CC. Metformin improves insulin sensitivity and decreases hepatic gluconeogenesis and, therefore, reduces hyperinsulinism, basal and stimulated LH levels, and free testosterone concentration. Consequently, the patient with PCOS becomes responsive to CC ovulation induction. Metformin is used as an insulin sensitizer. It helps in treating the root cause of PCOS and improves fertility by rectifying endocrine and metabolic functions.

Adverse effects of metformin include gastrointestinal intolerance, nausea, vomiting, and abdominal cramps. Weight loss has also been observed. The initial dose is 500 mg PO once a day for 7 days, then 500 mg BID for another 7 days, and finally 500 mg TID. Since patients can ovulate while on metformin treatment, pelvic ultrasonography is required for documentation of ovulation. In case ovulation does not occur, CC is started at the initial dose of 50 mg/day for 5 days.

TREATMENT OF ENDOMETRIOSIS

Treatment of subfertility in women with endometriosis involves stepwise application of various therapies:
- Surgical resection of endometriosis
- Ovulation induction (first with CC and if unsuccessful, gonadotropins) plus IUI
- ARTs (IVF)

For details regarding treatment of endometriosis, kindly refer to chapter 30.

TREATMENT OF UNEXPLAINED INFERTILITY

> Q. Write a long essay discussing unexplained infertility.

Initially, couples with unexplained infertility are managed expectantly. Next line of management comprises the use of drugs such as antiestrogens (usually CC) and IUI. If none of these options work, the final stage of management is IVF treatment.

ASSISTED REPRODUCTIVE TECHNIQUES

> Q. Discuss in detail the different methods of ART and the patient selection for each method.
>
> Q. Discuss in detail the recent advancements in the treatment of an infertile couple.
>
> Q. Write a long essay discussing the outcomes of ARTs.
>
> Q. Name the procedures used for ART and also enumerate their indications.

In Vitro Fertilization

In vitro fertilization consists of retrieving a preovulatory oocyte from the ovary, fertilizing it with sperm in the laboratory, and subsequently transferring the embryo within the endometrial cavity. With increasing developments in the field of science and technology, IVF is now being recognized as an established treatment for infertility.

Factors Affecting the Outcome of IVF Treatment

- *Woman's age:* Women should be informed that the chances of a live birth following IVF treatment reduce with an increase in the woman's age and that the optimal female age range for achieving a successful IVF treatment is 23–39 years. Chances of a live birth per treatment cycle are >20% for women aged 23–35 years, 15% for women aged 36–38 years, 10% for women aged 39 years, and 6% for women aged 40 years or older.
- *Number of embryos to be transferred:* The more the number of embryos transferred, greater would be the chances of success. However, in order to reduce the chances of multifetal gestation, number of embryos transferred has been limited to two at most of the IVF centers. The present trend is toward transferring a single high-quality embryo.
- *Number of previous treatment cycles:* The chances of conception greatly reduce after three cycles of IVF.
- *Pregnancy history:* Treatment is more effective in women who have previously been pregnant and/or had a live birth.
- *Alcohol, smoking, and caffeine consumption:* Couples should be informed that maternal and paternal smoking can adversely affect the success rates of assisted reproduction procedures, including IVF treatment.
- *BMI:* Women should be informed that a female BMI outside the normal range (19–30) is likely to reduce the success rate of assisted reproduction procedures.

Indications

Indications for IVF include the following:
- Uterine malformations (e.g., unicornuate uterus)
- Damage/absence of fallopian tubes

Infertility

- Severe pelvic adhesions
- Severe endometriosis, which is unresponsive to medical or surgical treatment
- Severe oligospermia or a history of obstructive azoospermia in the male partner
- Premature ovarian failure
- Gonadal dysgenesis including Turner's syndrome
- Bilateral oophorectomy
- Ovarian failure following chemotherapy or radiotherapy.

Procedure

In vitro fertilization consists of retrieving preovulatory oocytes from the ovary and fertilizing them with sperms in the laboratory, with subsequent embryo transfer within the endometrial cavity. The procedure of IVF comprises the following steps **(Figs. 34.16A to G)**, which are subsequently discussed in detail:

1. Pretreatment adjuvant strategies
2. Pituitary downregulation

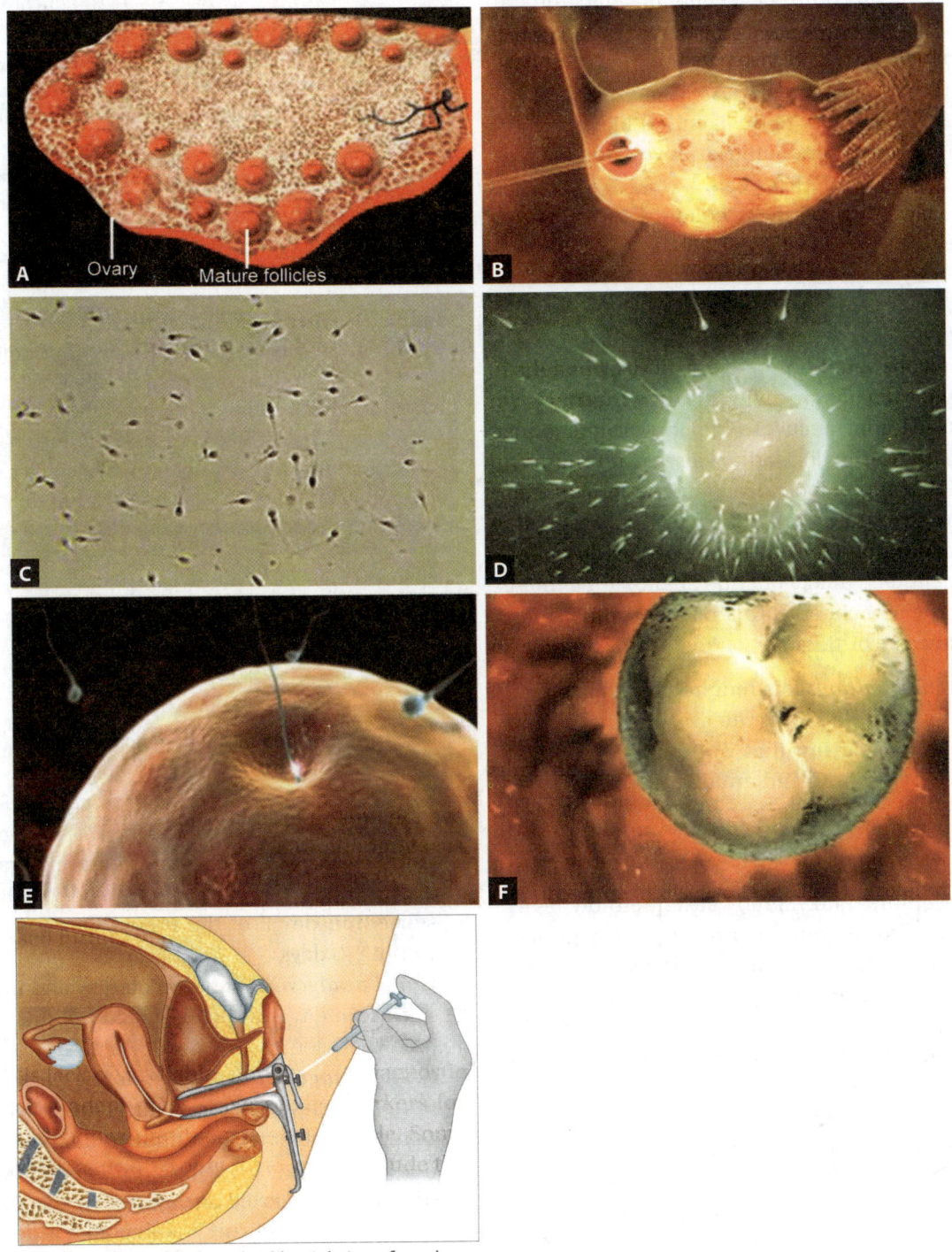

Figs. 34.16A to G: Process of IVF. (A) Follicular stimulation; (B) Follicular aspiration; (C) Sperm concentrate; (D) Oocyte insemination with multiple sperms; (E) Fertilization of the ovum with a single sperm; (F) Embryo culture; (G) Transfer of embryo inside the uterine cavity.

3. Controlled ovarian hyperstimulation
4. Final follicular maturation trigger
5. Oocyte and sperm retrieval
6. Oocyte classification
7. Sperm preparation and oocyte insemination
8. Embryology process [IVF or intracytoplasmic sperm injection (ICSI)]
9. Intrauterine embryo transfer
10. Luteal phase support.

1. *Pretreatment adjuvant strategies:* These may include the following:
   - *Hormonal pretreatment:* These may include the use of various hormonal agents such as OCPs, progestogen, and estrogen. The use of these agents is likely to help in follicular priming, endometrial development, and facilitating the timing of ART cycles.
   - *Surgical treatment of pelvic pathology:* Certain pelvic pathologies may require treatment because if left untreated they may negatively impact fertility and the success rate of ART. This would include surgical interventions such as salpingectomy in cases of hydrosalpinx, hysteroscopic septoplasty for uterine septum, myomectomy for cavity-distorting intramural fibroids >50 mm, polypectomy for polyps, adhesiolysis for intrauterine adhesions, laparoscopic treatment for superficial endometriosis, surgery if size of endometrioma >40 mm, and surgery for symptom relief in cases of deep infiltrating endometriosis.
   - *Other interventions:* Intake of antioxidant supplements are likely to be associated with a better rate of clinical pregnancy and live birth rate.

2. *Pituitary downregulation:* It is required for suppressing the endogenous gonadotropin release and premature ovulation, thereby ensuring that oocytes are available for retrieval. GnRH agonists and antagonists can be used for downregulation. Administration of GnRH agonists is associated with an initial flare-up response due to the stimulation of endogenous gonadotropins, resulting in depletion of receptors, and thereby sustained low levels of gonadotropins. On the other hand, GnRH antagonists directly inhibit the release of gonadotropins by binding competitively with the pituitary GnRH receptors. This is known as chemical hypophysectomy. Various GnRH agonists and antagonist preparations available are tabulated in **Table 34.10**.

Various protocols for pituitary downregulation are listed in **Box 34.5 and Figure 34.17**. These protocols are described next in detail.
   - *GnRH agonist long protocol:* GnRH agonists are administered starting either from the midluteal phase of the previous cycle (long luteal protocol) or the first day of cycle for approximately 14 days (long follicular protocol) before ovarian stimulation and until the administration of hCG.

TABLE 34.10: Various GnRH analogues.

GnRH analogue	Route of administration	Dosage
GnRH agonists		
Buserelin	Nasal spray	*150 µg/metered spray:* One nasal spray four times a day
Nafarelin	Nasal spray	*200 µg/metered spray:* One spray in each nostril
Goserelin	Injection	3.6 mg in a syringe applicator to be administered SC every 28 days
Leuprorelin	Injection	3.75 mg/vial or prefilled syringe to be administered SC or IM once every 28 days
Triptorelin	Injection	3 mg/vial (with dilutant) to be administered IM once every 28 days or 3.75 mg prefilled syringe to be administered IM or SC once every 28 days
GnRH antagonists		
Cetrorelix	Injection	250 µg vial (with solvent) to be administered in the dose of 250 µg IM/day
Ganirelix	Injection	500 µg/mL, 0.5 mL prefilled syringe, 250 µg/day

BOX 34.5: Various protocols for pituitary downregulation.
- GnRH agonist long protocol
- GnRH agonist short (flare) protocol
- GnRH agonist ultrashort protocol
- GnRH antagonist fixed protocol
- GnRH antagonist flexible protocol
- GnRH antagonist single bolus protocol

(GnRH: gonadotropin-releasing hormone)

   - *GnRH agonist short/flare protocol:* GnRH agonist is started in the early follicular phase of the cycle and continued until the time of hCG administration.
   - *GnRH agonist ultrashort protocol:* GnRH agonist is started on day 2 of the menstrual cycle and stopped within 2–3 days.
   - *GnRH antagonist fixed protocol:* GnRH antagonists are started on day 6 and continued until the administration of hCG trigger.
   - *GnRH antagonist flexible protocol:* GnRH antagonist is started when the leading follicle has reached the size of 14 mm diameter and continued until the hCG trigger.
   - *GnRH antagonist single bolus protocol:* Ovarian stimulation is started on day 2 or 3 of the menstrual cycle, and a single-dose GnRH antagonist is administered on day 8.

Choosing the appropriate pituitary downregulation protocol: In the long GnRH agonist protocols, administration of

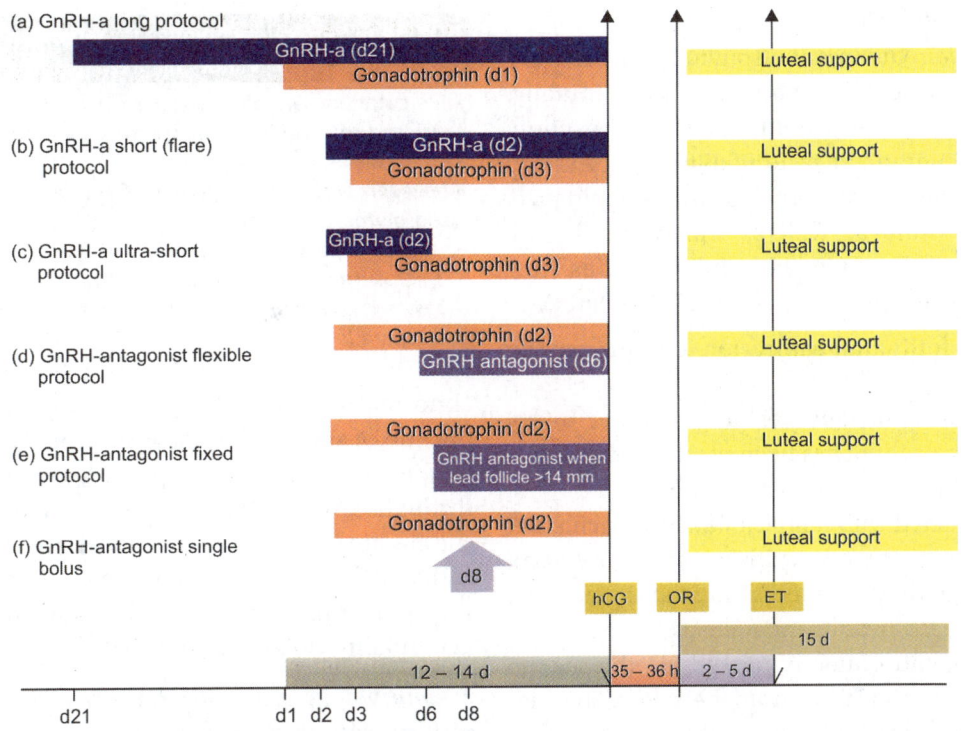

Fig. 34.17: Various protocols for pituitary downregulation.
(d: day; ET: embryo transfer; h: hour; hCG: human chorionic gonadotropin; OR: oocyte retrieval)

exogeneous gonadotropins is responsible for the recruitment, selection, and growth of the follicles. On the other hand, in case of GnRH antagonist cycles, endogenous gonadotropins are responsible for the initial recruitment and selection of follicles, whereas exogenous gonadotropins are responsible for augmenting their development. This may be responsible for the retrieval of lower number of growing follicles in GnRH antagonist cycles.

In women with normal ovarian reserve, the rates of pregnancy and live births are not significantly different in the GnRH agonist and GnRH antagonist protocols. However, the incidence of OHSS is significantly lower in GnRH antagonist cycles.

3. *Controlled ovarian hyperstimulation:*

> Q. Write a long essay discussing ovulation induction.
>
> Q. With the help of a long essay, discuss the newer concepts in ovulation induction.
>
> Q. Discuss briefly about the ovulation-inducing drugs.

In the menstrual cycles in a normal woman, a cohort of 10–20 ovarian antral follicles develops. Of these, only one follicle becomes the dominant follicle and eventually ovulates. However, in the IVF cycles, the use of FSH-containing gonadotropins for controlled ovarian stimulation aims at overriding the mechanisms which produce mono-ovulation. As a result, multifollicular development is achieved from which more than one oocyte can be harvested. Previously, CC was the first drug to be used for controlled ovarian stimulation. In the present times, gonadotropins have become the agents of choice for controlled ovarian stimulation.

To predict ovarian response to controlled ovarian stimulation, the NICE recommends testing the following markers of ovarian reserve:
- Serum AMH levels
- Ultrasound assessment of AFC
- Early follicular phase serum FSH levels.

Monitoring of controlled ovarian stimulation: This can be done using two-dimensional TVS scan and/or hormonal assessment. The aims of monitoring are as follows:
- Determination of appropriate timing for the final follicular maturation
- To decide on cycle cancellation in case of an under-response
- In case hyper-response is suspected, deciding between careful monitoring for OHSS and cycle cancellation.

4. *Final follicular maturation trigger:* Once satisfactory controlled ovarian stimulation is achieved, pituitary downregulation is discontinued. This is followed by the administration of a hormone, which mimics the midcycle LH surge in natural cycles. This is likely to facilitate final follicular maturation, cause resumption of meiosis, and initiate follicular luteinization to form a corpus luteum. Since many years, hCG, a functional analogue of LH, has been used for final follicular maturation trigger. Recombinant hCG (rhCG) and recombinant LH (rLH) preparations are also available for use.

5. *Oocyte and sperm retrieval:*
   - *Follicular aspiration:* Oocytes are aspirated from the ovary 35–36 hours following administration of hCG. Initially, all aspirations were performed under laparoscopic guidance. However now, follicular aspirations are commonly performed under ultrasonographic guidance, both transabdominal as well as transvaginal. The transvaginal route for follicular aspiration has now become the preferred procedure in most IVF programs.

The procedure of follicular aspiration comprises the following steps:
- Oocyte aspiration is usually performed under heavy sedation, while the patient has been placed in the dorsal lithotomy position.
- Vaginal wall is washed with saline, following which a 5–9 MHz ultrasonographic probe with a sterile cover and attached needle guide is inserted inside the vagina. This helps in localizing the ovaries and follicles.
- A 17 G needle is subsequently passed via the needle guide through the vaginal fornix into the ovaries in order to aspirate the follicular fluid.
- Once the fluid has been aspirated out, it is sent to the IVF laboratory as soon as possible.

6. *Oocyte classification:* Following their aspiration, the oocytes are graded according to the appearance of the corona–cumulus complex. The presence of a polar body (metaphase II stage) and/or germinal vesicle (prophase stage) is a determining factor for the short preincubation time prior to the insemination. The degenerated oocytes are those which are atretic or have a fractured zona. The last category constitutes fewer than 15% of the total oocytes obtained.

7. *Sperm retrieval:* A semen sample is obtained through masturbation in the laboratory after a 3–5-day period of sexual abstinence immediately prior to the oocyte retrieval. In case the sample is obtained at home, men should be advised to keep the sample at body temperature during transport and ensure that the sample reaches the lab within 60 minutes of ejaculation. Men in whom it is not possible to produce a semen sample by masturbation, special silastic condoms can be used for semen collection following intercourse. In men with ejaculatory dysfunction, sperms can be obtained through vibratory and electrical stimulation. In men with retrograde ejaculation, urine samples must be collected post masturbation and analyzed for the presence of vital spermatozoa, which can be used for treatment. Surgical techniques which can be employed to retrieve sperms in men with azoospermia or ejaculatory failure are listed in **Box 34.6.**

The procedure of sperm preparation involves the removal of certain components of the ejaculate (i.e., seminal fluid, excess cellular debris, leukocytes, and morphologically abnormal sperms) along with the retention of the motile fraction of sperms. For most specimens, the motile portion of sperms is separated via the process of centrifugation through a discontinuous density gradient system. The sperms are incubated for 60 minutes in an atmosphere of 5% carbon dioxide in air. Finally, the supernatant containing the motile fraction of sperm is removed. Sperm concentration and motility are determined.

> **BOX 34.6:** Surgical techniques for retrieving sperms in men with azoospermia or ejaculatory failure.
> - Percutaneous epididymal sperm aspiration
> - Microsurgical epididymal sperm aspiration
> - Testicular sperm aspiration
>
> *Above three procedures act as the first-line procedures for obstructive azoospermia and some men with ejaculatory failure*
> - Testicular sperm extraction
> - Microsurgical testicular sperm extraction
>
> *Above two procedures are used for men with nonobstructive azoospermia*

8. *Embryology procedure (IVF or ICSI):* Standard method of fertilization of gametes is IVF, which is initiated 4–6 hours following oocyte retrieval. It involves incubation of 25,000–50,000 capacitated sperms with a single oocyte. The inseminated oocytes are incubated in an atmosphere of 5% carbon dioxide in air with 98% humidity. The presence of two pronuclei and the extrusion of a second polar body are the criteria which ascertain fertilization and should occur approximately 18 hours following insemination.

The fertilized embryos are transferred into growth media and placed in the incubator. No further evaluation is performed over the next 24 hours. At four- to eight-cell stage, pre-embryo is observed approximately 36–48 hours after insemination.

The procedure of ICSI is discussed later in the text.

9. *Intrauterine embryo transfer:*

 Q. Write a short essay on embryo transfer.

Previously, the embryo transfer was done on day 2 or 3 when the embryos are at two- to eight-cell stage. The recent trend is toward transferring the embryo on day 5 or 6 when the embryo has reached 64-cell stage (blastocyst stage). By this time, the selected embryos have a better implantation potential due to self-selection. The transfer is usually performed transcervically under guidance of transabdominal ultrasound. The embryos should be loaded with 15–20 µL of culture media at the time of transfer. The catheter is advanced up to the fundus of the endometrial cavity, and then withdrawn slightly. The embryos are ejected into the miduterine cavity, approximately 1–2 cm away from the fundus. Subsequent to the embryo transfer, the patient must be on bed rest for 30–60 minutes. No more than two embryos must be transferred during any one cycle. As previously mentioned, the present trend is toward transferring a single high-quality embryo. The NICE recommends elective single embryo transfer when a top-quality blastocyst is available. Cryostorage of supernumerary embryos can be offered if there are more than two embryos.

10. *Luteal phase support:* Following 36–72 hours after oocyte retrieval, the endometrium must be supplemented with progesterone in order to maintain the luteal phase. Supplementation with exogenous progesterone is especially required because the superovulation and follicular aspiration at the time of oocyte retrieval are likely to have induced an abnormal endocrine milieu. Several progesterone preparations are available for use, for e.g., natural progesterone in oil base for IM injection, vaginal progesterone suppositories and gels, and capsules of micronized progesterone to be used vaginally or sublingually. Normally, progesterone supplementation is continued for approximately 2 weeks. In case the pregnancy test result is positive, progesterone must be continued until the 12th week of gestation.

Poor Responders to Ovarian Stimulation

Increasing attention is now being focused on women who are unable to produce an optimal number of follicles in response to ovulation induction. Such women are also termed as "poor responders." Though the definition of a poor responder has not been universally defined, it generally includes women who are unsuccessful in producing an optimal number of follicles (usually ≤3, having a diameter of ≥18 mm) in response to induction of ovulation. In a first practical attempt at standardizing the definition of poor ovarian responders (PORs), the ESHRE working group has proposed a standardized, simple, and reproducible definition for POR, also known as the Bologna criteria. In accordance with the Bologna criteria, at least two of the following three features must be present:

1. Advanced maternal age or any other risk factor for POR
2. Previous POR
3. Abnormal ovarian reserve test (ORT).

Apart from the above three criteria, in the absence of advanced maternal age or abnormal ORT, the patient can be defined as a poor responder if she has two episodes of poor ovarian response even after maximal stimulation. Although one stimulated cycle is necessary for diagnosing POR, patients with advanced age or abnormal ORT may be considered poor responders, because both the factors suggest the possibility of decreased ovarian reserve. They, therefore, serve as markers of poor stimulation cycle outcomes. Such patients should be classified as "expected poor responders." The group reached the conclusion that such a comprehensive criterion is likely to assist the researchers in selecting a homogenized population for future studies, having a lower bias due to spurious POR definitions. This would facilitate the comparison of results for reaching precise decisions.

Presently, there is inadequate evidence supporting the routine use of any particular intervention in the form of pituitary downregulation with either GnRHa or antagonists, ovarian stimulation, or adjuvant therapy for the management of poor responders to controlled ovarian stimulation in IVF.

However, there is an exception. A combination of long-acting gonadotrophin (corifollitropin alfa) with highly purified (HP) hMG in a GnRH antagonist regimen appears to be a promising approach. Better evidence from good-quality randomized, double-blinded multicentric trials would be required in future to arrive at a definite conclusion.

Assisted Fertilization Techniques

Previously, some of the techniques which help in facilitating fertilization such as partial zona dissection and subzonal sperm injection were commonly used. These techniques have now been largely replaced by procedures such as ICSI and assisted hatching (AH). Currently, only ICSI and AH are being used clinically. These procedures can be used on their own or as part of an IVF cycle for treatment of infertility.

Intracytoplasmic Sperm Injection

 Q. Write a short essay on ICSI.

Partial zona dissection and subzonal insemination (SUZI) are obsolete and have now been replaced by the ICSI procedure. ICSI has revolutionized the treatment of severe male factor infertility because only a single live sperm is required, which is injected directly into the ovum. It is commonly used in cases of male factor infertility such as obstructive azoospermia (due to congenital absence of the vas deferens). ICSI nowadays is also commonly being used as part of an IVF cycle.

Procedure: The sperm can be obtained through masturbation, epididymal aspiration, testicular biopsy, or needle puncture of the testes. The sperm is paralyzed by stroking the distal portion of its tail.

The oocyte is stripped from the cumulus using a solution of hyaluronidase.

To inject the sperm, first the oocyte is stabilized with a micropipette; then the sperm is loaded, tail first, into a microneedle **(Figs. 34.18A to E)**. The oocyte membrane is pierced with the microneedle and the oolemma is entered. The spermatozoon is released inside the oolemma, and the microinjected oocyte is kept in the incubator.

Indications: Indications for ICSI are as follows:
- Severe deficits in semen quality
- Obstructive azoospermia
- Nonobstructive azoospermia
- Failure of previous IVF treatment cycles.

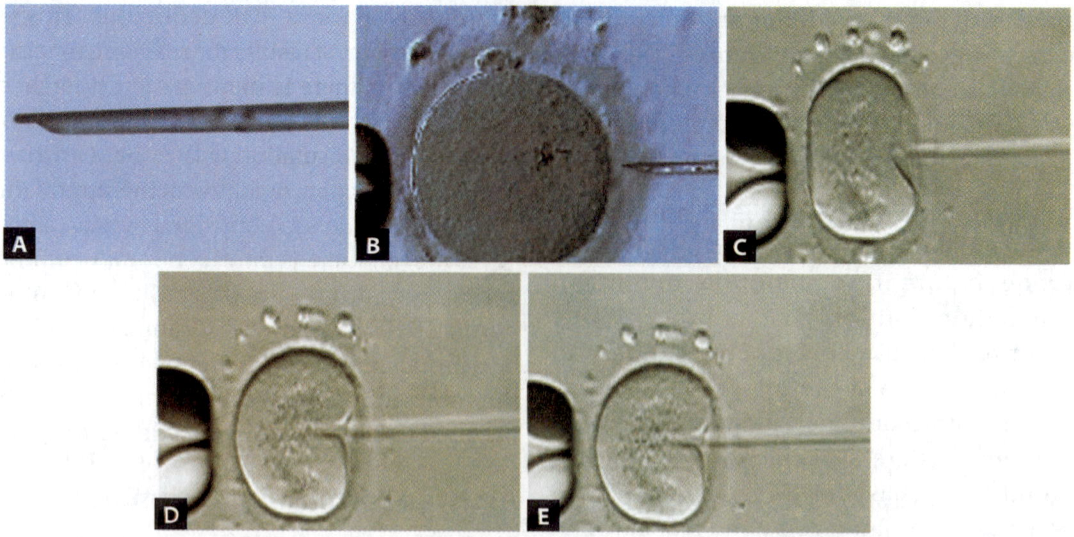

Figs. 34.18A to E: Intracytoplasmic sperm injection. (A) Microneedle is loaded with a sperm; (B) The microneedle approaches the oocyte; (C) The microneedle pierces the oocyte membrane; (D) The microneedle is advanced deeper inside the cytoplasm; (E) The spermatozoon is released inside the oocyte.

Where the indication for ICSI is a severe deficit of semen quality or nonobstructive azoospermia, the man's karyotype should be established. Men who are undergoing karyotype testing should be offered genetic counseling regarding the genetic abnormalities that may be detected. Couples should be informed that ICSI improves fertilization rates compared to IVF alone, but once fertilization is achieved, the pregnancy rate is no better than with IVF.

Success rate of ICSI depends on retrieving adequate number of spermatozoa or spermatids from the testes. Successful pregnancy has been reported even with injection of fresh or cryopreserved immature sperm cells, including spermatids, but not with spermatocytes. While the children conceived by IVF and/or ICSI are at increased risk for birth defects, the absolute risk is very low. Moreover, there is no risk difference between children conceived by IVF and/or ICSI. The rate of achieving pregnancy and live birth with ICSI is similar to that achieved during natural conception. New surgical techniques have been presented in order to retrieve spermatozoa from patients with nonobstructive azoospermia. Testicular sperm extraction (TESE) using microdissection is used for extraction of sperms from the seminiferous tubules in patients with nonobstructive azoospermia.

Assisted Hatching

Embryo hatching is an obligatory step in the process of embryo implantation. It has been observed that some of the IVF embryos may have a rather thick zona pellucida. This thickened zona may represent an obstacle for the normal embryo hatching, thereby interfering with the implantation. In order to facilitate the hatching of normal embryos, the procedure of AH is sometimes used for the embryos which show a thick zona pellucida. The procedure is usually performed a couple of hours before the embryo transfer. AH can be performed mechanically, using laser beams to create a microrent, or by chemical digestion of the zona using Tyrode solution (low pH). Both the procedures create a weak spot within the zona, facilitating the break of the zona and hatching of the embryo. AH is recommended for patients undergoing IVF who are older than 38 years, patients with multiple ART failures, and in all cryopreserved embryos.

In Vitro Fertilization-Related Procedures

In vitro fertilization-related procedures such as GIFT and zygote intrafallopian transfer (ZIFT) are sometimes used as alternatives to IVF. These would now be described in brief.

Gamete Intrafallopian Transfer

The procedure of GIFT comprises stimulating the ovaries, monitoring follicular development, and oocyte aspiration similar to IVF. This procedure is different from IVF in the sense that in IVF the embryo is transferred inside the endometrial cavity while in case of GIFT the gametes are transferred into the fallopian tube. Thus, in order to qualify for this procedure, the patient must have at least one normal-appearing and patent fallopian tube.

Following the oocyte aspiration and classification of oocytes, a laparoscopy or a minilaparotomy is performed. The oocytes, along with 150,000 sperms, are loaded into a special catheter in the laboratory under a microscope and then handed over to the surgeon in the operating room. Before the injection of the gametes into the fallopian tube, the fimbria must be gently picked up with an atraumatic grasping forceps. The ostium must be identified, following which the tip of the catheter is passed through the ostium and advanced up to the ampulla of the fallopian tube, where the gametes are eventually released. Fertilization therefore occurs inside the fallopian tube, unlike the procedure of IVF where fertilization occurs in the laboratory settings. Thus, this procedure is more physiologic and mimics the normal procedure of conception more closely than IVF. Nevertheless, a major disadvantage associated with GIFT procedure is that it does not allow for visual confirmation of fertilization because it occurs inside the body. Furthermore, if pregnancy does not occur, there is no way to determine whether the cause of failure was lack of fertilization or lack of implantation. Also, the procedure of GIFT requires a laparoscopy or minilaparotomy, both of which can be performed under general anesthesia. Both these factors are likely to increase the total cost of the procedure.

Zygote Intrafallopian Transfer

The ZIFT procedure is a combination of IVF and GIFT. Fertilization occurs in the IVF laboratory. However, the pre-embryo is transferred into the fallopian tube via laparoscopy at the two-pronuclei stage or 24 hours after oocyte retrieval.

Donor Insemination

Indications for Donor Insemination

The use of donor insemination is considered effective in managing fertility problems associated with the following conditions:

- Obstructive azoospermia
- Nonobstructive azoospermia
- Infectious disease in the male partner (such as HIV)
- Severe rhesus isoimmunization
- Severe deficits in semen quality in couples who do not wish to undergo ICSI
- Cases where there is a high risk of transmitting a genetic disorder to the offspring. Before starting treatment by donor insemination, it is important to confirm that the woman is ovulating. Women with a history that is suggestive of tubal damage should be offered tubal assessment before treatment. Couples using donor sperms should be offered IUI in preference to intracervical insemination because it improves pregnancy rates.

Women who are ovulating regularly should be offered a minimum of six cycles of donor insemination without ovarian stimulation to reduce the risk of multiple pregnancy and its consequences.

Oocyte Donation

Indications for Oocyte Donation

The use of donor oocytes is considered effective in managing fertility problems associated with the following conditions:

- Premature ovarian failure
- Gonadal dysgenesis including Turner's syndrome
- Bilateral oophorectomy
- Ovarian failure following chemotherapy or radiotherapy
- Certain cases of IVF treatment failure

- There is a high risk of transmitting a genetic disorder to the offspring.

All people considering participation in an egg-sharing scheme should be counseled about its particular implications.

COMPLICATIONS

Since PCOS and endometriosis are amongst the common causes for infertility, the complications associated with these two diseases would be primarily covered. Also, with the advent of ART, many complications can be associated with the procedure per se.

COMPLICATIONS RELATED TO POLYCYSTIC OVARIAN SYNDROME PER SE

The possible late sequela of PCOS includes development of complications such as type 2 diabetes mellitus, dyslipidemia, hypertension, cardiovascular disease, and endometrial cancer in future.

Complications Related to Medical Management

Complications related to the use of various medicines for PCOS are described next.

Clomiphene Citrate

- *Multiple pregnancy:* Women who are being prescribed CC should be informed that this drug might be associated with the risk of multiple gestation. Women undergoing treatment with CC should be offered ultrasound monitoring during at least the first cycle of treatment to ensure that they receive a dose that minimizes the risk of multiple pregnancy.
- *Thickening of cervical mucus:* Another important adverse effect associated with the use of this drug is the thickening of cervical mucus under the antiestrogenic effect of CC. This may create an iatrogenic cervical factor, which may be responsible for producing infertility in a patient who has otherwise ovulated.
- *Other adverse effects:* Other side effects, which may be rarely associated with CC, include hot flashes, scotomas, dryness of the vagina, headache, and ovarian hyperstimulation. The use of CC is contraindicated in cases of ovarian cyst, pregnancy, and liver disease. Its use is also controversial in patients with a history of breast cancer.

Gonadotropins

Side effects associated with the use of gonadotropins are as follows:

- Multiple adverse effects and complications that may occur following the use of the gonadotropins include polyfollicular response, multiple pregnancy, ectopic pregnancy, miscarriages, ovarian torsion and rupture, and OHSS. Due to the risk of various side effects, especially OHSS, the administration of hMG and its derivatives should be directly supervised by a reproductive endocrinologist under ultrasound guidance and daily determinations of estradiol, FSH, and LH levels. Moreover, it is an expensive, stressful, and time-consuming form of treatment, which usually needs intensive monitoring. Of these various complications, OHSS, being a life-threatening complication of ART, assumes importance and has been described in detail later in the chapter.

Complications Related to Surgical Management

Complications associated with LOD are enumerated as follows:

- Accidental injury to internal organs or major blood vessels from the laparoscope or other surgical instruments
- Internal bleeding
- Pain after the procedure as a result of pneumoperitoneum
- Problems caused by anesthesia
- *Adhesions:* Adhesion formation was a significant complication of bilateral ovarian wedge resection, which occurred as a result of tissue handling and serosal trauma at the time of laparotomy. Adhesions lead to nonavailability of ovarian surface for ovulation, thereby resulting in anovulation. Moreover, their presence may interfere with peritoneal ovum transport as well. As a result, the procedure, which had been performed with the intention of resolving the problem of infertility, may itself become responsible for producing infertility. On the other hand, LOD has a small but definite potential for causing tubal adhesions. The definite etiology of pelvic adhesion formation is not yet clearly known. However, there are some factors which are associated with an increased risk for the development of pelvic adhesions. Some of these factors include intra-abdominal infection, tissue hypoxia or ischemia, tissue drying, manipulation of tissues during surgery, presence of a reactive foreign body, or intraperitoneal blood.
- *Atrophy:* Ovarian atrophy and failure are rare complications of LOD. Rarely, the ovaries can undergo irreparable damage and experience atrophy. It appears that application of seven or more punctures per ovary represents an excessive amount of thermal energy used and therefore must be discouraged. Despite the absence of strong evidence regarding the association of premature ovarian failure with LOD, precautions should be taken to minimize the chances of causing irreversible damage to the ovaries. These include keeping the dose of ovarian cautery to the minimum effective level and avoiding putting any cautery points close to the ovarian hilum.

- *Hyperprolactinemia:* Hyperprolactinemia after ovarian cauterization can be considered as a possible cause of anovulation in women with polycystic ovaries and improved gonadotropin and androgen levels. The cause of hyperprolactinemia remains unknown. Therefore, determination of levels of prolactin in anovulatory patients after LOD is recommended.

COMPLICATIONS RELATED TO ENDOMETRIOSIS PER SE

For details regarding the complications associated with endometriosis, kindly refer to chapter 30.

COMPLICATIONS RELATED TO ASSISTED REPRODUCTIVE TECHNIQUE PER SE

Some disadvantages associated with the procedure include:
- High cost of the procedure
- Administration of certain medications to the woman and performance of certain procedures on her
- Increased rates of multiple pregnancy and other complications related to the procedure

Maternal morbidity and mortality rates directly related to IVF per se are low. Complications are primarily related to hormonal stimulation and egg retrieval, and include complications such as OHSS, thromboembolism, infection, abdominal bleeding, adnexal torsion, allergic reaction, anesthetic complications, ectopic pregnancy, and heterotopic pregnancy. If the IVF cycle proves to be successful, the woman is at risk of usual pregnancy-related complications (e.g., preeclampsia or eclampsia, hemorrhage, amniotic fluid embolism, thromboembolism, and sepsis). Some of the complications associated with ART or IVF are described next.

Ovarian Hyperstimulation Syndrome

Ovarian hyperstimulation syndrome is an iatrogenic condition that occurs in patients undergoing ovulation induction with hMG or controlled ovarian hyperstimulation for ARTs. OHSS has been discussed in detail later in the chapter.

Ectopic Pregnancy

Ectopic pregnancy is another complication which can occur as a result of ART with an incidence of 1–3% of pregnancies being ectopic following assisted reproduction. Kindly refer to chapter 32 for details related to ectopic pregnancy.

Iatrogenic Multiple Pregnancy

Widespread use of ART over the past few decades has been associated with an increase in iatrogenic multifetal gestations. Since multifetal gestations are associated with their own risks and complications, their occurrence in association with infertility treatment has to be regarded as an adverse outcome. Some fetal complications associated with multifetal gestations include a higher incidence of miscarriage, preterm deliveries, congenital malformations, discordancy, and IUGR, all of which increase the perinatal morbidity. Multifetal gestations may also be associated with a higher incidence of maternal complications such as preeclampsia, anemia, labor difficulties, postpartum hemorrhage, failed lactation, and psychological disturbances in a woman.

Strategies to Reduce the Risk of Multiple Pregnancies

Some of the strategies which have been adopted to reduce the risk of multiple pregnancies during ARTs are as follows:

- *Elective single embryo transfer:* Recently, transfer of a single, high-quality embryo has been found to be associated with a high chance of live birth. As a result, elective single embryo transfer has been recommended as the standard of care in the ART cycles.
- *Excess oocyte aspiration and vitrification:* Results of recent studies have shown that the cycles with three or four follicles do not result in any substantial gain in pregnancy rate but are associated with an increased rate of multiple pregnancies. A less aggressive ovarian stimulation serves as an effective method for preventing excessive multifollicular growth, therefore reducing the risk of multiple pregnancies in ovarian stimulation. The application of excess oocyte retrieval and vitrification (oocyte cryopreservation) may further improve the cost-effectiveness of stimulated IUI by effectively reducing the rate of multiple pregnancies, at the same time offering additional chances of pregnancy.
- *Multifetal pregnancy reduction (MFPR):* MFPR techniques have been promoted to reduce high-order pregnancies to twin gestation, with the aim of improving perinatal outcomes. The technique of MFPR appears to work as an effective treatment option by reducing the rate of pregnancy loss, antenatal complications, preterm birth, cesarean delivery, low birthweight babies, and neonatal death.
- *Other strategies:* Other strategies for prevention of multiple pregnancies as a result of ovulation stimulation include cycle cancellation, coasting, aspiration of follicles before the administration of hCG, and switching to IVF in an IUI cycle. Coasting is a method involving withdrawal of exogenous gonadotropins until there is a decline in serum estradiol levels.

Heterotopic Pregnancy

Heterotopic pregnancy is a complication of pregnancy in which both intrauterine and extrauterine pregnancies occur simultaneously. This is a relatively rare complication in case of natural pregnancy with the rate being about 1 in 30,000 cases. On the other hand, heterotopic pregnancies can occur in nearly 1% pregnancies conceived after IVF. A high index of suspicion is required in these cases. Repeated ultrasound examination and early intervention usually help in salvaging the viable intrauterine pregnancy and avoiding maternal mortality. The prognosis of a viable intrauterine pregnancy is usually good.

Oncogenic Risk

Recently, there have been reports showing increased prevalence of perinatal problems associated with ART. Evidence obtained from animal experiments raises concerns that infertility and its treatment with ART (processes such as ovarian stimulation and culture of gametes and embryos) may be associated with an increased oncogenic risk (ovarian cancer, breast cancer, etc.) in both women and their offspring. Although there appears to be a possible risk of ART treatment causing oncogenesis, this has not been proven. The oncogenic risks are minimal, especially with the use of short stimulation protocols nowadays. Nevertheless, long-term studies and follow-up are required to reach any definitive conclusion.

OVARIAN HYPERSTIMULATION SYNDROME

> Q. Write a long essay discussing ovarian hyperstimulation syndrome.
>
> Q. Write a long essay on prevention and treatment of ovarian hyperstimulation syndrome.

Ovarian hyperstimulation syndrome is an iatrogenic condition that occurs in patients undergoing ovulation induction with hMG or controlled ovarian hyperstimulation for ARTs **(Fig. 34.19)**. The incidence rate fluctuates from 0.1% to 30%. The pathophysiology of the disease is not well understood but is associated with massive

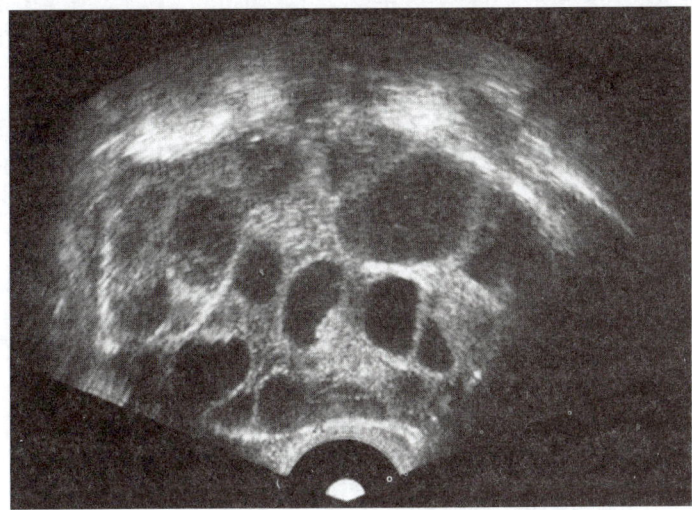

Fig. 34.19: Ovarian hyperstimulation syndrome showing "wheel-spoke appearance" on transvaginal examination.

TABLE 34.11: Features of ovarian hyperstimulation syndrome.

	Mild form
Stage A	• Symptoms such as abdominal heaviness, abdominal swelling, and pain. • *Chemical hyperstimulation:* 17β-estradiol levels of 1,000–1,500 pg/mL
Stage B	*Chemical hyperstimulation:* Ovaries enlarged up to 6 cm in diameter. Each ovary is characterized by the presence of multiple follicular and corpus luteum cysts
	Moderate form
Stage A	17β-estradiol levels > 4,000 pg/mL, ovaries enlarged up to 6–12 cm
Stage B	Presence of ascites on ultrasound examination, findings as in stage A with gastrointestinal symptoms such as vomiting and diarrhea
	Severe form
Stage A	17β-estradiol levels > 4,000 pg/mL, ovaries enlarged to >12 cm plus clinical manifestations including pleural effusion, pericardial effusion, breathing difficulties, hypovolemia, impairment of renal function, electrolyte imbalance, disturbance in liver function, thromboembolic phenomena, shock, tension ascites, and acute respiratory distress syndrome
Stage B	Presence of all the above plus change in the blood volume, increased blood viscosity due to hemoconcentration, coagulation abnormalities, and diminished renal perfusion and function

extravascular accumulation of fluid. This causes severe depletion of the intravascular volume, resulting in dehydration, hemoconcentration, and electrolyte imbalance (i.e., hyponatremia and hyperkalemia).

Schenker and Weinstein have classified OHSS into three main categories: (1) mild, (2) moderate, and (3) severe **(Table 34.11)**. Hematocrit value of >45% is categorized as severe OHSS, whereas hematocrit value of >55% is categorized as critical OHSS.

Risk Factors

Various risk factors for the development of OHSS include young age of the patient (<35 years), polycystic ovary-like appearance of ovaries, asthenic habitus, pregnancy, and hCG luteal supplementation. Exogenous hCG administration is critical for the development of OHSS. Severe OHSS is dependent on both exogenous administration of hCG and endogenous pregnancy-derived hCG. hCG is administered exogenously during ovarian stimulation for both triggering ovulation and luteal support.

Moreover, different protocols used for stimulation of ovaries in ART cycles may also affect the incidence and severity of OHSS. Stimulation of ovaries is likely to result in high serum estradiol levels and development of multiple follicles.

Pathogenesis

The exact pathogenesis of OHSS is not yet clear. It is thought to occur as a result of increased vascular permeability. The exact substances responsible for this have not yet been identified. Mechanism of fluid shift occurring in cases of OHSS is shown in **Flowchart 34.7**.

Prevention

Some of the methods for prevention of OHSS are as follows:
- *Patient monitoring:* Monitoring the patients for suspected signs of OHSS while they are undergoing various steps of ART procedures forms an important step for prevention. Urinary LH kit is a practical way to monitor these patients. Pelvic ultrasonography can be used once a week until the dominant follicle is detected.
- *FSH for ovulation induction:* Using pure FSH treatment for ovulation induction in PCOS patients who are clomiphene resistant. Pure FSH must be started at 37.5 IU/day subcutaneously. The dosage is increased slowly (i.e., by 37.5 IU q5d) until follicle development is detectable based on an elevation of the E2 levels and the presence of follicle development on sonograms. Using this small amount of FSH, the patient generally develops 1–2 follicles, decreasing the risk for multiple pregnancy and eliminating the risk of OHSS.
- *Final follicular maturation trigger:* Using GnRH trigger rather than hCG for final follicular maturation is likely to reduce the risk of OHSS.
- *Metformin:* The use of metformin is likely to reduce the risk of OHSS. Simultaneous use of cabergoline has also been shown to reduce the risk of OHSS.

Management of Ovarian Hyperstimulation Syndrome

No active form of treatment is required for mild OHSS. Patient observation and maintenance of hydration by the oral route usually work for such patients. Close observation and hospitalization are usually required for moderate-grade OHSS, since these patients may rapidly undergo a change of status, particularly when conception occurs. Patients with severe OHSS may require immediate hospitalization and treatment. During hospitalization, careful monitoring of hemodynamic stability is required.

Large-volume crystalloid infusion is recommended for renewal of the depleted intravascular volume. However, these patients must be closely monitored, as this can result

Flowchart 34.7: Mechanism of fluid shift occurring in ovarian hyperstimulation syndrome.

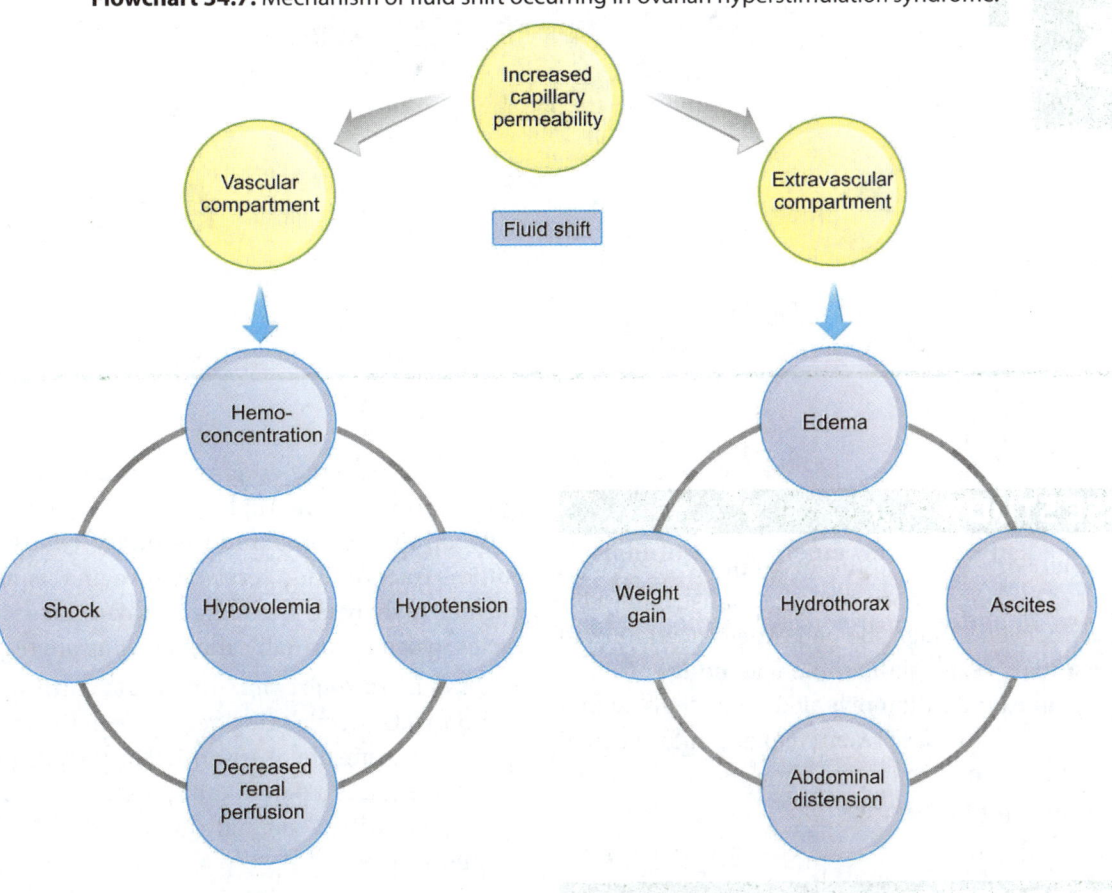

Flowchart 34.8: Management of ovarian hyperstimulation syndrome (OHSS).

Management of a patient with OHSS

Patient monitoring
Monitoring of the following:
- Vital signs
- *Fluid balance*: Fluid intake, urinary output
- Daily measurement of the patient's weight and abdominal girth
- Central venous pressure monitoring
- *Blood tests*: Complete blood count, hematocrit, serum electrolytes and proteins, liver function tests, coagulation profile, acid–base balance, blood gases
- Urine osmolarity
- *Imaging*: Ultrasonography (abdomen, chest), computed tomography (abdomen, chest)

Patient treatment
- *Maintenance of blood volume*: Plasma expanders
- *Reduction of capillary permeability*: Indomethacin, angiotensin-converting enzyme inhibitors
- *Prevention of thromboembolic phenomenon*: Heparin
- *Surgery*: Only in cases of torsion/rupture of ovarian cysts

in sequestration of fluid in the third space. Management of OHSS is summarized in **Flowchart 34.8**. Monitoring of induction of ovulation is the most reliable method in the prevention of OHSS. When the peak plasma estradiol levels are >2,000 pg/mL, or an abnormal increase in the serum estradiol levels (doubling during 2 or 3 days) occurs, hCG should be withheld.

Complications of Ovarian Hyperstimulation Syndrome

The most serious complications of OHSS are both arterial and venous thromboembolic phenomena. Arterial thromboembolic phenomena may result in cardiovascular accidents and sometimes even death.

 EVIDENCE-BASED CLINICAL TRIALS

 List of references can be scanned through QR code to enable the readers gain deeper insight of the subject by referring to the entire article or its abstract.

CHAPTER 35

Amenorrhea

CASE STUDY

A 15-year-old girl presented to the gynecology OPD with the complaint of absence of periods. The menstrual cycles had never begun, even though she had experienced normal breast and secondary sexual development at the age of about 13 years. Physical examination revealed an absent vaginal canal. A small depression was present in place of the vaginal introitus. An ultrasound examination showed absent uterus and the presence of normal ovaries.

INTRODUCTION

Amenorrhea implies the absence of menstrual periods. It can be of two types: primary and secondary. Primary amenorrhea is the absence of menstrual cycles in a woman who had never experienced menstrual cycles before. Secondary amenorrhea, on the other hand, is defined as the cessation of menstruation in a woman who had been previously experiencing normal menstrual bleeding. This cessation must last for at least 6 months or for at least three of the previous three-cycle intervals. Secondary amenorrhea is more common than primary amenorrhea. Primary amenorrhea can be defined as follows:

- Absence of menses by the age of 13 years with the absence of growth or development of secondary sexual characteristics or
- Absence of menses by the age of 15 years with normal development of secondary sexual characteristics

PATHOPHYSIOLOGY OF MENSTRUAL BLEEDING

As previously described in Chapter 22, circulating estradiol levels in the body stimulate the growth of uterine endometrium. Progesterone, which is produced by corpus luteum, is formed after ovulation. It transforms proliferating endometrium into a secretory one. If pregnancy does not occur, this secretory endometrium breaks down and sheds in the form of menstrual bleeding. A complex interaction between the hypothalamic–pituitary–ovarian axis and the outflow tract (uterus, cervix, and vagina) is required for the normal menstrual bleeding to take place. For menstrual cycles to occur normally, the following are required:

- *Intact outflow tract:* An intact outflow tract, which connects the bleeding occurring in the internal genitalia with the outside, is essential for normal menstrual flow. This requires a patent outflow tract and continuity of the vaginal orifice, vaginal canal, and endocervix with the uterine cavity.
- *Normal endometrial development:* Normal development of endometrial lining, which responds cyclically to stimulation by estrogen and progesterone
- *Normal-functioning ovaries:* Proper functioning of the ovaries is required for secretion and synthesis of estrogens and progesterone. The entire spectrum of follicle development, ovulation, and formation of corpus luteum occurs here.
- *Normal-functioning pituitary glands:* The stimulus for the production of ovarian hormones and ovarian follicles is provided by the hormones secreted from anterior pituitary including hormones such as FSH and LH.
- *Normal-functioning hypothalamus:* The secretion of these hormones by the pituitary is dependent on secretion of GnRH by the hypothalamus.

Any disruption of the interaction in the above-mentioned compartments can result in amenorrhea. The causes of primary amenorrhea are therefore related to defects in either of the four compartments as described below and shown in **Figure 35.1**.

- *Compartment I:* Outflow tract and the uterus
- *Compartment II:* Defect in ovulation
- *Compartment III:* Defect at the level of pituitary gland
- *Compartment IV:* Defect at the level of hypothalamus and CNS

Amenorrhea

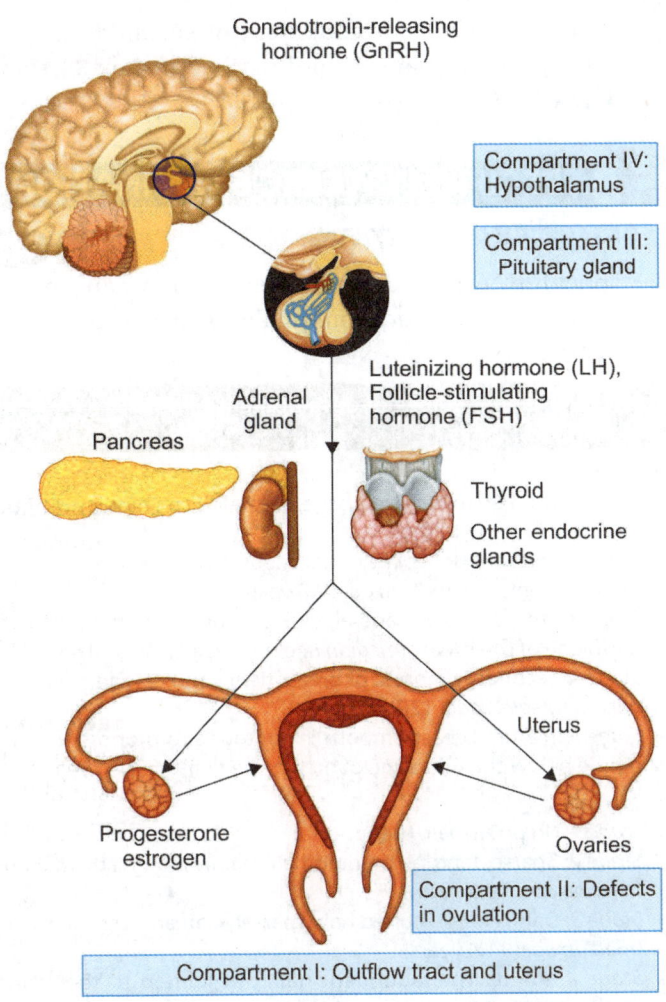

Fig. 35.1: Causes of primary amenorrhea related to defects in either of the four compartments.

HISTORY AND CLINICAL PRESENTATION

A good history can reveal the etiologic diagnosis in up to 85% of cases of amenorrhea. Clinicians should take a comprehensive patient history including the following points:

- History of exercise, excessive weight loss, current or previous chronic illness, and illicit drug use could be suggestive of hypothalamic amenorrhea. History of psychosocial stressors (recent emotional upsets and psychological dysfunction) and extreme dieting (anorexia or bulimia nervosa) can also be the cause for amenorrhea.
- History of irradiation or chemotherapy to the CNS could be another cause for hypothalamic amenorrhea.
- History of previous pelvic/abdominal radiation could result in premature ovarian failure (POF). The presence of vasomotor symptoms such as hot flashes and dryness of vagina could be suggestive of POF.
- History of galactorrhea, headache, and visual disturbances could be related to the presence of pituitary tumors.
- History of infertility needs to be specifically asked because in many cases infertility could be related to the history of amenorrhea, which the woman may specifically tend to hide.
- Symptoms suggestive of thyroid dysfunction
- Recent change in body weight, extreme dieting, and symptoms suggestive of anorexia nervosa

FAMILY HISTORY

- *Pubic hair pattern:* Androgen insensitivity syndrome (AIS), which shows autosomal recessive inheritance, is associated with breast development but no pubic or axillary hair development.
- Age of menarche and menopause and menstrual history show similarity amongst various family members (e.g., mother and sisters).
- Constitutional delay of growth and puberty shows a hereditary pattern.

MENSTRUAL HISTORY

It is important to ask the patient if she had been experiencing menstrual cycles previously in order to determine whether amenorrhea is primary or secondary. In case of secondary amenorrhea, the woman needs to be asked if there is any possibility of pregnancy, e.g., is the urine pregnancy test positive?

PREVIOUS OBSTETRIC HISTORY

If the woman has previously conceived, her amenorrhea is secondary in nature. It is important to take history regarding the use of OCPs in these cases.

Prolonged use of OCPs can result in postpill amenorrhea.

TREATMENT HISTORY

History of intake of drugs such as progestogens, combined oral contraceptive and chemotherapy drugs needs to be elicited. The use of these drugs can sometimes result in amenorrhea.

GENERAL PHYSICAL EXAMINATION

General physical examination involves the following steps:
1. *Assessment of the patient's nutritional status and BMI:* Increased BMI could be associated with PCOS.
2. *Anthropomorphic measurements and growth chart:* These measurements may detect abnormalities such as constitutional delay of growth and puberty.
3. Signs of androgen excess such as hirsutism or acne could be associated with PCOS.
4. Signs of virilization, e.g., deep voice and clitoromegaly, in addition to hirsutism, and acne could be related to the presence of androgen-secreting tumors.
5. *Clitoral measurement:* Measuring the clitoris is an effective method for determining the degree of

androgen effect. The clitoral index can be determined by measuring the glans of clitoris in the anteroposterior and transverse diameters. A clitoral index >35 mm² is an evidence of increased androgen effect. A clitoral index >100 mm² is evidence of virilization. Other features suggestive of virilization include labioscrotal fusion, breast atrophy, hirsutism, deepening of voice, increased muscle mass, etc.

6. *Dysmorphic features:* Diseases like Turners syndrome could be associated with specific dysmorphic features, which are described later in the chapter.
7. *Cushing's syndrome:* Symptoms suggestive of Cushing's disease such as striae, buffalo hump, central obesity, easy bruising, hypertension, or proximal muscle weakness
8. *Thyroid examination:* It is especially important to rule out hypothyroidism or hyperthyroidism. Thyroid diseases serve as a cause of amenorrhea and menstrual irregularities.
9. *Breast examination:* It is important to check for galactorrhea. If galactorrhea is present, it is important to evaluate whether it is spontaneous or present only after careful expression by the examiner, whether it is unilateral or bilateral and persistent or intermittent. Breast secretions due to hormonal imbalance come from multiple duct openings in comparison to pathological discharge, which comes from a single duct.
10. *Fundoscopy and assessment of visual fields:* This must be done if there is suspicion of pituitary tumor.
11. *Pubertal development:* A thorough physical examination must be conducted in patients with amenorrhea in order to assess normal female pubertal development.

Tanner stages of development of secondary sexual characteristics have been described in **Box 35.1** and **Figures 35.2A and B**.

SPECIFIC SYSTEMIC EXAMINATION

PELVIC EXAMINATION

Per speculum examination and inspection can help in detection of outflow tract abnormalities such as transverse

BOX 35.1: Tanner stages of development of secondary sexual characteristics.

Breast:
- *Stage 1:* No palpable breast tissue, areola <2 cm; nipples may be inverted, flat, and raised
- *Stage 2:* Breast budding with small mound of breast tissue; areola begins to enlarge (*median age*: 9.8 years)
- *Stage 3:* Further growth and elevation of breast nipple at/above midplane of the breast (*median age*: 11.2 years)
- *Stage 4:* Secondary mound of breast tissue, projected areola and papilla (*median age*: 12.1 years)
- *Stage 5:* Mature breast, smooth in contour and proportion with nipple below the midplane of breast (*median age*: 14.6 years)

Pubic hair:
- *Stage 1:* No pubic hair, prepubertal
- *Stage 2:* Sparse, long pigmented hair mainly along labia majora (*median age*: 10.5 years)
- *Stage 3:* Dark, coarse, curled hair, sparsely spread over the mons (*median age*: 11.4 years)
- *Stage 4:* Adult type, abundant hair, but limited to the mons (*median age*: 12.0 years)
- *Stage 5:* Adult type spread in quantity and distribution (*median age*: 13.6 years), i.e., spread occurs to the medial aspect of thighs

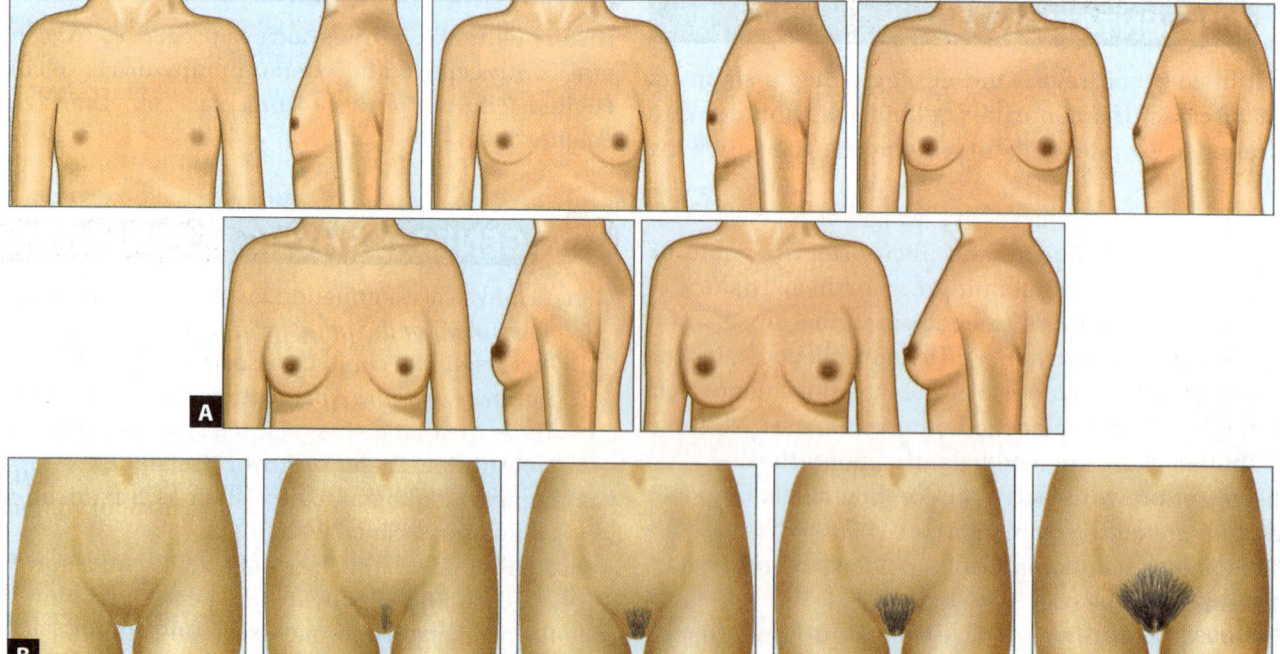

Figs. 35.2A and B: Tanner stages of development. (A) Breast; (B) Pubic hair.

Amenorrhea

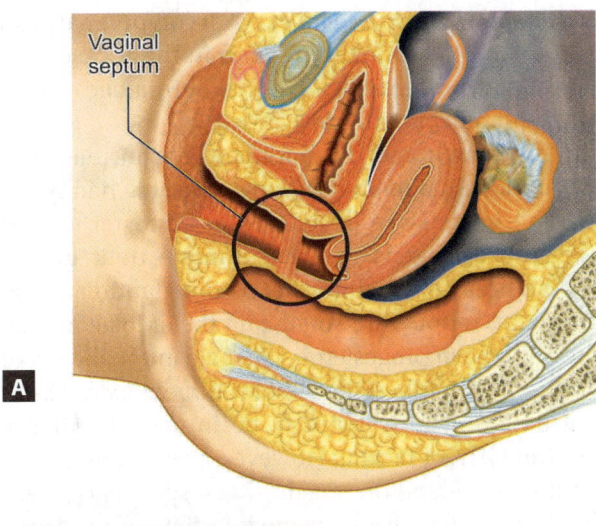

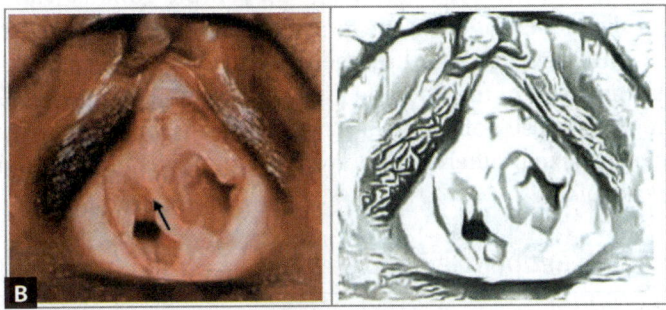

Figs. 35.3A and B: Vaginal septum. (A) Transverse vaginal septum; (B) Longitudinal vaginal septum.

vaginal septum **(Figs. 35.3A and B)** and imperforate hymen. The appearance of external genitalia and the distribution of pubic hair pattern may provide a clue regarding the presence of relevant pathology, for e.g., the typical absence of pubic hair pattern in patients with AIS. The Tanner stages of development of pubic hair must be established on inspection of external genitalia.

Rudimentary or absent uterus can be detected on bimanual examination.

■ DIFFERENTIAL DIAGNOSIS

The various causes of amenorrhea depending upon the compartment involved are described below.

Compartment I

Müllerian Agenesis (Mayer–Rokitansky–Küster–Hauser Syndrome)

Müllerian agenesis may be the probable diagnosis in an individual with primary amenorrhea and no apparent vagina. There is usually an absence or hypoplasia of the internal vagina and an absence of fallopian tubes and uterus. The syndrome occurs due to defect in fusion of the Müllerian ducts, resulting in the absence of proximal one-third of vagina with or without the uterus **(Figs. 35.4A and B)**. Since the ovaries are not Müllerian structures, they are normal.

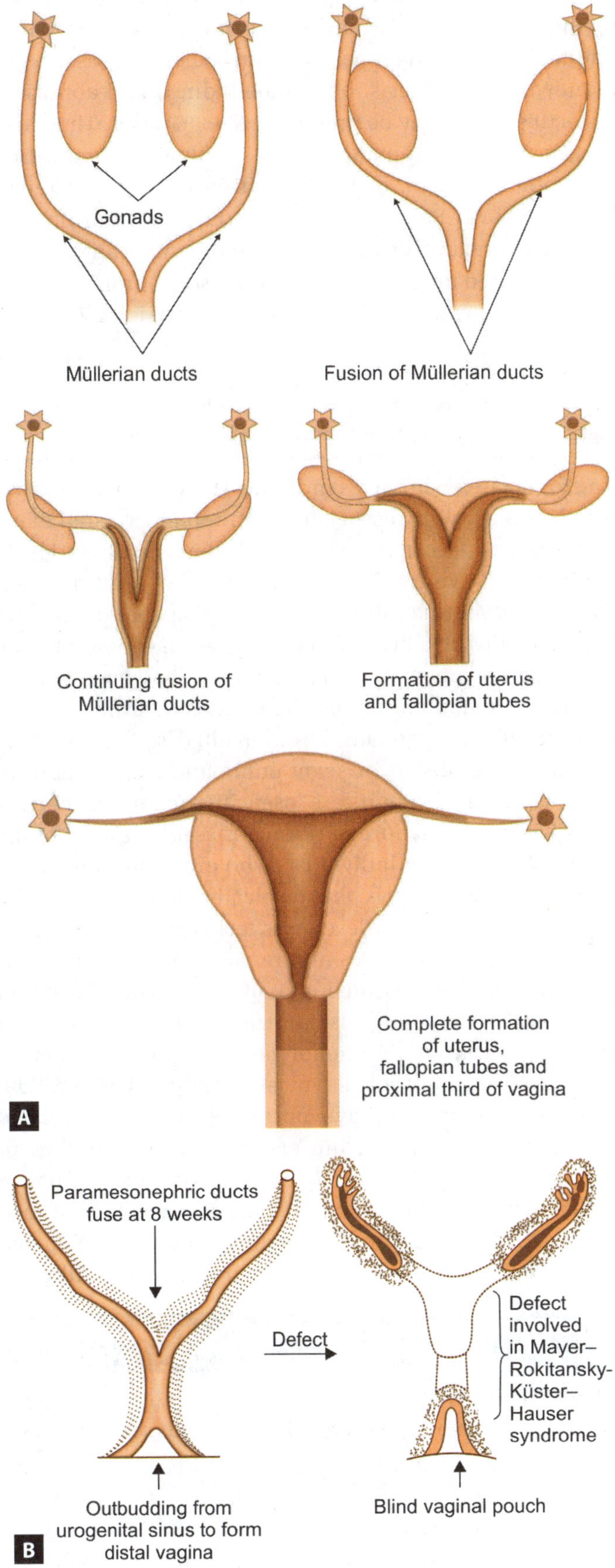

Figs. 35.4A and B: (A) Sequence of embryological development of female gonads; (B) Defect involved in Mayer–Rokitansky–Küster–Hauser syndrome.

The cause of this syndrome is unknown and is probably related to mutations in the gene for anti-Müllerian hormones or the gene for anti-Müllerian hormone receptor. Other anomalies including renal tract anomalies such as ectopic kidney, renal agenesis, horseshoe kidney, and abnormal collecting ducts may be present in 15–30% cases. There can also be skeletal anomalies such as scoliosis, sacralization of lumbar vertebra, or lumbarization of sacral vertebra, hemivertebra. Sometimes, there may be neurological defects. Extirpation of the Müllerian remnants, if any present, is not required unless they are causing some problems such as fibroid growth, hematometra, or endometriosis.

Androgen Insensitivity Syndrome

> **Q.** Write a short essay on testicular feminization syndrome.

Androgen insensitivity syndrome is another condition which is commonly associated with a blind vaginal canal and absent uterus. It was formerly known as testicular feminization syndrome. Patients with this syndrome are male pseudohermaphrodites. This implies that the patient is genetically a male, i.e., has a male karyotype (46XY). Since the karyotype is male, the patient has male gonads or testes. Pseudohermaphrodite implies that the genitalia are opposite of the gonads. The individual is phenotypically a female with absent or scant pubic and axillary hair. In these cases, the receptors are insensitive to androgens, due to which there is failure of normal masculinization of the external genitalia in individuals who are genetically male. As a result, the patient is phenotypically a female. The pubic and axillary hair fail to develop as testosterone is unable to exert its action. The testes may remain undescended. This syndrome can be classified into different grades based on the degree of genital masculinization, varying between grade 1 (normal male phenotype) and grade 5 (external genitalia are those of a typical female) **(Table 35.1)**. Affected individuals have normal testes with normal production of testosterone and normal conversion to dihydrotestosterone (DHT), unlike 5-alpha reductase deficiency (5-ARD), which is characterized by reduced levels of DHT. The transmission of this disease is via X-linked recessive inheritance. The gene responsible for androgen intracellular receptor is defective. A karyotype analysis is required to reach the proper diagnosis in these cases. The female child may present with inguinal hernia because the testes are frequently partially descended.

While the growth and development are normal, there may be a eunuchoidal tendency (long arms, big hands, and big feet). The breasts are developed as testosterone gets converted into estrogens, which stimulate their growth. However, the breasts are abnormal as the glandular tissue is not abundant, nipples are small, and the areolae are pale due to the absence of progesterone. Female internal genitalia (uterus and fallopian tubes) are either rudimentary or absent. In such a patient, the testes may be intra-abdominal or present in the form of hernia. However, even if present, the testes are immature and do not show any spermatogenesis. Due to high incidence of malignancy in the gonads with Y chromosomes, they must be removed at the age of 16–18 years once full development has been attained after puberty. The plasma levels of testosterone are within normal-to-high male range. As a result of failure of action of testosterone, the critical steps in sexual differentiation which require testosterone fail to take place.

5-Alpha Reductase Deficiency

> **Q.** Justify your management of a newborn who on examination is found to have ambiguous genitalia with the help of a long essay.

5-alpha reductase deficiency syndrome with autosomal recessive inheritance is characterized by inability to convert testosterone to the more physiologically active DHT. Since DHT is required for the normal masculinization of the external genitalia in utero, genetic males with 5-ARD are born with ambiguous genitalia (i.e., male pseudohermaphroditism). Some other causes of ambiguous genitalia are summarized in **Box 35.2**.

The condition affects only genetic males (having a Y chromosome) because DHT has no known role in female development. The clinical abnormalities of the disease range from individuals with normal male genital anatomy to underdeveloped male individuals with hypospadias to those with predominantly female external genitalia, most often with mild clitoromegaly. Since these patients have primary female characteristics, they are often raised as girls. At the time of puberty, these individuals often experience amenorrhea and virilization.

TABLE 35.1: Sinnecker's classification of androgen insensitivity syndrome.

Grade	Phenotype
1	Normal male phenotype with impaired spermatogenesis
2	Male genitalia with hypospadias, micropenis, and bifid scrotum (Reifenstein's syndrome)
3	Ambiguous genitalia
4	Female genitalia with virilization such as clitoromegaly and partial labial fusion
5	Complete androgen insensitivity syndrome

BOX 35.2: Causes of ambiguous external genitalia.

- *Congenital adrenal hyperplasia:* The most common cause of congenital adrenal hyperplasia, which can cause ambiguous genitalia, is 21-hydroxylase deficiency in a genetically female infant
- Androgen secreting tumor
- XX females with Mayer–Rokitansky–Küster–Hauser syndrome (absent vagina with or without the uterus)
- 5-alpha reductase deficiency

Asherman's Syndrome

Asherman's syndrome is an important cause of secondary amenorrhea occurring as a result of overzealous postpartum curettage, which can result in the destruction of endometrial lining due to the formation of intrauterine scars. These adhesions can completely obliterate the endometrial cavity, internal cervical os, and cervical canal. The condition can also occur following uterine surgery, including cesarean section, myomectomy, or metroplasty. Besides amenorrhea, patients with this syndrome can present with symptoms such as miscarriage, dysmenorrhea, or hypomenorrhea. The diagnosis and treatment of this condition are by hysteroscopic resection. Following the resection of adhesions, an intrauterine device is inserted inside the uterine cavity in order to prevent the adherence of the raw uterine walls. The uterine cavity can also be distended with the help of a pediatric Foley's catheter, distended with about 3 mL of fluid and removed after 7 days.

Imperforate Hymen

Imperforate hymen occurs as a result of abnormal or incomplete embryologic development.

This condition commonly causes amenorrhea, which is usually associated with cyclical abdominal pain, which tends to worsen over time. If a hematocolpos is present, bluish discoloration is visible behind the translucent membrane **(Figs. 35.5A to C)**.

Compartment II (Disorders of the Ovary)

Turner's Syndrome

> Q. Write a long essay on the diagnosis and management of Turner's syndrome.
>
> Q. Write a short essay describing clinical features and management in case of Turner syndrome.
>
> Q. Explain briefly about Turner's syndrome.

Turner's syndrome is associated with the absence of one X chromosome and is characterized by several dysmorphic features and hypergonadotropic hypoestrogenic amenorrhea **(Box 35.3 and Fig. 35.6)**. An absence of the short arm of X chromosome may be associated with phenotypic features of Turner's syndrome, whereas absence of the long arm may be associated with sexual infantilism. Due to the presence of streak gonads which lack ovarian follicles, no gonadal sex hormones are produced at the time of puberty, and patients present with primary amenorrhea. Karyotype analysis must be done in all cases with elevated gonadotropin levels. Such individuals are short-statured and may have a height below 5th centile.

Pure Gonadal Dysgenesis

As the name suggests, pure gonadal dysgenesis implies only atypical development of gonads in which the reproductive tissue is replaced by functionless tissue called streak gonad. Chromosomal composition is normal, either 46XX or 46XY. Such individuals do not have stigmata associated with Turner's syndrome, and their height is normal. In cases of XY karyotype (known as Swyer's syndrome), there is an abnormality of *SRY* gene. Due to this, there is a presence of dysgenetic or streak gonads, which fail to produce testosterone and Müllerian-inhibiting substance (MIS), thereby resulting in an entirely female phenotype. Such individuals are phenotypically female with sexual infantilism. Due to the risk of future development of carcinoma in the rudimentary gonads, gonadectomy is essential in these cases.

In cases with XX karyotype, streak ovaries are present, which are unable to produce estrogen. Lack of estrogen is unable to inhibit the secretion of FSH or LH. This hormonal imbalance causes failure to initiate puberty, due to which such individuals are unable to experience menstrual

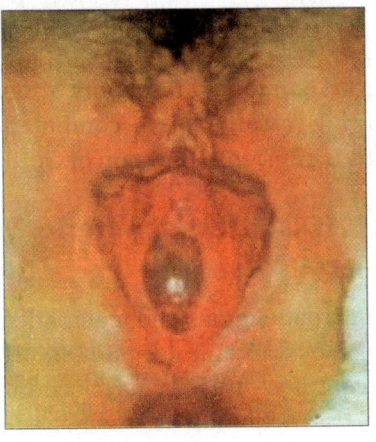
A

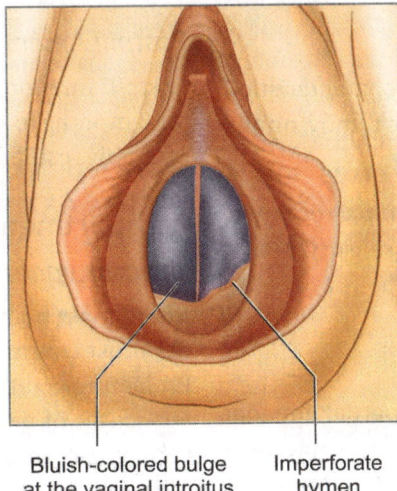
B
Bluish-colored bulge at the vaginal introitus — Imperforate hymen

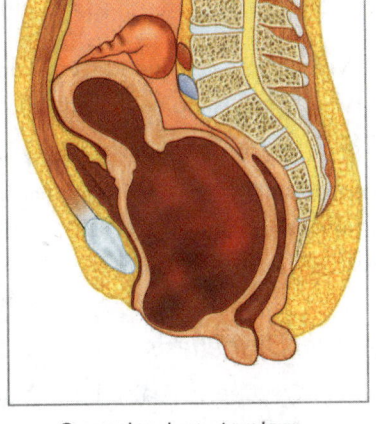
C
Secondary hematocolpos due to collection of menstrual blood behind an imperforate hymen

Figs. 35.5A to C: (A and B) Imperforate hymen; (C) Accumulation of blood in the uterine cavity as a result of imperforate hymen.

BOX 35.3: Stigmata of Turner's syndrome.

Eyes:
- Epicanthal folds
- Strabismus
- Red-green color blindness
- Ptosis
- Amblyopia

Ears:
- Low-set ears
- Sensory—neural hearing loss
- Otitis media

Head/neck/chest:
- Low hairline
- High-arched palate
- Webbed neck
- Shield-like chest
- Widely spaced nipples

Cardiovascular system:
- Coarctation of aorta
- Bicuspid aortic valves
- Aortic root dilatation
- Aortic aneurysm
- Aberrant right subclavian artery
- Persistent left superior vena cava
- Pulmonary venous abnormality
- Long arch of aorta
- Aortic dissection

Skeletal abnormalities:
- Cubitus valgus
- Genu valgum
- Wide carrying angle
- Scoliosis
- Fourth shortened metacarpal
- Dysplastic nails

Renal abnormalities:
- Horseshoe kidneys
- Duplicated renal pelvis
- Hydronephrosis
- Pelvic kidney
- Unilateral renal agenesis

Cancers:
- Endometrium
- Bladder
- CNS

(*Breast carcinoma is typically not seen in these cases*)

Autoimmune diseases:
- Hypothyroidism
- Type 1 diabetes mellitus
- Hepatitis
- Vitiligo
- Celiac disease
- Hashimoto's disease
- Thrombocytopenia

Others:
- Pigmented nevi
- Attention-deficit hyperactivity disorder
- Hypoplastic uterus
- Lymphedema
- Short stature

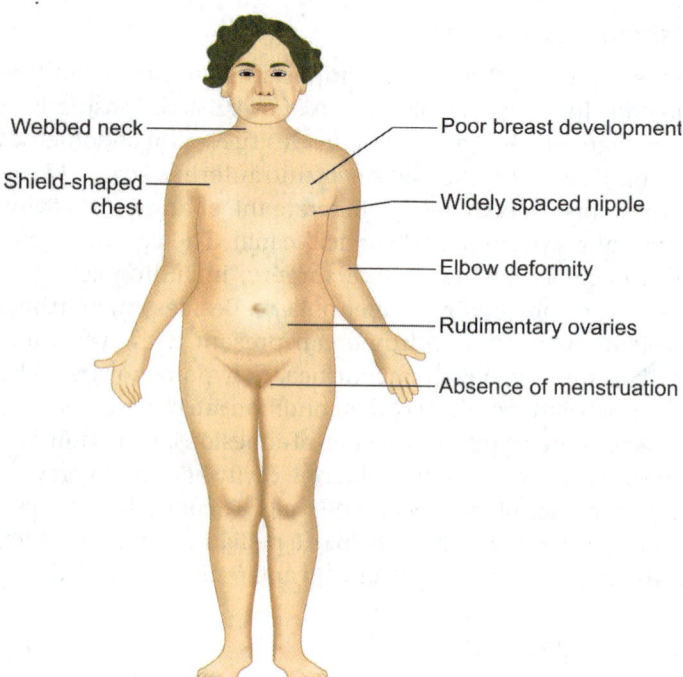

Fig. 35.6: An 18-year-old female with primary amenorrhea who was diagnosed to be suffering from Turner's syndrome.

cycles or development of secondary sexual characteristics. In these cases, there is no requirement for removing the dysgenetic gonad.

Perrault syndrome: This is a rare type of autosomal recessive, pure gonadal dysgenesis (46XX) along with sensory neural hearing loss.

Mixed Gonadal Dysgenesis

Mixed gonadal dysgenesis is also known as partial gonadal dysgenesis or XO/XY mosaicism. Such individuals may have two cell-lines and are characterized by varying degree of testicular dysgenesis, ambiguous genitalia, and the absence of regression of Müllerian structures.

Premature Ovarian Failure

In these cases, the failure of ovarian function occurs prematurely before the age of 40 years. Ovarian failure could also occur as a result of radiation therapy to the pelvis or chemotherapy. There is no risk of POF if the radiation field excludes the pelvis. Chemotherapy drugs, typically alkylating agents (cyclophosphamide, methotrexate, and fluorouracil), are very toxic to the gonads.

Polycystic Ovarian Syndrome

Polycystic ovarian syndrome may be associated with amenorrhea in about 15–20% cases and has been described in detail in Chapter 34.

Postpill Amenorrhea

Postpill amenorrhea is defined as the absence of menstruation for 6 months following cessation of the combined OCPs and probably results from transient inhibition of GnRH.

Compartment III (Disorders of Anterior Pituitary)

Hyperprolactinemia

Adenomas (both microadenomas and macroadenomas) are the most common causes of anterior pituitary dysfunction. Prolactin-secreting pituitary tumors may account for nearly 50% cases of pituitary adenomas. The increased dopamine concentration present in hyperprolactinemic women with pituitary tumors is likely to reduce pulsatile LH secretion and produce acyclic gonadotropin secretion, which most probably results in menstrual irregularities. Patients with pituitary adenomas having markedly elevated prolactin levels (especially those >100 ng/mL) often experience symptoms such as galactorrhea, headaches, and visual disturbances. Imaging with MRI must be done in these patients to rule out pituitary adenomas.

The treatment of these patients comprises the use of the drug bromocriptine (dopamine agonist), which is available in the form of 2.5 mg tablets. A total 5–15 mg of oral dose of bromocriptine may be required. Depot bromocriptine preparations are also available, which must be administered in the monthly dosage of 50–75 mg IM injection. The use of bromocriptine can be associated with numerous side effects such as nausea, headache, fainting due to orthostatic hypotension, dizziness, and fatigue.

Cabergoline is another ergot-derived selective dopamine receptor type-2 agonist, which is initially administered in the dosage of 0.25–0.5 mg once weekly. This can be increased to a maximum of 1 mg twice per week. It is associated with lower rates of side effects in comparison to those associated with bromocriptine. It also has greater potency and longer duration of action, thereby requiring only twice-weekly administration. This drug is effective in individuals who are tolerant or resistant to bromocriptine. In high doses (>3 mg/day), this drug can be associated with side effects such as causation of hypertrophic valvular heart disease. Therefore, cabergoline must be used in lowest possible doses required to normalize serum prolactin concentrations. In individuals who cannot tolerate oral treatment, vaginal treatment proves to be effective and is associated with fewer side effects.

Besides pituitary tumors, other important causes of hyperprolactinemia include the use of medications such as OCPs, antipsychotics, antidepressants, antihypertensives, and opiates. However, in these cases, prolactin levels are raised to levels of <100 ng/mL.

Compartment IV (Defects at the Level of Hypothalamus)

Anorexia Nervosa

Hypothalamic amenorrhea could be associated with anorexia nervosa. These patients with anorexia nervosa are characterized by weight loss of 25% or weight that is 15% below the normal for a particular age and height. Other important features of this disease include denial of the problem by the patient, distorted body image, unusual hoarding or handling of food, and amenorrhea. The patient may indulge in self-induced vomiting in order to lose weight. There are no other underlying medical or psychiatric disorders.

Athletes Amenorrhea

This type of amenorrhea may be encountered amongst women athletes who indulge in intense exercise or are elite athletes. Such women may suffer from a triad of menstrual dysfunction, low mineral density (osteopenia), and low energy availability (with or without an eating disorder).

Summary

The likely causes for primary amenorrhea are described in **Box 35.4** whereas the causes for secondary amenorrhea are described in **Table 35.2**.

BOX 35.4: Differential diagnosis in a patient with primary amenorrhea.

Presence of secondary sexual characteristics:
- *Genitourinary malformation*, e.g., imperforate hymen, transverse vaginal septum, and absent vagina with or without a functioning uterus
- *Müllerian agenesis* (Mayer–Rokitansky–Küster–Hauser syndrome)
- *Androgen insensitivity:* XY female or testicular feminization

Absence of secondary sexual characteristics:
- Resistant ovary syndrome
- Hypothalamic dysfunction, e.g., chronic illness, anorexia, weight loss, and stress
- Gonadotropin deficiency, e.g., Kallmann syndrome
- Tumors of the hypothalamus or pituitary gland
- Hypopituitarism
- Hyperprolactinemia
- Gonadal failure, e.g., ovarian dysgenesis/agenesis, premature ovarian failure
- Hypothyroidism

TABLE 35.2: Differential diagnosis of secondary amenorrhea.

No features of androgen excess	Features of androgen excess are present
• *Physiological*, e.g., pregnancy, lactation, and menopause • *Iatrogenic*, e.g., depot medroxyprogesterone acetate contraceptive injection, radiotherapy, and chemotherapy • *Systemic disease*, e.g., chronic illness and hypo- or hyperthyroidism • *Uterine causes*, e.g., cervical stenosis and Asherman's syndrome (intrauterine adhesions) • *Ovarian causes*, e.g., premature ovarian failure and resistant ovary syndrome • *Hypothalamic causes*, e.g., weight loss, exercise, psychological distress, chronic illness, and idiopathic • *Pituitary causes*, e.g., hyperprolactinemia, hypopituitarism, and Sheehan's syndrome • *Hypothalamic/pituitary damage*, e.g., tumors, cranial irradiation, head injuries, sarcoidosis, and tuberculosis	• Polycystic ovarian syndrome (PCOS) • Cushing's syndrome • Late onset congenital adrenal hyperplasia • Adrenal or ovarian androgen-producing tumor

MANAGEMENT

Q. What is the most likely diagnosis in the case study described in the beginning of the chapter? The karyotype analysis in this case revealed a female pattern (i.e., 46XX). How should the case be further managed?

PRIMARY AMENORRHEA

The first step of management in case of primary amenorrhea is to determine whether the patient has developed secondary sexual characteristics or not. In these patients, the presence or absence of secondary sexual development directs further course of evaluation. Evaluation of the patient with primary amenorrhea is described in **Flowcharts 35.1 and 35.2**.

Secondary Sexual Characteristics Have Developed

If a patient with amenorrhea has experienced normal breast development, but minimal or no pubic hair, the usual diagnosis is AIS (i.e., the patient is phenotypically female but genetically male with undescended testes). In case of genital tract abnormalities, a karyotype analysis is required in order to determine proper treatment **(Flowchart 35.3)**. If testes are present, they should be removed because of the high risk of malignant transformation after puberty.

If a patient has normal secondary sexual characteristics, including pubic hair, the clinician should perform MRI or ultrasonography to determine if a uterus is present. If ultrasound examination shows the presence of a normal uterus, outflow tract obstruction should be considered. An imperforate hymen or a transverse vaginal septum can cause congenital outflow tract obstruction. Imperforate hymen typically results in cyclic abdominal pain due to accumulation of the blood in the uterus and vagina.

If the outflow tract is patent, the physician should continue an evaluation similar to that for secondary amenorrhea. If the uterus is absent or abnormal, a karyotype analysis should be performed to determine if the patient is genetically female. If the patient is genetically a female (46XX), the cause of amenorrhea could be Müllerian agenesis, where there is congenital absence of vagina and abnormal (usually rudimentary) uterine development. If the karyotype is that of a genetic male (46XY), the patient is probably suffering from AIS.

Secondary Sexual Characteristics Have not Developed

If there is an absence of secondary sexual characteristics, estimation for serum gonadotropin levels must be performed. This test helps in diagnosis of two causes

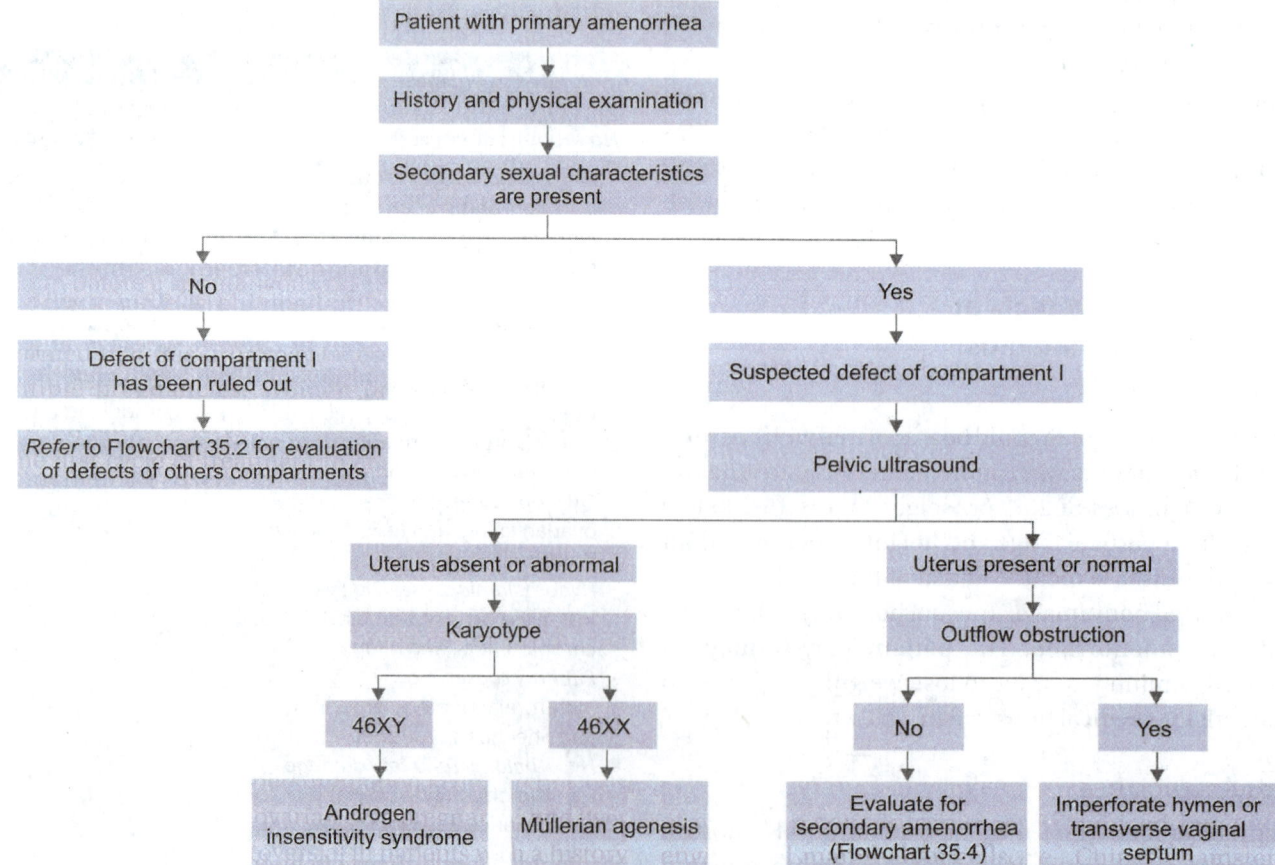

Flowchart 35.1: Evaluation of primary amenorrhea in cases with suspected abnormality of compartment.

Flowchart 35.2: Evaluation of primary amenorrhea in cases with suspected abnormality of compartments II–IV.

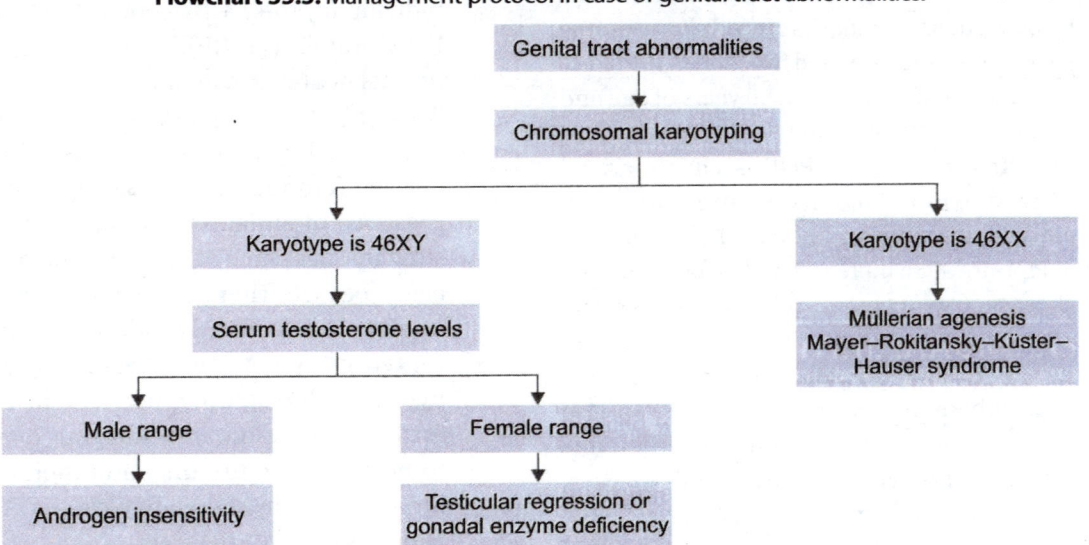

(FMR1: fragile X mental retardation 1; MRI: magnetic resonance imaging; PCOS: polycystic ovarian syndrome; TVS: transvaginal sonography)

Flowchart 35.3: Management protocol in case of genital tract abnormalities.

of amenorrhea: (1) hypogonadotropic hypogonadism and (2) hypergonadotropic hypogonadism. In cases of hypergonadotropic hypogonadism, a karyotype analysis must be performed to determine whether the cause of amenorrhea is related to POF (46XX) or Turner's syndrome (45XO).

Hypogonadotropic Hypogonadism

Hypogonadotropic hypogonadism is associated with low levels of FSH and LH, usually <5 IU/L. This could be related to the abnormalities in the secretion of GnRH, which is commonly due to disruption of the hypothalamic–pituitary–ovarian axis. The important causes for this include constitutional delay of growth and puberty and hypothalamic or pituitary failure. Hypothalamic amenorrhea is often caused by excessive weight loss, exercise, or stress. BMI of <19 (normal range 20–25) has been found to be associated with amenorrhea.

The mechanism by which stress or weight loss affects GnRH secretion is presently unknown.

Kallmann syndrome, which is associated with anosmia, can also cause hypogonadotropic hypogonadism.

Hypergonadotropic Hypogonadism

> **Q.** Write a short essay on fragile X syndrome.

Hypergonadotropic hypogonadism (elevated FSH and LH levels) in patients with primary amenorrhea may be caused by gonadal dysgenesis or POF. These two causes can be differentiated from one another by performing a karyotype analysis.

- *Gonadal dysgenesis:* Turner's syndrome (45XO karyotype) is the most common cause for female gonadal dysgenesis. About 50% have mosaic forms such as 45X/46XX or 45X/46XY. Characteristic physical findings of Turner's syndrome have been tabulated in **Box 35.3**. Individuals with the various forms of gonadal dysgenesis typically present with hypergonadotropic amenorrhea regardless of the extent of pubertal development and the presence or absence of associated anomalies or stigmata. It is well known that cytogenetic abnormalities of the X chromosome can impair ovarian development and function.
- *POF:* Normally, menopause occurs at 50 years of age and is caused by ovarian follicle depletion. Sometimes ovarian failure can occur prematurely. POF is characterized by amenorrhea, hypoestrogenism, and increased gonadotropin levels occurring before 40 years of age. Women with POF are at an increased risk of osteoporosis and heart disease. Two types of inherited enzymatic defects also may be associated with POF. These include 17 α-hydroxylase deficiency and deficiency of the enzyme galactose-1-phosphate uridyltransferase. POF can also sometimes be associated with autoimmune endocrine disorders such as hypothyroidism, Addison's disease, and diabetes mellitus. Therefore, fasting glucose levels, TSH, and, if clinically appropriate, morning cortisol levels should be measured. Diagnosis of ovarian failure is established in the presence of low ovarian estrogen and high serum FSH levels. A karyotype analysis must be performed because surgical removal of the gonads is indicated in any individual in whom a Y chromosome is identified. A karyotype analysis also helps in excluding genetic abnormalities such as chromosomal translocations, deletions, and mosaicism. Some tests for detection of genetic mutation, which need to be done in these cases, include the following:

> **BOX 35.5:** Typical features of fragile X syndrome.
> - Large testis or macroorchidism (in men)
> - Large ears, long narrow face, soft skin, poor eyesight
> - Large body size, square chin, frontal bossing
> - Developmental delays, mental retardation, learning disabilities
> - Delayed speech, rapid repetitive speech, poor conversational skills
> - Good verbal imitative skills
> - Premature ovarian failure (if present in women)

- *Testing for fragile X mental retardation 1 (FMR1) premutations:* Women with POF must be offered testing for FMR1 premutations. This syndrome runs in families and shows X-linked dominant inheritance pattern. It is associated with FMR1 mutations, which cause intellectual disabilities as well as result in typical physical features **(Box 35.5)**.

  Fragile X syndrome is the most common cause for mental retardation, autism. This syndrome results from abnormal expansion of an unstable trinucleotide [cytosine–guanine–guanine (CGG)] repeat sequence in *FMR1* gene located on the long arm of X chromosome. The gene normally contains about 30 CGG repeat sequences. However, in the presence of fragile X syndrome, the number of CGG repeats can be >200. There has been found to be an association between POF and fragile X premutations, characterized by 55–200 CGG repeats. In normal individuals, the *FMR1* gene makes a protein called FMR protein (FMRP). This protein is required for normal neural development.
- *Testing for antiadrenal antibodies (anti-CYP21):* Ovarian failure may be sometimes due to Addison's disease (autoimmune adrenal insufficiency). The presence of antiadrenal antibodies (antiCYP21) is strongly suggestive of autoimmune oophoritis as the cause of POF. Therefore, women with POF require careful evaluation to exclude adrenal insufficiency.
- *Imaging:* When no clear-cut explanation for hypogonadotropic hypogonadism can be found, further evaluation with imaging may be required to help exclude tumors and differentiate between pituitary and hypothalamic causes. The method of choice is usually MRI scan.

SECONDARY AMENORRHEA

The management plan of a patient with secondary amenorrhea is described in **Flowchart 35.4**. The first step

Flowchart 35.4: Management plan of a patient with secondary amenorrhea.

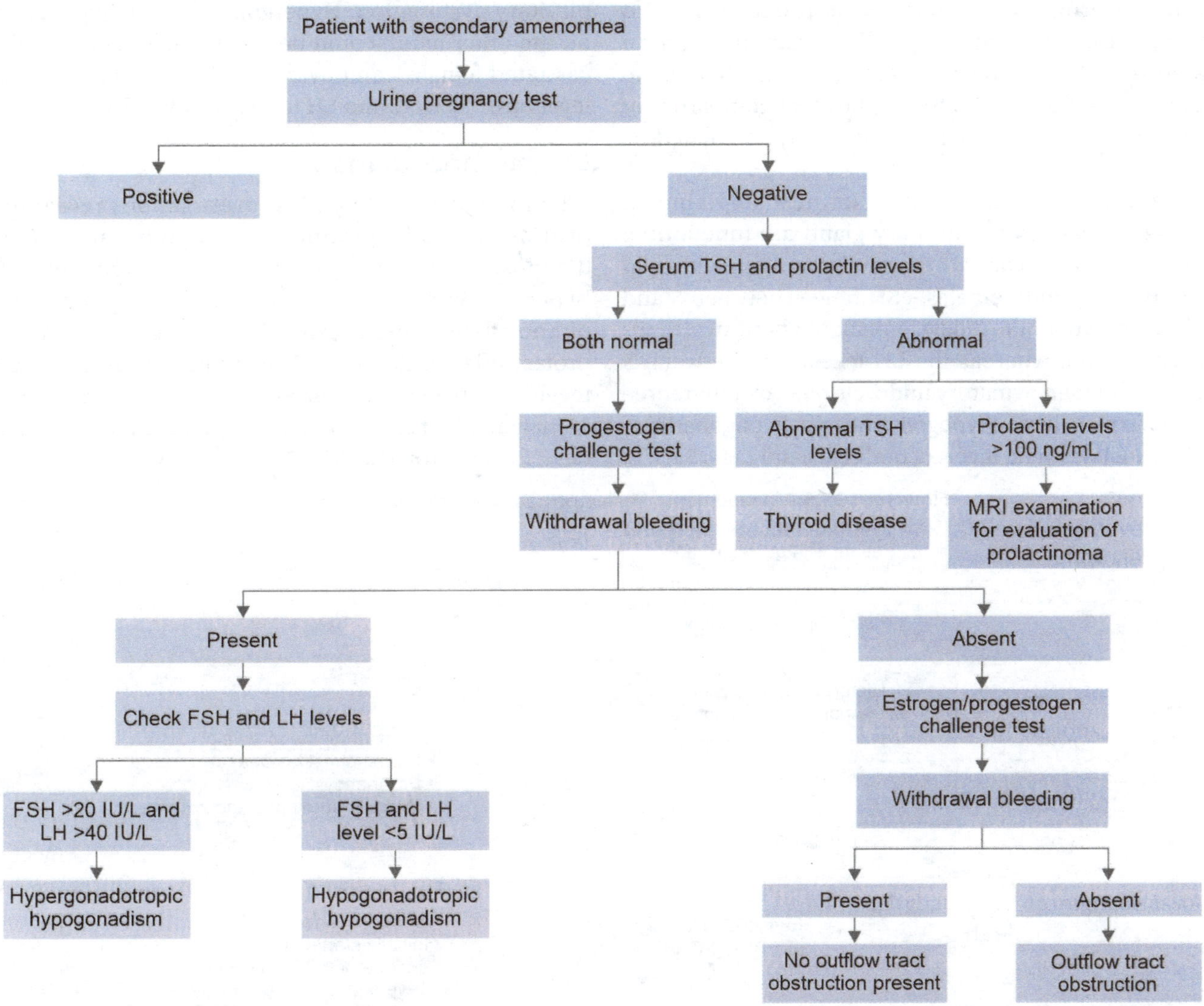

in the management of patients with secondary amenorrhea is to rule out pregnancy because that is the most common cause of secondary amenorrhea. Once the pregnancy has been ruled out, the initial workup involves measurement of TSH and prolactin levels and a progestin challenge test. In case the patient with amenorrhea also presents with galactorrhea, imaging of sella turcica may also be required. Hypothyroidism may also produce galactorrhea by reducing the levels of dopamine (a prolactin inhibitory substance). Hypothyroidism also causes unopposed thyrotropin-releasing hormone (TRH) production, resulting in stimulation of pituitary cells, which produce prolactin.

The progestin challenge test can be performed using the following:

- 200 mg of parenteral progesterone in oil
- Oral micronized progesterone in the dose of 300 mg daily
- Medroxyprogesterone in the dosage of 10 mg daily for 5 days
- *Micronized progesterone gel (4–8%):* Intravaginal application for at least six applications

Following 2–7 days of conclusion of a progestin challenge test, the patient either does or does not bleed. If the patient bleeds, the diagnosis of anovulation can be established. The presence of bleeding confirms the presence of a functional outflow tract and a uterus lined by reactive endometrium prepared by endogenous estrogens. Significant hyperandrogenemia associated with anovulation and PCOS is an important cause of amenorrhea, which responds to the progestin challenge test. Chronic unopposed exposure of the endometrium to endogenous estrogens can serve as a risk factor for the development of endometrial cancer. At the minimum, these women must be prescribed a progestational agent (5 mg daily) for the first 2 weeks of each month in order to reduce the risk of development of endometrial cancer. OCPs can be given in case contraception is desired.

If withdrawal bleeding does not occur in response to progestational medications, there can be two causes: (1) either the outflow tract is not patent or (2) the endometrium has not been adequately prepared by endogenous estrogens. In order to differentiate between the two, orally active estrogens (1.25 mg of conjugated estrogens) must be administered for at least 21 days. An orally active progestational agent (10 mg of medroxyprogesterone) can be added in the last 5 days to achieve withdrawal bleeding. If no withdrawal bleeding occurs even after the addition of estrogens, amenorrhea is probably related to a defect in compartment I (outflow tract and uterine endometrium). If withdrawal bleeding occurs, there is no defect in compartment I. It also implies that compartment I has normal functional activities, if properly stimulated by estrogens.

If withdrawal bleeding occurs, the next step aims at finding if the ovaries and pituitary gland are functioning normally or not. This involves the assay of serum gonadotropin levels. In normal adult females, FSH ranges between 5 and 20 IU/L, with ovulatory midcycle peak of about two times the baseline level, whereas the LH levels vary between 5 and 40 IU/L, with an ovulatory midcycle peak of about three times the baseline level. Hypogonadotropic hypogonadism, which is associated with levels of both FSH and LH < 5 IU/L, could be due to prepubertal state and hypothalamic or pituitary dysfunction. Hypergonadotropic hypogonadism, on the other hand, could be due to postmenopausal state, castrated females, and ovarian failure. In these cases, FSH levels are >20 IU/L and LH levels are >40 IU/L.

Chronic Anovulation

When the results of various investigations reveal normal ovarian estrogen production and normal FSH levels, diagnosis of chronic anovulation is established. Since hyperprolactinemia is one of the most common causes of anovulation and amenorrhea, measurement of serum prolactin levels is done. Measurement of serum prolactin levels is especially important in cases with galactorrhea. Management of an amenorrheic patient with galactorrhea is described in **Flowchart 35.5**.

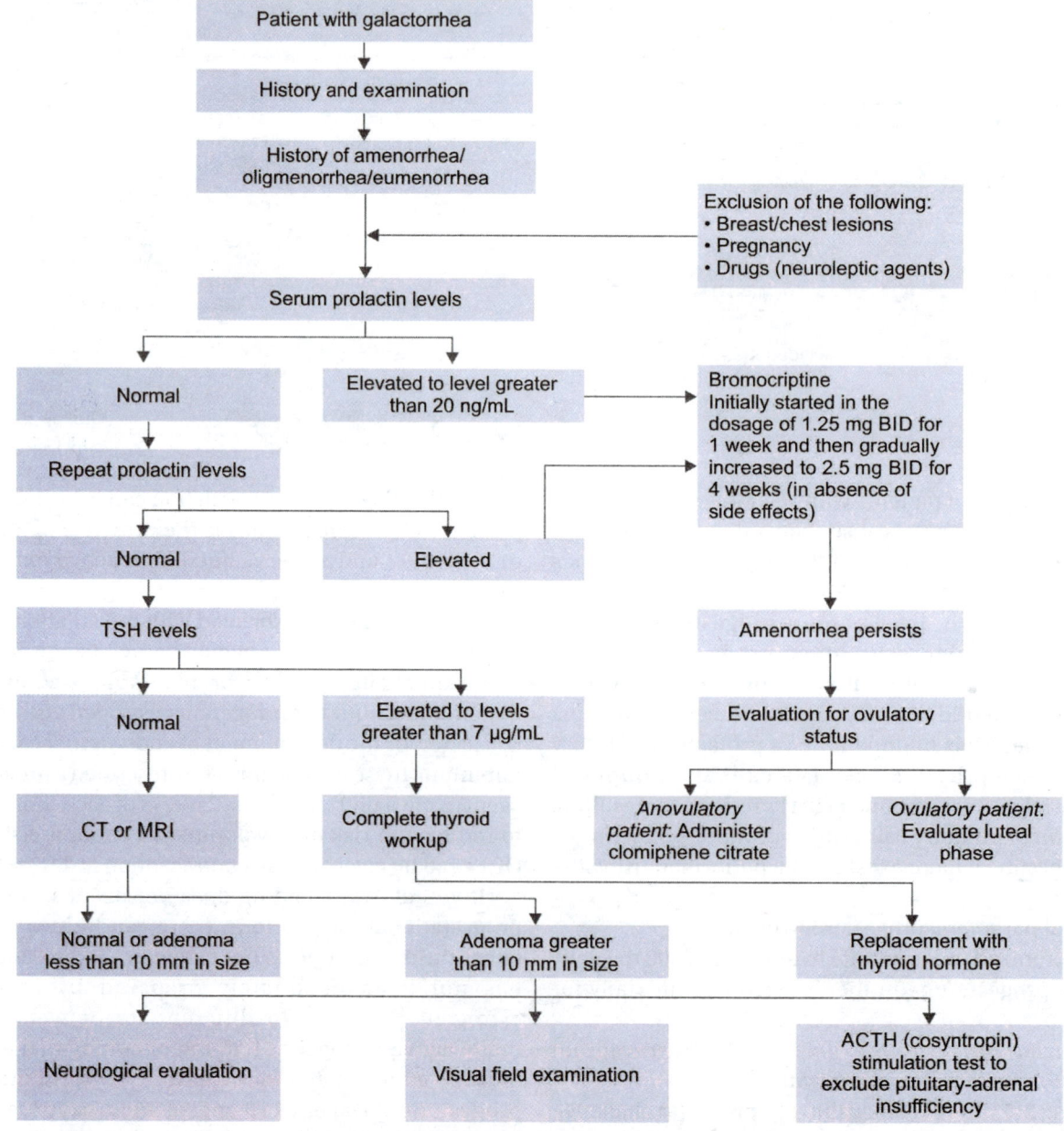

Flowchart 35.5: Management of galactorrhea in an amenorrheic patient.

(ACTH: adrenocorticotropic hormone; CT: computed tomography; MRI: magnetic resonance imaging; TSH: thyroid stimulating hormone)

Since thyroid disorders are also easily identifiable and treatable, measurement of serum TSH concentration is also justified in all women with amenorrhea. Other likely causes of anovulation, besides thyroid and prolactin disorders, include PCOS and obesity. Women with PCOS usually have signs of hyperandrogenism due to which they can easily be identified.

A normal random prolactin measurement of 15–20 ng/mL is helpful in excluding hyperprolactinemia. Mildly elevated prolactin levels (20–40 ng/mL) are best repeated and confirmed before the diagnosis of hyperprolactinemia is made. Once intake of some medicines (causing galactorrhea) have been ruled out as a cause of hyperprolactinemia, further evaluation with MR imaging is required in women with amenorrhea and hyperprolactinemia to exclude pituitary tumors or hypothalamic mass lesions.

Women with chronic anovulation are likely to progress to hyperplasia, atypia, and cancer within a short duration of time due to unopposed estrogen stimulation. At the minimum, these women require periodic treatment with progestins to induce menstruation and provide protection against the risk of developing endometrial cancer.

INVESTIGATIONS

Various investigations and the reasons for conducting them have already been discussed in the text. Those investigations would be merely enumerated here.

KARYOTYPING

Karyotype analysis is important for identifying the patient's genetic sex.

SERUM TESTOSTERONE/ANDROGEN LEVEL

Women with PCOS may have mildly raised level, while women with androgen-secreting tumors of the ovary or adrenal gland may have high levels of serum testosterone.

GONADOTROPIN LEVELS (FSH AND LH)

Measurement of gonadotropin levels helps in differentiating between hypogonadotropic and hypergonadotropic causes of hypogonadism. Low level of gonadotropins is associated with hypogonadotropic hypogonadism, while high level of gonadotropins is associated with hypergonadotropic hypogonadism.

SERUM PROLACTIN LEVELS

Serum prolactin levels may be raised in women with prolactinomas.

THYROID FUNCTION TESTS

Thyroid function tests are indicative of thyroid dysfunction, which could be the possible cause of amenorrhea.

EVALUATION OF OVARIAN FUNCTION

Abnormalities in ovarian function are the most common causes for amenorrhea. Some methods for assessing ovarian estrogen production include measurement of serum estradiol levels, bioassays of estrogen production (based on the amount and character of cervical mucus), progestin challenge test, or measurement of endometrial thickness using TVS.

Bioassay of Cervical Mucus Production

Assessment of ovarian function can be done through the evaluation of cervical mucus characteristics. Estrogenic cervical mucus is clear, watery, relatively abundant and suggests normal estrogen production.

Progestin Challenge Test

Administration of a pure progestational agent [medroxyprogesterone acetate (MPA) 10 mg daily for 5–7 days or progesterone in oil, 200 mg IM] will induce menses in women having normal circulating estrogen concentration. A positive test indicated by the presence of bleeding within 2–7 days after completion of progestin treatment implies normal estrogen production and ovarian function. Negative test, implying no withdrawal bleeding, suggests hypogonadism. Scant spotting suggests marginal levels of endogenous estrogen production by the ovaries.

Measurement of Endometrial Thickness using TVS

Endometrial thickness as determined by TVS is a measure of endometrial proliferation. This is reflective of the levels of estrogen produced by the ovaries. Also, measurement of endometrial thickness using TVS can help identify individuals with chronic anovulation at risk of having associated pathology such as endometrial hyperplasia or cancer.

Serum Follicle-stimulating Hormone Concentration

Normal or low FSH levels (**Table 35.3**) are indicative of functional ovarian follicles and may be observed in a variety of conditions associated with amenorrhea including chronic anovulation, (e.g., PCOS), pituitary diseases, and

TABLE 35.3: Interpretation of serum gonadotropin levels.

Clinical state	Serum FSH (IU/L)	Serum LH (IU/L)
Normal adult woman	5–20	5–40
Hypogonadotropic state	<5	<5
Hypergonadotropic state	>20	>40

(FSH: follicle stimulating hormone; LH: luteinizing hormone)

hypothalamic dysfunction. A high serum FSH concentration is a reliable indicator of ovarian follicular depletion or failure. One or more repeated measurements of FSH levels are warranted to confirm the findings of a single examination.

 TREATMENT/GYNECOLOGICAL MANAGEMENT

The treatment of primary and secondary amenorrhea is based on the causative factor, especially in cases of primary amenorrhea. It involves management of three aspects: menstrual function, sexual function, and reproductive function. Treatment goals include prevention of complications such as osteoporosis, endometrial hyperplasia, and heart disease; preservation of fertility; and, in case of primary amenorrhea, progression of normal pubertal development.

MAYER-ROKITANSKY-KÜSTER-HAUSER SYNDROME

Treatment of the condition usually involves progressive dilatation using Frank's dilators. Initially, the dilatation is begun in the posterior direction, and then after 2 weeks it is changed to the upward direction in the line of vaginal axis. This must be performed daily for 20 minutes to the point of modest discomfort. By utilizing increasingly larger-sized dilators, a functional vagina can be created within a period of several months. Operative treatment is used in patients in whom Frank's method is unacceptable or fails. It is important for the gynecologist to provide adequate reassurance and support in these cases.

Adequate counseling helps in avoiding problems with altered body image, which are likely to develop in these cases. The woman also needs to be counseled that she would not be able to have her periods. Creating an artificial vagina either through the use of Frank's dilators or surgical procedure (McIndoe's vaginoplasty) at the time the patient plans to get married helps in ensuring that she and her partner would be able to obtain adequate sexual enjoyment following their marriage. Having regular sexual intercourse helps in maintaining the patency of newly created artificial vaginal orifice. Though the patient remains infertile, she can lead an almost normal life. Genetic offspring can be achieved by collecting oocytes from genetic mother, fertilizing them with sperms obtained from genetic father, and their placement in a surrogate carrier.

McIndoe's vaginoplasty appears to the best option for creating a vaginal opening. In these cases, transverse incision is administered at the lower end of labia minora. Dissection is done below the plane of bladder and rectum, and the median raphe is cut to obtain a better depth of the vagina. A mold covered with split skin graft used to be placed in the original procedure. However, the modified McIndoe's procedure involves placing a mold covered with intercede (oxidized cellulose). Amongst the recently used laparoscopic techniques, the Davydov's procedure is one of the most common techniques used in which the vesicorectal space is coated with peritoneum. This appears to be a safe and effective surgical method for patients with MRKH syndrome, provided self-dilatation is practiced postoperatively. Vecchietti's technique is another procedure which has been tried and comprises laparoscopic pull-up technique wherein size of vagina is increased gradually by applying traction over the vaginal vault. Ileal vaginoplasty has also been tried but was associated with excessive vaginal discharge and risk of infection, therefore not being used commonly nowadays. William's surgery comprises suturing the labia together to create a pouch.

TURNER'S SYNDROME

Treatment of individuals with Turner's syndrome includes the following:

- *Hormone replacement therapy (HRT):* It helps develop the patient's uterus and achieve normal reproductive function with donor oocytes. Therapy with low-dose estrogen (0.025 mg/day of transdermal estradiol or 0.3–0.625 mg of conjugated estrogens or estradiol valerate, 0.5–1 mg orally) must be initiated. Progestins such as MPA in the dose of 5–10 mg or micronized progestogens in the dosage of 200 mg orally can be added for 12–14 days every 1–2 months to prevent endometrial hyperplasia.
- *Growth hormone:* Its use is likely to improve her height and is administered in the dosage of 0.375 mg/kg body weight (in seven divided doses). Growth hormone is usually administered prior to 8 years of age, before the closure of epiphysis. Once the epiphysis closes, growth hormones will usually not have much effect. Administration of growth hormone is stopped once height of 150 cm is achieved.
- *Donor ovum:* It can be used for attaining reproductive function.

ANDROGEN INSENSITIVITY SYNDROME

Vaginoplasty or creating an artificial vagina helps the patient attain sexual functioning. She will not experience menstrual cycles and would require adoption for reproductive function. Gonadectomy to remove the rudimentary testis will help prevent development of future malignancy. In complete AIS, gonadectomy must be done after 16–18 years of age to take complete benefit from the hormones produced. Testosterone produced by rudimentary gonads gets converted into estrogens, which help in breast development.

HYPOTHALAMIC AMENORRHEA

Treatment of hypothalamic amenorrhea depends on the etiology.

Anorexia nervosa: Women with excessive weight loss should be screened for eating disorders and treated accordingly if anorexia nervosa or bulimia nervosa is diagnosed. Menstrual cycles usually return after a healthy body weight has been achieved.

In patients with amenorrhea caused by eating disorders or excessive exercise, the use of OCPs or menopausal hormone therapy may decrease bone turnover and partially reverse bone loss. However, neither therapy has been shown to significantly increase the bone mass. Adequate calcium and vitamin D intakes are recommended for these patients.

Hyperprolactinemia: Microadenomas are slow-growing and rarely malignant. Treatment of microadenomas should focus on management of infertility, galactorrhea, and breast discomfort. A prolactin-producing microadenoma usually responds to treatment with dopamine agonists. A dopamine agonist can help improve the symptoms of amenorrhea and fertility. Bromocriptine, a dopamine agonist, is the most commonly used drug for treatment and has been discussed previously in the text. Trans-sphenoidal surgery may be an option for women with large macroadenomas (>3 cm) or those who are resistant to treatment with dopamine agonists.

POLYCYSTIC OVARIAN SYNDROME

Treatment of PCOS has been discussed in detail in Chapter 34.

THYROID DYSFUNCTION

Hypothyroidism is treated using thyroid preparations such as levothyroxine sodium (e.g., Eltroxin).

HYPOPITUITARISM

Hypopituitarism is associated with generalized deficiency of various hormones. In these cases, thyroid replacement therapy should not be instituted until adrenal function has been assessed and treated. Serum gonadotropin and gonadal steroid levels are typically low in cases of hypopituitarism. In cases with hypopituitarism where oocytes are still present, ovulation can be induced with exogenous gonadotropins when pregnancy is desired. Human menopausal gonadotropin (hMG) is the treatment of choice for patients with primary amenorrhea due to hypopituitarism. In order to prevent the risk of ovarian hyperstimulation syndrome, hMG should be started at the minimal dose (75 IU SC qd for 7 days). Exogenous pulsatile GnRH may also be used to induce ovulation if the disorder is hypothalamic. When pregnancy is not desired, signs and symptoms of estrogen deficiency can be prevented by instituting maintenance therapy with cyclic estrogen and progestogens.

PREMATURE OVARIAN FAILURE

Treatment in women with POF comprises the following:
- Psychological and emotional support
- Appropriate genetic counseling (especially in cases of FMR1 premutations)
- Appropriate monitoring in patients with autoimmune diseases
- *Treatment with exogenous estrogens:* In the absence of endogenous estrogens, women with POF are at an increased risk for developing complications such as osteopenia, osteoporosis, and early coronary heart disease. They may also develop symptoms of estrogen deficiency such as vasomotor flushes and genitourinary atrophy. Treatment with oral estrogens (micronized estradiol, 1–2 mg daily or conjugated equine estrogens 0.625–1.25 mg daily) or transdermal estrogens must be undertaken in these women. Since most of these women also have an intact uterus, cyclical treatment with progestogens (micronized progesterone, 200 mg daily or MPA 10 mg daily) for 12–14 days each month serves as a useful option for prevention of endometrial hyperplasia/malignancy, etc., in women still hoping to conceive.

COMPLICATIONS

Certain complications, which may be present in the patient with amenorrhea, are mentioned in the following text.

OSTEOPOROSIS

Women with amenorrhea associated with estrogen deficiency are at significant risk of developing osteoporosis. This increased risk persists even if normal menses are resumed. Estrogen deficiency is of particular concern in younger women as a desirable peak bone mass may not be attained. The use of HRT, calcium, and vitamin D preparations in these patients may prove to be useful.

CARDIOVASCULAR DISEASE

Young women with amenorrhea associated with estrogen deficiency may also be at an increased risk of developing cardiovascular disease, hypertension, and type 2 diabetes in future.

ENDOMETRIAL HYPERPLASIA

Women with amenorrhea having unopposed estrogen secretion (without an associated progesterone secretion) are at an increased risk of developing endometrial hyperplasia and endometrial carcinoma (see Chapter 23).

INFERTILITY

Women with amenorrhea generally do not ovulate and are usually infertile.

PSYCHOLOGICAL DISTRESS

Amenorrhea often causes considerable anxiety, because it may cause women to start having concerns regarding the loss of fertility, or loss of femininity. The diagnosis of Turner's syndrome, testicular feminization, or Müllerian agenesis can be traumatic for both the girls and their parents.

EVIDENCE-BASED CLINICAL TRIALS

List of references can be scanned through QR code to enable the readers gain deeper insight of the subject by referring to the entire article or its abstract.

Index

Page numbers followed by *b* refer to box, *f* refer to figure, *fc* refer to flowchart, and *t* refer to table

A

Abdomen 157, 694, 751
  general examination of 12
  inspection of 12, 66, 102*b*
  palpation of 103*b*
Abdominal circumference 297, 301, 302
  ultrasound measurement of 303*f*
Abdominal examination 12, 32, 61, 66, 102, 110, 114, 145, 158, 170, 190, 231, 257, 268, 299, 322, 340, 348, 365, 421, 452, 471, 495, 520, 670, 695, 717, 753
Abdominal hysterectomy 531, 532, 549, 550, 550*t*, 706
  types of 532
Abdominal lump 466, 685
  causes for 685*b*
Abdominal pain 99, 157, 193, 230, 374, 466, 500*f*, 594, 716, 727
  differential diagnosis for 159*b*
Abdominal palpation 13, 66, 90, 102, 299, 300, 341
  diagnostic accuracy of 299
  Leopold's maneuvers of 17
Abdominal sacral colpopexy 660, 660*f*
Abdominal skin incision, types of 215, 215*f*
Abdominal vaginal method 115, 115*f*
Abdominal wall 473
  mobility of 472
Abdominovaginal delivery 119, 119*f*
Ablation 679
Abnormal ovarian reserve test 785
Abnormal uterine bleeding 486, 487*t*, 497, 498, 499*b*, 501, 506, 507, 525, 546, 623, 689
  conservative management of 545
  differential diagnosis of 496*b*
  management of 497*fc*, 498*fc*, 526
ABO
  classification 187
  compatibility 147
  system 187, 187*t*
Abortion 4
  complete 718
  incomplete 718, 724
  recurrent 245
  septic 139, 751
  threatened 231
  tubal 714
  unexplained 260
Abruptio placentae 155, 161*fc*, 163, 381, 382
Abruption 268, 319, 367
  complications of 162*b*
  fetal complications of 162
  incidence of 165
  maternal complications of 162
  recurrence of 163

Acardiac fetus, umbilical cord of 185
Acardiac twin 184
  categories of 185
  types of 186
Accurate gestational age, estimation of 341, 343
Acid-fast bacilli, assessment of 503
Actaea racemosa 563
Actinomycin 241, 690
Activated partial thromboplastin time 165, 254, 262, 269
Acute ectopic pregnancy 716*b*
  diagnosis of 718
Add-back therapy, use of 528
Addison's disease 802
Adenocarcinoma 621, 687
  in situ 607, 636
  papillary 687
Adenofibroma 687
Adenoma 798
  malignum 621
Adenomyoma 739, 742
Adenomyosis 521, 523, 739, 745, 739*f*, 740-742, 742*f*
  diagnosis of 741, 742, 742*f*
  focal 521, 744
  histopathological appearance of 739*f*
  uteri 741
Adenosarcoma 621
Adherent placenta 225, 293
  management of 293
  types of 293*t*
Adhesions
  barriers, use of 536*f*
  development of 536
  lysis of 773
  prevention of 679
Adjuvant therapy 679
Adnexa 767
Adnexal lesion, evaluation of 696
Adnexal mass 520*t*
  scoring system 701*t*
Advanced epithelial ovarian cancer 696
Advanced glycation end product 389
Adverse reproductive outcomes, causes of 618*b*
Alanine
  aminotransferase 359, 363
  transaminase 356
Alcohol 27, 255, 780
  consumption, excessive 752
Alkali hematin method 267
Alkaline phosphatase 497
  levels of 557
Allen stirrups 540
Allergic reactions 439
Allis forceps 220*f*
Alloimmune factors 252
Alpha-fetoprotein 298, 335
  presence of 335

Alpha-hydroxyprogesterone caproate 326
Alpha-methyldopa 378
Alpha-reductase deficiency 796
Alzheimer's disease 554
Ambiguous external genitalia, causes of 796*b*
Amenorrhea 466, 689, 716, 750, 792, 796, 807, 808
  hypothalamic 793, 807
  postpill 798
  primary 798*f*, 799*b*, 800
  secondary 96, 122, 792, 802, 903*fc*
  type of 799
Amino metabolites, production of 576
Amniocentesis 183, 195, 196
Amniotic cavity 309*t*
Amniotic fluid 373, 402
  amount of 309
  analysis 196
  changes 339
  index 301, 342, 373, 406
  levels 309
    assessment of 181
  measurement of 309
  volume 28, 309, 309*t*
    assessment of 175
Amniotic sacs 173*f*
Amniotomy 63
Amnisure test 335
Amoxicillin 274, 326, 457, 583
Ampicillin 335, 457, 577, 586
Amsel's criteria 575*b*, 576
Anal incontinence 468
Anal sphincters, repair of 290*f*
Analgesia 275
  epidural 59, 101, 211, 329
Analgesics 676
Anaphylactoid shocks 439
Ancylostoma duodenale 431
Androblastomas 687
Androgen insensitivity syndrome 796, 796*t*, 806
Androgen
  levels 759, 777, 805
  signs of 753, 793
Androgenic agents 678
Android pelvis 100
Androstenedione 757
Anembryonic gestation 231
Anemia 145, 155, 180, 325*t*, 417, 418, 423, 425, 427, 427*t*, 471, 518
  adverse effects of 440
  causes of 421*fc*, 427
  correction of 432
  cytometric classification of 418*t*
  development of 420, 471, 520
  diagnosis of 270, 428*fc*
  dimorphic 423, 426
  grading of 417, 418*t*
  hemolytic 165*f*, 423, 426, 427, 430, 431*f*

identification of 214
macrocytic 425
management of 270
megaloblastic 425, 426, 430, 430f
microcytic 423
  hypochromic type of 427
mild 418
moderate 427
multifactorial etiology of 423f
normochromic normocytic 422
physiological 421
postpartum 436
prevention of 149
severe 427, 432
signs of 169, 520
Angiogenesis inhibitors, incorporation of 709
Angiogenic factors 368
Angioneogenesis 668
Angiotensin 377
  converting enzyme 3, 377
    inhibitors 445
  infusion test 367
  receptor blockers 375
Anisocytosis 429
Ankle clonus 365
Anogenital infection, uncomplicated 586
Anorexia nervosa 793, 799, 807
Anovulation, chronic 491, 804
Antenatal card 24, 42, 315, 454
Antenatal management 192, 454
Antenatal period 149, 175, 312, 401t
Antepartum fetal surveillance 27, 28fc, 341
Antepartum hemorrhage 142, 147, 180, 195, 208, 299, 315, 320, 348, 459
  causes of 142fc
  complications 152
  extraplacental causes of 147
Antepartum period 195
Antepartum vaginal bleeding 146
  causes of 158
Anterior anal laceration 290
Anterior colporrhaphy 656
  principles of 656
Anterior shoulder, delivery of 56f
Anterior vaginal mucosa 264f
Anterior vaginal wall
  points 650
  retractor 478f
Anthropoid, presence of 100
Antiadrenal antibodies, testing for 802
Antiangiogenetic drugs 668
Antianxiety agents 558
Antiarrhythmic medicines, use of 455
Antibiotic 407
  prophylaxis 214, 329, 457t, 766
  therapy 326
  use of 584
Antibody, measurement of 191
Anticardiolipin 253
  antibodies 252, 255, 259
Anticoagulants 491
  regimen, types of 459
Anti-D antibodies 192t
Anti-D immunoglobulins 138, 195b, 195t, 237
  mechanism of action of 195f
Antidepressants 558
Antifibrinolytics 276

Antifungal 578
  drugs 578
  therapy, topical 578t
Antiglobulin test 193f
Antihypertensive agents 370, 375
Antihypertensive drugs 372
  use of 375
Antihypertensive therapy 369, 386
Anti-Müllerian hormone 758
  receptor 796
Antioxidants 366, 367, 613
Antiphospholipid 253
  antibody 245, 252
    complete profile of 262
    syndrome 252f, 253, 254, 257, 261
  syndrome 255t, 257, 362
  classification of 255
Antiplatelet agents 312
Antiprogestins 529
Antiprogestogen 350, 678
Anti-Rh antibodies 188, 194
Antiseptic solutions, use of 291
Antithrombotic drugs 366
Antithrombotic therapy 312
Aorta, coarctation of 449, 453
Aortic clamp 289f
Aortic compression, application of 289f
Aortic regurgitation 445
Aortic stenosis 446, 453, 461
Aortocaval syndrome 444
Aortopathy 460
Apgar scores, low 85
Appendectomy 688
Appendicitis 551
Appendix 667
Appetite, loss of 518
Aquamocolumnar junction, identification of 597f
Arcus tendineus
  fascia 644
    pelvis 662
  rectovaginalis 644
Arm prolapse 96, 96f
Aromatase inhibitors 679, 744, 778
Arrhythmia 449, 460
Arterial perfusion 181
Arteriolar diameter 366
Arteriolar smooth muscles 377
Arteriovenous anastomosis 182f
Artery disease, coronary 448
Artificial intrauterine insemination 772
Arzoxifene 564
Ascaris lumbricoides 431
Ascites 550, 695
  presence of 473, 694, 695
Ascorbic acid 366
Asherman's syndrome 141, 248, 259, 285, 755, 767, 797
Ashkenazi jews 762
Aspartate aminotransferase 359, 363
Aspermia 764
Aspiration pneumonitis, prevention of 214
Aspirin 367
  high-dose 460
  low-dose 260, 262, 460
Assisted breech vaginal delivery 79
  steps of 77f

Assisted fertilization techniques 785
Assisted hatching 786
Assisted reproductive techniques 453, 684, 692, 716, 780, 788
  use of 169
Asthenozoospermia 764
Asynclitism
  anterior 53f
  posterior 53f
Atelectasis 347f
Atenolol 375, 381
Athletes amenorrhea 799
Atonic postpartum hemorrhage, management of 271, 274
Atonic uterus 267, 267f
  causes of 267
  medical management of 274
  treatment of 281
Atrial contraction 309f
Atrial fibrillation 458
Atrial septal defects 449
Atrophic vaginitis 581
Atrophy 550, 556, 788
Auscultation 102, 171, 474
Autoantibodies, target of 254
Autoimmune disease 362, 798
Autoimmune disorders 367
Axillary hair development 793
Ayre's spatula 601f
Azithromycin 583
  use of 584
Azoles 578
Azoospermia 763, 764, 785b
  diagnosis of 763

B

Back ache, severe 158
Bacteria
  adherence of 576
  anaerobic 139
  Calymmatobacterium granulomatis 586
Bacterial vaginosis 140, 574-576, 594
  Amsel's diagnostic criteria for 575b
  diagnosis of 576
  screening for 325
  treatment of 247
Baden-Walker halfway system 641, 641t, 649
Bagel's sign 721f
Balloon tamponade 278
Bandl's ring 114f, 121
  development of 121f
  presence of 114
Barium enema 702, 703
Basal body temperature 771
  method 771f
Basic PALM-COEIN classification system 487fc
Bearing down sensation 648
Benign ovarian tumor 521, 694
  diagnosis of 696
  management of 696
Benzodiazepines 380
Beta-2 glycoprotein 254
Beta-adrenoceptor agonists 406
Beta-agonists 333
Beta-blockers 375, 445, 458
  use of 455

Beta-human chorionic gonadotropin 497, 498, 719, 725, 728, 730
   discriminatory zone of 719
   levels 232
Betamethasone 406
Betamimetics 332
   drugs 403
   tendency of 403
Beta-receptor blockers 377
Beta-thalassemia, pathogenesis of 424f
Bethesda system 604b
Bevacizumab 709
Biguanide compound 399
Bimanual pelvic examination 590, 671
Bimanual uterine
   compression 274f
   massage 274
Bimanual vaginal examination 479, 480f
Bimastoid diameter 50
Biochemical markers, concentration of 448
Biophysical profile 27, 28, 175, 301, 302, 304, 310, 311, 342, 343
   components of 311f
   modified 311
Biophysical tests 303
Biopsy 502, 557, 558, 584, 624, 702
Biparietal diameter 50, 301, 302
   ultrasound measurement of 302f
Bipolar radiofrequency 548
Birth
   injuries 122
   mode of 402
   spacing 27
   trauma 345
   weight 5
Bishop's score 115
   assessment of 115
   modified 39t
Bisphosphonates 566, 567t
Bispinous diameter 46
Bitemporal diameter 50
Bituberous diameter 46
Bivalent cervarix 611
Björk–Shiley mitral valve, mechanical 456
Black cohosh 563
Bladder 154, 637
   catheterization 136
   edematous 97f
   injury 252
Blastocyst 229f
Bleeding 152, 419, 622
   absence of 518
   acute 242
   amount of 145, 488, 489
   anovulatory 490
   causes of 273
   cessation of 529
   disorders 194, 496
   duration of 139, 489
   episode of 143
   excessive 272
   extraplacental causes of 142
   higher risk of 461
   intraoperative 617
   intraventricular 317
   mechanism of 267
   nature of 488
   occurrence of 145
   pathophysiology of 155
   pattern of 490
   per vaginum 146
   postoperative 617, 618
   severe 149, 162
   types of 145
   uncontrollable 532
Bleomycin 690
Bloating, abdominal 694
Blocking antibodies 252
   absence of 253f
Blood
   accumulation of 797f
   adult unit of 201
   cellular indices 428
   characteristics of 145, 200, 201
   clotting disorders 158
   coagulation, homeostatic regulation of 253
   flow 288f, 309f
      redistribution of 418
   glucose
      assessment 395f
      levels 257, 395
      testing 404
      values 393
   group 187, 187t, 188t, 190, 230, 231, 190, 257
      A 187
      AB 187
      B 187
      O 187
      typing 718
   index 425, 429
   investigations 369, 395
   loss 269, 269t, 294, 419, 423, 516
      abnormal 520
      amount of 159, 266, 489
      excessive 155, 471, 493
      postpartum, estimation of 267
      total 237
      volume of 486
   pressure 190, 363, 363f, 450, 470, 471, 495
      diastolic 362f
      measurement of 556
      reading, measurement of 364
      systolic 362f
   smear, normal 430f
   sugar
      estimation of 557
      fasting 394
      transfusion 281, 386, 432
         indications of 432
         reaction 294
   urea 370, 652
   vessels
      appearance of 608f
      normal 608f
      vasoconstriction of 418
   volume 201, 444
      calculation of 200
      restoration of 273
B-lynch compression sutures 283, 284, 284f
   application of 284f
B-lynch square sutures, modified 284
Body
   mass index 25t, 299, 315, 321, 362, 410, 493, 519, 556, 631, 692
   surface area 730
Bone
   densitometry, process of 558f
   health 564
   marrow
      density 565f
      examination 431, 432b
      findings 432b
Bonney's approach 534
Bonney's hood 534
   approach 535f
Bonney's myomectomy clamp 533
Bony pelvis, deformities of 61
Borderline tumors, epidemiology of 688
Boric acid capsules 579
Bovine hemoglobin concentrate 435
Bowel mesentery 707
Bowl metastases 694
Brachial plexus
   anatomy of 415f
   injuries 414
   left-sided 411f
Brachytherapy 634
   application of 635f
Brain
   injury, ischemic 315
   sparing effect 306f
Braxton hicks contractions 8, 9
Breast 11f, 491, 695
   cancer 555, 561, 569
      high-risk factors for 558
   changes 716
   development, staging of 471
   exact site of 11
   examination 11f, 471, 495, 623, 752, 794
   lump, detection of 495
   ovarian cancer syndrome 692
   Tanner stages of 794f
Breastfeeding 27, 201, 579
Breathing exercises 222
Breathlessness 450
Breech
   complete 65
   delivery, spontaneous 76
   engagement of 76f
   extraction
      reverse 119, 119f
      total 76
   gestation 67f
   position of 65f
   presentation 65-68, 68fc, 86t
      causes of 66
      fetal risk factors for 66
      intrapartum management of 78fc
      types of 65f, 67, 86
   vaginal delivery 72b, 76, 79b
      mechanism of 76f
      types of 76
Brenner's tumors 686, 687
Brisk knee jerks 372
Broad ligament hematoma 715
Broad spectrum antibiotics 274
Brow presentation 109, 111, 111f
Bullous edema, presence of 509
Burns–Marshall technique 75, 81, 81f
Buserelin 528, 782
Butoconazole 578

C

Cabergoline 799
Caffeine 255
　consumption 780
Calcium 367, 559
　antagonist 381
　channel blockers 332
Caldwell and Moloy's classification 42f
Campylobacter jejuni 139
Cancer
　advanced stage of 623
　antigen 125 743
　　serum 673
　cachexia 623, 695
　cells, exfoliation of 691
　cervix 596, 619, 633f
　deposits 704f
　develops, type of 691
　genome atlas classification 510
　grading 628
　gynecological 465
　high-grade 705
　low-grade 705
　moderate-grade 705
　nonendometrioid 513
　ovaries 691, 697
　routes of spread of 628b
　stage 707fc
Cancerous lesions, previous history of 622
Candida
　albicans 579
　　wet mount preparation of 577f
　infection 577, 577b
　organisms, diagnosis of 593
　vulvovaginitis 578t
　　indications of 591
Cannon ball appearance 235, 236f
Capillary blood glucose levels 403
Captopril 381
Carbetocin 275
Carbohydrate metabolism 391t
Carbon dioxide
　embolism 550
　transportation of 417f
Carbonyl iron 437
Carboplatin 511
Carboprost 274
Carcinoma 777
　cervix 142
　　laparoscopic surgery in 634
　embryonal 687
　endometrium 513
　　management of 508
　　staging of 508
　　treatment of 513
　in situ 596, 604, 626
　ovaries, staging of 699t
Carcinosarcoma 621
Cardiac apex, point of 451
Cardiac complications 460b, 460t
Cardiac decompensation 442
　signs of 445
Cardiac disease 453, 453b, 460, 461
　severe 375
Cardiac dysfunction, preexisting 449
Cardiac lesions
　acquired 445
　congenital 445

Cardiac surgical interventions 453
Cardinal–uterosacral ligament complex 644
Cardiomyopathy, hypertrophic 458
Cardiorespiratory diseases 420
Cardiotocographic examination 160
Cardiotocography 28, 302, 304, 314
Cardiovascular disease 441, 567, 807
　development of 447
　high risk for 554
Cardiovascular disorders, acquired 447
Cardiovascular drugs 366, 458f
Cardiovascular health after maternal placental syndromes 447
Cardiovascular system 421, 443, 798
　examination 474
　exact site of 451
Carneous degeneration 551
Carnett's sign 670, 671f
Cefazolin 457
Ceftriaxone 121, 457
Cells
　free fetal DNA 196, 197
Cellular fibroids 552
Cellular hyperplasia, process of 295
Central nervous system 360, 458
　complications 338
Central venous pressure 273, 375
Cephalexin 457
Cephalic index 302
Cephalic presentation 341
　types of 40f
Cephalopelvic disproportion 112, 112t, 117b, 118, 176, 205
Cephalosporin, third-generation 121
Cerclage
　contraindications for 251
　indications for 251
　procedures, types of 327
Cerebral artery
　anterior 306
　Doppler analysis 373
Cerebral hemorrhage 381, 382
　development of 382
Cerebral palsy 202, 317, 337
Cerebroplacental ratio 297, 309, 314
Cervarix 611
　use of 612
Cervical biopsy 610f
Cervical canal 485
Cervical cancer 610, 619, 621f, 622f, 628, 629, 629fc, 630fc, 636, 638t
　changes, management of 624
　detection of 599
　downstaging of 628
　early-stage 629
　histologic diagnosis of 625b
　magnitude of 620
　morphological progression of 598f
　pathology of 619
　preinvasive 597
　prevention of 610
　screening 599, 604
　　protocol for 599
　　tools for 600fc
　specimen of 620
　spread of 628
　staging 626, 630
　　system for 626t

　treatment of 629, 636
　vaccination against 622
Cervical cells
　precancerous 599
　preparation of 607
Cervical cerclage
　classification of 327t
　role of 327
　use of 327
Cervical condylomata 599
Cervical conization 626
Cervical culture 504, 593, 673
Cervical cytology 703
Cervical dilatation 38, 38f, 61, 119
　normal 110
Cervical discharge 750
Cervical dysplasia 751
　progression of 597f
Cervical epithelium, normal 598f
Cervical erosions 146
Cervical extension 513
Cervical factor
　evaluation of 764
　infertility 754
　treatment of 772
Cervical fibroids 532
Cervical glandular intraepithelial neoplasia 602
Cervical incompetence 141, 245, 248, 251f, 263, 326, 334
　development of 250b
　management of 263
　presence of 320
　test for 260
　treatment for 250
Cervical inflammation 618
Cervical intraepithelial neoplasia 596, 597, 597f, 602, 604
　treatment of 617
Cervical lacerations 141, 416
Cervical length 326
　measurement of 322, 324f
　ultrasound assessment of 323
Cervical malformations 321
Cervical mass 624f
Cervical mucus 7
　ferning pattern of 755f
　production, bioassay of 805
　thickening of 787
Cervical pathology, screening for 468
Cervical plasticity, loss of 618
Cervical polyps 488
　presence of 142
Cervical pregnancy 737
　diagnostic criteria for 725b
Cervical punch biopsy forceps 610f
Cervical ripening 59
Cervical softening 9f
Cervical squamous epithelium 598
Cervical stenosis 618, 755
Cervical surgery 618b
Cervical tears 291, 467
Cervical trauma 136, 321
Cervical tuberculosis, diagnosis of 624
Cervicitis, severe 599
Cervicography 609
Cervicopexy, abdominal 658
Cervix 8, 9, 154, 622, 751, 766
　adenocarcinoma of 636

anatomical location of 620f
complications, adenocarcinoma of 637
fungating growth of 622f
incompetent 250
laser vaporization of 616f
malignant tumors of 621t
per speculum examination of 269f
premature dilatation of 618
pulling anterior lip of 264f
surface of 608f
transvaginal sonography of 625f
ulcerative growth of 622f
visual inspection of 604
Cesarean birth 205b
Cesarean delivery 95, 120, 145, 210b, 213t, 221b, 225t, 329, 382, 448
   advantages of 212b
   alternative techniques for 222
   classification of 213
   disadvantages of 212
   indications for 109b, 204, 344b, 403b
   previous 224t
   timing for 178, 212
Cesarean scar
   over abdomen, previous 13f
   pregnancy 725b, 737
   previous 224
Cesarean section 95f, 109, 119, 162, 178, 204, 204b, 205, 207fc, 220, 314
   classical 223
   hemostatic 222
   indications for 74b, 178, 204b, 374, 384b, 456b
   lower segment 153
   previous 204
   rate of 206
   second stage of 119
   steps of 217f, 219f
   surgery for 214
   time of 152b
Chadwick's sign 8
Chancroid 587
Chaperone 465
Chemoradiation 634
   therapy 631
Chemotherapy 238, 631, 635, 708
   drugs 752, 798
   high-dose 241
   indications for 240, 708b
   side effects to 712
   types of 709
Chest 798
   examination 695
   pain 450
     acute history of 450
     pleuritic 450
   X-ray 235, 236f
Chlamydia 140, 247, 256, 269, 335, 582, 590, 593, 760, 750
   antibody 768, 769
   trachomatis 136, 319, 573, 765, 769
     life cycle of 582f
     screening tests for 765
   treatment of 583
Chlamydial infection 582-584
   clinical features 582
Chlorpromazine 380
Chocolate cysts 666

Chorioadenoma destruens 242
Chorioamnionitis 63, 159, 267, 268, 334, 337, 594
Choriocarcinoma 228, 242, 687
   gestational 242
Chorioepithelioma 242
Chorionic sacs 172f
Chorionic villus sampling 261
Chromosomal abnormality 203
   presence of 245
Chromosomal defects 181
Chromosomal disorders
   occurrence of 175
   screening for 175
Chronic pelvic pain 665
   causes of 666t, 674
   management of 673fc
Cilial epithelium 761
Circulatory collapse 294
Cisplatin 241, 631, 690
   use of 632
Citalopram 559
Clamping cord 56
Claviceps purpurea 275
Clavulanate potassium 326
Cleidotomy 414
Clindamycin 577
   phosphate vaginal cream 594
   use of 584
Clomiphene 744
   citrate 265, 751, 775, 777, 780, 787
   use of 686
Closed mitral valvuloplasty 446, 447
Clostridium welchii 351
Clotrimazole 578
Clubfoot 181
Clue cells 592
   presence of 576
Coagulation 355
   disorder 492, 519
   factors, study of 496
   pathways 164fc
   profile 231, 269
     abnormal results of 165t
   restoration of 273
Coagulopathy 487
Coelomic epithelium 686
Coelomic metaplasia, theory of 667
Cold-knife conization 614
Coliforms 139
Colonoscopy 674, 703
Color Doppler ultrasound 87f
Colostrum, antenatal banking of 405
Colpocleisis
   advantages of 661b
   procedure of 662f
Colpoperineorrhaphy 656
Colporrhaphy, posterior 656
Colposcopic directed biopsy 599, 609
Colposcopic examination 607f, 625
Colposcopy 607, 617
   indications for 608b
   management 602fc
Columnar epithelial cells 585
Complete blood count 231, 255, 496, 497, 521, 673, 718, 729, 730
Complex tubal adnexal mass 721f

Computed tomography 239, 804
   examination 485
   scan 703f
Conception, abnormalities in 747
Condom
   catheter 280
     insertion of 280f
   tamponade 280
   use of 613
Cone biopsy 614, 614f, 615f, 631
Congenital malformations 181b, 407, 767
   screening for 401
Conization 617
Conjoined twins 170f, 171f, 185
   types of 170f
Conjugated equine estrogen 530, 807
Conjunctiva, lower palpebral 10f, 420f
Connective tissue
   disorders 460, 461
Constriction ring 114
Continuous maternal blood pressure monitoring 372
Contraception 27, 238, 454, 491, 558, 750
   types of 467
Contractions
   grading duration of 36t
   strength of 34
   stress test 28
Controlled cord traction 270, 271f
Controlled ovarian hyperstimulation 783
Contusions 416
Coombs test, indirect 349
Cor pulmonale 460
Cord
   accidents 348
   clamping 329
   entanglement 186, 186f
     risk of 71
   presentation 204
   prolapse 86, 86f, 87f, 337, 348
     causes of 86, 86t
     incidence of 86, 86t
     management of 86, 87fc
Cordocentesis 195, 198
   procedure of 199f
   risks of 198
Cornual block, bilateral 765f
Cornual ectopic pregnancy 722f
Cornual ostium 765
Cornual pregnancy 726b
Coronavirus disease vaccination 26
Corpus cancer syndrome 492, 494
Corpus luteum 468
   cysts 686
Corticosteroid 386, 391, 579
   therapy 329, 333
   use of 402
Corticotropin-releasing hormone 319
Coumadin 262
Couvelaire uterus 163, 163f
Coyne spoon 120
Cramp, abdominal 577, 637
Cranial bones, collapse of 349
Craniopagus twins, autopsy specimen of 170f
Creatinine, serum 370
Crown-rump length 301, 340
Cryosurgery 614
Cryptozoospermia 764

Cul-de-sac 671, 682f
  obliteration of 655, 667, 669
Culdocentesis 724
  procedure of 724f
Culdoplasty 655
Cullen's sign 472
Cusco's speculum 146, 477, 478, 478f
  insertion of 478
Cushing's syndrome 794
Cyanosis 450
Cyclical rectal bleeding 667
Cyclooxygenase 743
Cyclophosphamide 241, 690
Cyst
  functional 685, 701f
  stool examination for 430
Cystadenocarcinoma, papillary 687
Cystadenofibroma 687
Cystadenoma 687
  papillary 687
Cystic degeneration 551
Cystic fibrosis 408
  screening for 762
Cystic ovarian neoplasm 234
Cystitis, interstitial 666
Cystocele 556, 642f
  moderate 642f
  repair, procedure of 657f
Cystostomy 531
Cystourethritis 637
Cytoflowmetry 232
Cytokines 425
  role of 319t
Cytologic screening 599
Cytological analysis 603
Cytological tests 584
Cytomegalovirus 200, 298
Cytoreduction 707
Cytoreductive surgery 706, 708
  procedure of 707b
Cytosine 802

D

Dabigatran 459
Dactinomycin 240, 241
Daily fetal movement count 27, 300, 312, 342, 343, 371, 373
  chart 175
Danazol 527, 530, 678, 681, 743
Danish Osteoporosis Prevention Study 568
Das' four categories 185
Dawn phenomenon 399
Debulking surgery 706
Deep transverse arrest 104
  causes of 104b
Deep transverse perineal muscle 644, 645, 645f
Deep vein thrombosis 254, 458
Degenerated menstrual endometrium, reflux of 667
Dehydroepiandrosterone 758, 779
  sulfate 340, 757, 758, 779
Delivery 329
  deciding time of 327, 335
  decisions 314
  expected date of 3
  method of 5
  mode of 71, 152, 177, 316, 350, 370
  route of 647
  time of 177, 198, 199, 313, 330, 344, 373, 440
Delphi consensus criteria 296
Dementia 569
Denosumab 567
  binds 567
Deoxyribonucleic acid 581, 600, 608, 729
Dermoid cyst 700f
Desvenlafaxine 559
Detemir 398
Diabetes
  classification of 388
  control of 261
  education 397
  effect of 401b
  mellitus 246, 362, 388, 389fc, 392, 395, 402, 403t, 404t, 406, 802
    complications of 389fc
    disorders of 388t
    gestational 180, 388, 390, 393t, 394, 396, 398f, 399, 403b, 405, 405t, 406, 406t, 408b, 409
    insulin dependent 388
    noninsulin-dependent 388
  pregestational 407
  triad of 467
Diabetic ketoacidosis 388, 407
  development of 407b
  management of 407b
Diagonal conjugate, measurement of 45, 45f
Diamniotic dichorionic
  pregnancy 174f
  twins 172f, 173f
Diamniotic monochorionic monozygotic twin pregnancy 167
Diathermy 526, 679
Diazepam 380
  use of 380
Diazoxide 376, 377
Dichorionic diamniotic twin gestation 178
Dietary iron, absorption of 434b
Dietary salt restriction 455
Diethylstilbestrol 256, 258, 725, 750
Diffuse adenomyosis 744
  presence of 539
Digoxin 455, 458
Dihydralazine 380
Dihydrotestosterone 796
Dilatation and curettage 497, 498, 503, 505
  advantages of 504b
  complications of 504b
  indications for 504b
Dilated veins, presence of 471
Dilute Russell viper venom time 254
Dilute vasopressin 533
Dinoprostone, use of 210
Direct antiglobulin test 193f
Disseminated intravascular coagulation 156, 159, 163, 163fc, 164b, 165, 165f, 165t
  causes of 164
  common sign of 164
  treatment of 165
Distal tubal obstruction 774
Distant metastasis 699
Distress, psychological 808
Diuretics 455
  use of 376b
Dizygotic twin 166, 167t, 168f
  formation of 167f
Dominant follicle 756, 767
  presence of 484f
Donor insemination 787
  indications for 787
Donor ovum 806
Donovanosis 586
Dopamine
  agonist 799
  infusion 375
Doppler analysis, arterial changes on 309
Doppler blood flow 701t
Doppler study 304t
  types of 304
Doppler ultrasonography 28, 235
Doppler ultrasound 148, 196, 305f
  principle of 305f
Doppler waveforms, types of 28f
Double-rimmed gestational sac 22f
Douglas pouch 694, 707, 721f, 722f, 724, 724f, 753
Dowager's hump 565
Down's syndrome 26, 175
Doxycycline 583
Doyen's retractor, insertion of 216, 217f
Dual energy X-ray absorptiometry 558
Ductus venosus 302, 308f, 309f, 314
  blood flow in 308f
  Doppler 307
Dührssen's incision 85f
Dydrogesterone 260
Dye, bilateral spillage of 765f
Dyschezia 739
Dysfunctional uterine bleeding 486, 498
Dysgerminoma 687, 690
Dyskaryosis, low-grade 603
Dysmaturity syndrome 345
Dysmenorrhea 466, 518, 527
  congestive 466
  severe 684
Dyspareunia 467, 589, 739, 750
  severe 684
Dysphagia 419, 596
Dysplasia
  bronchopulmonary 318
  mild 596, 617
  moderate 597
  presence of 599
  severe 597
Dysplastic cervical changes, complication of 617
Dyspnea 363, 450
  acute onset of 450
  exertional 450
  severe 450
Dystocia 60, 204
  dystrophy syndrome 114
Dysuria 589

E

Early pregnancy 231
  symptoms of 169
Ears 798
Eclampsia 275, 365, 374, 381, 382, 384b
  complications of 381
  management of 382, 383fc

ominous features of 383, 384b
prevention of 382
treatment of 382
Ectopic adnexal mass, chronic 715
Ectopic endometrial glands, growth of 740f
Ectopic pregnancy 195, 482, 713, 713f, 714f, 715-718, 718t, 719, 721, 721f, 723, 724, 728fc, 738, 767, 788
classical 714
course of 714, 714f
diagnosis of 719fc, 722t
differential diagnoses of 717t
expectant management of 728b
implantation of 713t
laparoscopic management of 733
left-sided 722f
management of 727, 733
occurrence of 714f
persistent 737, 738
presence of 138
rupture of 733, 737
sac 731
treatment of 729b
tubal 722f, 734, 736f
types of 737t
unruptured 717, 724f
Edema 370
peripheral 450, 451
pitting 11f
presence of 451
testing for 11f
Eduard Gratacos criteria 314t
Edwards' syndrome 175
Ehlers-Danlos syndrome 460, 461
Eisenmenger's syndrome 453, 460
Ejaculatory failure 784b
Ejaculatory sexual dysfunction 771
Ejection fraction 453
Elective cesarean section 74, 206, 211, 213
preparations for 214
Elective single embryo transfer 789
Electrocoagulation 614
Electrosurgery, use of 536
Elemental iron, amount of 436, 437t
Elevated liver enzymes 360, 373, 374
Eltroxin 807
Embolism, pulmonary 255, 450
Embryo
culture of 789
number of 780
transfer 716, 783
Embryonic sex cords 688
Emergency cesarean section 75
indications for 152b, 316b
Emergency delivery, indications for 152
Empty uterine cavity 725
Empty uterus 721, 721f
Enalapril 381
Encephalopathy, neonatal 317
End-diastolic flow, absent 297
Endemic infection, management of 435
Endocarditis, infective 450
Endocervical canal 251f, 615, 765
Endocervical curettage 626
Endocervical glandular involvement 509
Endocervical mucosa 686
Endocervical stromal sarcoma 621
Endocervix 792

Endocrinopathy 495
Endodermal sinus tumor 687, 690
Endometrial ablation 530, 545-547, 547f, 549, 550b
indications for 546b
methods 548
procedures for 547b, 549f
techniques 545, 547
use of 547b
Endometrial adenocarcinoma 499f
Endometrial adhesions, laparoscopic excision of 683f
Endometrial aspiration 504, 504f, 558
procedure 504
Endometrial biopsy 501, 503-505, 767, 768
complications of 503, 503b
histological findings on 502
indications for 502b
Endometrial cancer 486, 492, 500b, 508-510, 511f, 512t, 525, 569, 694, 741
adjuvant therapy for 511
classification for 510
diagnosis of 488b, 741
differentiation of 510b
gynecological management of 508
management of 508, 511
pathology of 508
predisposing factors of 508
prognostic risk groups of 509
protective factors for 495b
risk factors for 493, 494b
screening for 505, 508
staging of 509, 509t
subgroups of 510
surgical management of 511t
syndromes, hereditary 492t
type 1 488t
type 2 488t
Endometrial carcinoma 467, 488, 494fc, 499f, 501, 509, 551, 552, 689
high-risk 510
Endometrial cavity 533, 675, 767
distortion of 756
Endometrial cycle, secretory phase of 468
Endometrial fertility index 680
Endometrial glands 469, 470
Endometrial histopathology 504
Endometrial hyperplasia 488, 505, 552, 569, 741, 777, 807
classification of 506t
diagnosis of 741
management of 507, 507fc
Endometrial inflammation 553
Endometrial malignancy 490
Endometrial polyp 488, 501f, 516, 523, 741
Endometrial resection 549, 550, 550t, 502, 542, 546, 557
Endometrial sampling 558
procedure of 502
Endometrial surface 682f
Endometrial thickness 485
measurement of 499, 805
Endometrial tumors 686
Endometrioid cancer 621
Endometrioid endometrial cancer 510
Endometrioid intraepithelial neoplasia, histopathological appearance of 506f
Endometrioid tumors 687

Endometrioma, malignant transformation of 667
Endometriosis 466, 468, 482, 666, 670, 672, 676fc, 680, 680b, 682b, 684, 715, 740, 741, 750, 760, 761t, 788, 796
associated pain 679
treatment for 676
deep infiltrating 684
development of 669
etiopathogenesis of 667
excision of 679
immunity for 667
indications of 682
infertility in 680
lesions of 674b
management of 668, 674
mild 761
minimal 761
moderate to severe 671
nonclassic 760
occurrence of 667
origin of 667
pathogenesis of 667
severe 761
small nodules of 674
staging of 675, 676t, 677f
surgery 679
treatment of 675, 684, 780
type of 761
Endometriotic lesions 666f, 669, 760
ablation of 683f
Endometritis 618, 755
postpartum 594
Endometrium 470, 503, 686
early proliferative phase 484
functional layer of 470
layer of 468, 546f
lumen of 485
proliferative 469f
secretory phase 470f
thickened 501t
transcervical resection of 545, 548, 548f
Endomyometrial ablation 745
Endothelial dysfunction 360, 368
Endothelium 355
Enterocele 641, 642f
Enzyme
aromatase 744, 778
linked immunosorbent assay 255, 583
Epidural analgesia 59, 101, 211, 329
administration of 60f
Epinephrine 439
Episiotomy 268, 290, 329
mediolateral 58, 268
Epithelial cell 592
abnormalities 604
adhesion molecule 492
Epithelial ovarian cancer 692, 694t, 708, 708b
diagnosis of 705
Epithelial ovarian carcinoma 696
Epithelial tumors 686
different types of 686
unclassified 687
Erb's palsy 415
Erectile dysfunction 752
Ergometrine 275
stimulant action of 275
Ergot alkaloids 275

Erythroblastosis fetalis 189, 202
   clinical manifestations of 202
Erythrocytes, escape of 407
Erythromycin 583, 586
Escherichia coli 544, 573
Estradiol levels 468
Estriol 391
Estrogen 560
   cardioprotective mechanisms of 568b
   cream 562
   deficiency 561
   dominance 740
   exogenous 488, 807
   levels of 647, 767
   measurement of levels of 558
   plus progestin trial 568
   replacement therapy 683
   secreting ovarian tumors 494
   status 589
   therapy 559
Ethamsylate 527
Etoposide 242
European Menopause and Andropause Society 568
European Society for Radiotherapy and Oncology 509
European Society of Hysteroscopy Classification of Myomas 538f
European Society of Pathology 509
Exablate 2000 system 545
Exchange transfusion 201
   procedure of 201
Exercise 25, 366, 397, 761
Exophytic endometrial cancer growth, hysteroscopic appearance of 505f
External anal sphincter 644
   repair, technique of 290
External aortic compression 288
   application of 289f
External ballottement 7, 7f
External beam radiotherapy 632
External cephalic version 68, 69t, 93
   complications of 71, 94, 95b
   contraindications for 93t
   prerequisites for 69, 93
   procedure 70, 93
   timing for 69
External parasitic twin 181
External radiation therapy 635
External suture, placement of 655f
External version score 71, 71t
Extraovarian primary cancers 696
Extrauterine pregnancy 10t
   diagnosis of 720
Extremities, exact site of 753
Eye 798
   examination 752

F

Face, edema of 363, 365
Fallopian tube 691, 697, 699t, 713, 715, 721f, 723f, 751, 753, 754, 760, 768, 796
   epithelium of 686
   patency of 259, 485, 765
Falloposcopy 768
Fallot, tetralogy of 449, 453, 460
Familial breast ovarian cancer syndrome 692
Familial gynecological cancer, risk reduction in 705
Fascia, posterior 662f
Fascial incision 215f
Febrile morbidity, incidence of 544
Federation of Gynecology and Obstetrics 628
Female external genitalia 796
   anatomy of 475f
   inspection of 477f
Female gonads, embryological development of 795f
Female infertility, causes of 754
Female internal genitalia 796
   anatomy of 475f
Female pelvic anatomy, normal 642f
Female pelvis, blood supply to 282
Female reproductive tract 764
Femininity, loss of 808
Femoral artery 542f
Femur length 297, 303
Ferning 335, 755f
Ferric carboxymaltose 438
Ferrous fumarate 437
Ferrous gluconate 437
Ferrous glycine sulfate 437
Ferrous succinate 437
Ferrous sulfate 437
   amount of 437
   anhydrous 437
   dry 437
Fertility 749
   effect on 544, 745
   preserving surgery 706
   sparing
      surgery 631
      therapy 513
      treatment 513, 513b
Fertilization, normal process of 229f
Fetal acidosis 63
Fetal acoustic stimulation 71
Fetal anemia 192b, 198f
   assessment of 196
   development of 196
   treatment of 199
Fetal ascites 203f
Fetal asphyxia 98
Fetal assessment
   method of 27
   rationale for 372
Fetal attitude 16
   types of 17f
Fetal bleeding diathesis 204
Fetal blood
   cells 189
   sampling 192
   small amounts of 188
Fetal body parts, palpation of 7
Fetal bradycardia 158, 445
Fetal circulation 308f
   persistent 317
Fetal complications 63, 64, 85, 98, 162, 165, 180, 181, 202, 317, 334, 337, 338, 344, 381, 406, 407, 414, 440, 461
Fetal congenital malformations, diagnosis of 324
Fetal death 155, 165, 350
Fetal descent, abdominal assessment of 34
Fetal disorders 340
Fetal distress 155, 165, 344, 374
Fetal dysmaturity syndrome 346b
Fetal echocardiography 455
Fetal erythroblastosis fetalis, pathogenesis of 202fc
Fetal face, direction of 413f
Fetal fibronectin 322, 325f
   levels 325
Fetal growth
   restriction 297t, 367
   stages of 296t
   ultrasound monitoring of 402
Fetal head 74b, 168
   anterior fontanels in 49f
   asynclitism of 51
   crowning of 55f
   delivery of 54, 55f, 219f
   diameter of 53f
   elevators 120
   engagement of 39, 51t
   entrapment 85
   extension of 67
   mobility of 114
   molding of 106, 106f
   occipitolateral position of 31f
   palpation of 103f, 299
   position of 61
   posterior fontanels in 49f
Fetal heart 309
   absent 349
   auscultation 20, 67, 91
   rate 54, 79, 205, 373
      location of 21f
      transient reduction of 95
   sound 7, 156, 159, 161, 171
Fetal hemoglobin 425, 428
Fetal hydrops 192, 203
   development of 203b
Fetal hypoglycemia
   development of 399
   pathogenesis of 404fc
Fetal hypoxemia 374
Fetal infection 320
Fetal inflammatory response 320
Fetal intrauterine blood transfusion 200
Fetal lie 15
   types of 15, 15f, 15t
Fetal macrosomia 267, 268, 337
   pathogenesis of 410fc
Fetal malpresentation 204, 374
Fetal middle cerebral artery 196
   Doppler velocimetry of 191
Fetal ponderal index 303
Fetal position 16, 39
Fetal presentation 15, 38
   abnormal 29
   diagnosis of 17
   types of 16f, 16t
Fetal problems 408t
Fetal red cells 192t
Fetal reduction, selective 184
Fetal scalp
   bones, molding of 41f
   electrode 329
Fetal shoulder 91f, 119
   and arm, delivery of 79, 80f
   presentation 91f
Fetal size, assessment of 32

Fetal skull 48, 50f
   bones of 48f, 350f
   diameters of 50, 50f
   molding of 41t
   parts of 49
Fetal sleep patterns 310
Fetal status, nonreassuring 204
Fetal surveillance 175, 196, 262, 312, 329, 343, 369, 401t, 454
   antenatal measures of 316
   measures of 303
   test of 343, 343t
Fetal trauma 337
Fetal weight
   estimated 295, 297, 301, 314
   ultrasound based estimation of 303t
Fetal well-being, tests for 341
Feto-fetal transfusion syndrome 183
Feto-maternal hemorrhage 188, 195
   estimating volume of 190
Fetopelvic disproportion, assessment of 114, 121
Fetus 95f
   descent of 106
   exact site of 13
   in-fetu 181
   intra-abdominal version of 95f
   management of 92fc
   normal 198f
   palpation of 15
   posterior shoulder of 413f
Fever, causes of 518b
Fibrin degradation products 165
Fibrinogen levels 350
Fibrinolysins 527
Fibrinolytic pathway 164fc
Fibroblast growth factor receptors 710
Fibroids 516, 518b, 552, 553, 553b, 751
   anatomical location of 756
   blocking blood supply of 543f
   destruction of 541
   development of 519
   FIGO classification of 516, 517f
   growth 796
   histological appearance of 516f
   large 520
   medical management of 526
   possible effects of 553
   presence of 231
   treatment of 544, 545f
   types of 516
   ultrasound appearance of 523f
   uterus 521, 522fc, 525fc
      management of 521, 526
Fibromas 688
Fibromyomas belonging 538
Fifth-line salvage therapy 579
FIGO classification system 487
FIGO revised cervical cancer staging 627f
Figure-of-eight 8, 9f
Fimbria 680
Fimbrial expression 732
Finger clubbing 450
Finger-Prick method 395f
First antenatal visit 3, 23
First-line salvage therapy 579
Fitz-Hugh-Curtis syndrome 583, 583f
Five-finger rotation 108

Flamm and Geiger scoring system 208, 208t
Flexion
   complete 17f
   moderate 17f
Flow cytometry 191
Fluconazole 578
Fluid
   thrill 474, 474f
Fluorescent treponemal antibody absorption 588
Fluorouracil 631
Fluoxetine 559
Focal endometrial vascular disturbance 553
Folate deficiency 426, 427t
Folic acid 230, 423, 435, 436f
   deficiency of 427
   regular intake of 396
Folinic acid 240, 241
Follicle-stimulating hormone 754, 757, 758, 762, 776, 805
   concentration, serum 805
Follicular aspiration 781f, 784
Follicular ovarian masses 686
Follicular stimulation 781f
Food, fortification of 435
Foot dorsiflexion 222
Footling breech 65
Forceps
   application of 82b, 83f
   rotation 109
   use of 268
Foul-smelling discharge 623
   causes of 623b
   per vaginum 491
Fourth-degree tear, repair of 290
Fourth-line salvage therapy 579
Fractures 566f
   risk assessment tool 565
Fragile X mental retardation 801
   testing for 802
Fragile X syndrome 802
   typical features of 802b
Frank's breech 65, 65f, 67f
Frank's dilators 806
Free vaginal mesh techniques 662
Fresh frozen plasma 460
Friedman's criteria 63
Friedman's labor graph 61t
Full-hand method 108
Functional murmur, characteristics of 451b
Fundal grip 18, 67, 90
Fundal height 13
   causes of 171
   estimation of 14
Fundoscopy 794
Furosemide 375

G

Gabapentin 559
Gait 114
Galactorrhea 491, 750, 793, 799
   management of 804fc
   presence of 496
Gamete
   culture of 789
   intrafallopian transfer 786
Gangrene, development of 550

Gardnerella mobiluncus 575
Gardnerella vaginalis 575
Gastrointestinal abnormalities 408
Gastrointestinal effects 637
Gastrointestinal malignancy 703
Gastrointestinal pathology 696
Gelatin microspheres 542
Gene mutation 492
Genetic disorders 340
Genetic syndromes 181, 203
Genital herpes 584
   treatment of 584
Genital hiatus 650f
Genital masculinization 796
Genital organs 8, 8t
Genital prolapse 467
Genital tract abnormalities 801fc
Genital trauma 491
Genital ulcer disease, management of 584
Genitourinary atrophy 807
Genitourinary fistula 98f
   development of 96, 122
Gentamicin 274
Germ cell tumors 686, 687, 689-691
   types of 689fc
Gestation
   abdominal measurement of 13f
   ectopic 242, 720
   neonatal 326
   period of 139, 150, 328, 329, 336, 371, 432
Gestational age 199t, 299, 314
   estimation of 301
   small for 295, 296, 296t, 299, 368
Gestational diabetes mellitus 180, 388, 390, 393t, 394, 396, 398f, 399, 403b, 405, 405t, 406, 406t, 408b, 409
   development of 393b
   diagnosis of 393t, 394
   management of 392, 394
   medical management of 394
   obstetric management of 394
   pathogenesis of 391
   screening for 392
   treatment of 399
Gestational hypertension 355-358, 368, 369, 369b, 447
   management of 368
Gestational sac 719, 721f, 721t, 722f
   tubal 721
Gestational trophoblastic disease 138, 227, 238b, 241b, 242
   classification of 228b
Gestational trophoblastic neoplasia 228
   development of 230, 230b
   diagnosis of 236, 237b
   FIGO staging of 240t, 241t
Gestrinone 678, 679
Girth, abdominal 340
Glibenclamide 398, 399
Globin levels 440
Glossitis 577
Glucose
   challenge test 392, 393
   intolerance, postpartum evaluation for 405t
   metabolism 390
   monitoring 399
   tolerance 390
Glyburide 398, 399
   efficacy of 399

Glycemic control, worsening of 402
Gonadal dysgenesis 802
Gonadorelin 777
Gonadotropin 777, 778, 787
    levels 805
    loss of 527
    releasing hormone 525-527, 546, 676, 682, 743, 777, 782
        agonist 527, 546, 678, 782
        analogs 681, 686, 743
        antagonists 528, 782
Gonorrhea 585, 585f, 593, 760
    diagnosis 585
    etiology 585
    investigations 586
    management 586
Goodell's sign 8, 9f
Goserelin 528, 678, 782
Grand multipara 4
Grandmother theory 195
Granulation tissue 586
Granulocyte colony-stimulating factor, employment of 241
Granuloma inguinale 586, 599
Granulomatous cervical conditions 599
Granulosa cells 468, 688
    tumor 688, 689
        histopathological pattern of 689f
Grasping protruding fundus 292f
Grey Turner's sign 472
Groin traction 84
Group B *Streptococcus*
    prophylaxis 326
    role of 319
Growth
    benign 686
    chart 793
    discordant 181
    hormone 806
    rapidity of 694
    restriction 373
        pathogenic 295, 296, 296t
Guanine 802
Guillain-Barré syndrome 254
Gynandroblastoma 687
Gynecologic oncology group 707
Gynecological malignancy, screening for 468
Gynecological management 508

H

Haemophilus
    ducreyi 587
    influenzae 139
    vaginalis 575
Halban's cul-de-sac closure 655
Halban's culdoplasty 655f
Hands
    edema of 363, 365
    palm of 10f
Haplotypes 188t
Hartmann's solution 273, 281
Hayman compression suture, application of 284f
Hayman technique 284
Head circumference 297, 301
Head of family, education of 6t
Headache 363, 577, 793
Healthy diet, components of 435f
Heart disease 442, 443b, 451t, 452, 453b, 454t, 457, 460, 460b
    clinical indicators of 451b
    congenital 408, 449, 460
    implications of 443
    incidence of 461
    rheumatic 443, 452
Heart failure 442
    chronic 458
    congestive 442, 445
    increased risk of 460
    rheumatic 452
    treatment of 454
Heavy menstrual bleeding 515, 517, 522
    causes of 515t
Hefner's cerclage 250, 265
Hegar's sign 8, 9, 9f
HELLP syndrome 373, 374, 384, 385t, 386fc
    classification 385
    complications 387
    diagnosis 384
    differential diagnosis 385
    hemolysis in 385
    Mississippi of 385t
    pathophysiology 384
    physical examination 385
    symptoms 384
    treatment 385
Helmet cells 165f
Hematochezia 667
Hematocrit 366, 370, 428, 433
    value 427
Hematologic malignancies 425
Hematoma 291
    infralevator 291
    prevent formation of 291
    supralevator 291
Hematometra 285, 796
Hematoperitoneum 716
Hemivertebra 796
Hemochromatosis 752
Hemodilution, physiological 422
Hemoglobin 417, 418, 428, 443, 652
    alpha 424, 425, 428
    concentration 418, 422
        restoration of 273
    electrophoresis 431
    estimation of 429f, 432t, 718
    glycosylated 246
    levels 727
    molecules, role of 417f
    oxygen dissociation curve 418
    production 422, 423
    routine determination of 433
    synthesis 434
Hemoglobinopathy 423, 427
Hemolysis 360, 373, 374
Hemolytic disorders 189
Hemophilia 496
Hemorrhage 419, 736
    accidental 551
    antepartum 142, 147, 180, 195, 208, 299, 315, 320, 348, 459
    cerebral 381, 382
    decidual 319
    intracranial 122
    intranatal 440
    intraperitoneal 472
    intraventricular 315, 318, 330
    life-threatening 736
    massive 281
    maternal 252
    postpartum 63, 120, 122, 163, 180, 266, 269b, 272, 272b, 273b, 274t, 294, 416, 423
    retroperitoneal 472
    severe 139
    warning 145
Hemostasis 456
Hemostatic compression sutures 283
Heparin 367
    unfractionated 262, 458
Hepatic failure 492
Hepatitis
    B 200
    C 200
Hernia, inguinal 753
Herpes
    genitalis 584
    simplex virus 247, 581
    viral infection 257
High-grade squamous intraepithelial lesion 596, 597f, 604, 622
Hingorani's sign 520
Hip
    bones 114
    delivery of 76f
    dislocation, congenital 181
Hirsutism 466, 749
    management of 779fc
Histrelin 528
Hockey-stick incision 223
Hodgkin's disease 622
Hoffman's exercises 12
Home uterine activity monitoring 324
Hookworm
    infection 435
    infestation 420
Horizontal uterine incision 534f
Hormonal contraceptives 677
Hormonal influence, independent of 468
Hormonal replacement therapy 561
Hormonal therapies 677, 681
Hormonal treatment, use of 681
Hormone
    adrenocorticotropic 340, 758, 804
    antidiuretic 275
    assays 497
    receptor status 513
    replacement therapy 238, 498, 507, 527, 561, 623, 636, 692, 806
        effect of 567f
        pills of 560f
    therapy 554, 559
Hot flushes 555
    treatment of 559
Hot Seitz bath, use of 562
Huhner test 764
Human chorionic gonadotropin 686, 718, 729, 730, 783
    levels of 468
Human epididymis protein 700
Human fertilization 174
Human immunodeficiency virus infection 622
Human leukocyte antigen 258

Human menopausal gonadotropin 686, 774, 776, 807
Human ovarian tumors 686
Human papillomavirus 599, 600, 602, 610, 611t
   high-risk 602, 619
   infection, prevention of 611
   test 613
     use of 603
   triage 602
   vaccination 611
Hyaline membrane disease 337
Hydatidiform mole 227, 228, 238, 359
   complete 227f, 229f
Hydralazine 376-378, 445, 449
   side effects of 378
Hydramnios 90, 158, 406
Hydrops fetalis 202, 203f
Hydrosalpinx
   laparoscopic appearance of 760f
   treatment of 774
Hyperandrogenemia 471
Hyperandrogenism 749, 757
   biochemical 757
   symptoms of 757
Hyperbilirubinemia 202
Hyperemesis gravidarum 180
Hyperextension 17f
Hyperglycemia 393, 403
   maternal 408t
Hyperkalemia 790
Hypermagnesemia 380
Hyperosmolar nonketotic diabetic coma 388
Hyperplasia 507
   benign endometrial 506f
   trophoblastic 236f
Hyperplastic trophoblastic tissue, presence of 236
Hyperprolactinemia 246, 758, 788, 798, 807
Hyperreflexia 370
Hypersegmented neutrophil 430f
Hyperspermia 764
Hypertension 405
   chronic 158, 355, 356, 358, 362, 377t, 420
   classification of 355, 358t
   degree of 358
   gestational 355-358, 368, 369, 369b, 447
   postpartum 380
   pregnancy induced 361
   primary pulmonary 460
   pulmonary 333
   refractory 375
   severe 355, 376t
     pulmonary 460
   treatment of 231
Hypertensive diseases 362
Hypertensive disorders, classification of 356fc, 356t
Hyperthermic intraperitoneal chemotherapy 711
   advantages of 711b
Hyperthyroidism 231
   symptoms of 231, 256b
Hypertriglyceridemia 317
Hypertrophic decidual vasculopathy 359, 361f
Hypertrophy, myometrial 739
Hyperviscosity syndrome 317

Hypocalcemia 317, 380
Hypoechogenic mass 552f
Hypofibrinogenemia, risk for 350
Hypogastric artery ligation 285
Hypoglycemia 317
   development of 403
   increased risk of 405
   risks of 400
Hypoglycemic therapy 396
Hypogonadism 752
   hypergonadotropic 802
   hypogonadotropic 802
Hypogonadotropic hypogonadic state 678
Hypoinsulinemia 317
Hyponatremia 790
Hypopituitarism 807
Hypoplasia, pulmonary 337
Hyporeflexia 380
Hypospermia 764
Hypotension 141, 493, 717
   prevention of 214
   sudden 377
Hypothalamic amenorrhea 793, 807
   causes for 793
Hypothalamic pituitary disease 754
Hypothalamus 470
   level of 799
   normal functioning 792
Hypothermia 317
Hypothyroidism 246
   maternal 246
Hypotonia 380
Hypovolemic shock 294
   evidence of 717
Hysterectomy 155, 153f, 238, 530, 531, 531f, 532, 549, 617, 655b, 656, 679, 683, 744
   advantage of 531
   disadvantages of 531b
   extrafascial 631
   indications for 531b, 656b
   obstetric 288
   technique of 532
   total abdominal 507, 688
   types of 633f
Hysterogram 225
Hysterosalpingo-contrast sonography 766, 769
Hysterosalpingogram 765, 765f, 766, 775
   normal 765f
Hysterosalpingography 259, 485
Hysteroscopic myomectomy 526, 530, 532, 533, 537, 538b
   indications for 537b
Hysteroscopy 260, 505, 537f, 767
   operative 261
Hysterotomy 541f
   closure 540

I

Idiopathic preterm labor 321
Idiopathic thrombocytopenic purpura 496
Iliococcygeus 645
Imidazoles 578
Immature teratomas 689
   management of 696
Immunity 622
Immunization 25

Immunoassay 583
Immunodeficiency 578
Immunoglobulin 439
Immunohistochemistry 510
Immunological defects 668
Immunological tests 584
Immunosuppressive agents, use of 578
Imperforate hymen 797, 797f
In vitro fertilization 261t, 299, 684, 725, 780, 781, 786
Inadequate trophoblastic invasion 359, 361f
Incision over uterine surface 540
Increta 153, 283
Indigo carmine dye 768
Indirect antiglobulin test 193f
Indomethacin 332, 406
Induction theory 668
Infections 140, 155, 226, 265, 268, 319, 337, 544, 550, 599, 618
   duration of 588
   recurrent 436
   screening for 26
   spread of 320b
Infectious disease 256
Inferior mesenteric artery 512
Infertile couple
   evaluation of 762
   management of 772b
   workup of 762b
Infertility 465, 466, 468, 552, 618, 680, 693, 749, 750, 761t, 793, 808
   causes of 680, 732, 749t, 761, 764
   duration of 750
   evaluation of 768
   female causes of 750f
   mechanisms for 680b
   primary 750
   secondary 750
   tubal factors of 773
   type of 750
   unexplained 780
Inflammation 756
Inflammatory cells 756
Inflammatory mediators, role of 391
Inflammatory pelvic masses 674
Inguinal lymph nodes, develop enlargement of 587
Inguinofemoral nodes 623
Injury 86, 157
Insulin 407
   glargine 398
   infusion, low-dose 403t
   injection 400f
     sites for 400
   preparation, types of 398, 398t
   resistance 777
   sensitizing agents, use of 265
   therapy 397
   types of 398
Interleukin 319, 425, 708
Intermenstrual bleeding 518
   causes of 518b, 623b
Internal anal sphincters, repair of 290
Internal artery ligation, time of 286f
Internal ballottement 7, 7f, 231
Internal iliac artery 287f
   ligation 287f, 294

Internal podalic version 94, 174
  complications 96
  technique of 95f, 179
Internal radiation therapy 634
Internal sutures, placement of 655f
Interstitial brachytherapy 635
Intervening membrane 173f
Intestinal glands 690f
Intra-abdominal tumor 473, 694
Intra-amniotic dye injection 335
Intracavitary brachytherapy 634
Intracavitary fibroid 524f
Intracytoplasmic sperm injection 785, 786f
Intraepithelial lesions, high-grade 599
Intraepithelial neoplasia 598, 626
Intramural fibroid 523f, 524f
Intramuscular injection 379
Intranatal period 440
Intrapartum antibiotic prophylaxis 456
Intrapartum care 76, 456
Intrapartum management 78fc, 105, 176fc, 198, 210, 329, 344, 384
Intrapartum monitoring 211
Intrapartum period 149, 176, 195, 313, 371, 402, 440
Intraperitoneal chemotherapy 709
Intraperitoneal transfusion 200
Intrathoracic tumors 203
Intrauterine abnormalities 485
Intrauterine adhesions 485
  visualization of 249f
Intrauterine clots 159
Intrauterine contraceptive device 496, 497, 726
  removal of 546
Intrauterine death 158, 315, 339, 348, 349, 402, 406
  causes of 348, 348t
  prevention 349
Intrauterine device 491, 504, 515, 581, 767
Intrauterine embryo transfer 784
Intrauterine fetal death 408
  evaluation of 349t
Intrauterine gestation 720
Intrauterine gestational sac 719, 720
Intrauterine growth restriction 28, 74, 178, 295, 297, 304, 312, 316, 317, 345, 360, 371, 374, 381, 410, 553
  classification of 296f
  diagnosis of 300
  fetuses, management for 315fc
  management of 300
Intrauterine infection 320b, 334, 594
  chronic 299
Intrauterine insemination 765, 773b, 778
Intrauterine pregnancy 10t, 22f, 718, 719, 789
  abnormal 720
  signs of 720
Intrauterine procedures 195
Intrauterine transfusion 197
  blood for 200
Intravascular blood transfusion 200
Intrinsic factor, deficiency of 426f
Introitus 37
Invasive cancer 629
  management of 624
Invasive carcinoma 626
Invasive cervical carcinoma, treatment of 630t

Invasive epithelial ovarian cancers, types of 686
Invasive hemodynamic monitoring 375
Invasive placenta 268
Invasive squamous cell carcinoma, histopathology of 598f
Inverted T-shaped incision 223
IOTA simple rules 700
Iron 417, 436f
  absorption 434b
  deficiency 423, 430
    anemia 419, 423, 423b, 425, 425t, 429, 429t, 430f, 432b, 432t, 433fc, 433, 435f, 530
  deficient diet 422
  dextran injections, use of 439
  folic acid supplementation 436
  formulations 437t
  medication 437b
  metabolism 430
    normal 431f
  parenteral forms of 437
  polysaccharide 437
  requirements 422t
  rich foods 434
  salts 437
  stores
    depletion of 423
    recovery of 422
  studies, serum 430
  sucrose 436, 438
  supplementation 434, 436
    exogenous 435
  therapy 432, 433b, 439
Irregular bleeding 499f, 500f, 529
Irritable bowel
  disease 674
  syndrome 666
Ischial spine 47, 644
  assessment of 47f
Isoflavones 563
Isometric exercise test 367
Isoxsuprine 333
Isthmus extension 513
Itching 589
Itraconazole 578

J

Jacquemier's sign 8, 8f
Jaundice 189
  development of 201
Jejunum 424
Jello sign 159
Joel-Cohen blunt incision 215
Johnson's method 292, 292f
Joshi's sling 659
J-shaped incision 223

K

Kahn's test 588
Kallmann syndrome 754
Kangaroo care 330f
Kaolin clotting time 254
Karman's cannula 138
Kegel exercises 652
Keratin pearls 621f
Ketoacidosis 403

Ketosis prone 388
Khanna's sling surgery 659
Kidney
  disease, chronic 362
  function test 366, 383, 524, 729, 730
  injury, acute 356
  transplant 622
Kielland's forceps 109
Kissing ulcers 587
Kleihauer–Betke test 190, 191f
Klumpke's palsy 415
Knee jerks 365
Koilonychia 420f
Kuppuswamy's socioeconomic scale, modified 6t
Kyphosis, maternal 101

L

Labetalol 376, 377, 381
Labia majora 37
Labor 37, 351
  abnormal progress of 61
  active management of 269
  classification of 33t
  dysfunctional 440
  dystocia 62
  failure of progress of 118
  first stage of 31, 105, 118, 440
  fourth stage of 270
  induction of 54, 59, 59b, 59t, 118, 314, 350, 402t, 456
  initiation of 340fc
  management in 402
  mechanism of 92
  normal 51, 52f
  onset of 109
  pain
    false 36, 36t, 340
    true 36, 36t
  premature 180
  prolonged 60, 122
  second stage of 106, 118, 440
  spontaneous onset of 350
  stage of 32t, 33f, 75
  third stage of 31, 179, 269, 270, 440, 457
  triad of 72, 117, 118t
Lactate dehydrogenase 689
Lactic acidosis 388
Lambda sign 174
Lambdoid suture 48
Laparoscopic assisted vaginal hysterectomy 531, 664
Laparoscopic examination 260, 723
Laparoscopic excision 683f
Laparoscopic myolysis 526
Laparoscopic myomectomy 535, 535f, 536, 536b
  advantages of 535, 536b
  complications of 536, 536b
  safety of 532
Laparoscopic ovarian drilling 777, 778, 779f
Laparoscopic salpingectomy 735
  procedure of 735f
Laparoscopic salpingotomy 736f
Laparoscopic surgery 679, 682, 732, 733b, 735
  advantages of 733b
Laparoscopic uterine
  artery ligation 544
  nerve ablation 684

Laparoscopy 618, 674, 679, 731, 762, 768, 773
   role of 705
Laparotomy 211, 618, 679, 731, 733
   emergency 737
   exploratory 703
   indications for 733*b*
Laryngopharynx 419
Laser
   ablation 614
      selective 184
   cervical conization 616*f*
   excision 615
Lash procedure 250, 265
Lasofoxifene 744
Last menstrual period 299
Latent syphilis 588
Late-onset fetal growth restriction, diagnosis of 295
Latex agglutination test 581
Laurence–Moon–Biedl syndrome 754
Le Fort colpocleisis 660
   indications for 661
Lecithin 150
Lee-Frankenhäuser plexus 684
Left ischial spine, assessment of 116*f*
Left low uterine vessel ligation 287
Left mentum 18
   anterior 18, 21
   transverse 18
Left ventricular ejection fraction 460
Leg elevation 222
Leiomyomas 482, 515, 516*f*, 518, 530, 741, 755
   management of 532, 532*b*
   types of 516*f*
Leiomyomatosis, cutaneous 519
Leiomyosarcoma 551, 552*f*, 621
Leopold's maneuvers 17-19, 20*f*, 66*f*, 67, 90, 90*f*, 91
Lesions 590
   recurrent 636
   types of 452
Letrozole 774, 776, 778
   advantages of 780*b*
Leukemia 425
Leukomalacia, periventricular 315
Leukoplakia 609
Leuprolide 678, 777
   acetate depot 528
Leuprorelin 528, 782
Levator ani muscle 644, 645, 645*f*, 646*f*
Levonorgestrel-releasing intrauterine system 506, 507, 529, 678, 743
Leydig cells 688
Lidocaine 458
Ligase chain reactions 583
Ligatures, placement of 288*f*
Light-headedness 450
Limbs, lower 76*f*, 114
Lincosamides 577
Linea nigra 12, 13*f*
Linear salpingostomy 732
Lipoprotein
   high-density 554
   low-density 554
Liquid-based cytology 605, 606*f*, 607*f*
Liquor
   adequacy of 67
   amount of 34, 35*t*
   meconium staining of 344*b*

Lithotomy position 476
Liver
   dullness 473
   function 381, 497
      test 366, 371, 383, 385, 729, 730
   Glisson's capsule of 363
Longitudinal vaginal septum 795*f*
Loop electrosurgical excision procedure 250, 616, 616*f*
Løvset's maneuver 80, 83, 84*f*
Low birth weight babies 594
Low uterine vessel ligation, right 287
Low vascular resistance, pregnancy induced 442
Lower genital tract 591*t*
   infection 334
      assessment of 324
Lower oculocerebral syndrome 754
Lower uterine segment 36, 143, 283
Low-grade squamous intraepithelial lesion 597*f*, 604
   treatment of 617*b*
Low-molecular-weight heparin 262, 316, 367, 442, 458
Lugol's iodine 600, 604, 606*f*
   application of 609
Lumbar vertebra 796
Lump, presence of 694
Lungs 242
   hyperexpanded areas of 347*f*
Lupron 678
Lupus anticoagulant 252, 255
   testing for 259
Luteal phase defect 246, 768
   treatment of 261
Lutein cells 688
Luteinizing hormone 527, 757, 758, 762, 776, 805
   hypersecretion of 246
Lymph node 514, 625, 707
   enlargement 624
   involvement 638*t*
   metastasis 513
   regional 699
   sampling 511
Lymphadenectomy 512, 632, 688
   indications for 512*fc*
   levels of 634*t*
Lymphadenopathy 471, 623
Lymphatic spread, metastatic theory of 668
Lymphedema 637
Lymphogranuloma venereum 586, 599
Lymphoma 425
Lymphovascular space 511
   invasion 510, 513, 629, 631
Lynch syndrome 493*f*, 494, 494*fc*, 692
   genetic screening of 493*b*

M

Macroadenomas 798
Macroalbuminuria 396
Macrosomia 209, 345, 408
   causes of 409*b*
   development of 409*f*
   management of 409
Magnesium
   levels of 379

   sulfate 330, 332, 375, 378, 379*t*, 380, 382, 386
      dose of 380
      mode of action of 378
      regimens 379
      use of 333*b*, 378
Magnetic resonance imaging 239, 801, 804
   examination 485
Malaria 420, 435, 716
Male genital organs 752
Male infertility
   causes of 754, 754*t*, 762
   treatment of 771, 772*fc*
Malena 419
Malignancy 465, 482, 485, 521
   detection of 685
   diagnosis of 623
   high clinical suspicion of 530
   index, risk of 701, 702*b*
   suspicion of 551
   symptoms suggestive of 589
Malignant ovarian tumor, management of 696
Malignant transformation, increased risk of 619
Mammalian cells 776
Manchester method 635*f*
Manchester repair 656, 657
   procedure for 657, 659*f*
Marfan's syndrome 453, 456, 460
Mari's chart 199*t*
Marijuana 761
Martin classification 385*t*
Mass
   abdominal 465, 472
   bilateral 473
   cancerous 686*f*
   causes of 495*b*
   classification of 701*t*
   consistency of 473, 694
   extrapelvic 685
   intra-abdominal 473
   margins of 472
Massive transfusion protocol, activation of 281
Mastodynia 7
Maternal cardiovascular hemodynamic status 297
Maternal chromosomes, set of 228
Maternal complications 88, 96, 180, 203, 334, 337, 406
Maternal death 162, 374, 407
Maternal early warning score 270*t*
Maternal fetal medicine unit 208
Maternal mirror syndrome 203
Maternal mortality rate, high 440
Maternal pelvis 42, 44*f*, 45*f*
   anterior rotation of 43*f*
Maternal perineum 411*f*
Maternal placental syndromes 447
Maternal serum 191
   creatine kinase 723
Maternal spiral arterioles, maladaptation of 359
Maternal syndrome 360
Maternal vitals, monitoring of 374
Maternal weight 372
   record 340
Maternal wellbeing, optimization of 62
Mature teratomas 689
   histological picture of 690*f*
Mauriceau–Smellie–Veit maneuver 75, 81, 82*f*

Mayer-Rokitansky-Küster-Hauser syndrome 795, 795f, 806
McCall's culdoplasty 655, 655f
McDonald cervical cerclage 263
McDonald procedure 250, 263, 263f
McIndoe's vaginoplasty 806
McRoberts maneuver 411, 412, 412f
Mean corpuscular hemoglobin 425, 429
    concentration 418, 425, 429
Mean corpuscular volume 418, 425, 427-429
Meconium
    aspiration 346f
        consequences of 347f
        syndrome 317, 344, 346, 347f
    staining 346
Medical disorders, presence of 30
Mefenamic acid 527
Megaloblastic anemia 425, 426, 430, 430f
    pathogenesis of 426f
Meigs' syndrome 688
Melasma 11f
Membranes
    artificial rupture of 161, 342
    assessment of 39
    management of premature rupture of 336fc
    premature rupture of 319, 322, 334, 594
    preterm
        premature rupture of 208, 406, 618
    ruptures, bag of 78
    stripping of 341
    sweeping 343
Mendelson syndrome 403
Menometrorrhagia 533
Menopausal hormone therapy 554, 559, 561b, 562, 562b, 566, 569b, 693
    use of 560, 561t
    use of 562
Menopause 554, 562
    anatomical changes 555
    clinical presentation 555, 557
    effects of 557f
    etiology 555
    hormone therapy 559
    physiology of 559
    premature 554, 637, 712
    treatment of 559, 563f
Menorrhagia 486, 521, 530, 744
    treatment of 527b
Menstrual bleeding 792
    abnormal 465, 466
    pathophysiology of 792
Menstrual blood loss, estimates of 489
Menstrual calendar 526
Menstrual cycle 669, 693, 767, 768, 771
    anovulatory 490, 490t
    infrequent 751
    irregular 751
    middle of 468
    normal 468, 469f
    ovulatory 490, 490t
    phases of 546f
    regular 751
    regulation of 468
Menstruation
    cessation of 6
    ectopic 466
    physiology of 468

Mentum, anterior rotation of 111
Mentzer's index 424
    lower 424
Mesenchymal tissue, tumors of 621
Mesosalpinx 734
Metabolic acidosis 122
Metabolic disorders 203
Metaplasia 514, 596, 712
    squamous 609
Metastasis, pulmonary 236f
Metastatic disease 235
    low-risk 240
    treatment of 240
Metformin 265, 398, 399, 780, 790
    adverse effects of 780
    use of 399
Methergine 274, 440
Methotrexate 240, 241, 727, 729-731
    adjuvant therapy, use of 155
    administration 731b
    multidose regime 730b
    single-dose 729, 730b
    therapy 729b
Methyldopa 369, 377
Methylergometrine 274, 275
Methylergonovine, dose of 275
Metoclopramide 407
Metoprolol 381
Metronidazole 121, 274, 576, 577, 581, 594
Metrorrhagia 486, 740, 744
Miconazole 578
Microadenomas 798
Microalbuminuria 396
Microaneurysm 407
Microcolon, congenital 408
Microhemagglutination assay 588
Micronized progesterone 803, 807
Micronormoblastic erythroid hyperplasia 432
Microseptostomy 184
Microsurgery 773
Microvillous cells 470
Micturition, frequency of 8
Middle cerebral artery 301, 304, 305, 306f, 314, 371
    Doppler studies 306
    index of 300
    peak systolic velocity 183, 197, 199, 200
Midpelvis 47
    assessment of 40
    contraction 112
    diameters of 47
Mifepristone 350, 529, 731
Migraine 254
Mild placental abruption 160, 162
Minimal small incisions 538f
Minimum invasive surgery 634, 731
Mirena 560
Miscarriage 139, 180, 250, 750, 788
    causes of 252f, 253f
    previous 256
    recurrent 256, 258fc, 260, 261t, 467
    spontaneous 195
    threatened 195
Misgav Ladach technique 222
Misoprostol 274, 276, 350, 384, 451
    dosage of 351t
Mitral balloon valvotomy, percutaneous 447
Mitral regurgitation 445

Mitral stenosis 445, 446f, 447, 453, 460
Mitral valve disease 443
Mixed epithelial tumors 687
Mixed gonadal dysgenesis 798
Mixter's forceps 287f
    placement of 287f
Molar gestation
    pathophysiology of 229f
    signs in 230b
    symptom of 230, 230b
Molar pregnancy
    complete 236f
    management of 233fc, 237
Molding
    diagnosis of 40
    grading degree of 40
Molecular markers 510
    clinical significance of 511t
Molecular tumor markers 514
Moles, complete 228t, 233
Monilial infection 577
Monoamniotic monochorionic monozygotic twin pregnancy 167
    twins 172f
Monochorionic diamniotic twin 173f
    gestation 178
Monochorionic monoamniotic twin 173f
    gestation 178
Monochorionic multifetal gestation, complications of 175
Monochorionic twins
    diagnosis of 171
    management of 171
Monozygotic twin 167, 167t, 168f, 181
    formation of 168f
    gestation 186
    pregnancy
        diamniotic dichorionic 169f
        diamniotic monochorionic 169f
        monoamniotic monochorionic 169f
    types of 167, 168f
Monsel's paste 609
Morcellation 540
Morison's pouch 722
Morphine sulfate, administration of 449
Morphological uterus sonographic assessment 742f
Morphology 763
Morris waste space 48, 48f
Moschcowitz culdoplasty 655, 655f
Motile trichomonads 581
Mucinous cystadenoma 688, 700f, 703f
Mucinous tumors 687, 688
Müllerian agenesis 795, 808
Müllerian anomalies 247
Müllerian defects 485
Müllerian inhibiting substance 797
Müllerian remnants 796
Müllerian rests 668
Müllerian structures 795, 798
Müller-Munro Kerr method 115
Multidose methotrexate regimen, protocol for 730
Multifetal gestation 90, 158, 166, 168, 181b, 789
    clinical presentation 169
    general physical examination 169
Multifetal pregnancy 275
    reduction 789
        procedure of 174

Multigravida 4
Multimodal spectroscopy 609
Multipara 4
Multiple drug allergies 439
Multiple gestation 145, 178t, 231, 367
Multiple placentas 172
Multiple pregnancy 204, 334, 359, 787
 complications of 180
 iatrogenic 788
 risk of 789
Multiple prosthetic valves 458
Multiple subserosal fibroids 531f
Multiple uterine 519
 fibroids 521
Muscle, abdominal 472
Musculoskeletal disease 666
Mutation 494
 analysis 510
Myasthenia gravis 333, 380
Mycobacterium tuberculosis 247
Mycoplasma 256
 genitalium 573
 hominis 319, 575
Myelitis, transverse 254
Myeloma 425
Myocardial infarction 388, 450, 458
 acute 448
Myolysis 541
Myoma 516, 526, 530b, 535f, 696
 coagulation 541
 enucleation of 540
 large 533
 location 540
 removal of 532, 540
 shelling out of 541f
Myomectomy 465, 525, 530, 532, 533, 533b, 756
 abdominal 533, 534f, 539, 539b
 immediate 533
 indications for 532b
 principles of 532
 route of 526
 type of 533
Myometrial invasion 513
 depth of 511
Myometrium 242, 740f
 hyperplastic 740
 mottled texture of 742f
 placental invasion of 153f
 thickness of 287
 upper segment of 275

N

Naegele's obliquity 53f
Naegele's pelvis 112, 113f
Naegele's rule 3
Nafarelin 528, 782
Nasopharyngeal symptoms 419
National Anemia Prophylaxis Program 435
National Chlamydia Screening Programme 583
National Diabetes Data Group Criteria 394t
National Health Service Cancer Screening Programme 601
National Health Service Trusts 393
National High Blood Pressure Education Program 377
Necator americanus 431
Necrotizing enterocolitis 318

Necrotizing fasciitis 550
Neglected arm prolapse, consequences of 97fc
Neisseria gonorrhoeae 136, 256, 335, 573, 583
Neoadjuvant chemotherapy protocol 710
Neonatal complications 317, 334, 337, 460
Neoplastic ovarian growths, histological classification of 687b
Neoplastic tissue 609
Nephropathy, diabetic 407
Neural tube defects 181, 408
Neurological injury 416
Neurontin 559
Neuropathic origin, pain of 665
Neuropathy, diabetic 407
Neuroprotection 333
Nifedipine 331, 332, 376, 377, 381
Nile blue sulfate 335
Nitrates 449, 458
Nitrazine paper test 335
Nitric oxide 361
 donors 332, 333
Nitroglycerin 376
Nocturnal leg cramps 419
Nodular endometrial lesions 682f
Nodules, pulmonary 236f
Nonadherent placenta 292
Nonendometrioid endometrial cancer 509, 510
Nonepithelial cell tumors 621
Nonepithelial ovarian cancer 686
Nonimmune hydrops, causes of 203t
Nonmetastatic disease, treatment of 240
Nonpolyposis colorectal cancer, hereditary 492, 494
Nonprostaglandin methods 211
Nonrapid eye movement, average period of 310
Nonreactive nonstress test, implications of 310
Nonreassuring fetal heart rate pattern 337
Nonresectoscopic endometrial ablation techniques 548
Nonsexually transmitted bacteria 715
Nonsteroidal anti-inflammatory drugs 221, 501, 525, 527, 676, 743
Nonstress test 27, 28, 175, 302, 304, 309, 311, 342, 343, 371
 procedure 309
Nontreponemal tests 588
Nontubal ectopic pregnancy
 diagnostic criteria for 724
 treatment of 736
 types of 724
Norepinephrine reuptake inhibitors 559
Normal cervical squamous epithelium, transformation of 598f
Normal uterine artery 305f
 blood flow 305f
Normocytic anemia 421
 causes of 421
Normozoospermia 764
Novasure device 549f
Novel angiogenesis inhibiting agents 710, 710t
Nuchal arms 79
Nuchal arms, delivery of 80f
Nuchal translucency, measurement of levels of 22f
Nuclear factor kappa B
 cells 319
 ligand 567

Nucleic acid amplification test 583, 586
Nulligravida 4
Nullipara 4
Nulliparity 362, 494
Nulliparous prolapse, management of 651
Nutrition 24, 613
Nystatin 578
 dose of 578

O

O'sullivan's method 292
Obesity 256
Obliterative procedures 660
Obstructed labor 64, 96, 97f, 112, 120
 diagnosis 121
 etiology of 121, 122t
 management 121
Obstructive pulmonary disease 752
Occipitoposterior position 17f, 99
 clinical presentation 102
 development of 100
 general physical examination 102
 investigations 103
 management 103
 maternal complications 109
 obstetric management 103
 specific systemic examination 102
 treatment 103
Offensive vaginal discharge 499f
Oligoasthenoteratozoospermia 764
Oligohydramnios 309, 349, 373
 causes of 35
Oligomenorrhea 486
Oligospermia 761
Oligozoospermia 764
 severe 763
Oliguria 363
Omental metastases 694
Oncovin 241
Oocyte 750, 784
 aspiration, excess 789
 classification 784
 cryopreservation 789
 donation 787
  indications for 787
 insemination 781f
 retrieval 783
Oogenesis 756
Oophorectomy 632, 683
 bilateral 683
Operative delivery 268
Optimal cytoreduction 707
Oral antiviral medications 584
Oral contraceptive
 agents 528
 pill 525, 573, 676, 693
  form of 491
 use of 590
Oral estrogens 807
Oral glucose tolerance test 257, 394f, 394t
Oral hypoglycemic agents 399
Oral iron
 dose of 437
 salt 437
 therapy 438b
  failure of 433b
Oral metronidazole 577

Organ transplant 622
Organic cardiac disease 275
Organisms, anaerobic 140
Orgasmic disorders 466
Ornidazole 577
Osada procedure 744
Osiander's sign 8
Ospemifene 564, 744
    oral tablet of 562
Osteochondral junction 114
Osteomalacic pelvis 112, 113f
Osteopenia 565
Osteoporosis 262, 554, 556, 564, 566f, 567f, 807
    complications of 564
    development of 565b
    diagnosis of 564
    maternal 459
    postmenopausal 564
    prevention of 562, 564, 567b
    treatment 559
Ouahba's technique 285
Ova, stool examination for 430
Ovarian cancer 685, 686, 691, 692t, 693b, 705, 711, 712, 712b
    grading of 705
    high-grade 708
    management for 696
    moderate 708
    risk of 702
    screening for 705
    serous 510
    spread of 692f
    syndrome, hereditary 692
    types of 691
Ovarian cycle 468
Ovarian cyst 468, 482, 551, 698fc, 700f
    development of 529
    excision of 467
    ruptured 724
    simple 697fc
Ovarian endometrioma 674
Ovarian factor 769, 776fc
    infertility 756
    treatment of 774
Ovarian function, evaluation of 805
Ovarian hilum 788
Ovarian hyperstimulation syndrome 770, 775, 778, 780, 788, 789, 789f, 790t, 791fc
    complications of 791
    management of 790, 791fc
    pathogenesis of 790
    signs of 790
Ovarian malignancy 703, 708
    presence of 685
    risk of 702
    screening for 705
    spread of 691
Ovarian masses 685
Ovarian neoplastic growth, types of 686
Ovarian pregnancy 726b, 737
Ovarian stimulation 785
Ovarian torsion 788
Ovarian tumors 231
    borderline 688
    different types of 696
    epidemiology of 685
    histogenesis of 686
Ovarian volume 770

Ovary 557, 680
    dermoid cyst of 689
    disorders of 797
    mesothelium of 686
    mucinous cystadenoma of 688
    normal 792
        functioning 792
        left-sided 235f
    postmenopausal 557
    removal of 637
    right-sided 235f
    thyroid tumor of 690
Ovasure test 702
Overdistended uterus 268
Ovulation 470
    disturbances of 553
    induction 265, 790
        medicines 768
    prediction kit 770
    trigger 777
Ovulatory bleeding 490
Ovulatory disorders 756
    classification of 757t
Ovulatory dysfunction 487, 749
    causes of 756
Ovum
    death of 726
    fertilization of 781f
Oxidative stress 368
Oxidized cellulose 806
Oxygen
    dissociation curve 419f
        sigmoid shape of 418
    hemoglobin for 418
    transportation of 417f
Oxytocin 63, 106, 274, 275, 384, 440
    administration of 276
    antagonists 332
    infusion 350
        contraindication of 106b
    use of 237

P

Packed cell volume 428
Paclitaxel 242, 511
Pain 518, 669
    abdominal 99, 157, 193, 230, 374, 466, 500f, 594, 716, 727
    acute 518b
    aggravating factors for 466
    anginal 453
    chronic 544
    diagnosis of 666
    duration of 669
    epigastric 370
    exact site of 466
    following treatment 731
    intensity of 466
    killers, use of 291
    localization 669
    lower back 648
    nature of 466
    persistent 544
    radiation of 466
    relieving factors for 466
    severe abdominal 211
    severity of 669
    treatment of 666

Painless bleeding, episode of 143
Pallor 10, 495
    development of 420fc
PALM COEIN classification system 487
Palmer's sign 8, 9
Palpation 171
    abdominal 13, 66, 90, 102, 299, 300, 341
Pancreatic beta cells 399
Papanicolaou smear 485, 504, 524, 599, 600, 604, 606, 762
    abnormal 594, 596
    examination 558
    kit 600, 600f
    previous 491
        history of 750
Papanicolaou stain 601
Papanicolaou test 485
Papilledema 365
Para-aortic lymph node dissection 509
    boundaries of 512
Para-aortic lymphadenectomy 512, 632
Paracervical block 767
Parametritis 139, 618
Paraneoplastic syndrome 694
Parathyroid hormone levels 565
Parental prostaglandins, administration of 276
Parenteral iron 438
    therapy 436
        use of 438b
    use of 439, 440b
Parietal bone, anterior part of 105
Parietal peritoneum 217f
Paroxetine 559
Paroxysmal nocturnal dyspnea 450
Partial hydatidiform mole 229f
    diagnosis of 227
Partial mole 228t, 235
    pathophysiology of 228
Partogram 54
Patau's syndrome 175
Patent ductus arteriosus 449
Paterson-Kelly syndrome 421
Pathological vaginal discharge 573, 590
    causes of 573t
Patwardhan's method 120
Pawlik's grip 18
Pedal edema 11f, 421, 421f, 623
Pedicle, torsion of 550
Pelosi's technique 222
Pelvic abscess 618
Pelvic adhesions 674, 715
Pelvic anatomy, normal 483, 484f
Pelvic assessment 40, 116f
Pelvic blood vessels 282f, 286f
Pelvic bones 114
Pelvic brim 67
    boundaries of 44f
Pelvic cavity 35f, 46, 768
    diameters of 46
Pelvic diaphragm, muscles of 644, 645f
Pelvic endometriosis, clinical features of 670
Pelvic examination 64, 115, 257, 474, 476, 476b, 495, 520, 542, 590, 649, 671, 695, 717, 740, 753, 794
    components of 476
    indications of 115
    prerequisites for 115
Pelvic exenteration 635

Pelvic floor
    deep perineal muscles of 644
    exercises 652
    muscles of 644, 645f, 647f
    superficial muscles of 644, 645f
Pelvic grip
    second 18
    third 103f
Pelvic hemorrhage 242
Pelvic infection 715, 751
Pelvic inflammatory disease 496, 582, 594, 618, 669, 692, 717, 760
    acute 573
Pelvic inlet 43, 76f
    assessment of 40
    contraction 112
    diameters of 44
    oblique diameters of 46
    superior view of 46f
    transverse diameter of 45
Pelvic lymph node dissection, boundaries of 512, 513t
Pelvic masses 651, 685
Pelvic organ 473
    prolapse 466, 468, 556, 641, 651, 651t
        evaluation of 641t
        surgery for 654
Pelvic outlet 43, 46
    assessment of 40
    diameters of 46
    evaluation 116f
Pelvic pain 465, 527, 665, 665, 670, 671f
    chronic 665
    early acute abdominal 544
    severe 684
Pelvic pathology
    diagnosis of 674
    surgical treatment of 782
Pelvic prolapse 466
    quantification of 649, 650f
Pelvic radiation 793
Pelvic scar tissue 715
Pelvic sepsis 242
Pelvic ultrasonography 762
Pelvis 42f, 113f, 751, 768f
    deep infiltrating endometriosis of 684
    false 42
    laparoscopic visualization of 779f
    true 43
    types of 43t
    ultrasound of 232
Percreta 153, 283
Pereira technique 285, 285f
Perianal area 584
Perigee system 663f
Perinatal deaths, previous 5
Perinatal morbidity 347
Perinatal mortality 72, 344, 347, 618
Perineal body 644, 645, 650f
    attachments of 646f
Perineal injury
    repair of 289
    severe 347
Perineal tear 645, 652
    degrees of 289f
    first degree 289f
    fourth degree 289f
    second degree 289f
    third degree 289f

Perineum
    central tendinous point of 645
    female 644f
Peripartum cardiomyopathy 448, 448b, 453
Peripheral smear 165f, 385, 426, 427, 429, 430, 430f, 521
Peritoneal defects 760
Peritoneal incision 215f
Peritoneum 216, 697
    closure of 220f
Peritubular adhesions 732
Perrault syndrome 798
Persistent corpus luteum cysts 767
Persistent disease
    ruling out presence of 238
    treatment of 239
Pessary, use of 653b
Petechiae 365
Pethidine 380
Pfannenstiel incision 216f
    closure of 220f
    sharp 215
Phenergan 380
Phenytoin 380
    use of 380
Phosphatase 492, 494, 506
Phosphate 407
Phytoestrogens 563
Pictorial blood loss assessment chart 489, 489f
Pinard's maneuver 85, 85f
Pitocin overdose 122
Pituitary gland 527
    normal functioning 792
Piver-Rutledge classification 633t
Placenta 143, 154, 273, 292
    accreta 153-155, 225t, 283
        spectrum, diagnosis of 154
    delivery of 179, 219f
    exact site of 349
    fundal implantation of 267
    increta 153f, 154f
    large 268
    manual removal of 293, 293f
    normal 155f
    percreta 154f
    previa 142, 143, 143f, 144, 145, 149b, 150fc, 151, 151b, 158, 159, 159t, 225, 268, 293, 374
        degrees of 143
        diagnosis of 146, 147
        low-lying 144f
        marginal 144f
        partial 144f
        presence of 78
        risk of 145, 225t
        total 144f
    region of 227
    rending asunder of 155
Placental abruption 147, 155, 155f, 156, 158, 159t, 160, 160f, 246, 447
    clinical classification of 156, 156t
    concealed type of 157f
    diagnosis of 159
    pathophysiology of 156fc
    prevention of 149, 160
    severe cases of 160
    signs of 157
    symptoms of 157

    treatment 160
    types of 157, 157f
Placental alkaline phosphatase 689
Placental alpha macroglobulin 336
Placental disease 297
Placental function 296, 345fc
Placental insufficiency 296, 348
Placental perfusion 367
Placental separation, degree of 157
Placental site trophoblastic tumor 243
Placental syndrome 359
Placental tissues
    develop 227
    exact site of 349
Plantar flexion 222
Plasma
    antibody 187
    cell endometritis 594
    glucose value 393
    protein-A 299, 315
    volume 443
Plasmapheresis 387
Platelet
    activation of 254
    count 231, 366, 370, 521
        low 360, 373, 374
        measurement of levels of 231
    derived growth factor receptors 710
Platinum resistant disease 711
Plummer-Vinson syndrome 421
Pneumothorax 347f
Poikilocytosis 429
Poliomyelitis 114
Polycystic ovarian syndrome 245, 246, 265, 468, 491, 494, 515, 692, 756, 757, 758, 776, 778, 780, 787, 798, 801, 807
    pathophysiology of 758fc
    treatment of 777
Polycystic ovary 767
    bilateral 759f
    disease 493
Polycythemia
    blood tests for 404
    secondary 518
Polyembryoma 687
Polyhydramnios 114, 180, 185, 192, 267, 309, 334, 406
    causes of 35
Polymaltose 437
Polymerase chain reaction tests 581
Polypoidal cancerous growth 704f
Polypropylene tapes 662
Polyurethane condoms 562
Polyvinyl alcohol 542
Pop-Q staging system 649, 650, 650f, 651t
Population-based screening program 603
Porcine dermis 662
Porcine small intestine submucosa 662
Positron emission tomography 485, 702
Postcoital bleeding 619
    causes of 623t
Postcoital test 764
Postdated pregnancy 339
    management of 341
Postembolization syndrome 544
Posterior arm, delivery of 414, 414f
Posterior shoulder, delivery of 56f, 84

Posterior vaginal wall 641
   mucosa 264f
   points 650
Postmaturity syndrome 337
Postmenopausal age group 490
Postmenopausal bleeding 487, 495b
   causes of 488t
   evaluation of 508fc
Postmenopausal estrogen therapy 494
Postnatal jaundice, mild degree of 189f
Postoperative adhesions, prevention of 536f
Postpartum hemorrhage 63, 120, 122, 163, 180, 266, 269b, 272, 272b, 273b, 274t, 294, 416, 423
   causes of 267, 267b
   control of 457
   etiology of 271
   management of 271, 272fc
   prevention of 270, 271
   secondary 266, 294
   severe 277
   traumatic causes for 267
Postpartum period 195, 372, 381, 384
Postpartum pituitary necrosis 751
Postpartum sterilization 495
Postprandial glycemic control 399
Post-term pregnancy 340, 341, 343, 345fc 347, 347f
   management of 341, 342fc, 343
Post-testicular defects 754
Potassium 407
   chloride 731
   hydroxide 576
      preparation 593
      Whiff test 593
Povidone iodine solution 766
Powder-burn lesions 682f, 760
Prader-Willi syndrome 754
Prague's maneuver 83f
   reverse 83
Precipitate labor 64
   complications 64
   diagnosis 64
   etiology 64
   management 64
Preconception period 395, 396
Preeclampsia 158, 180, 204, 230, 242, 320, 355, 357t, 361f, 362, 362b, 365, 372, 381t, 406
   atypical 356
   clinical
      classification of 358t
      features of 355, 357f
   complications of 381
   etiopathogenesis of 358
   increased risk of 362
   management of 369, 371fc
   mild 359t, 370
   pathophysiology of 358, 359, 359t, 360fc
   predictive tests for 367
   presence of 447
   recurrent 367
   risk for 246
   severe 275, 359t, 373, 373b, 374t, 375, 378, 382, 384b
   symptoms of 363
   treatment of 372

Pregnancy 11f, 30, 174, 231, 359b, 396, 396t, 399, 421, 443, 447, 452, 458, 458t, 470, 553, 584
   abdominal 726b, 737
   anticipation of 454
   complications 553, 594
   duration of 444f
   early 231
   ectopic 195, 482, 713, 713f, 714f, 715-718, 718t, 719, 721, 721f, 723, 724, 728fc, 738, 767, 788
   effect of 442
   fatty liver of 180
   first trimester of 6, 355
   heterotopic 727b, 737, 789
   hypertensive disorders of 180, 381
   location of 722
   loss 244t
      recurrent 257, 530
      second trimester 618
   management of 300
   medical termination of 453b, 467
   monochorionic 173, 174f
   normal 3
   onterstitial 725b, 737
   physiologic hemodilution of 428
   physiological effects of 390
   postmature 339
   post-term 340, 341, 343, 345fc 347, 347f
   previous 190, 321t
   primary abdominal 726
   related disorders 231
   second trimester of 7, 355
   symptoms suggestive of 491
   test 21, 459, 592
   therapeutic termination of 195
   trimesters of 408t
   triplet 178
Premarin 530
Premature birth 155
Premature ovarian failure 798, 807
Prematurity, retinopathy of 315
Prenatal folic acid 454
Presacral neurectomy 679
Pressure
   intra-abdominal 647
   symptoms, presence of 491
Preterm birth 85, 328
   classification of 318t
   severity of 318
Preterm delivery 618
   risk of 321t
Preterm intrauterine growth-restricted fetus 316
Preterm labor 318, 321, 322b, 324f, 327, 330, 330b, 332t, 334, 334t, 337, 406, 594
   absence of 406
   advanced 322
   clinical presentation 321
   complications 334
   differential diagnosis 322
   early 322
   etiopathogenesis of 318
   investigations 322
   management of 322, 323fc, 327
   obstetric management 326
   pathogenesis of 318, 319b, 319fc, 319t
   prediction of 318, 322

   presence of 406
   prevention of 175, 326b, 328fc
   risk factors for 319, 320f
   surgical management 334
   treatment 326
Previous miscarriages 256
   number of 245
Primary amenorrhea 798f, 799b, 800
   causes of 793f
   evaluation of 800fc, 801fc
Primigravida 4, 65
   management of 68
Primipara 4
Primordial prevention 610
Primrose 563
Procainamide 458
Progesterone 391, 491, 560, 723
   absence of 796
   only hormonal contraception 715
   only pills 743
   receptor modulators 529
   therapy 328
   use of 326
Progestin
   challenge test 805
   exogenous 528
   role 326
Progestogen 527, 678
   only pills 405
   routine 261
Prolapse
   degree of 649, 654
   laparoscopic surgery for 663
   pessary treatment for 652
   surgery 661, 662b
   symptoms of 648
   uterus 641, 656b
      third-degree 651
Prostaglandin 210, 276, 342, 343, 360, 384, 468, 731
   E 319
   E_2 210, 319
   F_2 alpha 319, 340
   preparations, role of 343
   synthetase inhibitors 331, 332, 527
Prosthetic heart valve 458, 459
Prosthetic material
   types of 662b
   use of 661
Prosthetic mitral valve 458
Protamine zinc insulin 398
Proteinuria 364
   grading of 365t
   measurement of levels of 364
   occurrence of 365
Prune juice 230
Pruritus vulvae 591
Pseudogestational sac 721t
   presence of 721
Pseudohermaphroditism, male 796
Pseudo-Meigs syndrome 520, 550
Psychiatric disorders 670, 799
Pubertal development 794
Pubic hair
   development 793
   pattern 793
   Tanner stages of 794f
Pubic symphysis 206, 412f
Pubocervical fascia 662f

Pubococcygeus 645
Puerperium 180
Pull method 118
Pulmonary artery
　catheter 375
　pressure monitoring 375
Pulmonary edema 374, 375, 381
　clinical signs of 375
　complications of 375
　prevention of 457
　treatment of 446b
Pulmonary maturity, assessment of 29
Pulmonary system, exact site of 474
Pulmonary valve stenosis 449
Pulmonary vascular obstructive disease 460
Pulsatility index 297, 301, 305, 314
Pulse 450
　dosage radiotherapy brachytherapy 635
　oximetry 456
Pure gonadal dysgenesis 797
Push method 119
Pyelography, intravenous 524, 703
Pyometra 285

Q

Quadrivalent gardasil 611
Quadrivalent vaccines 611

R

Radiation
　abdominal 793
　therapy 634, 708
　　primary 631
Radical hysterectomy 633t, 637, 637t
　modified 629
　type of 633
Radical surgery 684
Radical trachelectomy 631b
Radio-femoral delay, presence of 450
Radiologic pelvimetry 117
Radiotherapy 634b, 637
Raloxifene 530, 564, 744
Rapid plasma reagin 257, 588
Rapid-acting insulin analogs 398
Rash, development of 439
Raw uterine walls 797
Reactive nonstress test, implications of 310
Reactive oxygen species 360
Rectal bleeding 694
Rectocele 643f
Rectosigmoid colon 637
　resection of 706
Rectovaginal fistula 416, 573, 637
Rectovaginal septum 669, 672
Rectus sheath, closure of 219, 220f
Recurrent miscarriage 256, 258fc, 260, 261t, 467
　causes of 245f, 531
Recurrent pregnancy loss 257, 530
　causes of 245b
　management of 257
Red blood cell antigen 187
Red cell
　alloantibodies 25
　distribution width 429
Reid's colposcopic index 609
　modified 609t

Renal complications 338
Renal defects 408
Renal disease 362, 375
　end-stage 397
Renal failure 162, 294, 492
　acute 139
Renal function 381
　assessment of 625
　tests 497
Renal insufficiency 333, 752
Renshaw's classification 408t
Renshaw's staging system 409f
Reproductive tract malformations 749
Reserpine 377
Resistance index 305
Respiratory depression 380
Respiratory distress syndrome 317, 327, 337, 347
Respiratory rate 450
Resuscitation 272
Reticulocyte count 429, 439
Retinal arterioles, constrictions of 366
Retinal assessment 395, 396
Retinal vasculopathy 407
Retinopathy
　diabetic 407
　progression of 407
Retraction ring, formation of 97f
Retrieving sperms, surgical techniques for 784b
Retrograde menstruation 667
　basic anatomy of 668f
Retroperitoneal tissues, dissection of 287f
Retroplacental clot, presence of 160f
Rhabdomyosarcoma, embryonal 621
Rhesus
　alloimmunization 202fc
　antigens 188t
　blood grouping 25
　classification 187
　compatibility 147
　incompatibility disease 188
　isoimmunization
　　pathogenesis of 189fc
　　recurrence of 151
　sensitized pregnancy 193
　system 187, 188t
Rheumatic activity 442
Rheumatic heart valve disease 445, 460
Rh-negative pregnancy 187
　case study 187
　clinical presentation 190
　complications 202
　general physical examination 190
　history 190
　investigations 190
　management 190
　obstetric management 192
　specific systemic examination 190
　treatment 192
Riboflavin 434
Ribs 114
Right ischial spine, assessment of 116f
Ring of fire appearance 723f
Ritodrine 333
Robert's pelvis 113f
Robert's sign 350
Robertsonian translocations 246
Robotic myomectomy 538, 539, 541f

Robotic surgery 538f
Robotic system, cameras of 540f
Robotic technology
　advantages of 539
　over conventional laparoscopy, advantages of 539b
Robotic-assisted laparoscopic myomectomy 539
　advantages of 539b
Robson's ten group classification system 205, 205t
Roller ball endometrial ablation 548f
Roll-over test 367
Rosette test 191, 191f
Rotterdam's criteria 757
Rubella
　immunity for 762
　immunization status 454
Rubin maneuver 413, 413f
Rusch urological catheter 278

S

Saccharomyces cerevisiae 611
Sacral agenesis 408, 408t, 409f
Sacral promontory, assessment of 116f
Sacral vertebra 796
Sacroiliac joints, right 110
Sacrosciatic notch, evaluation of 116f
Sacrospinous ligament 661f
Sahli's apparatus 429f
Salbutamol 333
Saline
　adenine-glucose-mannitol 201
　infusion sonography 498, 499, 500, 500f, 501f, 523, 524f, 766
　transabdominal amnioinfusion of 71
Salpingectomy 723, 731, 734, 735b
　indications for 733b
　partial 734
　procedure of 734
Salpingitis 618
Salpingo-oophorectomy
　bilateral 507, 509, 707
　unilateral 706
Salpingo-ophoritis 552
Salpingostomy 734, 735b
Salpingotomy 723, 731, 734
　incision 736f
　tube-sparing 735
Salvage 579
　therapy
　　second-line 579
　　third-line 579
　treatment 579
Sapporo's classification, revised 255t
Scanzoni's double application 109
Scar
　absence of 12
　defects, visualization of 225
　integrity, assessment of 225
　marks over abdomen 472
　presence of 12
　rupture, recurrence of 224t
　thickness, measurement of levels of 225
Schiller's iodine 604
Schiller-Duval bodies 690
Schistosomiasis 599

Schoorel scoring system 208
Screening test, prerequisites for 600, 600b
Secondary amenorrhea 96, 122, 792, 802, 903fc
   differential diagnosis of 799t
Secondary postpartum hemorrhage 266, 294
   causes of 294
   management of 294
   treatment of 294fc
Secondary sexual characteristics 753, 799, 800
   development of 794, 794b
Seizures 365
Selective estrogen receptor modulators 530, 564, 566, 775
Selective progesterone receptor modulators 529
Sellheim spoon 120
Semen
   parameters 752, 763
   quality, poor 749
   volume, low 763
Semen analysis 762, 763
   abnormal 763
      results of 764t
   interpretation of 763
   normal parameters for 763t
   parameters for 763t
Semiconservative surgery 684
Sengstaken-Blakemore tube 278, 279f
Senile vaginal atrophy 561
Sensitization, process of 189
Sentinel lymph node biopsy 513
Sepsis 122, 139, 242, 315, 318, 544
   chances of 330
   late-onset 330
   puerperal 294
Septostomy 184
Serotonin 559
Sertoli cells 688
Sertoli-Leydig cell tumors 687
Serum
   alpha-fetoprotein 723
      levels 312
   beta-human chorionic gonadotropin levels 718
   glutamic pyruvate transaminase 497
   gonadotropin levels, interpretation of 805t
   human chorionic gonadotropin concentration 720
      levels 720
   progesterone 771
      levels 722, 770
   prolactin levels 257, 805
   testosterone 805
      levels, detection of 764
   uric acid 370
      levels 366
Severe anemia 427, 432
   management of 427, 430
Severe preeclampsia 275, 359t, 373, 373b, 374b, 375, 378, 382, 384b
   indications of 359b
   management of 372
   symptoms indicative of 370
Sex cord stromal cell tumors 686-688
Sexual arousal disorders 466
Sexual desire 466

Sexual dysfunction 466
Sexual history 590, 620, 750
Sexual intercourse 576
Sexual pain disorders 466
Sexual partners 576
   treatment of 579
Sexually transmitted disease 573, 581, 590, 591t, 669
   screening for 762
Sexually transmitted infections 562
Sheehan's syndrome 122, 751
Shirodkar's modification 657
Shirodkar's operation 250
Shirodkar's technique 263, 264f
Shock 122, 145, 440
   bacterial 139
   hemorrhagic 242
   hypovolemic 294
   index, calculation of 273
   maternal 162
   puerperal 294
   signs of 716
   symptoms of 716
Shoulder dystocia 120, 410, 411f, 412, 413b, 413f, 415f
   complications of 414
   development of 410, 410t, 411f
   management of 410, 412fc
   maternal complications of 416
   prediction of 410
   presence of 410
   unilateral 410
Shoulder, delivery of 55f, 56
Shrink fibroids 529
Siamese twin, types of 170, 170t
Sibai's regimens 379
Sickle cell anemia 431f
Sigmoid colon 667
Sigmoidoscopy 674
Silicone arabin pessary 327
Sim's speculum 137f, 477, 478f, 502
Sim's test 764
Single placenta, presence of 173f
Singleton gestation 25t
Sinnecker's classification 796t
Sinusoidal fetal heart rate pattern 198f
Skeletal abnormalities 798
Skin
   changes 7, 11f
   closure 219
   edema 203f
   exact site of 753
   preparation of 214
   vertical incision of 215f
Small for gestational age 295, 296, 296t, 299, 368
   fetuses, prevention of 312
Smooth triangular uterine cavity 259f
Snowstorm appearance 234
Society for Maternal Fetal Medicine 326
Sodium
   bicarbonate 407
   ferric ethylenediaminetetraacetate 435
   nitroprusside 376, 377
Soft sore 587
Soft tissue injuries 467
Somatic origin, pain of 665
Somogyi phenomenon 399

Sonography
   transabdominal 481, 483, 523, 700f, 701f
   transvaginal 150, 250, 303f, 323, 324b, 481, 500b, 502, 522, 674, 700f, 701f, 720, 725, 728, 730, 801
Sonohysterography 259
Soonawala's sling 660
Sore skin 637
Spalding sign 350, 350f
Speech problems 202
Sperm 760
   abnormal 784
   concentrate 763, 781f
   interaction 754
   preparation 773
      procedure of 784
   retrieval 784
   transport, disorders of 754
Sphingomyelin 150
Spinal cord segments, nerve roots of 414
Spine 114
   exact site of 471
Spiral vessels, intradecidual segments of 298
Spironolactone 752
Sporadic embryonic losses, half of 246
Squamocolumnar junction 609
   normal 601f
Squamous cell carcinoma 621
   histopathological appearance of 621f
Stallworthy's sign 146
Stargazing sign 67
Stem cell carcinoma 621
Stenosed mitral valves 446f
Sterile per speculum examination 334
Steroid
   anabolic 752
   hormones 391
Stillbirth 165, 346, 406
   exact site of 349
Stimulation 63
Stitching uterine incision 220f
Streptococcus infection 330
Streptomycin 586
Stress 256
Striae gravidarum
   over abdomen 13f
   presence of 12
Stroke 460, 569
   ischemic 562
   volume 443
Stroma 470
Stuck twin syndrome 183f
Stump 552
Sturmdorf sutures, application of 615f
Subcutaneous fat 215f
   loss of 346
Subepithelial connective tissue 585
Submentum 49
Submucosal fibroid 485, 516, 523, 526, 537f, 553
Submucosal myoma, appearance of 537f
Subserosal myoma, removal of 535
Subserous fibroid 535f
Suction cannula 277
   procedure 277
Sudden infant death syndrome 155
Sulfonylurea 399

Superficial transverse perineal muscle 644, 645, 645f
Supine hypotension syndrome 444
    pathogenesis of 445f
Suprapubic pain, severe 625f
Suprapubic pressure 411, 412
    application of 412f, 413f
Surgery
    abdominal 467
    conservative 732, 744
    indications for 242b, 530b, 682b
Surgical therapy, indications for 732b
Sutures, application of 617
Suturing anal sphincters, overlap method of 291f
Swelling, abdominal examination of 695
Swollen chorionic villi 236
Swyer's syndrome 797
Symphysiotomy 120
Symphysis fundal height 295, 315
Symphysis
    estimation of 300
    fundus
        growth curve 14, 14f, 300
        height, measurement of levels of 13, 14f
Syncytiotrophoblast 227
Syntocinon 275
Syntometrine 275
Syphilis 257, 587
    congenital 299, 588
    diagnosis 587
    serologic test for 255, 349
    stages of 588
    tertiary 588
Systemic chemotherapy 709
    benefits of 634
Systemic lupus erythematosus 245, 258

T

T sign 174
Tachyarrhythmia, supraventricular 449
Tachycardia 211, 493
Talipes equinovarus 181
Tamoxifen 494, 744, 778
    citrate 778
    therapy 494
Tamponade 277
Tanner stages 794, 794b
Teeth 556
Teletherapy 635
Tenaculum 502
Tenderness, abdominal 472
Teratomas 687, 690f
Teratospermia 764
Teratozoospermia 764
Terbutaline 333
Terconazole 578
Teriperatide 567
Testes 688
    acquired disorders of 754
    undescended 753
Testicular disease 754
Testicular feminization 808
Testicular seminoma 690
Testicular trauma 751
Tetanus toxoid 25

Tetracycline 577, 583, 586
Thalassemia 424, 425, 425t, 431f
Theca
    cells 688
    lutein cyst 235, 235f, 686
Third-degree tear, repair of 290
Thoracopagus twins, autopsy specimen of 170f
Three line sign 484
Three-finger rotation, procedure of 107
Thrombin 268
    time 165
Thrombocytopenia, heparin-induced 459
Thromboembolic complication
    development of 442
    prevention of 457
Thromboembolism 221, 226, 294
Thrombophilia
    inherited 252, 265
    screening 260
Thrombophilic state 253
Thromboprophylaxis 151, 214, 221
    peripartum management of 458
    regimes 262t
Thrombosis 254
    prevention of 261
    syndrome 459
Thyroid
    dysfunction 261, 750, 807
        symptoms of 492, 519
    examination 471, 752, 794
    function test 257, 496, 805
    gland 10
    stimulating hormone 258, 804
    storm 231
    testing 496
    tissue 690f
Tibolone 559, 564, 567
Tilt test 268
Tioconazole 578
Tiredness 637
Tissue 268
    abnormal 614
    destruction of 618
    protrusion of 648
Tocolysis 329, 330
Tocolytic agents 330, 331, 403
Tocolytic drug 406
Tocolytic therapy 328, 331b
    contraindications for 330b
    initiation of 327, 331
Tongue 10f
    burning of 419
Tonic uterine contractions 98
Topical azole antifungal agents 578
Toremifene 744
Torsion 550
Total iron
    binding capacity 425, 428
    requirement reflects 439
Total peripheral vascular resistance 443
Toxemia, preeclamptic 361
Toxic effects 761
Toxoplasma gondii 247
Trachelectomy, procedure of 631
Tranexamic acid 276, 360
Transabdominal cerclage 250, 265
Transabdominal imaging 148f, 523

Transcervical fibroid tissue passage 544
Transdermal skin patches 559, 560
Transformation zone 609
    large loop excision of 602, 615, 616f
Transobturator cystocele repair 663, 663f
Transobturator tension 662
Transvaginal examination 482
Transvaginal sacrospinous ligament fixation 660, 661f
Transvaginal sonography 150, 250, 303f, 323, 324b, 481, 500b, 502, 522, 674, 700f, 701f, 720, 725, 728, 730, 801
    advantages of 482
    disadvantages of 483
    technique of 483
Transvaginal ultrasound 269, 324f, 482, 483, 499, 499f, 522
    cervical length 328
Transvaginal uterine artery clamp 277, 278f
    application of 278f
Transverse diameter, measurement of levels of 47f
Transverse lie 89, 90, 92f
    management 91
Transverse lower uterine incision 95f
Transverse sutures around uterus 285f
Transverse vaginal septum 795f
Trauma 157, 226
    neonatal 86
Trendelenburg's position 520
Treponema
    organisms 588
    pallidum 587
Treponemal tests 588
Triazole 578
    agents 578
    antifungals 578
Trichofuran suppositories 581
Trichomonads 592
Trichomonas vaginalis 319, 573, 580f
    transmission of 580f
Trichomonas vaginitis 579
Trichomoniasis 574, 575f, 579, 593
    risk factors for 581
Tricuspid arteries 453
Triple stripe appearance 260f
Triptorelin 528, 782
Trisacryl gelatin 542
Trisomy 12 519
Trocar placement 540
Trophoblast 229f
    abnormal 242
Trophoblastic tissue
    embolization of 242
    neoplasm of 227
Trophotoxic substances 731
T-sign, presence of 174f
Tubal disease, treatment of 775fc
Tubal factors 759, 768
    infertility, treatment option for 775t
Tubal ligation 750
Tubal mole 714
Tubal obstruction 773
    causes of 760
Tubal ostium, hysteroscopic evaluation of 767f
Tubal patency 775t
    laparoscopic test for 769f
Tubal pregnancy, laparoscopic management of 732

Tubal ring sign 721
Tubal rupture 714, 715
Tubal surgery 715, 717
Tube, congenital abnormalities of 716
Tuberculosis 715
Tubo-ovarian
   artery 734
   mass 760f
Tubotubal anastomosis, steps of 774f
Tumor
   abdominal 203
   diagnosis of 473
   fixation of 694
   intraperitoneal 473
   monodermal 690
   necrosis factor 319
   node, and metastasis
      classification 697
      staging system 626
   nonmetastatic 240
   phenotype 492
   pituitary 799
   retroperitoneal 473
   serous 688
   size 513
   synchronous 696
   trophoblastic 228, 242
   volume reduction 524f
Tumor markers 698
   loss of 514
   types of 712t
Tunica albuginea 758
Turner's syndrome 781, 797, 798f, 801, 802, 806
   diagnosis of 808
   stigmata of 752, 798b
Turtle sign 410, 411f
Twin 174, 178
   breech, management of 73
   delivery of 174
   embolization syndrome 186, 186f
   in utero, designation of 171
   peak sign 174, 174f
   presentations, types of 179, 179t
   reversed arterial perfusion syndrome 184
   syndrome 169
   types of 177
Twin gestation 177, 177t, 178, 180, 181, 209
   etiology of 166
   incidence of 166
   types of 166, 177, 177t
Twin pregnancy 171
   occurrence of 174
   recurrence of 180
Twin-to-twin transfusion 181
   quintero stages of 183
   syndrome 178, 182f, 298, 348
      diagnosis of 183b
   ultrasound findings 182
Twinning, mechanism of 166
Two-finger vaginal examination 479f
Tyrode solution 786
Tzanck smear 584

U

Ulceration, benign 599
Ultrasonography 197, 299, 767
   transabdominal 148

transrectal 684
transvaginal 148, 684
Ultrasound 771
   Doppler flow velocimetry 303
   estimated fetal weight 303
   examination 22, 27, 103, 136, 159, 335, 340, 498, 522, 674, 741
      use of 4981
   imaging 225
   indicated cerclage 327
   parameters 341
   principle of 481, 481f
   probes 482f
   transabdominal 269, 498
   transperineal 117f
   transvaginal 269, 324f, 482, 483, 499, 499f, 522
   types of 482
Umbilical artery 297, 304, 315, 316
   blood flow patterns 307f
   circulation 306f
   Doppler analysis 306, 313
   waveform analysis 312, 313
Umbilical blood flow 308b
Umbilical cord 194
   blood sampling, percutaneous 196
   compression 122
Umbilical eversion 471
Umbilical inversion 471
Umbilical vein 302
   diameter 192
Upper gastrointestinal hemorrhage 419
Upper quadrant abdominal pain, right 363
Upper respiratory tract procedures 457t
Upper segment
   scar, strength of 223
   uterine scar 217
Ureaplasma urealyticum 319, 573
Ureters, peristalsis of 531
Urethra 561
Urethrocele 641, 642f
Urge incontinence 466
Urinalysis 269
Urinary catheter 214, 222
Urinary dysfunction 637
Urinary symptoms 7, 518, 556, 589, 648
Urinary tract 226
   infection 159, 389, 466
Urinary urgency 694
Urine 372, 718
   analysis 673
   culture 652, 673
   examination 652
   human chorionic gonadotropin 713
      levels 496
   pregnancy test 520, 718
      positive 793
   retention of 518
Urogenital atrophy
   mild 561
   moderate-to-severe 561
Urogenital diaphragm, muscles of 644, 645f
U-suturing technique 286f
   modified 285, 286f
Uterine 321
   abnormalities, diagnosis of 259f
   cancer, recurrence of 560
   distension, pathogenic 319

   environment 518
   evaluation 546
   exploration 211
   fundus 539
   hyperstimulation, increased risk of 343
   hypertonicity 158
   infection 139, 242, 291
   ischemia 544
   leiomyosarcomas, occurrence of 551
   mass 520, 520t
   massage 266
   obstruction, face of 121
   origin, pain of 466
   papillary serous carcinoma 510
   softening 716
   sound 502
   surface, appearance of 683f
   surgery 153
   suspension 660
   synechiae 773
   tone diminishes 348
   trauma 136, 740
   tumor 474f
   vault, descent of 641
   volume 741
   walls, strengthening of 537
Uterine anomalies 324
   classification of 248f
   congenital 247
   correction of 334
   structural 260
Uterine artery 282, 297, 304, 542f
   blood flow patterns 305f
   Doppler 304
      waveforms, abnormal 305f
   ligation 286
Uterine artery embolization 287, 294, 522, 524f, 525, 526, 531, 542, 543, 745
   complications 543
   contraindications of 542b
   investigations 542
   procedure 542
Uterine atony
   development of 267
   postpartum 163
Uterine bleeding 594
   abnormal 486, 487t, 497, 498, 499b, 501, 506, 507, 525, 546, 623, 689
   excessive 530
   normal 487t
Uterine cavity 293, 539, 753, 765
   distortion of 247
   size of 502
   transvaginal sonography 499
Uterine contractions 34, 158
   abnormal 101
   duration of 34
Uterine factor
   infertility 755
   tests for 765
   tubal factors of 773
Uterine fibroids 248, 468, 520, 740
   classification system of 517t
   symptomatic 465
Uterine incision 219f
   classical 223
   closure of 218
   double layered closure of 218

extension of 218f
single layered closure of 218
types of 217
Uterine inversion
    diagnosis 291
    treatment 292
Uterine leiomyomas
    cure for 531
    presence of 158
    treatment modality for 530
Uterine malformations 247, 780
    drug-induced 755
Uterine muscle 224, 534
    fibers, arrangement of 9f
Uterine myomas 515, 550
    treatment options for 525t
Uterine perforation 139, 550, 617
    recurrence of 139
Uterine prolapse 641, 642f, 647, 650f
    causes of 646
    development of 652
    diagnosis of 648, 651
    stages of 650f
    surgery for 661
    tubal factors of 653f
Uterine rupture 223, 224, 224b, 252, 416, 536b
    types of 224
Uterine scar 667
    lower segment 217
Uterine septa 260
    lysis of 773
Uterine septum 247, 249f
    resection of 249f
Uterine tamponade 277, 279f, 280f, 281
    application of 280
Uterine vessel 288
    ligation
        bilateral 287
        technique of 287
        unilateral 287
    low 288
Utero-ovarian vessel 288
    ligation, bilateral 287
Uteroplacental apoplexy 163
Uteroplacental dysfunction 358
Uteroplacental function, assessment of 304
Uteroplacental insufficiency 381
Uteroplacental pathology, indications of 175
Uteroplacental perfusion 378
Uterosacral ligaments 643, 671, 684
Uterotonics, use of 221
Uterus 8, 248, 274, 557, 671, 740, 767, 796
    abnormal hardness of 36b
    acute inversion of 291
    bicornuate 259, 521, 722f, 765, 767, 773
    blood supply to 282f
    brace sutures of 282
    curettage of 294
    cut specimen of 739f
    didelphys 765
    exact site of 13
    gentle repositioning of 292f
    inversion of 291
    medical evacuation of 195
    removal of 531
    rupture of 96, 122, 225, 289
    septate 259, 765, 767
    serosal surface of 667

shape of 260
size of 14, 479
supports of 643
surgical evacuation of 195
transvaginal ultrasound of 260f
T-shaped 755
ultrasound examination of 499
unicornuate 765, 780
visualization of 217f

V

Vacuum aspiration, procedure of 136
Vagina 242, 556, 584, 643
    appearance of 575f
    epithelial lining of 561
    lactobacilli in 575
    potential space of 643
    suspension of 655
Vaginal atrophy 561
Vaginal birth 75
    after cesarean 206, 207, 213
        delivery 206
    after cesarean section 206, 209, 210
        advantages of 209
        contraindications for 209
        prediction of 207
        recurrence of 209
    indications for 177
    previous 207
Vaginal bleeding 157, 211, 230, 716, 717
    abnormal 624f
    excessive 242
Vaginal breech delivery 72, 74
    indications for 74b
Vaginal clindamycin cream 577
Vaginal cuff 650
    removal of 617
Vaginal culture 593
Vaginal cysts 651
Vaginal delivery 54, 178, 178b, 456
    instrumental 250
    mechanism of 106, 107f
    normal 54
    operative 108, 109
    prerequisites for 79
    spontaneous 111
Vaginal discharge 466, 573, 588, 591, 592fc, 593f, 750
    causes of 589t, 591, 591t, 594t
    Gram's staining of 576
    management of 591
    pathological causes of 573t
    physiological causes of 573t
    types of 575f, 590
Vaginal douching 576
Vaginal dryness 528, 554, 555
Vaginal epithelial cells, exfoliation of 576
Vaginal estrogen 561, 562
    low-dose 561
    preparations 560
    ring 562
    tablet 562
Vaginal examination 21, 36, 37, 38b, 61, 67, 67f, 91, 91f, 102, 105, 110, 121, 146, 158, 171, 231, 322, 341, 465, 495, 713
    contraindications for 37
    indications for 37, 37b

preparation for 37
prerequisites for 36
Vaginal fluid sample 322
Vaginal hematomas 291
Vaginal hysterectomy 531, 664
Vaginal infection, history of 491
Vaginal injuries, repair of 289
Vaginal intraepithelial neoplasia 589
Vaginal introitus 41, 55f, 651
Vaginal irritation 589
Vaginal length, total 650f, 651
Vaginal lubricants 561
Vaginal moisturizing agents 561
Vaginal mucosa 289, 291, 649, 753
    thickness of 590
Vaginal mucosal inflammation, signs of 590
Vaginal pH 578, 581
Vaginal probe, use of 482
Vaginal prolapse 655b
Vaginal repair 661
Vaginal route 531
Vaginal secretions 335
Vaginal septum 795, 795f
Vaginal stenosis 637
Vaginal swab, high 257, 269, 652
Vaginal tears 290
Vaginal tissue, levels of support for 643t
Vaginal touch picture 110f
Vaginal vault 660
Vaginal walls 656
Vaginismus 466
Vaginitis 591b
    causes of 574t
    emphysematous 594
Vaginosis 575
Valium 380
Valvular heart disease 442
Vanishing twins 173
Varicocele 753
Varicosities 180, 471
Vasa previa 146, 147f, 180
    diagnosis of 147f
Vascular disease, peripheral 388
Vascular endothelial growth factor 708
    receptors 710
Vascular resistance 308b, 367
    Doppler evaluation of 175
Vascular spread, metastatic theory of 668
Vasectomy 750
Vasoactive substances, secretion of 553
Vasomotor symptoms, control of 564
Vasopressin 277
Vasospasm 360
Vault granulation tissue 573
Vault prolapse
    diagnosis of 660
    management of 660
    surgical management of 660
Vecchietti's technique 806
Vein, normal ratio of 366
Vena cava, inferior 302
Venereal disease research laboratory test 257, 588
Venlafaxine 559
Venous thromboembolism
    incidence of 564
    recurrence of 562

Ventricular septal defects 449
Vertex 15, 49
Vertical incision 215f
 closure of 220f
Vesicovaginal fistula 122, 252, 573
Vessels
 abnormal 609
 atypical 609
Vincristine 241, 690
Virilization, signs of 793
Virkud's composite sling operation 659
Visceral origin, pain of 665
Viscoelastic testing 281
Visual disturbances 793
Visual fields, assessment of 794
Visual inspection, method of 604
Vital signs 268, 450, 470
Vitamin
 A 230, 434
 B_{12} 426f, 434
  deficiency of 427, 427t
  supplementation 426
 C 366, 563
 D 366, 559
  deficiency of 565
  low levels of 565
 E 366, 563
 K, administration of 460
Vitrification 789

von Willebrand disease 268, 496
Vulva 556
 appearance of 575f
Vulvar cysts 651
Vulvar intraepithelial neoplasia 589
Vulvar pruritus, chronic 558
Vulvovaginal candidiasis 574, 575f, 577, 591
Vulvovaginal itching 574
Vulvovaginitis 574, 591, 594
 recurrent 577

W

Waiter's tip position 415
Warfarin 458-460, 491
 low-dose 459
Weak scar, causes of 225b
Weight gain 25, 365
 distribution of 25f
 extreme 761
Weight loss 518
 extreme 761
Weinstein scoring system 208, 208t
Wet mount 593f
 preparation 592
Wheel-spoke appearance 789f
Whiff test 576, 576f
White blood cells 592, 764
White's classification system 390, 390b

Willis circle 306f
Woods' screw maneuver 412, 413, 413f, 414
 reverse 412, 414, 414f
Worsening dysmenorrhea 751
Wurm's stitch, application of 265f

X

X chromosome 797, 802
Xenograft 662
X-ray abdomen 349
XY karyotype 797

Y

Yolk sac
 development 690
 tumor 690

Z

Zatuchni and Andros score 72t
Zavanelli maneuver 414, 415f
Zinc 423, 434
Zoladex 528, 678
Zoledronic acid 567
Zona pellucida 786
Z-score 565
Zuspan regimen 379
Zygote intrafallopian transfer 787